Netter's Internal Medicine

Netter's Internal Medicine

Edited by

Marschall S. Runge, MD, PhD
The University of North Carolina
School of Medicine, Chapel Hill

M. Andrew Greganti, MD
The University of North Carolina
School of Medicine, Chapel Hill

Illustrations by Frank H. Netter, MD

Contributing Illustrators

John A. Craig, MD
Carlos A. G. Machado, MD

Icon Learning Systems · Teterboro, New Jersey

Published by Icon Learning Systems LLC, a subsidiary of MediMedia USA, Inc.
Copyright © 2003 MediMedia, Inc.

FIRST EDITION

ISBN 1-929007-00-0

Library of Congress Catalog No 2001132777

Printed in the U.S.A.
First Printing, 2003

NOTICE

Every effort has been taken to confirm the accuracy of the information presented and to describe generally accepted practices. Neither the publisher nor the authors can be held responsible for errors or for any consequences arising from the use of the information contained herein, and make no warranty, expressed or implied, with respect to the contents of the publication.

Before prescribing pharmaceutical products, readers are advised to check the product information currently provided by the manufacturer of each drug to be administered to verify the recommended dose, the method and duration of administration, and the contraindications. It is the responsibility of the treating physician, relying on experience and knowledge of the patient, to determine dosages and the best treatment for the patient. Neither the publisher nor the editors assumes any responsibility for any injury and/or damage to persons or property.

Executive Editor: Paul Kelly
Editorial Director: Greg Otis
Managing Editor: Jennifer Surich
Editorial Assistant: Nicole Zimmerman
Art Production Manager: Jonna Armstrong
Media Project Editor: Karen Oswald
Graphic Artist: Colleen Quinn
Print Production Manager: Mary Ellen Curry

Binding and Printing by Banta Book Group
Digital Separations by R.R. Donnelly and Page Imaging

10   9   8   7   6   5   4   3   2   1

ACKNOWLEDGMENTS

Developing a new textbook of internal medicine was a major undertaking not only for us, but also for many other dedicated individuals.

First, we thank the contributing authors of the University of North Carolina School of Medicine, Chapel Hill. Without their intellect, dedication and drive for excellence, *Netter's Internal Medicine* could not have been published.

Special recognition goes to Drs. John A. Craig and Carlos A.G. Machado. They are uniquely talented physician-artists who through their work brought to life important concepts in medicine in the new and updated figures included in this text.

We also thank Jennifer Surich, Greg Otis, Kate Kelly, Paul Kelly, and their colleagues in the editorial and production offices of Icon Learning Systems, for their care and commitment in developing this new text.

We are also indebted to Ms. Angela C. Rego, whose superb organizational skills were invaluable.

We would especially like to acknowledge our families: our wives—Susan Runge and Susan Greganti—whose constant support, encouragement and understanding made completion of this text possible; our children— Thomas, Elizabeth, William, John and Mason Runge, and Paul, Taylor and Katie Greganti—who inspire us and remind us that there is life beyond the word processor; and finally our parents—whose persistence, commitment, and work ethic got us started on this road many, many years ago.

Marschall S. Runge, MD, PhD, was born in Austin, Texas and graduated from Vanderbilt University with a BA in General Biology and a PhD in Molecular Biology. He graduated from the Johns Hopkins School of Medicine and trained in internal medicine at the Johns Hopkins Hospital. He was a cardiology fellow and junior faculty member at the Massachusetts General Hospital. Dr. Runge's next position was at Emory University, where he directed the Cardiology Fellowship Training Program. He then moved to the University of Texas Medical Branch in Galveston where he was Chief of Cardiology and Director of the Sealy Center for Molecular Cardiology. He came to UNC in 2000 as Chairman of the Department of Medicine. Dr. Runge is board certified in internal medicine and cardiovascular diseases and has spoken and published widely on topics in clinical cardiology and vascular medicine. He maintains an active clinical practice in cardiovascular diseases and medicine, in addition to his teaching and administrative activities in the Department of Medicine.

M. Andrew Greganti, MD, was born in Cleveland, Mississippi, graduated from Millsaps College with a BS in Chemistry and later received his medical degree from the University of Mississippi School of Medicine. He trained in Internal Medicine at the University of Rochester School of Medicine, Strong Memorial Hospital. After two years on the faculty of the University of Mississippi School of Medicine, he joined the faculty at UNC in the Division of General Medicine and Clinical Epidemiology in 1977, and has been Professor of Medicine since 1990. During his tenure at UNC he has been Director of the Internal Medicine Residency Training Program and the Medicine-Pediatrics Residency Training Program, and has served as Division Chief of the Division of General Medicine and Clinical Epidemiology. He has also served as Associate Chairman and Interim Chairman of the Department of Medicine. He is currently Vice Chairman of the Department of Medicine and a member of the UNC Health Care System Board of Directors. He is board certified in internal medicine, and lectures as well as publishes on clinical topics in internal medicine and medical education. Known as the "doctor's doctor" at UNC, Dr. Greganti is one of the School of Medicine's busiest clinicians and a resource for many in the institution, regionally and nationally.

As all clinicians know, maintaining the currency of one's medical knowledge is an ever-increasing challenge, especially for those who practice the discipline of internal medicine. Our specialty has experienced an explosion of its information base over the past four decades, and the predicted doubling of the National Institutes of Health budget between 1995 and 2005 is a sign that this trend will continue and accelerate. Although we welcome these advances in our field, internists, both generalists and subspecialists, now must process a seemingly endless amount of information in their daily effort to provide their patients with the best possible care. This challenge is magnified by the demands of increasing patient volume and the attendant paperwork, which constrain the time to read. Responses to the need for access to up-to-date information include 2500-page, detailed textbooks like *Harrison's Principles of Internal Medicine,* easily accessible electronic databases like "Up-to-Date" and "Emedicine," innovative continuing education programs, and self-learning and assessment tools like the Medical Knowledge Self Assessment Program (MKSAP). Having utilized many of these over the years, most practitioners have come to realize that there is no single best way to "keep up" and that the efficient utilization of time is key.

Netter's Internal Medicine represents a substantially different approach. When presented with the possibility of using the artwork of one of medicine's greatest teachers, the late Frank H. Netter, MD, in a textbook of general internal medicine, we saw an ideal opportunity to provide a useful, practical resource for busy, time-pressured clinicians. Rather than publishing another exhaustive text that would only add to "data overload," we wanted to provide the essentials of clinical practice in a readable and understandable format. We began with the goal of making learning an easier process for our readers, whether they be students, house officers, or practicing physicians. We decided to cover, in concise yet complete chapters that can be read and understood in a short period of time, the most common clinical problems encountered by practicing internists. We then asked our authors to prepare text that would provide insight into complex medical problems so as to help clinicians make accurate diagnoses and select appropriate therapy. We have purposely avoided extensive discussions of pathobiology, focusing instead on the clinical concepts that must be understood in order to make practical decisions regarding patient care. This approach assumes a basic understanding of the topic and the ability to go elsewhere for more detail.

Is all of this really possible? We think it is, for two reasons.

First, to select the authors, we asked ourselves whom others in our institution, the University of North Carolina School of Medicine at Chapel Hill, considered the "person to call" to deal with a particular clinical problem. We then asked those experts to distill reams of information to the most important and useful facts and to write about their topic in a well-organized and logical format. Thus, this is a text written by authors from diverse clinical departments in a single institution, a medical school well known for its scholarly productivity in both research and clinical practice. All of the authors are practicing clinicians, many of them well known for their national and international contributions. We are convinced that keeping the text within our institution, in large part within the Department of Medicine, has allowed us to maintain our focus and accomplish our goals.

Second, as we have produced this book we have taken advantage of the magic of Dr. Netter's unique medical illustrations, during which process we have learned that thousands of words cannot describe what one of his plates depicts. His artwork has been a resource for physicians for decades and an inspiration to our authors. In each chapter, Dr. Netter's plates enhance the reader's understanding while serving as a pictorial outline of chapter content. In some cases

PREFACE

we have revised Dr. Netter's illustrations to assure that they reflect the newest concepts in the field, and in others we have called for the creation of new artwork by two artists, John A. Craig, MD, and Carlos A.G. Machado, MD, both worthy successors to Dr. Netter.

We believe we have created in *Netter's Internal Medicine* a highly useful resource for all physicians, both generalists and subspecialists, who need to remain current in internal medicine—from the young to the old, from trainees to experienced practitioners. Have we succeeded? We welcome the comments, suggestions, and criticism of readers, which will help us improve future editions of this work.

Marschall S. Runge, MD, PhD
Chairman, Department of Medicine
The University of North Carolina
  School of Medicine, Chapel Hill

M. Andrew Greganti, MD
Vice Chairman, Department of Medicine
The University of North Carolina
  School of Medicine, Chapel Hill

Frank H. Netter, MD

Frank H. Netter was born in 1906 in New York City. He studied art at the Art Student's League and the National Academy of Design before entering medical school at New York University, where he received his M.D. degree in 1931. During his student years, Dr. Netter's notebook sketches attracted the attention of the medical faculty and other physicians, allowing him to augment his income by illustrating articles and textbooks. He continued illustrating as a sideline after establishing a surgical practice in 1933, but he ultimately opted to give up his practice in favor of a full-time commitment to art. After service in the United States Army during World War II, Dr. Netter began his long collaboration with the CIBA Pharmaceutical Company (now Novartis Pharmaceuticals). This 45-year partnership resulted in the production of the extraordinary collection of medical art so familiar to physicians and other medical professionals worldwide.

Icon Learning Systems acquired the Netter Collection in July 2000 and continues to update Dr. Netter's original paintings and to add newly commissioned paintings by artists trained in the style of Dr. Netter.

Dr. Netter's works are among the finest examples of the use of illustration in the teaching of medical concepts. The 13-book Netter Collection of Medical Illustrations, *which includes the greater part of the more than 20,000 paintings created by Dr. Netter, became and remains one of the most famous medical works ever published.* The Atlas of Human Anatomy, *first published in 1989, presents the anatomical paintings from the Netter Collection. Now translated into 11 languages, it is the anatomy atlas of choice among medical and health professions students the world over.*

The Netter illustrations are appreciated not only for their aesthetic qualities but, more importantly, for their intellectual content. As Dr. Netter wrote in 1949, ". . . clarification of a subject is the aim and goal of illustration. No matter how beautifully painted, how delicately and subtly rendered a subject may be, it is of little value as a medical illustration if it does not serve to make clear some medical point." Dr. Netter's planning, conception, point of view, and approach are what inform his paintings and what makes them so intellectually valuable.

Frank H. Netter, MD, physician and artist, died in 1991.

CONTRIBUTORS

All the contributors are associated with the University of North Carolina School of Medicine at Chapel Hill.

Marschall S. Runge, MD, PhD
Marion Covington Distinguished Professor of Medicine
Professor and Chairman, Department of Medicine

M. Andrew Greganti, MD
John Randolph and Helen Barnes Chambliss Distinguished Professor of Medicine
Professor and Vice Chairman, Department of Medicine

Adaora A. Adimora, MD, MPH
Associate Professor of Medicine
Division of Infectious Diseases

Robert M. Aris, MD
Associate Professor of Medicine
Director, Pulmonary Transplant Program
Division of Pulmonary and Critical Care
  Medicine

Maria Q. Baggstrom, MD
Instructor of Medicine
Division of Hematology and Oncology

Christopher C. Baker, MD
Professor of Surgery
Chief, Trauma Surgery

Robert G. Berger, MD
Professor of Medicine
Director, Medical Informatics
Associate Chief of Staff
Division of Rheumatology and Immunology

Lee R. Berkowitz, MD
Professor of Medicine
Associate Chair for Education
Division of Hematology and Oncology
Lineberger Comprehensive Cancer Center

Stephen A. Bernard, MD
Professor of Medicine
Division of Hematology and Oncology
Lineberger Comprehensive Cancer Center

William S. Blau, MD, PhD
Associate Professor of Anesthesiology
Director, Anesthesiology Pain Management
  Center

Brian A. Boehlecke, MD, MSPH
Professor of Medicine
Co-Director, UNC Sleep Program
Division of Pulmonary and Critical Care
  Medicine

John F. Boggess, MD
Assistant Professor of Obstetrics and
  Gynecology
Division of Gynecologic Oncology

Mark E. Brecher, MD
Professor of Pathology and Laboratory
  Medicine
Director, Transfusion Medicine and Transplant
  Services,
McLendon Clinical Laboratories

Sue A. Brown, MD
Assistant Professor of Medicine
Division of Endocrinology and Metabolism

Elizabeth Bullitt, MD
Professor of Surgery
Division of Neurosurgery

M. Janette Busby-Whitehead, MD
Associate Professor of Medicine
Chief, Division of Geriatric Medicine
Director, Program on Aging

John B. Buse, MD, PhD
Associate Professor of Medicine
Chief, Division of General Internal Medicine
  and Clinical Epidemiology
Director, Diabetes Care Center

Debra L. Bynum, MD
Assistant Professor of Medicine
Division of Geriatric Medicine

CONTRIBUTORS

Lisa A. Carey, MD
Assistant Professor of Medicine
Division of Hematology and Oncology
Lineberger Comprehensive Cancer Center

Timothy S. Carey, MD, MPH
Professor of Medicine
Director, Cecil G. Sheps Center for Health
 Services Research
Division of General Internal Medicine and
 Clinical Epidemiology

Culley C. Carson III, MD
Professor of Surgery
Chief, Division of Urologic Surgery

David R. Clemmons, MD
Sarah Graham Kenan Professor of Medicine
Chief, Division of Endocrinology and
 Metabolism

Romulo E. Colindres, MD, MSPH
Professor of Medicine
Division of Nephrology and Hypertension

AnnaMarie Connolly, MD
Assistant Professor of Obstetrics and
 Gynecology
Division of Urogynecology and
 Reconstructive Pelvic Surgery

Benjamin J. Copeland, MD, PhD
Resident, Department of Otolaryngology,
 Head and Neck Surgery

Kathryn A. Copeland, MD
Instructor of Obstetrics and Gynecology
Division of Urogynecology and
 Reconstructive Pelvic Surgery

Shane Darrah, MD
Instructor of Medicine
Division of Cardiology

Cynthia J. Denu-Ciocca, MD
Assistant Professor of Medicine
Division of Nephrology and Hypertension

Thomas S. Devetski, OD
Assistant Professor of Ophthalmology

Darren A. DeWalt, MD
Instructor of Medicine
Division of General Internal Medicine and
 Clinical Epidemiology

Luis A. Diaz, MD
Professor of Dermatology
Chairman, Department of Dermatology

James F. Donohue, MD
Professor of Medicine
Chief, Division of Pulmonary and Critical Care
 Medicine

Mary Anne Dooley, MD, MPH
Associate Professor of Medicine
Division of Rheumatology and Immunology

Jean M. Dostou, MD
Assistant Professor of Medicine
Division of Endocrinology and Metabolism

Douglas A. Drossman, MD
Professor of Medicine and Psychiatry
Co-Director, UNC Center for Functional GI
 and Motility Disorders
Division of Digestive Diseases and Nutrition

Joseph J. Eron, MD
Associate Professor of Medicine
Director, Adult Clinical Trials Unit
Division of Infectious Diseases

Ronald J. Falk, MD
Doc J. Thurston Professor of Medicine
Chief, Division of Nephrology and
 Hypertension

Elizabeth A. Fasy, MD
Assistant Professor of Medicine
Division of Endocrinology and Metabolism

Alan G. Finkel, MD
Associate Professor of Neurology
Section of Adult Neurology

William F. Finn, MD
Professor of Medicine
Division of Nephrology and Hypertension

Carol A. Ford, MD
Associate Professor of Medicine and
  Pediatrics
Director, Adolescent Medicine Program

Wesley Caswell Fowler, MD
Instructor of Surgery
Division of Neurosurgery

Michael W. Fried, MD
Associate Professor of Medicine
Director, Section of Hepatology
Division of Digestive Diseases and Nutrition

Shannon Galvin, MD
Instructor of Medicine
Division of Infectious Diseases

J. C. Garbutt, MD
Professor of Psychiatry
Division of Adult Psychiatry

Susan A. Gaylord, PhD
Assistant Professor of Physical Medicine and
  Rehabilitation
Director, Program on Integrative Medicine

John H. Gilmore, MD
Associate Professor of Psychiatry
Division of Basic Psychobiology
Division of Adult Psychiatry

Paul A. Godley, MD, PhD
Associate Professor of Medicine
Assistant Professor of Epidemiology
Division of Hematology and Oncology
Lineberger Comprehensive Cancer Center

Lee R. Goldberg, MD
Instructor of Medicine
Division of Cardiology

Robert S. Greenwood, MD
Professor of Neurology
Chief, Section of Child Neurology

Ian S. Grimm, MD
Associate Professor of Medicine
Division of Digestive Diseases and Nutrition

Steven H. Grossman, MD
Associate Professor of Medicine
Division of Nephrology and Hypertension

Robert E. Gwyther, MD, MBA
Professor of Family Medicine
Director, Medical Student Programs

John J. Haggerty, MD
Associate Professor of Psychiatry
Director, Division of Social and Community
  Psychiatry

Colin D. Hall, MBChB
Professor of Neurology
Vice Chairman, Department of Neurology

William D. Heizer, MD
Professor of Medicine
Division of Digestive Diseases and Nutrition

David C. Henke, MD
Associate Professor of Medicine
Division of Pulmonary and Critical Care
  Medicine

Michael A. Hill, MD
Associate Professor of Psychiatry
Director, Adult Inpatient Program
Medical Director, Geropsychiatry Inpatient Unit

Alan L. Hinderliter, MD
Associate Professor of Medicine
Division of Cardiology

Albert R. Hinn, MD
Associate Professor of Neurology
Section of Adult Neurology

Gerald A. Hladik, MD
Associate Professor of Medicine
Division of Nephrology and Hypertension

Mina C. Hosseinipour, MD
Instructor of Medicine
Division of Infectious Diseases

James F. Howard, Jr, MD
Professor of Neurology
Chief, Section of Neuromuscular Disorders

CONTRIBUTORS

Xuemei Huang, MD, PhD
Assistant Professor of Neurology
Section of Adult Neurology

Burton R. Hutto, MD
Associate Professor of Psychiatry
Division of Adult Psychiatry

Kim L. Isaacs, MD, PhD
Associate Professor of Medicine
Associate Director, UNC Inflammatory Bowel
  Disease Center
Division of Digestive Diseases and Nutrition

Bruce F. Israel, MD
Instructor of Medicine
Division of Infectious Diseases

Heidi T. Jacobe, MD
Assistant Professor of Dermatology

Peter Lars Jacobson, MD
Professor of Neurology
Director, Palliative Care Program
Section of Adult Neurology

Sandra M. Johnson, MD
Assistant Professor of Ophthalmology

Beth L. Jonas, MD
Assistant Professor of Orthopedics and
  Medicine
Division of Rheumatology and Immunology

Joanne M. Jordan, MD, MPH
Associate Professor of Medicine
Division of Rheumatology and Immunology

Fathima Kabir, MD
Instructor of Medicine
Division of Rheumatology and Immunology

Kevin A. Kahn, MD
Assistant Professor of Neurology
Section of Adult Neurology

Andrew H. Kaplan, MD
Associate Professor of Medicine
Division of Infectious Diseases

Rachel Keever, MD
Instructor of Medicine
Division of Cardiology

Meera K. Kelley, MD
Associate Professor of Medicine
Division of Infectious Diseases

Shannon C. Kenney, MD
Professor of Medicine and Microbiology and
  Immunology
Division of Infectious Diseases
Lineberger Comprehensive Cancer Center

Raymond L. Kiser, MD
Instructor of Medicine
Division of Nephrology and Hypertension

John S. Kizer, MD
Professor of Medicine and Pharmacology
Division of General Internal Medicine and
  Clinical Epidemiology

Mark J. Koruda, MD
Professor of Surgery
Chief, Division of Gastrointestinal Surgery

James E. Kurz, MD
Assistant Professor of Medicine and Pediatrics
Division of General Internal Medicine and
  Clinical Epidemiology
Division of Community Pediatrics

Garrett K. Lam, MD
Instructor of Obstetrics and Gynecology
Division of Maternal-Fetal Medicine

Peter A. Leone, MD
Associate Professor of Medicine
Medical Director, Wake County Human
  Services STD Clinic
Division of Infectious Diseases

B. Anthony Lindsey, MD
Professor of Psychiatry
Associate Chair for Clinical Affairs

J. Douglas Mann, MD
Professor of Neurology
Section of Adult Neurology

William D. Mattern, MD
Professor of Medicine
Division of Nephrology and Hypertension

Travis A. Meredith, MD
Sterling A. Barrett Distinguished Professor of
Ophthalmology
Professor and Chairman, Department of
Ophthalmology

William R. Meyer, MD
Associate Professor of Obstetrics and Gynecology
Associate Director, Obstetrics and
Gynecology Residency Program
Division of Reproductive Endocrinology and
Infertility

William C. Miller, MD, PhD, MPH
Assistant Professor of Medicine and
Epidemiology
Division of Infectious Diseases

Beverly S. Mitchell, MD
Wellcome Distinguished Professor of Cancer
Research
Chief, Division of Hematology and Oncology
Associate Director, Lineberger
Comprehensive Cancer Center

Kenneth J. Moise, Jr, MD
Upjohn Distinguished Professor of Obstetrics
and Gynecology
Chief, Division of Maternal-Fetal Medicine

Stephan Moll, MD
Assistant Professor of Medicine
Director, Thrombophilia Program
Division of Hematology and Oncology

Douglas R. Morgan, MD, MPH
Assistant Professor of Medicine
Division of Digestive Diseases and Nutrition

Dean S. Morrell, MD
Assistant Professor of Dermatology

M. Cristina Muñoz, MD
Assistant Professor of Obstetrics and
Gynecology
Division of Women's Primary Health Care

Yoshihiko Murata, MD, PhD
Instructor of Medicine
Division of Infectious Diseases

Ringland S. Murray, Jr, MD
Instructor of Obstetrics and Gynecology

Patrick H. Nachman, MD
Associate Professor of Medicine
Division of Nephrology and Hypertension

Linda M. Nicholas, MD, MS
Associate Professor of Psychiatry
Chief, Division of Adult Psychiatry
Director, Outpatient Services
Medical Director, Crisis/Emergency
Services
Medical Director, Adult Diagnostic and
Treatment Clinic

E. Magnus Ohman, MB
Ernest and Hazel Craige Professor of
Cardiovascular Medicine
Chief, Division of Cardiology
Director, UNC Heart Center

David A. Ontjes, MD
Professor of Medicine
Division of Endocrinology and
Metabolism

Kevin O'Reilly, MD
Instructor of Medicine
Division of Nephrology and
Hypertension

Robert Z. Orlowski, MD, PhD
Assistant Professor of Medicine
Division of Hematology and Oncology
Lineberger Comprehensive Cancer Center

Valerie M. Parisi, MD, MPH
Robert A. Ross Professor of Obstetrics and
Gynecology
Professor and Chair, Department of
Obstetrics and Gynecology
Chief Obstetrician and Gynecologist
North Carolina Women's Hospital

CONTRIBUTORS

Cam Patterson, MD
Professor of Medicine, Pharmacology, and
  Cell and Developmental Biology
Director, Carolina Cardiovascular Biology
  Center
Division of Cardiology

Kristine B. Patterson, MD
Instructor of Medicine
Division of Infectious Diseases

Harold C. Pillsbury III, MD
Thomas J. Dark Distinguished Professor of
  Otolaryngology, Head and Neck Surgery
Professor and Chairman, Department of
  Otolaryngology, Head and Neck Surgery

John Powderly, MD
Instructor of Medicine
Division of Hematology and Oncology

Daniel S. Reuland, MD
Assistant Professor of Medicine
Division of General Internal Medicine and
  Clinical Epidemiology

Melissa Rich, MD
Instructor of Medicine
Division of Digestive Diseases and Nutrition

Yehuda Ringel, MD
Assistant Professor of Medicine
Division of Digestive Diseases and Nutrition

M. Patricia Rivera, MD
Assistant Professor of Medicine
Division of Pulmonary and Critical Care
  Medicine

Robert A.S. Roubey, MD
Associate Professor of Medicine
Division of Rheumatology and Immunology

David S. Rubenstein, MD, PhD
Assistant Professor of Dermatology

William A. Rutala, PhD, MPH
Professor of Medicine
Division of Infectious Diseases

Yolanda V. Scarlett, MD
Assistant Professor of Medicine
Division of Digestive Diseases and Nutrition

Nicholas J. Shaheen, MD, MPH
Assistant Professor of Medicine and
  Epidemiology
Division of Digestive Diseases and Nutrition

Thomas C. Shea, MD
Professor of Medicine
Division of Hematology and Oncology
Director, Bone Marrow and Stem Cell
  Transplantation Program
Lineberger Comprehensive Cancer Center

Richard G. Sheahan, MD
Associate Professor of Medicine
Director, Electrophysiology Laboratory
Division of Cardiology

William W. Shockley, MD
Professor of Otolaryngology, Head and Neck
  Surgery
Chief, Division of Facial Plastic and
  Reconstructive Surgery
Vice Chair, Department of Otolaryngology,
  Head and Neck Surgery

Roshan Shrestha, MD
Associate Professor of Medicine
Medical Director, Liver Transplantation
Division of Digestive Diseases and Nutrition

Linmarie Sikich, MD
Assistant Professor of Psychiatry
Division of Child Psychiatry

Ross J. Simpson, Jr, MD, PhD
Professor of Medicine
Director, Lipid and Prevention Clinics
Division of Cardiology

Sidney C. Smith, Jr, MD
Professor of Medicine
Director, Center for Cardiovascular Science
  and Medicine
Division of Cardiology

Mark A. Socinski, MD
Associate Professor of Medicine
Division of Hematology and Oncology
Director, Multidisciplinary Thoracic Oncology
  Program
Lineberger Comprehensive Cancer Center

P. Frederick Sparling, MD
J. Herbert Professor of Medicine and Chair
  Emeritus
Division of Infectious Diseases

Thomas E. Stinchcombe, MD
Practicing Oncologist
Alamance Cancer Center

George A. Stouffer, MD
Associate Professor of Medicine
Director, Cardiac Catheterization Laboratory
Division of Cardiology

Carla A. Sueta, MD, PhD
Associate Professor of Medicine
Division of Cardiology

Mark Taylor, MD
Instructor of Medicine
Division of Hematology and Oncology

Michael J. Thomas, MD, PhD
Assistant Professor of Medicine
Division of Endocrinology and Metabolism

Nancy E. Thomas, MD, PhD
Associate Professor of Dermatology

John M. Thorp, Jr, MD
McAllister Distinguished Professor of
  Obstetrics and Gynecology
Division of Maternal-Fetal Medicine
Co-Director, North Carolina Program on
  Women's Health Research

Robert S. Tomsick, MD
Associate Professor of Dermatology

Charles M. van der Horst, MD
Professor of Medicine
Associate Director, Division of Infectious
  Diseases

Bradley V. Vaughn, MD
Associate Professor of Neurology
Section of Adult Neurology

Pamela G. Vick, MD
Assistant Professor of Anesthesiology

James A. Visser, MD
Assistant Professor of Medicine and
  Pediatrics
Director, Medicine/Pediatrics Residency
  Program
Division of General Internal Medicine and
  Clinical Epidemiology
Division of Community Pediatrics

Robert J. Vissers, MD
Assistant Professor of Emergency Medicine

Lea C. Watson, MD
Robert Wood Johnson Clinical Scholar
Department of Psychiatry

David J. Weber, MD, MPH
Professor of Medicine
Medical Director, Hospital Epidemiology
Medical Director, Occupational Health
Division of Infectious Diseases

Robert S. Wehbie, MD, PhD
Practicing Oncologist
Raleigh, NC

Mark C. Weissler, MD
Joseph P. Riddle Distinguished Professor of
  Otolaryngology, Head and Neck Surgery
Chief, Division of Head and Neck Oncology

Ellen C. Wells, MD
Associate Professor of Obstetrics and
  Gynecology
Chief, Division of Urogynecology and
  Reconstructive Pelvic Surgery

Young E. Whang, MD, PhD
Assistant Professor of Medicine
Division of Hematology and Oncology
Lineberger Comprehensive Cancer Center

CONTRIBUTORS

David R. White, MD
Resident, Department of Otolaryngology,
  Head and Neck Surgery

Michelle C. Whittier, MD
Instructor of Medicine
Division of Nephrology and Hypertension

Park W. Willis IV, MD
Professor of Medicine and Pediatrics
Director, Echocardiography Laboratory
Division of Cardiology

David A. Wohl, MD
Assistant Professor of Medicine
Division of Infectious Diseases

Leslie P. Wong, MD
Instructor of Medicine
Division of Nephrology and Hypertension

TABLE OF CONTENTS

TABLE OF CONTENTS

TABLE OF CONTENTS

TABLE OF CONTENTS

TABLE OF CONTENTS

TABLE OF CONTENTS

IX. INFECTIOUS DISEASES

TABLE OF CONTENTS

TABLE OF CONTENTS

TABLE OF CONTENTS

TABLE OF CONTENTS

Section I

COMMON
CLINICAL
CHALLENGES

Chapter 1

Evaluation and Treatment of Chronic Pain

Pamela G. Vick and William S. Blau

Pain, as defined by the *International Association for the Study of Pain*, is an unpleasant sensory or emotional experience associated with actual or potential tissue damage, or described in terms of such damage. Pain is subjective; no one test can measure it. A patient's pain experience is a result of inter-related physical and psychologic factors. In the chronic setting, pain becomes a disease rather than merely a symptom. The best strategy for the management of chronic pain employs a multidisciplinary approach with pharmacologic, interventional, physical, and psychologic therapies. Each patient is unique, and response to therapy may be unpredictable, requiring sequential trials of alternative therapies to arrive at an optimal treatment plan. Some intractable pains are resistant to virtually every available therapy.

ETIOLOGY AND PATHOGENESIS

Pain transduction involves free nerve endings in the integument, viscera, and periosteum. Nociceptor responses are triggered directly by exogenous tissue trauma, but are also influenced by many endogenous factors whose precise mechanisms are unknown. Three classes of endogenous mediators are involved: 1) those that activate nociceptive afferents and produce pain by local application (e.g. bradykinin, acetylcholine, potassium); 2) those that facilitate pain by sensitizing nociceptors but are ineffective in evoking pain themselves (e.g. prostaglandins); 3) those that produce local extravasation (e.g. substance P). These mediators contribute to secondary hyperalgesia, where pain thresholds in proximity to traumatized tissue are lowered.

Nociceptive transmission involves primarily unmyelinated C and thinly myelinated A delta nerve fibers. The cell bodies are located in the dorsal root ganglia, with first order synapse within the marginal layers of the spinal cord dorsal horn. Substance P, glutamate, calcitonin gene related peptide, cholecystokinin, and vasoactive intestinal peptide have all been implicated in synaptic pain transmission. Spinothalamic, spinoreticular, and spinomesencephalic pathways are the primary routes of transmission to the brain, where pain is ultimately perceived. The hypothalamus, medial thalamus, and limbic systems are involved in the motivational and affective features of pain.

The periaqueductal gray and descending inhibitory pathways selectively inhibit pain transmission at the level of the spinal cord. Norepinephrine, serotonin, enkephalin, and endorphins are the predominant inhibitory neurotransmitters.

Chronic pain may involve ongoing peripheral nociception, as in osteoarthritis or pain associated with intervertebral disc degeneration. In many other cases, persistent neuropathic pain may result from pathological alteration in the pain signaling processes themselves, e.g., in diabetic or post-herpetic neuralgia.

PAIN CLASSIFICATION

Pain may be classified according to its severity using various scales such as verbal (mild, moderate, severe), numerical (0 to 10 where 0 = no pain and 10= worst imaginable), visual analogue, faces (most appropriate for pediatric assessment) or more elaborate questionnaires (e.g., McGill Pain Questionnaire). Ultimately, all clinically useful scales are subjective and rely upon the report of the patient.

Current schemes for classification of pain according to the underlying pathophysiology remain relatively unsophisticated. Nociceptive pain arises from ongoing stimulation of peripheral nociceptors as in the case of chronic/recur-

Table 1-1
Etiology of Painful Neuropathies: Major Categories

Toxic-metabolic	Endocrine (e.g., diabetic)
	Chemotherapy (e.g., isoniazid)
	Chemical exposure associated
	Nutritional (e.g., beriberi)
Posttraumatic	Complex regional pain syndromes
Compressive	Nerve entrapment syndromes (e.g. carpal tunnel syndrome)
Autoimmune	Vasculitic
	Demyelinating
	Paraneoplastic
Infectious	Parainfectious
	Viral (e.g., herpes zoster)
	Spirochetal (e.g., Lyme)
	Guillain-Barré disease
Hereditary	Fabry's
	Amyloid

Adapted from Hewitt D. Painful Peripheral Neuropathies. Abram SE and Haddox JD, eds. *The Pain Clinic Manual,* 2nd edition. LWW, 2000; 191–199.

rent trauma or degenerative disease; the source may be somatic or visceral. Neuropathic pain may be characterized by a paucity of physical findings, and yet it includes some of the most severe pain disorders (Table 1-1). Typical descriptors include burning, tingling, shooting, numbing, and constricting. Cutaneous sensory abnormalities may range from anesthesia to hyperalgesia or allodynia (painful response to a nonpainful stimulus). Some varieties of neuropathic pain depend upon tonic activity of the sympathetic nervous system (sympathetically maintained pain). Pain and others symptoms may be abolished by sympathetic blockade with local anesthetics.

Anesthesia dolorosa is the clinical finding that defines a deafferentation pain syndrome – spontaneous pain in an area otherwise devoid of sensation; for example, when a nerve is severed (e.g., phantom limb pain). The presence of pain in the absence of intact nerve conduction pathways implicates a problem with sensory integration at the level of the CNS either due to direct tissue injury to the CNS (post spinal cord injury pain, post thalamic stroke syndrome) or functional (psychogenic).

Cancer-related pain is sometimes considered a separate category, although this is somewhat artificial as it is defined by the context rather than the pathophysiology. Cancer pain can be caused by any one or more of the above categories of pain.

CLINICAL PRESENTATION

Patients may present with one or more types of pain, and the precise pain diagnosis may remain obscure. It is important to develop a stepwise approach to the evaluation and treatment of patients with chronic pain. A commonly accepted approach is for the primary care physician and other members of the health care team to utilize a 9-step plan (Table 1-2).

MANAGEMENT AND THERAPY

Chronic pain syndromes often involve significant emotional and behavioral issues, often lead to significant functional impairments, and are accompanied by significant sleep disturbance. It is often necessary to enlist the assistance of specialists in psychology, psychiatry, physiatry, physical/occupational therapy and others.

Pharmacologic Therapy

Medical treatment of the pain itself often begins with pharmacologic therapy. There are only two classes of general-purpose primary analgesics in

Table 1-2
Nine Steps to Evaluation

Localize source of pain	Muscle, vascular, ligamentous, osseous, neuropathic
Review previous treatment	Opiate and nonopiate (side effects or benefit), physical therapy, injection therapy
Look for signs of chemical dependency	Multiple drug allergies, multiple physicians, voluminous records documenting the need for controlled substances
Identify factors contributing to altered pain perception	Secondary gain, depression
Identify comorbid states	Coexisting cardiac, peripheral vascular, or pulmonary disease, diabetes, peptic ulcer disease
Define short- and long-term goals	Pain reduction, increasing functional independence, less focus on pain, improved sleep
Use diagnostic testing and consultation to further define pain	If patient has not responded to initial conservative therapies
Assume the role of coordinator	
Describe the treatment you feel comfortable providing	Plan based on goals felt appropriate and plausible

Dickerman J, McMartin S. A nine step program for chronic pain. Fam Pract Recert. 1992;14:62-75.

use: *nonsteroidals* and *opioids*. The utility of these classes of drugs is limited by toxicity, side effects, inefficacy, physical dependence, and risk of addiction or withdrawal.

Adjuvants such as antidepressants or anticonvulsants enhance the effectiveness of a primary analgesic, limit the side effects, treat concurrent symptoms that can increase pain, and provide analgesia for certain types of pain. They may be used alone or in combination with primary analgesics. Some adjuvants also have sedating or anxiolytic side effects that can be useful in treating insomnia or anxiety. Adjuvants should be started in low doses and titrated slowly to minimize side effects and maximize benefit. Sometimes maximal analgesic effects are not seen for 4 to 6 weeks after therapeutic levels are reached. Patients should be educated about the potential delay in action of these drugs and informed that serial drug trials might be required before an adequate combination is found.

Nonsteroidals/Acetaminophen

NSAIDs are most effective in mild to moderate inflammatory pain, post-surgical, trauma, arthritis, and cancer pain (Table 1-3). The analgesic effect is potentiated when used in conjunction with opiates or other adjuvants. NSAIDs differ from opiate analgesics in the following ways: (a) there is a ceiling effect to analgesia; (b) they do not produce tolerance, physical dependence, or psychological dependence; (c) there is the potential for significant end-organ toxicity; and (d) the primary mechanism of action is inhibition of cyclooxygenase preventing the formation of prostaglandins which sensitize peripheral nerves and central sensory neurons to painful stimuli. Cyclooxygenase-II specific inhibitors that theoretically decrease the risk of gastrointestinal bleeding and do not inhibit platelet aggregation may also be used for these pain syndromes.

Opiates

Opiate therapy is indicated when chronic cancer or nonmalignant pain does not respond to nonopiate therapy alone (Table 1-4). Opiates have a central and peripheral site of action particularly in the presence of inflammation. Many opiates are available in combination with nonopiates;, this latter component is the dose-limiting factor. For example, the upper dose limit for acetaminophen

Table 1-3
Adult Dosages of Commonly Used NSAIDs

Drug	Average Dose	Dosing Interval	Maximum Daily Dose	Comments
Aspirin	600–1500 mg	4–6 hours	2400–6000 mg	
Celecoxib	100–200 mg	12 hours	400 mg	COX-II inhibitor
Choline magnesium trisalicylate	500–1000 mg 750–1500 mg	8 hours 12 hours	1500–3000 mg	No effect on clotting time
Diclofenac sodium	50 mg 75 mg	6–8 hours 12 hours	150–200 mg	
Ibuprofen	200–800 mg	4–8 hours	1200–3200 mg	
Indomethacin	25–50 mg	8–12 hours	150 mg	
Nabumetone	500–1500 mg	12–24 hours	1500–2000 mg	Food increases absorption
Naproxen	250–500 mg	8–12 hours	500–1000 mg	
Rofecoxib	12.5–25 mg	24 hours	25 mg	COX-II inhibitor

Table 1-4
Commonly Used Long-Acting Opiates and Adult Doses

Drug	Equianalgesic Oral or Transdermal Dose[*]	Starting Dose	Comments
Fentanyl	25 mcg/hour (transdermal patch) roughly equals 45 mg/day of sustained-release morphine	25 mcg/hour	12-hour delay in drug onset and offset
Methadone	2.5–10 mg (oral); highly variable between patients; use extreme caution when converting	10–20 mg/day	Long plasma half-life (12+ hours) leads to drug accumulation. Escalate dose slowly.
Morphine	30 mg (oral)	15–30 mg/day	All opioids require extreme caution in patients with reduced respiratory function, increased intracranial pressure, liver failure.
Oxycodone HCl[†]	20 mg (oral)	20–40 mg/day	

[*] Equianalgesic dose may be lower with chronic use and varies between patients.
[†] In some products, combined with aspirin or acetaminophen.

preparations is 4000 mg daily in adults and 90 mg/kg daily in children under 45 kg. For daily pain, long-acting drugs or formulations are preferred.

The undertreatment of pain is often due to the misconception that opiate therapy will lead to unmanageable tolerance and physical and psychological dependence. Tolerance can occur but it is not the most likely cause of increased narcotic requirement. Disease progression or new pain syndrome should be excluded. Physical dependence and withdrawal symptoms can be prevented by careful monitoring, slow withdrawal, and tapering of narcotics. Psychological dependence is rare if narcotics are prescribed correctly. Pseudo-

Table 1-5
Commonly Used Antidepressants and Dose

Drug	Dose*	Side Effects
Tricyclic		
Amitriptyline	10–150 mg	Anticholinergic and alpha adrenergic blocking effects, cardiotoxicity,
Nortriptyline	25–75 mg	orthostatic hypotension, narrow angle glaucoma, lower seizure threshold
Desipramine	25–100 mg	
Doxepin	25–100 mg	
Atypical		
Trazodone	50–300 mg	Priapism, little anticholinergic effect
SSRIs		
Fluoxetine	20–60 mg	Insomnia, restlessness, GI distress, tremor, primary ejaculatory delay, nausea
Paroxetine	10–40 mg	
Sertraline	50–20 0mg	

*Once daily at bedtime.
Adapted with permission from Manning DC. Adjuvant Analgesics. Abram SE and Haddox JD, eds. The Pain Clinic Manual, 2nd edition. LWW 2000; 153.

addiction is a pattern of drug seeking behavior in an attempt to gain pain relief, and may be perceived as addiction. It is often the result of uncontrolled pain due to inadequate treatment. This behavior should stop once pain is adequately relieved.

The long-term use of opioid analgesics is often appropriate for the control of otherwise intractable pain, but it requires close monitoring and an ongoing patient-physician relationship.

Antidepressants

Tricyclic antidepressants have been used as first line therapy for a variety of neuropathic pain disorders, and may be helpful in managing sleep disturbance associated with chronic pain. Atypical antidepressants, serotonin reuptake inhibitors, and monoamine oxidase inhibitors may also have a role, although the results of clinical trials of their efficacy as analgesics have been equivocal (Table 1-5).

Anticonvulsants

Anticonvulsants may relieve lancinating pain arising from peripheral nerve syndromes such as trigeminal neuralgia, postherpetic neuralgia, diabetic neuropathy, cancer pain, and posttraumatic neuralgia. These drugs are also effective as mood stabilizing drugs and in migraine prophylaxis (Table 1-6).

Physical Interventions

Exercise, massage, applications of heat and cold, transcutaneous electrical nerve stimulation (TENS), and acupuncture are used in addition to medication therapy. These are particularly helpful in myofascial or localized pain disorders.

Various types of injections and nerve blocks can be employed as important diagnostic and therapeutic tools. Trigger point injections are effective in myofascial pain. Epidural steroid injection and selective nerve root blocks are effective for radicular neuropathic pain problems or spinal stenosis. Facet joint injections and medial branch nerve blocks are useful in mechanical back and neck pain.

Sympathetic nerve blocks (stellate ganglion, celiac plexus, lumbar sympathetic) can be diagnostic and therapeutic for sympathetically maintained pain, and can facilitate rehabilitation-oriented therapy. If a patient experiences profound but temporary benefit from nerve blocks, then he/she may be considered for chemical or surgical neurolysis. Such procedures are generally not permanent and not without risk; they are best considered only as a last resort, especially for patients with limited life expectancy.

More aggressive interventional pain therapies include radiofrequency denervation, spinal cord stimulation, and intrathecal pumps.

FUTURE DIRECTIONS

Until such time as we have the means to effectively eliminate chronic pain, newer cost-effective models of multidisciplinary assessment and care of patients are needed. Our understanding of neuropathic pain mechanisms and pathophysiol-

Table 1-6
Commonly Used Anticonvulsants and Dose

Drug	Daily Dose	Side Effects
Gabapentin	Start 300 mg qhs, titrate to 900–1200 mg TID	Sedation, ataxia, edema, tremor, psychomotor slowing, difficulty concentrating
Topiramate	Start 50 mg qhs, titrate to max dose 200 mg BID	Sedation, fatigue, psychomotor slowing, difficulty concentrating, paresthesias, kidney stones
Lamotrigine	Start 25 mg qhs, titrate to 300–500 mg BID	Rash, drug interaction with other anticonvulsants
Carbamazepine	Start 200 mg qhs, titrate to 400–1200 mg/day	Sedation, ataxia, hepatitis, aplastic anemia, slow intracardiac conduction
Valproate	Start 5–10 mg/kg/day, titrate to 15–60 mg/kg/day	Sedation, transient elevation SGOT/SGPT, thrombocytopenia, platelet dysfunction at higher doses

Adapted with permission from Manning DC. Adjuvant Analgesics. Abram SE and Haddox JD, eds. The Pain Clinic Manual, 2nd edition. LWW 2000; 152.

ogy is still in its infancy, but advancing rapidly; there are more novel analgesic drugs currently under investigation. Custom designed analgesics seek to impact pain processes on a cellular level—to block nociception, to counteract the processes of neuropathic pain, and to prevent central sensitization. New interventional techniques, such as intradiskal electrothermocoagulation for discogenic pain, continue to be developed and explored as means to treat the sources of intractable pain. Chronic pain prevention is an area ripe for research and clinical development.

REFERENCES

Dickinson BD, Altman RD, Nielsen NH, Williams MA. Use of opioids to treat chronic, noncancer pain. *West J Med.* 2000;172:107-115.

Fine PG, Rosenberg J. Functional neuroanatomy. In: Brown DL, ed. *Regional Anesthesia and Analgesia.* Philadelphia, Pa: WB Saunders Co; 1996:25-49.

Lipman AG. Analgesic drugs for neuropathic and sympathetically maintained pain. *Clin Geriatr Med.* 1996;12:501-515.

Raj PP. Management of patients with acute and chronic pain. *J Clin Anesth.* 1992;4(suppl 1):33S-44S.

Russo CM, Brose WG. Chronic pain. *Annu Rev Med.* 1998; 49:123-133.

Pain.com Web site. Pain library. Available at: http://www.pain.com/library. Accessed January 31, 2003.

Chapter 2

Drug Therapy in the Elderly

Debra L. Bynum

It is estimated that medication use by people over the age of 65 accounts for 25% to 30% of all prescriptions per year in the United States. The elderly living in the community take on average 3 to 4 medications at a time, and the institutionalized elderly are prescribed an average of 8 medications. Moreover, older people are at an increased risk for significant adverse drug reactions due to interactions between multiple medications and chronic disease states.

AGE RELATED CHANGES IN PHARMACOKINETICS AND PHARMACODYNAMICS

Pharmacokinetic processes are based upon bioavailability, distribution, and clearance. Bioavailability, the fraction of drug reaching the circulation after administration, is directly correlated with absorption for oral drugs. Although there is evidence that acid secretion and gut perfusion are decreased in aging, there is no evidence to suggest a clinically significant effect on overall rate and extent of absorption for most medications.

The distribution of a drug is mainly determined by plasma protein binding characteristics and tissue binding properties. In general, drugs that are highly protein–bound have a smaller volume of distribution. A decrease in lean body mass and total body water composition are important age–related changes that decrease the volume of distribution in the elderly, especially for women, and can lead to higher initial concentrations of water soluble drugs. Highly lipid soluble drugs such as diazepam may be more extensively distributed leading to a prolonged elimination time. Decreased serum albumin may lead to higher free drug levels of agents such as phenytoin and warfarin that are highly bound to albumin. Thus, age–related changes in distribution volumes and protein binding may affect free and total levels as well as elimination times for many drugs.

Elimination of drugs is mainly based upon renal and hepatic clearance. There is an age–related decrease in creatinine clearance. As muscle mass decreases, serum creatinine alone becomes an inaccurate marker for creatinine clearance and formulas commonly used to estimate clearance

are not always reliable. Drugs such as digoxin, gentamicin, lithium, and trimethoprim-sulfamethoxazole require care in the setting of impaired renal excretion. Age–related changes in renal clearance should be anticipated in the elderly, even with a normal serum creatinine.

Hepatic mechanisms, predominantly through the cytochrome P450 family of enzymes, clear drugs by inactivation with oxidative or conjugative reactions. This system is responsible for the metabolism of a multitude of drugs, including benzodiazepines, clarithromycin, calcium channel blockers, ketoconazole, lidocaine, warfarin, phenytoin, and many nonsteroidal anti-inflammatory agents. Induction or inhibition of these enzymes forms the basis of many drug-drug and drug-food interactions. Despite decreased hepatic blood flow and decreased hepatic size observed with aging, there is no evidence in human studies to suggest a clinically significant decrease in metabolic rates or enzyme activity. Apparent effects of impaired hepatic metabolism often reflects drug interactions that are more likely to occur in older patients who are taking several medications.

The elimination *half-life* is the time needed for the amount of drug in the body to decrease by half. It is also the amount of time needed to reach 50% of a steady state concentration after initiation of a drug. It takes 3.3 times the half-life of a drug to reach a 90% steady state concentration. Multiple drugs are reported to have an increased elimination half-life associated with aging, but these changes reflect mainly the changes in drug clearance and distribution as previously discussed. Allow an adjusted time between doses of medications in older patients and allow adequate time for drug elimination when drug toxicity is suspected.

Pharmacodynamic changes relate to variances in observed drug effects, given similar serum concentrations, between different individuals. In the elderly, these effects include more profound sedation seen with benzodiazepines, decreased beta-adrenoceptor blocking activity observed with propranolol, a greater decrease in blood pressure with calcium channel blockers, and an increased sensitivity to the anticoagulant effects of warfarin. A "therapeutic" level of drug may still have adverse effects, mandating lower initial doses of most drugs in the elderly patient and careful titration.

ADVERSE DRUG EFFECTS

Adverse drug reactions in the elderly are common and often unrecognized because they may appear as secondary to other disorders (falls, anorexia, fatigue, confusion, incontinence, constipation) (Table 2-1). Although the elderly are more likely to have adverse drug reactions, the average number of drugs taken by an individual, not age alone, appears to be the main risk factor.

Drug-drug interactions can be due to pharmacokinetic changes, in which one drug alters the concentration of another drug, as well as pharmacodynamic changes with one drug altering the physiologic response to a second drug. Interactions may be additive or antagonistic. Clinically important drug-drug pharmacodynamic interactions include the significant hypotension observed in some older patients when given the combination of vasodilators, anticholinergics, and diuretics.

Drug-disease interactions are also common. Observed interactions include the increased water retention seen in patients with congestive heart failure who are taking NSAIDs, increased urinary incontinence with diuretics, and the increased urinary retention in patients with prostatic hypertrophy given anticholinergics.

THE USE OF NONPRESCRIPTION DRUGS AND COMPLEMENTARY OR ALTERNATIVE THERAPIES AMONG THE ELDERLY

Multiple surveys have demonstrated that 35% to 60% of all adults in the United States have used some form of complementary/alternative medicine. In a survey of Californians enrolled in a Medicare supplemental program, 41% reported the use of some form of alternative medicine (24% reporting the use of herbal medications and 14% the use of acupuncture). Another survey of patients in a rheumatology and geriatric clinic found a prevalence of use rate of 66%. More than half of patients who reported using such therapies had not discussed this with their physicians.

Given an ample selection of nonprescription medications in addition to vitamins and medications considered complementary to standard care, there is an increasing need for physicians to be aware of the fact that many of their patients may be taking drugs that they are not aware of unless the patient is specifically queried.

SUMMARY

In general, the dosing of most drugs should be decreased in the elderly. Dosages should be titrated slowly, giving ample time to achieve a steady state. Common symptoms such as incontinence, confusion, constipation, falls and anorexia may be evidence for adverse drug reactions in the elderly. Nonprescription drugs, especially NSAIDs, and complementary therapies are popular and not commonly reported to physicians.

Polypharmacy is a difficult problem and is associated with an increased risk of adverse drug reactions. The number of medications, and not age alone, seems to be the main risk factor for such reactions in this age group. Polypharmacy has become increasingly difficult to avoid given current guidelines for the treatment of chronic diseases common to this population, such as diabetes, congestive heart failure, and coronary heart disease. Avoiding a tendency to undertreat conditions such as osteoporosis, depression, and chronic pain is equally important in the care of the older patient. Although there are risks with treatments for such diseases as atrial fibrillation, ischemic heart disease, and cerebrovascular events, we are recognizing that this group may be in a position for potential benefits from intervention. And while there are medications that many consider contraindicated for use in the elderly patient, it is not possible nor appropriate to create a list of "off limit" agents and apply this to each individual patient.

FUTURE DIRECTIONS

Prescribing medications for elderly patients is challenging and will become a problem faced by

Table 2-1
Clinical Examples of Adverse Drug Effects in the Elderly

Drug	Potential Effects
Aminoglycosides, once daily dosing concentrations	Possible increased nephrotoxicity, correlated with high peak
Diuretics	Incontinence, postural hypotension, hyponatremia, hypokalemia
Prazosin	Postural hypotension, incontinence
Digoxin	Nausea, confusion
Verapamil	Constipation
Theophylline	Nausea, tremor, confusion, arrhythmia
Cimetidine, Ranitidine	Confusion
Levodopa	Confusion, hallucinations, dystonia, postural hypotension
Bromocriptine	Confusion and postural hypotension
Phenytoin	Ataxia, falls, confusion
Phenothiazines	Confusion, parkinsonism, constipation, urinary retention, postural hypotension
Prochlorperazine and Metoclopramide	Most common cause of drug-induced parkinsonism in the elderly; confusion
Tricyclic antidepressants	Confusion, falls, hypotension, constipation, urinary retention
Benzodiazepines	Confusion, falls
Narcotics	Confusion, constipation
NSAIDS	Exacerbation of CHF or renal insufficiency
Nifedipine and Felodipine	Peripheral edema
Warfarin	Increased sensitivity with aging
Diphenhydramine	Agitation, confusion, urinary retention

physicians in nearly every field as this segment of the population continues to grow. Clinical trials, which have traditionally excluded women and the elderly, need to continue to expand eligibility requirements and even specifically examine this population. The balance between too much and too little medication in the older patient is something that will become increasingly challenging as the numbers of our elders, as well as our therapeutic options, continue to expand.

REFERENCES

Anderson DL, Shane-McWhorter L, Crouch BI, Andersen SJ. Prevalence and patterns of alternative medication use in a university hospital outpatient clinic serving rheumatology and geriatric patients. *Pharmacotherapy.* 2000;20:958-966.

Astin JA, Pelletier KR, Marie A, Haskell WL. Complementary and alternative medicine use among elderly persons: one-year analysis of a Blue Shield Medicare supplement. *J Gerontol A Biol Sci Med Sci.* 2000;55:M4-M9.

Avorn J, Gurwitz JH. Drug use in the nursing home. *Ann Intern Med.* 1995;123:195-204.

Hanlon JT, Schmader KE, Koronkowski MJ, et al. Adverse drug events in high risk older patients. *J Am Geriatr Soc.* 1997;45:945-948.

May FE, Stewart RB, Hale WE, Marks RG. Prescribed and non-prescribed drug use in an ambulatory elderly population. *South Med J.* 1982;75:522-528.

McLeod PJ, Huang AR, Tamblyn RM, Gayton DC. Defining inappropriate practices in prescribing for elderly people: a national consensus panel. *CMAJ.* 1997;156:385-391.

Montamat SC, Cusack BJ, Vestal RE. Management of drug therapy in the elderly. *N Engl J Med.* 1989;321:303-309.

Willcox SM, Himmelstein DU, Woolhandler S. Inappropriate drug prescribing for the community-dwelling elderly. *JAMA.* 1994;272:292-296.

Chapter 3

Nutrient Deficiencies

William D. Heizer

Nutrient deficiencies occur in various disease states and can contribute to morbidity and mortality, often in the absence of signs and symptoms of deficiencies. This chapter will focus on some of the nutrient deficiencies likely to be encountered in medical practice in developed nations. The important burden of nutrient deficiencies due to inadequate dietary intake in less-developed parts of the world is not included. Also, the possibility that ingestion of some nutrients in excess of currently recommended daily amounts may decrease the incidence or severity of some chronic diseases is beyond the scope of this chapter.

ETIOLOGY AND PATHOGENESIS

A nutrient deficiency can result from inadequate intake, decreased absorption, excessive loss, increased utilization, or genetically determined increased need. Up to one-third of individuals in developed countries ingest less than 70% of recommended amounts of calcium, iron, magnesium, vitamin A, and pyridoxine in their normal diet and are deficient or borderline deficient in one or more of these nutrients in the absence of disease. Deficiencies of those nutrients and of the water-soluble vitamins that have small body stores including folate, thiamine, niacin, and vitamin C should be suspected in patients with alcoholism, food fadism, prolonged anorexia, nausea, dysphagia, diarrhea, weight loss, advanced vital organ failure, and malabsorption. Deficiencies of the fat-soluble vitamins (A, D, E, and K) should be suspected with any form of chronic fat malabsorption including short bowel syndrome, pancreatic insufficiency, bacterial overgrowth, celiac sprue, Whipple's disease, and primary biliary cirrhosis.

Normal vitamin B_{12} absorption requires intrinsic factor from the stomach, proteolytic enzymes from the pancreas, a small bowel free of bacterial overgrowth, and specific receptors in the distal ileum. Because the liver stores a supply of vitamin B_{12} sufficient for 3 to 5 years, an otherwise normal individual eating a diet virtually devoid of vitamin B_{12} (e.g., a lacto-ovo vegetarian diet) would not become deficient sooner than in 3 to 4 years. Severe malabsorption of the vitamin can lead to deficiencies sooner because there is a substantial enteropatic circulation of vitamin B_{12}. Vitamin B_{12} deficiency is more prevalent than generally assumed. Risk factors include age greater than 60, total or subtotal gastrectomy, ileal resection (including ileal urinary conduit), ileoanal pull through, long-term suppression of gastric acid secretion, and small bowel bacterial overgrowth.

Zinc deficiency is most likely to occur in the setting of chronic diarrhea. Normally about one fifth of ingested zinc is absorbed along with a portion of the zinc present in pancreatic and other internal secretions. Excessive amounts of ingested and secreted zinc are lost in diarrheal stool. Poor iron absorption may contribute to iron deficiency in patients with celiac sprue, some other forms of malabsorption, Crohn's disease, and partial or complete gastrectomy.

CLINICAL PRESENTATION AND DIAGNOSTIC APPROACH

The classical signs and symptoms of vitamin and trace element deficiencies are well described in standard texts. Figures 3-1 to 3-4 illustrate deficiencies of thiamine, niacin, vitamin C, and vitamin A respectively. Patients at risk should be treated prophylactically before deficiency develops. Patients at risk of fat-soluble vitamin deficiency including those with short bowel syndrome, other forms of malabsorption, prolonged active Crohn's disease, and chronic weight loss should have yearly, measurements of bone density, 25-hydroxyvitamin D, vitamin A, vitamin E, and prothrombin time. Patients at risk for vitamin B_{12} deficiency should have measurements of serum vitamin B_{12} levels every 2 to 3 years. Elevated serum levels of homocysteine and methylmalonic acid are more sensitive measures of vitamin B_{12} status. Advanced

Figure 3-1

Thiamine Deficiency (Beriberi)

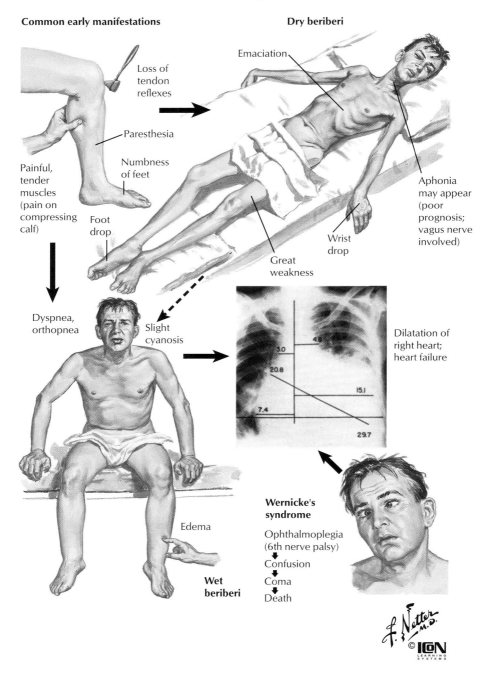

Common early manifestations

Loss of tendon reflexes

Paresthesia

Painful, tender muscles (pain on compressing calf)

Numbness of feet

Foot drop

Dyspnea, orthopnea

Slight cyanosis

Edema

Wet beriberi

Dry beriberi

Emaciation

Aphonia may appear (poor prognosis; vagus nerve involved)

Wrist drop

Great weakness

Dilatation of right heart; heart failure

Wernicke's syndrome

Ophthalmoplegia (6th nerve palsy)
↓
Confusion
↓
Coma
↓
Death

Figure 3-2

Pellagra

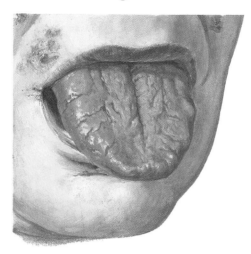

Pellagra tongue

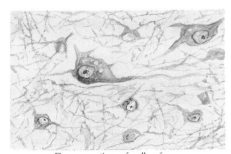

Degeneration of cells of
cerebral cortex

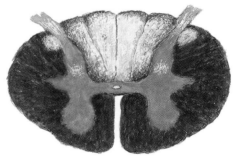

Degeneration in spinal cord

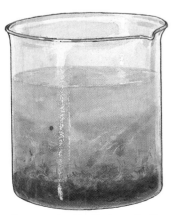

Aqueous stool in diarrhea of pellagra

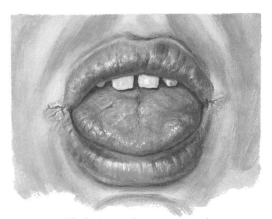

Cheilosis, angular stomatitis and
magenta tongue in ariboflavinosis

Figure 3-3

Vitamin C Deficiency (Scurvy)

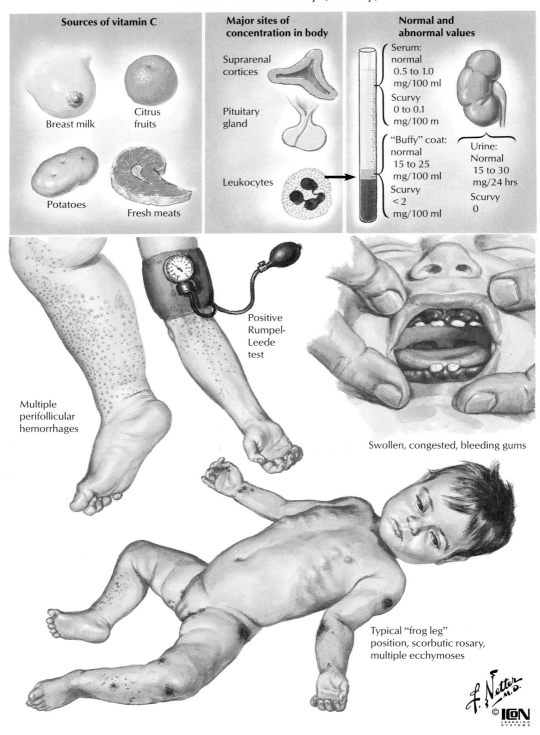

Sources of vitamin C

Breast milk

Citrus fruits

Potatoes

Fresh meats

Major sites of concentration in body

Suprarenal cortices

Pituitary gland

Leukocytes

Normal and abnormal values

Serum: normal 0.5 to 1.0 mg/100 ml
Scurvy 0 to 0.1 mg/100 m

"Buffy" coat: normal 15 to 25 mg/100 ml
Scurvy < 2 mg/100 ml

Urine: Normal 15 to 30 mg/24 hrs
Scurvy 0

Multiple perifollicular hemorrhages

Positive Rumpel-Leede test

Swollen, congested, bleeding gums

Typical "frog leg" position, scorbutic rosary, multiple ecchymoses

Figure 3-4

Vitamin A Deficiency

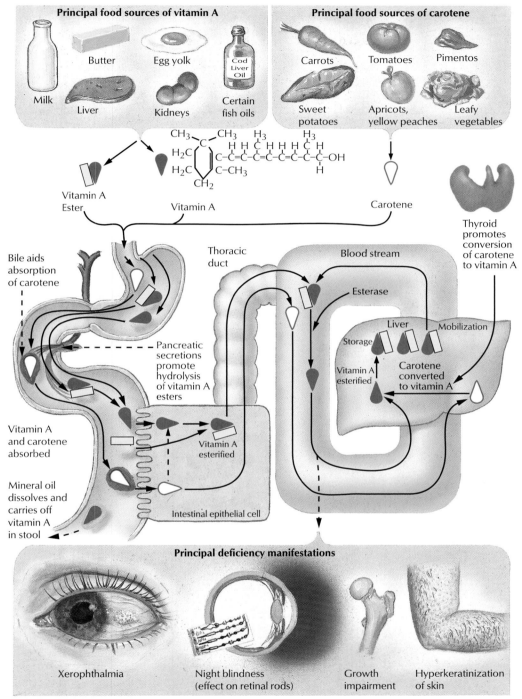

Principal food sources of vitamin A

Milk · Butter · Egg yolk · Liver · Kidneys · Cod Liver Oil · Certain fish oils

Principal food sources of carotene

Carrots · Tomatoes · Pimentos · Sweet potatoes · Apricots, yellow peaches · Leafy vegetables

Vitamin A Ester

Vitamin A

Carotene

Thyroid promotes conversion of carotene to vitamin A

Bile aids absorption of carotene

Thoracic duct

Blood stream

Esterase

Liver

Storage

Mobilization

Vitamin A esterified

Carotene converted to vitamin A

Pancreatic secretions promote hydrolysis of vitamin A esters

Vitamin A and carotene absorbed

Vitamin A esterified

Mineral oil dissolves and carries off vitamin A in stool

Intestinal epithelial cell

Principal deficiency manifestations

Xerophthalmia · Night blindness (effect on retinal rods) · Growth impairment · Hyperkeratinization of skin

vitamin B_{12} deficiency may cause megaloblastic anemia or neurologic abnormalities including subacute combined degeneration of the spinal cord, depression, or memory loss, all of which may be partially or completely irreversible. Vitamin B_{12} deficiency is often present in the absence of any specific hematologic or neurologic abnormality. Zinc deficiency can cause diarrhea, alopecia, skin rash especially on the face and groin, and decreased sense of taste. A serum zinc level may confirm deficiency but is not very reliable.

MANAGEMENT AND THERAPY
Vitamin D

The recommended daily intake (RDI) is 400 IU. Treatment of deficiency due to poor intake is 4000 to 8000 IU daily. For deficiency due to malabsorption, 50,000 IU orally from once daily to once weekly is usually required.

Vitamin A

The RDI is 5000 IU. Severe deficiency can be treated orally or intramuscularly with 100,000 IU daily for three days followed by 50,000 IU daily for two weeks, then 10,000 to 20,000 IU daily for two months.

Vitamin E

Deficiency can be treated with 300 mg of D-alpha-tocopherol (450 IU) daily orally or intramuscularly.

Thiamine

The RDI is 1.5 mg. Deficient patients should receive 25 to 50 mg orally or half that amount intramuscularly daily for seven days. Critically deficient patients may receive 50 to 100 mg intravenously plus the same amount intramuscularly daily for three days.

Niacin

The RDI is 20 mg. Patients with pellagra should be treated with 100 mg of nicotinic acid or nicotinamide orally three times daily. If necessary, 100 mg of nicotinamide can be given daily intramuscularly.

Folic Acid

The RDI is 0.4 mg. Replete body stores with 1 mg orally daily for 2 to 3 weeks.

Vitamin B_{12}

The RDI is 6 mcg but 2 mcg daily is sufficient for most normal adults. Most deficiency states can be treated with 500 to 1000 mcg orally daily. An intranasal preparation is also effective. Most prefer to treat with 1000 mcg subcutaneously or intramuscularly once a month. Severe deficiency should be treated with 100 to 1000 mcg subcutaneously or intramuscularly daily for 5 to 10 days.

Zinc

The RDI is 3 mg. Deficiency can be treated with 220 mg of zinc sulfate (50 mg elemental zinc) orally once or twice daily.

FUTURE DIRECTIONS

In developed countries, future research is likely to focus less on the impact of nutrient deficiencies and more on the possible use of supra physiological doses on chronic disease states. One example is the use of vitamin E, zinc, vitamin C, and beta-carotene in the prevention of macular degeneration. The development of cost effective approaches to the prevention and treatment of nutrient deficiency in developing countries will remain a challenge.

REFERENCES

Alpers DH, Klein S. Approach to the patient requiring nutritional supplementation. In: Yamada, T, Alpers DH, Laine L, Owyang C, Powell DW, eds. Textbook of Astroenterology. 3rd ed. Philadelphia, Pa: Lippincott Williams & Wilkins; 1999: 1080-1107

Nutrition.gov Web site. Available at: http://www.nutrition.gov. Accessed January 31, 2003.

Nutrition Navigator Web site. Available at: http://www.navigator.tufts.edu. Accessed January 31, 2003.

Subcommittee on the Tenth Edition of the RDAs Food and Nutrition Board Commission on Life Sciences National Research Council. Recommended Dietary Allowances. 10th ed. Washington, DC: National Academy Press; 1989.

WebMD Web site. Available at: http://www.webmd.com. Accessed January 31, 2003.

Bowman BA, Russell R, eds. Present Knowledge in Nutrition. 8th ed. Washington, DC: ILSI Press; 2001.

Chapter 4
Obesity

M. Andrew Greganti and Marschall S. Runge

Obesity is a complex multifactorial disorder that results in the accumulation of excess adipose tissue and increases the risk of morbidity and mortality (Figures 4-1 and 4-2). Definitions of the terms "overweight," "severe overweight," and "obesity" vary among authoritative sources. Using *National Center of Health Statistics* criteria, overweight individuals have a body mass index (BMI) (weight in kg/height in meters squared) greater than 27.3 for women and 27.8 for men. Obesity or severe overweight begins at a BMI of 32.3 for women and 31.1 for men. Based on *National Health and Nutrition Examination Surveys* (NHANES III) data, 35% of all Americans above age 20 are overweight or obese, representing a doubling in obesity between the 1970s and 1990s. This percentage varies depending on the ethnic group (e.g., 47% of African-American women are overweight) and prevalence increases with age. This epidemic in obesity and obesity–related illnesses likely represents the fastest–growing health risk for men, women, and children in the United States, and although most prevalent in the US, the rapid growth of obesity is becoming a worldwide problem, with similar trends in most European countries.

ETIOLOGY AND PATHOGENESIS

Obesity results from the complicated interaction of environmental and genetic factors. It is not simply a result of increased caloric intake and decreased exercise, but the obese person does consume more calories than expended through physical activity (Figure 4-3). While genetic factors are undoubtedly important, most experts believe that the marked increase in obesity in the US over the past 40 years is due to a convergence of two primary factors:

1) The increasing prevalence of obesity is explained, in part, by the fact that only 20% of the population exercises enough to be considered physically fit. Multiple influences have resulted in a generation of Americans who do not regularly exercise. These include the movement from a rural/agricultural to a metropolitan society, the reduced emphasis on exercise in the formative years (particularly primary and secondary school), and the ever-increasing "pace of life" cited by many Americans.

2) Dietary changes are equally important. The overwhelming influence of readily available high-fat foods through fast-food restaurants and vending machines (even in public schools), plus the emphasis on increased consumption of simple carbohydrates as exemplified by the traditional Food Pyramid of the *American Dietetic Association* have contributed to the imbalance between caloric intake and expenditure.

The increasing prominence of the role of genetic predisposition reflects the influence of recent studies of the molecular genetics of obesity in the mouse. Researchers have isolated 6 mouse genes associated with obesity. The most completely studied is the *ob* gene. The *ob* gene is expressed in adipose tissue and is responsible for the secretion of a protein, *leptin*. Increased leptin secretion occurs with increases in adipose tissue. Leptin stimulates a central feedback loop that increases energy expenditure and decreases appetite. In genetically engineered mice, inactivity of the leptin gene results in obesity owing to decreased energy expenditure and increased food intake. Researchers have defined a comparable gene in humans, *LEP*. It is not known whether leptin deficiency causes obesity in humans, nor whether administration of leptins will facilitate weight reduction. Indeed, leptin levels in humans seem to increase with increasing body weight, reflecting probable leptin resistance rather than leptin deficiency.

To compound the problem, obese people have great difficulty maintaining weight loss due to metabolic changes that accompany changes in weight. In effect, weight loss in a person predisposed to obesity triggers feedback mechanisms

OBESITY

Figure 4-1

Obesity I

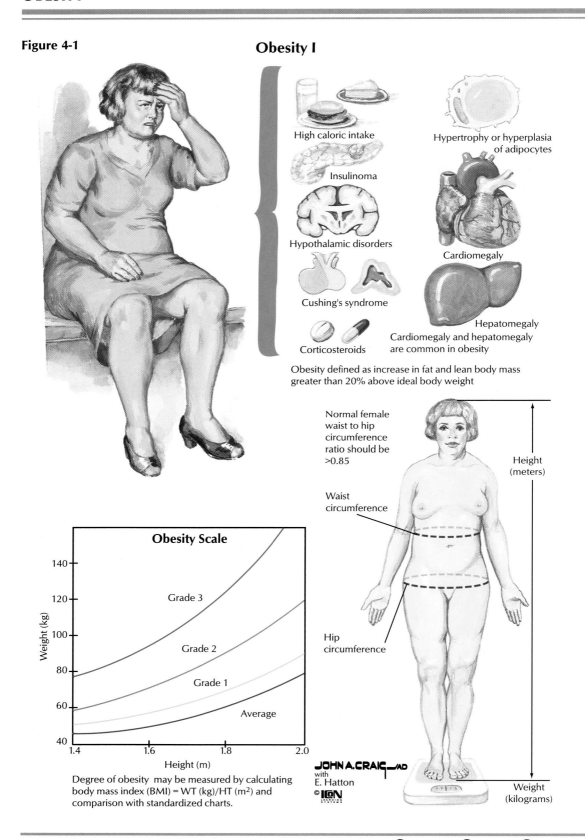

High caloric intake

Insulinoma

Hypothalamic disorders

Cushing's syndrome

Corticosteroids

Hypertrophy or hyperplasia of adipocytes

Cardiomegaly

Hepatomegaly

Cardiomegaly and hepatomegaly are common in obesity

Obesity defined as increase in fat and lean body mass greater than 20% above ideal body weight

Normal female waist to hip circumference ratio should be >0.85

Waist circumference

Hip circumference

Height (meters)

Weight (kilograms)

Obesity Scale

Grade 3

Grade 2

Grade 1

Average

Weight (kg): 140, 120, 100, 80, 60, 40

Height (m): 1.4, 1.6, 1.8, 2.0

Degree of obesity may be measured by calculating body mass index (BMI) = WT (kg)/HT (m²) and comparison with standardized charts.

JOHN A. CRAIG—AD
with
E. Hatton
© ICON

COMMON CLINICAL CHALLENGES

18

that increase appetite and lower energy expenditure as the body attempts to return weight to baseline. Studies have documented that total energy expenditure drops 15% more than the percentage decrease in body weight. One theory is that in earlier times, a physiological system may have protected humans when food accessibility was limited, leading to a survival advantage. Today, with high-fat food readily available, this physiology is clearly maladaptive, and it may explain the many frustrations faced by obese people who fail repeatedly in their attempts to sustain weight loss.

CLINICAL PRESENTATION/ DIAGNOSTIC APPROACH

Obesity presents in two predominant body adipose tissue distributions, each with a different health risk profile. *Abdominal*, or *viseral*, *obesity*, is marked by an increased deposition of fat in visceral areas. It is more common in men, manifests as an increased waist-to-hip circumference ratio, and is often referred to as having an "apple shape." Women most often have a "pear-shaped" fat distribution, with a preponderance of adipose tissue in the gluteofemoral areas and an associated decrease in waist-to-hip circumference (Figure 4-1). The well-known metabolic consequences and risks of increased visceral fat (abdominal obesity) include hyperinsulinemia, insulin resistance, glucose intolerance, adult-onset diabetes mellitus, an increase in very-low-density lipoproteins (VLDL), high low-density lipoproteins (LDL), low high-density lipoproteins (HDL), and hypertension. The prevalence of gallstones and cholecystitis also increases. In women with visceral obesity, there is associated hyperandrogenemia with anovulation and increased cortisol secretion (the polycystic ovary syndrome). The hyperinsulinemia associated with visceral obesity enhances the availability of androgens and manifests with hirsutism and other features of increased androgen levels. Risk correlates with a waist greater than 35 inches in women and 39 inches in men. In both men and women, the risk of visceral (abdominal) obesity is additive to that associated with an increased BMI.

In contrast, *gluteohumeral obesity* is associated with a lower prevalence of hyperinsulinemia, hypertension, and cardiovascular disease. Visceral fat is mobilized faster than peripheral fat and therefore has a greater negative impact on metabolism.

DIFFERENTIAL DIAGNOSIS

The differential diagnosis of obesity is very limited, and the overwhelming majority of obese individuals do not have an endocrinologic or other identifiable underlying cause. However, endocrine diseases, including hypothyroidism and hypercortisolism, warrant consideration. These causes are usually readily excluded on physical examination and routine laboratory testing. The gluteofemoral distribution of adipose tissue in hypercortisolism and associated buffalo hump, abdominal striae, and proximal muscle weakness provide helpful clues. Obesity is often associated with a positive history in multiple family members. Moreover, obese persons often trace their problem to early childhood or puberty.

MANAGEMENT AND THERAPY

The treatment of obesity is one of the most frustrating problems for patients and health care providers alike, reflecting the less than 10% rate of sustained response to therapy. It also reflects the unrealistic expectation of some patients who feel that they should lose 20% to 30% of total body weight. A goal of a 10% reduction in total body weight is probably more rational and likely to be achieved and sustained. This amount of weight loss will decrease the health risk profile of most patients, the primary goal of any therapeutic regimen. Finally, the concordance between body habitus and self-image can result in low self-esteem that only compounds the problem of obesity.

Diet and Exercise Therapy

Caloric restriction is an absolute requirement of any successful weight-reduction program, and may be achieved by following general guidelines for healthful eating or by adopting a more restrictive food or liquid diet. Successful weight reduction requires that total calories not exceed 1000 to 1200 kcal per 24 hours. Recent research has emphasized that low-fat foods often contain elevated levels of carbohydrate that produce hyperinsulinemia, increasing the risk for cardiovascular complications. Furthermore, the subtle swings in plasma glucose concentrations (in nondiabetics) that result from diets high in sugars and simple carbohydrates accentuate difficulties in appetite control in obese individuals. These observations have led to an emphasis on low-calorie, high-fiber, and high-protein

Figure 4-2

Obesity II

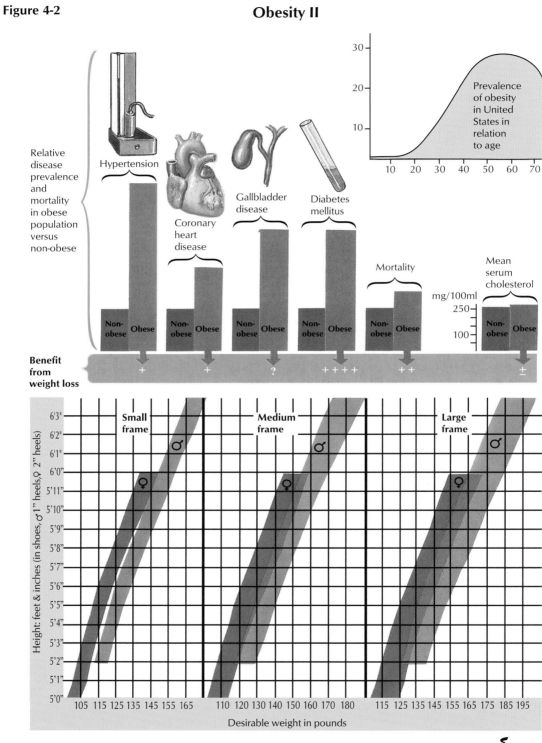

Figure 4-3

Obesity and Calories

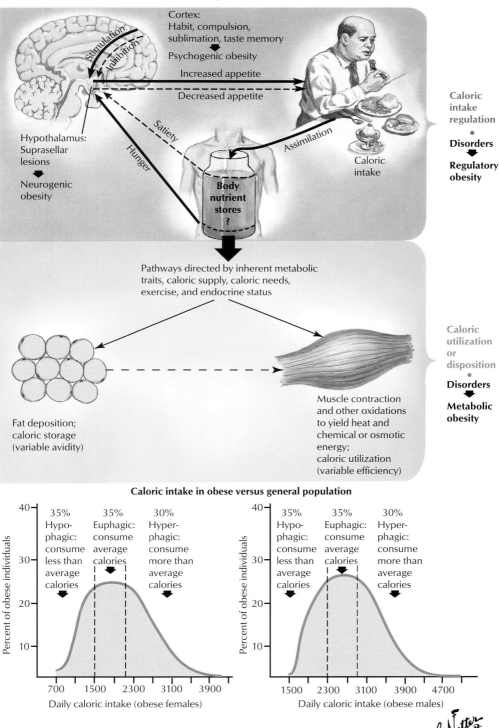

Cortex:
Habit, compulsion,
sublimation, taste memory
Psychogenic obesity

Stimulation

Inhibition

Increased appetite

Decreased appetite

Caloric
intake
regulation

• **Disorders**

**Regulatory
obesity**

Hypothalamus:
Suprasellar
lesions

**Neurogenic
obesity**

Satiety

Hunger

Assimilation

Caloric
intake

Body
nutrient
stores
?

Pathways directed by inherent metabolic
traits, caloric supply, caloric needs,
exercise, and endocrine status

Caloric
utilization
or
disposition

• **Disorders**

**Metabolic
obesity**

Fat deposition;
caloric storage
(variable avidity)

Muscle contraction
and other oxidations
to yield heat and
chemical or osmotic
energy;
caloric utilization
(variable efficiency)

Caloric intake in obese versus general population

35%
Hypo-
phagic:
consume
less than
average
calories

35%
Euphagic:
consume
average
calories

30%
Hyper-
phagic:
consume
more than
average
calories

Percent of obese individuals

700 1500 2300 3100 3900

Daily caloric intake (obese females)

35%
Hypo-
phagic:
consume
less than
average
calories

35%
Euphagic:
consume
average
calories

30%
Hyper-
phagic:
consume
more than
average
calories

Percent of obese individuals

1500 2300 3100 3900 4700

Daily caloric intake (obese males)

diets that do not stimulate high levels of insulin secretion. Whatever the regimen, patients should take a multivitamin to prevent vitamin deficiency.

Obese patients with a BMI over 30 may require a more aggressive approach to dietary restriction—to as low as 800 calories per day. There is no evidence that less than 800 calories per day is any more effective. The key to this degree of restriction is to assure a high biologic value protein intake of at least 1.5 grams per kg of ideal body weight and adequate amounts of vitamins, minerals, electrolytes, and essential fatty acids. These diets are contraindicated during pregnancy and lactation, in patients with bulimia, and in patients with anorexia nervosa. They are also relatively contraindicated in patients with chronic medical diseases: Type I diabetes mellitus, chronic liver disease, chronic renal disease, coronary disease manifested by arrhythmias or unstable angina, and in patients on chronic corticosteroid therapy. Complications include constitutional complaints of fatigue, weakness, and constipation/diarrhea. Gallstones and gout may also occur in the setting of rapid weight reduction. One advantage of the more restrictive diets (800 calories daily) is more immediate weight loss results, with accompanying positive feedback. In addition, there is evidence that appetite is more likely to be suppressed.

Caloric restriction is more likely to be successful when combined with behavioral therapy and exercise. Group-focused weight reduction programs have the advantage of peer support, especially if the group remains intact over time and is led by a professional who has experience dealing with the nuances of eating behaviors. Participation in a group program provides reinforcement when behavioral change is successful and support when it is unsuccessful. The group leader(s) must teach self-monitoring, including maintaining a diary of what is eaten under what circumstances and under which outside stressors. This allows more effective stimulus control, e.g., avoiding eating while watching television (or like activities) if doing both activities together predictably results in higher caloric intake. For many obese persons, stress is a major stimulus for overeating, a problem that necessitates the teaching of more productive approaches to stress control, such as exercise and meditation.

Exercise is key, but its impact is limited by the previously described tendency for the body to do everything possible to maintain weight in the setting of weight reduction. The energy expended for a given level of physical activity is less after weight loss occurs. Patients frequently become discouraged when they find that any weight decrease requires a disproportionately large amount of exercise. Aerobic exercise has remained a key component of successful programs, and is often supplemented by anaerobic strength training to build lean body mass. At least 30 minutes of exercise 3 days a week is recommended, with a maximum of 1 hour daily 6 days a week. Incorporating more exercise into daily activities, such as taking stairs rather than elevators, is also helpful.

While exercise alone rarely results in sustained weight loss, the importance of exercise should not be underemphasized. Exercise may be an important surrogate for an individual's motivation to lose weight. In a recent study of 32,000 dieters by *Consumer Reports*, individuals who lost at least 10% of their starting weight and kept it off for 1 to 5 years, credited exercise, not food deprivation, as the key to their sustained weight loss.

Pharmacologic Therapy

The use of drugs to treat obesity remains the hope for the future for many obese patients. The therapies that have been studied illustrate the limitations of current pharmacologic approaches to the treatment of obesity. In general, the literature documents a discouraging series of initial successes followed by failure, either because of poorly-sustained effectiveness or intolerable side effects.

Amphetamines were among the first drugs tried to suppress appetite and, although associated with short-term weight reduction, had an intolerable side-effect profile and a very high addictive potential. Trials of amphetamine-like appetite suppressants (phentermine and others) failed to show sustained benefits.

The short-lived enthusiasm for the combination of *phentermine* and *fenfluramine* (the "Phen-fen" diet) was based on reports of a 16.5% reduction in body weight compared with 4.3% in the placebo group over 34 weeks of therapy. Weight reduction leveled off after 6 months, and continuous therapy was necessary to prevent regaining what had been lost. No worrisome side effects were noted initially; in fact, proponents emphasized that the known side effects of one agent seemed to cancel those of the other. Initial questions about this therapy were raised by a 1997 report from the Mayo Clinic that described 24 cases of an unusual valvular disorder resembling the valvular disease associated with carcinoid syndrome. Despite early conflicting reports in the literature, valvular thickening, left-sided valvular regurgitation, and pulmonary hypertension are now believed to be related to this therapy. This led to the FDA recall of both fenfluramine and dexfenfluramine, another agent like fenfluramine that increases serotonin release and decreases reuptake. Dexfenfluramine had become one of the most commonly used agents outside of the United States and had enjoyed an anecdotal record of success in weight loss.

Noradrenergic agents like phenylpropanolamine and diethylpropion have been shown to be effective in short-term studies; however, a positive long-term benefit on health outcomes has not been demonstrated. Moreover, the question of an association of phenylpropanolamine with cerebrovascular disease has discouraged its use.

Antidepressants like sertraline and fluoxetine in the serotonin reuptake inhibitor group have shown short-term benefit in some patients, though weight is often regained after 6 months, even when the drugs are continued. Sibutramine, a norepinephrine and serotonin reuptake inhibitor, has shown encouraging results: an average weight loss of 5% in 65% of patients compared with 29% of placebo patients. Additional benefits include reductions in total and LDL cholesterol, triglycerides, and uric acid. There is also an associated increase in HDL. Negative effects include nausea, constipation, dry mouth, insomnia, and an increase in blood pressure in some patients. The hypertensive response is relatively mild and rarely requires withdrawal of therapy.

Orlistat is an inhibitor of pancreatic lipase that results in the malabsorption of 30% of all fat consumed. The associated negative gastrointestinal effects of fat malabsorption provide an added incentive to limit fat intake. In a 1-year placebo-controlled trial, 55% of orlistat-treated patients lost more than 5% and 25% lost more than 10% of body weight, compared with 33% and 15% in the placebo group. Positive benefits included reduced LDL, increased HDL, decreased fasting insulin levels, improved glycemic control, and

reduced blood pressure. Remarkably, the negative gastrointestinal effects did not result in a high dropout rate. The risk of malabsorption of fat-soluble vitamins requires supplementation with a multivitamin taken separately from orlistat.

Perhaps the most success has been seen in pharmacotherapy for obese patients with diabetes mellitus. *Metformin*, a commonly-used hypoglycemic agent, reduces hepatic gluconeogenesis, inhibits intestinal glucose transport, and enhances glucose uptake in muscle and adipose tissue. In contrast to exogenous insulin and insulin-stimulating oral agents, it causes weight loss, in part because it diminishes appetite. Glucose control in insulin-dependent and independent diabetics improves, as do lipid profiles. Lactic acidosis, a known risk, is very unlikely if patients with renal and hepatic dysfunction are excluded. The thiazolidinediones, including pioglitazone, have similar positive effects secondary to increasing insulin sensitivity in peripheral tissues. Patients are often able to reduce their insulin dose and have an associated reduction in body weight. However, long-term negative effects, including edema and hypertriglyceridemia, may complicate therapy with these agents.

Surgical Therapy

Surgery should only be considered in patients with a BMI over 40 who have failed other attempts at weight reduction and who have health complications including sleep apnea, cardiac failure, uncontrolled diabetes mellitus, or severe venous stasis. Noncompliant patients must be excluded, given the need for very careful adherence to a compulsory regimen of supplement vitamins and other critical nutrients. Small intestinal bypass procedures have been largely abandoned because of an unacceptable risk of life-threatening complications, and have been replaced by gastroplasty and gastric bypass procedures.

Gastric stapling (gastroplasty) reduces gastric reservoir size and restricts the gastric outlet. More than 50% of patients maintain a loss of 20% of total body weight at 5 years. The procedure fails in patients who gorge on carbohydrates, reversing weight loss in the process.

Gastric bypass is another approach involving the creation of a gastric pouch that empties into a gastrojejunostomy, thus excluding some small bowel absorptive area. Malabsorption of food and the dumping syndrome result in weight reduction but with the concomitant risk of vitamin and mineral malnutrition unless a careful supplemental regimen is followed.

Mortality in the hands of an experienced obesity surgeon is about 1%. Morbidity includes wound dehiscence/infection, anastamotic leaks, stomal stenosis, marginal ulcers, pneumonia, thrombophlebitis, and pulmonary emboli. At least some of the higher-than-expected risk relates to the risk of anesthesia and surgery in the morbidly obese. Refractory vomiting may occur with or without stomal stenosis. Esophageal dilatation, esophageal reflux/ulceration, and pouch ulceration may complicate gastroplasty. Folate, iron, B_{12}, and other micronutrient deficiencies are unique to gastric bypass and require careful followup and patient compliance. Even in the face of substantial morbidity risk, obesity surgery offers hope for a selected group of patients, and studies continue to show advantages over diet therapies.

FUTURE DIRECTIONS

Pharmacologic therapies will offer great promise in the coming years. Drug development based on new knowledge of the genetics of obesity perhaps offers the most hope for a practical and effective solution. Leptin and its congeners are currently under study and, although limited by the need for subcutaneous or intravenous administration, may prove useful in preventing weight regain in patients who have reduced via another therapy. The development of similar agents that provide for both short- and long-term success is key.

REFERENCES

Aronne LJ. Obesity. Med Clin North Am. 1998;82:161-181.

Bray GA. Health hazards of obesity. *Endocrinol Metab Clin North Am.* 1996;25:907–919.

Rosenbaum M, Leibel RL, Hirsch J. *Obesity. N Engl J Med.* 1997;337:396–407.

VanItallie TB. Prevalence of obesity. *Endocrinol Metab Clin North Am.* 1996;25:887–905.

West DB. Genetics of obesity on humans and animal models. *Endocrinol Metab Clin North Am.* 1996;25:801–813.

Williamson DA, Perrin LA. Behavioral therapy for obesity. *Endocrinol Metab Clin North Am.* 1996;25:943-954.

Yanovski SZ, Yanovski JA. *Obesity. N Engl J Med.* 2002;-346:591–602.

Zachwieja JJ. Exercise as treatment for obesity. *Endocrinol Metab Clin North Am.* 1996;25:965–988.

Chapter 5

Chronic Fatigue Syndrome

M. Andrew Greganti

The chronic fatigue syndrome (CFS) was first operationally defined in 1988 to describe patients who present, usually after a viral illness, with incapacitating fatigue of such severity that continuation of regular activities is impossible. Associated symptoms include generalized muscle pain, poor concentration, and irritability – all exacerbated after exertion. The onset is most often abrupt and disruptive of an otherwise productive life. Medical experts have not provided an acceptable explanation based on an underlying organic or "nonorganic" disease process such as anxiety or depression. The lack of a definitive explanation has led to the frustration of patients and physicians alike, and CFS has become one of several "medically unexplained" diseases.

Historical Overview and General Perspective

Medical authors have described patients with chronic fatigue at least since the late 1800s when the term "neurasthenia" defined a similar condition of uncertain cause ascribed to the impact of life stresses on the nervous system. Over time, the term "neurasthenia" has given way to a variety of others, each defining a similar clinical syndrome: Iceland disease, Royal-Free disease, epidemic neuromyasthenia, myalgic encephalomyelitis (ME), postviral fatigue syndrome, chronic brucellosis, chronic Ebstein-Barr virus infection, and Lake Tahoe disease, among others. CFS has become one of several highly prevalent conditions that defy a clearcut etiologic and pathogenetic explanation and challenge the dualistic model of medical illness. This model assumes that the mind and body are separate and categorizes every illness as mental or physical. The often-heated debate of recent years stems from moralistic prejudices that associate those illnesses characterized as "mental" with personal weakness and inferiority. In contrast, "physical" illnesses do not imply personal fault.

The dualistic model of illness has produced two approaches, each representing an attempt to explain the somatic and psychological symptoms that characterize CFS. The medical approach defines such syndromes as chronic fatigue, irritable bowel, and fibromyalgia as organic diseases with functional, rather than structural, abnormalities. The psychiatric approach regards these diseases as psychological disorders with somatic manifestations. Under this model, the somatic symptoms of CFS represent underlying depression and anxiety being manifest in an atypical "somatoform" manner. Whatever the case, the debate continues as patients and their physicians search for answers.

Epidemiology

Not surprisingly, the lack of consensus on the definition of CFS has produced great variability in prevalence estimates, ranging from 3 to 130 cases per 100,000 population. Using the most recent definition, the prevalence in persons greater than 18 years is 2.3 to 7.4 cases per 100,000. As in the case of irritable bowel syndrome and other similar entities, more aggressive case finding could lead to a higher estimate of prevalence.

ETIOLOGY AND PATHOGENESIS

A specific etiology has evaded investigators. Researchers have considered a number of mechanisms:

Viruses

Studies have implicated a number of viruses including enteroviruses, particularly Coxsackie B. Other viruses considered include herpes virus 6, herpes simplex, and retrovirus. Chronic Ebstein-Barr virus infection has received the most attention. Several epidemics of CFS have seemed to follow the pattern of an extended illness after acute infectious mononucleosis. This association has depended on the serologic markers of EBV infection. The common occurrence of infectious mononucleosis has produced a high prevalence of positive EBV markers, making interpretation of the association with CFS very difficult. It now seems unlikely that EBV will be the highly sought after underlying pathogen.

Chronic Lyme Disease

Initial excitement about the Lyme disease spirochete as a causative agent has also waned. As in the case of viral agents, investigators have had great difficulty confirming this association.

Immune System Dysfunction

The early literature documented a number of immune system abnormalities including: peripheral blood lymphopenia, abnormal numbers of T helper and T suppressor cells, impairment of delayed skin test sensitivity, decreased lymphocyte responses to mitogens, IgG subclass deficiencies, and excessive production of interferon alfa by mononuclear cells. Studies have not yielded consistent and reproducible results, and more data are needed in hopes of defining more specific associations.

Psychological Causes

Most CFS patients have a previous history of psychiatric disorders or symptoms compatible with depression and anxiety concomitant with their illness. The association with depression is especially notable and has led to debate about what is primary and what is secondary, i.e., is depression a reaction to the syndrome or is it the primary cause?

CLINICAL PRESENTATION

The most recent case definition, based on an international consensus of investigators, represents an attempt to provide a useful working definition pending the development of a better understanding of the etiology and pathogenesis of CFS. Table 5-1 lists the diagnostic criteria.

The overlap of the symptoms listed and those of depression and anxiety is obvious (Figure 5-1). Clinical diagnosis is complicated further by the fact that a large proportion of CFS patients have a previous history of major depression. In those patients who meet the criteria of both CFS and major depression, the onset of the two disorders commonly coincides. Despite this strong association, as many as 50% of patients with CFS cannot be categorized operationally under the diagnosis of a major

Table 5-1
Case Definition of Chronic Fatigue Syndrome

Inclusion Criteria:
- Clinically evaluated, medically unexplained fatigue of at least 6 months' duration that is:
  - Of new onset (not life long)
  - Not a result of ongoing exertion
  - Not substantially alleviated by rest
  - Has caused a substantial reduction in previous level of activity
- The occurrence of 4 or more of the following symptoms:
  - Subjective memory impairment
  - Sore throat
  - Tender lymph nodes
  - Muscle pain
  - Joint pain
  - Headache
  - Unrefreshing sleep
  - Postexertional malaise lasting more than 24 hours

Exclusion criteria:
- Active, unresolved, or suspected disease
- Psychotic, melancholic, or bipolar depression (but not uncomplicated major depression)
- Psychotic disorders
- Dementia
- Anorexia and bulimia nervosa
- Alcohol or other substance misuse
- Severe obesity

With permission from Fakuda K, Straus SE, Hickie I, et al. The Chronic Fatigue Syndrome: A Comprehensive Approach to Its Definition and Study. *Ann Intern Med.* 1994; 121:953.

depressive disorder. The consideration of anxiety as an underlying disorder in addition to depression still does not fully explain the full complement of symptoms experienced by many patients with CFS.

Most patients do not have definitively abnormal physical findings, at least ones that are specific. Some experience low-grade fever (37.6° to 38.6° C). Others have a nonexudative pharyngitis with palpable and/or tender cervical lymph nodes. Axillary adenopathy has also been observed.

DIFFERENTIAL DIAGNOSIS

Diseases that can present as fatigue include anemia, hypothyroidism, Addison's disease, chronic liver disease, hypercalcemia, low cardiac output states, neuromuscular diseases, sleep disorders, and depression.

Figure 5-1

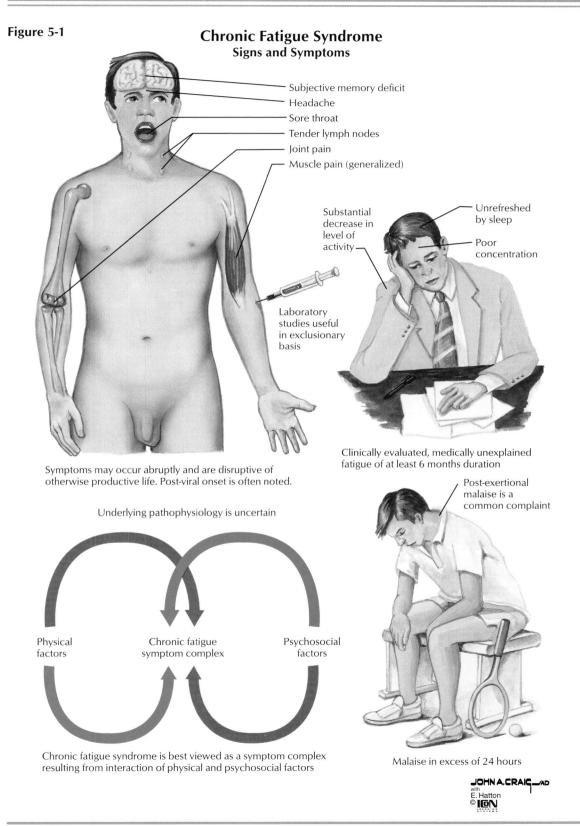

Chronic Fatigue Syndrome
Signs and Symptoms

Subjective memory deficit

Headache

Sore throat

Tender lymph nodes

Joint pain

Muscle pain (generalized)

Substantial decrease in level of activity

Laboratory studies useful in exclusionary basis

Unrefreshed by sleep

Poor concentration

Symptoms may occur abruptly and are disruptive of otherwise productive life. Post-viral onset is often noted.

Clinically evaluated, medically unexplained fatigue of at least 6 months duration

Underlying pathophysiology is uncertain

Physical factors

Chronic fatigue symptom complex

Psychosocial factors

Post-exertional malaise is a common complaint

Chronic fatigue syndrome is best viewed as a symptom complex resulting from interaction of physical and psychosocial factors

Malaise in excess of 24 hours

JOHN A. CRAIG_AD
with
E. Hatton
© ICON

DIAGNOSTIC APPROACH

The diagnosis depends on a careful review of the patient's history. In general, laboratory testing is not helpful given the lack of a sensitive and specific test and the associated poor likelihood ratios. The utility of lab testing lies in the need to exclude other diagnoses that can present as fatigue. Depression is an especially difficult diagnosis to exclude. Recommended testing includes the following: CBC, electrolyte profile, calcium, phosphorus, serum creatinine, urinalysis, glucose, liver function tests, TSH, and creatine kinase. Testing for adrenal insufficiency with am and pm cortisol levels should be considered. Evaluation for an underlying sleep disorder is also rational for unexplained fatigue, especially if there is evidence of daytime somnolence. Testing for antibodies to EBV and enteroviruses is not recommended. Similarly, immune function testing is of no diagnostic value given the variability of the results. The basic approach is to exclude other causes of fatigue first. This avoids labeling a patient with CFS prematurely.

MANAGEMENT AND THERAPY

Accepting the patient's symptoms and disability as "real" is an essential first step. Patients, after interacting with the medical system on several occasions, understand that medical science places them in an "unexplained" category, one that often questions whether they are really "sick." Discussion of possible underlying anxiety or depression regularly evokes overt hostility because such diagnoses equate with personal weakness and inferiority and, in effect, with the lack of "real" illness. It is helpful to emphasize that, in the face of insufficient knowledge about etiology, the patient and the physician must deal with a variety of possible underlying etiologies, but both must focus on treating the symptoms no matter what the cause. This requires them to abandon the dualistic model and to accept the inseparability of the mind and body in every disease process. Patients are much more willing to accept depression and anxiety as components of their disease process after being reassured that "it is not all in your head." They are also more willing to acknowledge that there is no "quick fix" given the complex interrelationships involved.

As is often the case for diseases without definitive etiologies, therapy must be individualized. It is essential to provide the patient and the family with educational materials about the nature of the syndrome, while avoiding unproductive arguments about what is and is not a likely etiology in the patient's case. Identifiable depression and anxiety must be treated with antidepressant drugs. Serotonin reuptake inhibitors with anxiolytic characteristics are often helpful. These agents may also help with insomnia that can only worsen fatigue. The physician should gently encourage the patient to return to normal functioning and to remain physically active. Exercise programs should be graded in intensity, allowing the patient input about what is and is not tolerated. Forcing poorly tolerated exercise can decrease rapport and patient self-confidence in the ability to recover function. Some studies have documented that cognitive behavioral therapy over extended intervals and with skilled therapists can help the patient develop coping skills in the face of a chronic illness.

Often, therapy is impaired by differences between the patient's and the physician's views on underlying disease mechanisms and therapy. Patients and their family members may have strong opinions based on the lay literature, Internet information, and information from self help groups. Differences arise when the provider has to complete an official report about disability and is torn between helping the patient and avoiding a self-fulfilling prophecy that CFS is a hopeless disease process. The physician should not immediately reject the patient's ideas in any of these areas. Special time must often be set aside to allow extended discussion with the patient and the patient's family. The need for such "special time" is one of many aspects that make the management of CFS patients challenging and leads to avoidance of this patient group by health care providers.

PROGNOSIS

The current literature does not provide reliable information about prognosis; however, there is clearly substantial variation among patients. The disease seems to be highly variable with day-to-day fluctuations and periods of incapacitating relapses occurring after periods of improvement. The duration of the disease is also variable, ranging from 1 to 5 years or more. The risk of morbidity is high, especially in patients who have the disease indefinitely. In contrast, mortality is rare.

Iatrogenic illness is a major risk brought on by frustrated attempts of both patients and their physicians to try any therapy, no matter how poorly documented. Patients fare worse when they insist that only an organic explanation is viable and fail to accept the biopsychosocial model of disease that espouses an intricate mind-body connection. This situation is greatly exacerbated by a health care system that insists on separating medical and psychiatric services, in effect catalyzing the dualistic approach. The exclusion of psychotherapeutic options by patients greatly limits what can be done to palliate their disease process. Unfortunately, the hesitancy of busy physicians, even those with the necessary training and experience, to take on "problem patients" also perpetuates the dualistic model.

FUTURE DIRECTIONS

The need to move from the highly descriptive term, chronic fatigue syndrome, which defines a very heterogeneous group of patients, to one or several that define a more homogeneous group(s), remains a central issue. Like other syndromes that are medically unexplained, CFS reminds us that our current classification model of disease perpetuates the dualistic mind/body separation and leads to the sub-optimal care of this large group of patients. The publicity surrounding CFS has made the need to move toward the biopsychosocial model more apparent to patients, their physicians, and, hopefully, to those who fund research. The need for more research that addresses underlying disease mechanisms and more useful ways to classify diseases that cross the mind/body divide is clear.

REFERENCES

Buchwald D. Fibromyalgia and chronic fatigue syndrome: similarities and differences. *Rheum Dis Clin North Am*. 1996; 22:219–243.

Fukuda K, Straus SE, Hickie I, Sharpe MC, Dobbins JG, Komaroff A. The chronic fatigue syndrome: a comprehensive approach to its definition and study. International Chronic Fatigue Syndrome Study Group. *Ann Intern Med*. 1994;121:953–959.

Schluederberg A, Straus SE, Peterson P, et al. NIH conference. Chronic fatigue syndrome research. Definition and medical outcome assessment. *Ann Intern Med*. 1992;117:325–331.

Sharpe M. Chronic fatigue syndrome. *Psychiatr Clin North Am*. 1996;19:549–573.

Straus SE. The chronic mononucleosis syndrome. *J Infect Dis*. 1988;157:405–412.

Chapter 6

Poisoning and Drug Overdose

Robert J. Vissers

Intentional overdoses in suicidal adults are the most common cause of poisoning that leads to hospitalization or death. Ingestion of substances in the home by children under age 6 accounts for the vast majority of reported poisonings; however, the morbidity is much lower. The incidence has more than doubled in the past decade, particularly in the teenage and elderly populations. Diagnosis can require the recognition of toxic syndromes and appropriate utilization of lab studies. Specific treatments using decontamination methods and antidotes may be required for some poisonings, although most are treated with supportive measures

ETIOLOGY AND PATHOGENESIS

Pharmaceuticals, particularly analgesics and over-the-counter preparations, are involved most frequently, followed by cleaning products, cosmetics, and plants. Ingestion is the most common route of exposure, but it may be dermal, inhalational, mucosal, parenteral, or envenomation.

The mechanism of toxicity varies with the substance. Effects may be limited to the site of exposure and represent nonspecific chemical reactions. Systemic effects are the result of interactions between the toxin and specific target sites, such as receptors or organs. Most deaths occur prehospital, often as a result of CNS and respiratory depression. Other life-threatening mechanisms include dysrhythmias, hypotension, and organ necrosis.

CLINICAL PRESENTATION

Presentations are extremely variable, not only between different substances but also for a specific toxin. Signs and symptoms depend on the time from ingestion, the amount taken, and the interaction of co-ingestants. This demands a thorough history and physical, and the consideration of a possible toxic ingestion in the differential of all patients with an unexplained sudden change in their physiologic status. Poisoned patients can deteriorate quickly, necessitating frequent reassessments and close monitoring.

Identification of potential toxins and the time of ingestion are critical for diagnosis and management (Figure 6-1). Most patients will admit to the substances ingested; however, the accuracy of the amount taken is notoriously unreliable. In addition, patients may be unable to give a history due to altered consciousness. Always assume a worst-case scenario regarding the amount taken (assume the bottle was full) and the probable presence of other co-ingestants. Collateral history from family members, friends and prehospital personnel is often helpful. Intentional overdoses are associated with a much higher potential mortality.

A complete physical examination of all systems, followed by frequently repeated vital signs and examinations, serves several purposes: 1) the identification of toxic syndromes or "toxidromes" and complications associated with the toxin; 2) the detection of underlying disease states or coexisting trauma; and 3) careful monitoring of the response to therapy (Figure 6-2, Table 6-1).

Both sympathomimetic and anticholinergic drugs can cause CNS excitation, mydriasis and an elevation of blood pressure, pulse rate, respiratory rate, and temperature. Anticholinergic agents may be distinguished by the findings of dry skin and mucous membranes, diminished bowel sounds, urinary retention, skin flushing, and decreased visual acuity. Poisoning with a cholinergic agent produces a mixture of muscarinic and nicotinic effects. The muscarinic effects produce a hypersecretory state of *s*alivation, *l*acrimation, *u*rination, *d*efecation, *g*astrointestinal hyperactivity and *e*mesis — thus the acronym "*sludge.*" Nicotinic effects include mydriasis, hypertension, tachycardia, muscle fasiculations, and weakness. Patients may present atypically when multiple toxins are involved.

Figure 6-1

Some Common Poisonous Plants

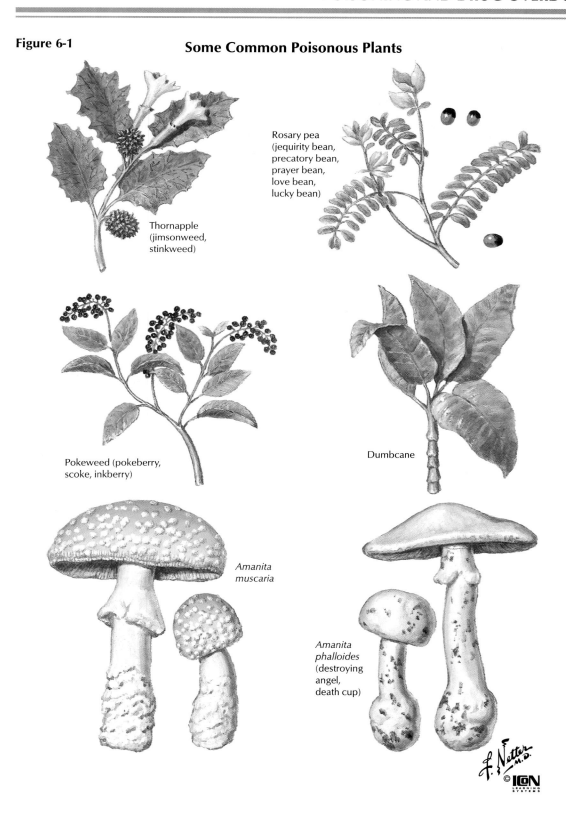

Thornapple
(jimsonweed,
stinkweed)

Rosary pea
(jequirity bean,
precatory bean,
prayer bean,
love bean,
lucky bean)

Pokeweed (pokeberry,
scoke, inkberry)

Dumbcane

*Amanita
muscaria*

*Amanita
phalloides*
(destroying
angel,
death cup)

Figure 6-2

The Pupils in Poisoning

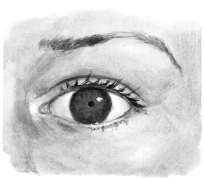

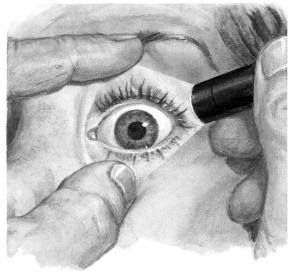

Miosis (pinhole pupils)
Seen in poisoning by morphine and morphine derivatives, some types of mushrooms, cholinesterase inhibitors, parasympathomimetics, nicotine, chloral hydrate, sympatholytics, and some other compounds

Mydriasis (pupils dilated and not reactive)
Seen in poisoning by barbiturates, carbon monoxide, methyl and other alcohols, oxalic acid, cocaine, belladonna derivatives, camphor, cyanide, sympathomimetics, parasympatholytics, and a number of other compounds

Table 6-1
Toxic Syndromes

Syndrome	Clinical Manifestations	Associated Toxins
Sympathomimetic	CNS excitation, seizures, tachycardia, hypertension, mydriasis, diaphoresis	Cocaine, caffeine, theophylline, amphetamines
Anticholinergic	Delirium, hallucinations, dry mucosa, mydriasis, decreased bowel sounds, dry skin, tachycardia, seizures	Atropine, tricyclic antidepressants, antihistamines, phenothiazines
Cholinergic	CNS excitation or depression, bradycardia or tachycardia, miosis or mydriasis, diarrhea, salivation, diaphoresis, lacrimation, paralysis	Organophosphates, pilocarpine, acetylcholine
Opiate	CNS depression, miosis, hypoventilation hypotension, response to naloxone	Heroin, codeine, propoxyphene, pentazocine, oxycodone
Serotonin	Altered mental status, increased muscle tone, hyperreflexia, hyperthermia, tremors	MAOI* + SSRI**, MAOI + meperidine, SSRI + tricyclic, SSRI overdose

*MAOI, monoamine oxidase inhibitor
**SSRI, selective serotonin reuptake inhibitor

DIFFERENTIAL DIAGNOSIS

The differential is very extensive and varies with the presentation. Poisonings need to be considered in patients with unexplained, acute alterations of mental status, seizures, or dysrhythmias.

DIAGNOSTIC APPROACH
Laboratory

Drug screens have limited utility in acute management. It is preferable to request specific drug assays in probable ingestions and when identification affects patient management. Specific quantitative toxicologic tests that may assist in management include: acetaminophen, carboxyhemoglobin, digoxin, ethanol, ethylene glycol, methanol, iron, lithium, methemoglobin, salicylates, and theophylline.

Acetaminophen should be routinely screened in all intentional overdoses because of its frequency, asymptomatic presentation, and preventable hepatic toxicity. A similar consideration may be given to screening for ASA and ethanol. The presence of some toxins may be suggested by an increased anion gap or an elevated osmolal gap (Table 6-2).

Liver function tests can be useful in acetaminophen toxicity. Calcium oxalate crystals in the urine are associated with ethylene glycol ingestion.

Electrocardiogram and Radiography

An EKG is rarely diagnostic but it can identify complications, particularly for toxins associated with sodium channel blockade. Widening of the QRS in tricyclic antidepressant overdoses is associated with seizures and dysrhythmias. Abdominal radiographs can occasionally demonstrate, but not rule out, some radiopaque ingestions (iron, phenothiazines, cocaine condoms, enteric coated tablets, heavy metals).

MANAGEMENT AND THERAPY

Most ingestions can be successfully treated through supportive care as opposed to specific antidotal therapy. Support of the airway, breathing, and circulation should take first priority. Ventilatory failure may be secondary to respiratory depression, pulmonary edema, bronchoconstriction, or paralysis. Endotracheal intubation may be needed to maintain the airway, and to facilitate oxygenation and ventilation. Hypotension usually

Table 6-2
Toxins Associated with Lab Abnormalities

↑ anion gap acidosis	↑ osmolal gap*
Ethanol	Ethanol
Methanol	Methanol
Ethylene Glycol	Ethylene Glycol
Paraldehyde	Mannitol
Iron	Isopropyl alcohol
Isoniazid	
Salicylates	

*Osmolal gap = measured osmolality − [2X Na (Meq/L) + glucose (mg/dL)/18 + BUN(mg/dL)/2.8 + ethanol (mg/dL)/4.3]

reflects venous pooling as opposed to myocardial depression; therefore, initial therapy consists of intravenous fluid boluses and Trendelenburg positioning. Norepinephrine is a good choice for inotropic support since alpha blockade is a common cause of hypotension in posionings.

Altered Mental Status and Coma

Altered mental status is a frequent complication of poisoning. Attributing the symptoms to alcohol alone is a potential pitfall, as many ingestions involve multiple toxins. CT scanning is indicated in patients with focal neurologic deficits or a history of head trauma. An immediate bedside glucose should be performed on all patients with coma or altered sensorium. Hypoglycemia may be treated with intravenous dextrose 50%. Intravenous thiamine 100 mg should be given to all malnourished and ethanol abusing patients. Intravenous naloxone 2 mg is recommended in all patients with coma of unknown etiology. Titrated doses of 0.4mg may be used in patients where withdrawal is anticipated. If an opioid overdose is strongly suspected (see toxidromes above), up to 10 mg may be required to reverse some opioids (propoxyphene, pentazocine, codeine). Flumazenil is a competitive antagonist of benzodiazepines. Intractable seizures and ventricular dysrhythmias may be precipitated in patients with a history of ethanol or benzodiazepine abuse, or a history of seizures. Its indiscriminate use in comatose patients is not recommended.

Figure 6-3

Emesis

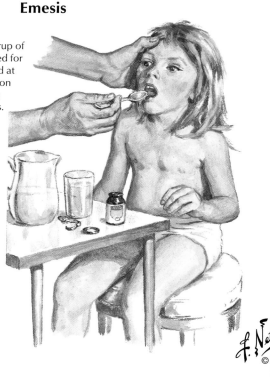

Vomiting induced by the emetic syrup of ipecac is occasionally recommended for pediatric ingestions, being managed at home, in consultation with the poison center. It no longer has a role in the hospital management of poisonings.

Surface Decontamination

Surface decontamination requires removal of clothing and flushing skin with copious amounts of water. There is no indication for using an acid or base neutralizing solution. Precautions must be taken to protect caregivers from secondary contamination.

Gastrointestinal Decontamination

This refers to interventions that empty the GI tract, remove the toxin from the GI tract, or bind to the toxin to prevent its absorption. Syrup of ipecac is an emetic agent which no longer has an indication in the hospital setting, but is still ocassionally recommended in cases of at-home pediatric ingestion in consultation with a poison control center (Figure 6-3). Orogastric lavage is utilized less frequently than in the past (Figure 6-4). It is indicated only in patients presenting after a recent ingestion (usually less than one hour) of a life-threatening toxin. It is contraindicated in alkali ingestions and nonintubated patients unable to protect their airway. It is performed through a large bore (36 to 40 French) tube. Patients should be placed in a left lateral decubitus, Trendelenburg position. Aspiration of the stomach is performed after confirmation of tube placement, and gastric lavage is repeated in 300cc aliquots until return is clear. Whole bowel irrigation uses large amounts of surgical bowel cleansing solution, administered through a nasogastric tube, to speed GI transit time and reduce absorption of the toxin. It is indicated for toxins poorly bound to charcoal (iron, lithium), sealed containers (body-packers), and sustained-release products. It is contraindicated in bowel ileus, obstruction, or perforation. Activated charcoal has a remarkable ability to bind toxins due to its large surface area. It is indicated in most poisonings, however it can obscure endoscopy in caustic ingestions and does not bind well to lithium, iron, alcohols, and strong acids and bases. The dose is one gram/kg po or per NG and may be combined with the cathartic sorbitol to reduce constipation and make the ingestion more palatable. Multiple dosing, every 4 hours, may be considered in sustained release products and toxins with an enterohepatic circulation (salicylates, digoxin, theophylline). Cathartics should not be used with repeated doses.

Figure 6-4

Gastric Lavage: Specialized Equipment

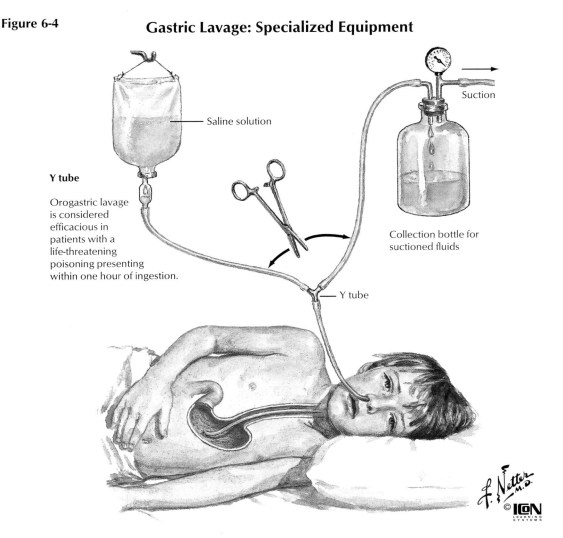

Saline solution

Suction

Y tube

Orogastric lavage is considered efficacious in patients with a life-threatening poisoning presenting within one hour of ingestion.

Collection bottle for suctioned fluids

Y tube

Enhanced Elimination

Forced diuresis is no longer recommended because of unproven efficacy and potential volume overload. Alkalinization of the urine (urine pH 7 to 8) may enhance the elimination of some toxins (salicylates, phenobarbital). Urinary acidification is not recommended for any poisoning because of the potential to exacerbate renal failure in the presence of rhabdomyolysis. Dialysis is useful only for a limited number of toxins, ideally those that are water-soluble and have a low volume of distribution and low protein binding (amphetamines, chloral hydrate, ethylene glycol, lithium, methanol, phenobarbital, salicylates, theophylline). The decision to dialyze is based upon serum levels, deterioration despite supportive care, the presence of renal failure and comorbidities.

Antidotes

Specific antidotal therapy is available for very few poisonings (Table 6-3). There are a few toxins for which antidotal therapy can be life-saving. The therapeutic half-life of the antidote may be shorter than the toxin, requiring repeat dosing or infusions (e.g., naloxone for a methadone overdose).

Management Resources

Regional poison center consultation is usually available 24 hours a day. Experienced nurses are commonly first line consultants; however, a

Table 6-3
Toxins with a Specific Antidotal Therapy

Toxin	Antidote
Acetaminophen	N-acetylcysteine
Beta Blockers	IV glucagons
Calcium channel blockers	IV calcium, glucagons
Cholinesterase inhibitors	Atropine, pralidoxime
Cyanide	Cyanide kit
Cyclic antidepressants	Sodium bicarbonate
Carbon monoxide	Oxygen
Digitalis	Digibind®
Ethylene glycol	Ethanol, 4-methylpyrazole
Fluoride	IV calcium, magnesium
Hypoglycemics	IV glucose
Isoniazid	IV pyridoxine
Iron	Deferoxamine
Methanol	Ethanol, 4-methylpyrazole
Methemoglobin producers	IV methylene blue
Narcotics	Naloxone, Naltrexone
Salicylates	Sodium bicarbonate

toxicologist is often on call and available for assistance with complex cases. The Poisondex® is a computer database available in most emergency departments and online. Nomograms are available for toxins such as acetominophen; however, specific criteria, such as accurate timing, a single ingestion, and no slow release, must be met for them to be clinically useful. Early administration of n-acetylcyseine may be life saving in acetaminophen overdose.

FUTURE DIRECTIONS

Fab fragment antidotes are drug specific antibody fragments which bind drug or protein antigen to prevent toxicity. The antibody-toxin is then excreted in the urine. Fab fragment therapy exists for digoxin and crotalid envenomations and is being developed for a number of other toxins. 4-methylpyrazole (4-MP), an alcohol dehydrogenase inhibitor, is available as an antidote to methanol and ethylene glycol poisoning. It does not cause the sedation that is associated with traditional ethanol therapy. Hallucinogenic designer drugs such as ecstasy (MDMA) and gamma-hydroxybutyrate (GHB) present new challenges in identification and management. Traditional herbal therapies can also be associated with significant toxicities, and databases are available to assist in their identification and management. There is a need for heightened disaster preparedness for mass toxin exposures associated with chemical warfare and terrorism.

REFERENCES

American Academy of Clinical Toxicology, European Association of Poisons Centres and Clinical Toxicologists: Position statements: ipecac syrup, gastric lavage, single-dose activated charcoal, cathartics, whole bowel irrigation. Clin Toxicol. 1997;35:699.

Jones AL, Volans G. Management of Self-Poisoning. BMJ. 1999;319:1414–1417.

Hoffman RS, Goldfrank LR. The poisoned patient with altered consciousness: Controversies in the use of a, coma cocktail., JAMA. 1995;274:562–569.

Chapter 7

Diagnostic Testing: The Example of Thromboembolism (PE/DVT)

John S. Kizer

Testing is a strategy to improve diagnostic certainty. It is necessary due to the statistical improbability of any disease presenting according to "classical" descriptions. The diagnostic certainty needed by a clinician depends on the seriousness of the illness in question and the hazards of therapy — the notion of an action threshold. For example, a benign illness with a benign therapy (viral pharyngitis-acetaminophen) requires little certainty to take action, whereas a more serious disease, thromboembolism (PE/DVT), with a more hazardous therapy, requires greater diagnostic certainty.

Typically, clinicians ask whether a test was positive or negative so that they may "rule out" or "rule in" a disease. Tests, however, are not dichotomous variables and convey increasing levels of information the further they deviate from "normal." For example, a patient with 4 mm ST segment depression and crushing chest pain during an ECG exercise test is much more likely to have coronary artery disease than a patient with 2 mm ST segment depression and no pain, even though both tests are "positive." Conversely, B_{12} deficiency is just as likely to be present at levels of 192 ng/ml and 194 ng/ml, even though the former is "abnormal" and the latter "normal" by laboratory nomograms. By extrapolation, one can never state that a patient does or does not have a disease, only the probability that the patient has a disease, and decide if a threshold for action has been crossed.

PE/DVT is particularly vexing because of the attendant morbidity, the difficulty in diagnosis, and the confusing array of diagnostic tests. Diagnostic algorithms have been proposed, but they are cumbersome, and still require the dichotomous notion of "cutoffs" (if "negative" go to A, if "positive" go to B). Diagnostic methods that permit one to acquire realistic estimates of disease and to decide if an action threshold has been crossed would be more useful. Such methods would circumvent cumbersome algorithms and enable clinicians to think of a continuum of risk. It is likely that concrete assessments of risk are understood more universally by clinicians than vaguer terms such as "low probability" and "high risk." For example, the perioperative risk of myocardial infarction in a "high risk" population is 4% to 5%.

GLOSSARY OF TERMS

Sensitivity: Rate of detection of those with disease, also true positive rate.

Specificity: Rate of detection of those without disease, also true negative rate.

False positive rate: (1-specificity).

False negative rate: (1-sensitivity).

Probability: or chance. Occurrence of given event expressed as fraction of all possible events. 2 heads, 2 tails. Probability of heads = 2/(2+2) = 2/4 = 50%

Odds: Number of occurrences of a one event expressed as a ratio to the number of occurrences of a second event. 2 heads, 2 tails = odds of 2/2 or 1/1 for heads. Thus, an odds of 1/1 = probability of 50%. (Note: odds may not be multiplied together).

Positive likelihood ratio: (+LLR) = True positive rate / False positive rate

Negative likelihood ratio: (-LLR) = False negative rate / True negative rate

Pretest probability of disease: The probability that a patient has a given disease before testing. The pretest probability of disease for a specific patient is also equal to the prevalence of the disease in a population of similar patients.

Pretest odds: As for pretest probability, but calculated as an odds.

Posttest probability: with positive test, also positive predictive value. Given a positive test, the probability that a patient has the disease for which he was tested.

Posttest probability with negative test, also negative predictive value.

Posttest odds with positive test. As for posttest probability, but expressed as an odds.

Posttest odds = pretest odds x LLR1 x LLR2 x LLR...n.

Posttest odds with negative test, similar to above.

THE CASE FOR LIKELIHOOD RATIOS (LLRS)

Traditionally, tests with high sensitivities have been advocated to "rule out" disease and tests with high specificities are considered to "rule in" disease. Consider, however, the following two tests: If the results are negative, which test best excludes disease in a patient with a 50% chance (pretest odds 1/1) of having the disease?

	Sensitivity	Specificity	+LLR	-LLR
Test A	90%	10%	1.0	1.0
Test B	80%	30%	1.1	0.7

Test A Pretest odds (1/1) x -LLR (1.0) = post test odds (1/1) = post test probability of 50% (no change).

Test B Pretest odds (1/1) x -LLR (0.7) = post test odds (0.7/1) = post test probability of 0.7 / 1.7 = 41%. Therefore, Test B is a better test.

Thus, a LLR can fully express the value of a test in a single number. As a guide, +LLRs near 10 and -LLRs near 1/10 are quite good and will affect decisions substantially.

Remember, according to Bayes Theorem, testing at a very high pretest probabilities of disease or at very low pretest probabilities may not greatly affect a clinical decision.

Example: What is the probability of breast cancer in a 40-year-old woman whose screening mammogram is read as suspicious? Pretest probability of breast cancer (prevalence) in 40 year-old = 1/4000 = pretest odds of 1/3999. +LLR for screening mammogram in 40 year-old = 80. Posttest odds = 1/3999 × 80 = 80/3999. Probability is 80/4079 or 1.9%. Thus 98% of women such as this do not have breast cancer even if they have a suspicious mammogram.

ESTIMATES OF PRETEST PROBABILITY OF THROMBOEMBOLISM (DVT/PE)
Pulmonary Embolism (PE)

In those few studies that have evaluated the operating characteristics of physical signs and symptoms in PE, authors have concluded from multivariate analyses that no single finding or group of findings substantially predicts the presence of PE. Clinicians seem to be reasonably adept at recognizing those at increased risk, however, because in the PIOPED study, the incidence of PE in those referred for V/Q scans was 33%.

Deep Venous Thrombosis (DVT)

Wells et al. enumerated 7 major and 5 minor findings that correlated with the presence of venographic DVT.

Major: (1) Cancer, (2) Paralysis or surgery in past month, (4) Tenderness along deep venous

Table 7-1
Testing for Thromboembolism

Test			+LLR	-LLR
Arterial blood gas, A-a gradient, etc.			~1	~1
	V/Q scan	High Probability	17	
		Intermediate	1.1	
		Low	0.7	
		Normal or near normal	0.1	
	Chest CT	Standard 3	2.8–90	0.6–0
		Dual section	Unknown	
	Chest MRI		Unknown	
	Pulmonary angiography		50	0.02
	D-dimer (SimpliRED)		2.5–3.0	0.06–0.48

Table 7-2
Testing for Deep Venous Thrombosis

Test (symptomatic patients)	+LLR	-LLR
Duplex & color flow ultrasonography	24	0.04
Impedance plethysmography	10	0.06
D-dimer	2.5–3.0	0.06–0.48

system, (5) Swollen leg and thigh by measurement, (6) Calf swelling >3 cm at 10 cm below the tibial tuberosity, and (7) Strong family history.

Minor: (1) Recent trauma to leg, (2) Pitting edema in affected leg, (3) Dilated varicosities in affected leg only, (4) Hospitalization past 6 months, (5) Erythema.

When 3 major or 2 major and 2 minor criteria were found in the face of no alternative diagnosis, the prevalence of DVT was 85%. The prevalence of DVT was only 5% when one major criterion and 2 minor were present with an alternative diagnosis or any lesser combination of findings. For combinations of findings between these extremes, the prevalence of DVT was 33%. At UNC in the absence of any major risk factors and the absence of unilateral calf swelling >2 cm compared to the asymptomatic leg, the incidence of DVT has been less than 2% where there is an alternative diagnosis.

Chest CT and the d-dimer test cannot be recommended to estimate the probability of PE because of the wide range of reported LLRs and lack of a large trial that has rigorously determined the clinical outcome of patients with negative CT scans or negative d-dimers. In the presence of chronic lung disease, the LLRs for V/Q scans are degraded, perhaps by half, due to the presence of more indeterminate scans. ABG's have no diagnostic utility.

STRATEGIES FOR TESTING

Strategies for the diagnosis of PE rely heavily on an understanding of the disease. First, immediate evidence of a proximal venous thrombosis is often lacking in those with PE, presumably because the clot is now in the lung. Second, in the stable patient with a recent PE, the goal of therapy is not to treat the current PE but to prevent a

Table 7-3
Pulmonary Embolism

High-risk patient (75% probability) and
· Positive V/Q scan - Odds (3/1) x +LLR (17) = post odds (51/1) or posttest probability 98%. Action-treat.
· Normal V/Q scan - (3/1) x (0.1) = posttest odds (0.3/1) or posttest probability 23%, well above action threshold. Action- test further for DVT (see below).

Moderate-risk patient (33% probability) and
· Positive V/Q scan - Odds (1/2) x +LLR (17) = posttest odds (17/2) or posttest probability 89%. Action - treat.
· Negative scan - (1/2) x (0.1) = posttest odds (0.1/2) = posttest probability 5%. Action - no treatment.

Low-risk patient (5%)
· Positive V/Q scan - Pretest odds (5/95) x +LLR (17) = posttest odds (85/95) or posttest probability of 47%. Action - test further for DVT since negative study can reduce probability below action threshold (see DVT below).
· Negative V/Q scan - (5/95) x (0.1) = posttest odds (0.5/95) or probability of 0.5%. Action - no treatment.

Low or intermediate probability scans have no impact on decision (LLR's near unity).

Table 7-4
Deep Vein Thrombosis

High-risk patient (85%)
· Positive ultrasound (US) - (85/15) x (24) = posttest odds (2040/15) or posttest probability of 99%. Action - treat.
· Negative US - (85/15) x (0.04) = posttest odds(3.4/15) or posttest probability of 18%. Action- further testing required.

Moderate-risk patient (33%)
· Positive US - (1/3) x (24) = posttest odds (24/3) or probability of 88%. Action - treat.
· Negative US - (1/3) x (0.04) = posttest odds (0.04/3) or posttest probability of 1.3%. Action - no treatment.

Low-risk patient
· Positive US- (5/95) x (24) = post\test odds (120/95) or probability of 56%. Action - treat. (Only venography can lower probability below action threshold.)
· Negative US - (5/95) x (0.04) = posttest odds (0.2/95) or probability of 0.2%.

Table 7-5
Further Testing for Equivocal Results

High-risk patient (75%) for PE, with negative V/Q scan (from above.) posttest probability 23%.
- If US now positive - Odds (0.3/1) x (24) = posttest odds (7.2/1) or probability 88%. Action - now treat.
- If US now negative - Odds (0.3/1) x (0.04) = posttest odds (0.012/1) or probability 1.2%. Action - no treatment.

High-risk patient (85%) for DVT, with negative US (from above) post test probability 18%.
- If US positive at one week - Odds (3.4/15) x (24) = posttest odds (81.6/15) or probability 84%. Action - treat
- If US negative at one week - Odds (3.4/15) x (0.04) = posttest odds (0.14/15) or probability 0.9%. Action - no treatment.

recurrence. Third, if the deep venous system (defined as the veins from the popliteal fossa proximally) remains empty of clot, the risk of recurrent PE is very low. These findings, coupled with the realization that calf vein thrombi rarely embolize unless they propagate proximally, have focused diagnostic strategies on proximal DVT in patients who cannot easily be proven to have a PE (Tables 7-1 to 7-5).

In the patient whose presentation suggests PE, the initial strategy is to perform a V/Q scan because the pretest probability of finding clot in the chest is higher than finding it in the leg. For similar reasons, in those suspected of DVT, investigation begins with studies of the leg.

For both PE and DVT, the calculated action threshold is about 5% because the goals of therapy are identical; therefore, the goal of testing is to reduce the probability of venous thromboembolism to below 5%. If this threshold cannot be reached by any combination of tests, then one is forced to treat.

FURTHER TESTING

When the V/Q scan or the initial US fails to lower the posttest probability below the action threshold of 5% to 10%, further testing is useful. If, on repetition of the US at one week, the proximal deep venous system can be shown to be empty of clot, the risk of DVT/PE is very low.

REFERENCES

Value of the ventilation/perfusion scan in acute pulmonary embolism. Results of the prospective investigation of pulmonary embolism diagnosis (PIOPED). The PIOPED Investigators. *JAMA.* 1990;263:2753–2759.

Farrell S, Hayes T, Shaw M. A negative SimpliRED D-dimer assay result does not exclude the diagnosis of deep vein thrombosis or pulmonary embolus in emergency department patients. *Ann Emerg Med.* 2000;35:121–125.

Hull RD, Raskob GE, Ginsberg JS, et al. A noninvasive strategy for the treatment of patients with suspected pulmonary embolism. *Arch Intern Med.* 1994;154:289–297.

Kline JA, Israel EG, Michelson EA, O'Neil BJ, Plewa MC, Portelli DC. Diagnostic accuracy of a bedside D-dimer assay and alveolar dead-space measurement for rapid exclusion of pulmonary embolism: a multicenter study. *JAMA.* 2001;284:761–768.

Rathbun SW, Raskob GE, Whitsett TL. Sensitivity and specificity of helical computed tomography in the diagnosis of pulmonary embolism: a systematic review. *Ann Intern Med.* 2000;132:227–232.

Wells PS, Hirsh J, Anderson DR, et al. Accuracy of clinical assessment of deep-vein thrombosis. *Lancet.* 1995:345:1326–1330.

Section II

DISORDERS OF THE UPPER RESPIRATORY TRACT AND OROPHARYNX

Chapter 8

Acute Otitis Externa

James A. Visser

Acute otitis externa, "swimmer's ear," is a disease state involving inflammation or infection of the auricle and external auditory canal. Commonly encountered in the outpatient setting, it ranges from mild drainage and discomfort due to inflammation to a life threatening infectious process requiring surgical intervention. It presents more frequently in hot, humid climates or warm summer months, and is indeed more prevalent in swimmers. The combination of moisture and warmth predispose to maceration of the outer layer of skin, a setup for initial stages of the disease.

ETIOLOGY AND PATHOGENESIS

The external ear is composed of the auricle and external auditory canal (Figure 8-1). The external auditory canal is 2.5 cm in length. The lateral 40% of the canal is cartilaginous, as is the auricle (pinna). The medial 60% is composed of bone. The osseous inner canal has a thin layer of skin containing no glands or hair. The cartilaginous skin is thick and contains hair sebum and apocrine glands (ceruminous). Cerumen (earwax) is a combination of apocrine and sebaceous gland secretions mixed with desquamated epithelium. Cerumen is hydrophobic and acidic, two defenses against infection. Sloughed epithelium with cerumen migrates laterally in the canal.

The skin of the external canal is colonized with similar bacteria to those that colonize skin elsewhere, including *Staphylococcus aureus, Staphylococcus epidermidis,* and *Corynebacterium.*

The external ear has several defense mechanisms to maintain its normal healthy state. Perturbations in the normal microenvironment of the external auditory canal predispose the canal to development of bacterial infections. Cerumen is an important defense mechanism; removal or dilution compromises its hydrophobic and acidic properties, two important protective barriers. The act of removing cerumen can damage the epithelial lining. Water (swimming) compromises the protective layer of cerumen and macerates the layer of skin. In warm, moist environments, invasive organisms including normal flora, but also hydrophilic organisms such as *Pseudomonas aeruginosa*, may invade the skin if the normal microenvironment is altered. Hearing aids, cerumen impaction or excessive hairs may function as barriers to the natural process of cerumen migration laterally and contribute to the initial infection. *Pseudomonas aeruginosa* and *Staphylococcus aureus* are the predominant pathogens in otitis externa.

CLINICAL PRESENTATION

Early stages of diffuse otitis externa present with pruritus and ear fullness. Progression of inflammation leads to ear pain, the most common presenting sign. The otalgia can be mild or severe and is exacerbated by manipulation of the auricle or tragus. Mastication also elicits pain. Pain is due to the heavily innervated skin connected to the periosteum and perichondrium of the external canal. Edema compresses these local nerves. With severe edema, the canal lumen is decreased, leading to conductive hearing loss. Ear drainage, another common symptom, leads to occlusion of the canal. Otorrhea is usually thick and white but can be thin or clear.

Physical exam findings include any or all of the following: erythema and edema of the external auditory canal, discharge, or pain with manipulation of the tragus or pinna. Otoscopy to visualize the tympanic membrane can be difficult due to debris in the canal, stenosis of the canal secondary to edema, and guarding by the patient when the examiner attempts to insert the speculum. Regional lymphadenopathy and fever may be present in advanced disease.

DIFFERENTIAL DIAGNOSIS
Acute Localized Otitis Externa

A painful external canal can be due to a pustule or furuncle of a hair follicle in the outer external

Figure 8-1

Acute Otitis Externa

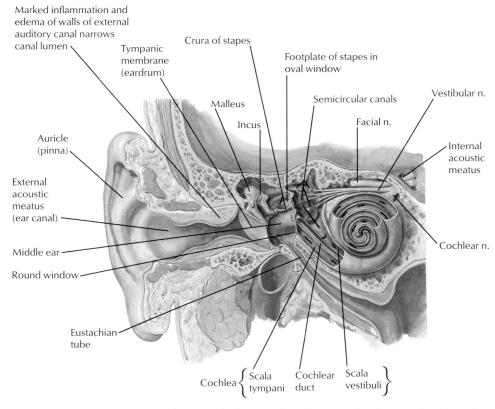

Marked inflammation and edema of walls of external auditory canal narrows canal lumen

Tympanic membrane (eardrum)

Crura of stapes

Footplate of stapes in oval window

Malleus

Incus

Semicircular canals

Facial n.

Vestibular n.

Internal acoustic meatus

Auricle (pinna)

External acoustic meatus (ear canal)

Middle ear

Round window

Cochlear n.

Eustachian tube

Cochlea { Scala tympani

Cochlear duct

Scala vestibuli }

In otitis externa, inflammation, edema, and discharge are limited to external auditory canal and its walls

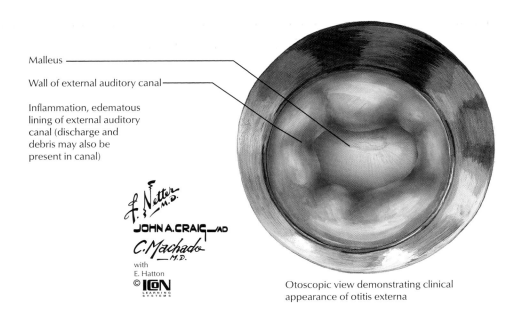

Malleus

Wall of external auditory canal

Inflammation, edematous lining of external auditory canal (discharge and debris may also be present in canal)

Otoscopic view demonstrating clinical appearance of otitis externa

canal. The pathologic organism is usually *Staphylococcus aureus.* Rarely, group A *Streptococcus* also can cause erysipelas in the canal. The exam demonstrates pain with manipulation of the auricle or attempted visualization of the canal. The furuncle may not easily be visualized if local edema is significant. There is no drainage unless the furuncle has ruptured, which will often relieve the pain. Treatment involves antistaphylococcal antibiotics and local heat. Incision and drainage may be necessary.

Acute Otitis Media with Tympanic Membrane Perforation

An acutely draining ear can be secondary to otitis media with perforation. The canal can be obscured with draining pus, making tympanic membrane visualization difficult. The history often consists of initial ear pain and sometimes fever, followed by a draining ear, often with concomitant pain relief. The tragus and auricle are not tender, nor is the canal edematous. The usual organisms that cause otitis media are *Streptococcus pneumoniae, nontypable Haemophilus influenza* and *Moraxella catarrhalis.* Treatment is oral antibiotics with coverage of these organisms.

Chronic Otitis Externa

A chronic otitis externa is often due to otorrhea from a persistent otitis media with tympanic membrane perforation. Chronic persistent middle ear infections with a draining ear are unusual. Infectious etiologies such as tuberculosis and syphilis, though rare, should be considered. Non-infectious etiologies include cholesteatoma. The underlying middle ear pathology needs to be addressed. These patients should be referred to otolaryngology.

Otomycosis

Fungal otitis externa is a less common etiology accounting for approximately 10% of the cases of otitis externa in the US. Otomycosis most commonly presents after a prolonged treatment of an external ear bacterial infection. Immunocompromised patients or those with diabetes are at an increased risk. Itching and drainage, more often than pain, are symptoms. The drainage is often thick white to black, resembling bread mold. Culture establishes the diagnosis. The most common organisms are *aspergillosis,* a saprophyte, and candida, a superficial pathogenic fungus; however, numerous other fungal organisms have also been identified as pathogens in otomycosis.

Non-infectious Otitis Externa

Several dermatologic conditions present with inflammation of the external ear. The chief complaint usually is pruritus. The examination shows scaling, erythema, crusting, lichenification, and fissuring of the ear. Etiologies include contact dermatitis and systemic dermatologic conditions such as psoriasis, seborrheic dermatitis, and systemic lupus. Carcinoma of the external canal can present as a non-resolving external otitis. Treatment is directed at removing the inciting agent or identifying and treating the underlying condition.

DIAGNOSTIC APPROACH

There are no published studies that address the diagnostic accuracy of acute otitis externa based on history, physical exam, or laboratory or radiologic studies. The diagnosis is based on the history and the typical clinical findings on physical exam.

MANAGEMENT AND THERAPY

Successful treatment of otitis externa is based upon restoring the environment of the external canal to its normal state. This is accomplished by cleansing the external canal and application of topical preparations.

Cleansing of the external canal (aural toilet) by removal of the desquamated epithelium is completed with the goal of visualization of the canal and tympanic membrane. Suctioning under microscopy is the standard approach used by otolaryngologists. A cotton swab can be used to dry-mop the ear. Cerumen spoons and curettes can cause additional trauma to the epithelium and should not be used. Flushing and irrigation of the ear should also be avoided because of further irritation of the canal and the usual poor visualization of the tympanic membrane prior to flushing. The cleansing process is often limited due to ear pain and external canal swelling.

Application of the topical preparation is the second component of treatment. Instillation of the drops into the canal is difficult if the canal is severely swollen. A wick or one-quarter inch sterile gauze placed in the external canal facilitates the topical medicine into the inner canal.

There are several different topical preparations available. Many are effective by acidifying the canal, thus inhibiting bacterial and fungal growth. The solutions and suspensions can be combined with antibiotics and topical steroids. The steroids decrease the inflammation in the canal. Controlled trials have shown equivalent results (80% to 90% efficacy) when comparing acidifying agents, antibiotic and steroid preparations, and quinolone drops. Otic suspension preparations are less acidic than solution preparations, and therefore may be preferred with tympanic membrane perforation because they are less irritating. Ophthalmic preparations are an alternative for patients who cannot tolerate the otic preparation. Ototoxicity with aminoglycoside, acetic acid, and polymyxin preparations is theoretically well established, particularly in animal models. However, the clinical importance is debatable as it is difficult to separate the underlying disease process from the topical medications. Recent small retrospective studies have shown ototoxicity, primarily vestibular rather than cochlear, with the use of topical aminoglycosides for a period greater than 7 days. The standard of care in the otolaryngology community is not to use aminoglycoside-based ototopical preparations with a perforated tympanic membrane. Topical quinolones provide an alternative with no evidence for ototoxicity.

In general, treatment length varies from 4 to 10 days. Some experts recommend using drops for 3 days after symptoms have abated. When a wick is placed in the canal, the patient should be seen every 2 to 4 days for ear cleansing until the edema resolves and the wick is no longer needed. Oral analgesics are often needed short-term for patients with otitis externa.

Several etiologies should be considered in a persistently draining ear despite treatment. Allergic dermatitis is associated with neomycin. Otomycosis after prolonged treatment of bacterial otitis externa is common. Treatment is directed at acidifying and drying the canal. Topical antifungal solutions (clotrimazole) and powders (nystatin or tolnaftate) are effective. Aspergillus may require the use of oral itraconazole.

Patients with recurrent attacks of otitis externa should be prescribed prophylactic treatment including acetic acid or drying agents such as 70% ethyl alcohol. Frequent ear cleaning should be avoided due to repeat alteration of the normal healthy canal.

The use of systemic antibiotics, oral or parenteral, is reserved for severe cases of otitis externa with spread to local soft tissues. *Necrotizing* (or malignant) *otitis externa* is a serious and life-threatening complication that occurs when infection extends from the external canal to the mastoid and base of the skull. Usual symptoms include a persistent draining ear with unrelenting pain. Fever and tachycardia are unusual. Exam usually shows granulation tissue in the canal. Seventh nerve paresis occurs in one third of those who present with necrotizing otitis externa. *Pseudomonas aeruginosa* is the bacterial etiology >96% of the time in a series of cases. The majority of patients are age 60 or older, and more than 90% have a history of glucose intolerance. However, diabetic severity does not correlate with the development of necrotizing otitis externa. Other immunocompromised patients, including those with malignancy and HIV infection, have been reported. CT or MRI may assist with the diagnosis by establishing involvement of the temporal bone. Parenteral antipseudomonal or β-lactam with aminoglycoside antibiotics and surgical intervention are indicated. Mortality is 10% to 20%.

FUTURE DIRECTIONS

As the population of the elderly increases, and patients with immunocompromised states such as diabetes, malignancy, and HIV live longer, the risk of necrotizing external otitis increases. Current diagnostic and therapeutic approaches for acute otitis externa are effective in most providers. However, a heightened awareness of the signs and symptoms of the disease is needed by clinicians that care for this population.

REFERENCES

Bojrab DI, Bruderly T, Abdulrazzak Y. Otitis externa. *Otolaryngol Clin North Am*. 1996;29:761–782.

Dibb WL. Microbial aetiology of otitis externa. *J Infect*. 1991;22:233–239.

Hirsch BE. Infections of the external ear. *Am J Otolaryngol*. 1992;13:145–155.

Rubin J, Yu VL. Malignant external otitis: insights into pathogenesis, clinical manifestations, diagnosis, and therapy. *Am J Med*. 1988;85:391–398.

van Asperen IA, de Rover CM, Schijven JF, et al. Risk of otitis externa after swimming in recreational lakes containing *Pseudomonas aeruginosa*. *BMJ*. 1995;311:1407–1410.

Chapter 9
Acute Otitis Media

James A. Visser

Acute otitis media (AOM) results from inflammation in the middle ear. Generally considered a disease of childhood, AOM is the most frequent diagnosis made in children younger than 15 who present to their pediatrician, accounting for about 25 million cases annually. In 1990, there were 24.5 million office visits for otitis media, an increase from 9.9 million visits in 1975. The peak incidence of the disease is age 3, but 16% of cases occur after age 15.

ETIOLOGY AND PATHOGENESIS

The development of middle ear fluid, inflammation, and the subsequent symptoms is best understood by considering the anatomy and function of the eustachian tube. The eustachian tube connects the middle ear to the nasopharynx, providing a conduit for drainage of secretions from the middle ear space to the nasopharynx. It also equilibrates air pressure with the external ear and protects the middle ear space from nasopharyngeal bacteria. Eustachian tube dysfunction, either anatomic or physiologic, plays a role in the development of middle ear effusions and acute infections.

The anatomy of the eustachian tube in children may be responsible for the high incidence of AOM in this age group (Figure 9-1). In young children, it is short, floppy, and horizontal, limiting draining by gravity and increasing access of the nasopharyngeal bacteria to the middle ear space. Stagnant fluid in the middle ear space increases the likelihood of bacterial infection. Dysfunction of the eustachian tube commonly occurs in viral upper respiratory infection. Inflammation and edema of the mucosa limit its ability to drain the middle ear. AOM in children and adults shows a seasonal variance correlating with viral URI, with peak incidences in winter. Other predisposing factors in children include ciliary dysfunction, cleft palate, immunodeficiency, tobacco smoke exposure, and absence of breast-feeding. A recent comparative study of twins demonstrates a heritable pattern of otitis media in children.

Streptococcus pneumonia (40%), non-typable *Haemophilus influenzae* (20%), *Moraxella catarrhalis* (10%), and group A *streptococcus* (5%) are the most common bacterial organisms responsible for AOM in children. Similar pathogens cause AOM in adults: *Streptococcus pneumonia (21%), Haemophilus influenzae (26%), and Moraxella catarrhalis (9%).* In both children and adults, 30% to 40% of cases represent viral etiologies or sterile effusions. Respiratory syncytial virus, parainfluenza, influenza, rhinovirus, enterovirus and adenovirus are the most commonly identified viral pathogens. Bacteria and viruses can be present at the same time in acute otitis media, and concomitant infection can lead to prolonged recovery from AOM.

CLINICAL PRESENTATION

Ear pain (89%) and decreased hearing (63%) are the most common symptoms in adults. Other symptoms include sore throat, vertigo, and otorrhea. Children may have these clinical symptoms but more often present with additional systemic symptoms including fever and diarrhea.

DIFFERENTIAL DIAGNOSIS
Otorrhea

In a patient presenting with a painful draining ear, it can be difficult to distinguish between acute otitis media with tympanic membrane rupture and otitis externa. The history in AOM is initially a painful ear, followed by drainage and relief of the pain with tympanic membrane rupture. Otitis externa presents more commonly in summer months. Often, the external ear, tragus, and auricle will be painful with movement in either AOM or otitis externa.

Otalgia

Pain in the ear can also be due to cerumen impaction or foreign body. If the canal and tympanic membrane appear normal, other etiologies for ear pain include dental caries, pharyngitis,

Figure 9-1

External Ear and Tympanic Cavity

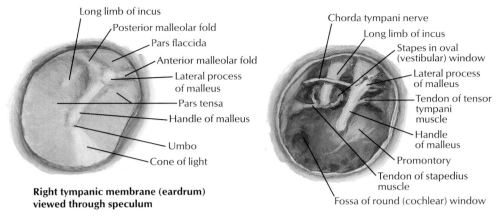

Right tympanic membrane (eardrum)
viewed through speculum

View into tympanic cavity after
removal of tympanic membrane

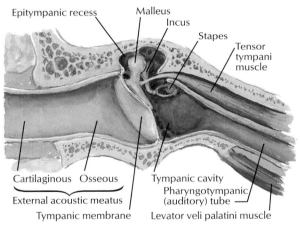

Coronal oblique section of external acoustic meatus and middle ear

parotitis, temporomandibular joint dysfunction, or mastoiditis.

DIAGNOSTIC APPROACH

The diagnosis of AOM is based upon clinical and otoscopic findings. Clinical signs and symptoms of acute inflammation and infection can supplement the otoscopic findings, but visualizing the tympanic membrane is fundamental in establishing the diagnosis. With AOM, it loses its normal translucent appearance and often is erythematous due to inflammation, or opaque secondary to purulent fluid in the middle ear (Figure 9-2). Under pressure, the tympanic membrane will lose normal landmarks

and may bulge. Pneumatic otoscopy can assist with diagnosis of middle ear fluid. A normal tympanic membrane moves easily with insufflation of air. An ear with middle fluid, pus, or high negative pressure has little mobility. Tympanometry provides objective evidence of fluid in the middle ear. Definitive bacteriologic diagnosis with tympanocentesis is not needed with the initial presentation of AOM.

MANAGEMENT AND THERAPY

The goal of treatment is to reduce the severity and duration of pain and other symptoms, prevent complications, and minimize adverse effects of treatment. The standard treatment in the US is oral

Figure 9-2

Acute Otitis Media

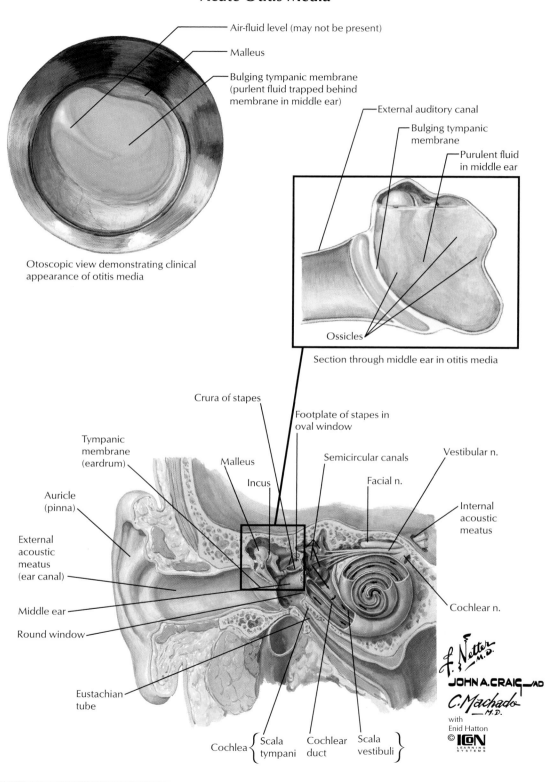

Air-fluid level (may not be present)

Malleus

Bulging tympanic membrane (purlent fluid trapped behind membrane in middle ear)

External auditory canal

Bulging tympanic membrane

Purulent fluid in middle ear

Ossicles

Section through middle ear in otitis media

Otoscopic view demonstrating clinical appearance of otitis media

Crura of stapes

Footplate of stapes in oval window

Tympanic membrane (eardrum)

Malleus

Semicircular canals

Vestibular n.

Incus

Facial n.

Auricle (pinna)

Internal acoustic meatus

External acoustic meatus (ear canal)

Middle ear

Cochlear n.

Round window

Eustachian tube

Cochlea { Scala tympani

Cochlear duct

Scala vestibuli }

with Enid Hatton

antibiotics, but this treatment has come under heightened scrutiny because of increased use overall, as well as the use of broader spectrum antibiotics. An association exists between antibiotic use and increased prevalence of resistant organisms, particularly penicillin-resistant *Streptococcus pneumoniae*. The Centers for Disease Control and Prevention and the Institute of Medicine have developed strategies that include decreased antibiotic prescribing.

The outcomes of the use of antibiotics in children with acute otitis media have been systematically reviewed. One major study reviewed the outcome of antibiotic therapy versus no treatment in acute otitis media in children. The findings were that by 24 hours two thirds of the children recovered whether they had received antibiotics or not. There was no reduction in pain at 24 hours. Antibiotics reduced the risk of pain at 2 to 7 days from 20% to 14.4 % (relative risk reduction 28% [95% CI: 15% to 38%]) for an absolute risk reduction of 5.6%. In this review, 17 children had to be treated for 1 additional child to receive complete resolution of symptoms. At age 1 to 3, there was no effect on hearing measured by tympanometry; however, audiometry was done in only 2 of the 6 studies, and the report was incomplete. Further, there were few complications, specifically only one report of mastoiditis in the 2,202 children pooled in this review.

This review and others do not resolve the controversy of the use of antibiotics in children with acute otitis media, although they show that early use has only modest benefit. One criticism is that the intervention group in several of the studies that were pooled used penicillin, an antibiotic that has long been held in the US to be inadequate therapy. Also, studies show that there are subgroups of children with severe symptoms that have greater benefit with antibiotic use than children with mild symptoms. The complication rate of mastoiditis in untreated children remains uncertain. It may be higher in developing countries.

Systematic reviews of antibiotic use in children with otitis media have concluded that antibiotics should be reserved for cases of purulent otitis media and severe symptoms. These recommendations seem reasonable for the adult population where visualization of the tympanic membrane is easier, allowing the clinician to better identify patients who may benefit from antibiotic therapy.

Antibiotics

The antibiotic agent for use should be active against the 3 common pathogens of AOM: *S. pneumoniae, M catarrhalis,* and *H influenzae*. Amoxicillin is the drug of choice based upon its low cost, limited side effects, adequate middle ear concentrations, and proven clinical success. It should be noted that amoxicillin is ineffective against β-lactamase–producing strains of *H. Influenzae (30%) and M catarrhalis (75%)*. The rationale for amoxicillin as a first-line agent is that *H. influenzae* and *M catarrhalis* account for about 40% of pathogens in AOM, of which 16% are caused by β-lactamase-producing organisms. At least 50% will clear spontaneously; therefore, fewer than 10% of first-line treatment failures are due to β-lactamase resistance to amoxicillin. Patients who do not respond to treatment in the first 48 to 72 hours are considered treatment failures. One should consider broadened coverage of β-lactamase-producing organisms in these patients. Second-line therapies include amoxicillin-clavulanate; oral cephalosporins (cefuroxime axetil, cefdinir, cefprozil, ceftibuten, cefpodoxime); macrolides (azithromycin and clarithromycin); and parenteral ceftriaxone.

Another consideration in amoxicillin treatment failure is inadequate coverage of penicillin resistant *S pneumoniae* organisms (intermediate and high level). Most experts recommend an increase in the dose of amoxicillin from 40 mg/kg/daily to 80mg/kg/daily. As an initial approach for amoxicillin treatment failure in the pediatric population, the high dose amoxicillin exceeds the MIC for intermediately resistant pneumococci. Other options include amoxicillin (40 mg/kg/daily) and amoxicillin-clavulanate (40 mg/kg/daily) combined therapy, clindamycin, and IM ceftriaxone. Higher doses of amoxicillin have not been studied in adults.

The usual duration of initial therapy is 10 days. Extended courses to 20 days have not shown benefit in children. Some studies show shorter courses (5 days) of antibiotics comparable to a 10-day course, based on 4 to 6 week outcomes in children older than 3 years.

Adjunct Therapies

Oral decongestants, antihistamines, and steroids have not been shown to be useful in AOM. Analgesics including oral ibuprofen and topical preparations (benzocaine and antipyrine) provide modest symptom relief.

Serous otitis media is a common occurrence after treatment of AOM with antimicrobials. Effusions may persist up to 10 weeks after treatment. Common features of serous otitis media are an effusion that impairs tympanic membrane mobility and eustachian tube dysfunction that limits drainage of the middle ear space. In children, hearing loss and the possibility of subsequent speech problems is of concern. Guidelines have been established for children 1 to 3 years old with persistent middle ear effusion (*American Academy of Pediatrics, American Academy of Family Physicians, American Academy of Otolaryngology*). The management options include observation without drug therapy, antimicrobials, or a combination of antimicrobials and corticosteroids. Ventilating tubes were recommended for children with persistent effusion for at least 4 months and a documented bilateral hearing impairment of 20 dB or more. Antihistamines and decongestants have not shown significant evidence of efficacy used alone or in combination for relief of signs of disease or resolution of serous effusions in children.

FUTURE DIRECTIONS

Efforts should be directed at identifying subgroups that clearly benefit from antibiotics and eliminating antibiotic use in those subgroups that do not derive significant benefit. The length of therapy is being studied to identify groups of patients that could receive equal benefit from short courses of treatment. Recently, a conjugate 7-valent pneumococcal vaccine has been recommended for all children less than 2 years old in the United States. The vaccine has been shown to prevent invasive pneumococcal disease. The efficacy in prevention of otitis media has been limited. This vaccine may change the epidemiology of pneumococcal disease for children and adults over the next decade.

REFERENCES

Managing otitis media with effusion in young children. American Academy of Pediatrics The Otitis Media Guideline Panel. *Pediatrics.* 1994;94:766–773.

Berman S. Otitis media in children. *N Engl J Med.* 1995;332:-1560–1565.

Bluestone CD, Stephenson JS, Martin LM. Ten-year review of otitis media pathogens. *Pediatr Infect Dis J.* 1992;11(suppl 8): S7–S11.

Celin SE, Bluestone CD, Stephenson J, Yilmaz HM, Collins JJ. Bacteriology of acute otitis media in adults. *JAMA.* 1991;266:2249–2252.

Glasziou PP, Del Mar CB, Hayem M, Sanders SL. Antibiotics for acute otitis media in children. *Cochrane Database Syst Rev.* 2000;CD000219.

McCaig LF, Hughes JM. Trends in antimicrobial drug prescribing among office-based physicians in the United States. *JAMA.* 1995;273:214–219.

Schappert SM. Office visits for otitis media: United States, 1975-90. *Adv Data.* 1992;214:1–19.

Chapter 10

Aphthous Ulcers and Other Common Oral Lesions

David R. White and William W. Shockley

The oral cavity, along with the nasal cavity, represents the initial point of contact for pathogens and irritants entering the respiratory and digestive systems. It extends from the vermilion border of the lips posteriorly to the junction of the hard and soft palate and the circumvallate papillae of the tongue. The oral cavity includes the lips, buccal mucosa, gingival mucosa, teeth, hard palate, floor of the mouth, retromolar trigone, and the anterior two thirds of the tongue. Complete examination of the oral cavity should include visualization of all mucosal surfaces and palpation of the buccal surfaces, the tongue, the palate, and the floor of the mouth.

APHTHOUS ULCERS

Recurrent aphthous ulcers (RAU) are the most common oral mucosal ulcers in North America, affecting 5% to 66% of the adult population (Figure 10-1). RAU are more common in higher socioeconomic classes and typically present in the second decade of life. Their etiology remains uncertain. Nutrient deficiency, hormonal influence, bacterial and viral infection, immunologically mediated responses, food hypersensitivity, and genetic predisposition have all been implicated in the pathogenesis of RAU.

Depending on the presentation, RAU are classified as minor, major, or herpetiform. All types are generally found on the nonkeratinized, mobile mucosa of the buccal region, lips, and floor of the mouth. RAU are not associated with fever or other systemic reactions. Recurrence is most frequent in younger patients, and 30% of patients may have constant disease for months to years.

Minor RAU are most common, accounting for 70% to 87% of all aphthous ulcers. Measuring less than 1 cm in diameter, they present as discrete, shallow, painful ulcers with central fibrous exudate surrounded by an erythematous border. Ulceration lasts 1 to 2 weeks, followed by spontaneous healing without scarring. Typically, *herpetiform* RAU comprises 7% to 10% of all RAU lesions, measure less than 5 mm, and occur in groups of 10 to 100. They may coalesce into larger ulcers and are found throughout the oral cavity. *Major* RAU, the most severe form, affects 7% to 20% of patients. Lesions greater than 1 cm in diameter may last for weeks to months. They may coalesce into large, irregular ulcers, producing scars when healed. Generally, the lips, soft palate, and tonsillar pillars are involved.

Differential diagnosis includes viral infection, syphilitic and fungal infections, autoimmune disease including Behçet's syndrome and pemphigus/pemphigoid lesions, cyclic neutropenia, and squamous cell carcinoma. Diagnosis is based primarily on a thorough history and physical exam. Patients with lesions that do not resolve after 2 to 3 weeks of therapy should be referred to a specialist for biopsy and further management.

Topical corticosteroids are the mainstay of treatment for RAU. When applied directly to the dried ulcer or area of prodromal pain and paresthesia, they reduce the duration of the lesion, but not the frequency of recurrence. Intralesional steroid injections and systemic corticosteroids are reserved for more persistent cases of major RAU. Tetracycline rinses may also reduce lesion pain and duration. Chlorhexidine 0.2% oral rinse has been shown to reduce duration of lesions and to lengthen the interval between lesions, but it may stain the teeth after long-term usage. Thalidomide has been shown to decrease lesion duration and disease-free time in refractory RAU, with remissions reported in up to one third of patients. However, the well-known side effects of teratogenicity and peripheral neuropathy have limited the widespread usage of thalidomide.

Figure 10-1

Common Oral Lesions

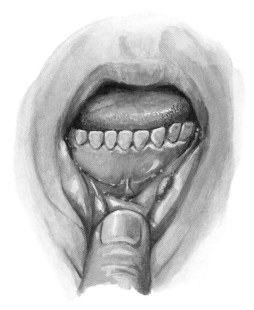

Recurrent aphthous ulcer

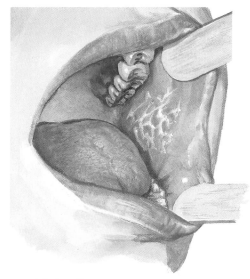

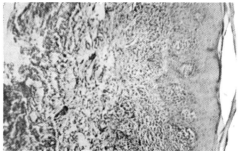

Lichen planus

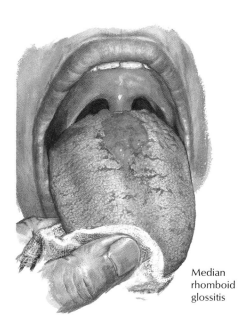

Median
rhomboid
glossitis

OTHER COMMON ORAL LESIONS
Viral Stomatitis

Herpes simplex is the most common organism causing viral stomatitis. Initial exposure to human herpesvirus-1 (HHV-1) usually occurs during childhood, after which the virus resides in the trigeminal ganglion. Primary infection is associated with fever and multiple 1 to 2 mm vesicles, which quickly rupture to form ulcers. These are found on the lips, gingiva, tongue, and hard palate. The ulcers undergo spontaneous healing in 10 to 14 days. Recurrent oral herpes is not associated with fever and may be initiated by trauma or sun exposure. The differential diagnosis is similar to that of aphthous ulcers. Diagnosis is generally clinical, but may be confirmed by a 4-fold rise in antibody titer to HHV-1 over a 2-week period, or a positive Tzanck test. Viral culture from lesions is the gold standard for diagnosis. Steroid treatment is contraindicated. Systemic acyclovir may shorten episodes and increase disease-free intervals. Topical acyclovir has not been shown to be effective. Topical anesthetic agents provide symptomatic relief.

Primary varicella-zoster virus (VZV) infection occurs during childhood when the human herpesvirus-3 causes chickenpox. The virus then remains dormant in sensory ganglia until it is reactivated, causing shingles. Shingles presents as an eruption of multiple 1 to 2 mm painful vesicles that soon burst to appear as ulcerative lesions. The classic unilateral dermatomal pattern is pathognomic. Eruptions generally indicate an immunosuppressed state, which may require further investigation. Treatment is generally supportive. Systemic acyclovir therapy may be indicated in severe cases in immunosuppressed individuals. Corticosteroids are contraindicated.

Herpangina and hand, foot, and mouth disease (HFM) are associated with Coxsackie A viruses (types A1 to 6, 8, 10, and 22 for the former, type A16 for the latter). Both diseases are accompanied by a viral prodrome followed by oral vesicular lesions. Lesions are seen in the anterior oral cavity as well as on the hands and feet in HFM, and on the soft palate and tonsillar pillars in herpangina. Pharyngitis is also present in herpangina. Both diseases are self-limited and require only supportive therapy.

Lichen Planus

Oral lichen planus (OLP) (Figure 10-1) is a common disorder affecting about 2% of adults. The etiology is unknown, but the final pathway is a T cell mediated immune response against the basal epithelial cell. Histologically, epithelial basal cell destruction and infiltration of the adjacent tissue with lymphocytes characterize OLP. The *reticular form*, the most common type of OLP, is seen most often as classic, lace-like striae of Wickham on the buccal mucosa. The *bullous form* is characterized by bullae of 0.5 to 4 cm diameter, which usually slough mucosa prior to presentation. *Asymptomatic OLP* also may present as a white plaque. *Erosive OLP* presents as painful, ulcerative lesions affecting the gingiva, buccal mucosa, and lateral tongue. Under magnification, each of these types of OLP typically demonstrates fine striae at the periphery of the lesion. Diagnosis is based on appearance in the case of reticular OLP. Inciting factors (e.g., ill-fitting dentures) should be removed. Candidal superinfection, present in 25% to 30% of OLP lesions, should be treated. *Reticular OLP* requires no further management. Bullous, *plaque-type*, and *erosive OLP* may require biopsy for diagnosis; erosive OLP can be a precursor to carcinoma in some patients. *Symptomatic OLP*, usually the erosive type, is treated first with topical steroids. Refractory cases usually respond to systemic steroids administered in a burst-and-taper fashion. Treatment with immunomodulating medications such as cyclosporine and azathioprine may be required in severe cases.

Oral Candidiasis

Candida sp., the most common cause of oral fungal infection, are present in the oral cavity of 30% to 60% of healthy adults; therefore, candida's presence is not considered pathologic. Candidal infections continue to be on the rise, primarily due to iatrogenic infections. Other factors predisposing to candidal infection include age extremes, immunocompromised state, malnourishment, concurrent infections, antibiotic treatment, radiation-induced mucositis, and xerostomia. Oral candidiasis classically presents as pseudomembranous candidiasis, or thrush. White, plaque-like lesions scrape easily away from the lesion, leaving a raw, hemorrhagic undersurface. *Hyperplastic candidiasis* presents as a white, plaque-like lesion that is not easily removed. *Chronic atrophic candidiasis*, the most common form of oral candidiasis is found in up to 60% of denture-wearing patients. It presents as an erythematous, cobblestone patch of denture-bearing mucosa. *Median rhomboid glossitis* (Figure 10-1), also called central papillary atrophy, is confined to the dorsal tongue. It presents as an asymptomatic, erythematous, well-demarcated area of papillary atrophy found just anterior to the circumvallate papillae. *Angular cheilitis* presents as painful, bleeding, ulcerative patches at the oral commissures. Diagnosis is based on clinical presentation. Differential diagnosis includes a wide range of oral lesions including squamous cell carcinoma. Failure of these lesions to respond to adequate therapy after 1 to 2 weeks should result in referral to a specialist for further management and possible biopsy.

Therapy consists of topical and systemic antifungals. Oral rinses with nystatin or clotrimazole solution 4 to 5 times per day is usually adequate for treatment of oral mucosal lesions. Denture-related lesions require treatment of the dentures with an antifungal soak or ointment as well as direct application of antifungal ointment or cream applied to the lesion. Angular cheilitis responds best to direct topical application of antifungal ointment to the lesion. Systemic fluconazole, ketoconazole, or itraconazole is indicated for severe or refractory lesions.

Hairy Tongue

Hairy tongue is a benign condition caused by accumulation of keratin and commensal bacteria on filiform papillae of the tongue. Hairy tongue has a characteristic appearance and is treated by reassuring the patient of the benign nature of the condition. Some improvement of appearance can be achieved by daily scraping of excess keratin and debris off the area (Figure 10-2).

Geographic Tongue

Geographic tongue, or *benign migratory glossitis*, is a benign condition characterized by areas of smooth atrophy on the tongue, with loss of papillae. The painless lesions spontaneously regress, only to appear on other parts of the tongue. Etiology is unknown, and no treatment is necessary (Figure 10-2).

Hairy Leukoplakia

Hairy leukoplakia is a benign mucosal lesion of the lateral tongue found in up to one third of HIV-positive patients. The painless lesions are caused by epithelial infection with the Epstein-Barr virus. It presents as irregular, white areas of mucosal thickening on the lateral tongue. Diagnosis is based on clinical presentation. Occasionally, biopsy is needed to confirm the diagnosis. No specific treatment is indicated, however, patients presenting with hairy leukoplakia should undergo testing for HIV.

Torus Palatinus and Torus Mandibularis

These are benign exostoses of the hard palate and mandible. Tori present as smooth, hard lesions of the midline hard palate or the lingual surface of the mandible. Patients are often unaware of their presence. Diagnosis is based on physical exam. No treatment is necessary, but tori occasionally must be removed to accommodate dentures (Figure 10-2).

Fordyce's Granules

These are ectopic sebaceous glands that appear as clusters of yellowish spots on the buccal mucosa, typically found just inside the oral commissure. Diagnosis is based on physical exam, and no treatment is necessary.

Amalgam Tattoo

Silver alloys used during dental procedures may become implanted in the surrounding gingiva, appearing as pigmented submucosal lesions. Differential diagnosis includes nevi and melanoma. Diagnosis is based on physical exam. Confirmation can be obtained with the appearance of fine, radio-opaque densities on dental films. Excisional biopsy should be performed for suspicious pigmented lesions.

Oral Papilloma and Verruca Vulgaris

These are easily recognized in the oral cavity. Both lesions are caused by infection with strains of HPV. Papillomas present as pedunculated, cauliflower-like masses of squamous epithelium similar to papillomas seen at other sites (Figure 10-3). Verrucae vulgaris present as hyperkeratotic, hard, round lesions similar to those seen on the skin of the hands and feet. Differential diagnosis includes

Figure 10-2

Common Oral Lesions

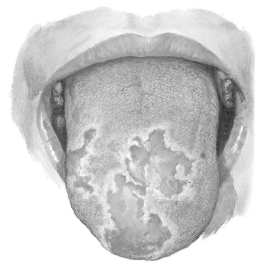

Geographic tongue

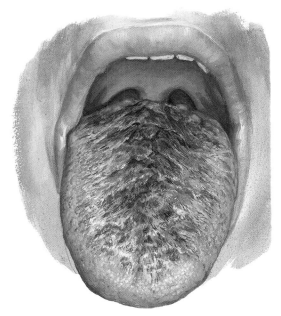

Hairy tongue

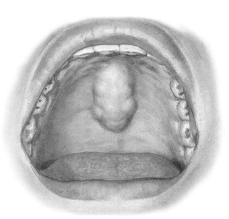

Torus palatinus

Figure 10-3 **Common Oral Lesions**

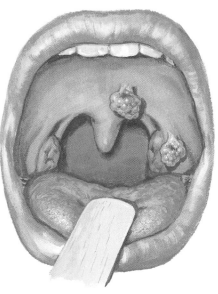

Papillomas of soft palate and anterior pillar

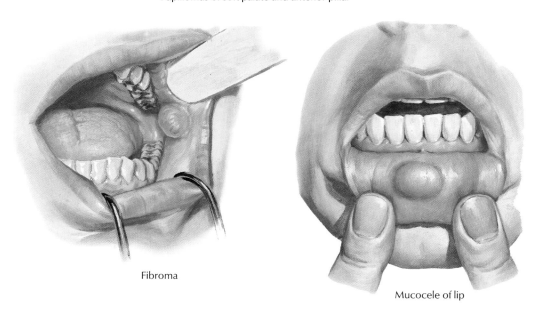

Fibroma

Mucocele of lip

condyloma acuminatum and verrucous carcinoma. Excisional biopsy is the treatment of choice.

Mucoceles

These form when saliva extrudes from a minor salivary gland into surrounding tissue. Trauma is thought to cause most mucoceles. They may present anywhere in the oral cavity, but are seen most commonly on the lower lip. They present as a bluish, round lesion with overlying smooth mucosa. They may burst and recur or become infected and purulent. Excision is the treatment of choice for persistent mucoceles. Marsupialization typically results in recurrence (Figure 10-3).

Fibromas

These are soft, tan or pink lesions found at sites of repetitive trauma, typically on the buccal mucosa or lateral tongue. Recurrent trauma results in chronic inflammation and fibrous hyperplasia. Excisional biopsy is diagnostic and therapeutic (Figure 10-3).

FUTURE DIRECTIONS

A careful physical examination of the oral cavity will remain the key element in the evaluation and treatment of patients with oral lesions. Research will continue in an attempt to define the specific etiology of aphthous ulcers, oral lichen planus, and other less well-understood lesions. The ultimate goal is to develop more specific therapies.

REFERENCES

Allen CM, Blozis GG. Oral mucosal lesions. In: Cummings CW, Fredrickson JM, Harker LA, et al, eds. *Otolaryngology–Head and Neck Surgery*. 3rd ed. St Louis, Mo: Mosby-Year Book Inc; 1998:1527–1545.

Bowers KE. Oral blistering diseases. *Clin Dermatol*. 2000;18:-513–523.

Lynch DP. Oral viral infections. *Clin Dermatol*. 2000;18:-619–628.

Miles DA, Howard MM. Diagnosis and management of oral lichen planus. *Dermatol Clin*. 1996;14:281–290.

Woo SB, Sonis ST. Recurrent aphthous ulcers: a review of diagnosis and treatment. *J Am Dent Assoc*. 1996;127:-1202–1213.

Chapter 11
Hoarseness

Mark C. Weissler

Hoarseness describes a rough or harsh voice caused by improper vibration of the epithelial covering of the vocal cord. Anything that causes stiffening or improper coaptation of the vocal cords will result in an abnormal voice. If the vocal cords do not coapt properly due to paralysis or bowing, there will often be a breathy and weak nature to the hoarseness. Any hoarseness persisting for 2 weeks or more warrants direct examination of the vocal cords by an otolaryngologist (Figure 11-1).

ETIOLOGY AND PATHOGENESIS/ CLINICAL PRESENTATION

Since hoarseness is the final common pathway for anything that impairs vocal cord vibration, a myriad of entities may cause it (Table 11-1 and Figures 11-2, 11-3, and 11-4). *Carcinoma of the glottic larynx* is of greatest concern in the adult patient. In otherwise healthy children, nodules of the vocal cords caused by excessive voice use (screamers' nodules) are common. An abnormal cry in the neonate warrants examination for a congenital or acquired abnormality of the vocal cords.

The threshold for what a patient identifies as hoarseness varies with how the voice is used. Professional voice users such as singers, teachers, ministers and actors may not tolerate even mild degrees of voice disturbance occurring only under certain circumstances.

DIAGNOSTIC APPROACH

Indirect laryngoscopy (Figure 11-1) is the

Table 11-1
Causes of Hoarseness

Inflammation, edema or swelling
· Tobacco smoking
· Gastroesophageal reflux
   — Alcohol use
   — Diet
   — Lifestyle
· Chronic rhinosinusitis/post-nasal drip
   — Allergy
· Chronic cough
   — Asthma
   — Associated with ACE inhibitors
   — Gastroesophageal reflux
   — Chronic rhinosinusitis
· Voice abuse/overuse
   — Screamers nodules in children
   — Amateur/professional singers without proper technique/coaching
· Myxedema
· Infections
   — Viral
   — Bacterial
   — Fungal
· Post-intubation

Stiffness
· Scarring from previous surgery
· Scarring from previous severe inflammation

· Due to any of the above inflammatory conditions

Mass lesion
· Nodule
· Cyst
· Granuloma
· Neoplasm
   — Squamous cell cancer
   — Granular cell tumor
   — Many others
· Certain fungal infections

Bowing of the vocal cords
· Presbylarynges
· Atrophy due to chronic inhaled steroid use

Paralysis or paresis
· Post-viral
· Lesion along coarse of vagus nerve from brainstem to arch of aorta.
   — Latrogenic
      Thyroidectomy
      Anterior approach to cervical spine for laminectomy
· Stroke
· Arnold Chiari malformation in neonates
· Other congenital malformations

Figure 11-1

Examination of the Larynx

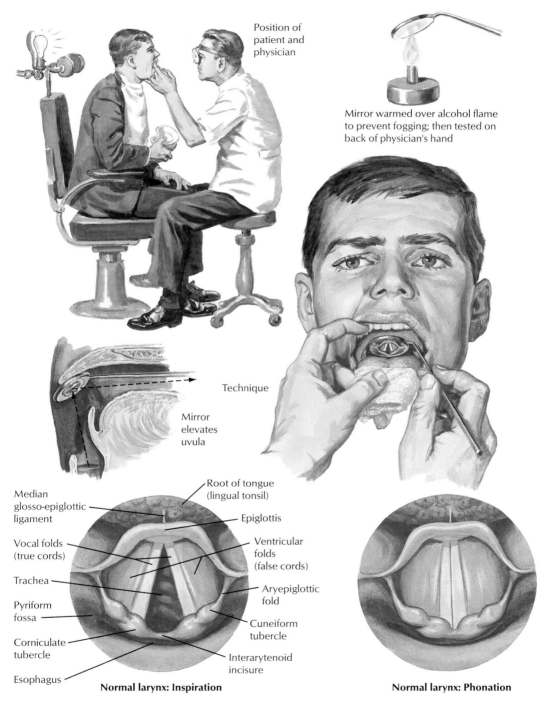

Position of patient and physician

Mirror warmed over alcohol flame to prevent fogging; then tested on back of physician's hand

Technique

Mirror elevates uvula

Median glosso-epiglottic ligament

Vocal folds (true cords)

Trachea

Pyriform fossa

Corniculate tubercle

Esophagus

Root of tongue (lingual tonsil)

Epiglottis

Ventricular folds (false cords)

Aryepiglottic fold

Cuneiform tubercle

Interarytenoid incisure

Normal larynx: Inspiration

Normal larynx: Phonation

Figure 11-2

Inflammation of the Larynx

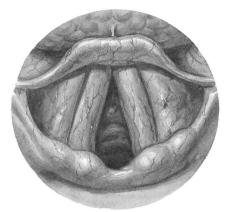

Acute laryngitis

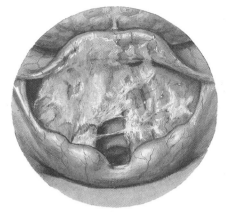

Membranous laryngitis

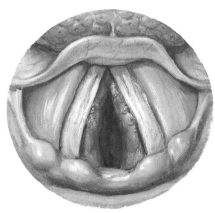

Subglottic inflammation and
swelling in inflammatory croup

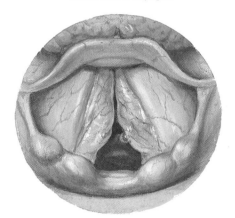

Edematous vocal cords
in chronic laryngitis

mainstay of evaluation. A mirror may be used, but a better examination can be performed using a flexible or rigid fiberoptic telescope. In this manner, the structure and function of the vocal cords can be evaluated in patients of all ages. For subtle cases, and most particularly for the professional voice user with subtle voice problems, fiberoptic laryngoscopy with videostroboscopy is essential. By timing a strobe light to the frequency of the vocalization, this examination allows visualization of the "mucosal wave" and is the only method that allows the examiner to appreciate subtle abnormalities in the vibration of the surface epithelium of the vocal cord.

When clinical examination reveals abnormalities that warrant a biopsy, direct laryngoscopy under general anesthesia in the operating room is indicated. Blood tests (e.g., TSH, thyroid function tests) and imaging (e.g., CXR, CT of the neck) may be appropriate in certain clinical situations. If the airway is in any way impaired, then emergent evaluation by an otolaryngologist is indicated.

Figure 11-3

Lesions of the Vocal Cords

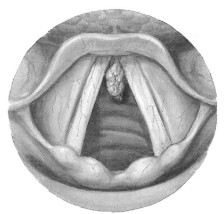

Pedunculated papilloma
at anterior commissure

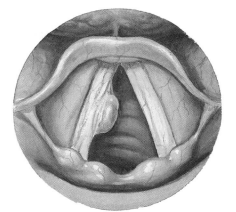

Sessile polyp

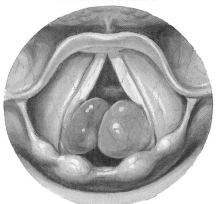

Large bilateral granulomas

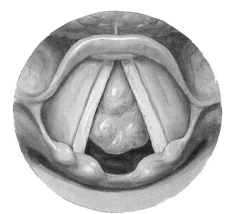

Subglottic polyp

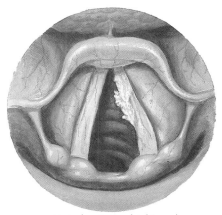

Hyperkeratosis of right cord

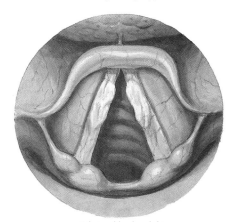

Bilateral leukoplakia

Figure 11-4

Cancer of the Larynx

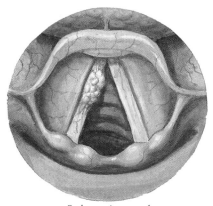

Early carcinoma of
left vocal cord

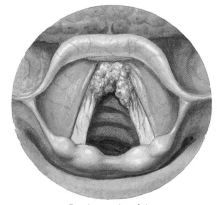

Carcinoma involving
anterior commissure

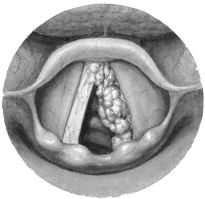

Extensive carcinoma of right vocal
cord involving arytenoid region

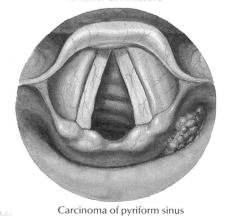

Carcinoma of pyriform sinus

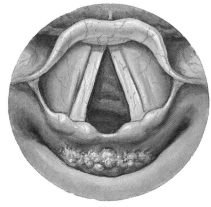

Postcricoid carcinoma

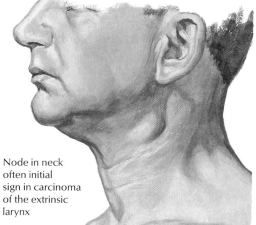

Node in neck
often initial
sign in carcinoma
of the extrinsic
larynx

MANAGEMENT AND THERAPY

Referral to an otolaryngologist for visualization of the vocal cords is indicated for any patient with hoarseness persisting longer than 2 weeks. Treatment depends on the specific clinical situation, but common interventions consist of voice rest; cessation of tobacco use; treatment for gastroesophageal reflux, chronic rhinosinusitis, and cough; and referral to a speech pathologist for therapy and vocal coaching. Most inflammatory conditions and those due to voice abuse are best treated non-surgically if possible. Biopsy may be necessary to exclude malignancy. Prior to therapeutic surgical intervention for benign disease, it is essential to control the underlying conditions causing the inflammation.

Smoking cessation is often difficult to achieve. The mainstay of treatment is to get all members of the household to stop smoking and do so together on a defined timetable. Nicotine substitutes can be helpful as can bupropion. Alternative medicine approaches such as acupuncture and hypnosis can benefit some patients.

Gastroesophageal Reflux Disease (GERD)

GERD is increasingly implicated in chronic inflammation of the upper aerodigestive tract. In up to 50% of cases, it is not associated with classic "heartburn." Initial therapy consists of lifestyle changes consisting of avoidance of substances known to exacerbate reflux such as caffeine, alcohol, peppermint and hot spicy foods or those that are associated with symptoms; avoiding eating for 3 hours before bedtime; elevating the head of the bed; regular exercise, and weight loss. If such measures are unsuccessful, addition of an over-the-counter H_2 receptor blocking antihistamine is indicated. If this is still not successful, initiation of prescription strength H_2 blockers and ultimately proton pump inhibitors is indicated. If the diagnosis remains in question, a 24-hour pH probe study with a concurrent diary performed while off anti-reflux medication can be helpful, though even this test is not absolutely accurate if the patient is not symptomatic at the time. Esophageal manometry and a barium swallow are also often performed. If these tests are positive, and medical therapy has been unsuccessful, then referral for consideration of surgical fundoplication, which can usually be performed laparoscopically, is indicated.

Chronic Rhinosinusitis and Post-Nasal Drip

Allergy and sensitivities to pollutants account for the majority of these cases. Treatment with avoidance, antihistamines, topical intra-nasal corticosteroids or antihistamines, and inhaled cromolyn form the basis of medical management. Antihistamines with a minimum anticholinergic effect are preferable for this indication, as the dryness associated with systemic antihistamines can aggravate vocal problems. In severe cases, formal intradermal allergy testing or radioallergosorbent testing (RAST) and subsequent desensitization may be indicated. Hypertonic buffered saline nasal irrigations and gargle can also prove beneficial. Ipratropium is the treatment of choice for vasomotor rhinitis with post-nasal drip. Patients not responding to medical management should undergo a CT scan of the paranasal sinuses and referral to an otolaryngologist (rhinologist). In some cases, endoscopic surgery to correct obstructions to drainage of the paranasal sinuses can be helpful.

Chronic Cough

The most frequent causes, after excluding chronic bronchitis/COPD, cardiac failure, pulmonary infection, and neoplasm, are gastroesophageal reflux, allergy, medications (especially angiotensin-converting enzyme inhibitors), chronic sinusitis with post-nasal drip, and reactive airways disease. A CXR should be performed on all such patients. If this is normal, institution of therapy for GERD, allergy, post-nasal drip, and asthma may be instituted one at a time, in a graduated and exploratory manner. Alternatively, formal allergy testing, a methacholine challenge test for reactive airways disease, 24-hour pH probe testing with manometry and a barium swallow, and CT scans of the paranasal sinuses can be undertaken also in a graduated and exploratory manner, searching for a cause.

FUTURE DIRECTIONS

There are many areas of ongoing active research. The neuromuscular control and reflex control of vocal cord function is under study and may lead to new treatment strategies for cough and vocal problems. The causes of GERD, including the physiology of gastric acid production and esophageal sphincter function and the precise substances that cause irritation, especially in the larynx and pharynx, are under intense study. An association between reflux and upper aerodigestive tract malignancy has recently been proposed and deserves further study.

REFERENCES

Banfield G, Tandon P, Solomons N. Hoarse voice: an early symptom of many conditions. *Practitioner*. 2000;244:267–271.

Berke GS, Kevorkian KF. The diagnosis and management of hoarseness. *Compr Ther*. 1996;22:251–255.

Garrett CG, Ossoff RH. Hoarseness: contemporary diagnosis and management. *Compr Ther*. 1995;21:705–710.

Maragos NE. Hoarseness. *Prim Care*. 1990;17:347–363.

Miller RH, Nemecheck AJ. Hoarseness and vocal cord paralysis. In: Bailey, BJ, Ed. Head and Neck Surgery: *Otolaryngology*. 2nd ed. Philadelpha, Pa: Lippincott-Raven; 1998:741–751.

Rosen CA, Anderson D, Murry T. Evaluating hoarseness: keeping your patient's voice healthy. *Am Fam Physician*. 1998; 57:2775–2782.

Chapter 12

Neck Masses in Adults

Mark C. Weissler

Neck masses may be due to any of a number of causes (Figure 12-1), including congenital disorders, infection, and neoplastic lesions. With careful attention to patient history, physical examination, and help from properly selected laboratory and imaging tests, the physician can usually arrive at a correct diagnosis quickly and efficiently.

ETIOLOGY AND PATHOGENESIS/ CLINICAL PRESENTATION
Age
The patient's age may give a clue to the diagnosis. Neck masses in infants and children are usually branchial cleft abnormalities, thyroglossal duct cysts, hemangiomas, lymphangiomas, or benign lymphadenopathy. Adolescents and young adults with significant cervical lymphadenopathy, malaise, and pharyngitis often have infectious mononucleosis. Single large, inflamed anterolateral neck masses in this age group that develop after upper respiratory infections suggest branchial cleft cysts. Multiple rubbery low neck masses, night sweats, fever, and malaise may indicate Hodgkin's disease.

Metastatic cancer, primary salivary gland infections or neoplasms, and lymphomas are common causes of neck masses in older adults.

History
The history helps to limit the differential diagnosis. Infectious processes usually develop over hours to days and have associated pain, redness, warmth, and fever. Patients often have preceding upper respiratory tract or dental infection. Infected congenital cysts may have enlarged on earlier occasions and resolved with antibiotic therapy. Submandibular gland infection often waxes and wanes, is exacerbated by eating, and causes a foul taste in the mouth as the gland decompresses. Hodgkin's disease is associated with night sweats, malaise, itching, and/or fever. Patients with cat-scratch disease give a history of cat contact.

Metastatic squamous cell carcinoma of the upper aerodigestive tract usually occurs in patients with a history of heavy smoking, many of whom also abuse alcohol. Odynophagia, dysphagia, dyspnea, voice change, and/or weight loss are indicative of the primary malignancy. Patients with metastatic disease from distant sites may report symptoms of the primary tumor, such as cough, hemoptysis, abdominal pain, hematochezia, abnormal uterine bleeding, or difficulty urinating. Salivary gland neoplasms are usually painless and grow slowly, though high-grade malignancies may enlarge rapidly. Parotid gland malignancies sometimes cause facial nerve paralysis. Schwannomas, paragangliomas, dermoids, and other benign neoplasms typically grow slowly, cause few symptoms, and are noticed only coincidentally.

Physical Examination
The head and neck exam should include thorough visualization of the ears, nose, oral cavity, oropharynx, nasopharynx, hypopharynx, and larynx; in children, general anesthesia may be required. The fiberoptic laryngoscope is helpful in patients with brisk gag reflexes. Auscultation of the chest and over the neck mass may yield important data. Palpation for cervical, axillary, and inguinal lymphadenopathy and for liver or spleen enlargement may strengthen a suspicion of lymphoma. Breast, rectal, and pelvic exams are appropriate in many cases.

Mass consistency and location are critical in the neck examination. *Metastatic squamous cell carcinoma* feels firm and becomes fixed when advanced. *Lymphoma* or *simple lymphadenopathy* feels rubbery or soft. Branchial and other cysts fluctuant. Infected lymph nodes or congenital cysts become tense. Infected masses become attached to the overlying skin as they begin to "point," are often warm and tender, and have erythematous overlying skin. Capillary hemangiomas are generally flat and appear pink to red, whereas cavernous hemangiomas are raised, purple to blue, and feel soft and cystic.

Thyroglossal duct cysts lie in or near the midline of the neck; most present below the level of the hyoid bone. Masses in the midline of the submental area can be dermoid cysts or teratomas; plunging ranulas may also present in this area. Masses in the submandibular region may represent sialadenitis, submandibular gland neoplasia, or enlarged submandibular lymph nodes from infection or metastatic tumor (most commonly squamous cell carcinoma of the oral cavity).

Posterior triangle lymph nodes suggest *squamous cell carcinoma of the nasopharynx*. The upper jugular lymph nodes are most commonly enlarged in cases of pharyngitis and are often the first site of metastasis for oropharyngeal cancers. Enlarged supraclavicular lymph nodes suggest *Hodgkin's disease* or metastases from the thorax or abdomen. Masses in the lower anterior neck often indicate *thyroid disease*.

DIFFERENTIAL DIAGNOSIS

The differential diagnosis of a neck mass is extensive. One helpful way to categorize possible pathologic processes combines tissue of origin and disease type.

Congenital Lesions

Congenital neck masses may become apparent in infancy or later in life. Branchial cleft anomalies and thyroglossal duct cysts are most common. Branchial sinuses, or fistulas, present at birth as small draining puncta along the anterior border of the sternocleidomastoid muscle or in the preauricular area. *Branchial cleft cysts* present in young adults, typically during or after an acute upper respiratory infection. The cyst develops as a painful, warm, soft, or fluctuant area in the neck along the anterior border of the sternocleidomastoid muscle; deep neck abscess or cellulitis may complicate this problem. Surgical excision is usually required. *Thyroglossal duct cysts* occur in or near the midline of the neck, slightly below the level of the hyoid bone, and move superiorly with tongue protrusion. They represent thyroid gland remnants left during the gland's descent from its origin near the foramen cecum of the tongue to its normal paratracheal location. *Der-

moid cysts often develop in the submental area. These congenital cysts may present acutely when they become infected (usually during or after an upper respiratory infection) or chronically (as cystic neck masses) during young adult life.

Capillary and *cavernous hemangiomas* are benign tumors, generally obvious at or shortly after birth. Capillary hemangiomas (port wine stains) do not regress significantly with age. Recently, pigment seeking laser therapy has yielded good results. Cavernous hemangiomas may regress significantly with age and therefore call for a "watch and wait" approach. Overly aggressive early treatment may result in unnecessary damage to involved normal structures. Surgery is reserved for bleeding lesions or lesions obstructing the airway or digestive tract and hemangiomas that have not regressed significantly by the preschool years.

Cavernous lymphangiomas, or cystic hygromas, appear as soft, fleshy masses. Although benign, lymphangiomas in infants are often infiltrative and may cause obstructive symptoms requiring surgical excision. Total extirpation is not usually possible, so involved normal structures should not be sacrificed at surgery. Adults often manifest less infiltration, permitting more definitive surgical excision.

Neoplastic Lesions

Squamous cell carcinoma of the upper aerodigestive tract metastatic to cervical lymph nodes is the most common cause of a unilateral neck mass in middle-aged or older men with a history of tobacco use. Other common neoplasms include tumors of the parotid and submandibular salivary glands, Hodgkin's and non-Hodgkin's lymphomas, neurogenic tumors (schwannomas and neurofibromas), and paragangliomas (carotid body tumors and glomus tumors).

Squamous cell carcinomas metastatic to the neck often originate in the oral cavity, pharynx, or larynx but may come from the skin or more distant sites. Involved lymph nodes usually feel firm and although initially mobile, they become fixed to surrounding structures as cancer breaks through their capsules. In advanced cases, there is multiple and/or bilateral node involvement. Usually, radical surgery is necessary (Figure 12-1).

Salivary gland tumors develop in older individuals. About 80% of parotid gland neoplasms, mostly pleomorphic adenomas, are benign. The most

Figure 12-1

Neck Masses in Adults

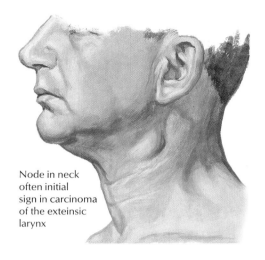

Node in neck
often initial
sign in carcinoma
of the exteinsic
larynx

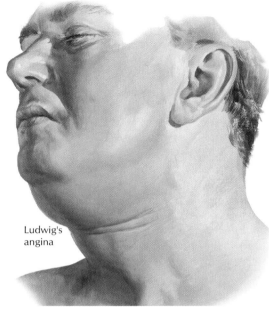

Ludwig's
angina

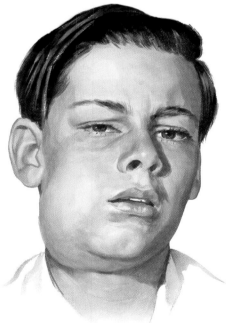

Abscess of the submandibular region

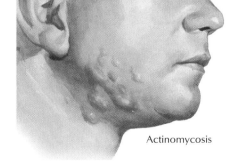

Actinomycosis

common malignant parotid gland tumor is the mucoepidermoid carcinoma. Approximately 50% of submandibular gland neoplasms are benign. The most common benign submandibular gland neoplasm is the *pleomorphic adenoma*; the most common malignant tumor is adenoid *cystic carcinoma*. Surgical excision is usually necessary, with additional postoperative radiation for high-grade malignancies.

Involved cervical lymph nodes in Hodgkin's disease feel softer and more rubbery than those of squamous cell carcinoma. This lymphoma often causes enlargement of multiple nodes in the lower neck. Non-Hodgkin's lymphoma generally presents in older patients. Enlarged nodes are often matted and multiple, again having a rubbery rather than a hard infiltrative feel. It sometimes involves the tissue of Waldeyer's ring (palatine tonsils, lingual tonsils, and adenoids). Diagnosis is confirmed by biopsy. Treatment consists of radiation therapy, chemotherapy, or both.

Schwannomas usually grow on the vagus nerve or cervical sympathetic trunk. Neural function usually remains normal, as the lesion enlarges very slowly over many years. Surgical removal is frequently recommended. Neurofibromas in the neck, often multiple, can coexist with neurofibromas elsewhere and may involve any nerve(s). Surgeons generally reserve excision for solitary lesions or those causing obstructive symptoms or severe deformity. Most neurogenic tumors are benign; however, malignant degeneration has been described, usually marked by a rapid growth phase or loss of nerve function.

Paragangliomas are usually benign and occasionally multiple; these highly vascular neoplasms often produce bruits. *Carotid body tumors* typically splay the internal and external carotid arteries. *Glomus jugulare* and *glomus vagale tumors*, originating in specialized paraganglion tissue along the internal jugular vein and the vagus nerve, respectively, often erode the temporal bone and present high in the neck behind the angle of the mandible. Surgical removal is generally recommended.

Infectious Neck Masses

These may be indolent or fulminant. *Simple lymphadenopathy* often occurs with acute viral or bacterial pharyngitis, sinusitis, or tooth infections. Generally, these nodes feel soft and shrink over days to weeks after the acute infection resolves. *Suppurative lymphadenopathy* occurs when the center of a node necroses and an abscess develops. Most abscesses require antibiotic therapy and surgical drainage; untreated suppurative lymphadenopathy can lead to deep neck infections, and spread to the mediastinum may be fatal.

Certain infection paths are common enough to have their own identity. *Ludwig's angina* begins with an infection in the oral cavity of dental origin. Sublingual inflammation and swelling retrodisplace and elevate the tongue, possibly leading to acute upper airway obstruction. (Figure 12-1) *Bezold's abscess* develops when a mastoid infection breaks out inferiorly into the deep neck. Deep neck space infections require emergency hospitalization, intravenous antibiotics, and usually surgical drainage.

The parotid and submandibular glands may become infected. *Acute parotid sialadenitis* afflicts elderly individuals most commonly, especially when they get dehydrated; it may also reflect sialolithiasis. Cystic degeneration of the parotid gland has been described in HIV infections. *Acute submandibular sialadenitis* often follows sialolithiasis. Patients often note intermittent submandibular swelling associated with eating. Parotitis is usually treated with hydration, intravenous antibiotics, local heat, massage, and sialogogues. *Recurrent submandibular sialadenitis* is usually treated with resection of the submandibular gland during a quiescent period (Figure 12-1).

Other infectious processes include atypical tuberculosis (scrofula), best treated by surgical excision of the involved lymph nodes; cat-scratch disease, which frequently requires surgical drainage; and actinomycosis, which often causes multiple chronically draining sinus tracts with "sulfur granules" of matted organisms (Figure 12-1). Many patients with HIV infection develop cervical lymphadenopathy; this complication does not generally require specific treatment unless rapid expansion suggests lymphomatous involvement.

Other Common Neck Masses

These include prominent normal structures, such as the (pulsatile) carotid bulb or the (hard) transverse process of the first cervical vertebra. Careful palpation should delineate these bilateral (although frequently asymmetric) structures.

Carotid aneurysm, although uncommon, should be suspected if the patient has an expanding neck mass or a history of cervical trauma. *Thyroid masses* are quite common. Diffuse nodular thyroid enlargement present for many years suggests simple goiter. Solitary thyroid nodules, although usually benign, may represent thyroid cancer and thus demand evaluation. Epidermal and dermal inclusion cysts are very superficial; they often result from recurrent cutaneous inflammation.

DIAGNOSTIC APPROACH
Laboratory Studies

A variety of studies may prove useful. A heterophil antibody test may reveal mononucleosis in the young patient with pharyngitis and cervical adenopathy out of proportion to that expected in cases of simple upper respiratory infection. Serologic tests for HIV infection may help in the evaluation of an at-risk patient with multiple enlarged cervical lymph nodes or parotid gland enlargement. Intradermal antigen testing for tuberculosis and a control substance, thyroid function tests, and a complete blood cell count with differential can each provide useful data in appropriate situations.

Imaging Studies

Chest X-rays may show lung carcinoma, metastases, findings consistent with lymphoma or tuberculosis, or tracheal deviation. CT scanning (or possibly MRI) can delineate cervical anatomic relationships and reveal pathology, such as a primary aerodigestive tract cancer. Thyroid scanning, although less frequent since the advent of fine-needle cytologic examination, still proves useful in some cases. Anteroposterior and lateral neck X-rays can show tracheal deviation or encroachment on the airway (before or instead of CT scans).

Further Diagnostic Workup

Patients should undergo complete clinical evaluation prior to any biopsy; the otolaryngologist with head-and-neck surgical training can best evaluate patients with neck masses of concern. Cytologic examination of neck masses via fine-needle aspiration is very helpful. More than 90% sensitive and specific, cytology often aids in counseling patients preoperatively or in directing further diagnostic maneuvers.

Patients with masses that represent metastases should undergo direct laryngoscopy, pharyngoscopy, esophagoscopy, and bronchoscopy under anesthesia prior to any excisional neck biopsy. If endoscopy reveals no obvious primary lesion, especially if previous cytologic evaluation documented squamous cell carcinoma in the neck, biopsies of the tongue base, the tonsils, and the nasopharynx should be obtained. If negative, the surgeon can perform an open neck biopsy and obtain frozen sections. If no primary tumor is found but the open neck biopsy reveals unequivocal squamous cell carcinoma, a neck dissection is performed at the time of biopsy. There is a 20% incidence of second primary tumors in patients with upper aerodigestive tract malignancies.

If open neck biopsy does not reveal squamous cell carcinoma, the surgeon and pathologist should be ready to thoroughly evaluate the tissue specimens. Cultures for aerobes, anaerobes, acid-fast bacteria, and fungi should be obtained, and material should be processed for immunohistochemical and/or electron microscopic study if indicated by the frozen section findings.

FUTURE DIRECTIONS

New treatment modalities for head and neck cancer are needed. The mainstay of treatment for many years has been surgical excision and radiation. New organ preservation protocols utilizing combinations of chemotherapy and radiation are becoming more popular. New treatments such as gene therapy, adenovirus vectors, antiangiogenesis factors, and immune modulators are on the horizon.

REFERENCES

Alvi A, Johnson JT. The neck mass. A challenging differential diagnosis. *Postgrad Med.* 1995;97:87-90, 93–94, 97.

Armstrong WB, Giglio MF. Is this lump in the neck anything to worry about? *Postgrad Med.* 1998;104:63–64, 67-71,75–76.

Park YW. Evaluation of neck masses in children. *Am Fam Physician.* 1995;51:1904–1912.

Schuller DE, Nicholson RE. Clinical evaluation and surgical treatment of malignant tumors of the neck. In: Thawley SE, Panje WR, Batsakis JG, Lindberg RD, eds. Comprehensive *Management of Head and Neck Tumors.* 2nd ed. Philadelphia, Pa: WB Saunders Co; 1999:1395–1415.

Sobol SM, Bailey SB. Evaluation and surgical management of tumors of the neck: benign tumors. In: Thawley SE, Panje WR, Batsakis JG, Lindberg RD, eds. *Comprehensive Management of Head and Neck Tumors.* 2nd ed. Philadelphia, Pa: WB Saunders Co; 1999:1416–1449.

Chapter 13

Pharyngitis

Daniel S. Reuland

Sore throat accounts for 1% to 2% of visits to outpatient clinics, physicians' offices, and emergency rooms. Identifying and treating the subset with *Group A beta hemolytic streptococci* (GABHS) *-associated pharyngitis* and its complications is the primary goal in clinical practice.

ETIOLOGY AND PATHOGENESIS

Adenovirus, rhinovirus, and other respiratory viruses cause most cases of sore throat. Other viral etiologies include Epstein-Barr virus, which causes pharyngitis in acute infectious mononucleosis, primarily in adolescents and young adults. Herpes simplex virus and coxsackie A viruses can cause oral and pharyngeal ulcers, at times mimicking GABHS infection.

Clinically, the most important common bacterial pathogen, GABHS or *Streptococcus pyogenes* ("strep"), is identified in 5% to 20% of subjects with sore throat in whom a throat culture is obtained. The organisms are spread by droplets from patients with pharyngitis or from asymptomatic nasopharyngeal carriers, and elaborate a variety of enzymes including streptolysins, streptokinase, deoxyribonucleases, and hyaluronidase that promote direct invasion of tissue, the most common way these organisms cause disease. GABHS also produce exotoxins, which are central in the pathogenesis of scarlet fever and the streptococcal toxic shock syndrome. Other streptococci from groups C and G can cause pharyngitis, though without the complications that can follow GABHS infection.

CLINICAL PRESENTATION

Patients present with sore throat often accompanied by one or more of the following: cough, congestion, swollen glands, difficulty swallowing, fever, or rigors. Cough and nasal congestion are usually absent in pharyngitis due to GABHS. The acute illness of streptococcal pharyngitis typically lasts 7 to 10 days.

Patients with streptococcal pharyngitis may develop suppurative complications such as peritonsillar or retropharyngeal abscesses, which occur in 1% to 2% of streptococcal pharyngitis cases. Streptococcal bacteremia with shock is a rare but serious complication of pharyngeal GABHS infection. Scarlet fever occurs primarily in children and is associated with certain toxin-elaborating strains of GABHS. It presents with a fine, erythematous, papular rash that starts on the trunk. Facial flushing with peri-oral pallor, petechiae, and, palmar desquamation may be seen.

Acute rheumatic fever (ARF) is the most serious of the non-suppurative complications of streptococcal pharyngitis infection. Antibiotics reduce the risk by more than two thirds. In the developed world, the incidence has declined so dramatically that antibiotic prescribing solely to prevent ARF is controversial given the extremely low absolute risk of this complication. *Post-streptococcal glomerulonephritis,* the other main non-suppurative complication, occurs with varying severity, although it is almost always self-limited. It is not known whether antibiotic treatment of GABHS reduces the risk of this complication.

DIFFERENTIAL DIAGNOSIS

Pharyngitis may be due to oropharyngeal candidiasis (thrush) in immunocompromised hosts and in those receiving antibiotics or inhaled corticosteroids. Gonococci occasionally cause pharyngitis in patients engaging in orogential sex. Though rarely diagnosed, other organisms associated with pharyngitis include *Mycoplasma pneumoniae, Chlamydia pneumoniae, Treponema pallidum* (primary or secondary syphilis), *Yersinia enterocolitica,* and fusobacteria. Certain spirochetes and anaerobes can cause a membranous pharyngitis associated with foul odor known as Vincent's angina. Diphtheria, caused by *Corynebacterium diptheriae,* presents with a grayish membrane on the tonsils, pharynx, uvula, and nares and requires prompt recognition and therapy (Figure 13-1). Outbreaks can occur in unimmunized populations. Pharyngitis is also part of the acute retroviral syndrome (along with fever, arthralgias, and lymphadenopathy) associated with primary infection with human immunodeficiency virus (HIV).

Other important diagnostic considerations in a patient with sore throat include retropharyngeal or peritonsillar abscesses. Symptoms are severe and typically include fever and systemic toxicity. The pain is such that patients are often unable to take liquids, resulting in dehydration. In peritonsillar abscess, the voice becomes altered and muffled, and there is swelling of the anterior tonsillar pillar and medial displacement of the tonsil (Figure 13-1). About one half of cases are due to GABHS, and antibiotics appear to reduce the incidence of these complications.

Ludwig's angina (see Chapter 12, Figure 12-1) describes other parapharyngeal space infections including the submandibular, sublingual, and submaxillary spaces. These are typically polymicrobial and associated with foreign bodies or poor dental hygiene. Epiglottitis is caused by GABHS or *H. influenzae*. It is rare, particularly in adults, but can progress rapidly and lead to airway obstruction. Suspicion for any of these conditions is an indication for urgent referral to an otolaryngologist.

Table 13-1
Suggested Office-Based Approach to Patient with Pharyngitis

Pre-test probability

Strep score*	%of GABHS	Action
0	1%	supportive care
1	4%	supportive care
2	9%	antigen testing (antibiotics if +)
3	21%	antigen testing (antibiotics if +)
4	43%	empiric antibiotic treatment

*Strep score is obtained by assigning one point for each of the following clinical findings: tonsillar exudates, history of fever, cervical lymphadenopathy, absence of cough.

DIAGNOSTIC APPROACH

No single clinical finding reliably distinguishes between sore throats caused by common viruses and those caused by GABHS. The prevalence of GABHS in a typical office practice is about 10%. In emergency departments, the prevalence is around 20%.

The Centor Criteria are used for estimating the clinical probability of strep pharyngitis and permit rational decision-making regarding "rapid" antigen testing and therapy for GABHS. A strep score is obtained by simply assigning one point for the presence of each of the following clinical findings: history of fever, tonsillar exudates, anterior cervical lymphadenopathy, and absence of cough.

Other predictive clinical factors include positive throat culture within the past year, exposure to family members with current documented strep infection, and temperature greater than 101° F. Once the probability has been estimated on clinical grounds, a rational decision on laboratory testing can be made.

Both antigen tests and throat cultures are used to diagnose GABHS. Antigen tests have sensitivities of about 85% and specificities of about 95%. Throat cultures, when performed by reference laboratories, have sensitivities of 90% and specificities approaching 99%. Office-based antigen testing offers rapid results and greatly improves the diagnostic accuracy over clinical assessment alone. This is especially true when the probability of strep is intermediate. Some controversy surrounds whether or not negative antigen tests should be confirmed by culture. A reasonable approach is to perform confirmatory throat culture when the clinical suspicion for strep is fairly high, (i.e., a strep score of 3) but the initial antigen test is negative.

MANAGEMENT AND THERAPY

In addition to those patients meeting treatment criteria as described in Table 13-1, empiric antibiotic therapy should be given to those patients with pharyngitis and a history of rheumatic fever and to those with a household contact with current documented strep throat. Penicillin is the antibiotic treatment of choice. Penicillin V taken 2 or 3 times daily for 10 days shortens the course of the illness. When adherence is a problem, benzathine penicillin given intramuscularly is highly

Figure 13-1

Infections of Pharynx

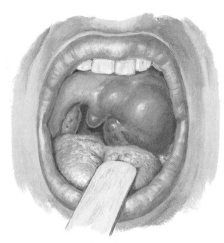

Peritonsillar
abscess (quinsy)

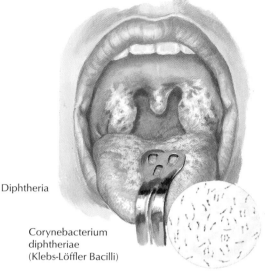

Diphtheria

Corynebacterium
diphtheriae
(Klebs-Löffler Bacilli)

effective, though the risk of anaphylaxis is higher. In penicillin-allergic patients, erythromycin, azithromycin, clarithromycin, clindamycin, or an oral cephalosporin are reasonable alternatives.

Symptomatic Treatment

Regardless of etiology, patients with pharyngitis require symptom relief. Acetaminophen, aspirin, and NSAIDs are probably similarly effective in relieving symptoms. There is limited evidence on the effectiveness of other treatments such as corticosteroids, pneumococcal or influenza vaccination, super colonization with alpha streptococcal bacteria, and benzydamine oral rinse. Routine use of these agents to treat or prevent GABHS is not presently warranted.

REFERENCES

Bisno AL. Acute pharyngitis. *N Engl J Med*. 2001;344:205–211.

Cooper RJ, Hoffman JR, Bartlett JG, et al, and the American Academy of Family Physicians, the American College of Physicians-American Society of Internal Medicine, and the Centers for Disease Control. Principles of appropriate antibiotic use for acute pharyngitis in adults: background. *Ann Intern Med*. 2001;134:509–517.

Del Mar CB, Glasziou PP, Spinks AB. Antibiotics for sore throat. *Cochrane Database Syst Rev*. 2000;CD000023.

Snow V, Mottur-Pilson C, Cooper RJ, Hoffman JR, and the American Academy of Family Physicians, the American College of Physicians-American Society of Internal Medicine, and the Centers for Disease Control. Principles of appropriate antibiotic use for acute pharyngitis in adults. *Ann Intern Med*. 2001;134:506–508.

Thomas M, Del Mar C, Glasziou P. How effective are treatments other than antibiotics for acute sore throat? *Br J Gen Pract*. 2000;50:817–820.

Chapter 14

Rhinitis: Allergic and Idiopathic

David C. Henke

Rhinitis presents clinically as nasal congestion. Symptoms include nasal discharge, itching, sneezing, and pressure. It often progresses to involve the paranasal sinus cavities and the eustachian tubes, producing frontal headaches and a "popping" sensation in the ears. The postnasal discharge of mucus can also cause cough. Most people will experience rhinitis symptoms during their lives. There are several syndromes associated with chronic rhinitis that can be grouped into allergic, idiopathic, and secondary rhinitis. Idiopathic rhinitis, previously called *vasomotor rhinitis* or *nonallergic noninfectious perennial rhinitis*, shares many features with allergic rhinitis, including nasal mucosal hyper-reactivity, but lacks the associated skin test sensitivity. *Acute and self -limited infectious rhinitis*, "the common cold," will not be reviewed here.

Allergic rhinitis is the fifth most prevalent chronic condition in the US, affecting more than 24 million people. The prevalence of allergic rhinitis has increased 25% in the past 2 decades. Related diagnoses such as nasal polyps, deviated nasal septum, and chronic disease of the tonsils and adenoids affect an additional 5.3 million Americans. The direct costs of allergic rhinitis in the US are estimated to be $1.23 billion annually. These figures do not include over-the-counter pharmacotherapy costs, nor do they allow for the costs associated with the introduction of new generations of antihistamines, diagnostic testing, or immunotherapy. In patients with asthma and allergic rhinitis as opposed to asthma alone, the cost of care increased by 46%.

ETIOLOGY AND PATHOGENESIS

Nonallergic and allergic rhinitis are associated with the release of histamine, prostaglandins, leukotrienes, and cytokines from mast cells, basophils, and eosinophils. In allergic disease, the release of mediators is associated with the cross-linking of IgE on the mast cell by allergen (Figures 14-1 and 14-2). A similar cellular reaction occurs in nonallergic rhinitis by an undefined mechanism.

The clinical expression of allergic rhinitis has been linked to whether the immune response is driven by Th1 or Th2 lymphocytes as determined by the interactions between the T cells and antigen-presenting cells (Figure 14-2). If the antigen-presenting (e.g., the dendritic cell) triggers the expression of Th2 cells, a number of factors, including interleukins (IL)-4, 5, 9, 13; histamine-releasing factor, and neuropeptides are released. These factors interact with other mediators including interferon gamma, IL-11, IL-12, and leukotrienes. The response leads to IgE production, the accumulation of eosinophils and basophils in the lung and upper airway, mast cell proliferation, airway hyperresponsiveness, mucus overproduction, and the exudation of bloodstream-derived proteins into the airways.

Both genetic and environmental factors appear to play a role in selecting for a Th2 inflammatory response. In nonatopic individuals, there is a switch to a Th1 response to allergen shortly after birth. There is an association between an allele of HLA-DR and a polymorphism for IgE and atopy. Atopic disease also appears to be associated with: 1) the Western life style, even when lived in a third-world environment; 2) "excessive" hygiene; 3) antibiotics in the first 2 years of life; and 4) vaccination (Figure 14-3).

There is some evidence to support the notion that microorganisms can influence T cell responses. For example, products of *Aspergillus fumigatus* evoke Th2-mediated IgE production. In contrast, interferon gamma from Th1cells and IL-18 from macrophages potentially inhibit the production of IgE. Immunotherapy and bacterial cytosine guanasine (C-p-G) DNA repeats, especially when used as adjuvants, may switch the Th2 to the Th1 phenotype.

Figure 14-1

Mechanism of Type 1 (Immediate) Hypersensitivity

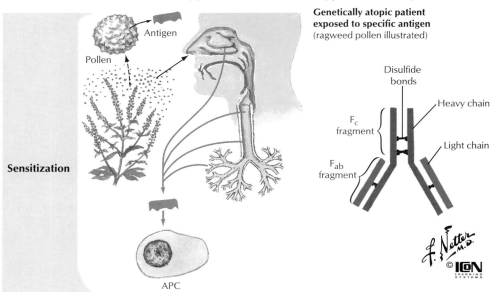

Genetically atopic patient exposed to specific antigen
(ragweed pollen illustrated)

Figure 14-2

Allergic Inflammation

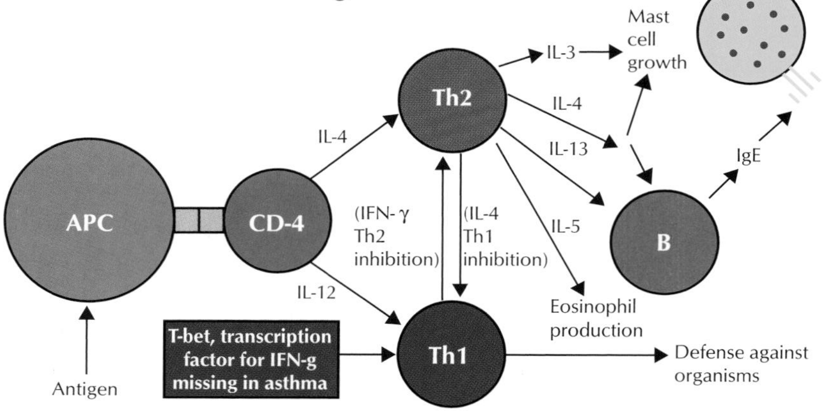

Adapted with permission from Kay AB. Allergy and allergic diseases. First of two parts. *NEJM*. 2001;344:30-37. Copyright ©2001 Massachusetts Medical Society. All rights reserved.

The increased prevalence in allergic rhinitis has also been linked to higher concentrations of pollen that in turn has been attributed to increase atmospheric CO_2. It has also been associated with the development of energy-efficient buildings that slow the exchange of outside air and promote the concentration of indoor allergens.

CLINICAL PRESENTATION

The various forms of rhinitis are diagnosed by recognizing the patient's symptom patterns and associations and to a lesser extent by physical examination and laboratory testing. Symptoms include: sneezing, watery eyes, pruritic eyes and ears, "popping" in the ears, sinus pain, and rhinorrhea. It is important to establish the duration, chronicity, and temporal patterns of the symptoms. Triggers such as exposures to flowering plants, mold-rich environments, animal danders, exacerbations during the spring and fall, and a positive family history suggest allergic rhinitis. But there are many other considerations when evaluating nasal congestion. Etiologies stemming from illicit drug use include upper airway irritation.

Figure 14-3

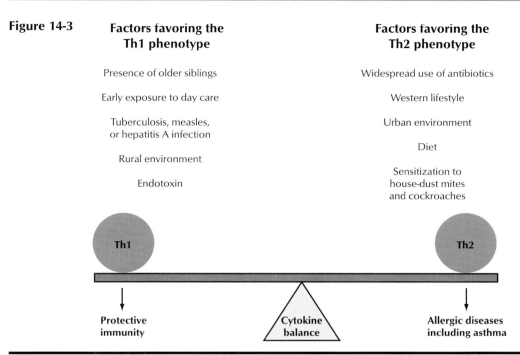

Factors favoring the Th1 phenotype	Factors favoring the Th2 phenotype
Presence of older siblings	Widespread use of antibiotics
Early exposure to day care	Western lifestyle
Tuberculosis, measles, or hepatitis A infection	Urban environment
Rural environment	Diet
Endotoxin	Sensitization to house-dust mites and cockroaches

Th1 — Protective immunity — Cytokine balance — Th2 — Allergic diseases including asthma

The frequent use of nasal decongestants may provide the clue to the diagnosis of rhinitis medicamentosa. Possible reactions to beta-blockers and nonsteroidal anti-inflammatory drugs (NSAID) in asthmatic individuals should be investigated. An occupational and hobby history may reveal exposure to nasal irritants and potentially carcinogenic wood dusts. Food allergies rarely cause adult rhinitis, but this etiology is more common in children. Upper airway resistance syndrome (UARS) leads to hypersomnolence and can be caused by allergic rhinitis. These patients may not have frank obstructive sleep apnea.

A physical examination revealing an "allergic crease" from frequent nose rubbing, reddened and inflamed upper airway mucosa, periorbital edema, and a bluish discoloration secondary to venous stasis ("allergic shiners") supports the diagnosis of chronic rhinorrhea. Polyps, foreign bodies, septal deviations or perforation, tumors, conjunctivitis, serous otitis, vasculitic rash, urticaria, and wheezing should be looked for since they suggest specific etiologies. Sinus pain, purulent drainage, and fever suggest complicating infection. The diagnosis of idiopathic rhinitis is one of exclusion.

Laboratory testing and physical examination are needed to diagnose local and systemic disorders that can mimic allergic rhinitis. Rhinitis has been linked to cystic fibrosis, tumors, foreign bodies, atrophic rhinitis, hypothyroidism, conditions associated with hormonal fluctuations such as pregnancy, Wegener's granulomatosis, and allergic granulomatosis of Churg-Strauss.

The diagnosis of allergic rhinitis is established by demonstrating specific IgE either by *in vivo* scratch skin testing or by *in vitro* radio adsorbent serum tests (RAST). Scratch skin testing is important when designing avoidance strategies and immunotherapy. A blood count differential demonstrating hypereosinophilia, an elevated IgE, and pulmonary function testing revealing reversible airflow obstruction, bronchial hyperreactivity, and an elevated diffusing capacity for carbon monoxide (DLCO) can be useful to confirm the diagnosis of allergic rhinitis associated with asthma.

MANAGEMENT AND THERAPY

Conservative interventions include topical or systemic decongestants, topical corticosteroids, anticholinergics, antihistamines, allergy and irritant avoidance strategies, immunotherapy, and mechanical devices such as CPAP when an UARS is diagnosed.

Decongestants

Topical decongestants are therapeutic but cause *rhinitis medicamentosa* when overused. Rhinitis medicamentosa is treated by slowly tapering the medication and topical nasal steroids. When employed as therapy, topical decongestants should be used sparingly and for no longer than 7 days. Systemic decongestants work well as nasal decongestants but are associated with tremor, oral dryness, palpitations, and insomnia. They also can aggravate cardiac disease, hypertension, diabetes, glaucoma, thyrotoxicosis, and bladder obstruction. Neither topical nor systemic decongestants significantly influence pruritus, sneezing, or rhinorrhea. The combination of decongestants and antihistamines is more effective than either agent alone (Table 14-1, see also page 77).

Corticosteroids

Corticosteroids reduce inflammation, promote vascular constriction, and diminish hyperactivity and vascular permeability. Topical application is the preferred route of administration because it avoids many of the unwanted systemic effects associated with oral and parenteral corticosteroids. The vasoconstrictive property of topical nasal steroids also provides a rapid therapeutic decongestant effect. However, mucosal drying can produce nasal irritation, bleeding, septal perforations, and candidiasis. Patients should titrate topical steroids to control symptoms and avoid excessive mucosal drying or use products available in aqueous formulation. Topical steroids are superior to antihistamines in controlling nasal symptoms.

Antihistamines

Oral H_1 blockers are employed in the therapy for allergic rhinitis (Table 14-1). H_1 blockers are in fact one of the most successful and widely used therapies. Sedation is a major limiting factor. The latest generation of antihistamines (acrivastine, cetirizine, fexofenadine, loratadine, and desloratadine) is less sedating and does not cause delayed cardiac repolarization OT prolongation by EKG), thus avoiding the potential complication of sudden cardiac death due to torsade de pointes asso-

Table 14-1
Antihistamines

Generic name

First generation
Chlorpheniramine
Diphenhydramine
Hydroxyzine
Triprolidine

Second generation
Cetirizine
Fexofenadine
Loratadine
Desloratadine

Topical
Azelastine (nasal)
Levocabastine (ophthalmic)
Olopatadine (ophthalmic)

Adapted with permission from *ENT–Ear, Nose and Throat Journal.* 2000; 79:700.

ciated with astemizole and terfenadine. The newer antihistamines (azelastine, levocabastine, and olopatadine) are available as topical medications. Azelastine inhibits histamine release, as well as other inflammatory mediator production, although use is associated with drowsiness. Levocabastine and olopatadine are available as topical ocular agents with a rapid onset of action and no sedating effects (Table 14-1).

Mast Cell Stabilizers

Cromolyn and its more potent derivative, nedocromil, increase intracellular cyclic AMP, thereby raising the threshold for mast cell degranulation and release of histamine. They ameliorate allergic symptoms, although to a less extent than topical steroids. Cromolyn is available OTC; nedocromil is available as an ophthalmic preparation but is not yet available in a topical nasal application. A drawback to the use of mast cell stabilizers is the need to use them multiple times each day.

Anticholinergics

Ipratropium bromide inhibits secretions from vagally innervated serous and seromucous glands by antagonizing acetylcholine at the cholinergic receptor. The drug is poorly absorbed, not associated

Antihistamine/Decongestant Combinations*

· Acrivastine and pseudoephedrine
· Azatadine and pseudoephedrine
· Fexofenadine and pseudoephedrine
· Loratadine and pseudoephedrine
· Triprolidine and pseudoephedrine

*Although phenylpropanolamine (PPA) was historically used as an oral decongestant, the Food and Drug Administration (FDA) has taken steps to remove phenylpropanolamine (PPA) from all drug products and has requested that all drug companies discontinue marketing products containing PPA. In addition, FDA has issued a public health advisory concerning phenylpropanolamine hydrochloride.

Adapted with permission from *ENT–Ear, Nose and Throat Journal.* 2000;79:698.

Topical Intranasal Steroids

· Beclomethasone
· Budesonide
· Fluticasone
· Mometasone
· Triamcinolone

Adapted with permission from *ENT–Ear, Nose and Throat Journal.* 2000;79:700.

with rebound rhinorrhea, and well tolerated. Ipratropium is effective in reducing rhinorrhea but not nasal congestion and sneezing.

Immunotherapy

Immunotherapy is reserved for patients with severe symptoms of allergic rhinitis who suffer much of the year or who cannot be managed with medications and avoidance strategies. The exact therapeutic mechanism is unknown. It is now thought that there is a switch in T-helper cell antigen processing away from pathways associated with IgE production. In general, this therapy is continued for about 6 years and then stopped. After discontinuing, there is often a "honeymoon" period, of variable duration, during which no therapy of any type is required. Patients with severe

asthma are considered at greatest risk of significant adverse reactions to immunotherapy, including anaphylaxis and death.

FUTURE DIRECTIONS

Discriminating between allergic and idiopathic rhinitis is difficult. Fas, a cell surface molecule that induces apoptosis, has been linked to rhinitis. The serum soluble Fas (sFas) level is "normal" in idiopathic rhinitis, a condition attributed to an imbalance in the autonomic nervous system. It is "reduced" in allergic rhinitis. Allergic rhinitis, to date, is the only disease associated with "reduced" levels.

Anti-IgE, now in clinical trials, has been demonstrated to have clinical efficacy in allergic rhinitis and asthma. Anti-IgE protocols have been successful, employing both intravenous and subcutaneous routes of administration. Agents that block interleukins are also of therapeutic interest. A soluble IL-4 receptor, for example, has demonstrated effectiveness in asthma and may prove useful in treating allergic rhinitis. Anti IL-5, while able to lower circulating eosinophils in asthmatics, had no clinical effect.

Future therapies may employ CpG bacterial DNA repeats as adjuvants with vaccines and in immunotherapy with the goal of altering allergen processing to avoid or cure an atopic condition.

REFERENCES

Borish LC, Nelson HS, Lanz MJ, et al. Interleukin-4 receptor in moderate atopic asthma. A phase I/II randomized, placebo-controlled trial. *Am J Respir Crit Care Med.* 1999;160:1816–1823.

Kato M, Hattori T, Ito H, et al. Serum-soluble Fas levels as a marker to distinguish allergic and nonallergic rhinitis. *J Allergy Clin Immunol.* 1999;103:1213–1214.

Kay AB. Allergy and allergic diseases. First of two parts. *N Engl J Med.* 2001;344:30–37.

Naclerio R, Solomon W. Rhinitis and inhalant allergens. *JAMA.* 1997;278:1842–1848.

Van Cauwenberge P, Watelet JB. Epidemiology of chronic rhinosinusitis. *Thorax.* 2000;55(suppl 2):S20–S21.

Weiss KB, Sullivan SD. The health economics of asthma and rhinitis. I. Assessing the economic impact. *J Allergy Clin Immunol.* 2001;107:3–8.

Yawn BP, Yunginger JW, Wollan PC, Reed CE, Silverstein MD, Harris AG. Allergic rhinitis in Rochester, Minnesota residents with asthma: frequency and impact on health care charges. *J Allergy Clin Immunol.* 1999;103:54–59.

Chapter 15

Rhinosinusitis

Daniel S. Reuland

Rhinosinusitis, characterized by inflammation of the maxillary and ethmoid sinuses, accounts for about 25 million office visits annually in the US. It is the fifth most common reason physicians prescribe antibiotics. Physicians tend to prescribe antibiotics about 90% of the time, even though most cases will resolve spontaneously. For practical purposes, "sinusitis" and "rhinosinusitis" are interchangeable terms, though many experts now prefer the latter because the nasal structures that are contiguous with the paranasal sinuses are also invariably inflamed along with the sinuses themselves.

ETIOLOGY AND PATHOGENESIS

Respiratory viruses are common causes of acute rhinosinusitis. *Acute bacterial rhinosinusitis* generally occurs as a secondary infection resulting from a viral upper respiratory infection. Cultures obtained via sinus puncture show the most common bacterial pathogens are *Streptococcus pneumoniae* and *Haemophilus influenzae*; however, other streptococci and *Moraxella catarrhalis* are sometimes isolated. Anaerobes have been associated with some cases of chronic sinusitis, though their pathologic role is unclear.

In patients with uncontrolled diabetes, neutropenia, or other immune–compromised states, etiologies such as *Aspergillus, Rhizopus (mucor), Candida, Alternaria, Pseudomonas, Nocardia, Legionella*, atypical mycobacteria, and certain parasites are unusual but important etiologic considerations. *Nosocomial sinusitis* associated with nasotracheal or nasogastric tubes is frequently polymicrobial. In this setting, *Staphylococcus aureus*, enteric gram-negative bacteria, and anaerobes, particularly anaerobic streptococci and *Bacteroides*, may be present.

The normal sterility of the sinuses is maintained by continuous mucociliary clearance. A variety of physiologic and anatomical abnormalities can lead to loss of patency of the sinus ostia and ostiomeatal complex, a mechanism common to the pathogenesis of most cases of *bacterial sinusitis* (Figure 15-1). Though viral URI is probably the most common antecedent, allergic and vasomotor rhinitis can also lead to bacterial sinusitis. Nose blowing can propel fluid and bacteria into the paranasal sinuses and may lead to sinusitis.

Anatomic factors include nasal polyposis, deviated nasal septum nasotracheal tubes, nasogastric tubes, and other foreign bodies.

Changes in altitude, underwater diving, and swimming are thought to play a role in some individuals. Cigarette smoking and certain intranasal drugs can impair ciliary action, predisposing to sinusitis. Any of these conditions may increase edema in or near the sinus ostia or impair clearance from the sinuses. A relatively distinct pathogenetic mechanism is the occasional extension of a dental abscess into the maxillary sinuses.

CLINICAL PRESENTATION

Facial pain and congestion are the most common historical features, though these symptoms are seen in other causes of nasal obstruction such as viral or allergic rhinitis. Maxillary toothache and purulent rhinorrhea are also common features of acute rhinosinusitis. A prolonged (> 10 days) "cold" with congestion and facial pain with or without purulent drainage often brings the patient to medical attention. Some patients will report a biphasic illness. Fever may be present, but is not typical. Some patients may have subacute (lasting 4 to 12 weeks) or chronic (lasting more than 12 weeks) symptoms.

Complications: Serious life-threatening complications of sinusitis are uncommon in the antibiotic era, but still occur. The bony orbits are surrounded on three sides by the paranasal sinuses; consequently, orbital infection can result from sinusitis, particularly ethmoid sinusitis with extension through the lamina papyracea. A swollen upper lid may be the initial sign, fol-

Figure 15-1

Histology and Physiology of Nasal Cavity and Sinuses

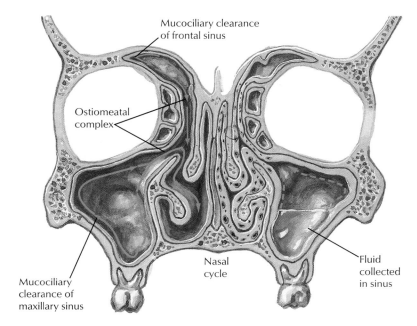

Mucociliary clearance of frontal sinus

Ostiomeatal complex

Mucociliary clearance of maxillary sinus

Nasal cycle

Fluid collected in sinus

Cilia drain sinuses by propelling mucus toward natural ostia (mucociliary clearance)

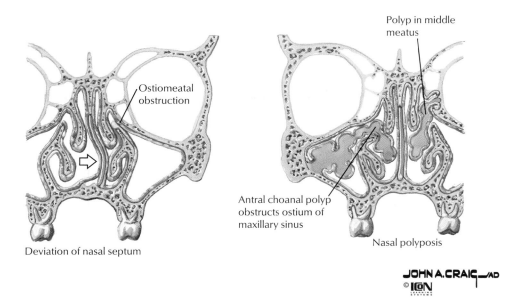

Ostiomeatal obstruction

Deviation of nasal septum

Polyp in middle meatus

Antral choanal polyp obstructs ostium of maxillary sinus

Nasal polyposis

JOHN A. CRAIG—AD
© ICON
LEARNING SYSTEMS

Figure 15-2

Physical Examination

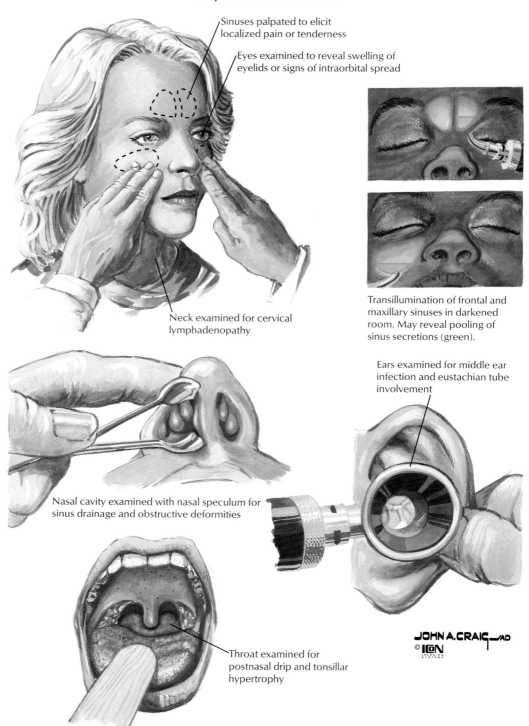

Sinuses palpated to elicit localized pain or tenderness

Eyes examined to reveal swelling of eyelids or signs of intraorbital spread

Neck examined for cervical lymphadenopathy

Transillumination of frontal and maxillary sinuses in darkened room. May reveal pooling of sinus secretions (green).

Ears examined for middle ear infection and eustachian tube involvement

Nasal cavity examined with nasal speculum for sinus drainage and obstructive deformities

Throat examined for postnasal drip and tonsillar hypertrophy

JOHN A. CRAIG_AD
©ICON

lowed by ptosis, conjunctival chemosis, proptosis, and ophthalmoplegia. Isolated infection of the frontal sinuses is rare, but potentially serious. Anterior spread of infection from the frontal sinus can lead to osteomyelitis of the frontal bone, which presents with headache, fever, and a palpable doughy edema of the frontal bone called a Pott puffy tumor. Retrograde migration of septic thrombi along venous channels can lead to thrombophlebitis of the cavernous sinus. Presenting findings include fever, toxicity, chemosis, proptosis, cranial nerve palsies involving nerves III (oculomotor), IV (trochlear), and VI (abducens). Cavernous sinus thrombosis may become bilateral because of spread via the intercavernous communications). Extension to the meninges or brain parenchyma can occur directly or through venous channels and can lead to epidural or subdural abscess, frontal lobe abscess, or meningitis.

DIFFERENTIAL DIAGNOSIS

Common causes of nasal and "sinus" symptoms include allergic rhinitis, acute viral upper respiratory infection, vasomotor rhinitis (idiopathic), abuse of nose drops (rhinitis medicamentosa), and deviated nasal septum. Less common causes include nasal polyps, Wegener's granulomatosis, drug-induced vasomotor rhinitis (from cocaine, prazosin, and angiotensin-converting enzyme inhibitors), foreign body, tumor, cerebrospinal fluid leak, and certain hormonal conditions (hypothyroidism, pregnancy).

DIAGNOSTIC APPROACH

Though no single sign or symptom is diagnostic of bacterial infection, several studies have indicated that certain clinical findings are helpful, particularly in combination. The following 3 symptoms—presence of purulent rhinorrhea, unilateral maxillary toothache, and poor response to decongestant therapy—along with purulent nasal secretion and abnormal transillumination are predictive of acute bacterial rhinosinusitis. The presence of 4 or more of these findings significantly increases the likelihood of acute sinusitis (tLLR = 6.4). The presence of 1 or none of these findings decreases the likelihood significantly (tLLR = 0.5 and 0.1), respectively.

Other diagnostic tests available to the generalist

include plain radiography and CT. Plain radiography is only moderately sensitive and specific for bacteriologically proven sinusitis, and a single Water's view correlates well with standard 4-view sinus series. Sinus CT is a highly sensitive test, but has poor specificity. Maxillary sinus radiographs of young adults with typical viral upper respiratory tract infections show mucosal abnormalities in about 40% of cases on the seventh day of illness, and computed tomographic scans are abnormal in about 85% of similar cases.

When cost considerations are factored in, the use of radiography or other imaging in the initial evaluation of suspected sinusitis is always much more expensive and not much more effective than other strategies such as empiric antibiotic treatment of patients with reasonably high clinical likelihood of bacterial rhinosinusitis and symptomatic therapy for others. For these reasons, radiography is recommended only when initial therapy is ineffective, or for cases of recurrent rhinosinusitis.

MANAGEMENT AND THERAPY

Acute rhinosinusitis resolves without antibiotic treatment in most cases. Non-toxic, immunocompetent patients with acute, uncomplicated rhinosinusitis should be treated with analgesics, decongestants, and topical heat for discomfort. Topical decongestants are felt to be important not only because they provide early symptomatic relief of congestion, but also because they decrease edema at the sinus ostia and ostiomeatal complex. The problem of short-term rebound is minimal when these medications are used for fewer than 4 days. Antihistamines are said to promote thickening of the secretions and therefore are discouraged, at least initially, though evidence for this is limited. Inhalation of warm, humid vapor may be helpful, as may nasal saline irrigation.

Selection of Patients for Antibiotic Therapy

It is important to emphasize that many, if not most, cases of acute "sinusitis" diagnosed in ambulatory practice are uncomplicated viral upper respiratory infections. Even when there is inflammation of the sinuses, bacterial and viral etiologies are difficult to distinguish on clinical grounds. Though antibiotics are clearly over-prescribed for this and other common upper respiratory tract infections, their use can be justified in a subset of patients with sinus complaints. Recent systematic reviews have examined the issue of antibiotic therapy for acute rhinosinusitis. When considered in aggregate, placebo-controlled studies of clinical response show an absolute benefit of about 15%, which means that approximately 7 patients need to be treated for each patient benefited. The degree of benefit is small, and most placebo-treated patients improve without antibiotic therapy. No serious complications have been reported in sinusitis trials among patients who received placebo. Thus, given the increasing problem of antibiotic resistance, most experts advocate reserving antibiotics for patients who have symptoms lasting longer than 7 days, maxillary pain or tenderness in the face or teeth, and purulent nasal secretions, as well as for those who fail to respond to decongestants or have severe symptoms. These recommendations apply to the majority of routine cases in immunocompetent patients. Early antibiotic therapy along with aggressive diagnostic evaluation and referral is indicated for any patient with signs of toxicity or evidence of complications. Referral to an otolaryngologist is also indicated when sinusitis is either recurrent or refractory to empiric treatment.

Choice of Antibiotic Agents and Duration of Therapy

Three recent meta-analyses have concluded that newer, broad-spectrum antibiotics are no more effective than narrow-spectrum agents. When an antibiotic is prescribed, it should be the agent with the narrowest spectrum that is active against the most common bacterial pathogens, *S. pneumonia* and *H. influenza*. Amoxicillin with or without clavulanate and trimethoprim/sulfamethoxazole (TMP/SMX) appear to be as effective as newer, more expensive agents when used as first-line therapies. Clarithromycin is an alternative for severely penicillin allergic patients. The optimal duration of therapy is unknown, but 7 to 14 day regimens are typically used. In one study, 3 days of TMP/SMX was as effective as 10 days of therapy. Given the rapid increase of antibiotic resistance among *S. pneumoniae* and *H. influenza*, the clinician may also want to consider current recommendations for therapy against these organisms when making treatment decisions, particularly if the prevalence of resistant organisms or the risk of complications is high.

FUTURE DIRECTIONS

More studies are needed to assess the prevalence of drug-resistant organisms and the implications for therapy. Because no simple, accurate office-based test is currently available to diagnose sinusitis, studies aimed at improving our ability to use clinical findings to make appropriate decisions would be helpful. Particular attention needs to be paid to assessing clinical outcomes at different time points, as well as incorporating symptom severity and patient-assigned utilities to help apply this increasing body of evidence to clinical practice.

REFERENCES

Diagnosis and treatment of acute bacterial rhinosinusitis. Evidence report/technology assessment: Number 9. 1999. Agency for Health Care Policy and Research, Rockville, Md. Available at: http://www.ahrq.gov/clinic/epcsums/sinussum.htm. Accessed February 2, 2003.

Hansen JG, Schmidt H, Rosborg J, Lund E. Predicting acute maxillary sinusitis in a general practice. *BMJ*. 1995;3111:233–236.

Hickner JM, Bartlett JG, Besser RE, Gonzales R, Hoffman JR, Sande MA, and the American Academy of Family Physicians, the American College of Physicians-American Society of Internal Medicine, the Centers for Disease Control, and the Infectious Diseases Society of America. Principles of appropriate antibiotic use for acute rhinosinusitis in adults: background. *Ann Intern Med*. 2001;134:498–505.

Williams JW Jr, Aguilar C, Makela M, et al. Antibiotics for acute maxillary sinusitis In: *The Cochran Library*, Issue 4, 2002. Oxford: Update Software.

Williams JW Jr, Simel DL. Does this patient have sinusitis? Diagnosing acute sinusitis by history and physical examination. *JAMA*. 1993;270:1242–1246.

Section III

DISORDERS OF THE CARDIOVASCULAR SYSTEM

Chapter 16
Angina Pectoris

George A. Stouffer

Angina is the sensation caused by the myocardial ischemia that results when cardiac metabolic demand exceeds supply. It is generally defined as "pressure," "discomfort," or "choking sensation" in the left chest that is precipitated by exertion, excitement, or cold weather, and relieved by rest or nitroglycerin. In some patients, the discomfort will radiate into the left arm, into the jaw, or, more rarely, into the right arm (Figure 16-1). When severe, it can be accompanied by dyspnea, diaphoresis, or nausea. Rather than these classic symptoms, myocardial ischemia can also cause jaw pain, fatigue, or upper abdominal pain, or myocardial ischemia can be "silent" (not associated with symptoms), especially in diabetics.

ETIOLOGY AND PATHOGENESIS

The most common cause of angina is obstruction of coronary arteries by atherosclerosis (Figure 16-2, 16-3). Atherosclerosis, the leading cause of death in the developed world, develops over a period of decades. Risk factors include hypertension, tobacco use, diabetes mellitus type I, insulin-resistant states (such as diabetes mellitus type II and obesity), hypercholesterolemia, family history of premature vascular disease, and hyperhomocysteinemia.

Angina can also result from other less common conditions in which cardiac metabolic demand exceeds supply. These include coronary artery anomalies, coronary artery spasm (Prinzmetal Syndrome), aortic stenosis, anemia, hyperthyroidism, cocaine use, carbon monoxide poisoning, and hypertrophic cardiomyopathy.

CLINICAL PRESENTATION

Coronary artery disease (CAD) generally manifests as chronic stable angina, unstable angina, acute myocardial infarction, unrecognized myocardial infarction, or sudden cardiac death. Patients with acute myocardial infarction can be further subdivided into those with ST elevation on ECG and those without (commonly called non Q-wave myocardial infarctions).

Chronic Stable Angina

Fixed, stable obstructive CAD causes a syndrome termed chronic stable angina that occurs when myocardial metabolic demand exceeds a fixed threshold of supply. Angina is commonly precipitated by exertion, emotional excitement, mental stress, or exposure to cold, and resolves after the precipitating event has ceased. Angina generally occurs at the same level of exertion but may vary depending upon time of day, recent meals, and ambient temperature.

The most commonly used classification for grading angina severity is the Canadian Cardiovascular Society scale. Patients in Class I experience angina with strenuous or protracted physical activity while those in Class II will occasionally have angina with normal daily activities such as climbing stairs or walking up a hill. Patients in Class III have marked limitation and commonly experience angina during activities of everyday living (e.g. walking across a room). Class IV symptoms occur at rest.

Unstable Angina/Non Q-Wave Myocardial Infarction

Unstable angina/non Q-wave myocardial infarction is generally due to formation of a non-occlusive thrombus at the site of rupture or erosion of the surface of an atherosclerotic plaque (Figure 16-3). This event exposes the blood to the highly thrombotic materials within the plaque, leading to thrombus formation. The thrombus can progress until it occludes the blood vessel or, alternatively, may embolize and occlude smaller, more distal vessels. Sudden onset of chest discomfort that is unrelated to a precipitating event is a hallmark of this syndrome. Other patients will initially have symptoms that occur with exertion but, over a period of days to weeks, the discomfort will occur with less and less exertion.

Figure 16-1

Angina Pectoris

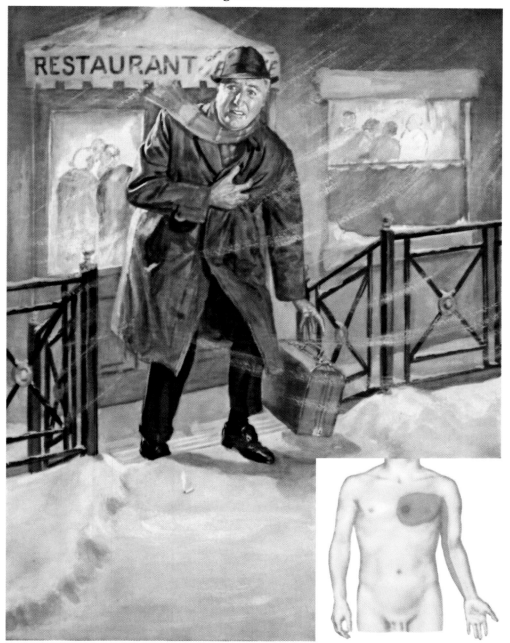

Common precipitating factors in angina pectoris:
heavy meal, exertion, cold, smoking

Characteristic distribution of
pain in angina pectoris

Figure 16-2

Types and Degrees of Coronary
Atherosclerotic Narrowing or Occlusion

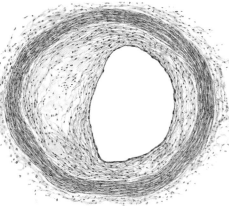

Moderate atherosclerotic narrowing of lumen

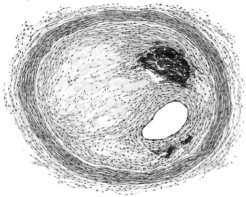

Almost complete occlusion by intimal
atherosclerosis with calcium deposition

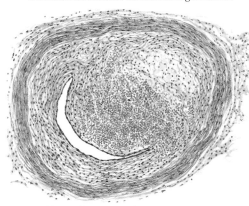

Hemorrhage into atheroma,
leaving only a slitlike lumen

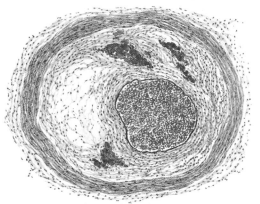

Complete occlusion by thrombus in
lumen greatly narrowed by atheroma

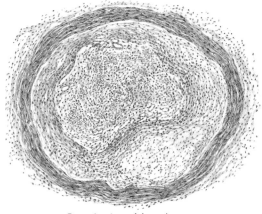

Organization of thrombus

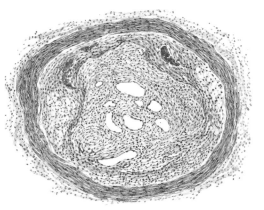

Organization with recanalization may occur

Figure 16-3

Atherogenesis: Unstable Plaque Formation

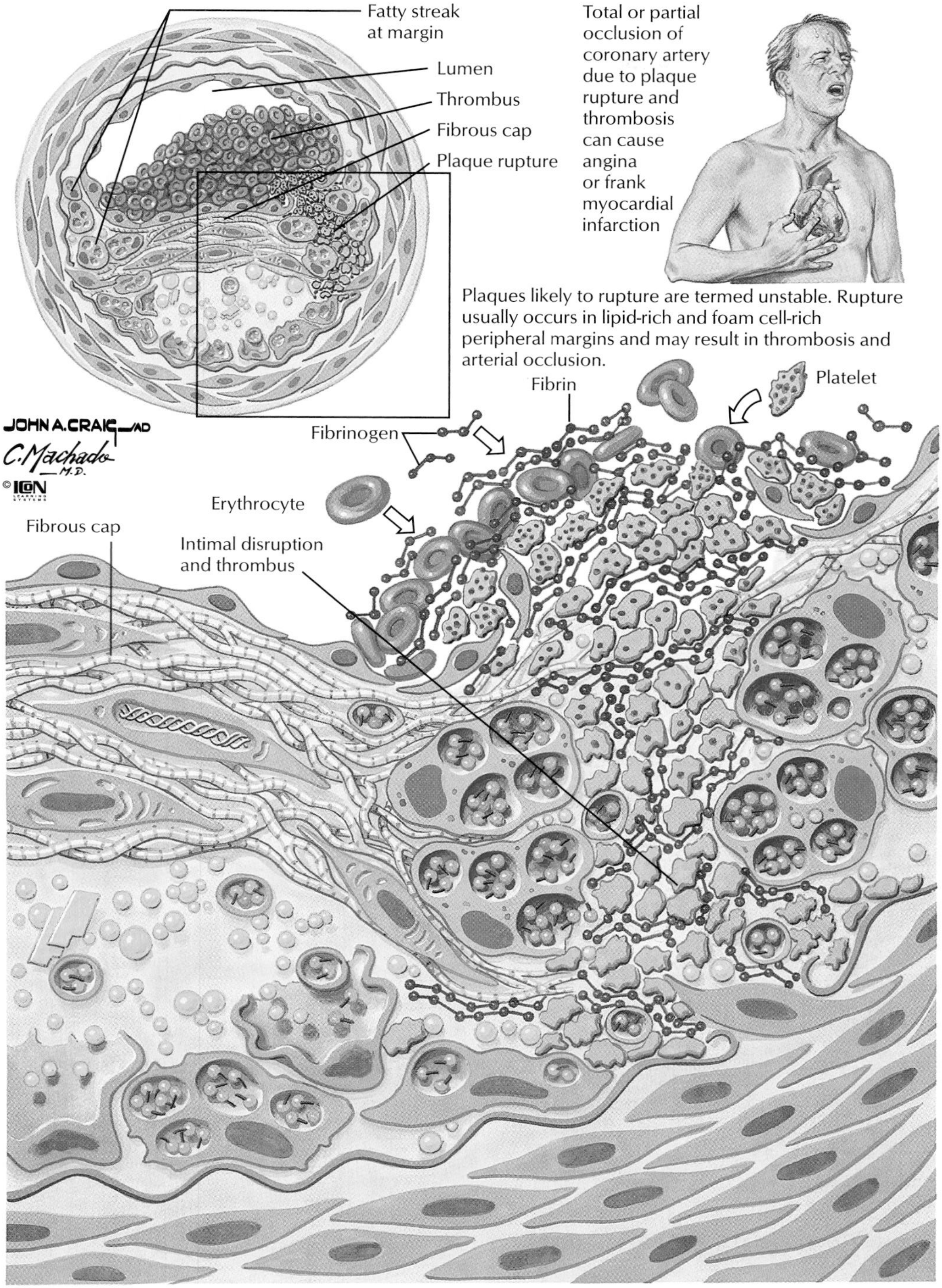

Fatty streak
at margin

Lumen

Thrombus

Fibrous cap

Plaque rupture

Total or partial
occlusion of
coronary artery
due to plaque
rupture and
thrombosis
can cause
angina
or frank
myocardial
infarction

Plaques likely to rupture are termed unstable. Rupture
usually occurs in lipid-rich and foam cell-rich
peripheral margins and may result in thrombosis and
arterial occlusion.

Fibrin

Platelet

Fibrinogen

JOHN A. CRAIG—MD
C. Machado
—M.D.
©ICON

Erythrocyte

Fibrous cap

Intimal disruption
and thrombus

Acute Myocardial Infarction with ST Segment Elevation

Acute myocardial infarction with ST segment elevation is characterized by the abrupt onset of unremitting chest discomfort, and is generally associated with dyspnea, diaphoresis and a "sense of doom." It is typically caused by abrupt occlusion of a coronary artery by thrombus at the site of a ruptured atherosclerotic plaque. The ECG shows ST elevation in two or more leads corresponding to the territory of a coronary artery. Patients who are not treated within 6 to 12 hours generally suffer significant myocardial damage.

Variant (Prinzmetal) Angina

In this uncommon disorder, coronary spasm develops, usually at the site of an atherosclerotic lesion. The hallmark is transient chest pain with ST elevation on ECG, often occurring at rest.

Syndrome X

Includes patients with angina, evidence of exercise-induced ischemia and normal epicardial coronary arteries. These patients are often female (approximately 70%), with an average age of 50 years. The pathophysiology of this syndrome is incompletely understood with various proposed etiologies including microvascular dysfunction, incipient cardiomyopathy, or altered pain perception.

DIFFERENTIAL DIAGNOSIS

A number of disease states can cause chest discomfort. In some cases, the symptoms can closely mimic angina, although a careful history can help distinguish between the various conditions. Exertional symptoms are common in diastolic dysfunction, exertional hypertension, asthma and pulmonary hypertension. Response to nitroglycerin can be observed in esophageal spasm and diastolic dysfunction. Other diagnoses mimicking angina include esophageal spasm, peptic ulcer, asthma, aortic dissection, mitral valve prolapse, pulmonary embolism, exertional hypertension, cholecystitis, musculoskeletal, anxiety (panic attack), pericarditis or pleuritis, congestive heart failure, diastolic dysfunction, and costochondritis.

DIAGNOSTIC APPROACH
Chronic Stable Angina

In chronic stable angina, typical history and pres-ence of risk factors are the most important information for diagnosis. The physical examination is usually not helpful but may provide evidence of left ventricular systolic or diastolic dysfunction (an S_3 or S_4 respectively). During an attack of angina, patients will tend to be still and may appear pale. The ECG is normal in more than half of the patients with coronary atherosclerosis, but there may be evidence of prior myocardial infarction or ischemia (e.g., ST depression). The three most important determinants of prognosis in patients with chronic stable angina are age, number of diseased coronary arteries, and left ventricular function.

An exercise treadmill test can diagnose CAD by the development of ECG changes with exercise. In addition, symptoms during exercise, blood pressure response, and duration of exercise are all important in determining the posttest probability of coronary artery disease and whether the patient needs further evaluation. The treadmill test can be enhanced by assessing left ventricular wall motion (with echocardiography) or myocardial perfusion (with nuclear imaging). Pharmacological stress testing can be used in patients who are unable to exercise.

Coronary angiography remains the gold standard for diagnosing CAD. This test, which involves direct injection of contrast dye into the coronary arteries, delineates the location and severity of obstructive coronary disease. As such, angiography is a necessary prerequisite for coronary revascularization via either percutaneous intervention or coronary artery bypass surgery. Left ventriculography, generally performed immediately before or after coronary angiography, provides important information regarding intracardiac pressures and left ventricular function.

Clinically assessing the functional importance of intermediate lesions (lesions which appear to obstruct 40%–60% of the coronary lumen) may be difficult using coronary angiography alone. This limitation can be partially overcome by using intracoronary ultrasound or by measuring coronary flow velocity or intracoronary pressure changes during maximal hyperemia.

Acute Coronary Syndromes

Patients with unstable angina, non Q-wave myocardial infarction or ST elevation myocardial infarction are considered to have acute coronary syndromes. The diagnosis is generally based on the constellation of typical symptoms (described above), ECG changes and elevated levels of cardiac enzymes (in the case of myocardial infarction).

The ECG is essential in differentiating unstable angina/non Q-wave myocardial infarction from ST-elevation myocardial infarctions. In unstable angina/non Q-wave myocardial infarction, the ECG may be normal or may demonstrate T-wave inversion or ST depression. ST depression often indicates multi-vessel CAD, and is associated with a worse prognosis in patients with unstable angina/non Q-wave myocardial infarction. In patients with ST-elevation myocardial infarctions, the ECG shows contiguous ST elevation involving the anterior (V1–V4), lateral (V5, V6, I, AVL), or inferior (II, III, AVF) walls.

Myocardial Infarction

Highly sensitive blood tests for myocardial proteins have greatly enhanced our ability to diagnose myocardial infarction. Troponins and creatine kinase-MB are intracellular cardiac proteins released into the blood stream upon the death of myocytes. Plasma levels of these proteins are useful both in detecting myocardial infarction and establishing prognosis. Troponins and creatine kinase-MB do not appear in plasma in significant levels until 8 or more hours after the onset of symptoms limiting their diagnostic value in the very early stages of an acute coronary syndrome.

MANAGEMENT AND THERAPY
Nonpharmacologic Interventions

Controlling risk factors for atherosclerosis is crucial. In particular, patients should be advised on the need to lower the intake of cholesterol and saturated fat in their diets, the importance of weight loss if obese, and the need to avoid tobacco. A regular exercise program should be prescribed for all patients in whom it is feasible. An exercise stress test can be used to determine safe levels of activity.

Pharmacologic Interventions

Pharmacological therapy for angina was traditionally directed at relieving symptoms. More recently, medications have been classified based on their effect on survival (Table 16-1). Medica-

tions that improve survival and decrease cardiovascular events in patients with CAD include aspirin, HMG-CoA reductase inhibitors ("statins"), and angiotensin-converting enzyme inhibitors. In patients with prior myocardial infarction or left ventricular dysfunction, beta-blockers also reduce mortality. Medications that treat symptoms without improving survival include nitrates and calcium channel blockers. The use of calcium channel blockers, with the exception of amlodipine and felodipine, should be avoided in patients with left ventricular dysfunction.

LDL cholesterol levels should be aggressively lowered, even in patients with ostensibly normal LDL levels, through the use of diet and statins. Recent guidelines suggest that LDL cholesterol should be less than 100 mg/dl in patients with CAD. Blood pressure should be closely monitored, with optimum levels below 140/90. In diabetics, optimum levels are even lower, with the goal of diastolic blood pressures at 80mmHg or less. Patients must be strongly encouraged to quit smoking and offered pharmacologic (e.g., nicotine patches, bupropion) or support group help as needed. Antioxidant vitamins have not been shown to be beneficial.

Therapies that interrupt thrombus formation have an important role in acute coronary syndromes. In unstable angina/non Q-wave myocardial infarction, aspirin and heparin reduce the rate of death and myocardial (re-)infarction. Glycoprotein IIb/IIIa inhibitors and low-molecular weight heparin are useful in patients with high-risk features (e.g., elevated troponins or ST depression) who are undergoing percutaneous coronary intervention. In ST-elevation myocardial infarction, the goal of therapy is rapid restoration of blood flow using either thrombolytic therapy or a percutaneous coronary intervention such as balloon angioplasty. Administration of streptokinase or tissue plasminogen activator (tPA), especially within 6 hours of the onset of symptoms, improves patient survival. Newer thrombolytic drugs derived from tPA, including reteplase (rPA), tenecteplase (TNK), and lanoteplase (nPA), have similar efficacy but are easier to administer (1 or 2 bolus injections). Primary angioplasty (angioplasty during acute myocardial infarction) achieves results that are at least equivalent to, and probably better than

Table 16-1
Summary of Pharmacologic Treatment of Patients with Chronic Stable Angina

Medication	Dosage	Which Patients?	Effect on Cardiovascular Clinical Endpoints
Aspirin	80–325 mg qD	All patients with vascular disease	Decreases the risk of death, myocardial infarction, and stroke
Statin drugs	Varies depending on particular drug	If LDL >130; all patients who have extensive vascular disease. In patients with known CAD, LDL >100	Decreases the risk of death in patients who have had a prior myocardial infarction
ACE Inhibitors	Varies depending on particular drug; initial dosage will depend on blood pressure	All patients with vascular disease (in particular, any patient with vascular disease and hypertension or diabetes)	In the HOPE trial, ramipril 10 mg/qD reduced the rate of death, MI, and stroke in patients with vascular disease
β-blockers	Begin at low dose (e.g, Metoprolol 6.25 or 12.5 mg BID) and titrate depending on heart rate and blood pressure	Patients with prior myocardial infarction or with cardiomyopathy (caution is needed when initiating b-blockers in patients with congestive heart failure)	Decreases the risk of death in patients who have had a prior myocardial infarction and improves outcomes in patients with dilated cardiomyopathy
Nitrates	Sublingual or buccal spray can be used prn; longer acting oral and transdermal formulations are available	Patients with anginal symptoms	None
Calcium channel blockers	Varies depending on particular drug; initial dosage will depend on blood pressure and heart rate	Patients with anginal symptoms	No beneficial effect; nifedipine worsens survival in acute coronary syndromes; diltiazem worsens survival in left ventricular dysfunction
Warfarin	Varies depending on response; needs continual monitoring	Useful in selected patients with vascular disease	A meta-analysis demonstrates reduction in the risk of death, MI, or stroke if INR >2 and used with concurrent ASA; bleeding increased by 1.9-fold

LDL, low-density lipoprotein; MI, myocardial infarction; INR, international normalized ratio; ASA, aspirin

thrombolytic therapy if the procedure is performed expeditiously by an experienced interventional cardiologist.

Revascularization

Revascularization reestablishes unobstructed blood flow via either percutaneous intervention, in which the atherosclerotic blockage is relieved by angioplasty balloon inflation and/or stent placement, or by coronary artery bypass grafting in which blood flow is diverted around atherosclerotic obstructions using an arterial (e.g., left internal mammary artery) or venous conduit. Revascularization prolongs survival in patients with significant left main coronary artery disease and multi-vessel CAD with impaired left ventricular function. The most common indication for revascularization, however, is relief of symptoms.

FUTURE DIRECTIONS

Plasma levels of C-reactive protein, a marker of inflammation, are useful in determining the prognosis of patients with unstable angina/non Q-wave myocardial infarction. Large, population-based studies have also shown a correlation between C-reactive protein levels and CAD. Electron–beam–computed tomography and 3-dimensional echocardiography may enhance the ability of noninvasive testing to detect CAD. In preliminary studies, inroads are being made into the identity of genetic polymorphisms that contribute to CAD. Further progress in this area may identify high-risk individuals who will benefit from specific, risk factor modifying therapy initiated early in life.

Several new pharmaceuticals are being evaluated for use in patients with angina, including potassium channel blockers and agents that enhance nitric oxide production. Large scale clinical studies are also testing the use of antibiotics and anti-inflammatory medications as means to slow the progression of atherosclerosis. New techniques such as transmyocardial revascularization, enhanced external counterpulsation, spinal cord stimulation, and sympathectomy are being evaluated in patients who have refractory angina despite optimal medical treatment. Finally, the stimulation of myocardial angiogenesis via intra-coronary injection of growth factors (e.g., vascular endothelial growth factor) or genes encoding angiogenic factors is an exciting area now entering clinical trials.

REFERENCES

Braunwald E, Antman EM, Beasley JW, et al. ACC/AHA guidelines for the management of patients with unstable angina and non-ST-segment elevation myocardial infarction: executive summary and recommendations. A report of the American College of Cardiology/American Heart Association Task Force on Practice Guidelines (Committee on the Management of Patients with Unstable Angina). *Circulation.* 2000;102:1193-1209.

Eagle KA, Guyton RA, Davidoff R, et al. ACC/AHA guidelines for coronary artery bypass graft surgery: executive summary and recommendations. A report of the American College of Cardiology/American Heart Association Task Force on Practice Guidelines (Committee to Revise the 1991 Guidelines for Coronary Artery Bypass Graft Surgery). *Circulation.* 1999;100:1464-1480.

Fletcher GF. How to implement physical activity in primary and secondary prevention. A statement for healthcare-professionals from the Task Force on Risk-reduction, American Heart Association. *Circulation.* 1997;96:355-357.

Fletcher GF, Balady G, Blair SN, et al. Statement on exercise: benefits and recommendations for physical activity programs for all Americans. A statement for health professionals by the Committee on Exercise and Cardiac Rehabilitation of the Council on Clinical Cardiology, American Heart Association. *Circulation.* 1996;94:857-862.

Gibbons RJ, Balady GJ, Bricker JT, et al, and the American College of Cardiology/American Heart Association Task Force on Practice Guidelines (Committee to Update the 1997 Exercise Testing Guidelines). ACC/AHA guideline update for exercise testing: summary article. A report of the American College of Cardiology/American Heart Association Task Force on Practice Guidelines (Committee to Update the 1997 Exercise Testing Guidelines). *Circulation.* 2002;106:1883-1892.

Gibbons RJ, Chatterjee K, Daley J, et al. ACC/AHA/ACP-ASIM guidelines for the management of patients with stable angina: executive summary and recommendations. A report of the American College of Cardiology/American Heart Association Task Force on Practice Guidelines (Committee on Management of Patients with Chronic Stable Angina). *Circulation.* 1999;99:2829-2848.

Grundy SM, Benjamin IJ, Burke GL, et al. Diabetes and cardiovascular disease: a statement for healthcare professionals from the American Heart Association. *Circulation.* 1999;100:1134-1146.

Grundy SM, Pasternak R, Greenland P, Smith S Jr, Fuster V. Assessment of cardiovascular risk by use of multiple-risk-factor assessment equations: a statement for healthcare professionals from the American Heart Association and the American College of Cardiology. *Circulation.* 1999;100:1481-1492.

Hennekens CH, Dyken ML, Fuster V. Aspirin as a therapeutic agent in cardiovascular disease: a statement for healthcare professionals from the American Heart Association. *Circulation.* 1997;96:2751-2753.

Krauss RM, Eckel RH, Howard B, et al. AHA dietary guidelines: revision 2000: a statement for healthcare professionals from the Nutrition Committee of the American Heart Association. *Circulation.* 2000;102:2284-2299.

Krauss RM, Winston M, Fletcher BJ, Grundy SM. Obesity: impact on cardiovascular disease. *Circulation.* 1998;98:1472-1476.

Kris-Etherton P, Daniels SR, Eckel RH, et al. Summary of the scientific conference on dietary fatty acids and cardiovascular health: conference summary from the Nutrition Committee of the American Heart Association. *Circulation.* 2001;103:1034-1039.

Malinow MR, Bostom AG, Krauss RM. Homocyst(e)ine, diet, and cardiovascular diseases: a statement for healthcare professionals from the Nutrition Committee, American Heart Association. *Circulation.* 1999;99:178-182.

O'Rourke RA, Brundage BH, Froelicher VA, et al. American College of Cardiology/American Heart Association Expert Consensus document on electron-beamcomputed tomography for the diagnosis and prognosis of coronary artery disease. *Circulation.* 2000;102:126-140.

Ryan TJ, Antman EM, Brooks NH, et al. 1999 update: ACC/AHA guidelines for the management of patients with acute myocardial infarction: executive summary and recommendations. A report of the American College of Cardiology/American Heart Association Task Force on Practice Guidelines (Committee on Management of Acute Myocardial Infarction). *Circulation.* 1999;100:1016-1030.

Scanlon PJ, Faxon DP, Audet AM, et al. ACC/AHA guidelines for coronary angiography: executive summary and recommendations. A report of the American College of Cardiology/American Heart Association Task Force on Practice Guidelines (Committee on coronary angiography) developed in collaboration with the Society for Cardiac Angiography and Interventions. Circulation. 1999;99:2345-2357.

Smith SC Jr, Blair SN, Criqui MH, et al. Preventing heart attack and death in patients with coronary disease. *Circulation.* 1995;92:2-4.

Tribble DL. AHA science advisory. Antioxidant consumption and risk of coronary heart disease: emphasis on vitamin C, vitamin E, and beta-carotene. A statement for healthcare professionals from the American Heart Association. *Circulation.* 1999;99:591-595.

Chapter 17

Cardiac Arrhythmias

Richard G. Sheahan

Cardiac arrhythmias are abnormal and usually symptomatic changes in heart rhythm. A palpitation is an awareness of a heart rhythm. Cardiac rhythm disturbances may involve abnormally fast (tachycardias) or slow (bradycardias) heart rates and may be either regular or irregular. In general, the diagnosis and treatment of tachyarrhythmias is more complex than that of bradyarrhythmias.

ETIOLOGY AND PATHOGENESIS

Tachycardias are divided into two broad categories, supraventricular or ventricular tachycardia, each of which represents multiple etiologies.

Supraventricular tachycardia (SVT) is often benign, and the majority require two discrete pathways or limbs with different conduction and refractory properties. Atrioventricular nodal reentrant tachycardia (AVNRT) has so-called "fast" and "slow" pathways. Atrioventricular reentrant tachycardia (AVRT) requires an accessory pathway in addition to the AV node. Atrial tachycardia arises from a more focal location. Atrial flutter occurs as a reentrant circuit in the right atrium. Atrial fibrillation is the most common arrhythmia, with incidence increasing with age. Once a patient develops atrial fibrillation, it is very likely to recur. A SVT becomes dangerous in settings where myocardial function is impaired at high heart rates, including coronary artery disease, congenital heart disease, and hypertrophic cardiomyopathy.

Ventricular tachycardia (VT) usually originates from scar tissue in patients with a previous myocardial infarction or from abnormal ventricular tissue found in various forms of cardiomyopathy, including dilated, hypertrophic, or infiltrative pathologies. Rarely, exercise-induced VT (the so-called verapamil- or adenosine-sensitive VT) can occur in patients with normal hearts. Ventricular fibrillation (VF) usually occurs in the setting of ongoing ischemia.

The long QT syndrome and Brugada syndrome are examples of arrhythmias resulting from inherited channelopathies. Brugada syndrome is characterized by ST elevation beginning at the terminal R wave with a slowly descending ST segment and continuing with a flat or negative T wave appearing spontaneously in leads V_1 to V_3. Both conditions are associated with sudden cardiac death.

CLINICAL PRESENTATION

In addition to palpitations, patients may present with other symptoms including: dyspnea, dizziness, lightheadedness, chest pain, syncope, weakness, fatigue, sudden death, or the consequences of injuries that result from the arrhythmia. Symptom severity depends upon a complex interaction between the hemodynamic consequences of the arrhythmia and the underlying cardiac function. Apart from sudden death, syncope does not distinguish a benign from a malignant arrhythmia. The occurrence of palpitations, syncope, or pre-syncopal during exertion requires urgent evaluation.

DIAGNOSTIC APPROACH
Patient Evaluation

In evaluating a cardiac arrhythmia, details of the presenting history, including the associated circumstances, family history of arrhythmia or sudden death, medications (including recent dose changes or additions), recent illnesses or surgeries, and physical examination are crucial (Table 17-1). A baseline electrocardiogram may help identify the abnormal arrhythmia, and may exclude AV conduction abnormalities, preexcitation of Wolff-Parkinson-White syndrome (delta wave, short PR interval, and a wider QRS complex), long QT syndrome, Brugada syndrome, and abnormalities in ventricular conduction. The laboratory tests chosen will vary from patient to patient, and should be tailored accordingly. For example, in a patient with bizarre behavior, consider blood alcohol and urine toxicology screening.

CARDIAC ARRHYTHMIAS

Table 17-1
Evaluation of a Patient with a Cardiac Arrhythmia

- History and physical examination: Family history of sudden death, medications
- Electrocardiogram: baseline and during event
- Laboratory may include complete blood cell count, electrolytes, blood glucose, serial cardiac enzymes, thyroid-stimulating hormone, digoxin, blood and urine drug screen, and alcohol levels
- Echocardiogram to document cardiac function and rule out valvular abnormality and cardiomyopathy
- Ambulatory Holter monitoring
- Patient-activated monitoring device: may include event, loop, or insertable loop recorder
- Procainamide provocative test
- Electrophysiology study

Adapted from Sheahan RG. Syncope and arrythmias: role of the electrophysiological study. *Am J Med Sci.* 2001;322:37-43.

Symptom Rhythm Correlation

A 12-lead electrocardiogram during the arrhythmia provides the gold standard of a symptom rhythm correlation. This is an elusive goal, because the symptoms are paroxysmal and occur infrequently. Holter monitoring over a 24- or 48-hour period can be used to document rhythms that occur almost daily. A loop recorder over a 1- to 2-month interval may record rhythms that occur once every 4 weeks. The use of these devices for longer periods is unlikely to yield a diagnosis due to decreasing patient motivation, and contact dermatitis caused by gel from the recording electrodes. An insertable loop recorder is a recording device that is implanted under the skin in the anterior chest well, and can be activated by the patient or automatically. The automated features record heart rates of less than 40 bpm or greater than 145 bpm, or ventricular asystole of greater than 3 seconds. The insertable loop recorder is an option for patients with infrequent but significant symptoms, after structural heart disease and other obvious causes have been excluded.

Ventricular arrhythmias require further evaluation of myocardial function to rule out significant coronary artery disease. An echocardiogram will detect segmental wall motion abnormalities, hypertrophic cardiomyopathy, dilated cardiomyopathy, right ventricular dysplasia, valvular abnormalities, and atrial dimensions (in atrial fibrillation).

In patients presenting with left ventricular dysfunction, undocumented palpitations or syncope, an electrophysiology study should be performed to identify those at a higher risk for sudden cardiac death. Revascularization, if required, should be performed before the electrophysiology study.

MANAGEMENT AND THERAPY
Acute Management of Arrhythmias

Rhythm recognition in conjunction with the hemodynamic consequences of the arrhythmia determines the immediate therapeutic approach to managing acute sustained arrhythmias (Table 17-2). If a patient has a supraventricular tachycardia with a blood pressure less than 80 mmHg and is pre-syncopal, then an immediate synchronized direct current (DC) cardioversion is required if an intravenous (IV) adenosine bolus does not terminate the arrhythmia. Similarly, if a patient has ventricular tachycardia, has a stable blood pressure, and is not pre-syncopal, then an antiarrhythmic agent can be safely initiated. Synchronized DC cardioversion is contraindicated in a symptomatic patient with sinus tachycardia and hypotension.

In patients who present with hemodynamically stable supraventricular tachycardia, the initial drug of choice is adenosine, infused as a rapid intravenous push in a large proximally located vein, followed by a fluid bolus. Intravenous diltiazem or metoprolol may also be used. One should avoid using an IV calcium channel blocker in a patient taking a scheduled dose of an oral beta-blocker, and vice-versa. In patients with known Wolff-Parkinson-White (WPW) syndrome and SVT, adenosine is the drug of choice.

Patients who present with hemodynamically unstable ventricular tachycardia require an urgent synchronized DC cardioversion under anesthesia or sedation, followed by IV amiodarone and IV magnesium for several hours. In hemodynamically stable ventricular tachycardia, consider IV lidocaine or IV amiodarone with IV magnesium. If several hours elapse without termination to sinus rhythm, then a synchronized DC shock should be performed.

Ventricular fibrillation requires an emergent asynchronous DC shock followed by infusion of intravenous amiodarone.

The acute management of atrial flutter and atrial fibrillation with rapid ventricular response in hemodynamically unstable patients requires a

Table 17-2
Acute and Long-term Management of Arrhythmias

Arrhythmia	Acute Care	Long-term Management
Sinus tachycardia (>100 bpm)	Treat underlying cause	If inappropriate, beta-blocker/calcium channel blocker. Persistent, consider RFA of the superior portion of the sinus node.
Sinus bradycardia (<60 bpm)	If asymptomatic, no intervention. If symptomatic and severe (rates <40/min) with nonreversible cause, consider temporary pacing.	If asymptomatic, no intervention. If symptomatic and severe (rates <40/min) with nonreversible cause, consider permanent pacing.
Premature atrial complexes	If asymptomatic, no intervention. Check potassium, magnesium.	If asymptomatic, no intervention. Check potassium, magnesium. If symptomatic, consider beta-blocker.
Premature ventricular complexes	If asymptomatic, no intervention. Check potassium, magnesium.	Echo to assess LV and RV function, and LV wall thickness. Normal echo: no intervention. Beta blocker for symptoms. Abnormal echo: Evaluate etiology and add beta-blocker.
Sinus node dysfunction	No intervention, unless unstable	Permanent pacemaker. Allows the use of beta-blocker in patients with tachybrady syndrome.
Prolonged PR interval	No intervention	No intervention unless symptomatic
Second degree AV block Mobitz Type 1 (Wenkebach)	No intervention, unless unstable	Symptomatic patient, consider permanent pacemaker
Mobitz Type 2 AV block	No intervention, unless unstable	Permanent pacemaker
Complete heart block	Possible temporary pacemaker	Permanent pacemaker
Supraventricular tachycardia (SVT)	Control SVT with adenosine	
Wolff-Parkinson-White syndrome and concealed accessory pathway	Control SVT with adenosine	WPW with SVT needs EPS and RFA, because of risk of sudden death
Atrioventricular nodal reentrant tachycardia	Control SVT with adenosine, metoprolol, diltiazem	Consider EPS and RFA for recurrent episodes
Atrial tachycardia	Control SVT with metoprolol, diltiazem	Consider EPS and RFA for recurrent episodes
Atrial fibrillation	Rate control	Warfarin with INR 2.0 to 3.0 in all at risk patients. Consider pharmacologic treatment and/or elective DC cardioversion

(continued)

Table 17-2
Acute and Long-term Management of Arrhythmias (continued)

Arrhythmia	Acute Care	Long-term Management
Paroxysmal	Rate control	Recurrent episodes need antiarrhythmic agent. Focal ablation for drug failures.
Persistent	Rate control	Cardioversion, addition of antiarrhythmic agent for recurrences. Focal ablation for drug failures.
Permanent	Rate control	Rate control. Unsuccessful AV node ablation and permanent pacemaker.
Atrial flutter	Rate Control	RFA for recurrent episodes
Ventricular tachycardia	DC cardioversion if unstable or refractory to antiarrhythmic drugs	Echo to assess LV function. Ischemic evaluation +/- revascularization. ICD placement. Normal echo, consider RVOT or LV VT and ablation.
Ventricular fibrillation	Emergent DC cardioversion	Rule out acute myocardial infarction. ICD placement in absence of acute myocardial infarction.
Nonsustained ventricular tachycardia (3 to 30 beats)	Rate control	Low ejection fraction, need electrophysiology study. If positive, needs ICD.
Left ventricular dysfunction	Primary prevention of sudden cardiac death	Previous myocardial infarction, LV ejection fraction <30% require, ICD placement
Hypertrophic cardiomyopathy	Treat as for arrhythmia	EPS for any ventricular tachycardia. If positive, needs IC.
Long QT syndrome	Resuscitate as for arrhythmia	Beta-blocker/permanent pacemaker at 85 bpm/ICD
Brugada syndrome	Resuscitate as for arrhythmia	ICD placement. Asymptomatic and abnormal EKG, EP Study +/- ICD

AV, atrioventricular; DC, direct current; EPS, electrophysiology study; ICD, implantable cardioverter defibrillator; INR, International Normalized Ratio; LV, left ventricular; RFA, radiofrequency ablation; RV, right ventricular; RVOT, right ventricular outflow tract; VT, ventricular tachycardia; WPW, Wolff-Parkinson-White syndrome.

synchronous DC shock. Intravenous diltiazem or esmolol are the drugs of choice because they provide graded, dose-related control of the ventricular response. Often they are not effective due to an inadequate dose. Slowing the ventricular response to less than 90 bpm increases the diastolic filling time and improves cardiac output.

In significant bradycardia due to sinus arrest or complete heart block, a temporary transvenous pacemaker should be placed in the right ventricle, until the condition resolves or a permanent pacemaker is placed (Figure 17-1). Patients, who present with second degree AV block Mobitz types I and II, should be monitored closely. Temporary pacing should be initiated only for hemodynamic instability or progression of the AV block (Figure 17-2).

A careful history and physical examination should provide clues as to the etiology of sinus tachycardia. These include, but are not limited to, dehydration, anemia, fever, pain, anxiety, medications including bronchodilators, vomiting, diarrhea, and illicit drug use.

Figure 17-1

Atrioventricular Conduction Variations I

A. Fixed normal PR interval
  Sinus rhythm

B. Fixed but short PR interval
  1. Junctional or coronary sinus rhythm
  2. Wolff-Parkinson-White syndrome

C. P wave related to each QRS complex, but variable PR interval
  1. Wandering atrial pacemaker
  2. Multifocal atrial tachycardia

D. Fixed but prolonged PR interval
  First-degree AV block

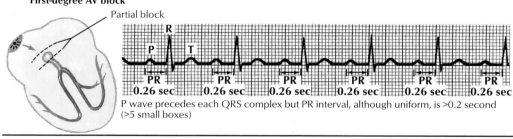

Partial block

P wave precedes each QRS complex but PR interval, although uniform, is >0.2 second (>5 small boxes)

E. Progressive lengthening of PR interval with intermittent dropped beats
  Second-degree AV block: Mobitz I (Wenckebach)

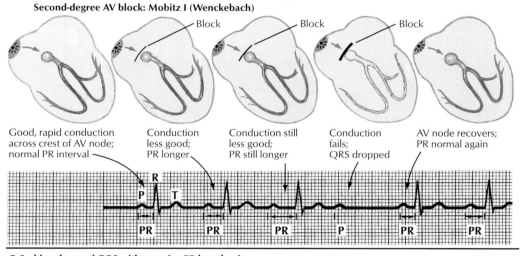

Block Block Block

Good, rapid conduction across crest of AV node; normal PR interval

Conduction less good; PR longer

Conduction still less good; PR still longer

Conduction fails; QRS dropped

AV node recovers; PR normal again

F. Sudden dropped QRS without prior PR lengthening
  Second-degree AV block: Mobitz II (non-Wenckebach)

AV block at level of bundle of His, or at bilateral bundle branches, or trifascicular

PR intervals do not lengthen

Sudden dropped QRS without prior PR changes

Figure 17-2

Atrioventricular Conduction Variations II

G. No relationship between P waves and QRS complexes: QRS rate *slower* than P rate

Third-degree (complete) AV block

1. Impulses originate at both SA node (P waves) and below site of block in AV node (junctional rhythm) conducting to ventricles

Block

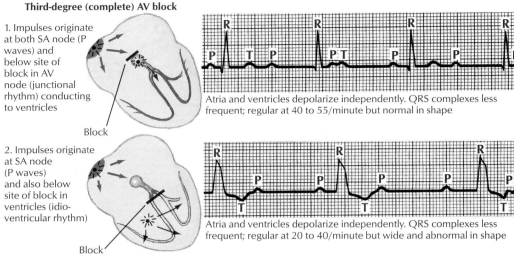

Atria and ventricles depolarize independently. QRS complexes less frequent; regular at 40 to 55/minute but normal in shape

2. Impulses originate at SA node (P waves) and also below site of block in ventricles (idio-ventricular rhythm)

Block

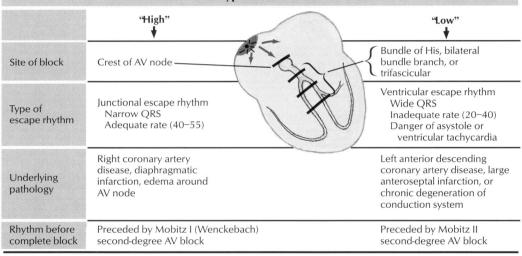

Atria and ventricles depolarize independently. QRS complexes less frequent; regular at 20 to 40/minute but wide and abnormal in shape

Features of two types of atrioventricular block

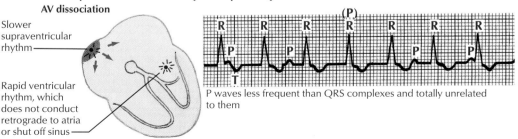

	"High"	"Low"
Site of block	Crest of AV node	Bundle of His, bilateral bundle branch, or trifascicular
Type of escape rhythm	Junctional escape rhythm Narrow QRS Adequate rate (40–55)	Ventricular escape rhythm Wide QRS Inadequate rate (20–40) Danger of asystole or ventricular tachycardia
Underlying pathology	Right coronary artery disease, diaphragmatic infarction, edema around AV node	Left anterior descending coronary artery disease, large anteroseptal infarction, or chronic degeneration of conduction system
Rhythm before complete block	Preceded by Mobitz I (Wenckebach) second-degree AV block	Preceded by Mobitz II second-degree AV block

H. No relationship between P waves and QRS complexes. QRS rate faster than P rate.

AV dissociation

Slower supraventricular rhythm

Rapid ventricular rhythm, which does not conduct retrograde to atria or shut off sinus

P waves less frequent than QRS complexes and totally unrelated to them

Long-term Management

Initial therapies for recurrent supraventricular tachycardia may include beta-blockers or calcium channel blockers (Table 17-2 and Figure 17-3). Initiation of these agents will depend on the frequency of the episodes and the presence of comorbid conditions. An electrophysiology study and radiofrequency ablation (RFA) should be considered for recurrent episodes, intolerance to medications, or women in childbearing years who wish to become pregnant. RFA successfully eliminates the supraventricular tachycardia in 90% to 95% of patients with a 5% recurrence rate.

For those with atrioventricular nodal reentrant tachycardia, the ablation target is the "slow pathway" which is occasionally located in close proximity to the AV node. Ablation in this location is associated with a 1% to 2% risk of heart block, which may require pacemaker placement. Other complications occur approximately 1% of the time.

Supraventricular tachycardia in the presence of Wolff-Parkinson-White (WPW) syndrome is associated with a risk for sudden death (Figure 17-3) in patients in whom atrial fibrillation develops with rapid conduction over the accessory pathway leading to ventricular fibrillation. In patients with pre-excited atrial fibrillation (a wide, rapid, irregular tachycardia) treatment options include IV procainamide or synchronized DC cardioversion. Blocking the AV node with agents such as verapamil and digoxin may accelerate the ventricular rate.

Patients who present with WPW syndrome and supraventricular tachycardia, should undergo a RFA to reduce the risk of sudden death. In WPW syndrome an accessory pathway allows antero-grade (antidromic) and retrograde (orthodromic) conduction. Most supraventricular tachycardias associated with WPW syndrome are orthodromic. Antidromic tachycardia presents with wide complexes that resemble ventricular tachycardia, and should be treated as such unless there is a clear history of WPW syndrome.

Patients may also have a concealed accessory pathway detectable only during an electrophysiology study. Tachycardia conducts retrograde over the accessory pathway and anterograde over the AV node.

Atrial tachycardia occurs in approximately 10% of supraventricular tachycardias. Ablation is more difficult. However, the latest mapping technology allows for accurate and early localization of the focus and facilitates ablation.

In atrial flutter, the atrial rate is usually 300 beats per minute with conduction occurring over the AV node at a 2:1, 3:1, 4:1, or 5:1 ratio. After the ventricular response is controlled, consider restoring sinus rhythm chemically or electrically. Antiarrhythmic agents may be used to treat recurrent episodes. New techniques allow successful and curative ablation for patients with refractory atrial flutter.

Atrial fibrillation is a lifelong condition, involving recurrent episodes (Figure 17-3). Atrial fibrillation presents in several ways: paroxysmal (terminates spontaneously), persistent (needs cardioversion to terminate), or permanent (cannot be maintained in sinus rhythm, i.e., chronic). Patients with nonvalvular heart disease who have any one of several risk factors (older than 65, hypertension, diabetes, congestive heart failure, previous embolic episode) have a higher risk (>5% per year) for stroke and require chronic anticoagulation.

Antiarrhythmic agents are indicated to prevent recurrences of either paroxysmal or persistent atrial fibrillation. Therapeutic choices include amiodarone, sotalol, propafenone, or dofetilide. The later three drugs have pro-arrhythmic effects and require close monitoring. Digoxin, beta-blockers (other than sotalol) and diltiazem do not convert atrial fibrillation to sinus rhythm, but conversion to normal sinus rhythm may occur with rate control. Focal ablation is a promising technique for drug failures or intolerance.

Permanent atrial fibrillation requires rate control using combinations of beta-blockers, calcium channel blockers, and digoxin. Patients in whom intermittent bradycardia develops (tachybrady syndrome) or who have a persistent tachycardia may require a permanent pacemaker with or without AV node ablation. If the ventricular response cannot be controlled or the medications cannot be tolerated, AV node ablation will prevent rapid ventricular response, and a permanent pacemaker will prevent bradycardia. After ablation and pacemaker placement, quality-of-life scores are greatly improved.

Inappropriate sinus tachycardia refers to sinus tachycardia occurring in the absence of provoking factors including hyperthyroidism. It is a frustrating and debilitating condition; patients complain of sudden rapid increases in heart rate with minimal

Figure 17-3 **Ventricular Rhythms I**

QRS <0.10 second

Supraventricular rhythm with normal intraventricular conduction

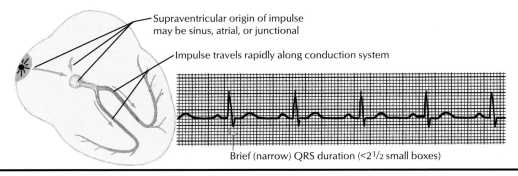

Supraventricular origin of impulse
may be sinus, atrial, or junctional

Impulse travels rapidly along conduction system

Brief (narrow) QRS duration (<2½ small boxes)

QRS >0.10 second

Intraventricular conduction defect (IVCD), including right or left bundle branch block

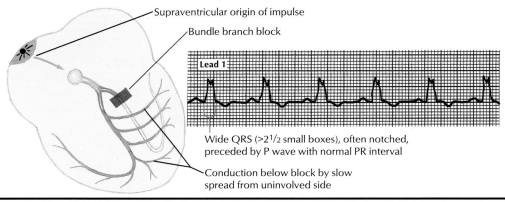

Supraventricular origin of impulse

Bundle branch block

Lead 1

Wide QRS (>2½ small boxes), often notched,
preceded by P wave with normal PR interval

Conduction below block by slow
spread from uninvolved side

Wolff-Parkinson-White (preexcitation) syndrome

Impulses originate at SA node
and preexcite peripheral
conduction system and ventricular
muscle via bundle of Kent
without delay at AV node.
(In type B, impulses may pass via
posterior accessory bundle)

After normal delay at AV node,
impulses also arrive at
ventricles via normal route to
continue depolarization

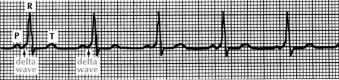

P wave is immediately followed
by short delta wave, producing
slurred upstroke on wide QRS
with short or no PR interval

R
P T
delta wave   delta wave

Figure 17-4

Ventricular Rhythms II

QRS > 0.10 second (continued)
    No P waves (ventricular impulse origin)
        Rate <40/minute: idioventricular rhythm

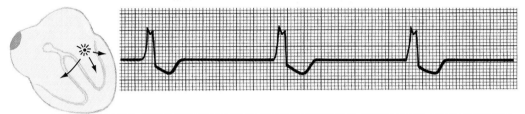

Rate 40 to 120: accelerated idioventricular rhythm (AIVR)

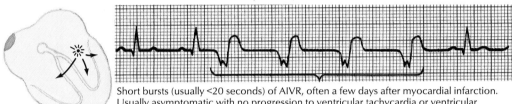

Short bursts (usually <20 seconds) of AIVR, often a few days after myocardial infarction. Usually asymptomatic with no progression to ventricular tachycardia or ventricular fibrillation

Rate >120: ventricular tachycardia

Infarct

Slowed conduction in margin of ischemic area permits circular course of impulse and reentry with rapid repetitive depolarization

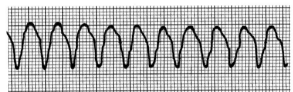

Rapid, bizarre, wide QRS complexes

Ventricular fibrillation

Chaotic ventricular depolarization

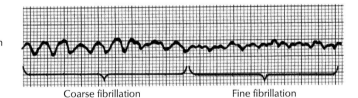

Coarse fibrillation   Fine fibrillation

Pacer rhythm

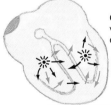

Transvenous pacemaker produces beat in right ventricle. Not supraventricular, and therefore wide QRS

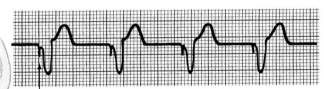

Pacemaker spike (may be small; sometimes missed)

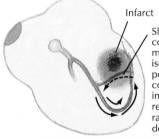

or no physical activity. Initially, either beta-blocker or calcium channel blocker alone or in combination may be used. If symptoms persist despite use of maximally tolerated doses, a RFA of the superior portion of the sinus node can be performed.

The use of internal cardiac defibrillators (ICDs) has significantly reduced arrhythmic death from ventricular tachycardia. The largest potential target group are patients with ventricular tachycardia due to prior myocardial infarction. Until recently, guidelines limited ICD infestation in this group of patients and were stringent, requiring demonstration of nonsustained ventricular tachycardia in the setting of left ventricular dysfunction due to a previous myocardial infarction, and a positive electrophysiology study for inducible ventricular tachycardia prior ICD placement. As a result of recent studies, ICD placement is now recommended in a much larger group of "at risk" patients. Primary prevention of sudden cardiac death has been confirmed with the publication of the Multicenter Automatic Defibrillator Implantation Trial II (MADET II) study. ICD placement is now recommended in patients with a previous myocardial infarction and a left ventricular ejection fraction of less than 30%.

Ventricular tachycardia usually presents in left ventricular dysfunction (Figure 17-4). If an abnormal ejection fraction is documented, the patient should have a cardiac catheterization with calculation of cardiac output and coronary angiography. Revascularization should precede electrophysiological evaluation. Many patients require placement of an ICD. Despite the use of antiarrhythmic agents and an ICD, some patients may also require RFA of the Ventricular Tachycardia circuit.

In patients with a normal echocardiogram, the ventricular tachycardia may originate from a focus located in the right ventricular outflow tract or the left ventricle, and may be verapamil- or adenosine-sensitive. RFA is a curative option. Patients presenting with syncope in the presence of left ventricular dysfunction should be considered to have ventricular tachycardia until proved otherwise by a negative electrophysiology study.

Patients with ventricular fibrillation that occurs outside the setting of an acute myocardial infarction should receive an ICD (Figure 17-4).

Patients with complete heart block, second-degree Mobitz type II AV block, and sinus pauses should receive a permanent pacemaker. Asymp-tomatic patients with prolonged PR intervals, sinus bradycardia, or second-degree Mobitz type I AV block (Wenkebach) should not receive a pacemaker (Figure 17-2).

Premature ventricular complexes without left ventricular dysfunction should be managed conservatively, as should premature atrial complexes. Exercise and a healthy lifestyle should be encouraged.

Congenital long QT syndrome is an inherited condition that presents with syncope or sudden death. Exercise-induced symptoms are a particular cause for concern. Frequently, a family history of similar episodes will be found. Management includes beta-blockers, dual-chamber pacemaker with a lower rate at 85 beats per minute, or an implantable cardioverter defibrillator.

Patients with the Brugada syndrome are at risk for sudden cardiac death. Symptomatic individuals should receive an ICD; asymptomatic individuals with an abnormal EKG pattern should undergo an electrophysiology study, and, if results are positive, should have an ICD placed.

FUTURE DIRECTIONS

Improvements in ablation technology for atrial fibrillation and other arrhythmias offer exciting hope for the future. ICD technology continues to evolve and improve the quality of life of patients who previously were at high risk for arrhythmic death. Cardiac resynchronization therapy with atrio-biventricular pacing in patients with congestive heart failure and prolonged intraventricular conduction (wide QRS complexes) is a promising technology in this group of severely impaired and debilitated patients.

REFERENCES

Brugada J, Brugada R, Antzelevitch C, Towbin J, Nademanee K, Brugada P. Long-term follow-up on individuals with the electrocardiographic pattern of right bundle-branch block and ST-segment elevation in precordial leads V1 to V3. *Circulation*. 2002;105:73-78.

Lee MA, Morady F, Kadish A, et al. Catheter modification of the atrioventricular junction with radiofrequency energy for control of atrioventricular nodal reentry tachycardia. *Circulation*. 1991;83:827–835.

Moss AJ, Zareba W, Hall WJ, et al, and The Multicenter Automatic Defibrillator Implantation Trial II Investigators. Prophylactic implantation of a defibrillator in patients with myocardial infarction and reduced ejection fraction. *N Engl J Med*. 2002;346:877–883.

Weber BE, Kapoor WN. Evaluation and outcomes of patients with palpitations. *Am J Med*. 1997;103:86.

Chapter 18

Congenital and Valvular Heart Disease

Lee R. Goldberg and Park W. Willis IV

Most patients with congenital or valvular heart disease come to medical attention when a routine examination detects cardiac abnormalities. Clinical presentation with symptoms of heart failure, an important arrhythmia, or infective endocarditis is less common. Although congenital heart disease is usually discovered in childhood, the diagnosis of atrial septal defect is occasionally made for the first time in an adult. The long-term followup and evaluation of patients with surgically corrected congenital heart disease is of increasing importance as the numbers of these patients reaching adulthood continue to grow. The incidence of rheumatic fever has declined, and acquired valvular disease is predominantly caused by progression of inherited conditions, or age-related degenerative change. To accurately define structural disease and quantify hemodynamic abnormalities, the diagnostic approach must include transthoracic echocardiography, appropriately focused according to clinical findings, in addition to standard chest radiography and electrocardiography. Transesophageal echocardiography and cardiac catheterization may be necessary in difficult cases. Antibiotic prophylaxis for infective endocarditis is indicated in almost all patients with congenital heart disease (the major exception being patients with uncomplicated secondary atrial septal defect). Those with rheumatic disease require prophylaxis for recurrent streptococcal infection. Participation in competitive athletics should be restricted in many conditions, and some patients require special consideration in the workplace. Family planning and management of pregnancy require a multidisciplinary approach.

AORTIC STENOSIS
Etiology and Pathogenesis

Congenital aortic stenosis is most commonly of valvular origin. Nonvalvular congenital causes include discrete subaortic membrane and supravalvular aortic stenosis. Congenitally bicuspid aortic valves, present in 1% to 2% of the general population, undergo accelerated degenerative change. Age-related calcification and rheumatic disease cause acquired stenosis of trileaflet valves.

Aortic stenosis causes fixed outflow obstruction and left ventricular pressure overload. Compensatory left ventricular hypertrophy increases myocardial oxygen demand, and ischemia can develop, even in the absence of coronary artery disease. Although contractile performance is preserved, hypertrophy causes decreased chamber compliance and diastolic left ventricular dysfunction. Consequently, atrial contraction can be critical to diastolic filling (Figure 18-1).

Clinical Presentation

Aortic stenosis causes a midsystolic murmur, loudest in the second right intercostal space and transmitted to the neck. Signs of moderate or severe aortic stenosis include a small and slow-rising arterial pulse, systolic thrill in the second right intercostal space or suprasternal notch, and sustained apical impulse. An aortic ejection sound is present in most patients with congenital valvular disease. The second heart sound is usually normal, but reversed splitting can occur with severe obstruction.

Important symptoms of moderate or severe aortic stenosis are angina pectoris, syncope, and left heart failure. The onset of atrial fibrillation can cause abrupt hemodynamic deterioration and precipitate symptoms.

Differential Diagnosis

Midsystolic murmurs can be innocent; pathological causes include any type of obstruction to ventricular outflow, dilation of the aortic root or main pulmonary artery, and high-output states such as pregnancy, anemia, fever, and thyrotoxicosis.

Hypertrophic cardiomyopathy causes dynamic left ventricular outflow obstruction. In these patients the carotid pulse is brisk and biferiens in

Figure 18-1

Valvular Stenosis and Insufficiency I

Aortic Stenosis

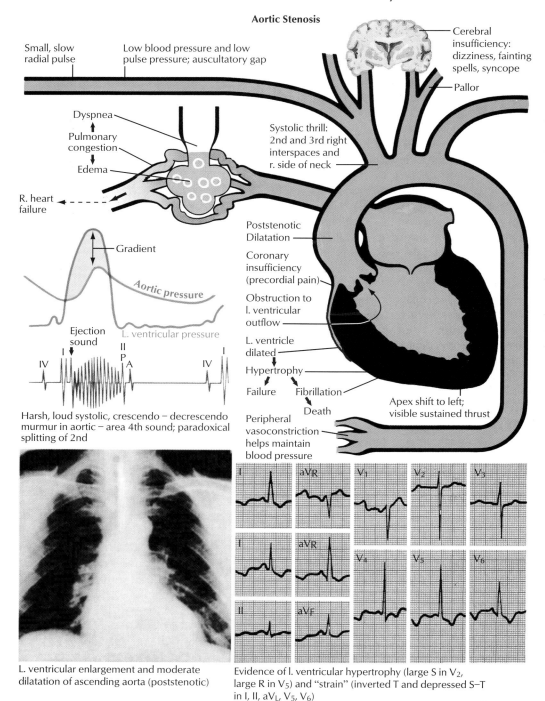

Small, slow radial pulse

Low blood pressure and low pulse pressure; auscultatory gap

Cerebral insufficiency: dizziness, fainting spells, syncope

Pallor

Dyspnea ↑ Pulmonary congestion ↓ Edema

R. heart failure

Systolic thrill: 2nd and 3rd right interspaces and r. side of neck

Posterstenotic Dilatation

Coronary insufficiency (precordial pain)

Obstruction to l. ventricular outflow

L. ventricle dilated ↓ Hypertrophy

Failure   Fibrillation

Death

Apex shift to left; visible sustained thrust

Peripheral vasoconstriction helps maintain blood pressure

Gradient

Aortic pressure

L. ventricular pressure

Ejection sound

I   II   P A   I

IV   IV

Harsh, loud systolic, crescendo – decrescendo murmur in aortic – area 4th sound; paradoxical splitting of 2nd

L. ventricular enlargement and moderate dilatation of ascending aorta (poststenotic)

Evidence of l. ventricular hypertrophy (large S in V_2, large R in V_5) and "strain" (inverted T and depressed S–T in I, II, aV_L, V_5, V_6)

I aV_R V_1 V_2 V_3

I aV_R V_4 V_5 V_6

II aV_F

contour, and the midsystolic murmur is characteristically loudest at the left sternal edge.

Diagnostic Approach

Precise quantification of aortic stenosis requires Doppler measurements of left ventricular outflow velocity and evaluation of left ventricular contractile performance, or invasive assessment in the cardiac catheterization laboratory.

Management and Therapy

In asymptomatic patients, *mild aortic stenosis* is an indication for annual evaluation and, in the absence of a change in clinical status or physical examination, repeat echocardiography every 2 or 3 years. Patients with *moderate aortic stenosis* require annual clinical examination and non-invasive studies. Those with *severe aortic stenosis* should be evaluated semiannually to determine whether the patient should undergo valve replacement.

Vasodilating drugs can alter well-compensated hemodynamics and should be used with caution in patients with severe aortic stenosis.

Valve replacement is indicated for patients with symptomatic severe aortic stenosis. Older patients require coronary angiography before aortic valve replacement. Left ventricular contractile dysfunction is not a contraindication to surgery, and operative results are satisfactory in symptomatic octogenarians. In selected cases, the Ross procedure is an alternative to valve replacement. Aortic balloon valvuloplasty is indicated in many children, but this technique is of limited utility in adults with calcified valves.

AORTIC REGURGITATION (INSUFFICIENCY)
Etiology and Pathogenesis

Congenitally malformed leaflets, rheumatic disease, age-related degenerative change, and infective endocarditis cause valvular aortic regurgitation. In long-standing hypertension and aging, aortic regurgitation may occur secondary to aortic root dilation. Congenital aortic valve disease and connective tissue abnormalities, including the Marfan syndrome, are associated with cystic medial necrosis of the aorta; complications include progressive aortic root dilation, aortic dissection, and aortic regurgitation.

Chronic aortic regurgitation causes left ventricular volume overload. These changes are compensatory initially, as left ventricular dilation enhances chamber compliance, and increasing end-diastolic volumes can be accommodated without a rise in filling pressure. In the long term, progressive left ventricular dilatation ultimately results in congestive heart failure. Acute aortic regurgitation, most commonly caused by infective endocarditis, does not allow time for left ventricular chamber dilation, and large regurgitant volumes result in rapidly increasing diastolic filling pressure, pulmonary edema, and shock (Figure 18-2).

Clinical Presentation

Most patients have a high-pitched, early diastolic decrescendo murmur at the left sternal edge. If the murmur is transmitted best to the right sternal border, aortic root disease is usually present.

Moderate or severe aortic regurgitation causes widened pulse pressure, systolic hypertension, biferiens carotid pulse, and displaced apical impulse. There is usually a midsystolic murmur caused by increased left ventricular stroke volume and turbulent flow though the outflow tract. A middiastolic (Austin Flint) murmur, mimicking mitral stenosis, can be audible at the mitral area. Symptoms of moderate or severe aortic regurgitation usually reflect left heart failure; angina pectoris is less common. Clinically silent aortic regurgitation can be detected by Doppler echocardiography.

In acute aortic regurgitation, left ventricular failure develops rapidly, and the physical signs of chronic disease are usually absent. In this circumstance, abnormal findings are limited to a soft first heart sound and short early diastolic murmur.

Differential Diagnosis

Pulmonary hypertensive pulmonic regurgitation causes an early diastolic decrescendo (Graham-Steel) murmur. Pulmonic regurgitation after complete repair for tetralogy of Fallot causes a relatively low pitched early diastolic decrescendo murmur.

Accurate measurement of left ventricular chamber size and contractile performance by echocardiography or radionuclide ventriculography is necessary for long-term management of patients with chronic aortic regurgitation.

Management and Therapy

In asymptomatic patients, *mild aortic regurgitation* calls for annual evaluation and, in the absence of a

Figure 18-2

Valvular Stenosis and Insufficiency II

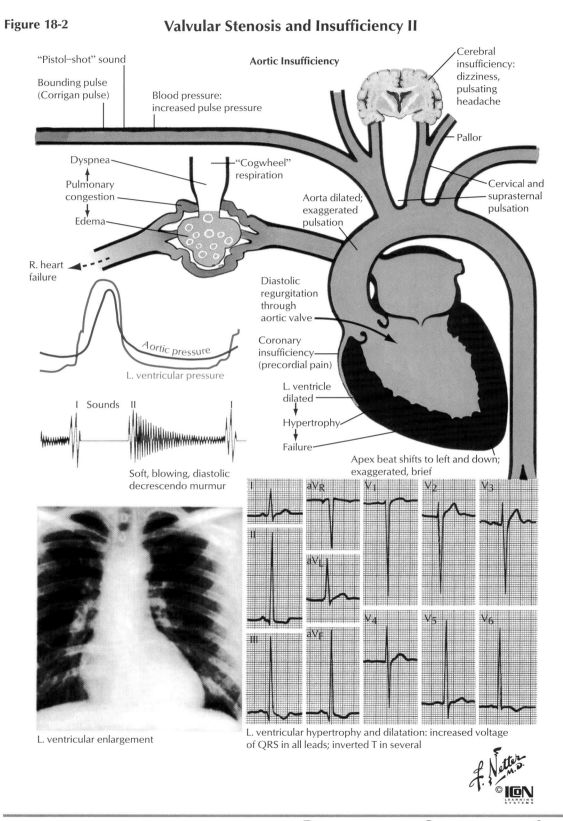

Aortic Insufficiency

"Pistol–shot" sound

Bounding pulse (Corrigan pulse)

Blood pressure: increased pulse pressure

Cerebral insufficiency: dizziness, pulsating headache

Pallor

Dyspnea

Pulmonary congestion

Edema

"Cogwheel" respiration

Aorta dilated; exaggerated pulsation

Cervical and suprasternal pulsation

R. heart failure

Diastolic regurgitation through aortic valve

Coronary insufficiency (precordial pain)

Aortic pressure

L. ventricular pressure

L. ventricle dilated

Hypertrophy

Failure

I Sounds II

Soft, blowing, diastolic decrescendo murmur

Apex beat shifts to left and down; exaggerated, brief

L. ventricular enlargement

L. ventricular hypertrophy and dilatation: increased voltage of QRS in all leads; inverted T in several

change in clinical status or physical examination, repeat echocardiography every 2 or 3 years. An interval change in left ventricular dimensions, or contractile performance, is an indication for 3- to 6-month followup to differentiate progressive disease from measurement variability. Patients with *moderate or severe aortic regurgitation* require annual examination and a noninvasive assessment of left ventricular function. For patients with symptoms of heart failure in addition to moderate or severe aortic regurgitation, aortic valve replacement is indicated. In acute aortic regurgitation, urgent surgical intervention is required.

Left ventricular contractile dysfunction can compromise long-term prognosis and operative results; even in the absence of symptoms, aortic valve replacement is indicated for patients with severe aortic regurgitation and echocardiographically-derived left ventricular end-systolic dimension 55mm or greater, or left ventricular ejection fraction 50% or less.

Patients with chronic aortic regurgitation secondary to disease of the aortic root, especially those with the Marfan syndrome, require annual echocardiographic evaluation. The timing of surgical intervention in these individuals is usually based on the degree and rate of root dilation rather than magnitude of regurgitant flow or left ventricular contractile performance.

Nifedipine can reduce excessive afterload and slow progression of chronic aortic regurgitation, delaying valve replacement. Beta-blocker therapy is indicated to prevent increasing aortic root dilation in patients with the Marfan syndrome.

MITRAL STENOSIS
Etiology and Pathogenesis

Mitral stenosis is usually a manifestation of rheumatic heart disease. Commissural fusion and degenerative change in the mitral apparatus obstruct left ventricular inflow. A rise in left atrial pressure helps to maintain left ventricular filling but causes left atrial chamber dilation, pulmonary venous congestion, and secondary pulmonary arterial hypertension. Irreversible pulmonary vascular disease can be a long-term complication of mitral stenosis (Figure 18-3).

Clinical Presentation

Abnormal physical findings precede the development of clinical symptoms. The earliest signs are increased amplitude of the first heart sound, an open-ing snap, and a mid-diastolic murmur at the mitral area. Approximately 50% of patients give a history of acute rheumatic fever. Symptoms of left heart failure commonly develop during pregnancy or other hemodynamic stress. The onset of atrial fibrillation can cause acute hemodynamic deterioration. The risk of systemic thromboembolism is high in patients with chronic, or paroxysmal, atrial fibrillation.

Differential Diagnosis

Congenital malformations of the mitral valve and papillary muscles, cor triatriatum and left atrial myxoma all can cause obstruction to left ventricular inflow and a mid-diastolic murmur at the mitral area. Mitral stenosis can mimic isolated severe pulmonary hypertension when decreased cardiac output causes the mid-diastolic murmur to be soft or absent.

Diagnostic Approach

The initial echocardiographic evaluation should include an estimate of mitral valve area and pulmonary arterial systolic pressure. A detailed assessment of the mitral apparatus for the degree and extent of degenerative change, leaflet mobility, magnitude of associated mitral regurgitation, and the presence or absence of a left atrial thrombus, is required before catheter-based or operative intervention.

Management and Therapy

Patients with mild left heart failure have a favorable prognosis and can be successfully managed with dietary sodium restriction and diuretic therapy. Beta-blocking drugs can improve diastolic filling of the left ventricle by slowing heart rate at rest and during exercise. Anticoagulation and antiarrhythmic drug therapy are required for patients with atrial fibrillation. Some studies suggest that surgery should be considered with the early onset of symptoms. Carefully selected patients with significantly limiting symptoms are candidates for percutaneous balloon valvuloplasty; for those with severe valvular calcification or significant mitral regurgitation, open commissurotomy or mitral valve replacement is required.

MITRAL REGURGITATION (INSUFFICIENCY)
Etiology and Pathogenesis

Congenital mitral regurgitation is rare as an isolat-

Figure 18-3

Valvular Stenosis and Insufficiency III

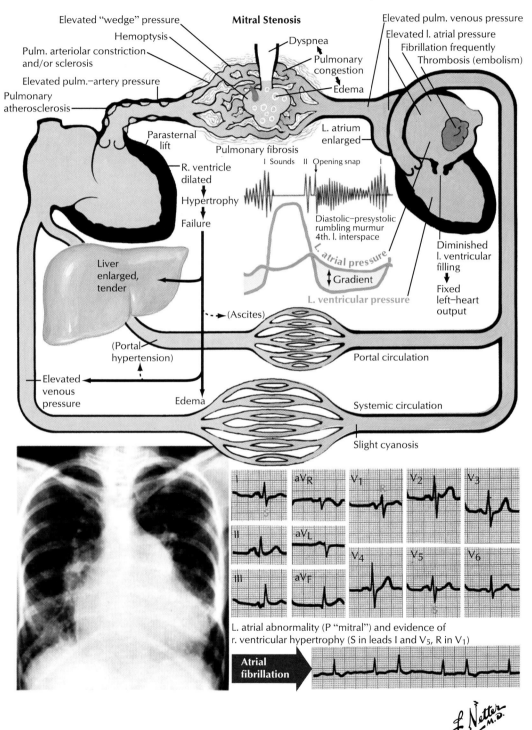

Mitral Stenosis

Elevated "wedge" pressure
Hemoptysis
Pulm. arteriolar constriction and/or sclerosis
Elevated pulm.–artery pressure
Pulmonary atherosclerosis

Dyspnea
Pulmonary congestion
Edema

Elevated pulm. venous pressure
Elevated l. atrial pressure
Fibrillation frequently
Thrombosis (embolism)

Parasternal lift
Pulmonary fibrosis

L. atrium enlarged

R. ventricle dilated
Hypertrophy
Failure

I Sounds   II   Opening snap   I

Diastolic–presystolic rumbling murmur 4th. l. interspace

L. atrial pressure
Gradient
L. ventricular pressure

Diminished l. ventricular filling

Fixed left–heart output

Liver enlarged, tender

(Ascites)

(Portal hypertension)

Portal circulation

Elevated venous pressure

Edema

Systemic circulation

Slight cyanosis

L. atrial abnormality (P "mitral") and evidence of r. ventricular hypertrophy (S in leads I and V_5, R in V_1)

Atrial fibrillation

Figure 18-4

Valvular Stenosis and Insufficiency IV

Mitral Insufficiency

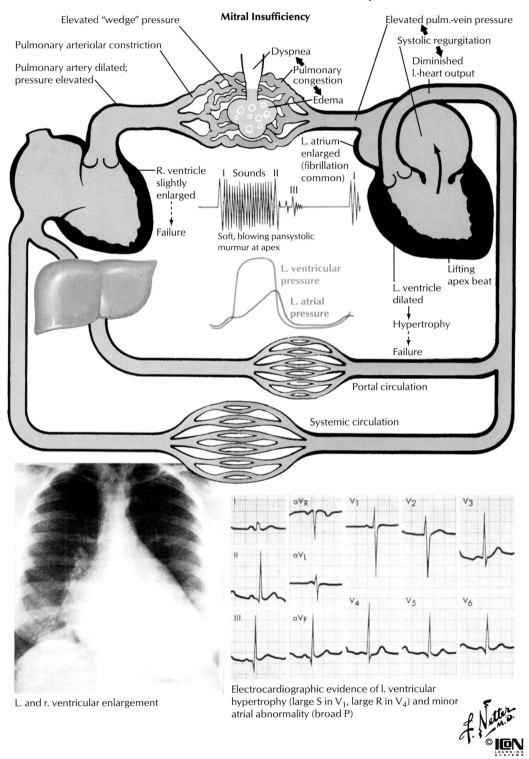

Elevated "wedge" pressure

Pulmonary arteriolar constriction

Pulmonary artery dilated; pressure elevated

Dyspnea

Pulmonary congestion

Edema

Elevated pulm.-vein pressure

Systolic regurgitation

Diminished l.-heart output

L. atrium enlarged (fibrillation common)

R. ventricle slightly enlarged

Failure

I Sounds II

III

Soft, blowing pansystolic murmur at apex

L. ventricular pressure

L. atrial pressure

Lifting apex beat

L. ventricle dilated

Hypertrophy

Failure

Portal circulation

Systemic circulation

L. and r. ventricular enlargement

Electrocardiographic evidence of l. ventricular hypertrophy (large S in V_1, large R in V_4) and minor atrial abnormality (broad P)

f. Netter M.D.

© ICON
LEARNING
SYSTEMS

ed abnormality. Acquired causes include papillary muscle dysfunction secondary to ischemic heart disease, myxomatous disease and prolapse of the mitral valve, rheumatic heart disease, spontaneous rupture of chordae tendineae, and infective endocarditis.

Chronic mitral regurgitation causes left atrial dilation, and large regurgitant volumes can be accommodated at normal pressure. With moderate or severe mitral regurgitation, there is progressive left ventricular dilation. Acute mitral regurgitation does not allow time for left atrial dilation, and pulmonary venous pressure rises precipitously, causing irreversible pulmonary edema and shock (Figure 18-4).

Clinical Presentation

The cardiac examination characteristically shows a pansystolic murmur, loudest at the mitral area, and commonly transmitted to the axilla or left sternal edge. Clinically silent mitral regurgitation can be detected by Doppler echocardiography. Moderate or severe chronic mitral regurgitation can cause lateral displacement of the apical impulse, wide splitting of S_2, and a third heart sound (S_3). Symptoms are related to left heart failure and atrial, or ventricular, arrhythmia. In acute mitral regurgitation, the systolic murmur is often abbreviated, and can be soft or entirely absent.

Differential Diagnosis

The pansystolic murmur of tricuspid regurgitation characteristically increases in amplitude on inspiration. A ventricular septal defect causes a pansystolic murmur, loudest at the left sternal border.

Diagnostic Approach

Chronic mitral regurgitation requires a thorough baseline assessment of left ventricular contractile performance by echocardiography, or radionuclide ventriculography for planning initial medical therapy and long-term follow-up.

Management and Therapy

In asymptomatic patients, *mild mitral regurgitation* calls for annual examination, but repeat echocardiography is not necessary unless there is a change in functional status or physical examination. Those with *moderate or severe mitral regurgitation* require annual examination and echocardiography or radionuclide ventriculography to assess left ventricular performance. Operative intervention is indicated

for symptomatic patients with moderate or severe mitral regurgitation. If the mitral apparatus is suitable, valve repair is the procedure of choice. Mitral valve replacement, with preservation of the chordal apparatus, is the next best option. Patients with chronic severe mitral regurgitation can develop subclinical left ventricular contractile dysfunction, which compromises operative results and long-term prognosis. For this reason, even in the absence of symptoms, operative intervention is indicated for those with echocardiographically derived left ventricular end-systolic dimension ≥45mm, or left ventricular ejection fraction of ≤60%.

Treatment of co-morbid conditions, especially systemic hypertension and coronary artery disease, can help to avoid unnecessarily accelerated progression of mitral regurgitation.

FUTURE DIRECTIONS

The number of patients with congenital and valvular heart disease will continue to grow. Improved medical management and evolving catheter-based interventions will delay, or replace, the need for cardiac surgery in some conditions. Evolving, less invasive operative techniques and increased utilization of autologous tissue, homografts, and more durable bioprosthetic valves will enhance surgical outcomes.

REFERENCES

26th Bethesda Conference: recommendations for determining eligibility for competition in athletes with cardiovascular abnormalities. January 6-7, 1994. *J Am Coll Cardiol.* 1994;24:845–899.

Brickner ME, Hillis LD, Lange RA. Congenital heart disease in adults. First of two parts. *N Engl J Med.* 2000;342:256-263.

Brickner ME, Hillis LD, Lange RA. Congenital heart disease in adults. Second of two parts. *N Engl J Med.* 2000;342:334–342.

Carabello BA, Crawford FA Jr. Valvular heart disease. *N Engl J Med.* 1997;337:32–41.

Dajani A, Taubert K, Ferrieri P, Peter G, Shulman S. Treatment of acute streptococcal pharyngitis and prevention of rheumatic fever: a statement for health professionals. Committee on Rheumatic Fever, Endocarditis, and Kawasaki Disease of the Council on Cardiovascular Disease in the Young, and the American Heart Association. *Pediatrics.* 1995;96:758–764.

Dajani AS, Taubert KA, Wilson W, et al. Prevention of bacterial endocarditis. Recommendations by the American Heart Association. *JAMA.* 1997;277:1794–1801.

Gutgesell HP, Gessner IH, Vetter VL, Yabek SM, Norton JB Jr. Recreational and occupational recommendations for young patients with heart disease. A Statement for Physicians by the Committee on Congenital Cardiac Defects of the Council on Cardiovascular Disease in the Young, and the American Heart Association. *Circulation.* 1986;74:1195A–1198A

Chapter 19
Heart Failure

Carla A. Sueta and Rachel Keever

Heart failure (HF) is the inability of the heart and circulation to meet peripheral metabolic demands while maintaining a normal filling pressure. *Systolic dysfunction* is the inability of the ventricle to empty normally, with reduced ejection fraction, usually accompanied by ventricular dilatation. *Diastolic dysfunction* is the inability of the ventricle to relax or fill normally, represented by an elevated end diastolic pressure and normal ventricular size and contraction.

HF affects 4.7 million Americans with an incidence of more than 550,000 cases per year, increasing significantly with age. It is the most common cause of hospitalization for patients 65 years and older. Annual health care cost exceeds 38 billion dollars.

Despite therapeutic advances, HF mortality remains high — 50% at 5 years. Possible explanations include increased survival of post-myocardial infarction patients in whom HF subsequently develops, undertreatment, and suboptimal risk factor modification. Recent trials demonstrate that treating hypertension, vascular disease, or high-risk diabetics significantly reduces the development of HF.

Risk factors include a history of hypertension, stroke, coronary artery disease, peripheral artery disease, or diabetes mellitus with increased total cholesterol, incresed low-density lipoprotiens, cigarette smoking, or microglobulinuria.

ETIOLOGY AND PATHOGENESIS

Coronary artery disease accounts for 50% of the cases of HF worldwide. In the US and western countries, this percentage is considerably higher. Patients with previous myocardial infarction can exhibit both decreased systolic performance and diastolic impairment due to interstitial fibrosis and scar formation.

Acute ischemia impairs ventricular relaxation and can produce transient systolic dysfunction. Hypertensive cardiomyopathy is a common cause of HF in African Americans and older patients. The most frequent cause of initially unexplained HF is idiopathic cardiomyopathy.

Other etiologies of dilated cardiomyopathies include: myocarditis, infection due to HIV, peripartum cardiomyopathy, diabetes mellitus, alcohol, cocaine, connective tissue disease, thyroid disease, doxorubicin therapy, and arrhythmias. Anemia or thiamine deficiency can cause high-output HF.

Systolic dysfunction results in a reduction in cardiac output that is perceived as hypovolemia by the kidneys. Activation of the renin-angiotensin-aldosterone system causes salt and water retention, increasing preload, transiently improving cardiac output but subsequently resulting in volume overload.

Decrease in blood pressure due to declining cardiac output triggers activation of the sympathetic nervous system and the renin-angiotensin-aldosterone system, creating systemic vasoconstriction; a compensatory response to preserve organ perfusion. However, vasoconstriction ultimately contributes to increased afterload and worsening HF. Sympathetic nervous system activation can also precipitate ventricular arrhythmias resulting in sudden death. Prolonged neurohormonal activation, also initially compensatory, is detrimental. Together, these physiologic responses to cardiac dysfunction trigger remodeling of the ventricle, increased preload, afterload, and wall stress; producing mitral regurgitation, and leads to worsening cardiac performance.

Diastolic dysfunction accounts for 30%–40% of HF cases and is more frequent in older patients, especially women. Ischemic heart disease and hypertension are the most common causes of isolated diastolic dysfunction.

Hypertension increases systolic wall stress and induces hypertrophy of the sarcomeres in parallel resulting in left ventricular (LV) hypertrophy. Elevated angiotensin and insulin levels may also contribute to the development of hypertrophy.

In restrictive cardiomyopathies, wall thickness is increased by infiltration or fibrosis due to amyloid, sarcoid, hemochromatosis, radiation therapy, and muscular dystrophy. Hypertrophic cardiomyopathy is characterized by myocardial fiber disarray and segmental or global hypertrophy. Constrictive pericarditis may also cause diastolic dysfunction related to the constraining effect of a thickened and rigid pericardium.

CLINICAL PRESENTATION

The initial presentation of patients with HF includes signs and symptoms of pulmonary congestion, systemic fluid retention, inadequate organ perfusion, or exercise intolerance. These same signs and symptoms do not distinguish whether the underlying etiology is systolic or diastolic dysfunction (Figure 19-1). Cardiomegaly can be due to ventricular dilatation or hypertrophy. Assessment of LV function is essential to correctly predict prognosis and devise treatment strategies.

Symptoms include dyspnea on exertion, exercise intolerance, orthopnea, paroxysmal nocturnal dyspnea, cough, chest pain, weakness, fatigue, nausea, abdominal pain, nocturia, oliguria, confusion, insomnia, depression, and weight loss. Physical examination findings that should be systematically assesssed include engorged neck veins, rales, pleural effusion, displaced point of maximal intensity, right ventricular heave, S_3, S_4, murmurs, hepatomegaly, low volume pulses, and peripheral edema.

Left heart failure is manifested by pulmonary edema and exercise intolerance, while right heart failure causes engorgement of neck veins and peripheral edema.

DIFFERENTIAL DIAGNOSIS

The difficulty in arriving at a new diagnosis of HF lies in its vague symptoms and exam mimickers. Symptoms of dyspnea and exercise intolerance can be attributed to many diagnoses: lung disease including thromboembolic disease, pulmonary hypertension, thyroid disease, arrhythmias, anemia, obesity, deconditioning, and cognitive disorders. Signs of volume overload are not specific to HF. Sodium avid states of nephrosis and cirrhosis, as well as pericardial disease, can manifest as jugular venous distension, hepatomegaly, and edema.

DIAGNOSTIC APPROACH

The diagnosis is made by taking a careful history, performing a directed exam, and assessing ventricular function. Laboratory evaluation and pulmonary function testing will eliminate the majority of other diagnoses.

Determine the Type and Degree of LV Dysfunction

Echocardiography is the best and most common method for initial assessment of HF. Ejection fraction, valve function, and hypertrophy are evaluated. Radionuclide ventriculography provides a more precise measurement of volumes and both left and right ventricular ejection fraction, and is the method of choice for obese patients or those with significant lung disease.

Define the Etiology

The degree of reversibility and, hence, the progress and management of HF, differs depending on the underlying etiology. Poor prognostic indicators include ischemic etiology, age, male gender, ejection fraction, and *New York Heart Association* (NYHA) class. Ischemic heart disease should be excluded in every patient with cardiac catheterization, exercise/pharmacologic stress testing, echocardiography, or nuclear sestamibi or thallium. Focal wall motion abnormalities do not always represent ischemic heart disease. Routine evaluation includes chest radiography, EKG, electrolytes, total protein, albumin, liver function tests, CBC, urinalysis, and measurement of thyroxine and thyroid-stimulating hormone levels.

> *NYHA classification is an important tool for assessing prognosis, medical management, and for longitudinal followup and evaluation of the response to treatment.*
> Class I: Symptoms at exertion levels similar to normal individuals.
> Class II: Symptoms with ordinary exertion.
> Class III: Symptoms with less than ordinary activity.
> Class IV: Symptoms at rest or with any physical activity.

MANAGEMENT AND THERAPY

As a first step, it is important to correct precipitating factors, such as dietary noncompliance, ischemia, uncontrolled hypertension, atrial fibril-

Figure 19-1

Left Heart Failure and Pulmonary Congestion

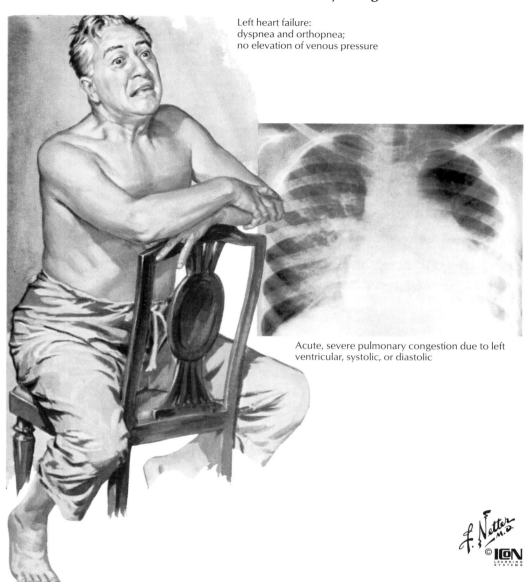

Left heart failure:
dyspnea and orthopnea;
no elevation of venous pressure

Acute, severe pulmonary congestion due to left
ventricular, systolic, or diastolic

lation, hypoxemia, thyroid disease, anemia, and the presence and causes of medical nonadherence including financial disability.

Revascularization should be considered in ischemic patients. Low ejection fraction and reversible ischemia indicate improved prognosis with revascularization.

Systolic Dysfunction

For systolic dysfunction (ejection fraction <40%), blockade of the renin angiotensin system with ACE-Inhibitor (ACE-I) therapy is the treatment of choice. ACE-I therapy improves survival and quality of life in patients with NYHA Class II-IV heart failure and in post-infarction patients at these target doses: enalapril 10 mg twice daily, captopril 50 mg 3 times daily (absorption is decreased by food), lisinopril 20 mg once daily, ramipril 5 mg twice daily, trandolapril 4 mg once daily, quinapril 20 mg twice daily. ACE-I therapy can also delay progression of HF in asymptomatic patients. Contraindications to ACE-I include moderate to severe aortic stenosis, renal artery stenosis and hyperkalemia > 5.5 mEq/dl.

If patients do not tolerate an ACE-I due to angioedema or intractable cough, angiotensin II receptor blocker, which has an equivalent effect on renal function, should be prescribed. In patients with significant renal dysfunction (potassium >5.5 mEq/dl), the combination of isordil (40mg three times a day) and hydralazine (75mg 3 to 4 times a day) is an alternative, although not as effective as ACE-I therapy. All patients with coronary artery disease should receive an aspirin unless there are contraindications.

Beta-blockers should be added in stable patients with NYHA Class II to IV symptoms. They significantly improve survival and ejection fraction while reducing sudden death and hospitalization in patients receiving an ACE-I. Contraindications include asthma, severe bradycardia, and advanced heart block. Beta-blockers should be started at a low dose (carvedilol 3.125 or 6.25mg twice daily, metoprolol XL 12.5 or 25mg) and up-titrated every 2 weeks. Beta-blockers should not be initiated or uptitrated in patients exhibiting volume overload; these patients should be treated for fluid overload first. Side effects (transient fatigue, weight gain, and diarrhea) are more common with the first few doses. Aim for the target dose: carvedilol 25mg twice daily (≤85 kg) 50 mg twice daily (>85 kg), bisoprolol 10mg once daily, metoprolol XL 200mg once daily. Although target doses should be the goal, a dose of carvedilol 6.25 mg bid also confers a mortality and morbidity benefit. As with ACE-I therapy, some studies support maximum "target doses" although uptitration should be continued with caution and stopped when adverse side effects occur.

Aldactone can be added to therapy in patients with Class III to IV HF. The potassium level generally rises, especially in diabetics, and monitoring is necessary.

Diuretics such as hydrochlorothiazide, furosemide, and bumetanide are prescribed in most patients to alleviate fluid overload. Because they activate the renin-angiotensin system, the minimal dose should be used. In patients with severe HF, combination therapy (a loop diuretic and hydrochlorothiazide or metolazone) can be used but potassium and magnesium levels must be carefully monitored.

Digoxin reduces hospitalization and improves symptoms. Serum concentrations of 0.8 to 1.2 ng/dL provide the same benefits as higher levels. *Nitrates* reduce preload and are prescribed as anti-anginal agents. At higher doses, systemic and pulmonary vasodilation occurs. Prevent nitrate tolerance acutely by increasing the dose and chronically by allowing a nitrate-free interval of at least 8 hours.

Trials with the newer *calcium channel blockers*, amlodipine and felodipine, show a neutral effect on mortality. These agents are used to treat hypertension and angina unresponsive to ACE-I and β-blockers. Because of their negative effect on contractility, nifedipine, verapamil, and diltiazem should not be used in these patients.

One should consider *intravenous diuretic therapy* in acute decompensation and refractory HF. Continuous furosemide infusion results in a steady diuresis. Hydrochlorothiazide and renal dose dopamine can be added in refractory cases. Nitrate therapy is particularly effective in acute myocardial infarction with pulmonary edema. Compared to acute nitroglycerin, nitroprusside is a more powerful afterload-reducing agent for the same degree of preload reduction. Dobutamine is an inotrope with limited chronotropic and no vasoconstrictor activity. Milrinone, a phosphodiesterase inhibitor, is both an inotrope and vasodilator.

Systolic Dysfunctions: Devices

Implantable defibrillators (ICD) are indicated in patients who have survived a cardiac arrest. ICDs have also been shown to reduce mortality in patients with a history of myocardial infarction and an ejection fraction ≤30%. Biventricular pacemakers can improve quality of life and reduce hospitalization but the effect on mortality is unknown. Left ventricular assist devices are used as a bridge to cardiac transplantation and have also been shown to prolong life in patients who are not transplant candidates.

Diastolic Dysfunction

There are no completed randomized trials indicating a medical regimen that improves survival in patients with diastolic dysfunction. Agents that reduce preload, such as diuretics and nitrates, are commonly prescribed. Nitrates are also used to treat ischemia. ACE-I, calcium channel blockers, angiotensin-receptor blockers, and beta-blockers cause regression of LV hypertrophy. Calcium channel blockers, particularly verapamil, improve ventricular relaxation. Agents that decrease heart rate (increasing diastolic filling time) including verapamil, diltiazem, and β-blockers, are beneficial.

Maintaining atrial contraction is very important. In patients with decreased compliance, atrial contraction contributes up to 50% of ventricular filling, explaining why the loss of atrial contraction in atrial fibrillation results in acute decompensation. Cardioversion and treatment with antiarrhythmic agents are options. Consider dual-chamber pacemakers in patients with junctional rhythm or heart block unresponsive to adjustment of medication.

Treatment of Comorbid Disease

Aggressive management of hyperlipidemia, hypertension, and diabetes mellitus are part of routine care.

Nonpharmacologic Strategies

These include daily exercise, salt restriction to less than 2.5 to 3 g daily, fluid restriction and daily weight measurement in the patient's care plan. Encourage weight loss, discontinuation of alcohol, and smoking cessation with nicotine replacement and bupropion if indicated. Educate the patient/family about the symptoms and signs of the disease, prognosis, medications, and when to contact a health professional.

Refer to an HF specialist if the patient remains severely limited on an optimized medical regimen, does not tolerate uptitration, or if the patient is a transplant candidate (refractory HF, LVEF <20%, without significant comorbid disease, age <65, compliant, psychologically stable and has good social support), or is a candidate for clinical trials.

FUTURE DIRECTIONS

Blockers of metalloproteinase that mediate tissue remodeling and vasopeptidase inhibitors are in development. Gene therapy approaches hold promise for the future with ongoing improvements in vector technology, cardiac gene delivery, and understanding of molecular pathogenesis. Disease prevention by aggressive modification of risk factors and early detection continue to have an enormous impact on cardiovascular disease leading to HF.

REFERENCES

Heart Failure Society of America (HFSA) practice guidelines. HFSA guidelines for management of patients with heart failure caused by left ventricular systolic dysfunction—pharmacological approaches. *J Card Fail.* 1999;5:357–382.

Adams KF Jr, Dunlap SH, Sueta CA, et al. Relation between gender, etiology and survival in patients with symptomatic heart failure. *J Am Coll Cardiol.* 1996;28:1781–1788.

Afridi I, Grayburn PA, Panza JA, Oh JK, Zoghbi WA, Marwick TH. Myocardial viability during dobutamine echocardiography predicts survival in patients with coronary artery disease and severe left ventricular systolic dysfunction. *J Am Coll Cardiol.* 1998;32:921–926.

Gomberg-Maitland M, Baran DA, Fuster V. Treatment of congestive heart failure: guidelines for the primary care physician and the heart failure specialist. *Arch Intern Med.* 2001;161:342–352.

Sueta CA, Chowdhury M, Boccuzzi SJ, et al. Analysis of the degree of undertreatment of hyperlipidemia and congestive heart failure secondary to coronary artery disease. *Am J Cardiol.* 1999;83:1303–1307.

Chapter 20

Hypercholesterolemia: Evaluation and Treatment

Ross J. Simpson Jr and Sidney C. Smith Jr

Cholesterol is a simple lipid component of cell membranes and a precursor of steroids and bile acids. It is a particularly important lipid because it is a major component of atherosclerotic plaques, and because elevated blood cholesterol concentration is a major, and reversible, cause of CHD.

Cholesterol is primarily synthesized in the liver and is excreted as bile salts (Figure 20-1). Individuals on the average Western diet absorb 20%-40% of their cholesterol or approximately 300-700 mg daily. Approximately 1000mg is recirculated each day by secretion and reabsorption as bile salts. Blood levels of cholesterol are determined by dietary intake of cholesterol, inheritance, physical activity, and intake of dietary fats, particularly saturated fats. Cholesterol is transported in the blood as macromolecules of lipoproteins, with the nonpolar lipid core surrounded by a polar monolayer of phospholipids, the polar portion of cholesterol and apoliproteins. Specific lipoproteins differ in lipid core content, the proportion of lipids in the core, and the proteins on the surface. Lipoproteins are commonly classified by density as chylomicrons, chylomicron remnants, VLDL, LDL, IDL, or HDL cholesterol.

Triglycerides are esters of glycerol and long-chain, saturated, and desaturated fatty acids. They are found in all plasma lipoproteins but are the major constituent of chylomicrons, chylomicron remnants, VLDL, and IDL. Most triglycerides are contained in VLDL, which comprises 10%-15% of the total cholesterol. If triglyceride-rich particles are present in sufficiently high concentration (>400mg/dL), the plasma is turbid or opalescent. Severe elevations of triglycerides (1000mg/dL) are associated with pancreatitis and eruptive xanthoma. However, the relationship of plasma triglycerides and atherosclerotic disease is still inconsistent due to the strong association of elevated triglycerides with low HDL as well as with other atherogenic factors (e.g., diabetes, smoking, and hypertension).

HDL encompasses a family of lipoproteins that usually comprises approximately 20%-30% of the total cholesterol and shows a strong inverse association with CHD risk. HDL may facilitate reverse cholesterol transport from tissue. HDL is decreased by diets high in polyunsaturated fats, obesity, smoking, diabetes, and drugs (diuretics, anabolic steroids, and progestins). Physical activity and alcohol increase HD. However, HDL concentration fluctuates considerably due to physiologic and analytic variation. Thus, a single measurement of the HDL is not sufficient to determine a patient's usual HDL.

LDL cholesterol comprises half to two-thirds of the total cholesterol and is thus the major determinant of the serum cholesterol. As commonly measured, LDL is not a unique molecule but a population of particles similar in chemical and physical properties. For example, IDL and lipoprotein (a), both of which appear to be atherogenic, generally comprise 2%-4% of the total cholesterol and are encompassed in the LDL cholesterol value.

LDL cholesterol shows a strong and consistent epidemiologic, experimental, and clinical link to the rate of coronary heart disease (Figure 20-2). Lowering of LDL cholesterol by diet, exercise, and/or pharmacologic therapy slows atherosclerotic vascular disease progression and lowers the risk of coronary events. This strong link of LDL cholesterol with coronary disease makes management of elevated LDL cholesterol a critical focus for medical treatment. While independent interventions to lower triglycerides and/or raise HDL cholesterol should also be considered, it should be noted that therapies that lower LDL cholesterol often positively impact triglycerides and HDL cholesterol.

ETIOLOGY AND PATHOGENESIS

Premature coronary heart disease may result from high LDL cholesterol levels in patients without other risk factors for coronary artery disease, particularly children and young adults who have inherited a lack of sufficient cell membrane receptors to remove LDL cholesterol from circulation. These forms of familial hypercholesterolemia, present in 1/500 who are heterozygous and 1/1,000,000 who are homozygous, are characterized by a 2-4 fold increase in LDL cholesterol levels in heterozygotes and even greater increases in homozygotes. Familial combined hypercholesterolemia occurs in approximately 1/100 people and is characterized by overproduction of apolipoprotein B. In all of these individuals, the coronary risk conferred by an elevated LDL cholesterol is further increased by the presence of additional coronary risk factors, as described below.

The mechanisms by which LDL cholesterol accelerate coronary atherosclerosis are complex. It appears to be part of an inflammatory response to endothelial injury in which monocytes infiltrate the arterial intima, promote cholesterol oxidation and conversion of monocytes into tissue macrophages and eventually to lipid-laden foam cells (Figure 20-2). These cells initially deposit in fatty streaks below the endothelial layer. With further accumulation, an eccentric lipid rich plaque develops. Smooth muscle cells form a fibrous cap over the lipid core that repeatedly fissures leading to thrombus formation and plaque growth. Eventually a major fissure occurs and a thrombus partially or completely obstructs the coronary artery, leading to unstable angina, myocardial infarction, or sudden cardiac death.

CLINICAL PRESENTATION

Individuals with lipid abnormalities may present in one of several ways. Most importantly, this is a diagnosis made by laboratory analysis. Given the efficacy of cholesterol-lowering interventions in reducing coronary risk, any individual presenting with chronic or acute coronary syndromes or deemed to be at increased risk because of a "high-risk" family history or who has diabetes mellitus or multiple cardiac risk factors should be screened. Historically, screening in these groups was underutilized, but with increased emphasis, this has improved substantially.

In some settings, patients not known to be at increased risk but with hypercholesterolemia can be identified. Patients with familial hypercholesterolemia may present with physical findings that reflect long-standing hypercholesterolemia. These include, subcutaneous cholesterol deposits, most frequently tendonous xanthomas or xanthelasmas. Arcus senilus, once thought to be indicative of hypercholesterolemia is far less specific, particularly in the elderly. Patients may also present after routine blood work reveals turbid serum.

DIFFERENTIAL DIAGNOSIS

Secondary causes of elevated cholesterol are common. These include poorly controlled diabetes, hypothyroidism, and the nephrotic syndrome. Estrogen replacement therapy may elevate triglycerides, and HDL may be dramatically lowered by progestins and anabolic steroids.

DIAGNOSTIC APPROACH

The primary blood test required for diagnosis and treatment of elevated cholesterol measures the fasting total cholesterol, triglycerides, and HDL. These values are then used to calculate the LDL cholesterol [total cholesterol − HDL-(triglycerides/5)]. This method is used only if the triglycerides are <400mg/dL. Direct measures of LDL cholesterol and estimation of LDL and other lipid fraction particle size and particle number are also available, but are not commonly necessary or used. Blood samples should be measured after a 12-hour fast, as chylomicrons interfere with the estimation of LDL.

Established coronary disease, and atherosclerotic vascular disease in other vascular beds dramatically increase the risk associated with elevated LDL cholesterol. In addition, diabetes mellitus has recently been defined as a "coronary risk equivalent", and patients with known diabetes should be evaluated and treated as if they have diagnosed coronary heart disease because of the increased risk associated with diabetes. These clinical situations require aggressive management of LDL cholesterol. For patients who are not in this highest-risk group, the goal of lipid management is to delay the complications of coronary artery disease and less aggressive therapy is warranted. For these reasons, a search for the major, established risk factors for coronary artery disease should be performed. A change in exercise capacity, chest pain, or angina should be assessed by appropriate historical information or diagnostic tests (e.g., treadmill, nuclear imaging, and cardiac angiography).

The accepted major risk factors for coronary disease include: age >45 in men and >55 in women, a history of premature coronary artery disease in first-degree relatives (sudden death or coronary disease onset before age 55 for men or 65 for women), current smoking, presence and severity of hypertension, physical inactivity, and dietary patterns. Life habit risk factors including obesity (body mass index ≥30), physical inactivity, and an atherogenic diet should also be assessed. Screening for elevated glucose may be particularly appropriate if the metabolic syndrome (central obesity, hypertension, glucose intolerance with low HDL cholesterol, elevated triglycerides, and modestly elevated LDL cholesterol) is suspected. Assessment of proteinuria, serum creatinine and liver function studies may also help guide therapy. Additional risk factors for coronary disease including lipoprotein (a), homocysteine, and prothrombotic and pro-inflammatory factors (C-reactive protein) are not routinely measured but may be helpful in situations where a family history or established CHD occurs in the absence of a markedly elevated LDL cholesterol. These risk factors are emerging as potentially important modifiable causes of coronary disease.

Lowering the LDL cholesterol should be the primary goal of therapy. For patients with CHD, other vascular disease, diabetes, or a 10-year Framingham risk of CHD events >20%, the target LDL cholesterol should be <100mg/dL. Ideal values of HDL cholesterol are >40 mg/dL, and triglycerides <150 mg/dL. For patients with increased triglycerides (>200 mg/dL), non-HDL cholesterol should be used to guide therapy, with a target level of 30 mg/dL greater than the recommended LDL cholesterol target.

MANAGEMENT AND THERAPY

Appropriate diet and exercise are the cornerstones of cholesterol management (Figure 20-3). All patients who have elevated cholesterol should receive dietary counseling and dietary reinforcement to help them achieve their cholesterol goals. Although there remains some controversy over the optimal diet to reduce coronary risk, the strongest data available today support either of two approaches. The modified step II American Heart Association diet of <7% of calories from saturated fat and <200 mg/day of dietary cholesterol focuses on reduction in cholesterol intake and low total fat intake. Plant sterols/stanols of 2g/day can be encouraged; these plant analogues of cholesterol displace cholesterol from bile salts and lower cholesterol, as do soluble fibers. The "Mediterranean Diet" encourages increased intake of fish and a variety of other foods that are low in saturated fats, but not as low as the American Heart Association diets in total fat. A planned program of physical activity should be started and reinforced. The routine use of high-dose vitamins or antioxidant supplements is not recommended.

Fish oil (epicosapentaenoic acid and docosahexaenoic acid) is a promising dietary intervention that appears to reduce hepatic triglyceride synthesis. Dietary supplements of fish oil containing 2g–5g of omega-3 fatty acid may decrease triglycerides by up to 30% and VLDL by 40%, with resulting modest decreases in LDL cholesterol and increases in HDL cholesterol. Gastrointestinal complaints (bloating, diarrhea), increased bleeding time, and effects of hypervitaminosis A and D (dermatitis or hypercalciumemia) may occur with high doses of fish oil.

Initiation of drug therapy is based on the absolute risk of a patient developing a coronary event and the LDL cholesterol value following diet therapy (Figure 20-3). If the ten-year Framingham risk is over 20% (according to paradigm described in the *Third Report of the National Cholesterol Education Program* referenced below) or the patient has a coronary risk equivalent, drug therapy should be initiated if the LDL cholesterol exceeds 100mg/dL. If the patient has a 10-year risk of <20% and has two or more risk factors, drugs should be considered if the LDL cholesterol exceeds 130mg/dL. If the patient has only one other risk factor and the 10-year risk is <10%, drugs are often initiated if the LDL cholesterol is 160mg/dL or higher.

Drug therapy with HMG Co-A reductase inhibitors (statins) is highly effective at lowering LDL. Statins inhibit cholesterol synthesis and increase LDL receptor uptake of LDL. In addition, statins lower triglycerides by up to 30% and can

Figure 20-1

Hypercholesterolemia
Cholesterol Synthesis and Metabolism

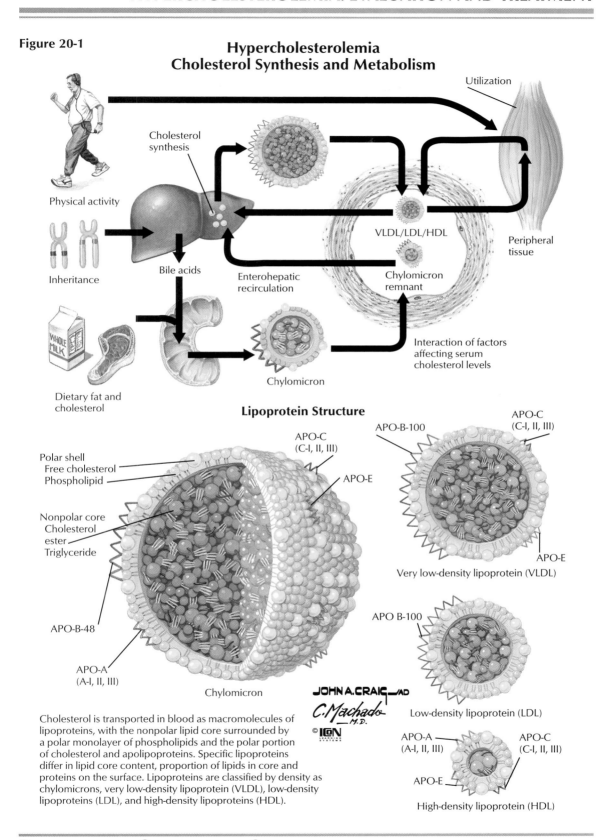

Utilization

Cholesterol synthesis

Physical activity

Inheritance

Bile acids

Dietary fat and cholesterol

Enterohepatic recirculation

VLDL/LDL/HDL

Chylomicron remnant

Peripheral tissue

Chylomicron

Interaction of factors affecting serum cholesterol levels

Lipoprotein Structure

Polar shell
Free cholesterol
Phospholipid

APO-C (C-I, II, III)

APO-E

Nonpolar core
Cholesterol ester
Triglyceride

APO-B-48

APO-A (A-I, II, III)

Chylomicron

APO-B-100

APO-C (C-I, II, III)

APO-E

Very low-density lipoprotein (VLDL)

APO B-100

Low-density lipoprotein (LDL)

APO-A (A-I, II, III)

APO-C (C-I, II, III)

APO-E

High-density lipoprotein (HDL)

JOHN A.CRAIG—MD
C.Machado
—M.D.
©ICN

Cholesterol is transported in blood as macromolecules of lipoproteins, with the nonpolar lipid core surrounded by a polar monolayer of phospholipids and the polar portion of cholesterol and apolipoproteins. Specific lipoproteins differ in lipid core content, proportion of lipids in core and proteins on the surface. Lipoproteins are classified by density as chylomicrons, very low-density lipoprotein (VLDL), low-density lipoproteins (LDL), and high-density lipoproteins (HDL).

Figure 20-2

Hypercholesterolemia as Risk Factor in Coronary Artery Disease

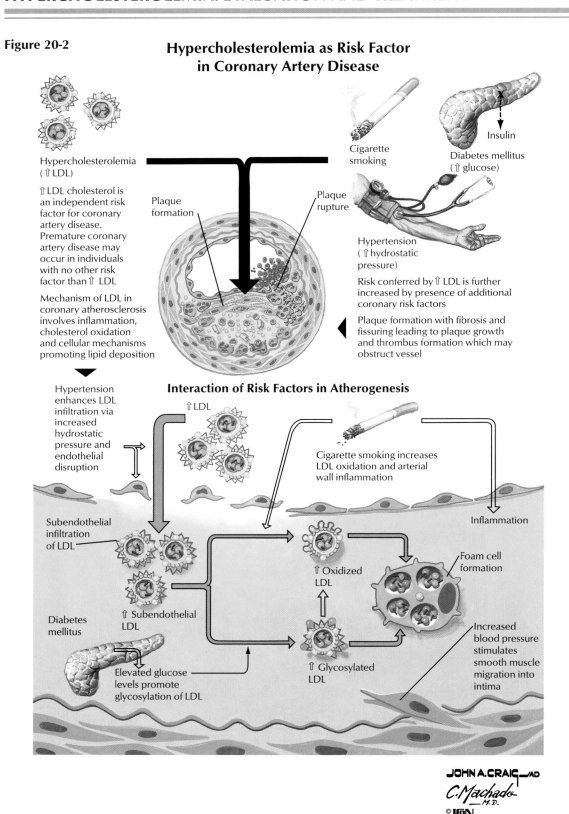

Hypercholesterolemia
(⇑ LDL)

⇑ LDL cholesterol is an independent risk factor for coronary artery disease. Premature coronary artery disease may occur in individuals with no other risk factor than ⇑ LDL

Mechanism of LDL in coronary atherosclerosis involves inflammation, cholesterol oxidation and cellular mechanisms promoting lipid deposition

Plaque formation

Plaque rupture

Cigarette smoking

Insulin

Diabetes mellitus
(⇑ glucose)

Hypertension
(⇑ hydrostatic pressure)

Risk conferred by ⇑ LDL is further increased by presence of additional coronary risk factors

Plaque formation with fibrosis and fissuring leading to plaque growth and thrombus formation which may obstruct vessel

Interaction of Risk Factors in Atherogenesis

Hypertension enhances LDL infiltration via increased hydrostatic pressure and endothelial disruption

⇑ LDL

Cigarette smoking increases LDL oxidation and arterial wall inflammation

Inflammation

Subendothelial infiltration of LDL

⇑ Oxidized LDL

Foam cell formation

Diabetes mellitus

⇑ Subendothelial LDL

Elevated glucose levels promote glycosylation of LDL

⇑ Glycosylated LDL

Increased blood pressure stimulates smooth muscle migration into intima

JOHN A. CRAIG—MD

C. Machado—M.D.

© ICON

Figure 20-3

Hypercholesterolemia
General Management Measures
Dietary Management

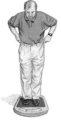 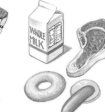 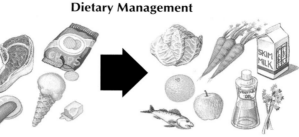 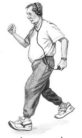

Weight control

Reduce consumption of foods high in cholesterol, saturated fat and *trans* fatty acids, and salt. Decrease total caloric intake.

Increase consumption of food low in saturated fat and high in fiber.

Increased exercise

Appropriate diet and exercise are cornerstones of cholesterol management. Dietary counseling and reinforcement and a planned program of physical activity are recommended.

Fish oil supplements

Actions of Lipid Lowering Medications

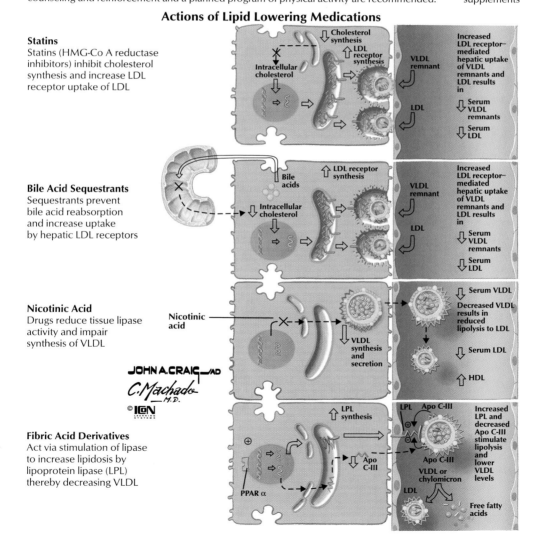

Statins
Statins (HMG-Co A reductase inhibitors) inhibit cholesterol synthesis and increase LDL receptor uptake of LDL

Bile Acid Sequestrants
Sequestrants prevent bile acid reabsorption and increase uptake by hepatic LDL receptors

Nicotinic Acid
Drugs reduce tissue lipase activity and impair synthesis of VLDL

Fibric Acid Derivatives
Act via stimulation of lipase to increase lipidosis by lipoprotein lipase (LPL) thereby decreasing VLDL

JOHN A. CRAIG—MD
C. Machado—M.D.
© ICN LEARNING SYSTEMS

be expected to raise HDL cholesterol by up to 15%. These drugs include lovastatin (20 mg–80 mg/daily), pravastatin (20 mg–40 mg/daily), simvastatin (20 mg-80 mg/daily), fluvastatin (20 mg–80 mg/daily), and atorvastatin (10mg–80 mg/daily). There is a predictable dose-response relationship with these drugs such that doubling the dose of the statin results in an approximate 6% additional LDL cholesterol reduction from the initial baseline level. The recommended starting doses for each statin are approximately equivalent in their ability to lower LDL. These drugs are, in general, well tolerated. There is a small risk of myopathy with higher doses or when statins are combined with fibrates or with drugs that interfere with metabolism of the statin. A modest but dose-dependent increase in the probability of elevated liver enzymes also occurs. Their benefit in lowering LDL cholesterol is potentiated by bile acid sequestrants.

Second-line medications include bile acid sequestrants: cholestryramine (4 grams–16 grams/daily, colestipol (5 grams–20 grams/daily) and colesevelam (2.6 grams–3.8 grams/daily). These drugs prevent bile acid reabsorption and increase uptake by liver LDL receptors. They can reduce LDL cholesterol by up to 30% in a dose-dependent manner and can increase HDL cholesterol by 5%, but may also increase triglycerides. They should not be used in patients with dysbetalipoproteinemia or elevated triglycerides. They are not systemically absorbed, and side effects are generally limited to their potential to interfere with decreased absorption of other drugs, constipation, dyspepsia, and bloating.

Nicotinic acid reduces tissue lipase activity and impairs VLDL synthesis. It lowers LDL cholesterol by up to 25%, decreases triglycerides up to 50%, and raises HDL cholesterol by up to 35%. Side effects include flushing, elevated blood glucose, hyperuricemia, abdominal pain and hepatotoxicity. Nicotinic acid should not be used in patients with severe gout, peptic ulcer disease, or liver disease, and should be used only with close monitoring in patients with diabetes or insulin resistance. Nicotinic acid is available in three forms: immediate release (1.5 grams–3 grams/daily), extended release (1 grams–2 grams), and sustained release (1 grams–2 grams). Although nicotinic acid is highly effective and has a demonstrated safety record, compliance is not good unless supportive counseling is provided.

Fibric acid derivatives [gemfibrozil (600mg twice daily), fenofibrate (160mg/daily)] decrease VLDL and triglyceride levels by increasing lipolysis by lipoprotein lipase, thereby increasing catabolism of triglyceride rich particles. They can be expected to lower LDL cholesterol by up to 20%, to raise HDL cholesterol by up to 20%, and to lower triglycerides by up to 50%. Side effects include dyspepsia, gallstones, and a propensity towards myopathy when combined with statins. These drugs are contraindicated in renal or hepatic disease.

Combination therapy may be required in patients with severely elevated LDL. In all cases, combination therapy should be carefully monitored. In particular, the combination of a statin with a fibric acid should be considered only in the most refractory circumstances since some such combinations carry an increased risk of serious side-effects including hepatic failure. In most patients, however, additional dietary considerations, or exercise or counseling to improve compliance will further improve their lipid management.

Specific Dyslipidemia

When LDL is extremely high (>190mg/dL) a genetic disorder should be suspected and family screening undertaken. Monogenetic familial hypercholesterolemia, familial defective apolipoprotein B100 synthesis, or polygenic hypercholesterolemia is likely. Therapy almost always requires a statin in high doses or a statin combined with another drug. Occasionally patients will require plasma apheresis, particularly in the rare homozygous forms of hypercholesterolemia.

Treatment of other lipid factors may also be required. Elevated triglycerides may be caused by obesity, physical inactivity, cigarette smoking, excess alcohol intake, failure to fast prior to the lipid test, a high-carbohydrate (>60% of energy intake) diet, type II diabetes, chronic renal failure, and nephrotic syndrome. Certain drugs (corticosteroids, estrogens, retinoids, high-dose beta blockers) and genetic dyslipidemia may also be implicated. However, when the triglycerides exceed 500 mg/dL, triglyceride-lowering therapy should be undertaken to avoid pancreatitis or eruptive xanthomas. Dietary counseling is essential and should focus on very low-fat diets (less than 15% of calories). Fibrates, nicotinic acid and fish oil dietary supplements, and tight diabetic control, can all be helpful in treatment of hyper-triglyceridemia.

FUTURE DIRECTIONS

New drugs and new therapies are rapidly being developed for managing cholesterol and diagnosing atherosclerosis earlier in its course. Diagnostic tests to more accurately predict the risk of developing coronary events include measurement of the C-reactive protein and measurement of lipid particle size and density as well as use of electron beam tomography to access calcium levels in the coronary arteries. Other noninvasive tests to assess the extent of atherosclerosis and establish risk of future events include carotid Doppler ultrasound to determine intima/media thickness ratio, and the ankle brachial index, a measurement of the extent of peripheral vascular disease that provides important cardiovascular prognostic information. Invasive techniques include intracoronary ultrasound to assess the plaque burden and lipid density and the possible propensity of coronary artery to plaque rupture.

Drugs that raise HDL and that selectively inhibit the absorption of cholesterol are also under development, as are increasingly potent statins. One example of a new approach is ezetimibe, a selective inhibitor of cholesterol absorption at the intestinal villi, which can reduce LDL by up to 17% and could potentially be combined with statins. Other promising therapies are in clinical trials and it is likely that in the future lipid disorders will be able to be managed more effectively with fewer side effects, thereby more effectively reducing cardiovascular risk.

REFERENCES

Executive Summary of The Third Report of The National Cholesterol Education Program (NCEP) Expert Panel on Detection, Evaluation, and Treatment of High Blood Cholesterol in Adults (Adult Treatment Panel III). *JAMA.* 2001;285:2486–2497.

MCR/BHF Heart Protection Study of cholesterol-lowering therapy and of antioxidant vitamin supplementation in a wide range of patients at increased risk of coronary heart disease death: early safety and efficacy experience. *Eur Heart J.* 1999;20:725–741.

Gotto, AM Jr. *Contemporary Diagnosis and Management of Lipid Disorders.* 2nd ed. Newtown, Pa: Handbooks in Health Care; 2001.

Keys AB. Seven Countries: A Multivariate Analysis of Death and Coronary Heart Disease. Cambridge, Mass: *Harvard University Press;* 1980.

Stamler J, Vaccaro O, Neaton JD, Wentworth D. Diabetes, other risk factors, and 12-yr cardiovascular mortality for men screened in the Multiple Risk Factor Intervention Trail. *Diabetes Care.* 1993;16:434–444.

The Working Group on Lipoprotein Measurement. *Recommendations on Lipoprotein Measurement.* Washington, DC: National Institutes of Health, National Heart, Lung, and Blood Institute; 1995. NIH publication 95–3044.

Chapter 21
Hypertension

Romulo E. Colindres and Alan L. Hinderliter

Hypertension is a major risk factor for atherosclerotic cardiovascular disease (Figure 21-1). Numerous large-scale prospective observational studies have demonstrated the risks of hypertension in 5 major areas. First, high blood pressure accelerates atherogenesis and increases the risk of cardiovascular events by two to threefold. Second, the level of systolic and diastolic blood pressure is associated with cardiovascular events in a continuous, graded, and apparently independent fashion. This relationship is tighter for systolic blood pressure than for diastolic blood pressure (Figure 21-1 and 21-2). Third, between a diastolic blood pressure of 110mmHg and 70mmHg, a persistently lower diastolic blood pressure of 5mmHg is associated with at least a 40% decrease in the incidence of stroke, and a 21% decrease in the incidence of coronary heart disease. Fourth, hypertension often occurs in association with other atherogenic risk factors, including dyslipidemia, glucose intolerance, hyperinsulinemia, and obesity. Fifth, the association of hypertension with other cardiovascular risk factors increases the risk of cardiovascular events in a multiplicative rather than additive fashion.

Pharmacologic treatment of hypertension reduces the incidence of stroke and coronary artery disease, and decreases mortality from cardiovascular causes in middle aged and older adults (Figure 21-3). Furthermore, the results from randomized trials may underestimate the favorable cardiovascular effects of blood pressure lowering because numerous patients assigned to active therapy stopped their treatment, while others assigned to placebo were prescribed medications. In addition, the average duration of treatment was only about 5 years, and most patients enrolled were at low risk for developing cardiovascular disease.

DEFINITION OF HYPERTENSION

Blood pressure is a continuous variable, and any level of blood pressure chosen to define hypertension will be arbitrary. Nevertheless, an operational definition of hypertension has long been advocated by clinicians as a guideline for treatment. The report of the *Sixth Joint National Committee* on the Prevention, Detection, Evaluation, and Treatment of High Blood Pressure (JNC VI) recommended the classification of blood pressure for adults shown in Table 21-1.

Epidemiology of Hypertension

The Third National Health and Nutrition Survey (NHANES III) defined hypertension in the population of the US. Trends in awareness, treatment, and control of high blood pressure in subjects 18 to 74 years of age between 1976 and 1994 in the US (Table 21-2) are similar to those found worldwide. The percentage of patients with controlled hypertension is lower in some Western countries such as Canada and England, and is less than 10% in developing countries—a disappointing figure given the medications available to treat hypertension and efforts made to educate the public and physicians about the risks of high blood pressure. Hypertension is therefore a major worldwide public health problem and a

Table 21-1
Classification of Blood Pressure for Adults Age 18 and Older

Category	Systolic (mmHg)	Diastolic (mmHg)
Optimal	<120	<80
Normal	<130	<85
High normal	130–139	85–89
Hypertension		
Stage 1	140–159	90–99
Stage 2	160–179	100–109
Stage 3	>180	>110

Figure 21-1

Hypertension as Risk Factor for Cardiovascular Disease*

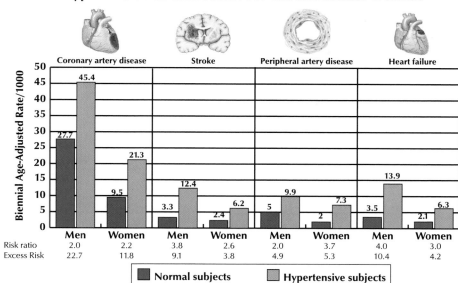

	Coronary artery disease		Stroke		Peripheral artery disease		Heart failure	
	Men	Women	Men	Women	Men	Women	Men	Women
Risk ratio	2.0	2.2	3.8	2.6	2.0	3.7	4.0	3.0
Excess Risk	22.7	11.8	9.1	3.8	4.9	5.3	10.4	4.2

■ **Normal subjects**   ■ **Hypertensive subjects**

Y-axis: Biennial Age-Adjusted Rate/1000

Values shown in bars: Coronary artery disease — Men 27.7 / 45.4, Women 9.5 / 21.3; Stroke — Men 3.3 / 12.4, Women 2.4 / 6.2; Peripheral artery disease — Men 5 / 9.9, Women 2 / 7.3; Heart failure — Men 3.5 / 13.9, Women 2.1 / 6.3

* According to Hypertensive status in subjects 35-64 years of age from the Framingham at 36 year follow-up. Adapted from : *JAMA* 1996;275:1
571–6. Adapted from Kannel, WB. Blood pressure as a cardiovascular risk factor: prevention and treatment. *JAMA*. 1196;275:1571–1576.

Level of blood pressure is associated with cardiovascular events in a continuous, graded, and apparently independent fashion**

Stroke

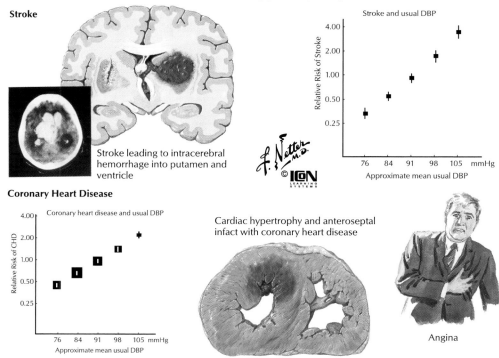

Stroke leading to intracerebral hemorrhage into putamen and ventricle

Stroke and usual DBP

Relative Risk of Stroke vs. Approximate mean usual DBP (76, 84, 91, 98, 105 mmHg)

Coronary Heart Disease

Coronary heart disease and usual DBP

Relative Risk of CHD vs. Approximate mean usual DBP (76, 84, 91, 98, 105 mmHg)

Cardiac hypertrophy and anteroseptal infact with coronary heart disease

Angina

** Relative risk of stroke and coronary heart disease as a function of usual diastolic pressure in 420,000 individuals 25 years or older with a mean follow-up period of 10 years. Adapted from MacMahon S, Peto R, Cutter S, et al. Blood pressure, stroke, and coronary heart disease: part one. *Lancet.* 1990;335:765-767.

Figure 21-2 Risk of Cardiovascular Events by Level of Systolic Blood Pressure:
38 Year Follow-Up for Framingham Subjects 65 to 94 Years Old

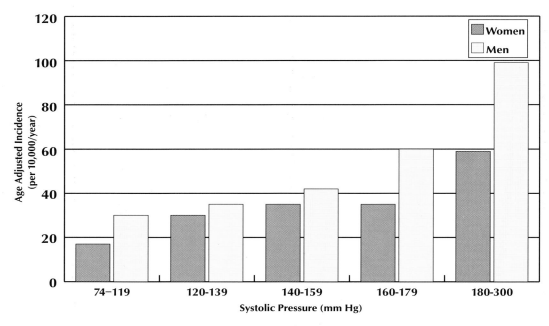

Figure 21-3 Effects of Antihypertensive Treatment on Stroke,
Coronary Heart Disease, Total Cardiovascular Deaths, and All Other Deaths*

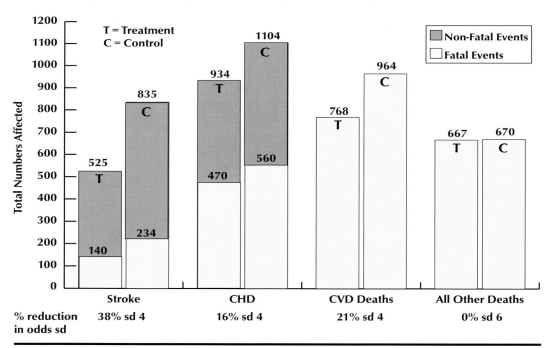

*Data from combined results of 17 randomized trials including 47,653 patients; sd, standard deviation
Adapted from Kannel WB. Blood pressure as a cardiovascular risk factor: prevention and treatment. *JAMA*. 1996;275:1571-1576
and Cutler, SA etal. In: Laragh. JH, Bremmer, BT eds. Hypertension. 2nd ed. *Raven Press*, New York. 1995:225.

Figure 21-4 Prevalence of High Blood Pressure by Age and Race/Ethnicity for Men and Women in US 18 Years or Older

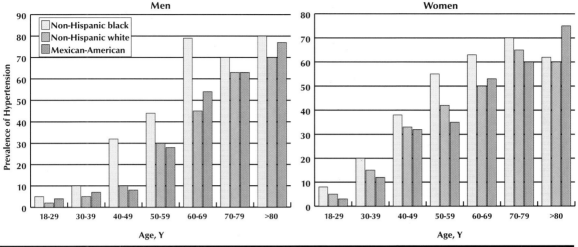

Adapted from Cutler, SA et al. In: Laragh. JH, Bremmer, BT eds. Hypertension. 2nd ed. *Raven Press*, New York. 1995:225.

Table 21-2
Trends in the Awareness, Treatment, and Control of High Blood Pressure in Adults in the United States

	NHANES II 1976-1980	NHANES III 1988-1991	NHANES III 1991-1994
Awareness	51	73	68.4
Treatment	31	55	53.6
Control	10	29	27.4

Data are for adults 18 to 74 years of age with a systolic blood pressure equal to or greater than 140mmHg and/or a diastolic blood pressure equal to or greater than 90mmHg. Control is defined as a systolic blood pressure <140mmHg and a diastolic blood pressure <90mmHg. NHANES II and III: Second and Third National Health and Nutrition Surveys. Phase 2 of the third survey was conducted between 1991 and 1994. With permission from The sixth report of the Joint National Committee on Prevention, Detection, Evaluation, and Treatment of High Blood Pressure. *Arch Intern Med*. 1997;157:2413-2446.

highly prevalent major cardiovascular risk factor, the prevention and treatment of which should be prioritized (Figure 21-4).

ETIOLOGY AND PATHOGENESIS

Hypertension is a disorder of blood pressure regulation that most often results from an increase in total peripheral vascular resistance. A common feature of essential hypertension is that cardiac output is usually normal, although increased cardiac output plays an etiologic role. This has been explained by the phenomenon of autoregulation, whereby an increase in cardiac output causes a persistently elevated peripheral vascular resistance, with a resulting return of cardiac output to normal. Figure 21-5 shows the mechanisms that can lead to hypertension. Inappropriate activation of the renin angiotensin system, decreased renal sodium execution, or an increase in sympathetic nervous system activity, individually or in combination, are most likely involved in the pathogenesis of all types of hypertension. Hypertension has both genetic and environmental causes, including excess sodium intake, obesity, and stress. The inability of the kidneys to optimally excrete sodium, and thus regulate the plasma volume, leads to a persistent increase in blood pressure regardless of the specific underlying etiology.

Many elderly patients with elevated blood pressure have isolated systolic hypertension—a systolic pressure that exceeds 140 mmHg with a normal diastolic pressure. Isolated systolic hypertension correlates with stiffening of large arteries, an increase in systolic pulse wave velocity causing an increase in systolic blood pressure, and increased myocardial work with decreased coronary perfusion (Figure 21-6).

CLINICAL PRESENTATION

Most patients with early hypertension have no

Figure 21-5 ## Factors Involved in the Control of Blood Pressure

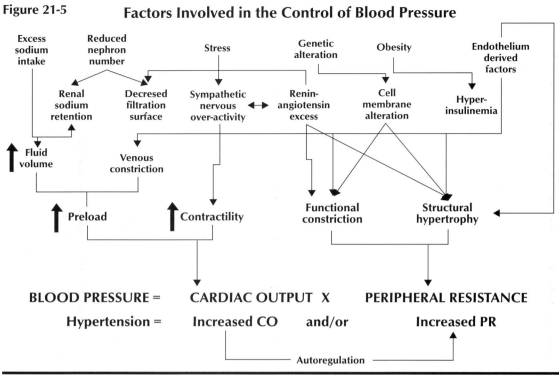

With permission from Kaplan NM, *Kaplan's Clinical Hypertension.* 8th ed. Philadelphia, Pa: Lippincott, Williams & Wilkins; 2002.

symptoms attributable to high blood pressure. Long-term blood pressure elevation, however, frequently leads to hypertensive heart disease, atherosclerosis of the aorta and peripheral vessels, cerebrovascular disease, and renal insufficiency.

The cardiac manifestations of hypertension result from both the hypertrophic effects of increased afterload and acceleration of coronary atherosclerosis. Left ventricular hypertrophy is a powerful and independent risk factor for cardiovascular morbidity and mortality. Most hypertensive patients with left ventricular hypertrophy have concentric hypertrophy—an increase in wall thickness relative to chamber dimensions. In addition, myocardial fibrosis, stimulated in part by increased angiotensin II and aldosterone levels, causes decreased ventricular compliance and diastolic dysfunction, and may result in congestive heart failure despite normal left ventricular systolic function. Sustained blood pressure elevations may ultimately lead to left ventricular decompensation and diminished cardiac output.

Hypertension is also an independent risk factor

for coronary artery disease. The incidence of coronary events increases proportionally with increase in systolic or diastolic blood pressure. The hypertrophic and atherosclerotic consequences of hypertension may combine to greatly enhance the risk of congestive heart failure and cardiovascular death (Figure 21-7).

Occasionally, asymptomatic hypertension may enter a phase called malignant or accelerated hypertension. This syndrome is characterized by greatly elevated systolic and diastolic blood pressures, severe neuroretinitis, proteinuria, microscopic hematuria, impairment of renal function, and a variety of symptoms caused by proliferative endarteritis and fibrinoid necrosis of small arteries and arterioles.

DIFFERENTIAL DIAGNOSIS

Approximately 95% of patients with elevated arterial pressure have essential hypertension. The remaining 5% have secondary hypertension (Figure 21-8). Although patients with secondary hypertension are few in number, it is important to identify such patients since their hypertension can often be cured or significantly improved by an

Figure 21-6

Wave Reflection and Isolated Systolic Hypertension

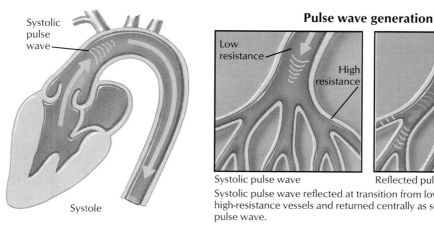

Systolic pulse wave

Systole

Pulse wave generation

Low resistance

High resistance

Systolic pulse wave

Reflected pulse wave

Systolic pulse wave reflected at transition from low- and high-resistance vessels and returned centrally as secondary pulse wave.

Normal diastolic return

Reflected (secondary) pulse wave

Pulse wave velocity

Abnormal systolic return

Summation of systolic and reflected pulse waves

Pulse wave velocity

JOHN A. CRAIG—MD
C. Machado—M.D.
© ION

ECG

Systolic pulse wave

Secondary pulse wave

Brachial artery

Ascending aorta

Arterial pressure (mmHg)

ECG

Systolic hypertension

Brachial artery

Ascending aorta

Amplitude of reflected wave greatest in periphery, accounting for higher systolic pressures in extremities than in aorta. Diastolic return of reflected wave to heart increases coronary perfusion and decreases afterload.

Stiffening of arterial wall increases pulse wave velocity and results in systolic return of reflected wave with increase in systolic pressure (isolated systolic hypertension), decresed diastolic pressure, increased afterload, and left ventricular hypertrophy.

Figure 21-7

The Development of Congestive Heart Failure (CHF) in Patients with Hypertension

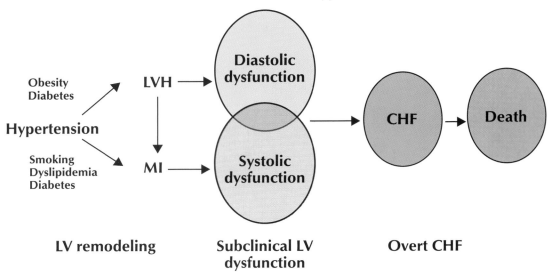

Adapted from Vasan RS, Levy D. The role of hypertension in the pathogenesis of heart failure. A clinical mechanistic overview. *Arch Intern Med.* 1996;156:1789–1796.

interventional procedure, a specific drug therapy, or stopping a culprit drug.

Evidence of identifiable causes of hypertension should be sought in the initial history, physical examination, and laboratory studies. Further diagnostic evaluation for causes of secondary hypertension should be pursued when the presentation is atypical for essential hypertension, or when the initial evaluation suggests an identifiable cause (Table 21-3). Diagnostic methods used in evaluating specific causes of secondary hypertension are discussed in Chapters 22 and 23.

DIAGNOSTIC APPROACH

The initial evaluation of the hypertensive patient should include:
- Confirmation of the presence of hypertension;
- Determination of the presence and extent of target organ disease;
- Identification of cardiovascular risk factors and co-existing conditions that influence prognosis and therapy; and
- Exclusion or detection of identifiable causes of elevated blood pressure.

These goals can usually be achieved with a comprehensive history, a thorough physical examination, and selected laboratory studies.

A comprehensive history is essential, and should include:
- The duration and severity of elevated blood pressure, and the results of prior medication trials;
- The presence of diabetes, hypercholesterolemia, tobacco use, and other cardiovascular risk factors;
- A history or symptoms of target organ disease, including coronary heart disease and heart failure, cerebrovascular disease, peripheral vascular disease, and renal disease;
- Symptoms suggesting identifiable causes of hypertension;
- The use of drugs or substances that may raise blood pressure;
- Lifestyle factors, such as diet, leisure time physical activity, and weight gain, that may influence blood pressure control;
- Psychosocial and environmental factors, such as family support, income, and educational level, that influence the efficacy of antihypertensive therapy;
- Any family history of hypertension or cardiovascular disease.

The physical examination should focus on

Figure 21-8

Causes of Hypertension

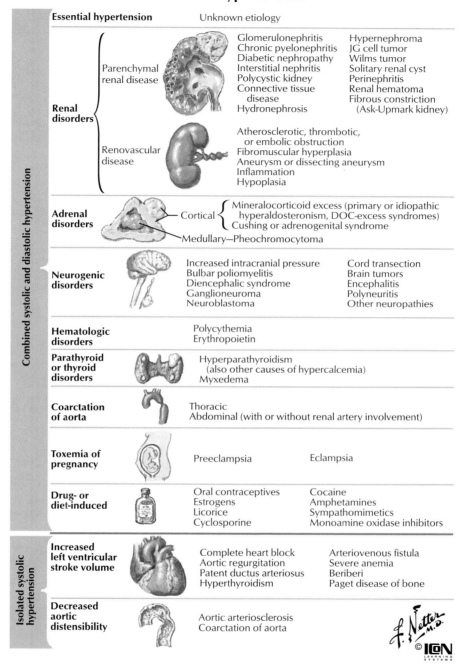

Combined systolic and diastolic hypertension

Essential hypertension — Unknown etiology

Renal disorders

Parenchymal renal disease

Glomerulonephritis
Chronic pyelonephritis
Diabetic nephropathy
Interstitial nephritis
Polycystic kidney
Connective tissue
  disease
Hydronephrosis

Hypernephroma
JG cell tumor
Wilms tumor
Solitary renal cyst
Perinephritis
Renal hematoma
Fibrous constriction
  (Ask-Upmark kidney)

Renovascular disease

Atherosclerotic, thrombotic,
  or embolic obstruction
Fibromuscular hyperplasia
Aneurysm or dissecting aneurysm
Inflammation
Hypoplasia

Adrenal disorders

Cortical — Mineralocorticoid excess (primary or idiopathic
  hyperaldosteronism, DOC-excess syndromes)
  Cushing or adrenogenital syndrome
Medullary—Pheochromocytoma

Neurogenic disorders

Increased intracranial pressure
Bulbar poliomyelitis
Diencephalic syndrome
Ganglioneuroma
Neuroblastoma

Cord transection
Brain tumors
Encephalitis
Polyneuritis
Other neuropathies

Hematologic disorders

Polycythemia
Erythropoietin

Parathyroid or thyroid disorders

Hyperparathyroidism
  (also other causes of hypercalcemia)
Myxedema

Coarctation of aorta

Thoracic
Abdominal (with or without renal artery involvement)

Toxemia of pregnancy

Preeclampsia   Eclampsia

Drug- or diet-induced

Oral contraceptives
Estrogens
Licorice
Cyclosporine

Cocaine
Amphetamines
Sympathomimetics
Monoamine oxidase inhibitors

Isolated systolic hypertension

Increased left ventricular stroke volume

Complete heart block
Aortic regurgitation
Patent ductus arteriosus
Hyperthyroidism

Arteriovenous fistula
Severe anemia
Beriberi
Paget disease of bone

Decreased aortic distensibility

Aortic arteriosclerosis
Coarctation of aorta

determining the level of blood pressure and searching for evidence of target organ disease or identifiable causes of hypertension. Important facets of the examination include:

· Careful measurement of blood pressure;

· Measurement of height and weight;

· Fundoscopic examination for hypertensive retinopathy;

· Examination of the neck for carotid bruits, elevated jugular venous pressure, and thyromegaly;

- Examination of the heart for abnormalities of the apical impulse or the presence of extra heart sounds or murmurs;
- Examination of the abdomen for bruits, enlarged kidneys, and other masses; and
- Examination of the extremities for diminished arterial pulsations or peripheral edema.

Laboratory studies are recommended to determine the presence of target organ damage and other cardiovascular risk factors, and to exclude identifiable causes of hypertension. These include:

- Complete blood count;
- Serum concentrations of potassium, creatinine, thyroid stimulating hormone, fasting glucose, and high density lipoprotein and total cholesterol;
- Urinalysis for blood, protein, glucose, and microscopic examination;
- An electrocardiogram.

Detection and diagnosis of hypertension begin with the accurate measurement of blood pressure. Measurements should be acquired at each health care encounter, with follow-up determinations at intervals based on the initial blood pressure level. Accurate equipment and utilization of a standardized technique are critical. In many patients, home blood pressure monitoring may help in establishing baseline blood pressure levels or evaluating the response to therapy. Twenty-

Table 21-3
Indications for Considering Testing for Identifiable Causes of Hypertension

- Age of onset of hypertension <20 years or >50 years
- Target organ damage at presentation
  - Serum creatinine concentration >1.5 mg/dl
  - Left ventricular hypertrophy by electrocardiography
- Presence of features indicative of secondary causes
  - Hypokalemia
  - Abdominal bruit
  - Labile pressures with tachycardia, sweating, and tremor
  - Family history of renal disease
- Poor response to generally effective therapy

four-hour ambulatory blood pressure monitoring may be useful in cases of unusual variability between visits, suspected "white-coat" hypertension, symptoms suggesting hypotensive episodes, or hypertension resistant to medication.

MANAGEMENT AND THERAPY

The principal goal in treatment of hypertension is to reduce the risk of cardiovascular morbidity and mortality. The approach to therapy in an individual should be determined largely by the absolute risk of a cardiovascular event, based on

Table 21-4
Risk Stratification and Treatment of Hypertension in Adults

Blood pressure stage (mmHg)	Risk Group A	Risk Group B	Risk Group C
High normal 130-139/85-89	Lifestyle modification	Lifestyle modification	Drug therapy if heart failure, diabetes, or renal insufficiency; lifestyle modification
Stage 1 140-159/90-99	Lifestyle modification for up to 12 months	Lifestyle modification for up to 6 months; consider drugs as part of initial therapy in patients with multiple risk factors	Drug therapy and lifestyle modification
Stages 2 and 3	Drug therapy and lifestyle modification	Drug therapy and lifestyle modification	Drug therapy and lifestyle modification

Risk group A – no risk factors, target organ damage, or clinical cardiovascular disease.
Risk group B – at least one risk factor (not including diabetes), no target organ damage or clinical cardiovascular disease.
Risk group C – target organ damage and/or clinical cardiovascular disease and/or diabetes, with or without other risk factors.
With permission from The sixth report of the Joint National Committee on Prevention, Detection, Evaluation, and Treatment of High Blood Pressure. *Arch Intern Med.* 1997;157:2413-2446.

the presence of major cardiovascular risk factors, clinical cardiovascular disease, or target organ damage. Table 21-4 shows recommended hypertension treatment strategies based on the presence or absence of cardiovascular risk factors or target organ damage.

Patients with diabetes mellitus, clinical cardiovascular disease, or target organ damage are at highest risk of cardiovascular events. Pharmacological therapy should be considered for these individuals when blood pressure is mildly elevated or in the high normal range, with a treatment goal of normalizing the pressure (i.e., <130/80 mmHg). Lower-risk patients may benefit from a period of observation and lifestyle modification, using medical therapy if the average systolic pressure exceeds 140 mmHg or diastolic pressure exceeds 90 mmHg over months of monitoring.

Lifestyle modifications are an important component of the therapy for high blood pressure. All patients with hypertension, high normal blood pressure, or a strong family history of hypertension should be encouraged to participate in regular aerobic exercise, limit alcohol intake, lose weight if overweight, and adjust diet for appropriate levels of sodium and potassium. These lifestyle changes are proven to lower blood pressure, and may reduce the need for drug therapy, enhance the effectiveness of antihypertensive drugs, and favorably influence other cardiovascular risk factors. Other measures, including smoking cessation and reduced intake of saturated fats, may further reduce cardiovascular risk.

Drug therapy is indicated if lifestyle modifications do not bring the blood pressure into the desired range. Thiazide diuretics, beta-adrenergic receptor blockers, angiotensin-converting enzyme (ACE) inhibitors, angiotensin-receptor blockers (ARBs), and calcium antagonists are appropriate first-line agents for the treatment of hypertension. Diuretics and beta-blockers are effective, well-tolerated, inexpensive, and of demonstrated efficacy in preventing cardiovascular events. They are recommended by expert panels as the drugs of choice in uncomplicated hypertension. In many patients, however, the choice of an agent is influenced by co-morbid conditions. Table 21-5 lists agents that are preferred or relatively contraindicated in specific circumstances.

In general, medical therapy should be initiated

Table 21-5
Choice of Anti-hypertensive Agent Based on Co-existent Illnesses

Indications for specific drugs

Diabetes mellitus	ACE-inhibitor or ARB
Congestive heart failure	ACE-inhibitor or ARB, beta-blocker, diuretic
Myocardial infarction	ACE-inhibitor, beta-blocker
Chronic coronary artery disease	ACE-inhibitor, beta-blocker
Renal insufficiency	ACE-inhibitor, ARB

Contraindications to specific drugs

Pregnancy	ACE-inhibitors, ARB
Renal insufficiency*	Potassium-sparing agents
Peripheral vascular disease	Beta-blockers
Gout*	Diuretics
Depression*	Beta-blockers, central alpha agonists
Reactive airway disease	Beta-blockers
2nd or 3rd degree heart block	Beta-blockers, non-dihydropyridine calcium antagonists
Hepatic insufficiency	Labetalol, methyldopa

*Relative contraindications

at low doses in an effort to minimize side effects. Based on the patient's response, the dose of the initial agent can be slowly titrated upwards, or a small dose of a second agent can be added. Effective drug combinations utilize medications from different classes and result in additive blood pressure lowering effects, while minimizing dose-dependent adverse effects. Diuretics potentiate the effect of beta-blockers, ACE-inhibitors, and ARBs; other useful combinations include dihydropyridine calcium antagonists and beta-blockers, or calcium antagonists and ACE-inhibitors. Long-acting formulations with 24-hour efficacy are preferred over shorter-acting agents because of greater patient adherence to once-daily dosing regimens, and more consistent blood pressure

Table 21-6
Agents Used for Intravenous Drug Therapy of Hypertensive Emergencies

- Nitroprusside: Preferred agent in most instances except acute coronary syndromes or pregnancy. Should be combined with beta blocker in some instances.
- Nitroglycerine: Use in acute coronary syndromes alone or combined with metoprolol or labetalol.
- Labetalol: Use as adjunctive therapy with nitroprusside or nitroglycerine. Use alone in less intensely monitored situations or treatment of postoperative hypertension.
- Enalaprilat: Use for scleroderma crisis or as adjunctive therapy in some high renin states.
- Hydralazine: May use for treatment of preeclampsia, eclampsia.
- Fenoldopam: Same indication as for nitroprusside. Useful in postoperative or post-procedure hypertension in closely monitored situations.
- Esmolol: Use in case of need for immediate, very short-acting beta blocker effect. Use for supraventricular tachycardia.

control during the course of the day.

The goal of preventing cardiovascular morbidity and mortality is usually achieved with a slow, gradual reduction of blood pressure, maintained over many years. Occasionally, a hypertensive crisis may occur and blood pressure must be reduced urgently. A hypertensive crisis is defined as acute organ dysfunction of the cardiovascular or nervous system accompanied either by a marked absolute elevation of blood pressure, or an abrupt increase in blood pressure in a previously normotensive individual. The initial therapy for hypertensive crisis may involve use of intravenous medications in an intensive care unit setting (Table 21-6).

FUTURE DIRECTIONS

The past half-century has witnessed remarkable advances in the understanding of the pathophysiology, epidemiology, and natural history of hypertension, as well as dramatic advances in therapy. Nevertheless, many patients with hypertension are undiagnosed or inadequately treated, and high blood pressure remains an important contributor to coronary events, congestive heart failure, stroke, and end-stage kidney disease.

Future research and public health initiatives should be directed at achieving the following objectives:

- To ascertain the most effective antihypertensive agents in reducing cardiovascular end points in patients with uncomplicated hypertension.
- To more accurately define treatment thresholds and optimal target blood pressures in patients with diabetes mellitus or with target organ damage.
- To determine the treatment threshold and optimal target blood pressure in elderly patients with isolated systolic hypertension.
- To develop more effective drugs for treating elderly patients with isolated systolic hypertension.
- To develop better strategies to improve patient compliance.
- To decrease the content of sodium and fat in American diets.
- To improve screening techniques and care delivery systems.

REFERENCES

The sixth report of the Joint National Committee on Prevention, Detection, Evaluation, and Treatment of High Blood Pressure. *Arch Intern Med.* 1997;157:2413–2446.

1999 World HealthOrganization-International Society of Hypertension Guidelines for the Management of Hypertension. Guidelines Subcommittee. *J Hypertens.* 1999;17:151–183.

Kannel WB. Blood pressure as a cardiovascular risk factor: prevention and treatment. JAMA. 1996;275:1571-1576.

Kaplan NM, Lieberman E, Neal W. *Kaplan's Clinical Hypertension.* 8th ed. Philadelphia, Pa: Lippincott Williams & Wilkins; 2002.

Neal B, McMahon S, Chapman N, and the Blood Pressure Lowering Treatment Trialists' Collaboration. Effects of ACE inhibitors, calcium antagonists, and other blood-pressure-lowering drugs: results of prospectively designed overviews of randomized trials. Blood Pressure Lowering Treatment Trialists' Collaboration. *Lancet.* 2000;356:1955–1964.

Psaty BM, Smith NL, Siscovick DS, et al. Health outcomes associated with antihypertensive therapies used as first-line agents. A systematic review and meta-analysis. *JAMA.* 1997;277:739–745.

Chapter 22

Hypertension in the Elderly

Debra L. Bynum and M. Janette Busby-Whitehead

Hypertension is extremely common in the elderly population, with a prevalence of 54% in persons between the ages of 65 and 74. Isolated systolic hypertension is present in 65% of all hypertensive patients older than 60 and has a prevalence of 10% in those older than 70 and up to 20% in those older than 80. In the elderly, data indicate that systolic blood pressure and "pulse pressure" (difference between the systolic and diastolic pressures) are better indicators of future cardiovascular events than diastolic blood pressure alone. Thus, in the elderly, systolic hypertension is as important a contributor to end organ damage as combined systolic and diastolic hypertension.

The increased overall risk of cardiovascular events in the elderly and the absolute risk reductions achieved with treatment underscore the importance of diagnosing and treating hypertension in this age group.

ETIOLOGY AND PATHOGENESIS

Differences in the etiology of hypertension in the elderly compared with younger age groups are not clear, particularly in regard to isolated systolic hypertension. Most cases of combined systolic and diastolic hypertension occur by the age of 55, suggesting that the pathophysiology of this type of hypertension is similar in these two age groups. Differences seen in the elderly include lower renin levels, higher sensitivity to sodium, and increased peripheral vascular resistance resulting from blood vessels that are less compliant with a loss of elasticity and increased atherosclerotic changes. Diminished beta-adrenergic responsiveness, reduced baroreceptor sensitivity, reduced glomerular filtration rates, and decreased ability to maximally excrete sodium contribute to the development of hypertension and affect treatment responses to specific agents in an older population.

CLINICAL PRESENTATION

Many patients do not manifest specific clinical symptoms; in fact, most are asymptomatic. Those with end organ damage may experience dyspnea or chest pain on exertion. Some present with transient ischemic attacks, which reflect damage to the cerebrovascular circulation (Figure 22-1).

DIFFERENTIAL DIAGNOSIS

"Pseudohypertension," falsely high sphygmomanometer readings secondary to decreased arterial wall compliance and increased vascular stiffness, is due to advanced atherosclerotic changes in the upper extremities. This condition should be considered in older persons with persistently elevated blood pressure measurements, no evidence of end-organ damage, and near-syncopal symptoms with therapy. The diagnosis of "pseudohypertension" requires invasive testing with intra-arterial measurement of blood pressure.

In addition, there is evidence of an increased prevalence of "white-coat" hypertension in the elderly, especially among women. Blood pressure measurements taken during clinic visits may greatly exceed those taken at home or after the patient has had time to relax. The noncompliant aging vascular tree probably makes elders more susceptible to labile blood pressure swings. Vigilance for this condition helps to avoid unwarranted pharmacologic treatment.

Secondary causes of hypertension are uncommon and account for only 1% to 5% of all cases within this group. Further evaluation for secondary causes is indicated with documented new onset and pronounced hypertension, difficulty in controlling blood pressure (especially diastolic) despite use of 3 or more drugs, or evidence of accelerated hypertension with end-organ damage. Renal artery stenosis (RAS) is the most common of the secondary causes in this age group (Figure 22-2).

Figure 22-1

Hypertension in the Elderly

The diagnosis of hypertension for all adults is based on the finding of systolic blood pressure of over 140 mmHg with diastolic blood pressure of over 90 mmHg, after two or more readings. Each reading must be performed after the person has been sitting for 3 minutes. A single reading with systolic blood pressure of over 210 mmHg or diastolic blood pressure of over 120 mmHg is consistent with hypertension

Etiology and pathogenesis

Clinical presentation

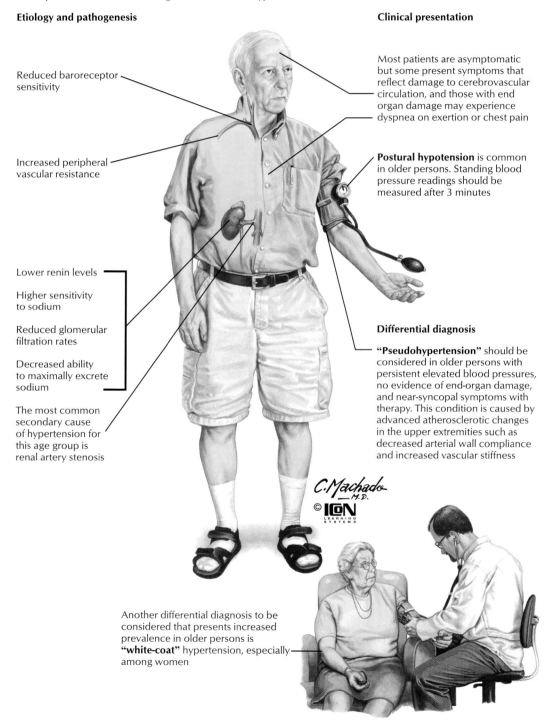

Reduced baroreceptor sensitivity

Increased peripheral vascular resistance

Lower renin levels

Higher sensitivity to sodium

Reduced glomerular filtration rates

Decreased ability to maximally excrete sodium

The most common secondary cause of hypertension for this age group is renal artery stenosis

Most patients are asymptomatic but some present symptoms that reflect damage to cerebrovascular circulation, and those with end organ damage may experience dyspnea on exertion or chest pain

Postural hypotension is common in older persons. Standing blood pressure readings should be measured after 3 minutes

Differential diagnosis

"Pseudohypertension" should be considered in older persons with persistent elevated blood pressures, no evidence of end-organ damage, and near-syncopal symptoms with therapy. This condition is caused by advanced atherosclerotic changes in the upper extremities such as decreased arterial wall compliance and increased vascular stiffness

Another differential diagnosis to be considered that presents increased prevalence in older persons is **"white-coat"** hypertension, especially among women

C.Machado
—M.D.
© ICON
LEARNING SYSTEMS

Figure 22-2

Varieties of Renal Artery Disease Which May Induce Hypertension

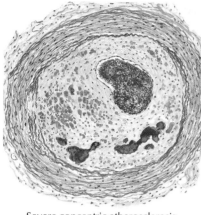

Severe concentric atherosclerosis of renal artery with lipid deposition and calcification, complicated by thrombosis (composite, x 12)

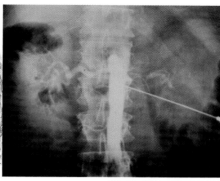

Translumbar aortogram and renal arteriogram, revealing atherosclerotic and thrombotic occlusion of r. renal artery

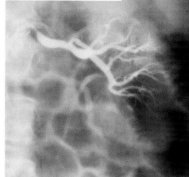

Selective arteriogram demonstrating asymmetrical narrowing of proximal l. renal artery by atherosclerotic plaque

Intimal fibroplasia in renal artery close to aorta in an infant (Verhoeff–Van Gieson stain, x 55)

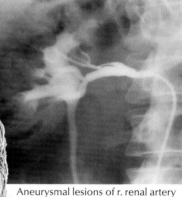

Aneurysmal lesions of r. renal artery

Intimal fibroplasia in branch of renal artery:
L=Lumen of artery
A=Cavity of dissecting aneurysm
(Verhoeff–Van Gieson stain, x 18)

DIAGNOSTIC APPROACH

The diagnosis of hypertension is based on the classification system used by the Joint National Committee for all adults (systolic blood pressure measurement greater than 140 mmHg with a diastolic blood pressure measurement greater than 90 mmHg). Isolated systolic hypertension is a systolic blood pressure measurement greater than 140 mmHg with a diastolic blood pressure measurement less than 90 mmHg. Hypertension is diagnosed based on two or more readings with an appropriately sized cuff, after the person has been sitting for 3 minutes. A single reading with a systolic blood pressure measurement greater than 210 mmHg or a diastolic blood pressure measurement greater than 120 mmHg indicates hypertension. Multiple readings are important in elders, because variations seem to be more common than in younger persons. Postural hypotension is common in elders, so blood pressure should be measured after the patient has been standing for 3 minutes; those measurements should be considered in initiating or altering treatment.

MANAGEMENT AND THERAPY

Nonpharmacologic management includes lifestyle modifications such as weight loss, decreased alcohol intake, exercise, reduced dietary sodium intake to less than 2.4 g/daily, and adequate potassium intake (90 mmol/daily). Health-care providers should emphasize control of cardiovascular risk factors including smoking cessation and cholesterol reduction.

There is strong evidence that pharmacological treatment of hypertension, including isolated systolic hypertension, reduces cardiovascular events including strokes and heart failure. Several large clinical trials and meta-analyses demonstrate reductions in cardiovascular events in the elderly with treatment. A 1994 meta-analysis by Insua et al found an overall reduction in all-cause mortality of 12%, with a 36% reduction in stroke mortality, a 25% reduction in coronary heart disease mortality, a 15% decrease in coronary morbidity, and a 35% reduction in stroke morbidity.

Staessen et al recently did a meta-analysis examining the risks and benefits of treatment for isolated systolic hypertension in the elderly. Treatment decreased total mortality by 13%, cardiovascular mortality by 18%, all cardiovascular complications by 26%, stroke by 30%, and coronary events by 23%. Greater benefits were seen in men, patients older than 70, and in those with prior cardiovascular complications.

The treatment of hypertension in the very old has been an area of controversy. Gueyffier et al performed a subgroup meta-analysis of randomized controlled trials in patients older than age 80. They found that treatment was associated with a lower risk of stroke, preventing one stroke per every 100 patients treated for 1 year. Rates of major cardiovascular events and heart failure decreased by 22% and 39%, respectively. No mortality benefit was observed; however, the benefit observed for nonfatal events more than justifies treatment of hypertension in the very elderly. Quality of life and the reduction in stroke events in this age group are as important as a reduction in all-cause mortality.

Diuretics, beta-blockers, and angiotensin-converting enzyme inhibitors are first-line agents, and selection depends on the patient's risk profile and other co-morbidities. Angiotensin receptor blockers tend to be well tolerated and can also be useful for the treatment of hypertension in elderly patients. A stepwise approach to treatment and target blood pressure goals are similar to those recommended for younger adults.

FUTURE DIRECTIONS

Knowledge of how to best treat hypertension in the elderly will grow as the prevalence of the disease within this age group is recognized and trials are designed specifically for these patients. Several large trials, including the Systolic Hypertension in the Elderly trial, the European Working Party on High Blood Pressure in the Elderly, Hypertension in Elderly Patients in Primary Care, and the Swedish Trial in Old Patients with Hypertension are ongoing and should help answer questions about effective treatment.

REFERENCES

Bennet NE. Hypertension in the elderly. *Lancet.* 1994;344:447–449.

Chrysant SG. Treatment of white coat hypertention. Current *Hypertension reports.* 2000 2(4):412–417.

Gueyffier F, Bulpitt C, Boissel JP, et al. Antihypertensive drugs in very old people: a subgroup meta-analysis of randomized controlled trials. INDIANA Group. *Lancet.* 1999;353:793–796.

Insua JT, Sacks HS, Lau TS, et al. Drug treatment of hypertension in the elderly: a meta-analysis. *Ann Intern Med.* 1994;121:355–362.

Staessen JA, Gasowski J, Wang JG, et al. Risks of untreated and treated isolated systolic hypertension in the elderly: the meta-analysis of outcome trials. *Lancet.* 2000;355:865–872.

Chapter 23

Hypertension Secondary to Renovascular Diseases

Romulo E. Colindres and Steven H. Grossman

Up to 20% of middle-age men and women in the United States have high blood pressure. In 90% to 95% of these patients the cause of the hypertension is unknown. This is termed essential or primary hypertension. The remaining 5% to 10% of the general population who have hypertension have an identifiable cause for the elevated blood pressure, with a defined pathophysiology and, in some instances, unique clinical or laboratory findings. This is called secondary hypertension. There is a strong incentive for diagnosing secondary forms of hypertension, since in many instances the cause of the hypertension can be eliminated or treated with a specific drug, procedure, or surgical intervention. Furthermore, early diagnosis of these conditions is of paramount importance, since most studies have shown that the longer secondary hypertension remains untreated, the less likely the hypertension can be cured. Secondary hypertension is more common in older people because of the higher incidence and prevalence of two frequent forms of secondary hypertension: renal parenchymal disease and atherosclerotic renal artery stenosis (ARAS).

There are several primary diseases of the renal artery that cause renal artery stenosis (RAS); the most common are atherosclerosis and fibromuscular dysplasia (FMD). The former accounts for approximately 80% to 90% of cases of RAS, while FMD accounts for 10% to 20% of such cases. Atherosclerotic RAS is associated with atherosclerosis of the abdominal aorta and other arteries. The atheroma usually narrows the lumen of the proximal third of one or both renal arteries; the ostium is involved in approximately 75% of cases. FMD is characterized by fibrous changes in the wall of the distal two-thirds of one or both renal arteries and their branches. This condition affects the media of the arteries in the majority of subjects, although in some individuals the disease involves only the intima or the adventitia of the vessel wall.

ETIOLOGY AND PATHOGENESIS

Atherosclerotic RAS is caused by the same factors that cause generalized atherosclerosis obliterans: smoking, dyslipidemia, hypertension, glucose intolerance, genetic predisposition, and other factors. The etiology of the fibrous changes that occur in the young patients with FMD are unknown. Possible causes include diseases of the vasa vasorum, genetic predisposition, and hormonal factors. There is evidence that smoking can worsen this condition. Hypertension caused by atherosclerotic RAS or FMD is caused by a decrease in renal perfusion pressure and is termed renovascular hypertension (RVH). Renovascular hypertension occurs in the presence of one or more high-grade stenoses, defined as a 60% or greater reduction of the lumen of the main renal artery or its branches and accounts for about 3% of cases of hypertension. High-grade RAS does not always cause hypertension, and even when hypertension and high-grade RAS coexist, the RAS may be incidental and the subject may have essential or another type of secondary hypertension. RAS is more common than renovascular hypertension. Figure 23-1 depicts the events leading to hypertension in the presence of high-grade unilateral RAS. Bilateral atherosclerotic RAS, or atherosclerotic RAS in a solitary kidney, can cause a decrease in excretory function of the kidney with the development of chronic renal failure. This is called ischemic nephropathy.

CLINICAL PRESENTATION

Atherosclerotic RAS may be silent, or may cause renovascular hypertension, ischemic nephropathy or both. Ischemic nephropathy can occasionally occur in the absence of hypertension. A syndrome related to renovascular hypertension and ischemic

Figure 23-1

Pathophysiology of Renovascular Hypertension in Unilateral Renal Artery Stenosis

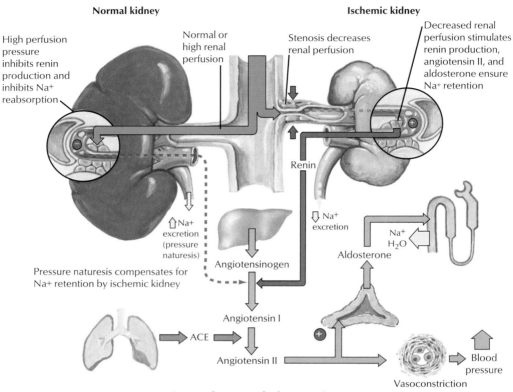

Normal kidney

High perfusion pressure inhibits renin production and inhibits Na⁺ reabsorption

Normal or high renal perfusion

Stenosis decreases renal perfusion

Ischemic kidney

Decreased renal perfusion stimulates renin production, angiotensin II, and aldosterone ensure Na⁺ retention

Renin

$\uparrow$Na⁺ excretion (pressure naturesis)

$\downarrow$ Na⁺ excretion

Na⁺ H₂O

Aldosterone

Pressure naturesis compensates for Na⁺ retention by ischemic kidney

Angiotensinogen

Angiotensin I

ACE

Angiotensin II

+

Vasoconstriction

Blood pressure

Causes of renovascular hypertension

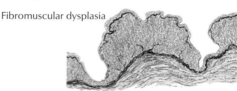

Atherosclerotic renal artery stenosis (RAS)

Fibromuscular dysplasia

Severe concentric atherosclerosis of renal artery with lipid deposition, calcification and thrombosis

Longitudinal section fibromuscular dysplasia demonstrating variations in mural thickness

Atherosclerosis is most common cause of renal artery stenosis

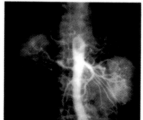

Renal arteriogram is "gold standard" in diagnosis and assessment of severity of renal artery stenosis

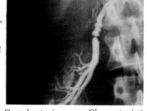

Aortorenogram. Atherosclerotic narrowing and poststenotic dilation of both renal arteries

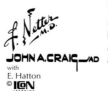

Renal arteriogram. Characteristic beaded appearance caused by alternate stenosis and aneurysmal dilations.

F. Netter M.D.

JOHN A. CRAIG—AD

with
E. Hatton
© ICON
LEARNING SYSTEMS

Figure 23-2

Captopril Renogram

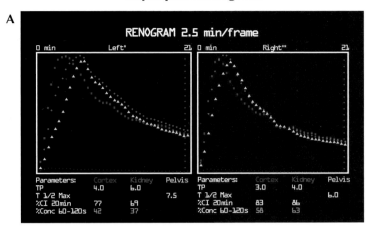

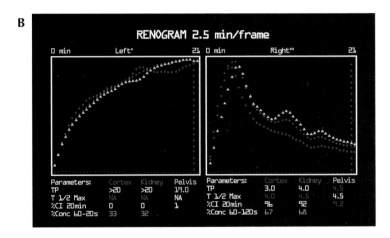

Uptake and excretion of Tc-99m mertiatide, given I.V., by the left and right kidney before (panel A), and after (panel B), oral administration of 50 mg of captopril. Panel B shows slow uptake and no excretion of the radiopharmaceutical, suggesting functionally significant stenosis of the left renal artery. Panel C shows a high grade atherosclerotic RAS of the left renal artery with poststenotic dilation in the same patient. The right renal artery is normal. Note the atherosclerotic changes of the abdominal aorta.

* Left kidney
** Right kidney

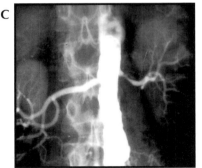

nephropathy is "flash" pulmonary edema, acute pulmonary edema that develops abruptly.

Atherosclerotic RAS occurs in older patients. Approximately 90% of patients are or have been heavy smokers. Most have evidence of atherosclerosis in other vascular beds. There may be abrupt onset of hypertension, or worsening of existing hypertension, or development of malignant hypertension after the age of 50 years. Physical examination may show advanced retinopathy, an abdominal or flank bruit, and pulse deficits or bruits over major arteries. Laboratory studies

Figure 23-3

Evaluation for Renal Artery Stenosis
in Subjects with Compatible Clinical Picture
and Predicted Benefit of Revascularization

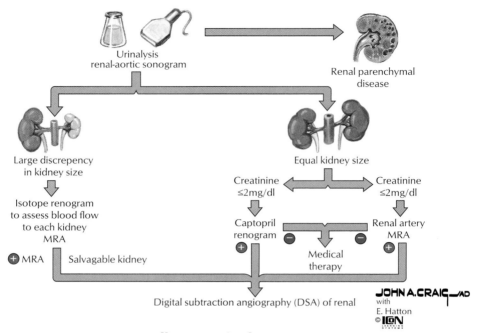

Urinalysis
renal-aortic sonogram

Renal parenchymal
disease

Large discrepency
in kidney size

Equal kidney size

Isotope renogram
to assess blood flow
to each kidney
MRA

Creatinine
≤2mg/dl

Creatinine
≤2mg/dl

⊕ MRA   Salvagable kidney

Captopril
renogram
⊕ ⊖

Medical
therapy

Renal artery
MRA
⊖ ⊕

Digital subtraction angiography (DSA) of renal

JOHN A. CRAIG—AD
with
E. Hatton
© ICN

Figure 23-4

Balloon Angioplasty
of Stenotic Renal Arteries

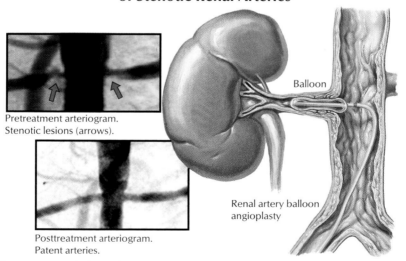

Pretreatment arteriogram.
Stenotic lesions (arrows).

Balloon

Posttreatment arteriogram.
Patent arteries.

Renal artery balloon
angioplasty

Patients with hypertension and atherosclerotic renal artery stenosis most likely to respond to balloon angioplasty are those with onset of hypertension within the past 5 years those without primary renal disease, and middle-aged men with atherosclerotic renal artery stenosis and malignant hypertension not caused by primary renal disease. A positive captopril renogram predicts cure or improvement of hypertension after revascularization.

C. Machado
—M.D.
© ICN

may show hypokalemia caused by elevated plasma renin activity (secondary aldosteronism) and elevation of serum creatinine concentration caused by ischemic nephropathy or other associated kidney diseases. There may be a large discrepancy in kidney size.

Renal artery stenosis caused by FMD presents as renovascular hypertension starting at a young age. The disease is more common in women younger than 50, and also occurs in children. An abdominal bruit may be present, but peripheral pulses are normal. Laboratory studies may show hypokalemia. A large discrepancy in kidney size is unusual. Fibromuscular dysplasia does not cause ischemic nephropathy or "flash" pulmonary edema.

DIFFERENTIAL DIAGNOSIS

The main differential diagnosis of renovascular hypertension caused by atherosclerotic RAS is essential and other types of secondary hypertension, particularly renal parenchymal disease. In older people with peripheral vascular disease or abdominal aortic disease, the prevalence of atherosclerotic RAS is as high as 38% to 55%. The prevalence of essential hypertension in this population is approximately 60%. Therefore, it is often difficult to establish whether atherosclerotic RAS in this setting is causing the hypertension or is an incidental occurrence, perhaps related to longstanding hypertension with consequent atherosclerosis. Correction of the stenosis in the latter situation would not lead to cure or improvement of hypertension. Renal failure caused by atherosclerotic RAS must be distinguished from renal failure resulting from renal parenchymal disease such as small vessel disease (nephrosclerosis or atheroembolic disease), or other diseases such as diabetic nephropathy. Characteristics of ischemic nephropathy are minimal proteinuria, scant urine sediment, and frequently a large discrepancy in kidney size.

The differential diagnosis of renovascular hypertension caused by FMD includes other causes of hypertension in children or young women: essential hypertension, subtle renal disease, obesity-related hypertension, endocrine hypertension, and coarctation of the aorta.

DIAGNOSTIC APPROACH

The gold standard for the diagnosis of RAS is a renal arteriogram, which permits an assessment of the degree of stenosis and shows the characteristic atherosclerotic involvement of the proximal third of the renal artery in atherosclerotic RAS. The most common form of FMD, medial fibroplasia (75%), has characteristic areas of stenoses alternating with aneurysmal dilatations ("string of pearls" image) in the distal renal artery, sometimes extending to the branches of the main renal artery. A renal arteriogram is an expensive and invasive test with associated discomforts and risks, and generally provides no information about the functional significance of the lesion. In view of these limitations, several screening tests for the detection of RAS or assessment of its functional significance have been developed (Table 23-1).

None of the anatomical screening tests is adequate to evaluate the distal renal artery; therefore, there is no adequate screening test for FMD, although a captopril renogram may suggest the presence of functionally significant RAS (Figure 23-2). Figure 23-3 shows a diagnostic scheme to evaluate subjects suspected of having RAS. Look for unsuspected renal parenchymal disease with renal sonography and urinalysis as a first step in the evaluation. Screening evaluation is limited to patients who have a compatible clinical picture *and* who are likely to benefit from revascularization of the renal artery(ies). There is no functional test that predicts improvement of renal function after revascularization.

MANAGEMENT AND THERAPY

The treatment of RAS can be divided into medical treatment and surgical or endovascular revascularization. Endovascular revascularization consists of balloon angioplasty with or without placement of a vascular stent (Figure 23-4). Medical treatment consists of antihypertensive therapy, smoking cessation, aspirin, and lipid-lowering drugs. The treatment of choice for young people with FMD is balloon angioplasty. If the balloon can reach the lesion, dilatation is usually successful and hypertension is cured or greatly improved in about 90% of patients. Randomized clinical trials of older patients with atherosclerotic RAS and hypertension have suggested that medical therapy is as effective as angioplasty and stent placement for treating hypertension. The patients with atherosclerotic RAS most likely to respond to balloon angioplasty with cure or marked improvement are

Table 23-1
Screening Tests for Renal Artery Stenosis

Test	Type of Assessment	Features
Captopril renogram	Functional: ACE-inhibitor induced reduction of GFR	High sensitivity/specificity. If kidneys equal size, SCr <2 mg/daily. Prognosis value for improvement of HTN.
MRA-renal arteries	Anatomical: proximal renal arteries	No nephrotoxicity
Doppler ultrasound of renal arteries	Anatomical: proximal renal arteries	Highly variable results; technically difficult; operator-dependent
Spiral computed tomographic angiography	Anatomical: proximal renal arteries	Large volume of contrast dye

Abbreviations: MRA, resonance angiography; ACE, angiotensin converting enzyme; GFR, glomerular filtration rate; SCr, serum creatinine concentration; HTN, hypertension

those who have had onset of hypertension within the past 5 years and do not have primary renal disease, and middle-aged men with atherosclerotic RAS and malignant hypertension not caused by primary renal disease. A positive captopril scan is a good predictor of cure or improvement of hypertension after revascularization.

Atherosclerotic RAS may be a cause of end-stage renal disease. Several studies have suggested that 11% to 22% of older people reaching end-stage renal disease have high-grade atherosclerotic RAS in at least one renal artery. No major clinical trials have compared medical treatment to balloon angioplasty of the renal artery for preserving or improving renal function. Only a minority of patients with atherosclerotic RAS and renal failure appear to benefit long-term from relief of the stenosis with angioplasty. Therefore, identify those subjects who are not likely to benefit from the procedure or who may be harmed by it. Factors that predict lack of improvement, or worsening of renal function with correction of high-grade atherosclerotic RAS are: 1) low grade stenosis with reduction in luminal diameter of less than 50% in at least one renal artery; 2) unilateral RAS unless the artery supplies a solitary kidney; 3) kidney length less than 8 cm; 4) presence of diabetic nephropathy or other known kidney diseases, or severe proteinuria accompanied by an "active" urine sediment suggestive of a primary renal disease; and 5) a high resistive index as determined with Doppler ultrasonography.

FUTURE DIRECTIONS

We believe that continued progress in the diagnosis and treatment of atherosclerotic RAS in the coming years will require:

· Continued technical improvement of balloon angioplasty and vascular stents;
· Development of noninvasive imaging techniques for assessment of the distal renal artery and its branches;
· Development of better functional tests to predict the effects of renal artery revascularization on blood pressure and renal function;
· Development of markers to detect diseases of the small arteries and arterioles of the kidney;
· Randomized clinical trials to compare the effect of revascularization of the renal arteries with medical therapy on the progression of chronic renal failure; and
· Development of new drugs to treat atherosclerosis and continued promotion of public health measures to decrease risk factors for atherosclerosis.

REFERENCES

Alcazar JM, Rodicio JL. Ischemic nephropathy: clinical characteristics and treatment. *Am J Kidney Dis.* 2000;36:883-893.

Pedersen EB. New tools in diagnosing renal artery stenosis. *Kidney Int.* 2000;57:2657–2677.

Radermacher J, Chavan A, Bleck J, et al. Use of Doppler ultrasonography to predict the outcome of therapy for renal-artery stenosis. *N Engl J Med.* 2001;344:410–417.

Safian RD, Textor SC. Renal-artery stenosis. *N Engl J Med.* 2001;344:431–442.

Chapter 24

Hypertension Secondary to Diseases of the Adrenal Gland

Romulo E. Colindres and Steven H. Grossman

Diseases of the adrenal gland are clinically important causes of secondary hypertension. In this chapter, we review their clinical presentation, evaluation, and therapy. Renovascular hypertension, another cause of secondary hypertension, is reviewed in Chapter 23.

The adrenal cortex can cause hypertension through overproduction of aldosterone, deoxycorticosterone (DOC), and cortisol. The first two are mineralocorticoid hormones that cause increased salt and water retention by the kidney. Cortisol is a glucocorticoid. When hypersecretion is marked, it can stimulate mineralocorticoid receptors and can be associated with release of DOC and vasoconstrictors. Pheochromocytoma is a tumor of the adrenal medulla that produces excessive quantities of catecholamines.

Identifying causes of adrenal hypertension is important because:
- Many of these disorders are curable or responsive to specific therapy;
- These conditions, particularly pheochromocytoma, are associated with the risk of severe hypertension and major cardiovascular complications, including sudden death;
- The prevalence of primary aldosteronism among individuals with hypertension may be higher than the 1% or less previously estimated;
- New syndromes of mineralocorticoid hypertension have been described or defined in the past few years; and
- Diagnostic tests for primary aldosteronism have been simplified.

PRIMARY ALDOSTERONISM/ MINERALOCORTICOID HYPERTENSION
Etiology and Pathogenesis
Table 24-1 shows the causes of mineralocorticoid hypertension and its associated syndromes, the most common of which is primary aldosteronism. The normal physiologic control of aldosterone secretion is by the renin-angiotensin system. Corticotropin (ACTH) and serum potassium concentration are less important. Hyperaldosteronism is caused by autonomous secretion of the hormone, totally or largely independent of the control of the renin-angiotensin system.

Hypertension caused by aldosterone results from increased stimulation of mineralocorticoid receptors in the collecting ducts of the kidney. This causes opening of sodium channels leading to increased tubular reabsorption of sodium, and secondary reabsorption of water. There is also increased secretion and urinary excretion of potassium and hydrogen ions. Salt and water retention causes an increase in plasma volume, and an increase in cardiac output, resulting in increased blood pressure and suppressed renin production. Total exchangeable sodium is increased, but the process is limited by a subsequent decrease in sodium reabsorption from the proximal tubule and the terminal part of the nephron under the influence of atrial natriuretic peptide and other natriuretic factors, an effect known as "aldosterone escape." The "escape" explains the lack of edema in primary aldosteronism and related syndromes. Other factors that may contribute to mineralocorticoid hypertension include central nervous system effects of aldosterone, increased sympathetic nerve activity and release of vasoconstrictive agents such as antidiuretic hormone (Figure 24-1).

Approximately 65% of patients with primary aldosteronism have a surgically curable aldosterone-producing adenoma (APA), while one-third have bilateral adrenal gland hyperplasia, a condition termed idiopathic hyperaldosteronism. Very rarely the hyperplasia can be unilateral, a condition

Figure 24-1

Primary Hyperaldosteronism/ Mineralocorticoid Hypertension

Mechanisms in Primary Aldosteronism

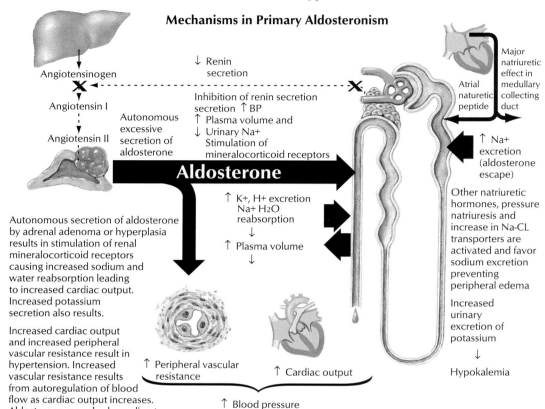

↓ Renin secretion

Angiotensinogen

Angiotensin I

Angiotensin II

Autonomous excessive secretion of aldosterone

Inhibition of renin secretion
secretion ↑ BP
↑ Plasma volume and
↓ Urinary Na+
Stimulation of mineralocorticoid receptors

Aldosterone

↑ K+, H+ excretion
Na+ H₂O reabsorption
↓
↑ Plasma volume
↓

Major natriuretic effect in medullary collecting duct

Atrial natriuretic peptide

↑ Na+ excretion (aldosterone escape)

Other natriuretic hormones, pressure natriuresis and increase in Na-CL transporters are activated and favor sodium excretion preventing peripheral edema

Increased urinary excretion of potassium
↓
Hypokalemia

Autonomous secretion of aldosterone by adrenal adenoma or hyperplasia results in stimulation of renal mineralocorticoid receptors causing increased sodium and water reabsorption leading to increased cardiac output. Increased potassium secretion also results.

Increased cardiac output and increased peripheral vascular resistance result in hypertension. Increased vascular resistance results from autoregulation of blood flow as cardiac output increases. Aldosterone may also have direct effects on the vasculature.

↑ Peripheral vascular resistance

↑ Cardiac output

↑ Blood pressure

Clinical Features

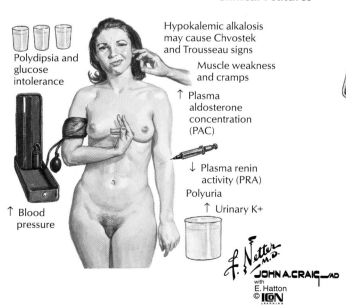

Polydipsia and glucose intolerance

Hypokalemic alkalosis may cause Chvostek and Trousseau signs

Muscle weakness and cramps

↑ Plasma aldosterone concentration (PAC)

↓ Plasma renin activity (PRA)

Polyuria

↑ Urinary K+

↑ Blood pressure

Primary aldosteronism

Plasma aldosterone concentration (PAC)   >20ng/dl

+

PAC/PRA   ≥30 : Aldosterone Renin ratio

Purpose of serum screen is to distinguish between primary aldosteronism and low renin essential hypertension

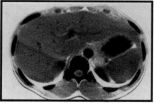

CT or MRI of adrenal glands used to select between surgically remedial APA and idiopathic hyperaldosteronism

F. Netter M.D.
JOHN A. CRAIG—AD
with
E. Hatton
© ICON

called primary adrenal hyperplasia. In glucocorticoid-remediable aldosteronism (GRA), ACTH controls secretion of aldosterone. This is an autosomal dominant disorder caused by a mutation in chromosome 8, so that aldosterone secretion is no longer under the control of angiotensin II but under the control of normal concentrations of ACTH. If ACTH secretion is inhibited with the glucocorticoid dexamethasone, aldosterone secretion decreases. Primary aldosteronism can also be caused by aldosterone-producing adrenal or ovarian carcinomas.

Clinical Presentation

The typical clinical features of primary aldosteronism are: hypertension, hypokalemia, excessive urinary excretion of potassium, suppressed plasma renin activity (PRA) and metabolic alkalosis. The symptoms of hypokalemia may include polyuria, polydipsia, muscle cramps, muscle weakness, and glucose intolerance. The hypokalemia is more severe in patients with APA than in those with idiopathic hyperaldosteronism.

The disease usually presents in middle-aged people and may be more common among women. The presence of the above symptoms in younger patients, or those with a family history of hyperaldosteronism, suggests a congenital type of mineralocorticoid-hypertension such as GRA or Liddle's syndrome. In most series, 10% to 20% of patients with primary aldosteronism may present with normokalemia. Patients with GRA frequently have a normal serum potassium concentration.

Differential Diagnosis

Primary aldosteronism should be suspected in the following circumstances:

· Hypertension with spontaneous (unprovoked) hypokalemia;
· Hypertension with severe and refractory diuretic-induced hypokalemia (serum potassium concentration <3mEq/L);
· Family history of hyperaldosteronism;
· Unexplained hypertension, refractory to treatment;
· Unexplained hypertension in children and young adults; and
· Incidentally discovered adrenal tumor.

Table 24-1
Differential Diagnosis of Mineralocorticoid Hypertension

Cause	Pathophysiology
Primary aldosteronism*	↑ Aldosterone secretion
Deoxycorticosterone-secreting tumors†	↑ DOC secretion
Congenital adrenal hyperplasia†	Congenital deficiency of enzymes needed for cortisol synthesis. ↑ ACTH secretion: ↑ DOC.
Liddle's syndrome†	Congenital upregulation of sodium channels in collecting ducts. ↑ Sodium reabsorption by kidney.
11β-hydroxysteroid dehydrogenase† deficiency/inhibition	Congenital deficiency (syndrome of AME) or inhibition (licorice) of the enzyme that converts cortisol to cortisone. ↑ Cortisol levels stimulate mineralocorticoid receptors.
S81OL mutation in minerolocorticoid receptor (MR)†	MR constitutively activated by steroids lacking 21 (OH) groups → progesterone
Ectopic ACTH syndrome**	1. ↑ Secretion of DOC 2. ↑ Cortisol: cannot all be degraded to cortisone 3. ↑ Vasoconstrictors, ↓ Vasodilators

* Causes of primary aldosteronism are discussed in the text.
Abbreviations and symbols: ↑, increased; ↓, decreased; DOC, deoxycorticosterone; ACTH, corticotrophin; AME, apparent mineralocorticoid excess; Ectopic ACTH Syndrome, production of corticotrophin by a tumor outside the pituitary gland. † aldosterone secretion inhibited, plasma renin activity suppressed. ** Aldosterone secretion inhibited, plasma renin activity variable.

Patients with hypokalemia and hypertension should have measurement of PRA. A PRA of >3ng/mL/hr suggests secondary hyperaldosteronism as seen with malignant hypertension, primary renal disease, reninoma, and estrogen use. A value of <1ng/mL/hr suggests low-renin essential hypertension or mineralocorticoid-hypertension. Under these circumstances, screening and confirmatory tests for the presence of primary aldosteronism should be performed.

Diagnostic Approach

Figure 24-2 shows a diagnostic approach for subjects with hypertension and unprovoked or severe diuretic-induced hypokalemia. The same approach can be used in evaluating difficult-to-treat hypertension of unknown etiology with normal serum potassium concentration.

The first step of the evaluation is to distinguish primary aldosteronism from low-renin essential hypertension. The measurement of plasma aldosterone concentration (PAC) and PRA in peripheral venous blood has become the most useful screening test for primary aldosteronism. A PAC >20ng/dL combined with an aldosterone: renin ratio (ARR) >30 has a sensitivity and specificity >95% for primary aldosteronism in subjects with normal renal function. A very high ARR but with normal PAC can be seen in some patients with low-renin essential hypertension; therefore, the test can only be considered to be indicative of primary aldosteronism if a high ARR coexists with a PAC >20ng/dL. False-positive results with high PAC are seen in patients with chronic renal failure and those who are taking large doses of spironolactone. Severe hypokalemia can cause a false-negative test by decreasing PAC. PAC and PRA can be measured while patients are on conventional antihypertensive medications, although diuretics and inhibitors of the renin-angiotensin system may produce false-negative results because of an increase in PRA.

The diagnosis of primary aldosteronism can be confirmed by demonstrating that secretion of aldosterone is not suppressed after an infusion of a solution of isotonic sodium chloride or ingestion of a high-salt diet. However, this confirmatory test is cumbersome and involves discomfort and risk for the patient. Most centers now consider a positive screening test enough evidence of primary aldosteronism to proceed with a CT scan or magnetic resonance imaging (MRI) of the adrenal glands to distinguish between surgically curable APA and idiopathic hyperaldosteronism.

Patients with APA have a high serum concentration of the aldosterone precursor 18-hydroxy-corticosterone [18-(OH)-B.] Thus, in addition to a CT or MRI scan, a blood sample should be obtained for measurement of 18-(OH)-B. The presence of a radiolucent adrenal adenoma, larger than 1cm in diameter on CT or MRI and a serum concentration of 18-(OH)-B >65 ng/dL is diagnostic for APA and is an indication for an adrenalectomy. Ambiguous findings in the adrenal glands or low serum levels of 18-(OH)-B require measurement of ACTH-stimulated aldosterone concentration from each adrenal vein to look for increased unilateral production of aldosterone indicative of surgically-curable primary aldosteronism. If GRA is suspected, genetic testing should be done.

Management and Therapy

The treatment of primary aldosteronism depends on the etiology of the condition as ascertained by diagnostic studies.

Surgery

Patients with APA, or with unilateral hyperplasia, should undergo adrenalectomy. For most patients this can be done by a laparoscopy approach. Patients should be treated with spironolactone, 100 to 200 mg/daily for 6 to 8 weeks before surgery, permitting correction of the hypertension and hypokalemia. This therapy also decreases extracellular fluid volume and restores the responsiveness of the renin-angiotensin system. A decrease in blood pressure predicts a good response to surgery. Approximately 65% to 70% of patients with an APA are cured of their hypertension; the remainder show improvement. The main postoperative complication is transient hypoaldosteronism with inability to conserve sodium, hypotension and mild hyperkalemia. This can be prevented by prior treatment with spironolactone and can usually be treated with a high salt intake. Persistent hypertension suggests superimposed essential hypertension or nephrosclerosis caused by long-standing hypertension.

Figure 24-2

Diagnostic Approach to Patients with Suspected Primary Aldosteronism

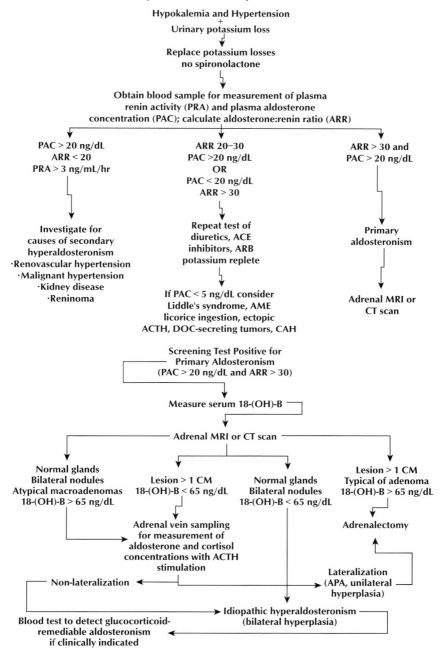

AME, syndrome of apparent mineralocorticoid excess; serum 18-(OH)-B, serum concentration of 18-hydroxycorticosterone; DOC, deoxycorticosterone; APA, aldosterone-producing adenoma; CAH, congenital adrenal hyperplasia; CT, computerized tomographic scan; ectopic ACTH, production of corticotropin by a tumor outside the pituitary gland.

Definition: lateralization=aldosterone: cortisol concentration ration in an adrenal vein 4 times greater than that in the other adrenal vein, and/or an aldosterone: cortisol concentration ratio from the vein of the unaffected adrenal that is less than the ratio in the vena cava. Urinary loss of potassium can be documented by measuring potassium excretion in a 24-hour collection of urine; excretion of more than 30 mEq per day in the presence of hypokalemia indicates potassium wasting. An alternative and simpler approach is to obtain a random sample of urine to calculate fractional excretion of potassium. A fractional excretion greater than 10% when hypokalemia is present indicates potassium wasting.

Medical Treatment

Medical treatment of bilateral adrenal hyperplasia is initiated with spironolactone, 100 to 200mg/daily, with a maximum dose of 400mg. However, painful gynecomastia and impotence in men, and menstrual irregularities in women are common at high doses. Therefore the goal should be to reduce the dose of spironolactone to 50mg/daily, with the addition of amiloride, 5 to 15mg/daily, or triamterene, 75 to 150mg/daily.

Many patients will require additional antihypertensive therapy. Drugs of choice are thiazide diuretics, calcium channel blockers, and angiotensin-converting enzyme inhibitors. The diet should be low in sodium and rich in potassium. Patients with GRA or apparent mineralocorticoid excess can be treated with 1 to 2 mg/daily of dexamethasone to suppress ACTH secretion; however, this may cause side effects and may not adequately control the hypertension. Patients with Liddle's syndrome do not respond to spironolactone, and should be treated with amiloride or triamterene and other antihypertensive drugs combined with salt restriction and potassium supplementation, as needed.

PHEOCHROMOCYTOMA
Etiology and Pathogenesis

Pheochromocytoma is a tumor, arising from adrenomedullary chromaffin cells, that produces excess secretion of catecholamines causing intermittent or sustained hypertension (Figure 24-3). These tumors account for less than 0.5% of causes of hypertension. Although rare, pheochromocytomas are important because of their potential lethality.

Clinical Presentation

Hypertension is the most common presenting feature, occurring in greater than 90% of patients. The hypertension may be severe and is usually sustained, but may be paroxysmal and associated with spells, or may present as a hypertensive emergency. The paroxysms may cause the classic symptom triad of headache, sweating, and palpitation. Other common symptoms are pallor, nausea, tremor, weakness, anxiety, epigastric pain, chest pain, flushing, and dizziness. The paroxysms may be fleeting or last for hours, and may occur spontaneously or be precipitated by activities such as lifting, straining, or stretching. The hypertension is sometimes resistant to pharmacological treatment but usually responds to alpha-adrenergic blocking agents.

Pheochromocytomas may occur at any age. Ninety-eight percent of pheochromocytomas are in the abdomen or pelvis, and 90% are in the adrenal gland; 5% to 10% are multiple, less than 10% are malignant and 10% are familial. Bilateral tumors are more likely to be familial. When extra-adrenal, the tumors are associated with chromaffin cells in paraganglia and are called paragangliomas (Figure 24-3). Pheochromocytomas may be inherited as part of the multiple endocrine neoplasm (MEN) syndromes. In MEN 2A, the pheochromocytoma is associated with medullary carcinoma of the thyroid gland and with parathyroid adenoma or hyperplasia. In MEN 2B, pheochromocytomas are also associated with neuromas of the lip and tongue, corneal nerve thickening, and marfanoid body features.

Pheochromocytomas may range in size from microscopic to kilograms in weight. The tumors are usually encapsulated. Only 10% of adrenal pheochromocytomas invade local structures or metastasize, whereas approximately 40% of extra-adrenal pheochromocytomas invade or metastasize.

Pheochromocytomas most often secrete norepinephrine and epinephrine, but rarely only one of these catecholamines. The finding of excess dopamine secretion suggests the presence of malignancy.

Differential Diagnosis

Pheochromocytoma should be considered in patients with essential hypertension and hyperadrenergic symptoms such as tachycardia, palpitations, sweating, anxiety, and panic attacks. Other syndromes with increased sympathetic nervous system activity and hypertensive crises include use of monoamine oxidase inhibitor antidepressants, clonidine or beta blocker withdrawal, ingestion of drugs with sympathomimetic effects, increased intracranial pressure, thyrotoxicosis, and angina pectoris.

Diagnostic Approach

The key to diagnosis is a high index of suspicion. Most patients who have a pheochromocytoma with a typical clinical presentation will have

Figure 24-3

Pheochromocytoma

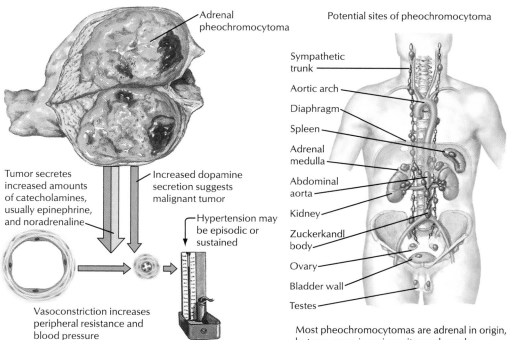

Adrenal pheochromocytoma

Potential sites of pheochromocytoma

Sympathetic trunk
Aortic arch
Diaphragm
Spleen
Adrenal medulla
Abdominal aorta
Kidney
Zuckerkandl body
Ovary
Bladder wall
Testes

Tumor secretes increased amounts of catecholamines, usually epinephrine, and noradrenaline

Increased dopamine secretion suggests malignant tumor

Hypertension may be episodic or sustained

Vasoconstriction increases peripheral resistance and blood pressure

Pheochromocytoma is a chromaffin cell tumor secreting excessive catecholamines resulting in increased peripheral vascular resistance and hypertension

Most pheochromocytomas are adrenal in origin, but can occur in various sites and may be associated with multiple endocrine neoplasia (men) syndromes. Most are sporadic, but some are hereditary.

Clinical features of pheochromocytoma

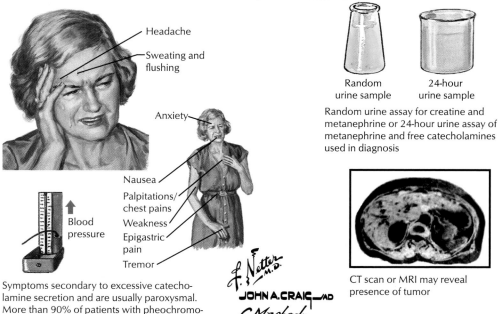

Headache

Sweating and flushing

Anxiety

Random urine sample

24-hour urine sample

Random urine assay for creatine and metanephrine or 24-hour urine assay of metanephrine and free catecholamines used in diagnosis

Nausea
Palpitations/chest pains
Weakness
Epigastric pain
Tremor

Blood pressure

Symptoms secondary to excessive catecholamine secretion and are usually paroxysmal. More than 90% of patients with pheochromocytoma have headaches, palpitations and sweating alone or in combination.

CT scan or MRI may reveal presence of tumor

Diagnostic Approach to the Patient With Suspected Pheochromocytoma

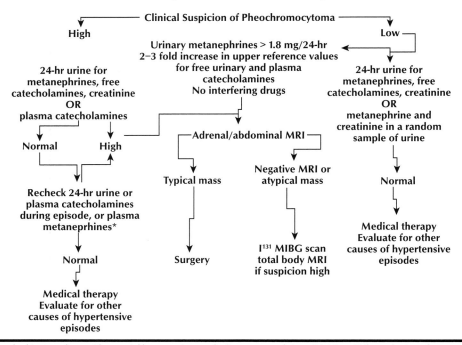

Values in normal subjects or those with essential hypertension: total urinary metanephrines=0.3-1.2 mg/24h; total urinary free catecholamines=less than 100 micrograms/24h; total urinary free catecholamines=less than 100 micrograms/24h; total plasma catecholamines=200-500 pg/ml; random urine metanephrine=0.5-1 mg/g creatinine; a value greater than 1 mg/g creatinine merits investigation with a 24 hour urine collection for measurement of total metanephrines.

MRI, magnetic reaonance imaging; −I¹³¹-MIBG scan, I¹³¹-labeled metaiodobenzylguanidine scan. *Alternative approach: when available measure plasma metanephrine levels, a test that appears to have a very high sensitivity and specificity even for small pheochromocytomas (www.catecholamine.org/labprocedures).

a positive biochemical test result. However, one third of pheochromocytomas are found incidentally. The approach to screening tests depends on the level of clinical suspicion (Figure 24-4). If there is any suspicion, and screening test results are equivocal, a different screening test should be considered. Larger tumors (greater than 1g) tend to produce more catecholamine metabolites. Measurement of 24-hour urinary metanephrine and free catecholamine levels have a diagnostic sensitivity of 70% to 90% and specificity of 80% to 100%. The adequacy of the urine collection should be ascertained by measuring creatinine excretion.

A more convenient screening test is the measurement of metanephrine and creatinine in a random, untimed urine sample. A value of >1 mg/g of creatinine is abnormal. In limited comparisons the diagnostic accuracy of this test is similar to that of 24-hour measurements of metanephrine.

Plasma catecholamines are highly specific but inconvenient to perform and somewhat less sensitive than urinary measurements. The lower sensitivity may be related to episodic secretion in most patients. However, a value of >2000 pg./mL is rarely seen in the absence of a pheochromocytoma. Values between 1000 and 2000 pg./mL require further investigation. Plasma metanephrine measurement has been reported to be highly sensitive but the assay is not yet widely available.

Once a pheochromocytoma is suspected clinically and biochemically, a radiographic approach to localization is initiated. CT or MRI depicts most pheochromocytomas; MRI is preferred because of higher specificity on T2 weighted images (Figure 24-3). Nuclear scanning with Iodine-131-metaiodobenzylguanidine (MIBG), or total-body MRI may be used when CT or abdominal-pelvic MRI results are negative in the presence of suggestive biochemical results.

Management and Therapy

Surgical removal is the definitive treatment for pheochromocytoma. During anesthesia and surgery, blood pressure may fluctuate widely. Blockade of alpha-adrenergic receptors blocks the effects of the high circulating catecholamine levels. Before elective surgery, oral phenoxybenzamine is prescribed and switched to parenteral phentolamine the day of surgery, and titrated to maintain blood pressure stability. Metyrosine has recently been approved for the short-term management of pheochromocytoma before surgery, for long-term management when surgery is contraindicated, or for treatment of chronic malignant pheochromocytoma. The drug blocks the conversion of tyrosine to dihydroxyphenylalanine, the rate-limiting step in the catecholamine biosynthetic pathway.

Once blood pressure control is attained, beta-adrenergic blocking drugs are administered to control heart rate and prevent arrhythmias, but they should not be used as the only therapy, as this would allow unopposed alpha-adrenergic stimulation. Patients with pheochromocytoma tend to be volume-depleted due to pressure natriuresis. Therefore, volume repletion is important before and during surgery.

CUSHING'S SYNDROME
Clinical Presentation

Hypertension is present in 80% of patients with Cushing's syndrome (Figure 24-5). The hypertension may be severe, and target organ damage is common. Most cases of Cushing's syndrome are caused by the administration of exogenous glucocorticoids, but hypertension is more common with the endogenous causes of hypercortisolism: primary hypersecretion of ACTH by the pituitary gland (Cushing's disease); adrenal adenoma, carcinoma, or hyperplasia; and ectopic secretion of ACTH by a non-endocrine tumor. ACTH secretion in this situation is greater than that with pituitary hypersecretion. Severe hypertension with hypokalemia and metabolic alkalosis is common with ectopic ACTH secretion.

The possible mechanisms of hypertension associated with glucocorticoid excess include stimulation of mineralocorticoid receptors with plasma volume expansion, increased cardiac output, and sodium shifts from the intracellular to the extracellular space. There is also an increase in peripheral vascular resistance caused by decreased production of vasodilator substances (nitric oxide, prostaglandins, atrial natriuretic peptide), and increased production of vasoconstrictor factors (angiotensinogen, adrenergic agents, endothelin). Increased levels of DOC and very high levels of cortisol are seen, particularly with ectopic ACTH secretion (Figure 24-5).

Differential Diagnosis

Patients presenting with hypertension, hypokalemia, and typical clinical features should be considered for evaluation. Patients with ectopic ACTH syndrome do not usually display the physical features associated with glucocorticoid excess. The main differentiation is from other causes of mineralocorticoid-associated hypertension. The approach to the diagnosis of Cushing's syndrome is presented in Chapter 29.

Management and Therapy

Medical management of the hypertension associated with glucocorticoid excess is the same as that for low-renin essential hypertension, pending possible surgical approaches. Diuretics, including potassium-sparing diuretics, are first-line therapy. Additions or substitutions are based on the blood pressure response and individual patient characteristics. The management of Cushing's syndrome is discussed in Chapter 29.

FUTURE DIRECTIONS

The next few years will see rapid advances in the diagnosis, localization, management, and genetics of adrenal hypertension. The following are key areas of interest:

- Developing imaging studies to distinguish functional from nonfunctional masses of the adrenal cortex;
- Determining the prevalence of normokalemic hyperaldosteronism;
- Continuing the study of genetic types of primary hyperaldosteronism and pheochromocytoma;
- Confirming the recently reported high sensitivity of plasma metanephrine concentrations for detecting pheochromocytoma; and
- Optimizing cost effectiveness of diagnostic imaging for pheochromocytoma and determining the role of new techniques such as positron emission tomography in the diagnostic evaluation.

Figure 24-5

Cushing's Syndrome/Mineralocorticoid Hypertension

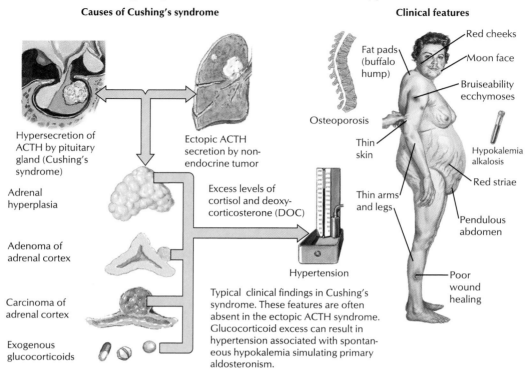

Causes of Cushing's syndrome

Hypersecretion of ACTH by pituitary gland (Cushing's syndrome)

Ectopic ACTH secretion by non-endocrine tumor

Adrenal hyperplasia

Excess levels of cortisol and deoxy-corticosterone (DOC)

Adenoma of adrenal cortex

Hypertension

Carcinoma of adrenal cortex

Exogenous glucocorticoids

Typical clinical findings in Cushing's syndrome. These features are often absent in the ectopic ACTH syndrome. Glucocorticoid excess can result in hypertension associated with spontaneous hypokalemia simulating primary aldosteronism.

Clinical features

Fat pads (buffalo hump)

Red cheeks

Moon face

Bruiseability ecchymoses

Osteoporosis

Thin skin

Hypokalemia alkalosis

Thin arms and legs

Red striae

Pendulous abdomen

Poor wound healing

Possible Mechanisms of Hypertension Associated with Glucocorticoid Excess

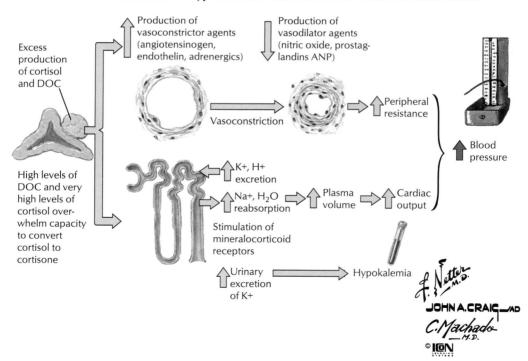

Excess production of cortisol and DOC

Production of vasoconstrictor agents (angiotensinogen, endothelin, adrenergics)

Production of vasodilator agents (nitric oxide, prostaglandins ANP)

Vasoconstriction

Peripheral resistance

Blood pressure

High levels of DOC and very high levels of cortisol overwhelm capacity to convert cortisol to cortisone

K+, H+ excretion

Na+, H_2O reabsorption

Plasma volume

Cardiac output

Stimulation of mineralocorticoid receptors

Urinary excretion of K+

Hypokalemia

F. Netter M.D.

JOHN A. CRAIG AD

C. Machado M.D.

© ICN

REFERENCES

Bornstein SR, Stratakis CA, Chrousos GP. Adrenocortical tumors: recent advances in basic concepts and clinical management..*Ann Intern Med.* 1999;130:759–771.

Lenders JW, Packa K, Walther MM, et al. Biochemical diagnosis of pheochromocytoma: which test is best? *JAMA.* 2002;-287:1427–1434.

Pacak K, Linehan WM, Eisenhofer G, Walther MM, Goldstein DS. Recent advances in genetics, diagnosis, localization, and treatment of pheochromocytoma. *Ann Intern Med.* 2001;134:315–329.

Stewart PM. Mineralocorticoid hypertension. *Lancet.* 1999;-353:1341–1347.

Pheochromocytoma and primary aldosteronism: diagnostic approaches. *Endocrinol Metab Clin North Am.* 1997;26:-801–827.

Chapter 25

Myocardial Infarction

Shane Darrah and E. Magnus Ohman

In 2002, more than 1 million Americans will have a myocardial infarction (MI). Nearly 650,000 of these will be new MIs and 450,000 will be a recurrent MI. Over 40% of people who have a MI in a given year will die from it. Up to one third of patients with acute MI will die suddenly, before reaching the hospital. This chapter will provide an overview of identification, management, and prognosis of acute MI. For a more comprehensive review, please refer to the reference section at the end of this chapter and the American Heart Association (www.americanheart.org) or the American College of Cardiology (www.acc.org) Web sites.

ETIOLOGY AND PATHOGENESIS

The vast majority of MIs are caused by atherosclerosis of the coronary arteries (Figure 25-1). Rupture of a vulnerable atherosclerotic plaque leading to thrombus formation and either complete or partial occlusion of a coronary artery at the site of the rupture has been demonstrated in numerous angiographic and autopsy studies. However, the exact mechanism leading to the rupture of an atherosclerotic plaque within the vessel lumen has yet to be established. Important events after plaque rupture that lead to thrombotic occlusion include platelet activation and thrombin generation leading to fibrin propagation. With coronary thrombosis, myocardial tissue distal to the occlusion immediately becomes ischemic due to the sudden mismatch in oxygen delivery and consumption. The physiological consequence of the anaerobic metabolism that follows include: diastolic and systolic dysfunction leading to decreased myocardial contractility and changes in conduction in the area of ischemia.

The process, if left unabated, will lead to myocardial necrosis. The longer the occlusion of the coronary artery, the more complete the necrosis. The 12-lead ECG is an invaluable tool in individuals with suspected MI, and changes in the ECG reflect the physiologic effects of myocardial ischemia. Typical changes include ST segment elevation, prolongation of conduction (QRS widening), development of Q waves, and either tachyarrhythmias or bradyarrhythmias. It is likely that arrhythmic events account for the sudden cardiac death that occurs in acute MI. In the absence of collateral blood flow, within 4 hours of the initial thrombotic event the myocardium supplied by the occluded coronary artery undergoes irreversible necrosis.

Thrombus formation can also be incomplete, resulting in diminished (but not completely absent) flow in the coronary artery involved. Although the physiological consequences are less severe they frequently also lead to reduced myocardial contractility. In this circumstance, ECG changes most commonly include ST depression and T-wave inversion rather than ST elevation. Necrosis tends to be less severe, oftentimes patchy and subendocardial rather than transmural. Severe life-threatening arrhythmias are less frequent with subendocardial infarctions.

CLINICAL PRESENTATION

The clinical presentation of myocardial infarction can range from very severe chest pain with associated symptoms to mild nonspecific symptoms, particularly in the elderly or in individuals with diabetes. In these groups, because atypical symptoms are common and the prevalence of coronary atherosclerosis is high, myocardial infarction should be considered even in the presence of minor or atypical symptoms.

The most typical presentation is of chest discomfort that is described as intense, retrosternal pressure (Figure 25-2). This pain often radiates to the left arm, or it may radiate to both arms as well as to the jaw or neck. Occasionally patients will present with pain in one of the previously-described areas without chest discomfort. Other

Figure 25-1

Atherogenesis: Unstable Plaque Formation

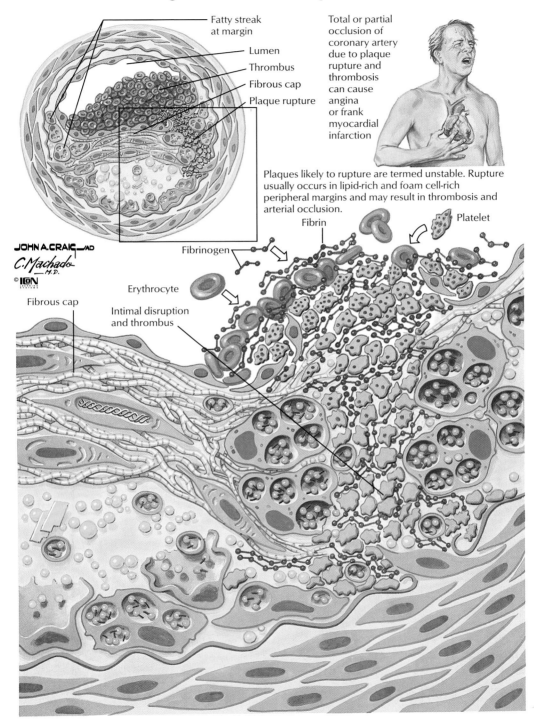

Fatty streak at margin

Lumen

Thrombus

Fibrous cap

Plaque rupture

Total or partial occlusion of coronary artery due to plaque rupture and thrombosis can cause angina or frank myocardial infarction

Plaques likely to rupture are termed unstable. Rupture usually occurs in lipid-rich and foam cell-rich peripheral margins and may result in thrombosis and arterial occlusion.

Fibrin

Platelet

Fibrinogen

Erythrocyte

Fibrous cap

Intimal disruption and thrombus

JOHN A. CRAIG—MD

C. Machado M.D.

©ICON

Figure 25-2

Pain of Myocardial Ischemia

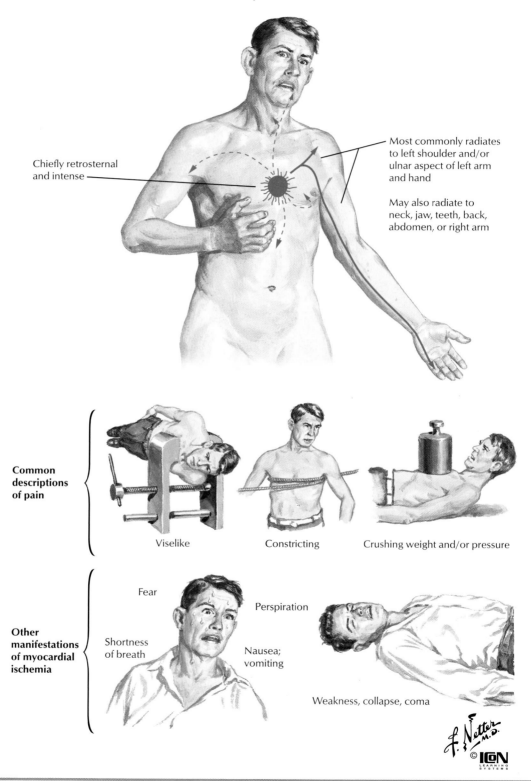

Chiefly retrosternal and intense

Most commonly radiates to left shoulder and/or ulnar aspect of left arm and hand

May also radiate to neck, jaw, teeth, back, abdomen, or right arm

Common descriptions of pain

Viselike

Constricting

Crushing weight and/or pressure

Other manifestations of myocardial ischemia

Fear

Perspiration

Shortness of breath

Nausea; vomiting

Weakness, collapse, coma

symptoms accompanying chest discomfort may include dyspnea, diaphoresis, nausea or vomiting, and palpitations, and in some cases these symptoms, rather than chest discomfort, may predominate.

Physical Examination

The physical examination is often unremarkable in an uncomplicated myocardial infarction. Clues to the diagnosis of a suspected myocardial infarction include assessment of cardiac risk factors such as: xanthelasma (indicative of hypercholesterolemia), nicotine stains on fingers (indicative of a smoking history), evidence of hypertension on ophthalmologic examination or the presence of left ventricular hypertrophy, and obesity or male gender in patients under the age of 55. Blood pressure, heart rate, and respiratory rate may all be elevated secondary to pain. An S_4 is often heart in patients with infarction, and is a sign of the reduced left ventricular compliance associated with ischemia. The presence of signs of congestive heard failure—including an S_3, crackles in the lung fields, and engorged neck veins—can be harbingers of cardiogenic shock, as can hypotension. Bradycardia is often seen in inferior myocardial infarctions due to ischemia of the atrioventricular (AV) node, while at least initially, tachycardia is more commonly seen. Rarely, mechanical complications of myocardial infarction may also be evident with a systolic murmur indicating mitral valve incompetence or a ventricular septal defect.

DIFFERENTIAL DIAGNOSIS

Many conditions can mimic myocardial infarction. The two most important are aortic dissection and acute pulmonary emboli, both of which have symptoms that can be identical to acute myocardial infarction. The symptoms of aortic dissection are more likely to radiate through to the back and have characteristics of stabbing nature. The diagnosis can frequently be suspected by a wide mediastinum on a chest radiography and a difference in blood pressure between the right and left arm. The diagnosis is confirmed by computerized tomography (CT) scan, MRI, or transesophageal echo. Acute MI can occur concurrently with aortic dissection as a result of dissection into a coronary ostium (most commonly the right coronary ostium)

and resulting coronary occlusion. When in doubt, aortic dissection should be excluded before consideration of thrombolytic therapy or use of potent antithrombotic therapy for acute MI (see below).

Acute pulmonary embolus should be suspected when symptoms of shortness of breath are the predominant complaint. The diagnosis can be suspected with a rightward axis shift on the ECG and findings of right ventricular strain or new right bundle branch block (RBBB). Frequently, oxygen saturation is reduced and there may be hypercapnia. The diagnosis is confirmed by testing for D-dimer in blood and ventilation perfusion scanning or helical CT scanning for evidence of proximal pulmonary emboli.

Other less serious conditions include pericarditis and a variety of gastrointestinal disorders, including esophageal spasm, gastroesophageal reflux, and peptic ulcer disease, even including gastrointestinal bleeding. This diagnosis should always be considered, as thrombolytic therapy or antithrombotic therapies can be devastating in a patient with active bleeding.

DIAGNOSTIC APPROACH

All patients with symptoms suggestive of acute MI should have 12-lead ECG and measurement of baseline cardiac markers within 10 minutes of arrival at the hospital. Patients with evidence of an evolving Q-wave MI, such as ST elevation, new left bundle branch block, or anterior ST depression indicative of a posterior MI, should immediately be considered for reperfusion therapy, such as fibrinolytic therapy or primary angioplasty (see therapeutic strategies below). In the remaining patients, obtain a serial ECG and cardiac markers (creatinine kinase-MB [CK-MB], myoglobin, or troponin) in the first 24 hours. For patients in whom cardiac markers indicate ongoing myocardial necrosis (non-ST-elevation MI), antithrombotic/anticoagulant and/or invasive therapies should be initiated.

The guidelines for defining MI have recently been updated. The following criteria satisfy the diagnosis of an acute, evolving, or recent MI.

Typical rise and gradual fall (troponin) or more rapid rise and fall (CK-MB) of biochemical markers of myocardial necrosis with at least one of the following: ischemic symptoms, development of pathologic Q waves on the ECG, ECG changes indicative of ischemia (ST segment elevation or depression), or coronary artery intervention (e.g., coronary angioplasty or coronary artery bypass grafting [CABG]).

The following criteria satisfy the diagnosis of established MI:

· Development of new pathological Q waves on serial ECGs. The patient may or may not remember previous symptoms. Biochemical markers of myocardial necrosis may have normalized, depending on the time since the infarct developed.

· Pathologic (including imaging studies) findings of a healed or healing MI.

Electrocardiography

ECG changes alone are not sufficient to diagnose MI. Only 30% to 60% of patients with acute myocardial infarction have classical ST elevation, and 5% to 10% of patients with ST elevation do not have measurable changes in cardiac markers, either due to an aborted infarct or ST elevation resulting from pericarditis or early repolarization changes (Figure 25-3). However, the ECG changes can be minimal in the early stages of infarction. The majority of ECG changes reflect myocardial ischemia as indicated below.

Patients with ST segment elevation: New or presumed ST elevation at the J point in 2 or more contiguous leads with the cut-off points greater than 0.2mV in anterior leads V_1 to V_6 and in limb leads greater than 0.1mV (lateral: I and aVL; inferior: II, III, and aVF) (Figure 25-3).

Patients without ST segment elevation: a) ST segment depression; b) T-wave abnormalities only; c) new LBBB, or d) ECG confounders including paced or idioventricular rhythm, severe left ventricular hypertrophy with strain, or any wide-complex tachycardia.

Electrocardiographic changes in established MI include any QR in leads V_1 through V_3 greater than 30 msec, or abnormal Q waves in leads I, II, aVL, aVF or V_4 through V_6 in any two contiguous leads and at least 1mm in depth.

Many findings on the ECG can obscure the diagnosis of myocardial infarction, including paced rhythms, left bundle branch block, left ventricular hypertrophy, and Wolff-Parkinson-White syndrome. ST depression, even when not associated with a true posterior MI, also has important prognostic information.

Serum Cardiac Markers

The use of cardiac-specific markers such as CK-MB, troponin T, or troponin I in the first 24 hours after admission to the hospital is currently the most accurate way to detect myocardial necrosis. Each marker has specific characteristics that should be considered.

The troponins and CK-MB typically become elevated 3 to 4 hours after the onset of myocardial infarction. Thus, it is not unusual to see normal cardiac markers among patients who arrive early after onset of symptoms. This underscores the importance of serial testing for all patients with suspected infarction. CK-MB peaks at approximately 12 to 24 hours and remains elevated for 36 to 48 hours. Troponin I and T remain elevated for 7 to 14 days after infarction, and have 2 peaks; one early at approximately 24 hours and one later at 5 to 10 days. The troponins are therefore useful as "late" markers, where an individual patient event may have occurred more than 48 hours before admission. Normal troponin concentrations do not exclude acute MI until at least 10 hours after the onset of symptoms.

Serum myoglobin has been used as an "early" marker, as it becomes elevated within 1 hour of symptom onset and peaks at about 6 hours. However, this marker is not cardiac-specific, it is found abundantly in noncardiac muscle. Myoglobin has been found to have a role for early detection when used with multiple other cardiac specific markers (CK-MB and troponin). This serum cardiac panel testing approach has been found to be superior to a single cardiac marker for detecting acute myocardial infarction and risk stratification.

Other Diagnostic Tools

Although the ECG and cardiac markers are the most important tests for suspected myocardial infarction because of their broad availability, other diagnostic tests such as the two-dimensional echocardiogram and nuclear imaging have been used as complementary tests for detection of other important prognostic factors such as size of infarct, left ventricular function, and area of jeopardized myocardium. The echocardiogram is particularly useful in electrocardiographically "silent" areas such as those in the circumflex artery distribution, where the sensitivity of the

Figure 25-3

Localization of Myocardial Infarcts

Anterior Infarct

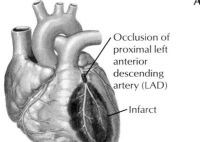
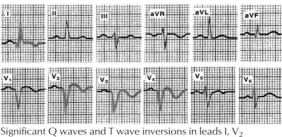

Occlusion of proximal left anterior descending artery (LAD)

Infarct

Significant Q waves and T wave inversions in leads I, V_2 V_3, and V_4

Anterolateral Infarct

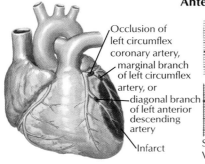
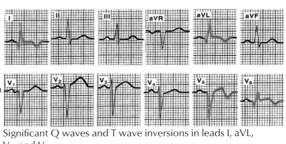

Occlusion of left circumflex coronary artery, marginal branch of left circumflex artery, or diagonal branch of left anterior descending artery

Infarct

Significant Q waves and T wave inversions in leads I, aVL, V_5, and V_6

Diaphragmatic or Inferior Infarct

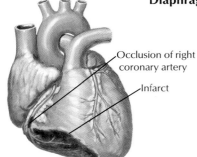
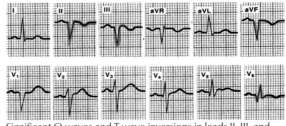

Occlusion of right coronary artery

Infarct

Significant Q waves and T wave inversions in leads II, III, and aVF. With lateral damage, changes also may be seen in leads V_5 and V_6.

True Posterior Infarct

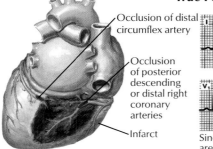
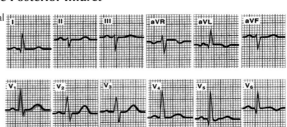

Occlusion of distal circumflex artery

Occlusion of posterior descending or distal right coronary arteries

Infarct

Since no ECG lead reflects posterior electrical forces, changes are reciprocal of those in anterior leads. Lead V_1 shows unusually large R wave (reciprocal of posterior Q wave) and upright T wave (reciprocal of posterior T wave inversion).

MYOCARDIAL INFARCTION

ECG in detecting ST-MI is less than 25% with standard techniques. Nuclear imaging such as perfusion imaging or infarct-avid scintigraphy are useful in suspected MI, particularly if used during ongoing chest discomfort. This technique, although useful, is limited by the need to have nuclear isotopes and personnel available at all times. If the clinical presentation suggests acute MI but the initial ECG does not demonstrate myocardial ischemia, bedside echocardiography is very useful. Normal left ventricular (LV) function, without wall motion abnormalities suggest that ongoing ischemia is unlikely. New wall motion abnormalities are diagnostic of ischemia. If baseline LV function is unknown, a wall motion abnormality may indicate ischemia or previous injury.

Risk Stratification

Over the past several years a variety of risk models have been developed to identify high-risk patients who would benefit from more invasive management. The details and characteristics of these models are outside the scope of this text, but a few key components should be emphasized.

The presence of congestive heart failure is one of the most important high-risk features. It is usually identified by physical findings, with evidence of low oxygen saturation and pulmonary edema on the chest radiograph. Cardiogenic shock is one of the highest-risk features, with signs of heart failure and evidence of clinical hypoperfusion with tachycardia (heart rate >100) and hypotension (systolic blood pressure <100 mm Hg). Cardiogenic shock has a mortality rate of 60% to 80% in the first 30 days after myocardial infarction. Other baseline characteristics that predict higher mortality include advanced age, tachycardia, low systolic blood pressure, anterior infarct location, female gender, previous MI or heart failure, and the presence of co-morbid illness such as diabetes mellitus or renal dysfunction. These characteristics are usually associated with more extensive significant coronary artery disease and worse left ventricular function, both of which have been shown to be the most important prognostic markers of long-term mortality among patients with coronary artery disease. These anatomic characteristics can most easily be defined by diagnostic cardiac catheterization.

MANAGEMENT AND THERAPY
Basic Principles

Ideally, patients with suspected acute myocardial infarction should be evaluated in a specific area of the emergency department with a set protocol and standardized pathways. This is most easily accomplished by having standardized order forms that provide a checklist for all appropriate tests and therapeutic strategies. Patients with suspected MI should be evaluated with a targeted history and physical examination and have an ECG performed and interpreted within 10 minutes of arrival to the emergency department. An intravenous line should be placed and oxygen administered through nasal prongs (routine administration to all patients with uncomplicated MI during the first 3 hours of treatment, and continued if either arterial desaturation <90%, or pulmonary congestion is present). Patients should also be placed on continuous cardiac telemetry monitoring for cardiac arrhythmias.

Once the initial evaluation has been completed and the diagnosis of acute MI has been made, an aspirin (160 to 325 mg orally or chewed) should be given. This simple therapy has been associated with a 24% reduction in early mortality. In addition, intravenous morphine (2 to 8 mg repeated at intervals of 5 to15 minutes) and sublingual nitrates (0.2 mg) should be given to relieve chest discomfort. Beta-blockers are known to reduce infarct size and improve survival in myocardial infarction. They should be given initially intravenously followed by oral therapy in the majority of patients with suspected myocardial infarction. Caution should be taken in patients with bradycardia (heart rate <60), hypotension (systolic pressure <100 mm Hg), cardiogenic shock or heart failure, and in those with severe asthma or chronic obstructive airway disease. Patients with confirmed infarction should be admitted to a coronary care unit or intermediate observation unit where serial ECGs and cardiac markers can be obtained while continuous cardiac telemetry is ongoing for at least the first 24 hours. The remaining treatment strategies are defined by the presence of ST elevation MI (including patients with a new LBBB) or non-ST elevation MI (all other ECG criteria with positive cardiac markers).

ST Elevation Myocardial Infarction

All patients with ST elevation or new LBBB on the ECG should be considered for immediate reperfusion therapy. Outcomes are time-dependent – the more rapidly reperfusion is obtained, the greater the preservation of LV function and the lower the mortality. Reperfusion therapy is most effective within 1 to 2 hours after the onset of symptoms. Numerous studies have demonstrated benefit, albeit decreasing with the time to reperfusion, up to 12 hours after the initial onset of symptoms. Reperfusion of the infarct-related artery can be established either with fibrinolytic (thrombolytic) agents that dissolve the thrombus in the coronary artery, or by primary angioplasty.

Commonly-used fibrinolytic agents include intravenous streptokinase (SK), or recombinant tissue plasminogen activators such as t-PA (alteplase), r-PA (retevase), or TNK-tPA. Each agent has advantages – SK is less costly; the recombinant agents are more efficacious; and in the case of r-PA and TNK-tPA, more easily administered. All have been associated with a significant reduction in both 30-day and long-term mortality. Low-molecular-weight heparin (for example, enoxaparin, 1mg/kg twice daily) has recently been found to be superior to unfractionated heparin when combined with TNK-tPA in reducing the rate of reinfarction after thrombolysis. Contraindications to fibrinolysis should be excluded before treatment. Absolute constraindications include: history of recent bleeding, stroke, intracranial hemorrhage, or major surgery. In addition, caution should be exercised among patients taking chronic antcoagulation with coumadin.

Primary percutaneous coronary intervention (PCI) (with or without intracoronary stenting) of the infarct-related artery has been found to be associated with lower early mortality compared with intravenous fibrinolytic therapy, particularly in centers with high PCI volumes. Primary PCI is also safer than thrombolysis, with a negligible rate of intracranial hemorrhage (0.1% vs. approximately 1%). Primary PCI is limited by the availability of qualified physicians and staff and in many institutions is not available 24 hours a day. Adjunctive intravenous glycoprotein IIb/IIIa (for example, abciximab or eptifibatide) inhibition has been found to enhance the outcome of primary PCI, with lower rates of death, reinfarction, and the

need for urgent repeat intervention during follow-up. Primary PCI also shortens hospital stay and is the preferred reperfusion strategy, along with aortic counterpulsation, in cardiogenic shock.

Non-ST Elevation Myocardial Infarction

This condition is seen in all subgroups of patients, but most commonly in older patients or those with co-morbid illnesses. Recent studies have highlighted several new treatment strategies that reduce the rate of death and non-fatal myocardial infarction. There is less time-dependency with initiating therapy for non-ST-MI as there is no evidence that the amount of myocardial damage can be reduced with earlier therapy. Studies on the benefit of early aggressive versus noninvasive strategies have produced mixed results, but the most recent studies suggest a benefit to early coronary angiography and intervention.

The cornerstone of the management of non-ST-MI is comprehensive anticoagulation and antithrombotic therapies. Until recently, aspirin and intravenous unfractionated heparin were the mainstays of therapy. Enoxaparin (1mg/kg twice daily) reduces death and non-fatal MI compared with unfractionated heparin. Furthermore, for high-risk patients (age >65 years, heart failure, ongoing refractory ischemia, troponin-positive, ST depression, or intermittent ST-T wave changes with chest pain), intravenous glycoprotein IIb/IIIa inhibitors in addition to aspirin and heparin reduce the rate of death and nonfatal infarction. In large prospectively randomized clinical trials, the efficacy of glycoprotein IIb/IIIa inhibitors in non-ST segment elevation MI was most evident in patients undergoing early PCI. The benefit of glycoprotein IIb/IIIa inhibitors in reducing platelet aggregation is also consistent with a significant reduction in death and MI among patients undergoing PCI with either abciximab or eptifibatide. Abciximab has not been found to be of value for medical stabilization in a large prospective trial.

Other Pharmacologic Agents

The antiplatelet agent *clopidogrel* (300 mg loading dose, 75 mg twice daily orally) has been extensively studied in conjunction with PCI and found to be essential for prevention of stent thrombosis. While clopidogrel was found to be marginally

Figure 25-4

Nondrug Therapy

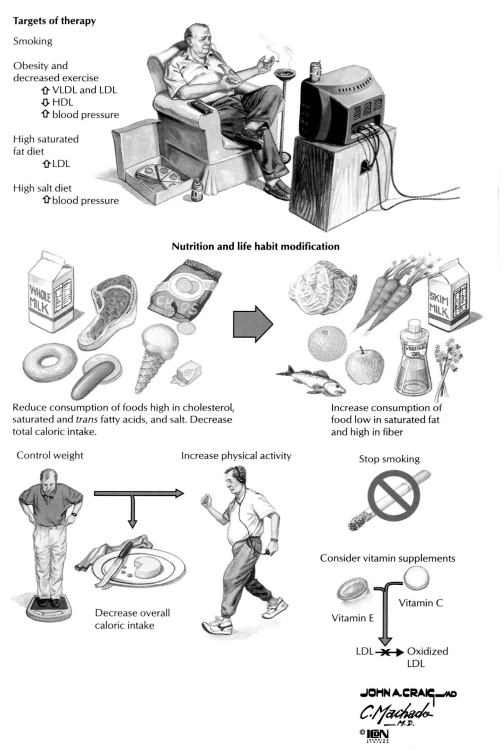

Targets of therapy

Smoking

Obesity and
decreased exercise
⬆ VLDL and LDL
⬇ HDL
⬆ blood pressure

High saturated
fat diet
⬆ LDL

High salt diet
⬆ blood pressure

Nutrition and life habit modification

Reduce consumption of foods high in cholesterol, saturated and *trans* fatty acids, and salt. Decrease total caloric intake.

Increase consumption of food low in saturated fat and high in fiber

Control weight

Increase physical activity

Stop smoking

Decrease overall caloric intake

Consider vitamin supplements

Vitamin C

Vitamin E

LDL ⤫→ Oxidized LDL

JOHN A. CRAIG—MD

C. Machado
—M.D.

©ICON

superior to aspirin alone in reducing vascular events (9% relative reduction), the combination of aspirin and clopidogrel was associated with a significant reduction (20%) in cardiovascular death, MI, and stroke at 12 months. The combination of aspirin and clopidogrel was associated with a small increase in bleeding (3.7% v. 2.7% with placebo).

Angiotensin converting enzyme (ACE) inhibitors improve survival in post-MI patients with heart failure and/or low ejection fraction (<40%), and in patients with hypertension. ACE inhibitors should not routinely be started in the first 24 hours of MI unless the patient has hypertension, because a profound decrease in blood pressure could result in the recurrent myocardial ischemia.

A fasting lipid profile (total cholesterol, low density liopprotein [LDL], and high density lipoprotein [HDL] cholesterol) should be measured in the first 24 hours after admission. Patients with increased total (>200 mg/dL) or LDL cholesterol (>100 mg/dL) should be started on a lipid lowering regimen. Although the best timing for starting agents such as HMG-Co-A reductase therapy (statins) has not been established, the majority of physicians favor starting these agents in the hospital to enhance compliance. Reduction in subsequent cardiac events has been demonstrated for numerous statins including simvastatin, or pravastatin in patients after myocardial infarction.

In-Hospital Management and Cardiac Catheterization

The treatment strategy for patients who undergo primary PCI for ST elevation MI is simplified because the extent of coronary artery disease in the noninfarct-related arteries is revealed during the acute cardiac catheterization. During left ventricular angiography the ejection fraction and any valvular disease will also be evident. For patients not having primary PCI, left ventricular function can be evaluated via echocardiogram and the extent of coronary artery disease can be indirectly evaluated with noninvasive stress testing. Patients who are unable to undergo a stress test, for whatever reason, are among those at highest risk for subsequent cardiac events. This has led many physicians to choose a more invasive approach with cardiac catheterization, although there is no clear evidence that this strategy is associated with an improved survival for ST-MI.

For patients with non-ST segment elevation MI, recent clinical trials have suggested that a more invasive approach is associated with improved survival. In patients with elevated troponin in the first 24 hours after admission who were randomized to cardiac catheterization or treatment with dalteparin (a LMWH), those undergoing early cardiac catheterization had a lower mortality at 1 year. The invasive strategy is also associated with a shorter initial in-hospital stay and a lower risk of readmission during follow-up.

Improvement of Cardiac Risk Factors and Secondary Prevention

For patients who present with an acute MI there is a tremendous opportunity to prevent further morbidity and mortality by altering poor cardiac habits. Advice and recommendations on smoking cessation and a heart-healthy diet can be helpful. In addition, referral to a cardiac rehabilitation program can reinforce these habits long term and improve exercise tolerance (Figure 25-4).

Patients should also be discharged on a "cardioprotective" combination of therapies. In the absence of specific contraindications, the list includes aspirin, beta-blockers, ACE inhibitors, and a lipid-lowering agent. Although these therapies have not been studied in combination, individually all have proven efficacy and it is likely that they work well in aggregate.

FUTURE DIRECTIONS

The most important development for patients with myocardial infarction has been the identification of patients with a high-risk of sudden cardiac death due to significant ventricular arrhythmia. Recent randomized clinical trial data have suggested that implantation of a defibrillator can improve survival for patients with recent MI, an ejection fraction less than 35%, and no contraindication to implantable defibrillators. The selection of those who will definitively benefit from defibrillator placement, as well as the cost-effectiveness of this therapy, are the topic of ongoing studies.

REFERENCES

Alpert JS, Thygesen K, Antman E, Bassand JP. Myocardial infarction redefined—a consensus document of The Joint European Society of Cardiology/American College of Cardiology Committee for the Redefinition of Myocardial Infarction. *J Am Coll Cardiol.* 2000;36:959–969.

Antman EM, Braunwald E. Acute myocardial infarction. In: Braunwald E, Zipes DP, Libby P, eds. *Heart Disease: A Textbook of Cardiovascular Medicine*. 6th ed. Philadelphia, Pa: WB Saunders Co; 2001:1114–1219.

Braunwald E, Antman EM, Beasley JW, et al, and the American College of Cardiology/American Heart Association Task Force on Practice Guidelines (Committee on the Management of Patients with Unstable Angina. ACC/AHA guideline update for the management of patients with unstable angina and non-ST-segment elevation myocardial infarction—2002: summary article. A report of the American College of Cardiology/American Heart Association Task Force on Practice Guidelines (Committee on the Management of Patients with Unstable Angina). *Circulation*. 2002;106:-1893–1900.

Ohman EM, Harrington RA, Cannon CP, Agnelli G, Cairns JA, Kennedy JW. Intravenous thrombolysis in acute myocardial infarction. *Chest*. 2001(suppl 1):253–277S.

Ryan TJ, Antman EM, Brooks NH, et al. 1999 update: ACC/AHA guidelines for the management of patients with acute myocardial infarction. A report of the American College of Cardiology/American Heart Association Task Force on Practice Guidelines (Committee on Management of Acute Myocardial Infarction). *J Am Coll Cardiol*. 1999; 34: 890–911.

Topol EJ, Van de Werf FJ. Acute myocardial infarction: early diagnosis and management. In: Topol EJ, Califf RM, Isner J, et al, eds. *Textbook of Cardiovascular Medicine*. 2nd ed. Philadelphia, Pa: Lippincott Williams & Wilkins; 2002:-385–419.

Chapter 26
Peripheral Vascular Disease

Leslie P. Wong and Marschall S. Runge

In most affected individuals, the development and progression of atherosclerosis is a diffuse process affecting not only the coronary arteries, but also arteries that supply blood to the brain, kidneys, and intestinal organs, and arteries supplying the lower extremities. Arterial occlusion in the heart, brain, kidneys, or intestinal organs leads to end-organ damage and loss of function (Figure 26-1). Arterial stenosis or occlusion in the lower extremities results in peripheral vascular disease (PVD), in a spectrum ranging from mildly symptomatic disease to severe symptoms to limb ischemia.

An estimated 60% of patients with PVD have coronary artery disease, cerebrovascular disease, or both. As a consequence, the patient with PVD has an increased risk of myocardial infarction, stroke, death, and disability. PVD is largely an affliction of age, with a negligible prevalence in young adulthood increasing to 10% to 12% in subjects aged 70 years or older. Exceptions to this rule are found in individuals with systemic illnesses that lead to abrupt thrombotic occlusion of a major peripheral artery. Otherwise, the same factors that predispose to coronary atherosclerosis also increase the likelihood of PVD. These include male gender, smoking, diabetes, hypertension, and hypercholesterolemia. Of these, the strongest association is between cigarette smoking and PVD.

Peripheral vascular disease produces symptoms of claudication. Derived from the Latin word *claudatico,* "to limp," claudication describes pain in the lower extremities produced by inadequate blood flow during exercise. As arterial occlusion worsens, critical limb ischemia may lead to amputation. However, more patients with claudication suffer myocardial infarction and stroke than limb loss. Recognizing the link between peripheral vascular disease of the extremities and atherosclerosis elsewhere has led to the integration of therapies that target not only claudication, but also cardiovascular death and morbidity.

ETIOLOGY AND PATHOGENESIS

Atherogenesis begins with injury to the vascular endothelium and formation of an atherosclerotic plaque. This process is potentiated by a local leukocyte-mediated inflammation and oxidized lipoprotein species, particulary low-density lipoproteins. The precise molecular mechanisms by which smoking, hypercholesterolemia, diabetes, and hypertension accelerate atherosclerosis are the subject of ongoing investigation.

The presence of endothelial dysfunction and fatty streaks (the predecessor of atherosclerotic plaques) is ubiquitous in western countries, as documented by autopsy studies on young adults dying of other causes. According to current theories, plaques probably expand in increments owing to subclinical episodes of plaque rupture, although plaques likely also undergo gradual enlargement with accretion of cells and noncellular material in the lipid-rich core. Most commonly, the plaque core is surrounded by a complex fibrotic cap composed of calcium, connective tissue, and smooth muscle cells. Stable symptoms, such as those of claudication, result from an inability to increase blood flow at times of increased demand. Plaque rupture exposes the highly thrombogenic core to circulating blood elements, resulting in platelet activation and aggregation, along with activation of fibrinogen.

As noted above, plaque rupture often only worsens an existing lesion without causing arterial occlusion or clinical symptoms. However, more significant episodes of plaque rupture result in worsening limb ischemia with effort, or ischemia at rest. These symptoms result either from thrombotic occlusion of a peripheral artery, or embolization of a thrombus with occlusion of small distal arteries.

Claudication is most commonly "stable" and

Figure 26-1

Carotid Artery Stenosis

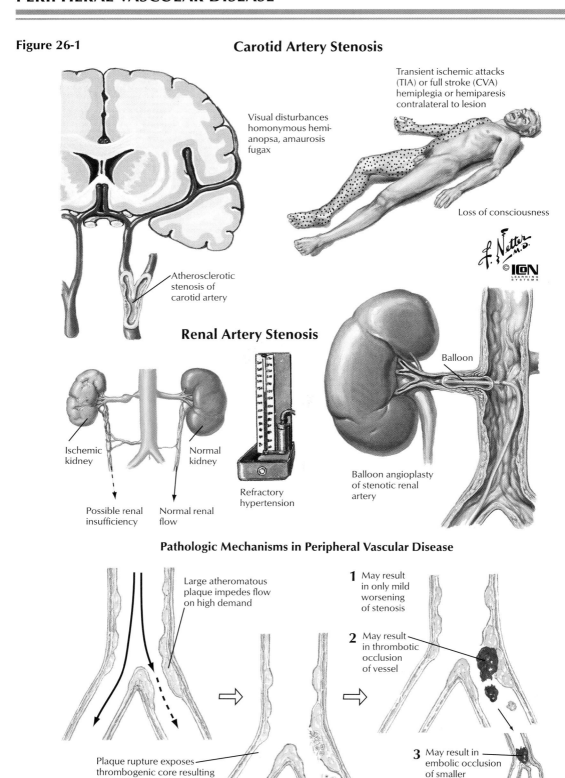

Visual disturbances
homonymous hemi-
anopsia, amaurosis
fugax

Transient ischemic attacks
(TIA) or full stroke (CVA)
hemiplegia or hemiparesis
contralateral to lesion

Loss of consciousness

Atherosclerotic
stenosis of
carotid artery

Renal Artery Stenosis

Ischemic
kidney

Normal
kidney

Possible renal
insufficiency

Normal renal
flow

Refractory
hypertension

Balloon

Balloon angioplasty
of stenotic renal
artery

Pathologic Mechanisms in Peripheral Vascular Disease

Large atheromatous
plaque impedes flow
on high demand

Plaque rupture exposes
thrombogenic core resulting
in platelet aggregation and
activation along with
fibrinogen activation

1 May result
in only mild
worsening
of stenosis

2 May result
in thrombotic
occlusion
of vessel

3 May result in
embolic occlusion
of smaller
distal vessels

quite reproducible. In these circumstances, despite the reduction in arterial lumen diameter, adequate blood flow to the tissues of the distal extremities is preserved at rest or with minimal exertion. However, when cardiac output and tissue oxygen demands increase with exercise, the luminal stenosis prevents sufficient blood flow to the extremities, and exercise-induced local vasodilation to facilitate increased tissue perfusion is also impaired. This combination results in local ischemia and production of lactic acid and other metabolites which are responsible for the pain associated with claudication.

CLINICAL PRESENTATION

Claudication is manifested by cramping pain in the lower extremites or buttocks that is reliably produced by a threshold level of exercise. This pain is relieved by a few minutes of rest. Elevation of the limb can worsen claudication, while holding the limb in a dependent position may help. Symptoms may be unilateral or bilateral, depending on the extent and location of atherosclerotic disease. Calf claudication represents femoral disease, while foot involvement suggests popliteal or proximal tibioperoneal disease. Thigh and buttock pain are indicative of aortoiliac involvement. As PVD worsens in severity, claudication may occur at night and at rest.

Despite the existence of PVD, classic claudication occurs in only about one-third of patients. Some patients may experience only mild leg discomfort with exercise and not communicate this to their physician, misinterpreting this as a normal consequence of aging. Because even asymptomatic patients with peripheral vascular disease still incur a higher relative risk of adverse cardiovascular events, it is important to maintain a high index of suspicion for atypical symptoms of claudication.

The physical exam usually demonstrates diminished or absent peripheral pulses. Loss of femoral and all distal pulses bilaterally is caused by occlusion at the aortoiliac bifurcation, referred to as Leriche's syndrome. Capillary refill is usually delayed. While it is important to perform auscultation over the femoral, renal, and carotid arteries in patients with risk factors or a clinical history suggestive of vascular disease, bruits are often absent even in patients with severe PVD. The skin may demonstrate pallor, a shiny texture, and coolness. Loss of body hair and thickened toenails may be present. Ischemia and symptom-related disuse may result in muscular atrophy. Ulcers, poor wound healing, and frank gangrene can develop with chronic critical ischemia (Figure 26-2).

DIFFERENTIAL DIAGNOSIS

Distinguishing true claudication from its mimic, pseudoclaudication (or spinal stenosis), by clinical symptoms is very important, because the diagnostic approach and treatment for the two entities are completely different. In distinction from the symptoms of claudication, pseudoclaudication is characteristically less reproducible based on a specific effort level. Rather than being relieved by cessation of exercise, pseudoclaudication typically is only relieved with sitting or other lumbar flexion maneuvers that increase spinal canal volume (spinal stenosis is discussed in more detail in Section XVI on "Disorders of the Immune System, Connective Tissue and Joints").

Alternative diagnoses should be actively sought in patients less than 50 years old and without predisposing risk factors. The extensive differential diagnosis includes:

· Osteoarthritis
· Deep venous thrombosis
· Ruptured Baker's cyst
· Atheroembolism
· Chronic venous insufficiency
· Diabetic neuropathy
· Reflex sympathetic dystrophy
· Chronic compartment syndrome
· Popliteal artery entrapment
· Restless leg syndrome
· Remote trauma
· Radiation injury
· Ergotamine abuse
· Vasospasm
· Vasculitis (e.g., Thromboangiitis obliterans, Takayasu's disease)

DIAGNOSTIC APPROACH

Careful history and physical exam are essential for the correct diagnosis of PVD, and should include a thorough elicitation of symptoms. Once PVD is suspected, an ankle-brachial index (ABI) should be measured. This is done by recording the systolic blood pressure by Doppler ultrasound in

Figure 26-2

Lower Extremity Arterial Occlusive Disease

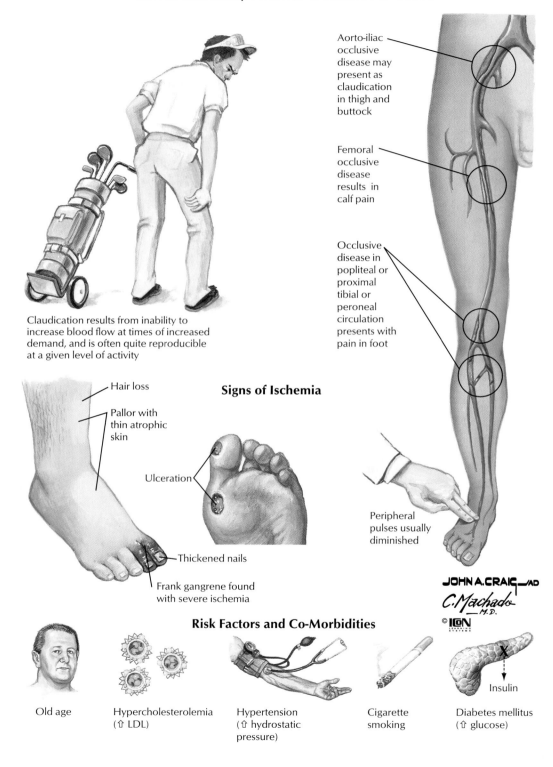

Aorto-iliac occlusive disease may present as claudication in thigh and buttock

Femoral occlusive disease results in calf pain

Occlusive disease in popliteal or proximal tibial or peroneal circulation presents with pain in foot

Claudication results from inability to increase blood flow at times of increased demand, and is often quite reproducible at a given level of activity

Signs of Ischemia

Hair loss

Pallor with thin atrophic skin

Ulceration

Peripheral pulses usually diminished

Thickened nails

Frank gangrene found with severe ischemia

JOHN A. CRAIG — MD
C. Machado — M.D.
© ICON

Risk Factors and Co-Morbidities

Old age

Hypercholesterolemia (⇧ LDL)

Hypertension (⇧ hydrostatic pressure)

Cigarette smoking

Insulin

Diabetes mellitus (⇧ glucose)

the brachial artery and comparing it with the pressure in the dorsalis pedis and posterior tibial arteries (Figure 26-3). The ratio of the highest measurement of the lower extremity divided by arm pressure for each side of the body is calculated. An ABI less than 0.9 is consistent with peripheral vascular disease. Values less than 0.4 suggest severe arterial occlusion.

Sensitivity may be increased by measuring the ABI following exercise treadmill testing. Elderly patients or those with diabetes or renal insufficiency may have significant vessel calcification resulting in an artifactually elevated ABI >1.3. These patients are better evaluated with toe brachial pressure index measurements. Arterial Doppler ultrasound studies and plethysmography are noninvasive modalities that are often useful in diagnosing PVD.

Contrast angiography remains the gold standard for complete assessment and definition of the arterial vasculature (Figure 26-3). It is necessary if revascularization is being considered, but not essential for clinical diagnosis. The severity of symptoms or objective evidence of effort-related or rest ischemia should be considered before proceeding with percutaneous or surgical revascularization. Because of the risks, however small, of arterial injury and contrast-induced nephrotoxicity, angiography should only be considered if revascularization is a viable option.

Computed tomographic angiography (CTA) and magnetic resonance angiography (MRA) have been touted as alternatives to angiography. A recent meta-analysis showed high accuracy in assessing lower extremity arterial disease, particularly with three-dimensional gadolinum-enhanced images. While neither CTA nor MRA has supplanted traditional arteriography in the preoperative mapping of vessels, these promising tools merits further study (Figure 26-3).

MANAGEMENT AND THERAPY

Medical management of claudication and reduction of cardiovascular risk factors are the cornerstones of treatment of peripheral vascular disease. Revascularization is usually only indicated for rest ischemia or in cases of effort-induced ischemia that are refractory to maximal medical therapy.

Medical Management

Smoking is strongly related to the progression of atherosclerosis and is associated with a higher risk of amputation. Tobacco use is also linked to increased cardiovascular death and events. Smoking cessation programs and treatment with nicotine replacement or bupropion should be emphasized.

Diabetes is a major cardiovascular risk factor and important in patients with PVD, as diabetics have a uniformly worse prognosis. Although large prospective trials have not shown a direct effect on peripheral vascular disease or macrovascular events with intensive glycemic control in diabetes, given the benefit in reducing microvascular complications, a goal HbA1C less than 7% is warranted. Tight glycemic control may delay the development of peripheral neuropathy, which can complicate the treatment of PVD.

Hypertension is closely linked to development of atherosclerosis. Although lowering of blood pressure has not been clearly shown to reduce claudication, the mortality benefit in cardiovascular disease is clear. The recommendations of the sixth Joint National Committee on Hypertension outline a goal blood pressure of <130/85 for most patients with PVD. Angiotensin converting enzyme inhibitors should be considered first-line agents, along with diuretics and beta-blockers. In recent years, the proposed detrimental effect of beta-blockers on claudication has been shown to rarely present a problem.

Hypercholesterolemia is a key component of atherogenesis. Lipid-lowering therapy has been shown to improve claudication, induce regression or stabilization of atherosclerotic lesions, and provide effective secondary prevention of cardiovascular events. Treatment of elevated cholesterol with a diet, exercise, and HMG CoA reductase inhibitors (statins) is warranted, with a goal serum LDL less than 100 mg/dL. Recent studies indicate that statin therapy not only reduces cardiac events, but also reduces the risk of stroke and death from stroke. Early reports suggest statins will improve outcomes in patients with PVD.

Hyperhomocysteinemia is associated with a higher risk of atherosclerosis and thrombosis. Due to a lack of prospective controlled trials, the benefit of vitamin supplementation to reduce homocysteine levels is unclear.

Antiplatelet agents are recommended in peripheral vascular disease. Treatment with aspirin (81 to 325 mg daily) reduces death and disability from

Figure 26-3

Peripheral Vascular Disease

Doppler analysis of peripheral vascular disease

Ankle-brachial index (ABI)

Doppler ultrasound measurements of systolic blood pressure in brachial artery compared with pressures in dorsalis pedis and posterior tibial arteries

$$ABI = \frac{\text{Lower extremity}}{\text{Upper extremity}}$$

Normal ≥ 1.0
PVD   < 0.9

Doppler wave form analysis

Analysis of wave forms of Doppler studies may help in identification and localization of lesion

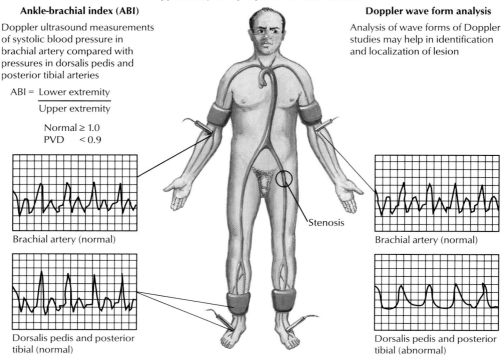

Stenosis

Brachial artery (normal)

Dorsalis pedis and posterior tibial (normal)

Brachial artery (normal)

Dorsalis pedis and posterior tibial (abnormal)

Contrast angiography

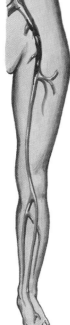
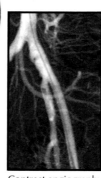

Contrast angiography showing stenosis of the proximal femoral artery

CT angiogram

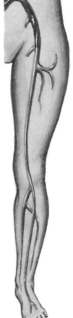
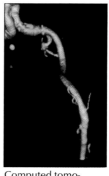

Computed tomographic angiogram demonstrating stenosis of the proximal left femoral artery

JOHN A. CRAIG—AD
with
E. Hatton
© ICON

stroke and myocardial infarction. The combination of aspirin and dipyridamole is not clearly better than aspirin alone. Ticlopidine is effective for reducing claudication severity and adverse cardiovascular events, but its use has declined due to its association with thrombotic thrombocytopenic purpura. Clopidogrel is slightly superior to aspirin in reducing ischemic complications related to vascular disease, but the absolute risk reduction is small, and the cost-effectiveness of clopidogrel versus aspirin is uncertain. In patients who cannot tolerate aspirin, clopidogrel is an excellent alternative.

Exercise is extremely important in treating claudication. The benefits of exercise seem to occur exclusive of a significant improvement in blood flow. With training, skeletal muscle oxidative capacity increases, and exercise-related inflammation decreases. Exercise also improves overall cardiorespiratory efficiency, reduces insulin resistance, and has a beneficial effect on lipids. This leads to increased functional capacity as measured by improved walking distance and quality of life.

Anticlaudicatory agents are used to improve symptoms. Two drugs are approved for claudication: pentoxifylline and cilostazol. Trials of pentoxifylline have shown mixed results and presently pentoxifylline is not routinely recommended. Cilostazol has demonstrated benefits in symptom relief, exercise capacity, and quality of life compared to placebo and pentoxifylline. The clinical benefits are modest relative to its cost, and cilostazol should probably be reserved for patients with disabling symptoms who are not candidates for revascularization. Cilostazol is contraindicated in congestive heart failure. Gingko biloba may have some small benefit. Vasodilators, chelation, vitamin E, testosterone, and estrogen have not shown any effect, and are not currently indicated.

Revascularization

Revascularization should be considered for patients who have symptoms refractory to comprehensive medical management or in individuals who cannot tolerate medical therapy due to medication side-effects. Two approaches are used: percutaneous intervention and surgical bypass. The choice depends on the length of the obstruction and location of the diseased arterial segment. Regardless of the technique chosen, early referral to an experienced interventional radiologist or cardiologist, or a vascular surgeon is prudent. Perioperative medical consultation is also wise.

Percutaneous Angioplasty

Percutaneous angioplasty (with or without endovascular stent placement) of the diseased vessel has become more common in recent years as an alternative to traditional surgical bypass. Endovascular intervention is the treatment of choice for focal stenoses less than 3 cm long. Stenoses 3 to 5cm long are also often amenable to percutaneous approaches (Figure 26-4).

Percutaneous Revascularization

Percutaneous revascularization for PVD remains controversial in several areas. First, the comparison of percutaneous versus surgical revascularization is understudied. Second, the use of stents has revolutionized coronary revascularization and will likely also improve percutaneous revascularization for PVD, although few studies have directly compared balloon angioplasty and stenting. Third, as for percutaneous revascularization in the coronary vasculature, technical improvements have greatly improved outcomes and safety. Finally, the degree to which the treating physician should push medical therapy is often subject to considerable input from patients who increasingly consider reports in the lay literature as a part of their decision.

These factors, along with more rapid recovery from surgery, have led to a dramatic increase in the use of percutaneous approaches. Until prospective, randomized studies are conducted, there will undoubtedly be considerable variation in practice for treating individuals with limiting symptoms from PVD.

Surgical bypass of the atherosclerotic vessel should be considered for carefully selected patients. Because operative mortality ranges from 1% to 3%, the benefits of surgery must be carefully weighed against the risk involved. Ideally, candidates should be younger than 70 years, nondiabetic, and have little distal arterial involvement. Bypass is the intervention of choice for multifocal stenoses and segments >5cm in length. Aortofemoral bypass for iliac disease results in >90% patency at 5 years. Infrainguinal procedures such as femoral-popliteal bypass share high

Figure 26-4

Percutaneous Peripheral Angioplasty

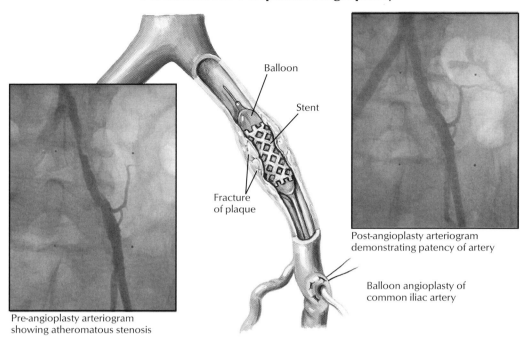

Balloon

Stent

Fracture of plaque

Pre-angioplasty arteriogram showing atheromatous stenosis

Post-angioplasty arteriogram demonstrating patency of artery

Balloon angioplasty of common iliac artery

Surgical Bypass Procedures

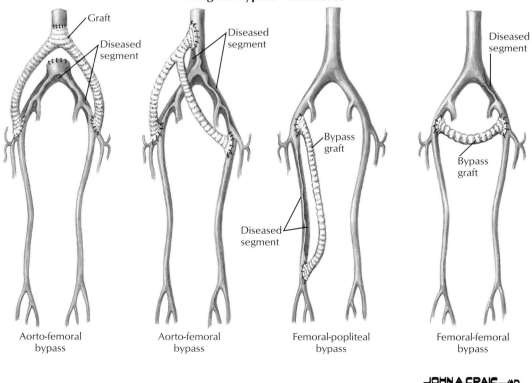

Graft

Diseased segment

Aorto-femoral bypass

Diseased segment

Aorto-femoral bypass

Bypass graft

Diseased segment

Femoral-popliteal bypass

Diseased segment

Bypass graft

Femoral-femoral bypass

JOHN A. CRAIG—AD
©ICON

long-term patency rates. Localized stenosis may be corrected by endarterectomy. Patients with PVD necessitating surgery often have co-existing coronary artery disease and must be screened appropriately before surgery.

FUTURE DIRECTIONS

Many new medications are currently under investigation. Levocarnitine, prostaglandins, naftidrofuryl, defibrotide, and angiogenic factors may someday be added to the armamentarium for treatment of claudication. Advances in the prevention and treatment of cardiovascular events will improve the prognosis of the patient with peripheral vascular disease. A growing body of experience with endovascular stenting may help clarify its role in therapy. Coated stents, laser recanalization, endoluminal radiation, and photoangioplasty are promising experimental modalities which may improve endovascular outcomes if proven in clinical trials. Because of these advances, individuals with symptomatic PVD will likely fare better in the coming years.

REFERENCES

The Cochrane Collection Web Site. Available at: http://www.cochrane.org.

Comerota AJ. Endovascular and surgical revascularization for patients with intermittent claudication. *Am J Cardiol.* 2001; 87:34D-43D.

eMedicine Web Site. Available at: http://www.emedicine.com.

Hiatt WR. Medical treatment of peripheral arterial disease and claudication. *N Engl J Med.* 2001;344:1608-1621.

Koelemay MJ, Lijmer JG, Stoker J, Legemate DA, Bossuyt PM. Magnetic resonance angiography for the evaluation of lower extremity arterial disease: a meta-analysis. *JAMA.* 2001;285:1338-1345.

Ouriel K. Peripheral arterial disease. *Lancet.* 2001;358:1257-1264.

Schmieder FA, Comerota JA. Intermittent claudication: magnitude of the problem, patient evaluation, and therapeutic strategies. *Am J Cardiol.* 2001;87:3D-13D.

UpToDate Web Site. Available at: http://www.uptodate.com.

Chapter 27

Preeclampsia and Eclampsia in Pregnancy

Garrett K. Lam and Valerie M. Parisi

Preeclampsia is a pregnancy-specific syndrome of reduced organ perfusion related to vasospasm and activation of the coagulation cascade. The syndrome is defined by a collection of signs and symptoms exhibited by the patient. It has many different clinical presentations. The classical definition of preeclampsia, the triad of hypertension, proteinuria, and edema, has been modified recently by the *National High Blood Pressure Working Group* to include a gestational blood pressure elevation of >140 mmHg systolic and >90 mmHg diastolic, measured over 2 separate occasions at least 6 hours apart. Proteinuria, on the order of ≥0.3 g protein excreted in a 24-hour sample, is usually seen. As most pregnant women become edematous to some extent during pregnancy, edema has been dropped as a diagnostic criterion. In most instances, preeclampsia occurs after 20 weeks' gestation, although earlier onset is seen in conjunction with triploid or molar pregnancies.

Pregnancy induced hypertension (PIH), which includes both pre-eclampsia and eclampsia; chronic hypertension, defined as increased blood pressure of various etiologies with onset predating the pregnancy; and chronic hypertension with superimposed pre-eclampsia are recognized as the 3 major types of hypertensive disorders of pregnancy by the *American College of Obstetrics and Gynecology* (ACOG). A fourth entity, "gestational hypertension," which includes transient hypertension of pregnancy without the presence of preeclampsia, has also been included as a hypertensive disorder of pregnancy by the *National High Blood Pressure Education Program*.

Considered as a whole, these hypertensive disorders of pregnancy are responsible for a large part of both the maternal and fetal morbidity and mortality seen in pregnancy. A recent review showed that 20% of maternal deaths over a 4-year period were directly related to a hypertensive complication of pregnancy. It is estimated that 7% to 10% of all pregnancies will be affected with some type of hypertensive problem, the majority of cases (70%) stemming from PIH/preeclampsia. As preeclampsia/eclampsia seem to be the major component of maternal morbidity, a closer look at its pathophysiology, clinical characteristics, and treatment is warranted.

ETIOLOGY AND PATHOGENESIS

Although the etiology of preeclampsia is unclear, its effects on organ systems have been well documented through pathologic inspection. Renal biopsies from preeclamptic patients reveal a characteristic glomerular capillary endothelial swelling (Figure 27-1). Proteinaceous deposits of fibrinogen derivatives are seen accompanying the endothelial cells. This condition has been labeled glomerular capillary endotheliosis. These glomerular changes usually resolve within several weeks postpartum. Hepatic involvement is seen in patients who develop the "HELLP" syndrome, a variant of severe preeclampsia. These patients exhibit *Hemolysis, Elevated Liver* function tests and *Low Platelet* counts. Pathologic exam of the liver reveals periportal hemorrhagic necrosis, which leads to the elevated liver enzyme levels (Figure 27-2). Bleeding from these lesions leads to subcapsular hematomas and subsequent swelling, which is manifested in the complaints of right upper quadrant pain from many preeclamptic patients.

Inspection of the placentas of affected gestations reveals gross areas of nodular ischemia, and if severe enough, areas of infarct (Figure 27-3). These changes are the result of compromised blood flow through the constricted spiral arterioles of the placenta. Histologic exam reveals the

Figure 27-1

Toxemia of Pregnancy

Preeclampsia; characteristic electron microscopic findings in renal glomerular capillaries: marked swelling of endothelial cells (**E**) compressing capillary lumen (**L**); basement membrane (**B**) essentially normal; dense proteinaceous deposits (**D**) between basement membrane and endothelial cell; foot processes (**P**) of epithelial cells (**EP**) normal or focally fused; mesangial cells (**M**) swollen, mesangial matrix (**MM**) unchanged

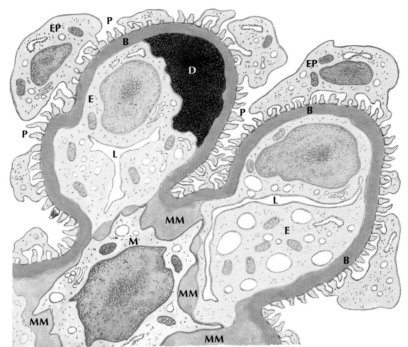

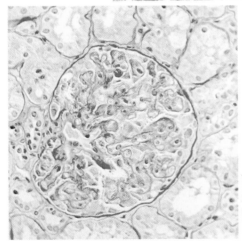

Light micrograph of typically avascular glomerulus with cytoplasmic swelling and prominence of mesangium; no cellular proliferation; urinary space diminished but not obliterated; capillary walls, Bowman's capsule, and surrounding tubules normal (pas stain)

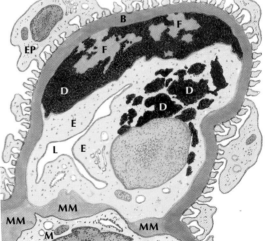

Occasional dense proteinaceous deposits (**D**) both within endothelial cells and between endothelium and basement membrane; very rare fatty deposits (**F**) within subendothelial proteinaceous deposits

Figure 27-2

Acute Toxemia of Pregnancy
Visceral Lesions in Preeclampsia and Eclampsia

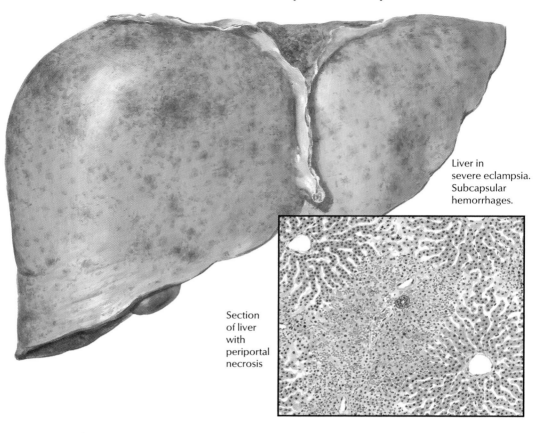

Liver in severe eclampsia. Subcapsular hemorrhages.

Section of liver with periportal necrosis

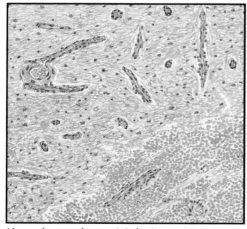

Hemorrhage and necrosis in brain

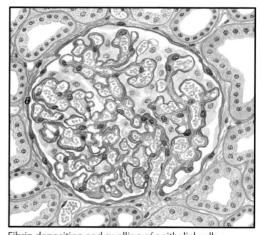

Fibrin deposition and swelling of epithelial cells in glomerulus

presence of endothelial cell damage, basement membrane disruption, platelet deposition, intimal cell proliferation, and smooth muscle hyperplasia, which all lead to decreased villous capillary lumen size, and compromised blood flow.

CLINICAL PRESENTATION

In the hypertensive gravida, blood pressure changes may result from other medical conditions, and proteinuria may not be consistently present. Therefore, careful scrutiny for other clinical signs and symptoms of preeclampsia is necessary. Findings such as an increased serum creatinine (>1.2 mg/dl), increased uric acid (>5.5 mg/dl), and decreased platelet count (<100,000 cells/mm), indicate multi-organ system involvement and usually define severe preeclampsia. Affected patients may also complain of right upper quadrant abdominal pain, which is manifested by abnormally elevated values of ALT/AST and may portend subcapsular hematoma or acute rupture of the liver (Figure 27-2). Severe preeclamptic disease is further characterized by oliguria, pulmonary edema or cyanosis, and cerebral disturbances such as unremitting headache, scotomata, or blurred vision. Fetal effects, such as intrauterine growth restriction and oligohydramnios, are also hallmarks of severe disease.

Older texts describe a unique examination of the ocular fundi (Figure 27-4). Specifically, preeclamptic patients may exhibit vasospasm of the retinal vessels. A series of spindle-shaped, sausage-linked constrictions may be seen, especially in the terminal part of retinal vessels, in the nasal branches, and in the portion close to the optic disc. A rapid proliferation of retinal veins may be seen, such that the ratio of arterioles to veins changes from a normal 2:3 ratio to 1:2 or 1:3. In actuality, examination of the eyegrounds is rarely, if ever done, in the contemporary workup of preeclamptic patients. However, in view of these retinal vascular changes, it is understandable why affected patients will often report symptoms of persistent headache, blurry vision and scotomata.

DIFFERENTIAL DIAGNOSIS AND DIAGNOSTIC APPROACH

In some cases, eclampsia – a more malignant disease associated with hypertension – develops. Eclampsia is defined as the occurrence of convulsions, not caused by any coincidental neurologic condition (i.e., epilepsy), in a woman who meets the diagnostic criteria for preeclampsia. The incidence of eclampsia is estimated at 1/1600 to 2000 pregnancies, with the frequency increasing as the gestation approaches term. In general, eclampsia is not necessarily a progression of preeclampsia. The signs and symptoms of severe preeclampsia, such as proteinuria and severe hypertension, are not necessary for the development of eclampsia. Some studies have demonstrated that only 40% of patients with eclampsia had severe hypertension and 20% had blood pressures below 140 mmHg systolic and 90 mm Hg diastolic. In essence, Sibai's data implies that eclampsia is a separate disease manifestation of a hypertensive disorder of pregnancy, and not necessarily a representation of the "next, worse step" of preeclampsia.

Any incidence of convulsions during the antepartum period of pregnancy, delivery, or in the immediate postpartum period should carry the diagnosis of eclampsia until proven otherwise. Other causes of seizure (i.e., epilepsy, intracranial hemorrhage, infectious states) must be ruled out.

MANAGEMENT AND THERAPY

Management of the preeclamptic patient is primarily restricted to seizure prophylaxis and delivery. In cases of mild preeclampsia, recent literature has shown that a combination of strict home bedrest with frequent outpatient checks of blood pressure and fetal monitoring is a viable alternative to strict hospitalization. There is no definitive evidence to support the use of antihypertensives or diuretics to prevent the development of preeclampsia or to prolong the duration of a preeclamptic gestation.

Recent trials have studied the use of calcium supplementation to prevent the development of preeclampsia. Preliminary evidence hinted that calcium might reduce blood pressure and therefore decrease the incidence of preeclampsia. However, in a prospective study of 4600 patients, calcium supplementation was not shown to alter the incidence of preeclampsia in healthy nulliparas. Thus, calcium is not recognized as a preventative agent for preeclampsia. Recent trials have also examined the use of low-dose aspirin to inhibit the platelet production of thromboxane, based on the idea that unequal amounts of throm-

Figure 27-3

Acute Toxemia of Pregnancy
Placental Lesions in Preeclampsia and Eclampsia, Infarcts

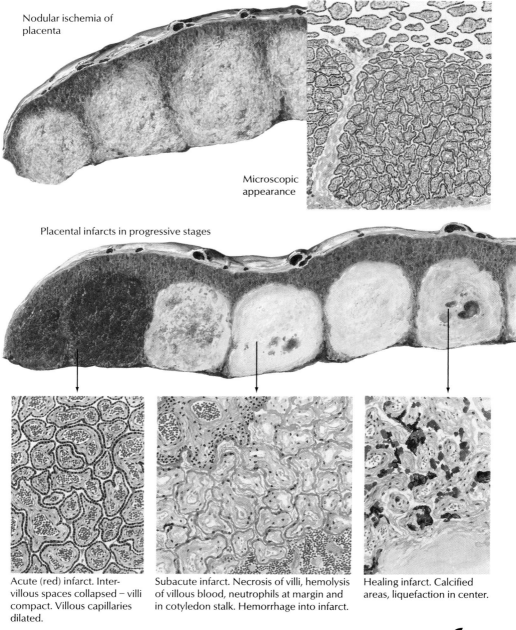

Nodular ischemia of placenta

Microscopic appearance

Placental infarcts in progressive stages

Acute (red) infarct. Intervillous spaces collapsed – villi compact. Villous capillaries dilated.

Subacute infarct. Necrosis of villi, hemolysis of villous blood, neutrophils at margin and in cotyledon stalk. Hemorrhage into infarct.

Healing infarct. Calcified areas, liquefaction in center.

Figure 27-4

Acute Toxemia of Pregnancy
Eyegrounds in Preeclampsia and Eclampsia

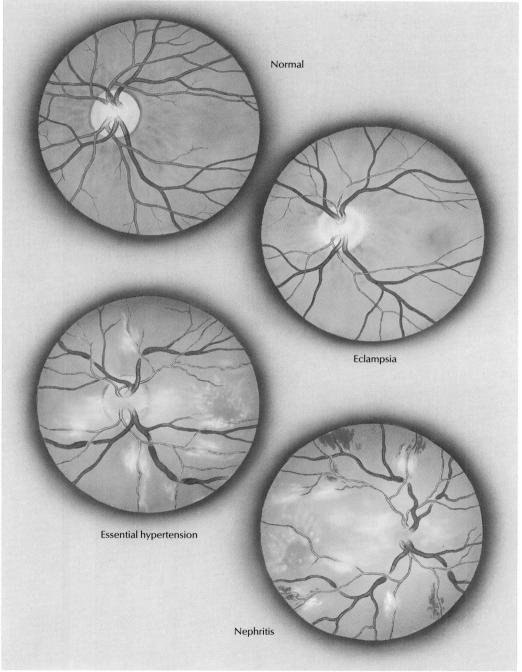

Normal

Eclampsia

Essential hypertension

Nephritis

boxane (vs. prostacyclin) are responsible for the development of preeclampsia. However, a small number of randomized multicenter trials have demonstrated that aspirin therapy does not decrease perinatal morbidity from affected mothers, and can lead to an increased risk of placental abruption. Thus, the routine use of low-dose aspirin as a prophylactic treatment for the prevention preeclampsia is not recommended.

The only known cure for preeclampsia is delivery. An effective medical treatment remains unknown, partly because the etiology of preeclampsia is not known. The basis of current antepartum treatment is seizure prophylaxis, most commonly with magnesium sulfate. Parenteral magnesium sulfate is given, usually as a continuous intravenous infusion, over the course of labor and 24 hours postpartum. This covers the highest risk interval for the development of eclampsia.

After delivery, affected patients must be counseled as to their risk for future problems. A recent study confirmed that women with prior preeclampsia are more likely to have severe preeclampsia in subsequent pregnancies, have a higher risk for placental abruption, and have a higher risk for chronic hypertension.

FUTURE DIRECTIONS

Currently, there are ongoing investigations examining the use of Vitamin E and Vitamin C to prevent preeclampsia, based on the theory that preeclampsia is associated with oxidative stress from lipid peroxides. Studies have shown a correlation between increased lipid peroxide levels and increased blood pressure in preeclamptic patients. Vitamin E is the major lipid-soluble antioxidant, and it is thought that dietary supplement may correct for the increased oxidative stress. This notion is supported by recent findings that normotensive pregnancies have increased ratios of vitamin E to lipid peroxides with advancing gestation, and that vitamin E levels are decreased in severe preeclampsia. A major therapeutic trial is yet to be published.

Preeclampsia is a complex and vexing disease. It is one of the most studied diseases of obstetrics, yet an understanding of its precise etiology continues to elude investigators. Despite our progress in its characterization, the only certain conclusion is that medical care providers will continue to struggle with the maternal and fetal mortality and morbidity caused by this disease until its cause(s) can be identified.

REFERENCES

American College of Obstetricians and Gynecologists. *Hypertension in Pregnancy*. Washington, DC: American College of Obstetricians and Gynecologists; 1996. Technical bulletin 219.

Report of the National High Blood Pressure Education Program Working Group on High Blood Pressure in Pregnancy. *Am J Obstet Gynecol*. 2000;183:S1–S22.

Hallak M. Hypertension in pregnancy. In: James DK, Steer PJ, Weiner CP, Gonik B, eds. *High Risk Pregnancy*. 2nd ed. London, England: WB Saunders Co; 1999:639–660.

Kaunitz AM, Hughes JM, Grimes DA, Smith JC, Rochat RW, Kafrissen ME. Causes of maternal mortality in the United States. *Obstet Gynecol*. 1985;65:605–612.

Sibai BM. Hypertension. In: Gabbe SG, Niebyl JR, Simpson JL, eds. *Obstetrics: Normal and Problem Pregnancies*. 4th ed. New York, NY: Churchill Livingstone; 2002:945–1004.

Sibai BM. Preeclampsia-eclampsia. *Curr Probl Obstet Gynecol Fertil*. 1990;13:1–45.

Section IV

DISORDERS OF ENDOCRINOLOGY AND METABOLISM

Chapter 28

Diabetes Mellitus and its Complications

John B. Buse

Diabetes mellitus (DM) affects approximately 17 million people in the United States and hundreds of millions of people worldwide. The lifetime risk of developing DM or its form *fruste*, impaired glucose tolerance, in Western society is 30% to 50%. There is a burgeoning epidemic of DM with increases in incidence rates of more than 6% per year, driven by increasing obesity and progressively sedentary lifestyles. DM is a major cause of morbidity and mortality. Premature vascular disease is the eventual cause of death in 80% of people with DM, leading to a loss of 7 to 10 years of life. The costs involved in the treatment of people with DM are staggering, accounting for 17% of all health-care expenditures in the United States.

We are in the midst of multiple revolutions in DM management. Evidence that lifestyle interventions and patient self-management education are effective has driven improved insurance coverage for these services. Therapeutic targets have been established on the basis of outcomes trials not only for glycemia but for common comorbidities—hypertension and dyslipidemia. There are new developments in glucose monitoring technology. Multiple new classes of pharmacological agents are available to treat DM. Together, these advances create the possibility that the early death and disability associated with DM can be avoided.

ETIOLOGY AND PATHOGENESIS

Type 1 DM (previously known as insulin-dependent DM) can occur at any age but is more common among children and young adults. It is characterized by insulin deficiency resulting from autoimmune destruction of insulin secreting beta-cells within the pancreatic islets of Langerhans. Other autoimmune endocrine disease such as hypothyroidism, ovarian failure, adrenal insufficiency, pernicious anemia, and vitiligo often co-exist in patients with type 1 DM. Though classically considered a disease of children, adolescents, and young adults, it is estimated that up to 10% of adults with new-onset DM have a slowly evolving form of type 1 DM. Islet cell antibodies, antibodies to glutamic acid decarboxy-

lase, and others are often present at diagnosis. The risk of DM is genetically determined and involves several genetic loci, the most important of these being genes within the human leukocyte antigen system. Only 10% of people with type 1 DM exhibit a family history; the risk of future DM in the first-degree relative of a patient with type 1 DM is 2% to 5%. There are likely environmental triggers to the development of this autoimmune process, although these are poorly understood.

Type 2 DM (previously known as noninsulin-dependent DM) generally occurs in adulthood, although it can develop at any age. Most patients have a first-degree relative with DM, and most are overweight, generally with a central pattern of obesity. Type 2 DM is more common in all ethnic minority groups and tends to occur at an earlier age in these high-risk groups as well as in women. From recent prospective studies of high-risk groups such as the Pima tribe of Native Americans in Arizona, we understand that type 2 DM develops as the result of progressive loss of insulin secretory capacity on the background of insulin resistance. Insulin resistance is defined as an inadequate response of metabolic processes to physiological insulin concentrations.

A number of clinical phenotypes are associated with insulin resistance and are sometimes discussed together as the metabolic (or dysmetabolic) syndrome. These features include obesity with a central pattern of weight distribution, dyslipidemia, hypertension, hypercoagulability, endothelial dysfunction, and accelerated atherosclerosis. The dyslipidemia is characterized by increased triglycerides, low HDL, and although the absolute concentration of LDL is the same as the population average, the LDL particles are generally small and dense and more atherogenic. The pathophysiology of these associations is unknown. Nevertheless, a substantial portion of the increased cardiovascular morbidity in DM is likely related to this syndrome and its associated features.

The pathophysiology of the microvascular complications is even less clear. There are genetic predispositions to retinopathy, nephropathy, and neuropathy. Putative mechanisms for the development of complications include the intracellular accumulation of sorbitol, overactivity of protein kinase C, and the development of advanced glycosylation end products. These advanced glycosylation end products result from the non-enzymatic glycosylation of amino groups in proteins and subsequent molecular reorganizations. This tendency is taken advantage of, in the case of the glycosylation of hemoglobin, as an index of the average level of glucose in the circulation for the previous 3 months. When such glycosylation occurs in structural proteins with long half-lives, these glycosylated proteins can cross-link and results in changes in structure and function.

CLINICAL PRESENTATION

In Type1 DM, clinical deterioration can be quite rapid and patients can transition from being completely asymptomatic to having rampant polyuria, polydipsia, and polyphagia with weight loss and blurred vision over a matter of days to weeks. Affected individuals generally have fairly widely fluctuating blood sugars. Diabetic ketoacidosis can occur when one or more insulin doses are missed or with physiological stress. Hypoglycemia is quite common as a complication of therapy. In type 2 DM, patients may be completely asymptomatic for years. Some present with classic symptoms of microvascular or macrovascular complications (Figures 28-1, 28-2 and 28-3). More often, subtle symptoms may be present for years as well such as fatigue, problems with recurrent cutaneous infections, or intermit-

tent nocturia. If hyperglycemia is allowed to progress unchecked, life-threatening problems, such as diabetic ketoacidosis or hyperosmolar states, can develop.

Diabetic retinopathy is generally asymptomatic although as late manifestations, patients may note a change in their visual field with retinal detachments or blurred vision in the setting of intraocular hemorrhage or macular edema (Figure 28-3). Diabetic nephropathy is likewise generally asymptomatic until late stages when patients present with fatigue, edema, symptoms of fluid overload, or in hypertensive crisis (Figure 28-3). Diabetic neuropathy has multiple manifestations as a result of involvement of peripheral motor and sensory nerves, cranial nerves, and the autonomic nervous systems. The most common of these is peripheral neuropathy, which can present with numbness or dysesthesias such as burning or tingling (Figures 28-1 and 28-2). In general, these symptoms proceed from distal sites proximally and can be associated with motor dysfunction. Motor, sensory, or cranial nerves can be afflicted by mononeuropathies where the function of a single nerve is affected. Entrapment syndromes such as carpal tunnel syndrome are quite common. Autonomic neuropathies can be disabling and can present with decreased night vision, facial sweating with meals, postprandial bloating, nausea, vomiting, diarrhea, constipation, orthostasis, dyshidrotic skin, urinary retention, and sexual dysfunction (Figure 28-1). With regard to macrovascular disease, the classic presentations of angina, myocardial infarction, stroke, transient ischemic attacks, or claudication are quite common (Figure 28-3). As is true in nondiabetic individuals, many - afflicted with life-threatening vascular disease have no symptoms at all.

DIFFERENTIAL DIAGNOSIS

Generally, DM is a primary disorder; however, it is worth noting the much less common secondary causes. Among these, pancreatic disorders are the most common, including chronic pancreatitis, cystic fibrosis, and pancreatic cancer. Although for years it was considered that these disorders were the result of destruction of the majority of functioning beta-cells, the pathophysiology of DM in these disorders is more complex, probably involving ill-defined humoral factors. There are iatrogenic syndromes and syndromes associated with hormonal overproduction of glucocorticoids, growth hormone, glucagon, and catecholamines that can produce DM.

Diabetic retinopathy is pathognomonic of DM, although it can be similar to retinopathy associated with acromegaly. Diabetic nephropathy characteristically is associated with protein excretion, initially only detected with a very sensitive assay for microalbuminuria progressing to nephrotic syndrome. In a patient with proteinuria and evidence of retinopathy, it is most likely that the kidney disease is related to DM. In the absence of retinopathy or significant proteinuria, renal insufficiency may more likely be related to other forms of kidney disease, particularly hypertensive kidney disease. There is a substantial differential diagnosis for each of the peripheral and autonomic neuropathies. Excluding reversible causes such as vitamin B_{12} deficiency, tertiary syphilis, hypothyroidism, heavy metal intoxication, and monoclonal gammopathies by history, physical examination, and selected laboratory tests is prudent. If physical examination findings are asymmetric or associated with back pain or other neurologic findings, consideration of spinal or central nervous system pathology is essential. In the evaluation of painful extremities, characteristically the pain of diabetic neuropathy is worst at rest. Subcritical peripheral vascular disease should be considered as it is fairly common and similarly sometimes associated with worsening in the supine position.

DIAGNOSTIC APPROACH

Approximately one third of cases of DM in the United States are undiagnosed. In some studies, 20% to 50% of people with DM have one or more complications of the disease at the time that a diagnosis is made. Estimates suggest that the diagnosis of DM could be made 7 to 12 years earlier. Current recommendations suggest screening for DM using a fasting plasma glucose starting at age 45 and repeat screening every 3 years. It is recommended that screening for DM should start at an earlier age and at shorter intervals in people with one or more risk factors. These risk factors include a family history of DM in a first-degree relative; obesity defined as a BMI >27 or 120% of ideal body weight; belonging to a

high-risk ethnic group (essentially all ethnicities except Caucasians of western European extraction), most particularly Native Americans, Latino Americans, African Americans and Asian and Pacific Islanders; hypertension; dyslipidemia (high triglycerides or low high density lipoproteins); birth of a child greater than 9 pounds; and prior abnormality of glucose tolerance, particularly prior gestational DM or a prior fasting glucose greater than or equal to 110 mg/dL. Other indications of high risk include the presence of acanthosis nigricans or a history of polycystic ovarian syndrome or ovarian hyperandrogenism. A normal fasting glucose value is <110 mg/dL. People with a fasting plasma glucose ≥126 mg/dL (7.0 mM) would have a tentative diagnosis of DM, which needs to be confirmed on a separate day (see below). People with intermediate levels (fasting plasma glucose 110 to 125 mg/dL) have impaired fasting glucose or prediabetes and are at high risk for the development of DM and early cardiovascular disease.

Recent studies have suggested that the onset of DM can be prevented or delayed in high-risk populations with diet and exercise aimed at producing a 7% loss of body weight and 30 minutes of physical activity at least 5 days per week or with certain medications including metformin, acarbose, and orlistat.

MANAGEMENT AND THERAPY

Glycemic control is a central issue in the management of both type 1 and type 2 DM (Figure 28-4). There are adequate prospective randomized clinical trial data documenting that treatment policies associated with more stringent glycemic targets are associated with decreased rates of retinopathy, nephropathy, and neuropathy. Epidemiological studies support the potential of intensive glycemic control to reduce cardiovascular risk. For most patients, premeal plasma glucose targets between 90 and 130 mg/dL, 1 to 2 hour postprandial glucose levels less than 180 mg/dL, and hemoglobin A1c levels below 7% would be associated with low risk for complications. Less stringent treatment goals may be appropriate for patients with limited life expectancies (<6 years). There are no adequately powered clinical trial data available to document the benefit of glycemic control in the setting of advanced

Figure 28-1

Peripheral Vascular Disease

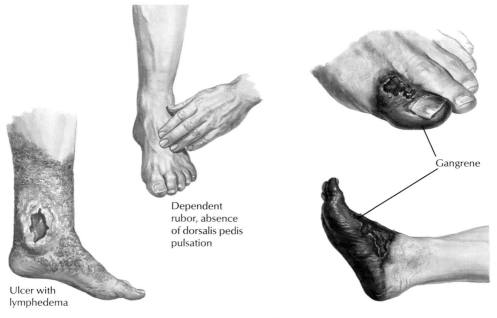

Dependent rubor, absence of dorsalis pedis pulsation

Gangrene

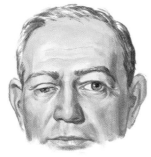

Ulcer with lymphedema

Neuropathy

Autonomic dysfunction

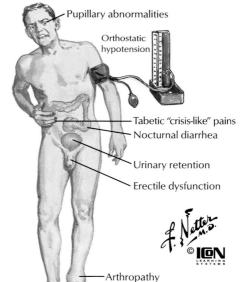

Pupillary abnormalities

Orthostatic hypotension

Tabetic "crisis-like" pains

Nocturnal diarrhea

Urinary retention

Erectile dysfunction

Arthropathy (Charcot's joints)

Extra-ocular muscle paralysis (ptosis, strabismus, diplopia)

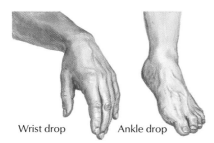

Wrist drop   Ankle drop

Figure 28-2

Neuropathy/Fungal Infection

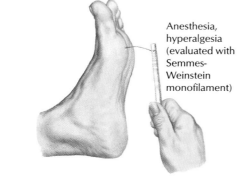

Anesthesia, hyperalgesia (evaluated with Semmes-Weinstein monofilament)

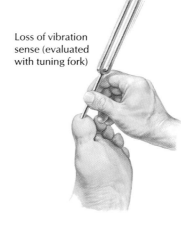

Loss of vibration sense (evaluated with tuning fork)

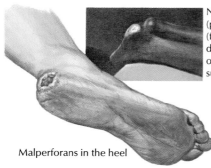

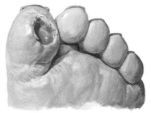

Neuropathic (painless) ulcers (fluorescein demonstration of good blood supply)

Malperforans in the heel

Malperforans in the first toe (one of the most frequent presentations)

Fungal Infection

Fungal infections of the nails and skin are common in patients with diabetes. With foot involvement, accompanying minor skin lesions can be the portal of infection which can result in chronic wounds and even amputations. Excellent foot care and antifungal therapy are important preventative measures in the setting of advanced diabetic neuropathy.

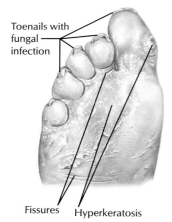

Toenails with fungal infection

Interdigital tinea pedis and fissures under the toes

Fissures   Hyperkeratosis

Dysfunction of sweat glands, observed among patients with autonomic neuropathy can cause local changes to the skin that can favor the occurance of cracks, fissures and ulcers that are potential portals of entry for bacteria

Toenail with fungal infection, showing sharp irregular edges

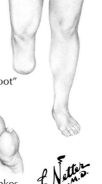

Amputation, the most disabling consequence of diabetic neuropathy results from deep infection which develops in the setting of the "insensate foot"

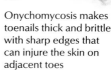

Onychomycosis makes toenails thick and brittle with sharp edges that can injure the skin on adjacent toes

Figure 28-3

Micro- and Macrovascular Complications

Diabetic retinopathy

Diabetic retinopathy can be easily detected during a dialated eye exam and is the leading cause of blindness among adults in the United States. Visual loss can be prevented with early recognition and treatment of retinopathy.

Nonproliferative retinopathy (early stage)

- Microaneurysms
- Hemorrhages
- Cotton-wool spots
- Hard exudate
- Narrowed arterioles

Proliferative retinopathy (late stage)

Massive hemorrhage

Retinitis proliferans

Diabetic nephropathy

Histologic view of diabetic glomerulo-sclerosis

Diabetes mellitus is the leading cause of end-stage renal disease in the Western world

Cerebrovascular disease

The high incidence of vascular complications among patients with diabetes is related not only to blood glucose elevations, but also to the frequent association of dyslipidemia, hypertension, a procoagulant state and the tendency to form unstable plaques in the arterial wall.

Ischemic stroke due to in situ thrombosis, usually triggered by plaque rupture in the carotid or cerebral artery

Myocardial infarction and related heart disease account for 70% of the mortality in people with diabetes

Myocardial infarction

Atheromatous aorta and branches

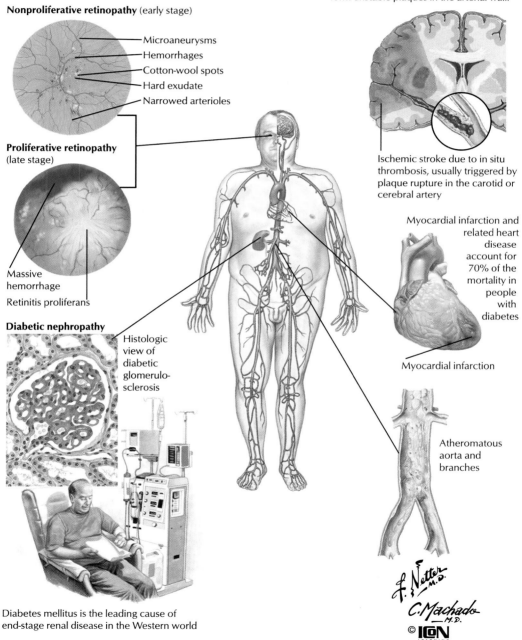

Figure 28-4

Non-Pharmacologic Therapy
Lifestyle Changes

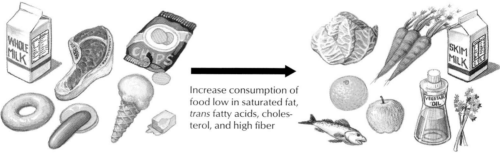

Control weight

Regular exercise

Stop smoking

Control blood pressure

Increase consumption of food low in saturated fat, *trans* fatty acids, cholesterol, and high fiber

Matching Pharmacology to Pathophysiology

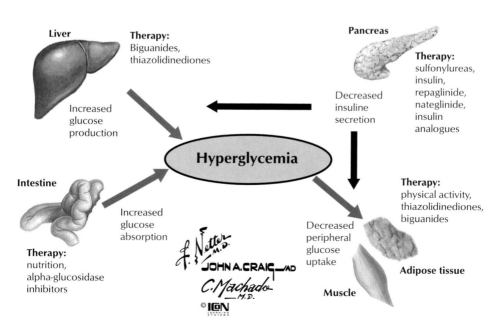

Liver

Therapy: Biguanides, thiazolidinediones

Increased glucose production

Pancreas

Therapy: sulfonylureas, insulin, repaglinide, nateglinide, insulin analogues

Decreased insuline secretion

Hyperglycemia

Intestine

Increased glucose absorption

Therapy: nutrition, alpha-glucosidase inhibitors

Therapy: physical activity, thiazolidinediones, biguanides

Decreased peripheral glucose uptake

Adipose tissue

Muscle

complications, in the elderly (over age 65), and in young children (less than 13). Severe or frequent hypoglycemia is an indication for modification of treatment regimens, including targeting higher glucose levels. Self-monitoring of blood glucose, lifestyle modification, and self-management education are integral parts of intensive glucose management strategies that have been associated with a lower risk of complications.

Management of type 1 DM requires replacement of insulin in a physiological fashion. Novel insulin analogues allow this to be achieved to a greater extent than older insulin preparations. In general, most patients with type 1 DM require a multiple daily injection regimen in which they administer a long-acting insulin, such as insulin glargine, to control fasting glucose and prevent the rise in glucose between meals. A fast-acting insulin analogue (lispro or aspart) is administered with each meal in proportion to carbohydrate intake, taking into account planned activity and current levels of glucose. Using this regimen or a continuous subcutaneous insulin infusion (insulin pump) minimizes glycemic excursions. Such intensive regimens generally require substantial commitment on the part of the patient as well as a team of health-care providers, including DM educators, dietitians, and physicians, to be effectively implemented.

There are inadequate clinical trial data to allow dogmatic statements regarding optimal approaches to the management of type 2 DM. A generally reasonable overall approach is to first work on lifestyle issues (diet and exercise) with patients, preferably with the help of a dietitian or DM educator (Figure 28-4). The major tenets of lifestyle management are to promote consistent carbohydrate intake in the context of a low saturated/polyunsaturated fat diet and regular aerobic exercise. The initial goal should generally be premeal blood glucose levels around 100 mg/dL. In patients with higher levels of glucose, a single pharmacological agent should be administered to reduce plasma glucose expeditiously. In general, metformin monotherapy has the greatest evidence based on outcomes studies to support its use as monotherapy, although there are a number of contraindications to its use that must be carefully considered. Sulfonylureas are very effective glucose-lowering agents and quite inexpensive. The thiazolidinediones (sometimes referred to as

glitazones) hold tremendous promise to reduce cardiovascular risk, but they have not been available long enough to complete efficacy studies. Long-acting insulins, primarily NPH and glargine, are also very effective agents to decrease premeal glucose levels. If a single agent is inadequate to achieve fasting and premeal glucose targets, additional agents should be added sequentially. There is some evidence to suggest that monitoring and specifically treating to achieve postprandial glucose targets may be associated with greater overall control and perhaps lower risk of weight gain and hypoglycemia. Most patients can achieve the glucose targets above using combinations of agents that improve insulin sensitivity (metformin and the thiazolidinediones) with agents that increase insulin levels (sulfonylureas, repaglinide and nateglinide, and insulin) as well as combinations of agents that primarily decrease fasting and premeal glucose levels (metformin, glitazones, sulfonylureas, and long-acting insulins) with agents that decrease postprandial glucose (alpha glucosidase inhibitors, repaglinide and nateglinide, and rapid-acting insulin).

Because more than 80% of patients with DM die of cardiovascular disease, aggressive management of other cardiovascular risk factors (smoking, blood pressure, and lipids) is at least as important as DM management. Current recommendations suggest that most patients with DM should take aspirin, reduce blood pressure to <130/80 mm Hg with a blood pressure regimen that generally includes an angiotensin-converting enzyme inhibitor, reduce low density lipoprotein level to <100 mg/dL, reduce triglycerides to <200 mg/dL, and optimize high density lipoprotein cholesterol.

FUTURE DIRECTIONS

There is a huge pipeline of drugs in development including agents aimed primarily at blocking the development of complications. An exciting possibility for the future is that new islet growth can be fostered. Better glucose monitoring and insulin delivery devices are under development, including approaches that combine these two techniques to create a closed loop or artificial beta-cell capable of administering glucose based on continuous monitoring of plasma glucose. There are a number of trials underway to explore

tighter glycemic targets and their risks and benefits. There is a growing body of evidence to suggest that prevention of type 2 DM is possible.
Additional studies are underway to demonstrate
the effectiveness of such approaches to improve
outcomes. Similarly, studies are underway regarding cardiovascular risk reduction in the setting of
DM, and it seems likely that broader and more
stringent targets will be adopted. A broad-based
public health approach to deal with the epidemic
of obesity and DM is necessary to avoid almost
unimaginable morbidity and expense in managing the metabolic consequences of overnutrition
and underactivity.

REFERENCES

American Diabetes Association: clinical practice recommendations 2003. *Diabetes Core.* 2003; 26 (suppl 1).

Atkinson MA, Eisenbarth GS. Type 1 diabetes: new perspec-
tives on disease pathogenesis and treatment. *Lancet.*
2001;358:221-229.

Weyer C, Bogardus C, Mott DM, Pratley RE. The natural history of insulin secretory dysfunction and insulin resistance in
the pathogenesis of type 2 diabetes mellitus. *J Clin Invest.*
1999;104:787-794.

Chapter 29
Diseases of the Adrenal Cortex

David A. Ontjes

Adrenocorticotropic hormone (ACTH) is the chief determinant of the secretion of cortisol and androgenic steroids by the adrenal cortex. ACTH secretion is controlled by corticotropin-releasing hormone (CRH) from the hypothalamus (Figure 29-1). At any given moment, ACTH secretion represents a balance between the stimulatory effects of the central nervous system, mediated by CRH, and negative feedback control exerted by circulating glucocorticoids. The secretion of both CRH and ACTH is subject to a diurnal rhythm, reaching a peak at about the time of awakening in the morning, and a nadir in the evening before sleep. Stressful stimuli such as trauma, infection, hemorrhage, or hypoglycemia normally activate CRH and ACTH secretion, causing cortisol levels to rise.

Aldosterone secretion is governed by the renin-angiotensin system (Figure 29-1). The chief determinant of aldosterone secretion is angiotensin II, which is generated under the influence of renin. Reduced systemic blood pressure and reduced renal perfusion are responsible for causing the release of renin. In humans, the synthesis of aldosterone is confined to the outer glomerulosa layer of the adrenal cortex; cortisol and androgens are produced by the fasciculata and reticularis layers.

The steroid products of both the adrenal glands and the gonads are derived from a series of biosynthetic steps beginning with cholesterol (Figure 29-2). The glucocorticoid, cortisol, and the mineralocorticoid, aldosterone, are the most active and important hormones produced by the adrenal cortex. The enzymes involved in steroidogenesis are members of a family of cytochrome P450 oxidases. Each individual enzyme is capable of handling more than one substrate. As a result, a few distinct enzymes are capable of catalyzing transformations leading to over a dozen steroid products. In the testes, an additional enzyme is present that converts the weak adrenal androgen androstenedione into testosterone. In the ovaries, an aromatase enzyme converts testosterone to estradiol. These terminal steps in the gonads do not occur to an appreciable extent in normal adrenal glands.

ADRENAL INSUFFICIENCY

Adrenal insufficiency arises whenever the quantity of circulating cortisol is insufficient to meet the needs of the body. Under basal conditions, cortisol is needed to maintain normal vascular tone, normal hepatic gluconeogenesis, and normal glycogen stores (hence the name glucocorticoid). Higher concentrations are needed during stress. Lack of adequate cortisol can lead to hypotension, shock, and hypoglycemia. Patients with cortisol deficiency may have variable deficiencies of aldosterone and adrenal androgens as well. Mineralocorticoid deficiency leads to renal wasting of sodium, retention of potassium, and a reduced intravascular volume. Adrenal androgen deficiency leads to a significant reduction of the overall androgen supply in women and can result in a loss of body hair and libido. In men who maintain normal testosterone production from the gonads, loss of adrenal androgens does not lead to an overall androgen deficiency.

Etiology and Pathogenesis

Any disease process causing direct injury to the adrenal cortex can cause *primary adrenal insufficiency*. Diseases affecting the hypothalamus or pituitary cause *secondary adrenal insufficiency* by reducing the secretion of ACTH (Table 29-1).

Primary adrenal insufficiency (Addison's disease) is the result of *chronic autoimmune destruction* of the adrenal cortex most commonly. Lymphocytic infiltration is the usual histologic feature. The adrenal glands are small and cortical cells are largely absent, although the medulla is preserved. Antibodies to cellular components of the adrenal cortex are present early in the disease process.

Figure 29-1

Control of the Secretion of Cortisol and Aldosterone

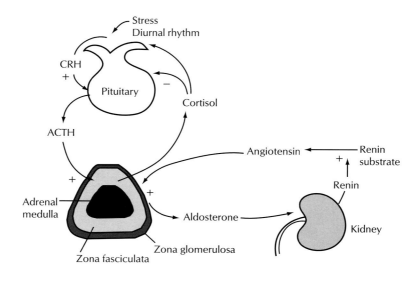

Figure 29-2

Synthetic Pathways for the Adrenal Steroids

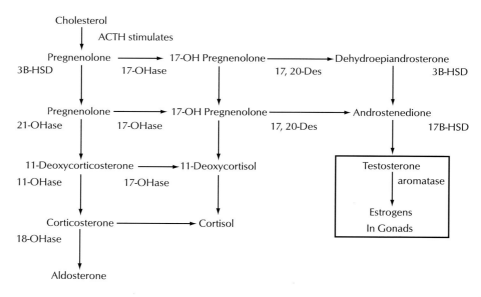

Patients with autoimmune adrenal disease are more likely to have autoimmune processes causing deficiency of other endocrine glands, including the thyroid, parathyroids, gonads, and pancreatic beta cells.

Several other mechanisms can cause primary adrenal insufficiency. Bilateral *adrenal hemor-rhage* occurs in critically ill patients who are taking anticoagulants or who have coagulopathies. The primary antiphospholipid antibody syndrome (lupus anticoagulant) is a common cause of adrenal hemorrhage. The importance of *tuberculosis* as a cause of adrenal insufficiency has waned in the United States, but not in other parts of the

Figure 29-3

Chronic Primary Adrenal Cortical Insufficiency
(Addison's Dieases)

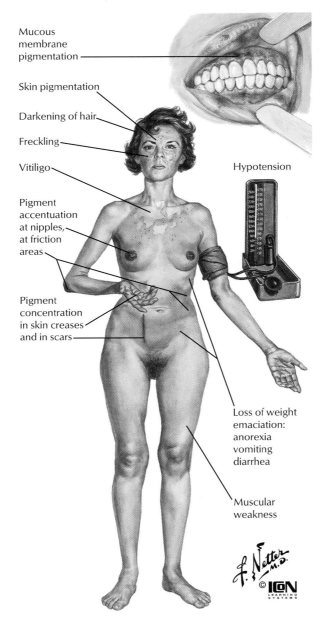

Mucous membrane pigmentation

Skin pigmentation

Darkening of hair

Freckling

Vitiligo

Pigment accentuation at nipples, at friction areas

Pigment concentration in skin creases and in scars

Hypotension

Loss of weight emaciation: anorexia vomiting diarrhea

Muscular weakness

world where it is common. Up to 5% of patients with terminal AIDS may have evidence of adrenal insufficiency, usually due to superinfection with agents such as cytomegalovirus.

The *congenital hyperplasia syndromes* are due to inherited defects in specific enzymes involved in the biosynthetic pathway for cortisol produc-

tion (Figure 29-2). The mode of inheritance is usually autosomal recessive. The most common inherited deficiency is 21-hydroxylase, followed by 11-hydroxylase. These disorders may cause a deficiency of cortisol, aldosterone, or both, and present in infants and children with acute adrenal insufficiency. There is a characteristic overpro-

Table 29-1
Causes of Adrenal Insufficiency

Primary Insufficiency	Secondary Insufficiency
Autoimmune destruction	Pituitary or hypothalamic tumors
Infectious diseases (tuberculosis, histoplasmosis, HIV)	Iatrogenic ablation (hypophysectomy, radiation therapy)
Iatrogenic destruction (bilateral adrenalectomy)	Pituitary infarction (post-partum necrosis or apoplexy)
Infiltrative diseases (metastatic tumors, amyloidosis, hemochromatosis)	Infection (tuberculosis, syphilis)
Acute bilateral adrenal hemorrhage	Sarcoidosis and granulomatous diseases
Adrenal leukodystrophy	Idiopathic hypopituitarism
Congenital adrenal hyperplasias	Withdrawal of high dose glucocorticoid therapy

duction of steroid precursors before the defective enzyme step. In 21-hydroxylase deficiency, these precursors give rise to excessive production of adrenal androgens.

Clinical Presentation

Acute adrenal insufficiency or adrenal crisis should be suspected in patients with unexplained volume depletion and vascular collapse, often accompanied by hyperkalemia, acidosis, or hypoglycemia. Chronic insufficiency usually develops more insidiously with symptoms such as weakness, weight loss, anorexia, and postural hypotension. Increased skin pigmentation develops in patients with primary, but not secondary, chronic insufficiency due to the melanocyte stimulating activity of chronically high levels of ACTH and related peptides (Figure 29-3).

Differential Diagnosis

Volume depletion and vascular collapse can occur with a large number of other conditions causing hypotension, including hemorrhage or sepsis. There are fewer conditions that mimic chronic adrenal insufficiency. Among these are chronic starvation (anorexia nervosa); chronic gastrointestinal disease (inflammation or malignancy); other diseases causing hyperpigmentation (drugs and heavy metals); or fatigue and lassitude (chronic fatigue syndrome). A high level of clinical suspicion is the key to correct diagnosis of both acute and chronic adrenal insufficiency.

Diagnostic Approach

Confirmation of a suspected clinical diagnosis consists of demonstrating inappropriately low cortisol secretion, determining whether the low cortisol level is due to a deficiency of ACTH, and seeking a treatable cause. Baseline measurements of plasma cortisol and ACTH are best obtained in the early morning when levels of both are normally high. A very low morning cortisol of less than 3 µg/dL strongly suggests adrenal insufficiency, while a level of less than 10 µg/dL should arouse suspicion. Administration of synthetic ACTH (cosyntropin) helps in defining adrenal insufficiency in borderline situations and in distinguishing primary from secondary adrenal insufficiency. Normal subjects will show a peak cortisol response to greater than 20 µg/dL after cosyntropin, while patients with both primary and secondary adrenal insufficiency will not. Primary and secondary insufficiency may then be distinguished by the baseline levels of ACTH, which will be high in primary insufficiency only (Figure 29-4). In addition, patients with primary insufficiency will fail to respond to repeated administration of cosyntropin, while patients with secondary insufficiency will show an increasing response to repeated testing.

Patients suspected of having adrenal insufficiency due to *congenital adrenal hyperplasia* may be diagnosed with the aid of cortisol and ACTH measurements, but further measurement of specific steroid intermediates is essential to identify the specific enzyme defect. For example, in patients with the common form of 21-hydroxylase deficiency, plasma levels of 17-hydroxyprogesterone will be markedly elevated (Figure 29-2).

Management and Therapy

Treatment of primary adrenal insufficiency consists of replacement of both glucocorticoids and mineralocorticoids. A combination of hydrocortisone, to meet the glucocorticoid requirement, and fludrocortisone, to meet the mineralocorticoid requirement, is often used. Patients with secondary insufficiency may not require a mineralocorticoid because aldosterone production remains responsive to control by renin and angiotensin. In monitoring therapy, signs and symptoms of adrenal sufficiency should be sought. Periodic laboratory measurement of serum electrolytes, cortisol, and ACTH may also be helpful. During periods of acute illness or stress, the requirement for glucocorticoids typically increases by twofold to tenfold. In this situation, the dose of glucocorticoid must be adjusted appropriately to avoid the risk of acute adrenal insufficiency.

The goal in treating congenital hyperplasia is to suppress the production of excessive steroid byproducts as well as to provide for basic glucocorticoid and mineralocorticoid requirements. To suppress excessive androgen production in 21-hydroxylase deficiency, it may be necessary to give high doses of glucocorticoids initially to suppress ACTH and reduce the degree of adrenal hyperplasia. Once control is achieved, the glucocorticoid dose can be reduced for physiologic maintenance.

ADRENOCORTICAL HYPERFUNCTION: CUSHING'S SYNDROME

Chronic glucocorticoid excess leads to a constellation of findings known as Cushing's syndrome. Chronic mineralocorticoid excess leads to a different set of findings, primarily hypertension and hypokalemia.

Etiology and Pathogenesis

Cushing's syndrome is classified as being either ACTH-dependent or ACTH-independent (Table 29-2).

Approximately 70% of reported cases are due to excess ACTH secretion by a *pituitary adenoma* (also known as Cushing's disease). These adenomas contain basophilic granules and tend to be smaller than adenomas secreting growth hormone or prolactin.

Larger tumors may appear chromophobic on histological study. ACTH-secreting pituitary tumors usually continue to exhibit feedback suppression by glucocorticoids, but require higher than normal levels. Certain malignant tumors of non-pituitary origin (small cell lung carcinomas, carcinoid tumors, pancreatic islet cell tumors, medullary carcinoma of the thyroid, and pheochromocytomas) have the capacity to secrete ACTH. Ectopic ACTH production accounts for approximately 10% of all cases of Cushing's syndrome. Typically, these tumors do not exhibit suppression of their production of ACTH even at very high glucocorticoid levels. Rarely, a tumor produces ectopic corticotropin-releasing hormone, causing increased ACTH secretion by the normal pituitary gland.

Among the ACTH-independent causes, administration of high doses of exogenous glucocorticoids is the most common. Excess production of cortisol by an adrenal tumor is the most common endogenous cause, accounting for approximately 15% of all spontaneous cases. Food-induced Cushing's syndrome is mediated by gastric inhibitory peptide, which is normally released upon eating and stimulates the adrenal cortex in a few individuals.

Clinical Presentation

Obesity is the most common complaint, occurring in 90% of cases. The distribution of excess fat is typically central, with thin arms and legs. (Figure 29-5). Other features due to chronic glucocorticoid excess include weakening of the connective tissues in the skin (striae, easy bruising), osteoporosis, glucose intolerance, psychiatric disturbances, and increased susceptibility to infections. The manifestations of mineralocorticoid excess include hypertension, edema, hypokalemia, and metabolic alkalosis. Androgen excess in females causes hirsutism, acne, and amenorrhea.

Differential Diagnosis

Most patients with obesity, hypertension, and

Figure 29-4

Outline of Tests for the Differential Diagnosis
of Adrenal Insufficiency

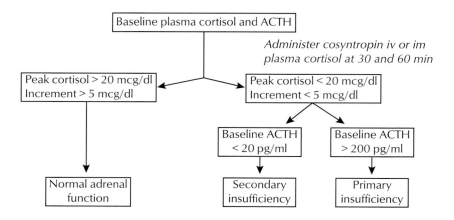

Table 29-2
Causes of Cushing's Syndrome

ACTH*-Dependent	ACTH-Independent
ACTH-secreting pituitary tumor (Cushing's disease)	Cortisol-secreting adrenal tumor; adenoma or carcinoma
ACTH-secreting non-pituitary tumor (ectopic ACTH syndrome)	Nodular adrenal hyperplasia
CRH†-secreting tumor	Food-dependent (GIP†† mediated)
	Exogenous glucocorticoids (iatrogenic or factitious)

*ACTH, adrenocorticotropic hormone; †CRH, corticotropin-releasing hormone; ††GIP, gastric inhibitory peptic.

diabetes mellitus do not have Cushing's syndrome, but exogenous obesity, which is far more common. Most women with obesity, hirsutism, and amenorrhea have the polycystic ovary syndrome, not hypercortisolism. Some patients may have increased secretion of cortisol secondary to another disorder. Examples include patients with primary depression or alcoholism.

Diagnostic Approach

The first step is to demonstrate the presence of inappropriately high cortisol secretion; the second step is to determine the cause of hypercortisolism (Figure 29-6). The initial step is collection of a 24-hour urine sample for measurement of free cortisol. If this value is normal, the patient is unlikely to have Cushing's syndrome. If the initial cortisol value is elevated, the patient is given a low dose of dexamethasone (2 mg/day for 2 days), and the urine collection is repeated during the second day. If urinary free cortisol is suppressed by more than 50%, the patient is unlikely to have Cushing's syndrome. If the low dose does not suppress the urinary free cortisol by 50%, the suppression test should be repeated with a higher dose of dexamethasone (8 mg/day for 2 days). Patients with an ACTH-producing pituitary tumor will usually suppress at the higher dose, while patients with adrenal tumors or the ectopic ACTH syndrome will not suppress. The latter two diagnoses may then be distinguished by the baseline ACTH level. In the ectopic ACTH syndrome, ACTH will be elevated. In Cushing's syndrome due to functioning adrenal tumors, the ACTH will be suppressed.

Magnetic resonance imaging allows visualization of a pituitary tumor in approximately 80% of cases. In cases where a tumor is not obvious, direct catheterization of the petrosal sinuses draining the pituitary bed may reveal an ACTH gradient, confirming a pituitary source. If baseline

Figure 29-5

Cushing's Syndrome (Clinical Findings)

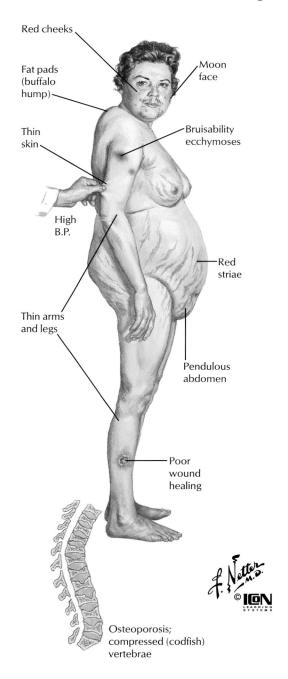

Red cheeks

Fat pads (buffalo hump)

Thin skin

High B.P.

Thin arms and legs

Moon face

Bruisability ecchymoses

Red striae

Pendulous abdomen

Poor wound healing

Osteoporosis; compressed (codfish) vertebrae

ACTH levels are suppressed, suggesting an adrenal tumor, it is possible to visualize the tumor in 90% of cases with a computed tomography scan of the abdomen.

Management and Therapy

An accurate diagnosis of the cause of Cushing's syndrome is essential for appropriate therapy. ACTH-secreting pituitary tumors are treated ini-

Figure 29-7

Outline of Tests for the Differential Diagnosis of Cushing's Syndrome

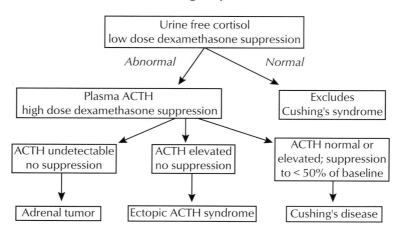

tially by resection, usually via a transsphenoidal surgical approach. The cure rate ranges from 60% to 85%. If surgery fails in removing the entire tumor, external pituitary radiation combined with drug therapy to inhibit cortisol synthesis induces remissions in most patients. Ketoconazole is the inhibitory drug used most frequently.

Cortisol-secreting adrenal tumors are primarily treated by surgical resection. The cure rate for adenomas is high, but it is much lower for carcinomas because metastases are commonly present at surgery. Second-line therapy for an inoperable tumor involves the use of blockers of cortisol synthesis. Tumors producing ectopic ACTH are almost always malignant. If they are not surgically resectable, they may be controlled with radiation therapy or chemotherapy.

FUTURE DIRECTIONS

Refinements in the management of adrenal insufficiency are constantly being proposed and tested. The replacement of adrenal androgens, as well as glucocorticoids and mineralocorticoids, may be important in women with adrenal insufficiency. Management of the hyperandrogenism in congenital adrenal hyperplasia continues to be a challenge because the higher doses of glucocorticoids required for full suppression often induce Cushing's syndrome. Drugs capable of blocking

androgen receptors may be useful adjuncts in this case. Virilization of the external genitalia in female infants may be reduced by treatment of the mother with dexamethasone during the first trimester of pregnancy.

The accurate diagnosis of ACTH-dependent Cushing's syndrome remains difficult in cases where a pituitary tumor cannot be depicted by current radiologic methods. Improved imaging techniques and petrosal sinus catheterization should identify the correct source of ACTH in all but a few cases.

REFERENCES

Aron DC, Findling JW, Tyrrell JB. Glucocorticoids & adrenal androgens. In: Greenspan FS, Gardner DG, eds. *Basic & Clinical Endocrinology.* 6th ed. Los Altos, Calif: Lange Medical Publications; 2001:334-376.

Boscaro M, Barzon L, Fallo F, Sonino N. Cushing's syndrome. *Lancet.* 2001;357:783-791.

Collett-Solberg PF. Congenital adrenal hyperplasia: from genetics and biochemistry to clinical practice, part 1. *Clin Pediatr (Phila).* 2001;40:1-16.

Don-Wauchope AC, Toft AD. Diagnosis and management of Addison's disease. *Practitioner.* 2000;244:794-799.

Stewart PM. The adrenal cortex. In: Larsen PR, Kronenberg HM, Melmed S, Polonsky KS, eds. Williams *Textbook of Endocrinology.* 10th ed. Philadelphia, Pa: WB Saunders Co; 2002.

Vaidya B, Pearce S, Kendall-Taylor P. Recent advances in the molecular genetics of congenital and acquired primary adrenocortical failure. *Clin Endocrinol (Oxf).* 2000;53:403-418.

Chapter 30
Disorders of Puberty

James E. Kurz

Puberty is defined as the development of secondary sexual characteristics, first apparent as breast budding in girls and testicular enlargement in boys, with the subsequent attainment of fertility. Puberty begins with the increase in pulsatile secretion of gonadotropin-releasing hormone (GRH) from the hypothalamus that stimulates the pituitary gland to increase production of the gonadotropins leuteinizing hormone (LH) and follicle-stimulating hormone (FSH).

The hormonal effects of GRH, LH, and FSH lead to the development of somatic secondary sex characteristics as described by Tanner (Tables 30-1 and 30-2). The sequence of development is as important as the age of onset, which can vary. Under normal circumstances, the transition to puberty proceeds at Tanner stage 2.

SEXUAL MATURATION

Breast budding (Tanner stage 2) is the first sign of puberty in most females; pubic hair develops soon after but sometimes precedes breast budding. According to recent data on female development, females in the United States are developing at a younger age compared to previously established norms. On average, African American girls begin puberty between 8 and 9 years of age with age 6 now accepted as the lower limit of normal. White girls begin puberty at 10 years of age on average with age 7 now accepted as the lower limit of normal. The average age of menarche is 12.2 years in African American girls and 12.9 years in Whites. Menarche usually occurs during Tanner stage 3 or 4 breast and pubic hair

Table 30-1
Sexual Maturity Ratings in Females

Tanner stage	Breast Development	Pubic Hair Growth
1	Prepubertal. No glandular tissue. Areola conforms to chest line. Elevation of papilla only.	None.
2	Breast bud with small amount of glandular tissue. Areola still flat but enlarges in diameter.	Small amount of pigmented downy hair mainly along the labia.
3	More elevation of breast and areola but no separation of contours.	Hair is darker, coarser and more curled. Spreads laterally and over the pubes.
4	Areola and papilla form a mound projecting from the breast contour.	Hair of adult quality, spreads further over pubes but spares medial thighs.
5	Adult breast tissue. Areola recedes to same contour as breast and papilla projects above areola.	Hair of adult quality spreading to medial thighs. Further hair growth up the linea alba is considered stage 6.

Adapted from Marshall WA, Tanner JM. Variations in pattern of pubertal changes in girls. *Arch Dis Child.* 1969;44:291.

Table 30-2
Sexual Maturity Ratings in Males

Tanner stage	Breast Development	Pubic Hair Growth
1	Prepubertal. Testes and scrotum childlike.	None.
2	Enlargement of testes to 2.5 cm in long axis. Scrotum reddens. No penile enlargement yet.	Small amount of pigmented downy hair at base of penis.
3	Enlargement of penis, primarily in length, and further growth of testes and scrotum.	Hair is darker, coarser and more curled. Spreads laterally and over the pubes.
4	Further enlargement of penis in breadth and length. Further enlargement of testes and scrotum.	Hair of adult quality, spreads further over pubes but spares medial thighs.
5	Adult genitalia.	Hair of adult quality spreading to medial thighs.

Adapted from Marshall WA, Tanner JM. Variations in the pattern of pubertal changes in boys. *Arch Dis Child.* 1970;45:13-23.

development. Menarche follows the peak growth spurt, and by age 15 most females have reached their adult height.

Testicular enlargement is the first sign of puberty in the male. Tanner stage 2 testes measure 2.5 cm in length along the long axis. Puberty in males begins on average at age 11.5 years with a range of 9 to 14 years. The growth spurt begins just before testicular enlargement and lasts longer than in females. Spermatogenesis, heralded by nocturnal emissions, occurs on average at age 13 and usually occurs with the appearance of pubic hair.

VARIANTS OF NORMAL DEVELOPMENT
Adolescent Gynecomastia

Physiologic pubertal gynecomastia occurs to some degree in almost two thirds of boys during mid-puberty. The gynecomastia is subareolar and can either be soft or can feel like a rubbery, firm nodule or mass. It is often asymmetrical and sometimes tender. The tissue usually recedes in 6 to 12 months. If breast tissue is excessive and persistent, or is so painful that it interferes with activities, it can be resected surgically. It is advisable to wait until after age 15 to treat because most cases resolve by then.

Breast Anomalies

Breast asymmetry in females is fairly common in early adolescence and usually corrects itself by age 15. Any asymmetry after age 15 or late into puberty will likely persist. Breast masses in males are usually physiologic gynecomastia. Most "masses" in females are due to physiologic swelling during the menstrual cycle. Of true breast masses in females during puberty, 99% are benign. Fibroadenomas comprise 80% of these masses; they are rubbery, mobile, and well demarcated and usually occur in the upper outer or lateral quadrants of the breast. Malignant tumors, rare in adolescents, are usually subareolar, hard, and fixed to the underlying tissue. Ultrasound can help distinguish the two. Mammograms are not helpful in this age group. Biopsy before the completion of breast development can permanently impair breast growth and should only be done for the most suspicious masses.

Penile Disorders

Micropenis is defined as a penis with a stretched length less than the tenth percentile for age. This correlates to a minimum of 4 cm in early adolescence. In most cases, the child has a normal sized penis that is buried in pubic fat; therefore, it is important to compress the pubic fat pad when taking a measurement. Causes of true micropenis include hypopituitarism, Klinefelter's, Noonan's, or Prader-Willi syndromes.

DELAYED PUBERTY

In females, puberty is delayed if there are no physical signs by age 13 or if menarche has not occurred by age 16. In competitive athletes, puberty may be delayed to age 14. Pubertal progression is delayed if menarche has not occurred within 5 years of the onset of puberty. In males, puberty is delayed if there are no physical signs of puberty by age 14.

Etiology and Differential Diagnosis

The most common cause of delayed puberty, particularly in males, is constitutional delay of growth and maturation. It is a variation of normal caused by a physiologic delay in the GRH surge. The pituitary gland remains in its prepubertal state and gonadotropin levels are low. Unlike males, females with delayed puberty are more likely to have a pathologic problem.

Pathologic causes of delayed puberty are categorized as *hypogonadotropic hypogonadism*, associated with low levels of LH and FSH, or *hypergonadotropic hypogonadism*, associated with elevated levels of LH and FSH. One cause of hypogonadotropic hypogonadism in boys and girls is Kallmann syndrome, which combines the features of impaired GRH release and impaired sense of smell. Hypogonadotropic delay can also be caused by suppression of the hypothalamus from chronic illness such as Crohn's disease, renal failure, cardiac disease, or severe asthma. Strenuous physical exercise, malnutrition, and anorexia can delay or halt the progression of puberty by the same mechanism. Pituitary tumors such as craniopharyngioma, prolactinoma, or adenoma can impair gonadotropin release.

Hypergonadotropic states are generally due to gonadal failure. Turner syndrome (45XO) is the most common cause in girls, and Klinefelter's syndrome (47XXY), the most common cause in boys. Chemotherapy or radiation injury can also cause secondary gonadal failure in boys or girls.

Clinical Presentation

In children younger than 16 years with an otherwise normal history and physical examination,

it may be difficult to distinguish those with constitutional delay from those with hypogonadotropism. Those with constitutional delay usually have a family history of "late bloomers." Stature is usually in the third to 25th percentile for age, and body habitus is typically thin. In contrast, those with endocrine disorders are often below the third percentile in height and tend to be overweight compared to height.

Stature can often provide clues as to the cause of pathologic delay. Delayed puberty associated with short stature occurs in hypopituitarism; Turner's, Noonan's, or Prader-Willi syndromes; glucocorticoid excess (iatrogenic or Cushing's disease); and chronic disease such as Crohn's. Delayed puberty with normal or tall stature is found in Kallmann syndrome, Klinefelter's syndrome, and chronic disease states. Children with CNS tumors may be short or tall depending on the effects on the pituitary gland.

Turner's syndrome occurs in 1 of 2,500 live female births and is characterized by short stature, webbed neck, widely spaced nipples on a shield chest, high arched palate, and congenital heart disease. These findings can be subtle or even missing, especially in cases of mosaicism. Turner's syndrome should always be considered in any female with delayed puberty (Figure 30-1).

Klinefelter's syndrome occurs in 1 of 1,000 live male births and is characterized by gynecomastia, small genitalia, and sparse facial hair (Figure 30-2). Puberty can commence at a normal age, but its progression is often delayed. Affected children often have cognitive and social difficulties. As adults they take on a feminine body habitus and often are plagued by varicose veins and venous insufficiency. They are at risk for osteoporosis and breast cancer. Given the wide variation in phenotypic expression, this diagnosis often goes undetected until well into adolescence or adulthood once infertility becomes an issue.

Diagnostic Approach

The history and physical examination should focus on finding any evidence of chronic disease, malnutrition, or CNS disease. The neurologic examination should focus on sense of smell, - visual fields, and the funduscopic examination. In most cases, CNS tumors will be associated with headaches, visual disturbances, or other focal

Figure 30-1

Turner's Syndrome

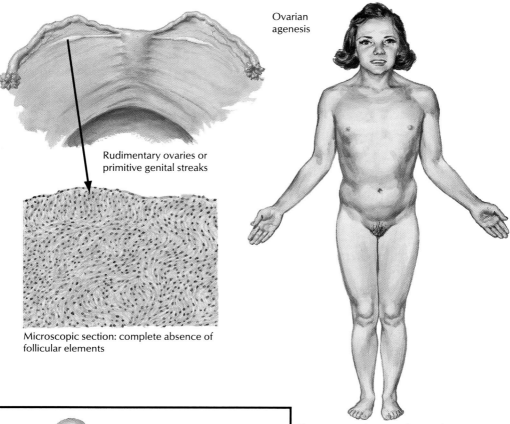

Ovarian agenesis

Rudimentary ovaries or primitive genital streaks

Microscopic section: complete absence of follicular elements

Short stature, absence of secondary sex characteristics, infantile genitalia, sparse pubic hair, high gondadotropin level, estrogen deficiency and multiple congenital abnormalities (web neck, shieldlike chest, cubitus valgus)

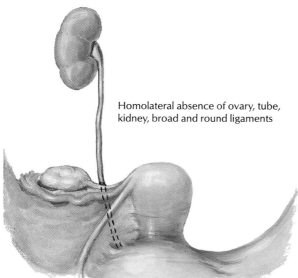

Homolateral absence of ovary, tube, kidney, broad and round ligaments

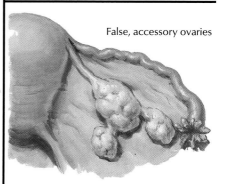

False, accessory ovaries

Figure 30-2

Klinefelter's Syndrome

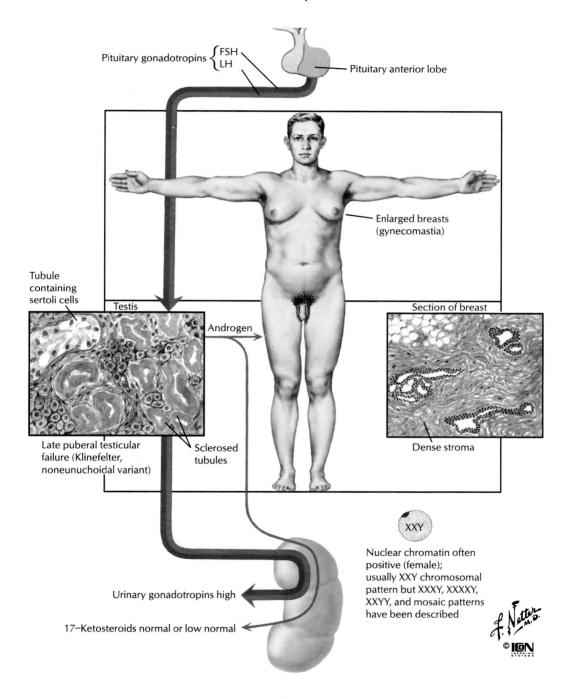

Pituitary gonadotropins $\begin{cases} FSH \\ LH \end{cases}$

Pituitary anterior lobe

Enlarged breasts (gynecomastia)

Tubule containing sertoli cells

Testis

Androgen

Section of breast

Late puberal testicular failure (Klinefelter, noneunuchoidal variant)

Sclerosed tubules

Dense stroma

XXY

Nuclear chromatin often positive (female); usually XXY chromosomal pattern but XXXY, XXXXY, XXYY, and mosaic patterns have been described

Urinary gonadotropins high

17−Ketosteroids normal or low normal

neurological deficits. Any disparity in androgen effects and secondary sexual characteristics are important. Boys with Klinefelter's syndrome, for example, will have small genitalia despite a fair amount of pubic hair.

A sedimentation rate, blood cell count, urinalysis, and measurement of thyroid function will rule out most occult chronic disease. If there is no evidence of chronic illness or a CNS lesion, then the investigation is organized based on levels of LH, FSH, and a bone age. Short females should undergo karyotype analysis to verify Turner's syndrome.

Hypogonadotropic states

If LH and FSH are low and bone age is slightly delayed, the child most likely has constitutional delay. If bone age is markedly delayed (more than 2 years), there is likely an endocrinopathy such as hypothyroidism. If bone age is appropriate for chronological age and the child is short, then a karyotype is needed. Head imaging is indicated, preferably with magnetic resonance imaging (MRI) of the pituitary region, if gonadotropin levels are low and there are any symptoms or signs of CNS disease. CT scanning of this region often lacks sensitivity because of interference from bony structures.

Hypergonadotropic states

Elevated levels of LH and FSH indicate gonadal failure. Unless there is some history of damage to the testes or ovaries that would explain the problem, a karyotype analysis is indicated. A karyotype analysis is diagnostic for either Turner's syndrome or Klinefelter's syndrome, both of which can present without the typical stigmata.

Management and Therapy

When pubertal delay is associated with low gonadotropin levels, the child can be observed unless the delay causes psychosocial problems for the child. Teenagers, usually boys, suffering emotional distress should be promptly referred for counseling and consideration of hormonal therapy even if the correct diagnosis cannot yet be determined. Treatment with exogenous androgens will increase phallic size and help with stature. Counseling is important to prevent problems with self-esteem and peer interaction.

Girls with Turner's syndrome can be treated with growth hormone to promote linear growth and estrogens to promote the development of secondary sexual characteristics. In all cases, hormone therapy should be directed under the careful guidance of an endocrinologist experienced in treating pubertal problems. Too rapid correction can lead to premature epiphyseal closure and decreased adult height.

PRIMARY AMENORRHEA IN PUBERTAL FEMALES

Primary amenorrhea is defined as no episode of uterine bleeding by age 16. Menarche usually occurs with Tanner stage 4 breast and pubic hair development. If there is no menarche within 5 years after the onset of breast development, an investigation is warranted. This section covers primary amenorrhea in females who are otherwise progressing through puberty normally. Any female who has not shown signs of puberty by age 13 should be considered to have delayed puberty.

Etiology and Differential Diagnosis

Pregnancy is always first on the differential diagnosis in amenorrheic pubertal females, even in primary amenorrhea. The differential is further divided into endocrine problems or genital tract abnormalities. Emotional or physical stress can cause hypothalamic suppression. Polycystic ovary disease, hypopituitarism, and ovarian damage due to autoimmune disease, chemotherapy, or radiation therapy can all cause amenorrhea. Abnormalities of the genital tract include imperforate hymen, testicular feminization (46XY), and vaginal agenesis (46XX).

Clinical Presentation

The presentation depends on the cause. Amenorrhea is one of the diagnostic criteria of - anorexia. In this circumstance, the body mass index will be near or below 18. Hirsutism is found in polycystic ovary disease. Imperforate hymen is associated with cyclic abdominal pain and a bluish mass at the vaginal opening. Adolescents with testicular feminization have female breast development but will have no pubic hair or uterus.

Diagnostic Approach

A pregnancy test is needed unless there are no

signs of puberty. Further testing includes LH, FSH, and estradiol. A high LH or FSH indicates ovarian failure, and a karyotype analysis is warranted. Low gonadotropin levels with a low estradiol indicate hypothalamic suppression or pituitary disease. In this case, a prolactin level is needed to rule out prolactinoma, and the pituitary region may need to be imaged by MRI if there is no other obvious explanation for the clinical picture (such as anorexia nervosa). Pelvic imaging with ultrasound or CT is needed in cases of primary amenorrhea associated with abnormal pelvic anatomy.

Management and Therapy

There is strong evidence that peak bone mass may be reduced in amenorrheic athletes and those with eating disorders; therefore, some endocrinologists recommend that these patients be placed on oral contraceptives. Patients with Turner's syndrome or some other type of ovarian failure require hormone replacement therapy under the direction of an endocrinologist. Oral contraceptives help regulate cycles and may help diminish hair growth and acne in girls with polycystic ovary syndrome.

FUTURE DIRECTIONS

The milieu of hormonal interactions that invoke normal pubertal development is complex and not completely understood. With better understanding of these hormonal changes, as well as more knowledge of what triggers the initiation of puberty, there will be better ways to differentiate those with constitutional delay from those with true delayed puberty and decisions on treatment can begin earlier before the patient suffers emotionally from the delay. Likewise, a better understanding of the pubertal process is needed to identify the unique causes of delayed or precocious puberty among those with chronic diseases such as renal failure, those with genetic disorders such as Turner's syndrome, and those treated for cancer with chemotherapy or radiation therapy. Once these hormonal interactions are better understood, the normal pubertal process can be better replicated to help those affected by pubertal disorders of any cause.

REFERENCES

Braverman PK, Sondheimer SJ. Menstrual disorders. *Pediatr Rev.* 1997;18:17-25.

Herman-Giddens ME, Slora EJ, Wasserman RC, et al. Secondary sexual characteristics and menses in young girls seen in office practice: a study from the Pediatric Research in Office Settings Network. *Pediatrics.* 1997;99:505-512.

Kulin HE, Muller J. The biological aspects of puberty. *Pediatr Rev.* 1996;17:75-86.

Styne DM. New aspects in the diagnosis and treatment of pubertal disorders. *Pediatr Clin North Am.* 1997;44:505-529.

Tanner JM. *Growth at Adolescence.* 2nd ed. Springfield, Ill: Charles C Thomas; 1962.

Chapter 31
Hirsutism

Jean M. Dostou

Hirsutism, which affects 5% to 10% of adult women, is characterized by the presence of terminal hairs that occur in a male-like pattern. Most cases are benign, although the condition can be extremely distressing to affected patients. The physician must distinguish benign from serious causes, and counsel the patient with regard to the efficacy and availability of treatment options.

ETIOLOGY AND PATHOGENESIS

Hirsutism results from increased production of androgens by the ovary, adrenal glands, or both, or from increased sensitivity of hair follicles to normal circulating levels of androgens (Figure 31-1). The latter is frequently caused by increased 5α-reductase activity, which converts testosterone to dihydrotestosterone (DHT), a more potent metabolite. Hyperandrogenism, resulting from any of these factors, prolongs the anagen (growth) phase of androgen-sensitive hairs, resulting in their conversion from fine, light, "vellus" hairs to coarse, dark, "terminal" hairs.

In women, *testosterone* is derived mainly from the ovary. Approximately 25% of the total pool is secreted directly by the ovary, and the remainder is produced by peripheral conversion from ovarian-derived precursors. *Androstenedione*, a less potent androgen, is produced in equal quantities by both the adrenal gland and ovary. *Dehydroepiandrosterone sulfate* (DHEAS), also a weak androgen, is secreted almost exclusively by the adrenal gland. Increased testosterone levels indicate ovarian hyperandrogenism; increased DHEAS levels imply adrenal hyperandrogenism. If neither is elevated, and other causes are excluded, increased peripheral conversion is generally assumed.

Circulating androgen levels also affect the concentration of sex hormone-binding globulin (SHBG). SHBG binds testosterone in the circulation. In general, approximately 80% of testosterone is bound to SHBG, 19% is bound to albumin, and 1% circulates free. Hyperandrogenism can reduce SHBG concentrations, with the result that a greater percentage of the total testosterone is present as the "free" unbound, active hormone.

CLINICAL PRESENTATION

The presentation of hirsutism varies according to the underlying etiology. The universal feature is an abnormal quantity and quality of sexual hair in the midline body areas. Most commonly, the face, chest, areola, linea alba, buttock, sacrum, inner thigh, and external genitalia are affected (Figure 31-1). The severity of hirsutism is quantified based on the Ferriman and Gallwey system, which evaluates 9 body areas for absent to severe hirsutism with scores of 0 to 4. A score greater than 7 (of a possible 36) is considered abnormal.

Other androgen-dependent symptoms that occur frequently include acne, menstrual irregularity, temporal recession, and frontal alopecia. Classically, hirsutism is distinguished from virilization, which also encompasses "masculinizing" symptoms such as increased muscle mass, loss of female body contour, flattening of breasts, deepening of the voice from laryngeal hypertrophy, and clitoral enlargement (greater than 1 cm if measured transversely at base of shaft). This extreme manifestation of hyperandrogenism rarely occurs unless androgen levels are very elevated (more than 2.5 times the upper limit of normal).

Hirsutism in adult women is due most commonly to polycystic ovary syndrome (PCOS) (~80%) or idiopathic hirsutism (IH) (15% to 20%). These conditions generally begin in the perimenarcheal or late teen years and progress in a gradual fashion. In contrast, neoplasms of the ovary or adrenal gland present abruptly, progress rapidly, and are frequently associated with virilization. Obesity, acanthosis nigricans, or both imply insulin resistance and suggest PCOS. Facial plethora, violaceous abdominal striae, easy bruising, and a suboccipital fat pad

Figure 31-1

Clinical Manifestations of Hyperandrogenism

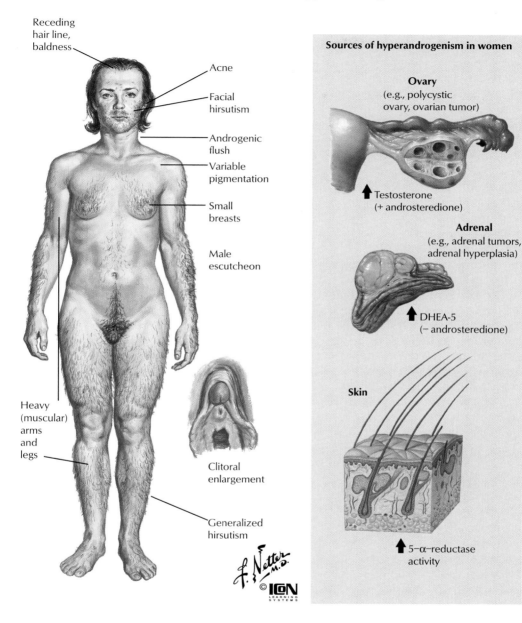

Receding hair line, baldness

Acne

Facial hirsutism

Androgenic flush

Variable pigmentation

Small breasts

Male escutcheon

Heavy (muscular) arms and legs

Clitoral enlargement

Generalized hirsutism

Sources of hyperandrogenism in women

Ovary
(e.g., polycystic ovary, ovarian tumor)

↑ Testosterone
(+ androsteredione)

Adrenal
(e.g., adrenal tumors, adrenal hyperplasia)

↑ DHEA-5
(− androsteredione)

Skin

↑ 5−α−reductase activity

suggest Cushing's syndrome. A history of infertility and hirsutism may suggest late onset congenital adrenal hyperplasia (NCAH). A history of galactorrhea suggests hyperprolactinemia as the cause.

DIFFERENTIAL DIAGNOSIS
Polycystic Ovary Syndrome

The criteria for the diagnosis of PCOS were defined by 1990 National Institutes of Health (NIH) consensus to include: (1) hyperandrogenism, which may be based on clinical findings such as hirsutism or other androgen-dependent features, *or* based on biochemical evaluation showing increased androgen levels; (2) oligomenorrhea (generally less than 8 menses/year); and (3) exclusion of other potentially causative conditions. Insulin resistance may affect ovarian androgen production by dysregulating an ovarian P450 cytochrome-oxidase17α-dependent pathway involving the conversion of progesterone to androstenedione. Insulin-mediated abnormalities of pituitary luteinizing hormone (LH) secretion may also contribute.

Although it is commonly associated with obesity, cases of PCOS in thin women who are also insulin resistant have been well documented.

Idiopathic Hirsutism

A uniform definition of IH is evolving, and a recent review suggests the inclusion of (1) hirsutism, (2) normal androgen levels, and (3) regular menses with normal ovulatory function. Confirmation of normal ovulatory function by basal body temperature measurement or midluteal phase progesterone measurement is required. If there is evidence of anovulation despite regular menses, the patient is considered to have PCOS. Pathogenesis of IH involves increased 5α-reductase activity as well as a possible alteration in androgen receptor function, resulting in increased sensitivity of the hair follicle to normal androgen levels.

Adrenal Hyperplasia

Classic congenital adrenal hyperplasia, an autosomal recessive condition, is generally diagnosed in childhood because it may cause ambiguous genitalia in infants. A partial form of this condition, nonclassic (late onset) congenital adrenal hyperplasia (NCAH), may present as a slowly progressive form of hirsutism in adulthood. The pathogenesis involves an enzymatic deficiency in adrenal steroidogenesis, resulting in accumulation of androgen precursors, most commonly 17-hydroxyprogesterone. The prevalence of congenital adrenal hyperplasia is less than 3%.

Cushing's Syndrome

This condition presents with hypercortisolemia caused by a cortisol-secreting pituitary adenoma (Cushing's disease), an adrenal adenoma, or an ectopic adrenocorticotropic hormone. It is a rare finding (<1%) in the evaluation of hirsutism unless induced iatrogenically by glucocorticoid administration.

Ovarian Tumor

Epithelial tumors, which are generally malignant, can cause hyperandrogenism by stimulating adjacent stroma. Androgen-secreting "functional" ovarian tumors include Sertoli-Leydig (arrhenoblastoma), lipoid cell, and hilus cell tumors. Together, these tumors have a prevalence is less than 1%.

Adrenal Tumor

Adrenal adenomas and carcinomas usually secrete DHEAS, although they can also co-secrete testosterone, cortisol, or both. This is also unusual, with a prevalence of less than 1%.

Hyperprolactinemia

This condition presents with galactorrhea, amenorrhea, and hirsutism. Prolactin can stimulate adrenal androgen secretion (mechanism poorly understood). This is also unusual, with a prevalence of less than 1%.

Drugs

Phenytoin, minoxidil, danazol, anabolic steroids, glucocorticoids, cyclosporin A, progestins (norgesterol and levonorgesterol) present in certain oral contraceptive pills can cause hirsutism.

DIAGNOSTIC APPROACH

The evaluation should focus on the age of onset, pattern of progression, severity (evidence of virilization), menstrual history, ethnicity (women of Mediterranean, Middle Eastern, Ashkenazi Jewish, and Indian subcontinent origins are more prone to hirsutism), and family history of hirsutism (PCOS, NCAH, and IH all have a familial tendency). A drug/medication history should be obtained, as well as a history about the extent of mechanical methods (frequency of shaving, tweezing, depilation, or electrolysis) used by the patient to control the condition.

Laboratory assessment for severe hirsutism is indicated to exclude neoplasm and to clarify the source of hyperandrogenism (ovary, adrenal gland, or peripheral conversion), which may direct therapy. For less severe hirsutism associated with amenorrhea or oligomenorrhea, laboratory evaluation to assess for hyperprolactinemia or thyroid dysfunction, for which treatment is not directed at androgen levels, is indicated. For mild hirsutism and a normal menstrual history, laboratory evaluation may reassure the patient and be used to follow the response to treatment. Recommended laboratory tests for all patients are testosterone and DHEA-S. Prolactin and thyroid-stimulating hormone may be added if hirsutism is associated with amenorrhea or oligomenorrhea. A morning cortisol level after 1 mg dexamethasone suppression or measurement of 24-hour urinary free cortisol should be done if features of Cushing's syndrome are present. More extensive laboratory evaluation is seldom indicated because the findings rarely influence treatment. However, additional tests can include 17-hydroxyprogesterone to diagnose NCAH, 3α-androstenediol glucuronide (a metabolite of testosterone used as a marker of 5α-reductase activity), and measurements of free testosterone or SHBG concentrations.

MANAGEMENT AND THERAPY

If the laboratory evaluation suggests an ovarian tumor (testosterone levels greater than 150 to 200 ng/dL) or an adrenal gland tumor (DHEA-S greater than 700 µg/dL or 2.5 times the upper limit of normal), abdominal and pelvic imaging with ultrasound, CT, or MRI is indicated, with surgical referral if a mass is detected. In other cases, medical therapy is directed at the underlying causative factors. Most agents require 3 to 6 months to achieve a noticeable effect on hirsutism, and patients should be counseled accordingly.

Androgen Suppression

Combination oral contraceptives decrease LH−dependent ovarian androgen production, and estrogen (30 to 35 µg is sufficient) increases the production of SHBG. The most effective agents have the least androgenic progestins. Ethynodiol diacetate 1/35 is the least androgenic and is a longstanding recommended treatment of hirsutism. Newer agents containing the progestin desogestrel are also effective. The most androgenic progesterone is norgestrel. Formulations that contain it are best avoided in this condition.

Glucocorticoids are indicated for adrenal sources of androgen excess, but are generally to be avoided unless satisfactory results cannot be achieved with other methods of androgen suppression. If necessary, dexamethasone, 0.125 to 0.25 mg given at bedtime, has been documented to suppress adrenal androgen secretion.

Androgen Receptor Blockers

Spironolactone blocks androgen action peripherally at the level of the hair follicle. The overall response is favorable with 60% to 70% of patients showing improvement at 6 months. Doses of 50 to 200 mg/daily have been used, and the effect is generally dose-related, with more than half of patients requiring the maximal dose to benefit. Side effects include a transient initial diuresis and occasional gastrointestinal symptoms. Hyperkalemia occurs but is rare in healthy patients. Spironolactone should be used only in conjunction with adequate contraception because of theoretical concern of feminizing a male fetus.

Flutamide at doses of 125 to 250 mg twice daily is similar in efficacy to spironolactone. The potential side effect of liver toxicity and high cost limit its feasibility for routine treatment.

Finasteride, a 5α-reductase inhibitor (at a dose of 5 mg daily), is similar in efficacy to spironolactone and flutamide. It is also costly and because of its ability to induce ambiguous genitalia in a male fetus, appropriate contraceptive measures are mandatory.

Cyproterone acetate, a progestin with antiandrogenic activity, is used extensively in Europe for the treatment of hirsutism. In Germany, this approach has been widely used with an approximate 70% response rate. It is not approved for use in the United States because of concerns of it causing cancer in laboratory animals at high doses.

Insulin sensitizers are agents that improve hyperandrogenism and anovulation associated with PCOS, but their effects on hirsutism tend to be milder than those achieved with antiandrogens. *Metformin* is first-line therapy for PCOS at doses of 500 mg 3 times daily to 1,000 mg two times a day (dose titration by 500 mg at weekly intervals to limit gastrointestinal side effects is recommended). *Troglitazone,* a thiazolidinedione, was withdrawn because of reports of severe liver toxicity, improved hirsutism and anovulation, hyperandrogenism, and insulin resistance in PCOS. To date, there are no published data on the newer thiazolidinediones (rosiglitazone, pioglitazone) in the treatment of hirsutism or PCOS, therefore, they are not recommended for this purpose. The investigational agent, d-chiroinositol, a phosphoglycan mediator that is deficient in insulin-resistant patients, improves hyperandrogenism and anovulation in PCOS, although data are lacking with regard to its effects on hirsutism.

Topical and Mechanical Treatments

Eflornithine hydrochloride cream 13.9% became available in 2001 for the treatment of facial hirsutism. Its mechanism of action is to inhibit keratin protein synthesis in the hair follicle, which slows the rate of hair growth. It may reduce the frequency of mechanical treatments, although it will not enhance the conversion of terminal to vellus hair, as will some of the androgen suppression treatments. It is applied twice daily, and effects occur within 4 to 8 weeks; 30% to 60 % of patients achieve some degree of clinical improvement. Minor skin irritation, generally infrequent, is the most common side effect.

Electrolysis removes hair permanently by deploying an electrical current through a fine needle to destroy the dermal papilla at the base of the hair. The procedure can be costly and time-consuming because only a small number of follicles can be treated in a single session.

Laser treatment has been used recently for the treatment of hirsutism. The most consistent data are with the use of the ruby laser, which targets melanosomes and delivers red light at a wavelength of 694 nm. Results tend to be best in light-skinned women with dark hair because the con-trast improves efficacy. The procedure is generally well tolerated although it can be extremely costly because several treatments are usually necessary to achieve complete and permanent hair removal.

Optimum Treatment

A combination of pharmacologic agents and cosmetic measures are usually required to achieve a satisfactory result. For PCOS, metformin is recommended as initial therapy with the addition of OCP +/- spironolactone +/-eflornithine hydrochloride cream, depending on therapeutic response. For IH, OCP +/- spironolactone +/- eflornithine hydrochloride cream is recommended as initial therapy. Response to treatment often requires 4 to 6 months, and it is reasonable to wait that long to assess the need for additional agents. Mechanical measures are more effective after hormonal therapy has been used to reduce androgen levels or decrease androgen action. Without mechanical treatments, most patients relapse after withdrawing from pharmacologic treatment.

FUTURE DIRECTIONS

With the availability of multiple agents that exert their effects on hirsutism by different mechanisms, additional data are needed regarding the most successful and cost-effective treatment combinations. Recognition and treatment of this syndrome early in its course diminishes the psychologic burden, the need for mechanical treatments, and the potential of chronic anovulation.

REFERENCES

Azziz R, Carmina E, Sawaya M. Idiopathic hirsutism. *Endocrine Rev.* 2000;21(4):347–362.

Hock D, Seifer D. New treatments of hyperandrogenism and hirsutism. *Obstet Gynecol Clin North Am.* 2000;27(3):567–581.

Moghetti P, Tosi F, Tosti A, et al. Comparison of spironolactone, flutamide, and finasteride efficacy in the treatment of hirsutism: a randomized, double blind, placebo-controlled trial. *J Clin Endocrinol Metab.* 2000;85(1):89–100.

Chapter 32
Hyperparathyroidism

Sue A. Brown

Hyperparathyroidism is characterized by an elevation in serum parathyroid (PTH) levels. The parathyroid glands synthesize and secrete PTH, which elevates calcium levels to maintain ionized calcium within a narrow physiologic range. PTH stimulates renal conversion of 25-hydroxyvitamin D to 1,25-dihydroxyvitamin D (calcitriol), which increases intestinal calcium absorption. PTH also acts to stimulate bone turnover, thereby releasing calcium and phosphorus from the bone matrix (Figure 32-1). Appropriate homeostatic increases in PTH can occur from secondary causes; however, this chapter focuses on the inappropriate PTH levels that occur in primary hyperparathyroidism.

ETIOLOGY AND PATHOGENESIS

Primary hyperparathyroidism results when the parathyroid glands hypertrophy and secrete excess PTH. Most individuals have 4 parathyroid glands, located in proximity to the thyroid gland. However, a wide range of variation exists. Two to 8 glands may be found throughout the neck or mediastinum in normal individuals. The majority of individuals with primary hyperparathyroidism have a solitary parathyroid adenoma (80% to 85%). The remainder have diffuse hyperplasia (12% to 15%), double or triple adenomas (2%), or rarely, parathyroid carcinoma (<1%).

Although most cases are sporadic, there are familial forms of hyperparathyroidism that occur as part of the multiple endocrine neoplasia (MEN) syndromes. Approximately 95% of individuals with MEN 1 have primary hyperparathyroidism along with pituitary and pancreatic tumors. Hyperparathyroidism occurs to a lesser extent in MEN 2a (20% to 30%) in conjunction with pheochromocytomas and medullary thyroid cancer. MEN 2b, which includes neuromas, does not generally have primary hyperparathyroidism as a feature. These familial forms have 4-gland hyperplasia and require bilateral neck dissection for therapy.

CLINICAL PRESENTATION

Primary hyperparathyroidism is usually asymptomatic (75% to 80%) and diagnosed when biochemical screening reveals hypercalcemia. Symptoms vary depending on the level and duration of hypercalcemia (Figure 32-2). Common symptoms include fatigue, constipation, polyuria, polydipsia, bone pain, or nausea. Neuropsychiatric symptoms (depression, memory loss, headaches) are reported frequently, but their relation to hypercalcemia is less clear because they do not always reverse with its correction. Nephrolithiasis is the most frequent overt complication, occurring in 15% to 20% of individuals. Nephrocalcinosis occurs infrequently. Bone disease is a prominent feature with osteopenia or osteoporosis and rarely, osteitis fibrosa cystica. Cortical bone (e.g., the distal radius) is affected more often than cancellous or trabecular bone (e.g., the vertebral column). Thus, bone loss is greater at the distal radius than in the spine. The hip is a mixture of both types of bone and is intermediate in its bone density. Despite decreased bone density, the fracture risk has not been adequately characterized. Cardiovascular manifestations include hypertension, left ventricular hypertrophy, and myocardial and valvular calcifications. Neuromuscular symptoms occur but are less prominent, and proximal muscle weakness with type II muscle cell atrophy is quite rare. Occasionally pancreatitis or peptic ulcer disease may be found. Gout and pseudogout may also be related to primary hyperparathyroidism.

DIFFERENTIAL DIAGNOSIS

The diagnosis is usually made after hypercalcemia is identified. Primary hyperparathyroidism and malignancies account for approximately 90% of cases of hypercalcemia. Malignancies include multiple myeloma, lymphomas, and prostate,

Figure 32-1

Physiology of the Parathyroid Glands

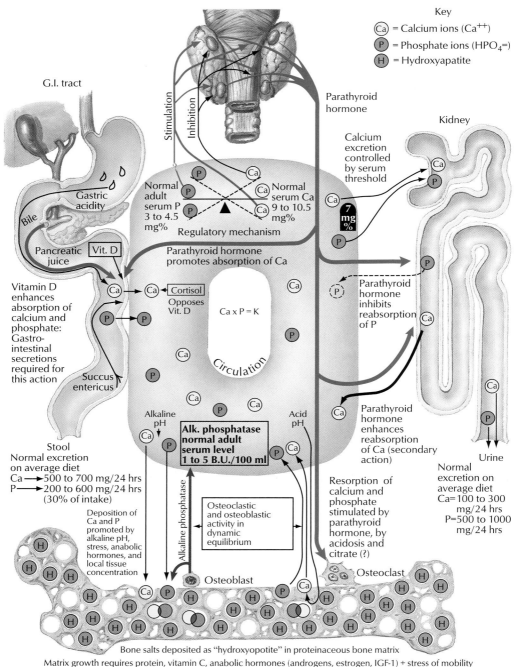

Key
Ca = Calcium ions (Ca^{++})
P = Phosphate ions ($HPO_4^=$)
H = Hydroxyapatite

G.I. tract

Stimulation
Inhibition

Parathyroid hormone

Kidney

Calcium excretion controlled by serum threshold

Gastric acidity

Bile

Normal adult serum P 3 to 4.5 mg%

Normal serum Ca 9 to 10.5 mg%

Regulatory mechanism

7 mg %

Pancreatic juice

Vit. D

Parathyroid hormone promotes absorption of Ca

Vitamin D enhances absorption of calcium and phosphate: Gastrointestinal secretions required for this action

Cortisol Opposes Vit. D

$Ca \times P = K$

Circulation

Parathyroid hormone inhibits reabsorption of P

Succus entericus

Alkaline pH

Acid pH

Parathyroid hormone enhances reabsorption of Ca (secondary action)

Stool
Normal excretion on average diet
Ca ⟶ 500 to 700 mg/24 hrs
P ⟶ 200 to 600 mg/24 hrs
(30% of intake)

Alk. phosphatase normal adult serum level 1 to 5 B.U./100 ml

Urine

Normal excretion on average diet
Ca=100 to 300 mg/24 hrs
P=500 to 1000 mg/24 hrs

Deposition of Ca and P promoted by alkaline pH, stress, anabolic hormones, and local tissue concentration

Osteoclastic and osteoblastic activity in dynamic equilibrium

Resorption of calcium and phosphate stimulated by parathyroid hormone, by acidosis and citrate (?)

Alkaline phosphatase

Osteoblast

Osteoclast

Bone salts deposited as "hydroxyopotite" in proteinaceous bone matrix

Matrix growth requires protein, vitamin C, anabolic hormones (androgens, estrogen, IGF-1) + stress of mobility
Matrix resorption favored by catabolic hormones (11-oxysteroids [cortisol], thyroid), parathyroid hormone + immobilization

Figure 32-2

Pathology and Clinical Manifestations of Hyperparathyroidism

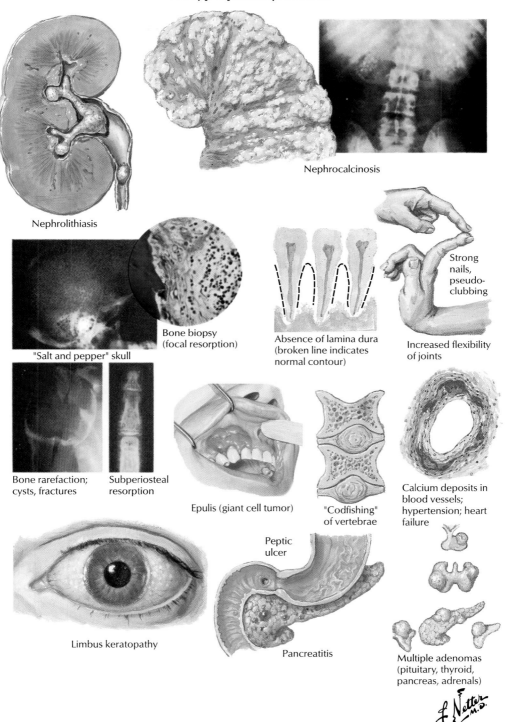

Nephrolithiasis

Nephrocalcinosis

"Salt and pepper" skull

Bone biopsy (focal resorption)

Absence of lamina dura (broken line indicates normal contour)

Strong nails, pseudo-clubbing

Increased flexibility of joints

Bone rarefaction; cysts, fractures

Subperiosteal resorption

Epulis (giant cell tumor)

"Codfishing" of vertebrae

Calcium deposits in blood vessels; hypertension; heart failure

Limbus keratopathy

Peptic ulcer

Pancreatitis

Multiple adenomas (pituitary, thyroid, pancreas, adrenals)

breast, and squamous cell lung carcinomas. Malignant tumors rarely secrete PTH, more often secreting PTH-related peptide, which does not cross-react on the current intact PTH assays. Certain medications cause hypercalcemia and may unmask underlying primary hyperparathyroidism. Thiazide diuretics decrease urinary calcium excretion and may affect the responsiveness of target cells to PTH. Lithium also increases urinary calcium retention and may directly promote secretion of PTH. Additional causes include other endocrine disorders (hyperthyroidism, primary adrenal insufficiency, and, less commonly, hypothyroidism and pheochromocytoma), milk alkali syndrome, excessive vitamin A or D intake, granulomatous disorders (sarcoidosis, tuberculosis), and immobilization. Generally, these conditions have suppressed PTH levels and can be readily distinguished from primary hyperparathyroidism. Benign familial hypocalciuric hypercalcemia is an autosomal dominant condition that causes asymptomatic hypercalcemia with low urinary calcium excretion (<100 mg/day) and usually normal PTH levels. A common primary abnormality is an inactivating mutation of the calcium receptor gene, and this should be suspected in individuals with a strong family history of hypercalcemia. It is important to diagnose this condition with a 24-hour urinary calcium measurement because these individuals do not require any surgical therapy.

Secondary hyperparathyroidism occurs commonly but is characterized by low or normal serum calcium levels. The elevated PTH often occurs as a physiologic response to conditions that cause hypocalcemia, such as vitamin D deficiency and acute hyperphosphatemia (tumor lysis syndrome, acute renal failure, and rhabdomyolysis). It is seen most commonly in renal insufficiency, particularly when renal 1,25-dihydroxyvitamin D production is impaired with subsequent decreased intestinal calcium absorption. In longstanding renal failure, the parathyroid glands become autonomous, and a condition of tertiary hyperparathyroidism can develop with PTH levels often greater than 2 to 3 times normal.

DIAGNOSTIC APPROACH

The diagnosis is usually straightforward with the demonstration of elevated PTH levels in the set-

ting of hypercalcemia. The calcium level should be confirmed because it can be falsely elevated from venipuncture alone. An intact PTH determination should be performed using the 2-site immunoassay. Radiologic studies are not necessary to confirm the diagnosis, but they are important when considering surgical management. PTH can be in the normal range in some individuals, which is inappropriate for an elevated calcium level. Less commonly, the calcium level remains normal while the PTH level is elevated. A search for a secondary cause should be considered in these cases, particularly ruling out vitamin D deficiency by measuring 25-hydroxyvitamin D levels. In primary hyperparathyroidism alone, 25-hydroxyvitamin D levels tend to be at the lower end of the normal range with 1,25-dihydroxyvitamin D levels being normal or even elevated (PTH drives the conversion of 25-hydroxyvitamin D to 1,25-di-hydroxyvitamin D).

Although phosphorus is released from bone, there is an increase in urinary phosphorus excretion induced by hyperparathyroidism. Serum phosphorus is, therefore, usually low or at the lower end of normal range. Typically, total urinary calcium excretion is at the upper end of normal with up to 40% of patients being hypercalciuric (>300 mg/day). Other bone turnover markers (e.g., alkaline phosphatase, urinary N-telopeptides, deoxypyridinoline) tend to be elevated, but usually do not aid in the diagnosis or management of primary hyperparathyroidism.

MANAGEMENT AND THERAPY

Primary hyperparathyroidism can be cured by surgical removal of the parathyroid glands. An experienced surgeon performing a bilateral neck exploration can achieve cure rates of over 90% (defined as a reduction in serum calcium and PTH levels) with a less than 1% operative mortality rate. Surgical morbidity is low (<5%) but can include bleeding, recurrent laryngeal nerve damage, and rarely, hypoparathyroidism. Many symptoms or signs may improve after parathyroidectomy. For instance, there is a significant reduction in recurrent nephrolithiasis after surgery, although no significant improvement in renal insufficiency occurs. Bone mineral density (BMD) also improves consistently by 6% in the first year and up to 10% to 12% after 10 years. Interestingly, BMD gains are usually greatest in cancellous bone and less so in cortical bone. There are conflicting data regarding reduction in fracture risk with some retrospective studies suggesting a decreased risk and others showing no change. Classic symptoms of osteitis fibrosa cystica and neuromuscular disease are rare today and can be reversed by surgery. In contrast, cardiac manifestations do not necessarily reverse after surgery, causing some to question their causal association. Specifically, hypertension does not usually improve after parathyroidectomy. Left ventricular hypertrophy may or may not regress after surgery, and cardiac calcifications usually remain unchanged. Neuropsychiatric symptoms also do not improve consistently after surgical therapy. Current accepted surgical indications in symptomatic patients include nephrolithiasis or nephrocalcinosis, osteitis fibrosa cystica, classic neuromuscular disease, or an acute episode of severe hypercalcemia.

The role of surgery in asymptomatic individuals is less clear and continues to be debated. The NIH convened a consensus conference in 1990 on surgical indications for asymptomatic primary hyperparathyroidism. The recommendations were largely based on expert opinion and were revised in an NIH workshop held in 2002. The updated recommendations for surgical intervention include the following: total serum calcium levels >1mg/dL above normal reference ranges; urinary calcium excretion >400 mg/day; reduced creatinine clearance by 30% without other causes; age less than 50 years; and decreased bone mineral density at any site less than 2.5 standard deviations below peak bone density (T score < −2.5).

Since the 1990 NIH consensus conference, a longitudinal observational study of mild primary hyperparathyroidism was completed. Sixty-one subjects who underwent parathyroidectomy and 60 subjects who did not were observed for 10 years. Surgical management resulted in normalization of biochemical parameters (calcium, PTH, and urinary calcium excretion) that persisted on 10-year follow-up study. There were no recurrences of nephrolithiasis. Subjects had sustained improvements in BMD at the femoral neck and spine throughout the study period (14% and 12% increases over 10 years, respectively). The untreated group also did well overall, with remarkable stability in their disease parameters

over 10 years. There was little progression of hypercalcemia or worsening of biochemical profiles. BMDs in the spine, hip, and distal radius were unchanged, which was unexpected given the average age of subjects was 58 and more than half of the subjects were postmenopausal women. Subgroup analysis suggested that perimenopausal women did continue to lose bone mass at rates similar to those of normocalcemic healthy women. Additionally, 27% had the development of one or more new indications for parathyroidectomy (calcium >12 mg/dL, increased urinary calcium excretion or distal radius Z score <-2.0). Taken together, these data demonstrate that surgery results in lasting improvements in biochemical parameters and BMD changes, whereas untreated groups overall did not have significant progression. Both sides of the debate have used these data to support their positions. In general, it is felt that additional factors favoring surgical management should include recent fracture in the absence of major trauma; vitamin D deficiency (<15 ng/mL); and perimenopausal women.

The traditional initial surgical approach is bilateral neck dissection. This approach is favored by many experienced surgeons. Because most individuals have a solitary adenoma, surgical techniques for localized exploration have been developed. These are dependent on adequate preoperative or intraoperative localization of the adenoma. Preoperative localization studies include ultrasound, nuclear imaging with technetium-sestamibi scans, CT, MRI, and selective venous catheterization for PTH measurements. Intraoperative techniques for localization include rapid PTH assays as well as use of sestamibi gamma probes, which allow less extensive and shorter operations. The impact of this approach on surgical cure rates is not proven. Local preferences are important because individual surgeons and institutions have variable expertise in these techniques. For persistent or recurrent disease, there is little debate that bilateral neck dissection is necessary. In this setting, preoperative localization increases the cure rate from approximately 60% to more than 90%.

Medical therapy should be considered for symptomatic patients awaiting surgery and in those for whom surgery is not an option. Outpatients with mild-to-moderate hypercalcemia should consume

1 to 1.5 L of fluid per day. Although moderate calcium intake should be maintained, medications such as vitamin D and thiazides, which exacerbate hypercalcemia, should be discontinued. Furosemide (20 to 40 mg orally once daily) may also be added provided adequate hydration is maintained. Oral bisphosphonates can be used to decrease bone turnover and lower the calcium level. However, they often increase the PTH level and, therefore, their long-term efficacy has not been established. Intermittent intravenous pamidronate is another alternative (30–60 mg intravenously every 3 months). Estrogen and progestin therapy has been given to reduce bone resorption, particularly in perimenopausal women, without adversely affecting PTH levels. All patients should be encouraged to exercise to maintain bone mass. Calcium levels should be assessed every 4 to 6 months with PTH and creatinine measured at least yearly.

FUTURE DIRECTIONS

Surgical approaches will continue to be refined and data will be forthcoming comparing various techniques. A better understanding of fracture risks and surgical indications for cardiac and neuropsychiatric manifestations in primary hyperparathyroidism will result from ongoing clinical studies. Calcimimetic agents have been developed that act on the calcium-sensing receptor to downregulate PTH secretion. Their use will aid in the medical management of primary and, in particular, secondary hyperparathyroidism due to renal insufficiency.

REFERENCES

Consensus development conference statement. *J Bone Miner Res.* 1991;6(suppl 2):S9-S13.

Bilezikian JP. Primary hyperparathyroidism. When to observe and when to operate. *Endocrinol Metab Clin North Am.* 2000;29:465-478.

Eigelberger MS, Clark OH. Surgical approaches to primary hyperparathyroidism. *Endocrinol Metab Clin North Am.* 2000;29:479-502.

Silverberg SJ, Shane E, Jacobs TP, Siris E, Bilezikian JP. A 10-year prospective study of primary hyperparathyroidism with or without parathyroid surgery. *N Engl J Med.* 1999; 341:1249-1255.

Strewler GJ. Medical approaches to primary hyperparathyroidism. *Endocrinol Metab Clin North Am.* 2000;29:523-539.

Chapter 33
Hyperthyroidism

Elizabeth A. Fasy

Thyrotoxicosis is the constellation of clinical findings that arise when the peripheral tissues are presented with and respond to an excess of thyroid hormone—free thyroxine (T4), and free triiodothyronine (T3). Hyperthyroidism refers to sustained increases in thyroid hormone synthesis and secretion by the thyroid gland.

Common symptoms of thyrotoxicosis include nervousness, emotional lability, fatigability, heat intolerance, weight change (usually weight loss), appetite change (usually increased), myopathic symptoms, increased frequency of bowel movements, sweating, menstrual irregularities (usually oligomenorrhea), and central nervous system disturbance. Common signs include hyperactivity; tachycardia or atrial arrhythmias; systolic hypertension; warm, moist, smooth skin; stare and eyelid retraction; tremor; hyperreflexia; and muscle weakness. Palpitations are a prominent symptom in the elderly, as is cardiac failure. Generally, elderly patients present with less florid features of thyrotoxicosis and commonly exhibit cardiac symptoms or dementia.

The most common causes of thyrotoxicosis in Western society are Graves' disease, autonomous single nodules (also known as toxic hot nodules), or multiple functioning nodules (also called toxic multinodular goiter), and thyroiditis. The pathogenesis in each of these conditions is different (Table 33-1). However, the initial therapy is similar and focuses on blocking the peripheral effects of thyroid hormone excess and reducing thyroid hormone overproduction where present.

ETIOLOGY, PATHOGENESIS, AND DIFFERENTIAL DIAGNOSIS
Graves' Disease

Graves' disease is the most common cause of hyperthyroidism in patients younger than 40 years old (Figure 33-1). The pathophysiology represents one of the classic receptor antibody disease states due to thyroid-stimulating hormone (TSH) receptor autoantibodies that continuously stimulate the thyroid gland as TSH

agonists. Intrathyroidal lymphocytic infiltrate is the initial abnormality (Figure 33-2). As in other autoimmune disease states, females are more commonly affected than males. A triad of manifestations define the disease: (1) hyperthyroidism and goiter; (2) ophthalmopathy, clinically evident in 10% to 25% of patients with a higher prevalence in men and in those who smoke; and (3) dermopathy in the form of localized myxedema, which is a skin thickening typically limited to the pretibial area. Approximately 4% of patients with clinically evident ophthalmopathy have thyroid dermopathy.

The onset of the disease is usually insidious. Some patients may notice the gradual development of goiter and its associated symptoms, including difficulty in fastening the collar button, fullness in the neck, or a choking sensation. Slightly more than one half of the patients experience symptoms of ophthalmopathy (i.e., grittiness and tearing of the eyes, retroocular pressure, photophobia, a staring appearance, and the development of diplopia) (Figure 33-3).

Toxic Multinodular Goiter and Toxic Hot Nodule

Autonomously functioning thyroid nodules are discrete and function independently of the pituitary-thyroid negative feedback loop. The nodules appear hyperfunctioning (hot) on radionuclide imaging, concentrating the radioiodide to a greater extent than the surrounding atrophic thyroid tissue (Figure 33-4). Thyroid nodules are the most common cause of thyrotoxicosis in the elderly. The disease onset is also insidious and the thyrotoxicosis is usually mild. The goiter may have been diagnosed many years previously. Because these disorders

Figure 33-1 — Hyperthyroidism with Diffuse Goiter (Graves' Disease)

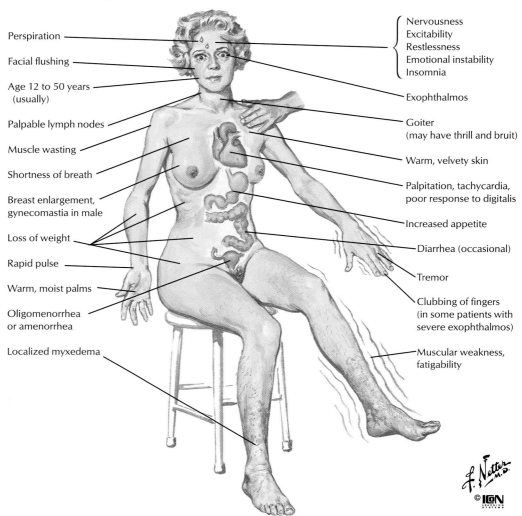

Perspiration

Facial flushing

Age 12 to 50 years (usually)

Palpable lymph nodes

Muscle wasting

Shortness of breath

Breast enlargement, gynecomastia in male

Loss of weight

Rapid pulse

Warm, moist palms

Oligomenorrhea or amenorrhea

Localized myxedema

Nervousness
Excitability
Restlessness
Emotional instability
Insomnia

Exophthalmos

Goiter (may have thrill and bruit)

Warm, velvety skin

Palpitation, tachycardia, poor response to digitalis

Increased appetite

Diarrhea (occasional)

Tremor

Clubbing of fingers (in some patients with severe exophthalmos)

Muscular weakness, fatigability

more commonly present in elderly patients, cardiac manifestations, such as tachycardia, atrial fibrillation, precipitation of angina, or cardiac failure, tend to predominate.

Iodine-Induced Hyperthyroidism

Iodine-induced hyperthyroidism is commonly an iatrogenic disorder occurring after patients with multinodular glands are exposed to large iodine loads. For unexplained reasons, the normal autoregulatory systems of the thyroid gland fail and the patient is rendered hyperthyroid. The most common sources of iodine are radiocon-

trast agents and amiodarone. Amiodarone may cause thyrotoxicosis by causing a specific form of focal thyroiditis. The presenting features are similar to those of a toxic multinodular goiter, except they are extremely resistant to antithyroid therapy.

Subacute Thyroiditis (De Quervain's Disease)

Subacute thyroiditis is characterized by granulomatous and giant cell inflammation. Patients present with transient symptoms of thyrotoxicosis. Usually, the thyroiditis follows a viral-like

Figure 33-2   Thyroid Pathology in Hyperthyroidism with Diffuse Goiter
(Graves' Disease)

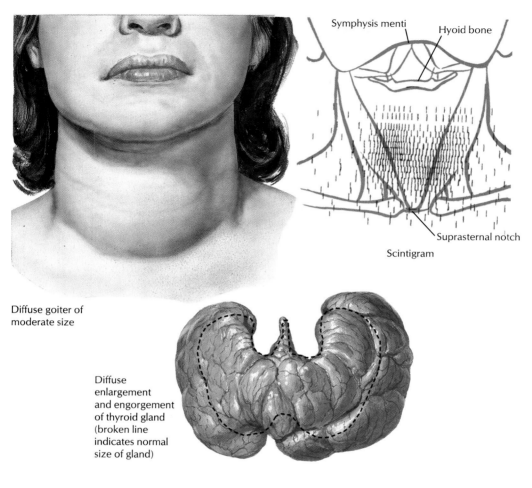

Symphysis menti

Hyoid bone

Suprasternal notch

Scintigram

Diffuse goiter of moderate size

Diffuse enlargement and engorgement of thyroid gland (broken line indicates normal size of gland)

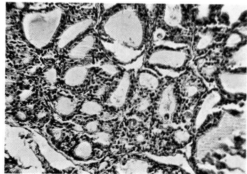

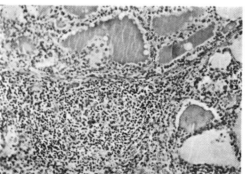

Diffuse hyperplasia

Hyperplasia with lymphocytic infiltration

Figure 33-3   Ophthalmopathy of Graves' Disease

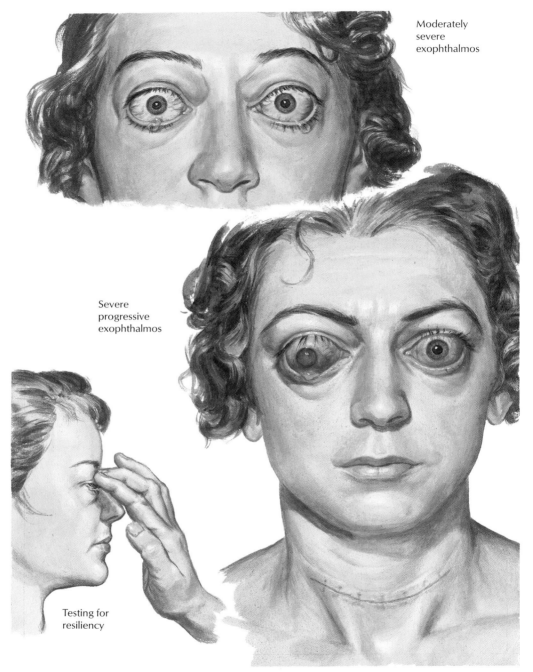

Moderately
severe
exophthalmos

Severe
progressive
exophthalmos

Testing for
resiliency

Figure 33-4   ## Pathophysiology of Hyperfunctioning Thyroid Adenoma

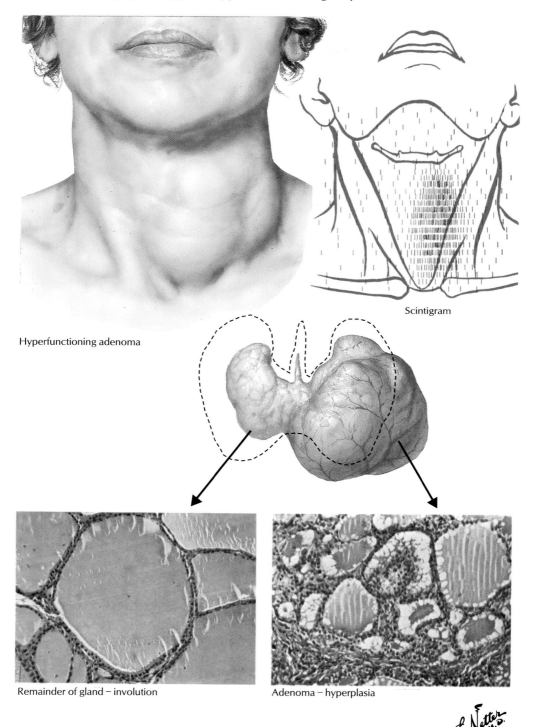

Scintigram

Hyperfunctioning adenoma

Remainder of gland – involution

Adenoma – hyperplasia

Table 33-1
Disorders Associated With Thyrotoxicosis

Disorder	Pathogenic Mechanism
High thyroid radioiodine uptake	
Graves' disease	Stimulating antibody to TSH receptor
Toxic multinodular goiter	Multiple foci of functional autonomy
Toxic hot nodule	Single focus of functional autonomy
TSH* hypersecretion	Thyrotroph adenoma/ thyrotroph resistance to T4
Trophoblastic tumor	Chorionic gonadotropin
Hyperemesis gravidarum	Chorionic gonadotropin
Low thyroid radioiodine uptake	
Silent/subacute thyroiditis	Leakage of stored hormone
Drug-induced thyroiditis (amiodarone, interferon-a)	Leakage of stored hormone
Radiation thyroiditis	Leakage of stored hormone
Infarction of thyroid adenoma	Leakage of stored hormone
Thyrotoxicosis factitia	Hormone ingestion in medication or food
Struma ovarii	Toxic adenoma in a dermoid tumor of ovary
Iodine, iodine-containing drugs, and radiographic contrast agents	Iodine plus thyroid autonomy

*TSH, thyroid-stimulating hormone.

illness and presents as a tender, enlarged thyroid gland. The pain radiates to the jaw, ears, and occipital area. Systemic symptoms may be present. Episodes are usually self-limiting, although temporary or permanent hypothyroidism can occur. Relapses are common.

Silent Thyroiditis
Silent (painless) thyroiditis is a lymphocytic thyroiditis associated with transient thyrotoxicosis and transient hypothyroidism. The pathophysiology is the same as that of postpartum thyroiditis. The duration of symptoms is short and confirmed by low thyroid radioactive iodine uptake. It has a self-limited course of a few weeks to months, and transient hypothyroidism occurs during recovery. One half of patients will have persistent autoantibodies, goiter, and hypothyroidism.

DIAGNOSTIC APPROACH
The diagnosis of thyrotoxicosis is established by demonstrating an elevated free T4 (FT4) level accompanied by a suppressed serum TSH level. All patients with thyrotoxicosis have a low or undetectable TSH level (<0.1 mU/L), except for TSH-induced thyrotoxicosis. FT4 levels have generally replaced total T4 levels, T3 resin uptake, and corrected measures of free T4 (e.g., free T4 index), as the tests for thyrotoxicosis. Free T3 levels are elevated in all patients and are used to monitor response to therapy or in mild states of hyperthyroidism (T3 toxicosis) where serum FT4 levels are normal. In Graves' disease and toxic multinodular goiter, T3 levels typically are higher than T4 levels (T3[ng/dL]: T4[ug/dL] ratio >20).

Thyroid Antibody Testing
Anti-thyroglobulin and *anti-microsomal antibodies* are directed toward the detection of cytoplasmic antibodies. These antibodies are usually present in patients with autoimmune thyroid disease, Graves' disease, and Hashimoto's thyroiditis. They are rarely present in patients with other types of thyroiditis. The TSH receptor-binding inhibitory immunoglobulins (TBII) radioreceptor assay and thyroid stimulating immunoglobulins (TSI) bioassay detect antibodies to the TSH receptor, which, if present, are indicative of Graves' thyrotoxicosis.

Imaging
In general, radioisotope imaging of the thyroid is not necessary in all patients with thyrotoxicosis.

Scanning may be useful to assess the function of a single nodule in the presence of biochemical evidence of hyperthyroidism, assess the function of nodules in toxic multinodular goiter, diagnose subacute thyroiditis when other clinical features are absent (i.e., absent uptake in the presence of hyperthyroidism), confirm the diagnosis of thyrotoxicosis factitia, or differentiate between silent or postpartum thyroiditis and Graves' disease in the postpartum patient (Table 33-1).

MANAGEMENT AND THERAPY
Pharmacologic Agents

The *thionamide antithyroid drugs* propylthiouracil (PTU) and methimazole act as competitive inhibitors of thyroid peroxidase to effectively reduce thyroid hormone production. PTU in higher doses may also have the advantage of inhibiting peripheral conversion of T4 to T3. These agents may also possess inherent immune-modulating effects that modify the disease pathophysiology, particularly in autoimmune thyroid disease. The usual starting doses are propylthiouracil 100 mg every 8 hours or methimazole 10 to 30 mg initally 3 times daily, in equal dosages. In most patients, therapy can be halved within 6 to 8 weeks and reduced to a once- or twice-daily maintenance dose after 3 months. For compliance reasons, evidence of increased potency, and lower complication rates, methimazole is preferred. The major side effects of the agents are agranulocytosis; hepatic dysfunction; a lupus-like syndrome; vasculitis; and, more commonly, skin rash, fever, urticaria, and arthralgia. The side effects are idiosyncratic and usually develop within the first 3 months of therapy. Patients should be warned about symptoms of fever and sore throat, which are typically seen with agranulocytosis. A baseline CBC with differential is recommended before initiating therapy.

β-Adrenoceptor antagonists block the peripheral effects of thyroid hormone excess and the peripheral conversion of T4 to T3. They are contraindicated in patients with asthma or chronic lung disease. Cardiac failure secondary to thyrotoxicosis is a relative contraindication. Most experience is with propranolol, 40 mg every 8 hours. These agents are given in conjunction with thiourea agents as first-line therapy to provide symptomatic relief of tremor, palpitations, anxiety, and heat intolerance.

Iodide is usually given just before surgery to reduce the vascularity of the gland or, rarely, as adjunctive therapy for a thyroid crisis. Three to 5 drops of iodine or a drop of saturated solution of potassium iodide in a glass of milk or water are given 3 times daily. The use of iodide is of short-term benefit only and precludes the use of radioactive iodine therapy in the short term.

Iodinated radiocontrast agents (e.g., iopanoic acid) are useful second-line agents. They have the additional advantage over iodide of inhibiting the conversion of T4 to T3.

Lithium carbonate acts by inhibiting thyroid hormone release into the circulation. This is a second-line agent and has the advantage of not blocking iodine 131 (^{131}I) uptake.

Optimum Treatment
Graves' Disease

Graves' disease is an autoimmune disorder characterized by spontaneous remission and relapse. Antithyroid drugs (e.g., thiourea and β-blockers) are given at appropriate dosages and are the recommended treatment for pregnant women, children, and adolescents. The length of treatment is variable but treatment for approximately 18 months results in long-term remission in 30% to 40% of cases. Patients with milder disease and small goiters are more likely to fully respond to a course of antithyroid medications and remain in disease remission. Therapy may be discontinued if the patient has been euthyroid for 18 months and the serum TSH is not suppressed. Most relapses occur within the first 6 months. Follow-up intervals of 2 months, 6 months, and 1 year are advised. A high dose of thiourea agents plus thyroxine replacement technique may result in a higher rate of sustained remission.

For patients with more significant hyperthyroidism and larger goiters, radioactive iodine therapy or surgery should be considered (usually subtotal thyroidectomy). The decision to proceed to more definitive therapy is governed by the preference of the patient and the treating clinician. Radioactive iodine will provide an effective cure after a single dose of therapy in 70% to 90% of patients. Most centers give a moderate dose of iodine (15 mCi) to ensure adequate ablation of the thyroid gland. The patient is instructed to cease antithyroid therapy 4 to 7 days before the dose of radioactive iodine and then to recommence therapy 2 days after the therapy. Most patients may experience a dry mouth and transient pain in the thyroid and salivary glands during therapy and for a short time afterward and may be rendered hypothyroid 4 to 12 weeks after therapy. The patients must understand that they will become permanently hypothyroid and will require lifelong thyroid hormone replacement. The effectiveness of radioactive iodine and antithyroid agents has diminished the role of surgery. Nodular or very large goiters are preferably treated with surgery. Radioactive iodine is not contraindicated in younger patients or women of childbearing age unless they are pregnant. A pregnancy test is required in women of childbearing age before the administration of therapy.

Autonomous Functioning Nodule(s)

Radioactive iodine is the therapy of choice with a toxic multinodular goiter. Higher doses (in the order of 30 mCi) are usually used to achieve euthyroidism. Radioactive iodine therapy is also successful in patients with a single hot nodule, but repeated doses are often required. An antithyroid drug may be considered to reduce the risk of treatment-induced thyrotoxicosis and to attain euthyroidism faster. Surgery is also an option.

Iodine-induced Hyperthyroidism

This is an extremely difficult condition to treat. Higher doses of thiourea agents are needed to control the hyperthyroidism. If possible, iodine consumption should be reduced and perchlorate may in addition be useful to block iodine uptake into the gland. Steroid therapy may be useful in amiodarone-induced thyrotoxicosis. Radioactive iodine uptake assessments are useful to determine the degree of uptake before ^{131}I therapy. Early surgery should be considered if no other option is available and the patient is not responding to other therapeutic approaches.

Subacute Thyroiditis

This is a self-limiting disease in which the hyperthyroidism results from the release of stored thyroid hormone into the circulation. Pain is treated with aspirin, if mild, or with steroids (prednisone 30 mg daily, rapidly tapered over a few days) if severe. The hyperthyroidism is treated with beta-blockers if necessary.

FUTURE DIRECTIONS

Recently, it was discovered that hereditary nonautoimmune hyperthyroidism is caused by activation of germline mutations in the TSH receptor gene in kindred with thyrotoxicosis, goiter, suppressed TSH, elevated FT3 and FT4 concentrations, and the absence of TSH receptor antibodies. This molecular diagnosis leads to consideration of genetic counseling and primary thyroid ablation in individuals found to have the activated TSH receptor germline mutation.

REFERENCES

The American Thyroid Association Web Site. Available at: http://www.thyroid.org. Accessed February 8, 2003.

Cooper D. Treatment of thyrotoxicosis. In: Braverman LE, Utiger RD, eds. *Werner & Ingbar's the Thyroid: A Fundamental and Clinical Text.* 8th ed. Philadelphia, Pa: Lippincott Williams & Wilkins; 2000:691-715.

Fuhrer D, Warner J, Sequeira M, Paschke R, Gregory J, Ludgate M. Novel TSHR germline (Met463Val) masquerading as Graves' disease in a large Welsh kindred with hyperthyroidism. *Thyroid.* 2000;10:1035-1041.

Reinwein D, Benker G, Lazarus JH, Alexander WD. A prospective randomized trial of antithyroid drug dose in Graves' disease therapy. European Multicenter Study Group on Antithyroid Drug Treatment. *J Clin Endcrinol Metab.* 1993; 76:1516-1521.

Roti E, Gardini E, Minelli R, Bianconi L, Braverman LE. Sodium ipodate and methimazole in the long-term treatment of hyperthyroid Graves' disease. *Metabolism.* 1993; 42: 403-408.

Thyroid Disease Manager Web site. Available at: http:// www. thyroidmanager.org. Accessed February 8, 2003.

Weetman AP. How antithyroid drugs work in Graves' disease. *Clin Endocrinol (Oxf).* 1992;37:317-318.

Chapter 34

Hypogonadism in the Male

David A. Ontjes

Hypogonadism in a male refers to a deficiency of either testosterone production or sperm production, or both. Disorders causing hypogonadism may result from direct damage to the testes (primary hypogonadism) or to the hypothalamus or pituitary gland (secondary hypogonadism).

The adult male testis consists of 2 main components: seminiferous tubules and Leydig or interstitial cells. The seminiferous tubules, which comprise over 80% of the total testicular mass, contain Sertoli cells and germ cells or sperm. Sertoli cells, in response to stimulation by pituitary follicle-stimulating hormone (FSH), secrete an androgen binding protein that increases the concentration of testosterone in the tubular lumen (Figure 34-1). They also provide an environment necessary for germ cell differentiation into mature sperm. Leydig cells produce testosterone and related steroids in response to stimulation by pituitary luteinizing hormone (LH). Testosterone acts locally on seminiferous tubules to promote sperm formation.

In the adult male, more than 95% of available testosterone is secreted by Leydig cells. The testes also secrete smaller amounts of the weak androgens dehydroepiandrosterone (DHEA) and androstenedione, as well as small amounts of estradiol and estrone. In peripheral tissues, a portion of the secreted testosterone is converted into dihydrotestosterone (DHT). Most target cells for testosterone contain an enzyme, 5α-reductase, that converts testosterone to DHT. Thus DHT, rather than testosterone itself, is responsible for many of the androgenic effects of testosterone. Testosterone can also be converted into the potent estrogen, estradiol, in tissues possessing an aromatase enzyme. Adipose tissue and the central nervous system are capable of converting androgens into estrogens by this mechanism.

Most of the activities of the testis, including sperm formation and secretion of testosterone, are controlled by the pituitary gonadotropins, LH and FSH. These hormones are in turn controlled by a peptide hormone produced by the hypothalamus, called gonadotropin-releasing hormone, or GnRH. The hormonal control of testicular function is shown in Figure 34-1. GnRH binds to gonadotropin-producing cells in the pituitary gland and stimulates the secretion of both LH and FSH. Receptors for LH are located on Leydig cells. The testosterone produced by Leydig cells exerts a negative feedback on both the pituitary gland and the hypothalamus to reduce the release of GnRH, LH, and FSH. Receptors for FSH are located on Sertoli cells, where production of an androgen binding protein is stimulated. Under the influence of FSH, the Sertoli cell also secretes proteins called inhibins. These proteins are capable of selectively inhibiting the secretion of FSH by the pituitary gland. Thus, any process leading to damage of seminiferous tubules will result in a rise of serum FSH, while damage to the Leydig cells will result in a rise of both FSH and LH.

ETIOLOGY AND PATHOGENESIS
Primary Hypogonadism

Patients with primary hypogonadism have reduced testosterone secretion, reduced sperm production, and increased serum gonadotropins. The disease processes causing primary hypogonadism may damage the seminiferous tubules and Leydig cells to varying degrees. In general, there is greater damage to sperm production than to testosterone secretion (Figure 34-2, Table 34-1).

Klinefelter's syndrome, the most common congenital cause of primary hypogonadism in males, is due to the presence of an extra X chromosome. The most common genotype, 47XXY, is due to nondisjunction of the maternal oocyte, yielding an egg with 2 X chromosomes. Other chromosomal patterns having extra X chromosome material

Figure 34-1

Hypogonadism

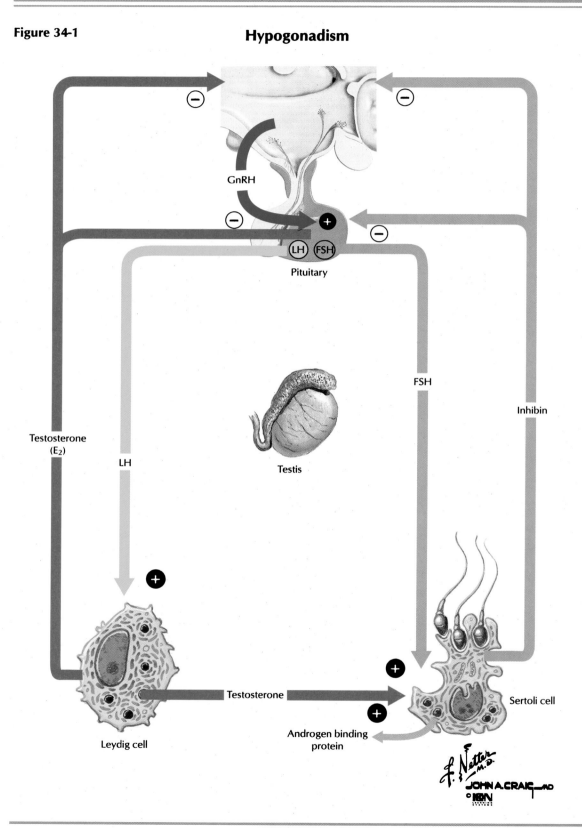

GnRH

Pituitary

LH FSH

FSH

Inhibin

Testosterone
(E₂)

LH

Testis

Testosterone

Androgen binding
protein

Leydig cell

Sertoli cell

Figure 34-2

Testicular Failure
Primary or Hypergonadotropic Hypogonadism, Prepubertal Failure

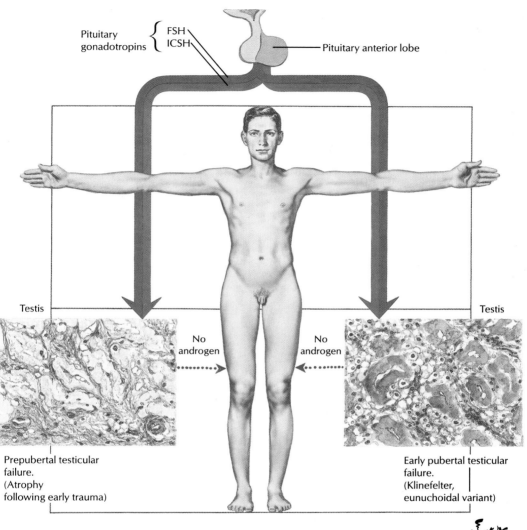

Pituitary gonadotropins { FSH / ICSH

Pituitary anterior lobe

Testis

No androgen

No androgen

Testis

Prepubertal testicular failure.
(Atrophy following early trauma)

Early pubertal testicular failure.
(Klinefelter, eunuchoidal variant)

may include 48XXXY, 49XXXXY, or mosaics such as 46XY/47XXY. Klinefelter's syndrome occurs in one of every 1,000 live births. Its likelihood increases with increasing maternal age. The chromosomal germ cell defect causes severe damage to the seminiferous tubules and variable damage to the Leydig cells. Individuals usually appear normal at birth and may experience normal pubertal development (Figure 34-3). As adult males, they have small, firm testes, azoospermia, gynecomastia, and usually low testosterone levels. Body proportions are affected, as shown in Figure 34-2, where there is prepubertal deficiency of testerone. Other abnormalities not directly related to testosterone deficiency occur more frequently, including chronic bronchitis, germ cell tumors,

Figure 34-3

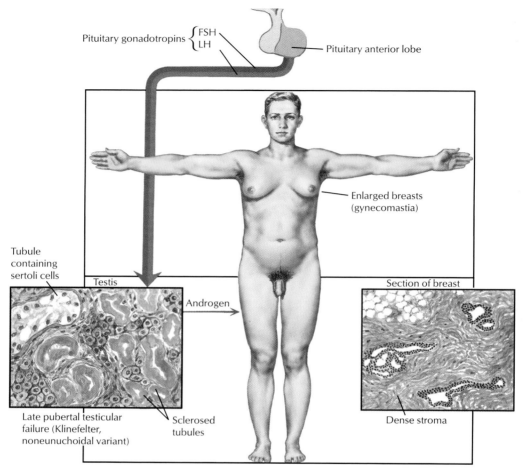

Testicular Failure
Seminiferous Tubular Dysgenesis (Klinefelter's Syndrome)

Pituitary gonadotropins { FSH LH

Pituitary anterior lobe

Enlarged breasts (gynecomastia)

Tubule containing sertoli cells

Testis

Androgen

Section of breast

Late pubertal testicular failure (Klinefelter, noneunuchoidal variant)

Sclerosed tubules

Dense stroma

Nuclear chromatin often positive (female); usually XXY chromosomal pattern but XXXY, XXXXY, XXYY, and mosaic patterns have been described

varicose veins, and diabetes mellitus.

Cryptorchidism refers to testes that have not descended from the abdominal cavity into the scrotum by 1 year of age. One or both testes may be involved. Approximately 5% of males have undescended testes at birth, but in 90%, descent occurs during the first year. The testis may fail to descend because of prenatal androgen deficiency, often due to defective testicular development in utero. In unilateral cryptorchidism, the descended testicle often exhibits abnormalities, including a low sperm count. The undescended

Table 34-1
Causes of Primary Hypogonadism in Males

Congenital Abnormalities	Acquired Abnormalities
Klinefelter's syndrome and other chromosomal abnormalities	Infections (mumps)
Cryptorchidism	Radiation
Myotonic dystrophy	Drugs and environmental toxins
Disorders of androgen biosynthesis	Trauma
Mutation of the FSH* receptor gene	Autoimmune disease
Spermatic duct obstruction or dysplasia	Acute and chronic systemic diseases
Varicocele	Idiopathic

*FSH, Follicle-stimulating hormone

testicle may be damaged further because of exposure to higher temperatures inside the abdomen.

Myotonic dystrophy, an autosomal dominant disorder leading to muscle atrophy, is accompanied by hypogonadism that usually develops after puberty. Congenital deficiencies in specific enzymes essential for androgen biosynthesis are rare autosomal recessive disorders that lead to testosterone deficiency during the first trimester of pregnancy, and hence to incomplete virilization of the male infant.

Spermatic Duct Obstruction or Dysplasia

Defects of the epididymis or vas deferens can cause absence of sperm in the semen (azoospermia), while spermatogenesis and testosterone secretion by the testes may be normal. Disorders of sperm transport may be either congenital or acquired. Most males with cystic fibrosis have congenital absence of the vas deferens. Acquired obstruction may result from infection (gonorrhea, chlamydia, tuberculosis) or surgical ligation (vasectomy).

Varicoceles are dilatations of the venous plexus

in the scrotum that exist in 10% to 15% of normal men. Because varicoceles exist in an even higher proportion of infertile men, they have long been proposed as a cause of infertility, perhaps by increasing temperatures within the scrotum. Whether or not fertility can be improved by ligation of varicoceles remains controversial.

Acquired diseases affecting the testes typically cause greater damage to the seminiferous tubules than to Leydig cells. The infection most commonly associated with testicular damage is mumps orchitis. Radiation and certain chemotherapeutic drugs used in the treatment of cancer can cause seminiferous tubule damage proportionate to the exposure. Alkylating agents such as cyclophosphamide and chlorambucil commonly cause oligospermia and elevations in serum FSH. Cisplatin or carboplatin can also decrease the sperm count, but at least partial recovery is usually seen. Many chronic systemic illnesses can cause hypogonadism, both by direct testicular injury and by causing reduced gonadotropin secretion. Cirrhosis, chronic renal failure, and AIDS are all associated with reduced testosterone secretion and variable levels of LH and FSH.

Secondary Hypogonadism

Patients with secondary hypogonadism have reduced sperm production, reduced testosterone secretion, and low or normal serum gonadotropin levels. Sexual differentiation is normal because Leydig cell function during the first trimester is stimulated by chorionic gonadotropin from the placenta. In contrast, penile growth during the third trimester is dependent on testosterone stimulated by LH from the fetal pituitary gland (Table 34-2).

Most cases of congenital hypogonadotropic hypogonadism are due to a lack of GnRH, as evidenced by a normal response of serum LH after repetitive administration of synthetic GnRH. In some cases, there are other associated abnormalities, as in the Prader-Willi syndrome, where hypogonadism is associated with mental retardation and obesity. Kallmann's syndrome is caused by a deletion in a gene on the short arm of the X chromosome that codes for an adhesion molecule, KALIG-1. Lack of this gene product leads to a failure of GnRH-secreting neurons to migrate during embryogenesis from the olfactory placode

Table 34-2
Causes of Secondary Hypogonadism in Males

Congenital Abnormalities	Acquired Abnormalities
Isolated idiopathic hypogonadotropic hypogonadism	Benign tumors and cysts Hyperprolactinemia
Hypogonadotropic hypogonadism associated with mental retardation	Malignant tumors
Hypogonadotropic hypogonadism associated with other pituitary abnormalities	Inflammatory and infectious diseases · Sarcoidosis · Langerhans cell histiocytosis · Tuberculous meningitis
Kallmann's syndrome	Hemochromatosis
Abnormal forms of LH* and FSH†	Pituitary apoplexy
	Trauma

*LH, luteinizing hormone; †FSH, Follicle-stimulating hormone

to the olfactory bulb and arcuate nucleus of the hypothalamus. The consequences are anosmia and hypogonadotropic hypogonadism. Most cases are sporadic, but familial inheritance also occurs. Inheritance is usually X-linked.

Any acquired disease affecting the hypothalamic-pituitary axis can cause hypogonadotropic hypogonadism. Mass lesions in the pituitary gland or hypothalamus are more likely to diminish the secretion of gonadotropins than that of ACTH or TSH. Thus, affected men may have hypogonadism without evidence of adrenal or thyroid deficiency. As a rule, most masses are large enough to cause dysfunction by compressing and damaging surrounding structures in the hypothalamus or pituitary. Prolactin-secreting pituitary adenomas may be an exception. High concentrations of prolactin produced by these tumors can act to inhibit production of GnRH in the hypothalamus. If prolactin concentrations are lowered by appropriate drugs, such as bromocriptine, gonadotropin secretion may resume even though the tumor remains.

Meningitis is a rare cause of hypogonadism in the United States, but tuberculous meningitis is seen in countries where tuberculosis is common. Inflammatory diseases such as sarcoidosis and Langerhan's cell histiocytosis (eosinophilic granuloma) impair GnRH secretion by damaging the hypothalamus, while hemochromatosis damages the pituitary gland by iron deposition.

Hypogonadism due to pituitary apoplexy occurs with sudden hemorrhage into the pituitary gland, usually from a preexisting pituitary tumor. Trauma to the base of the skull, as in a basilar skull fracture, can damage the pituitary stalk and impair the movement of GnRH from the hypothalamus to the pituitary gland. Both apoplexy and basilar skull fracture are usually associated with a deficiency of other pituitary hormones in addition to gonadotropins.

CLINICAL PRESENTATION

The clinical manifestations of impaired spermatogenesis are infertility and decreased testicular size. In a normal adult male, both testes should be from 4.0 to 7.0 cm in length. The clinical manifestations of testosterone deficiency depend on age at the onset of the deficiency. During embryonic life, testosterone acts to promote differentiation of the external genitalia along male lines. A lack of testosterone in a male infant during early uterine life will result in differentiation along female lines. If the deficiency is complete, the external genitalia may consist of a clitoris and labia, with the vagina ending in a blind pouch. Partial deficiencies lead to incomplete virilization, ranging from posterior labial fusion when the deficiency is more severe to hypospadias when it is mild. Insufficient testosterone late in pregnancy will not prevent normal differentiation of the external genitalia but will result in a very small penis (micropenis).

Lack of testosterone before puberty will result in failure of pubertal development. In the absence of testosterone, the epiphyses of the long bones may fail to close at the usual time so that linear growth may be prolonged, leading to an eunuchoidal body habitus (Figure 34-2). The lower body segment (floor to pubis) is characteristically more than 2 cm greater than the upper body segment, and the arm span more than 2 cm greater than total height. Testosterone deficiency occurring during adult life results in a loss of libido and

Figure 34-4

Approach to the Differential Diagnosis of Primary and Secondary Hypogonadism

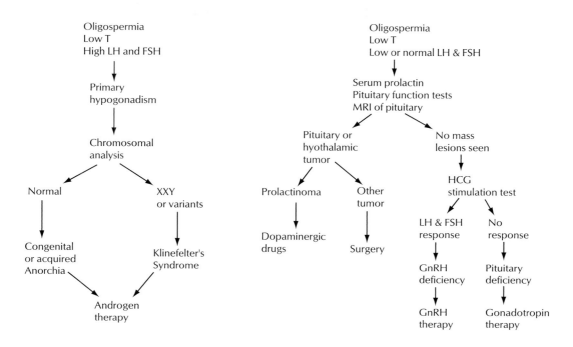

potency, as well as decreased muscle mass and diminished growth of body hair. Long- term effects also include a loss of bone mass, or osteoporosis.

DIFFERENTIAL DIAGNOSIS

Depending on the results of the patient's history, physical examination, semen analysis, and baseline measurements of testosterone and gonadotropins, other tests may be undertaken to arrive at a specific etiologic diagnosis. A simplified scheme for differential diagnosis is shown in Figure 34-4. In the teenage boy who is not undergoing pubertal changes at an expected rate, it may be difficult to distinguish constitutionally delayed puberty from one of the pathologic causes of secondary hypogonadism. A history of constitutional short stature, delayed dental maturation, or a family history of delayed puberty make a diagnosis of delayed puberty more likely.

DIAGNOSTIC APPROACH

Once a diagnosis of hypogonadism is made, it is important to determine whether it is primary or secondary. This is often apparent from the history

and physical examination. For example, a patient with secondary hypogonadism from a large pituitary or hypothalamic mass often has neurologic abnormalities such as visual field defects and evidence of a deficiency of other pituitary hormones. Men with primary hypogonadism are more likely to have breast enlargement (gynecomastia) due to the effects of elevated LH in stimulating testicular aromatase activity.

Laboratory Tests

The diagnosis is confirmed by finding decreased production of sperm or decreased production of testosterone. Semen analysis involves the measurement of the number of sperm in an ejaculated specimen, as well as their motility. Normal men produce more than 20 million sperm per milliliter of ejaculate, or 40 million per total ejaculate, and more than 60% are motile. Serum total testosterone measurement, which includes free plus protein-bound hormone, is a suitable test for testosterone secretion. Exceptions occur in very obese men, where the concentration of sex hormone—binding globulin is frequently low, and in elderly men where it may be high. In such individuals, measurement of the free (unbound) fraction of serum testosterone is a more accurate means of assessment. Serum gonadotropins, LH and FSH, should also be measured to interpret the significance of a low or borderline testosterone level. Elevated gonadotropin levels confirm the diagnosis of primary hypogonadism even when testosterone is in the low-normal range. Normal gonadotropin levels in the presence of a low testosterone level indicate secondary hypogonadism.

MANAGEMENT AND THERAPY

Testosterone replacement is indicated in most adult men with low serum testosterone levels, except in those cases where the underlying cause may be reversible. The preferred testosterone preparations are either testosterone esters for intramuscular injection or special formulations for transdermal administration. In the United States, testosterone enanthate and testosterone cypionate are the most frequently used intramuscular forms. Doses of 200 mg every 2 weeks or 300 mg every 3 weeks will maintain serum levels within the normal range throughout most of the dosing interval. Longer dosing cycles will result in subnormal serum levels toward the end of the interval. Transdermal formulations are available via skin patches that deliver 5 mg of testosterone every 24 hours and maintain serum testosterone level within the normal range. The patch must be changed daily. Testosterone is also available in a hydroalcoholic gel applied in doses of 50 to 100 mg, enough to maintain normal serum levels for 24 hours. Normalization of serum testosterone can lead to virilization in hypogonadal men and pubertal development in prepubertal boys. Libido, energy, bone mass, and muscle strength should all improve. If no improvement in hypogonadal symptoms is seen after a suitable interval, other causes for the symptoms should be considered. Adverse effects can include an increase in acne and aggressive behavior in adolescent boys, and exacerbation of benign prostatic hyperplasia, or, possibly, prostate cancer in older men. Testosterone therapy can also induce erythrocytosis and exacerbate sleep apnea. Monitoring in adults includes an annual prostate examination, measurement of hemoglobin and hematocrit, and inquiry about symptoms of sleep apnea.

Gonadotropin replacement, generally used for cases of secondary hypogonadism where fertility is the objective, is more complex and expensive than testosterone replacement. Some patients are stimulated to produce sufficient sperm for fertilization by injections of human chorionic gonadotropin (hCG), which replicates the effects of LH. Others require combination therapy with hCG and human menopausal gonadotropin, which contains both FSH and LH activity. The efficacy can be monitored by repeated semen analysis and measurement of the serum testosterone.

FUTURE DIRECTIONS

Improved recognition of the adverse effects of drugs and environmental toxins on testicular function should reduce the incidence of male hypogonadism worldwide. For example, exposure to the nematocide dibromodichloropropane is known to decrease spermatogenesis in farm workers using it in the fields. It is severely restricted in the United States, but it is still exported to and used in other countries. In men undergoing cancer chemotherapy with alkylating agents and other toxic drugs, concurrent suppression of gonadotropins with testosterone or inhibitory analogs of GnRH may protect gonadal function.

Rapid progress in assisted reproductive technology may enable men with severe oligospermia or low sperm motility to be fertile. Intracytoplasmic sperm injection (ICSI) involves the direct injection of a single spermatozoon into the cytoplasm of an oocyte previously collected from follicles produced under controlled ovarian stimulation. When there are no sperm in the ejaculate but there are germ cells in the testes, this technique can be performed using spermatozoa isolated from testicular biopsy specimens. ICSI has been successful in a few men with Klinefelter's syndrome. Germ cell transplantation has been accomplished in mice where the testes have been previously depleted of germ cells, and this technique may become a treatment for male infertility.

REFERENCES

Basaria S, Dobs AS. Hypogonadism and androgen replacement therapy in elderly men. *Am J Med.* 2001;110:563-572.

Braunstein GD. The testes. In: Greenspan FS, Gardner DG, eds. *Basic and Clinical Endocrinology.* 6th ed. New York: McGraw-Hill; 2001:422-452.

Griffen JE, Wilson JD. Disorders of the testes and the male

reproductive tract. In: Wilson JD, Foster DW, Kronenberg HM, Larsen PR, eds. *Williams Textbook of Endocrinology.* 9th ed. Philadelphia: WB Saunders; 1998:819–876.

Hargreave T, Ghosh C. Male fertility disorders. *Endocrin Metab Clin North Am.* 1998;27:765–782.

Mathur R, Braunstein GD. Gynecomastia: pathogenetic mechanisms and treatment strategies. *Horm Res.* 1997;48: 95–102.

Zitzmann M, Nieschlag E. Hormone substitution in male hypogonadism. *Mol Cell Endocrinol.* 2000;161:73–88.

Chapter 35
Hypothyroidism

Michael J. Thomas and Sue A. Brown

Hypothyroidism is a common condition that occurs when the thyroid is unable to produce enough thyroid hormone to meet the body's needs. Onset can occur at any age and is more common in women with a prevalence of approximately 2% in some age groups (compared with 0.1% for men). Congenital hypothyroidism is one of the most common endocrine abnormalities present at birth (about 1 in 5,000 births).

ETIOLOGY AND PATHOGENESIS

The synthesis and secretion of thyroid hormones by the thyroid are stimulated by thyroid-stimulating hormone (TSH, or thyrotropin), a glycoprotein produced by pituitary thyrotrophs. TSH binds to a plasma membrane receptor on thyroid follicular cells and activates adenylate cyclase. It stimulates every facet of thyroid iodine metabolism and promotes thyroid growth. TSH biosynthesis and secretion is inhibited by triiodothyronine (T3) and thyroxine (T4) forming a sensitive feedback loop to keep free thyroid hormone concentrations constant. TRH is a hypothalamic tripeptide that stimulates TSH release. TRH appears to set the level by which the negative feedback loop maintains thyroid hormone levels. Disturbances in the TRH-TSH-thyroid axis can lead to hypothyroidism.

Primary hypothyroidism, the most common cause of thyroid failure, results in low serum thyroid hormone with elevated TSH levels. Loss of functional thyroid tissue and interference of thyroid hormone production are the major causes of primary hypothyroidism (Figure 35-1).

Loss of functional thyroid tissue is usually due to autoimmune thyroid dysfunction (e.g., Hashimoto's or chronic lymphocytic thyroiditis) (Figure 35-1). It is sometimes associated with polyglandular autoimmune syndromes, a family history of thyroid dysfunction. High titers of antithyroid antibodies (antithyroid peroxidase and antithyroglobulin antibodies) are common, although titers are sometimes low, particularly in elderly patients. Cell-mediated (T-lymphocyte) destruction of the thyroid probably plays a more significant role in thyroid damage than thyroid antibodies. Pathologic study shows lymphocytic infiltration and fibrosis with destruction of follicles resulting in an atrophic thyroid gland or a firm, non-tender diffuse goiter. Gradually, T4/T3 synthesis is impaired, prompting a compensatory rise in TSH, and a "subclinical" phase that may precede the onset of frank hypothyroidism. Usually, hypothyroidism is chronic, but transient hypothyroidism as well as hyperthyroidism can occur. Silent ("painless") thyroiditis is a common cause of transient hyperthyroidism, hypothyroidism, or both in the postpartum period (approximate 5% prevalence). Procedures that remove or destroy functional thyroid tissue, such as surgery or radioactive iodine, can render a person permanently hypothyroid. Finally, congenital agenesis or dysgenesis of the thyroid gland can occur.

Interference with thyroid hormone production is often drug-induced. Iodine and lithium inhibit thyroid hormone secretion, particularly in patients with mild autoimmune thyroiditis. Endemic iodine deficiency can lead to goiter, cretinism, and hypothyroidism. Overtreatment with thionamides used for hyperthyroidism can also produce hypothyroidism. Amiodarone, an antiarrhythmic drug containing iodine, can block production of thyroid hormone. Rarely, congenital defects in T4 biosynthesis or maternal treatment with antithyroid drugs or iodine causes congenital hypothyroidism and goiter.

Secondary hypothyroidism (low TSH or inappropriately normal TSH with low thyroid hormone levels) is usually the result of hypothalamic or pituitary dysfunction due to tumors, trauma, surgery, or irradiation (Figure 35-1).
. TSH deficiency occurs when the anterior pituitary thyrotropes are unable to secrete adequate amounts of TSH to regulate thyroid hormone pro-

Figure 35-1

Adult Myxedema
Clinical Manifestations and Etiology

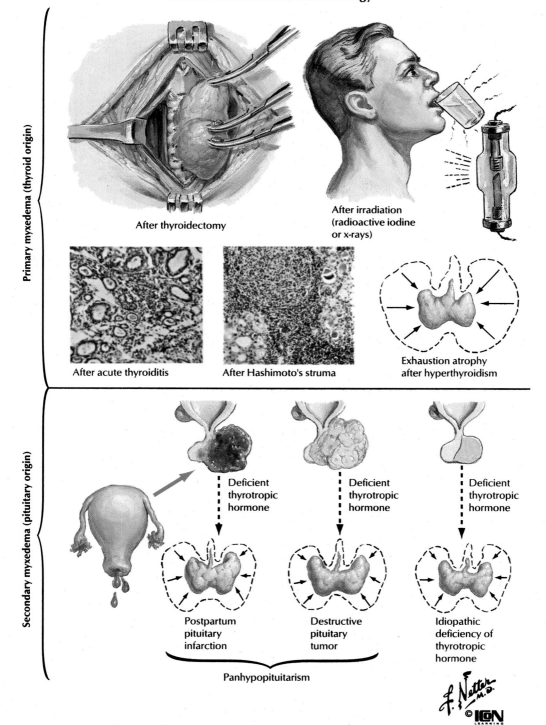

Primary myxedema (thyroid origin)

After thyroidectomy

After irradiation
(radioactive iodine
or x-rays)

After acute thyroiditis

After Hashimoto's struma

Exhaustion atrophy
after hyperthyroidism

Secondary myxedema (pituitary origin)

Deficient
thyrotropic
hormone

Deficient
thyrotropic
hormone

Deficient
thyrotropic
hormone

Postpartum
pituitary
infarction

Destructive
pituitary
tumor

Idiopathic
deficiency of
thyrotropic
hormone

Panhypopituitarism

duction. Hypothalamic defects lead to TRH deficiency.

Rare familial syndromes exist in which clinical hypothyroidism occurs despite elevated levels of T4/T3 and sometimes an elevated level of TSH. Resistance to thyroid hormone can be due to a mutation in one of the thyroid hormone receptors that binds T3, yielding the receptor unable to activate target DNA sequences, or the pituitary gland resistant to feedback inhibition of thyroid hormone.

CLINICAL PRESENTATION

The clinical spectrum of hypothyroidism is broad, ranging from "subclinical" with few or no manifestations to myxedema coma (Figure 35-2). The onset of symptoms can be insidious and is often overlooked in the elderly. Cold intolerance is the most specific symptom, and delayed relaxation of deep tendon reflexes is the most specific sign. Some clinical findings are explained by known thyroid hormone effects. Decreased metabolic rates lead to cold intolerance and a tendency to increased weight. The failure to metabolize glycosaminoglycans results in their accumulation in subcutaneous tissue, causing non-pitting edema (myxedema) (Figure 35-3). A goiter can be present in Hashimoto's thyroiditis or in iodine deficiency, whereas the thyroid gland may be normal size, small, or absent in post-procedural hypothyroidism, congenital thyroid agenesis, or dysgenesis. Mild pituitary gland enlargement occurs in some cases. Laboratory abnormalities often include hypertriglyceridemia, which can be reversed with adequate thyroid hormone replacement.

DIFFERENTIAL DIAGNOSIS

Hypothyroidism is accurately and easily diagnosed with thyroid function tests; however, these tests can be abnormal in sick, but apparently euthyroid patients ("non-thyroidal illness" or "euthyroid sick syndrome"). These changes are not believed to indicate abnormal thyroid function because TSH levels are usually normal and thyroid test results are normal after the underlying illness resolves. The biological importance of the euthyroid sick syndromes is not understood, and it may represent an adaptive stress response. The existence of these syndromes emphasizes the importance of exercising sound clinical judgment before ordering diagnostic tests. There are three

---

Major Clinical Findings of Hypothyroidism

- Constitutional: Malaise, cold intolerance, lethargy, fatigue, hoarseness.
- Skin: Thickened, coarse, dry, cool, non–pitting edema (myxedema), hair loss, decreased sweating.
- Cardiovascular: Cardiac contractility and rate, cardiac dilatation, pericardial/pleural effusions, increased peripheral resistance.
- Gastrointestinal: Decreased appetite, constipation, mild weight gain.
- Musculoskeletal: Myalgias, arthralgias.
- Hematologic: Mild anemia (usually children).
- Neurologic: Delayed relaxation phase of deep tendon reflexes, slowing of physical and/or mental activity, poor memory, somnolence, rarely dementia and/or anxiety.
- Thyroid gland: May be large, "normal," or absent.
- Suggestive Laboratory Abnormalities: Hypercholesterolemia, increased creatine kinase, hyponatremia, hyperprolactinemia, EKG changes (prolonged PR interval, low voltage), normochromic anemia, ± mild increase in MCV.
- Neonatal/Pediatric Hypothyroidism: Delayed growth and development, umbilical hernia, prolonged neonatal jaundice, protruding tongue, poor feeding, delayed bone age.

---

major patterns of abnormalities in patients with nonthyroidal illness.

Low T3 syndrome with impaired T4 to T3 conversion is seen in most acute and chronic diseases, trauma, surgery, and starvation. T3 levels are decreased, and reverse T3 levels are increased, while T4 and TSH concentrations are normal. Although common, this syndrome is seldom a diagnostic problem because T3 levels are not routinely measured.

Low (total) T4 syndromes, also seen in severe illnesses, often are due to very low levels of plasma-binding proteins. The T4 index is often low as well, but free T4 measured by equilibrium dialysis is normal. Normal TSH levels are seen in most patients and provide the best evidence against hypothyroidism.

High T4 syndromes are seen occasionally and

Figure 35-2

Hypothyroidism

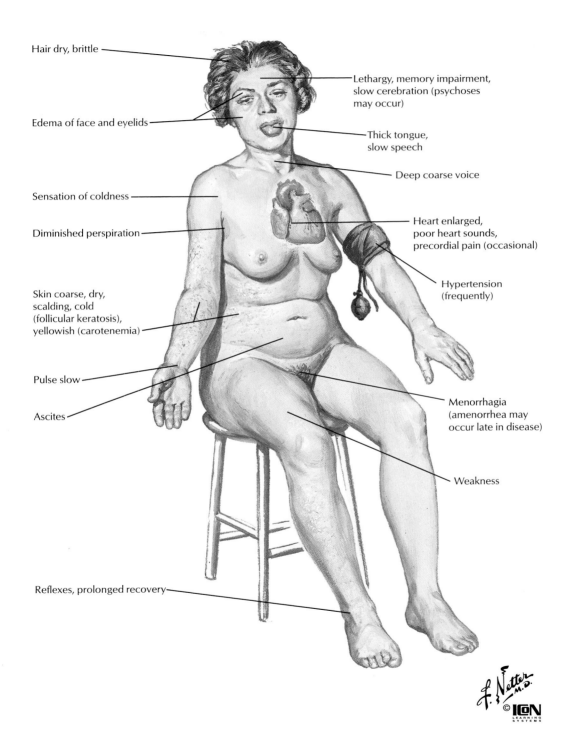

Hair dry, brittle

Lethargy, memory impairment, slow cerebration (psychoses may occur)

Edema of face and eyelids

Thick tongue, slow speech

Deep coarse voice

Sensation of coldness

Heart enlarged, poor heart sounds, precordial pain (occasional)

Diminished perspiration

Hypertension (frequently)

Skin coarse, dry, scalding, cold (follicular keratosis), yellowish (carotenemia)

Pulse slow

Menorrhagia (amenorrhea may occur late in disease)

Ascites

Weakness

Reflexes, prolonged recovery

may be due to increased plasma-binding proteins. These are usually transient, and normal TSH levels indicate that these patients do not have hypothyroidism.

DIAGNOSTIC APPROACH

An elevated TSH level confirms the diagnosis of primary hypothyroidism. The thyroxine level will be low and can be measured directly with a free T4 assay or estimated by a free T4 index (FTI). If the total T4 is decreased and T3 uptake is increased, the patient has decreased plasma–binding proteins, not hypothyroidism. The FTI is usually normal, and a normal TSH level confirms that the patient is euthyroid. If the total T4 and the FTI are decreased, but TSH is not elevated, the patient may have secondary hypothyroidism and evidence of other pituitary hormone deficits should be sought. In most cases, this combination of laboratory findings is due to abnormal plasma hormone binding or the effects of non-thyroidal illness on thyroid tests. A decreased serum free T4 (by equilibrium dialysis) verifies true T4 deficiency in the presence of binding protein changes or severe illness.

Diagnosis of the distinct cause of hypothyroidism is usually not necessary because most cases are either iatrogenic or due to autoimmune thyroiditis. Antithyroid antibodies, thyroid scans, and uptake measurements are rarely necessary because they do not change the management of the hypothyroidism. If secondary hypothyroidism is suspected, it is more important to assess the function of other pituitary hormones and obtain an MRI of the pituitary gland and hypothalamus, than it is to perform a TRH stimulation test.

MANAGEMENT AND THERAPY

Levothyroxine (L-T4) is the drug of choice. It has supplanted desiccated thyroid extract, which has variable potency and purity. L-T4 is deiodinated and peripherally converted to T3, producing normal plasma levels of both T4 and T3. Therapy begins with average replacement doses of 100 to 125 μg per day (approximately 1.6 μg/kg/day) and varies depending on age. In elderly patients or those with cardiac disease, therapy should be initiated with smaller doses (25 to 50 μg/day) and increase gradually to avoid precipitating myocardial ischemia or heart failure due to increased metabolic rate and cardiac output. Infants can be treated immediately with full doses (25 to 50 μg/day). The half-life of T4 is approximately 7 days, so most symptoms gradually resolve within several days to weeks of initiating therapy.

T3 is used infrequently for replacement due to its short half-life and slightly higher cost. Similarly, combination L-T4/T3 preparations offer no pharmacological advantage because T4 naturally undergoes deiodination in peripheral tissues once absorbed. The role for low supplements of T3 in patients with persistent fatigue, depression, or cognitive problems despite normalization of thyroid function tests is under investigation.

Parenteral L-T4 is indicated for myxedema (Figure 35-3) coma or severe life-threatening hypothyroidism, which is rare and occurs most often after an intervening illness. Glucocorticoids are also given in suspected cases because adrenal insufficiency commonly coexists with severe hypothyroidism.

In pregnancy, maternal thyroid requirements increase approximately 25%, and the increase in total T4 is accompanied by rising levels of thyroid-binding globulin (an effect of increased estrogen). Placental transfer of thyroid hormones is limited, and TSH does not cross the placenta. However, iodine and maternal antibodies readily cross the placenta. Recent studies suggest that maintaining euthyroidism in pregnancy is important for producing a normal intelligence quotient in offspring. Antithyroid drugs cross the placenta in limited amounts, but usually do not cause fetal hypothyroidism or goiter unless taken in large doses.

Subclinical hypothyroidism (an increased TSH level with normal T4 levels) is common, occurring in approximately 7.5% of women and approximately 3% of men. Treatment is controversial and usually not indicated. However, low doses of thyroid hormone can be given to normalize thyroid function tests and ascertain whether there is an improvement in symptoms.

The maintenance dose of L-T4 should be adjusted in primary hypothyroidism to normalize the TSH level. Because of T4's long half-life and the delayed decrease of chronically elevated TSH levels, dose adjustments are made no more often than every 5 to 6 weeks. It is important to avoid overtreatment because it is associated with accel-

Figure 35-3

Adult Myxedema
Clinical Manifestations and Etiology

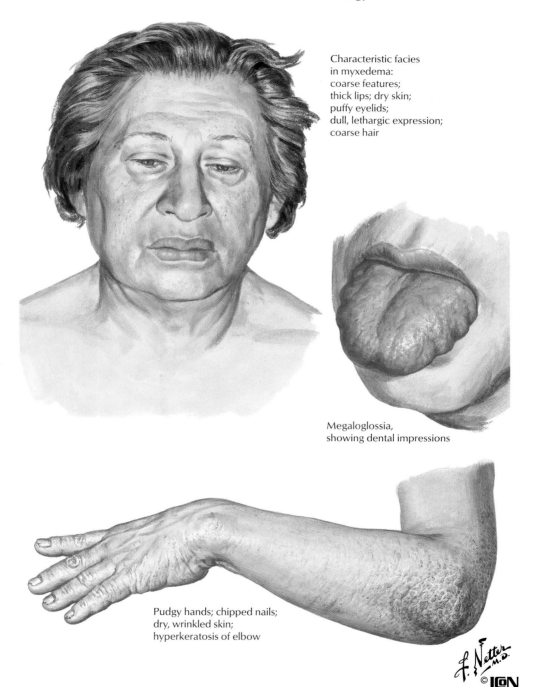

Characteristic facies
in myxedema:
coarse features;
thick lips; dry skin;
puffy eyelids;
dull, lethargic expression;
coarse hair

Megaloglossia,
showing dental impressions

Pudgy hands; chipped nails;
dry, wrinkled skin;
hyperkeratosis of elbow

erated loss of bone mass and a higher prevalence of arrhythmias.

In patients with secondary hypothyroidism, TSH is not regulated normally and cannot be used to adjust the dose. T4 or free T4 levels should be maintained within the normal range. If adrenal insufficiency is present, glucocorticoids should be administered before replacing thyroid hormone to avoid precipitating symptomatic adrenal crisis.

FUTURE DIRECTIONS

Further studies clarifying the role of combination L-T4/T3 therapy are forthcoming. Studies are also underway regarding the long-term outcome and appropriate treatment of patients with subclinical hypothyroidism. Prenatal screening of hypothyroidism will receive more attention given recent evidence of loss of cognitive ability in offspring of untreated mothers.

REFERENCES

Bunevicius R, Kazanavicius G, Zalinkevicius R, Prange AJ Jr. Effects of thyroxine as compared with thyroxine plus triiodothyronine in patients with hypothyroidism. *N Engl J Med.* 1999;340:424-429.

Hak AE, Pols HA, Visser TJ, Drexhage HA, Hofman A, Witteman JC. Subclinical hypothyroidism is an independent risk factor for atherosclerosis and myocardial infarction in elderly women: the Rotterdam Study. *Ann Intern Med.* 2000;132:270-278.

Lindsay RS, Toft AD. Hypothyroidism. *Lancet.* 1997;349:413-417.

Singer PA, Cooper DS, Levy EG, et al. Treatment guidelines for patients with hyperthyroidism and hypothyroidism. Standards of Care Committee, American Thyroid Association. *JAMA.* 1995;273:808-812.

Toft AD. Thyroxine therapy. *N Engl J Med.* 1994;331:174-180.

Chapter 36

Osteoporosis

David A. Ontjes

Osteoporosis is the most common bone disease and a major risk factor for fractures. In the United States, there are more than 1.5 million osteoporotic fractures each year with an annual cost of $15 billion in health care and disability expenses. The average 50-year-old white woman in the United States has a 50% chance of suffering at least one osteoporotic fracture during her remaining lifetime. With the aging of our population and the increased occurrence of osteoporosis in the elderly, the incidence of osteoporotic fractures could double over the next 30 years unless better methods for prevention and treatment are developed.

Osteoporosis is defined as low overall bone mass together with disruption of normal bone architecture, leading to fractures after minimal trauma. Histologically, there is an equivalent decrease in both bone mineral (composed of calcium and phosphorus) and bone matrix (composed of collagen and other bone proteins). The normal three-dimensional structure of trabecular bone is altered (Figure 36-1). In osteoporotic bone, there are fewer connecting bony spicules or "struts," and they are thinner than normal. Thus, both the radiologic density and mechanical strength of osteoporotic bone are diminished. The World Health Organization defines osteoporosis in terms of bone density measurements. Osteoporosis is present when the measured bone density is more than 2.5 standard deviations below the mean for a normal young individual. This amounts to a loss of 25% to 30% from normal peak bone mass. Osteopenia refers to a lesser degree of bone loss, in which the measured density is between 1.0 and 2.5 standard deviations below normal peak bone mass, leading to a loss of 10% to 25%.

Bone is a dynamic tissue in which new mineral is constantly being laid down, while previously mineralized sections are being resorbed (Figure 36-2). The cells governing the process are osteoblasts and osteoclasts. Osteoblasts are bone-forming cells derived from connective tissue stem cells that also give rise to fibroblasts. Mature osteoblasts synthesize collagen and other bone matrix proteins such as osteocalcin. They produce alkaline phosphatase, an enzyme that is believed to play a role in the mineralization process. Osteoclasts are the most important cells involved in bone resorption. They are derived from bone marrow stem cells and resemble macrophages. Mature osteoclasts are large, multinucleated cells located adjacent to mineralized bone surfaces. These cells contain lysosomes capable of releasing enzymes that can degrade bone matrix proteins.

ETIOLOGY AND PATHOGENESIS

A variety of inherited and acquired factors can predispose to low bone mass. Inherited or congenital risk factors include gender (female > male), race (White > African American), body build (thin with small frame), and family history. Acquired risk factors are age, a diet low in calcium and vitamin D, early menopause, a sedentary lifestyle, and cigarette smoking. Osteoporosis results when there is too much bone resorption, too little bone formation, or a combination of both. Estrogen deficiency associated with menopause in normal women is the most common cause of increased bone resorption. Accelerated bone loss continues for approximately 10 years after menopause, then the rate of decline subsides to the rate associated with normal aging. Estrogen replacement in the postmenopausal period reduces the rate of resorption and stabilizes bone mass. Men with hypogonadism have accelerated bone loss similar to that of postmenopausal women. Hyperparathyroidism and hyperthyroidism can also cause increased bone resorption.

Figure 36-1

Structure of Trabecular Bone

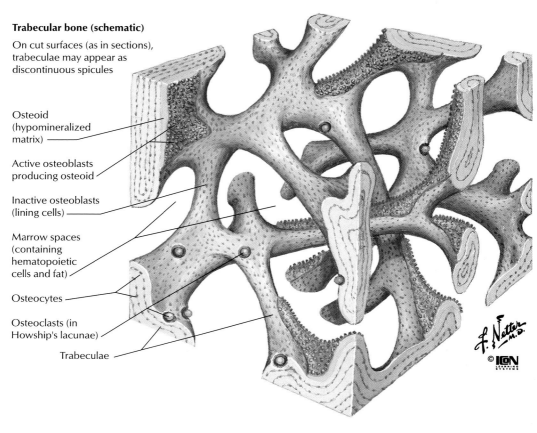

Trabecular bone (schematic)

On cut surfaces (as in sections), trabeculae may appear as discontinuous spicules

Osteoid (hypomineralized matrix)

Active osteoblasts producing osteoid

Inactive osteoblasts (lining cells)

Marrow spaces (containing hematopoietic cells and fat)

Osteocytes

Osteoclasts (in Howship's lacunae)

Trabeculae

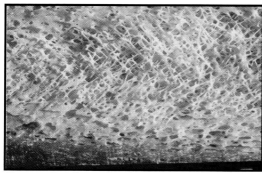

Cross section of cancellous bone (marrow elements removed). Trabecular bone in center; thin cortical bone at bottom

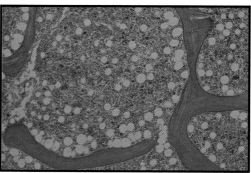

Photomicrograph of decalcified trabecular bone showing relationship of trabeculae to marrow. (Hematoxylin-eosin stain, x35)

Age-related bone loss affects both men and women and may be due in part to decreased dietary calcium absorption. In very elderly individuals, the rate of bone formation is often low. Exposure to certain drugs, such as glucocorticoids, and immobilization or lack of mechanical stress on bone itself can cause impaired bone formation.

Genetic factors play a major role in determining both the peak bone mass of young adults and the rate of bone loss in older individuals. In

Figure 36-2

Bone Remodeling

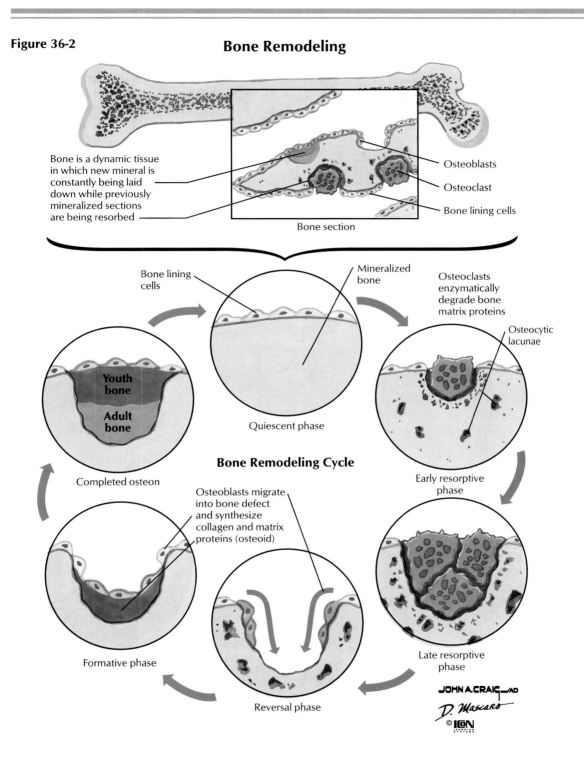

Bone is a dynamic tissue in which new mineral is constantly being laid down while previously mineralized sections are being resorbed

Osteoblasts

Osteoclast

Bone lining cells

Bone section

Bone lining cells

Mineralized bone

Osteoclasts enzymatically degrade bone matrix proteins

Osteocytic lacunae

Youth bone

Adult bone

Quiescent phase

Bone Remodeling Cycle

Completed osteon

Early resorptive phase

Osteoblasts migrate into bone defect and synthesize collagen and matrix proteins (osteoid)

Formative phase

Late resorptive phase

Reversal phase

JOHN A. CRAIG—MD

D. Mascaro

© ICN

population-based studies, natural variations (polymorphisms) in genes for the vitamin D receptor, the estrogen receptor, and for type 1 collagen matrix protein all appear to affect bone mass.

CLINICAL PRESENTATION

As bone is lost, there are no symptoms until fractures occur, typically with minimal trauma. Compression fractures of the vertebra are most common, followed by fractures of the proximal femur and the distal radius (Colles' fracture). As a result of vertebral compression with anterior wedging, patients will lose height and develop a kyphosis deformity of the spine (Figure 36-3). Patients who have experienced vertebral compression fractures often have chronic back pain. Proximal femur (hip) fractures are the most disabling, often leading to immobilization and a loss of independent living in elderly men and women. Because the entire skeleton is fragile, fractures are more likely to occur at other sites as well, including the pelvis, ribs, and long bones.

DIFFERENTIAL DIAGNOSIS

Other metabolic bone diseases that can cause structural weakness of bone include osteomalacia and osteitis fibrosa. Osteomalacia occurs when bone mineral fails to be deposited in normally formed bone matrix. Rickets in children is the equivalent of osteomalacia in adults. Osteitis fibrosa is due to high circulating levels of parathyroid hormone, causing increased bone resorption.

Several specific diseases can cause secondary bone loss and should be considered in the differential diagnosis of any patient presenting with low bone mass. It is important to identify these conditions, since appropriate treatment of the primary problem can often lead to improvement in bone mass as well. (Table 36-1)

DIAGNOSTIC APPROACH

Plain radiographs of bone can show several types of abnormalities that suggest osteoporosis or another metabolic bone disease. The most common finding is nonspecific osteopenia, or reduced radiographic density. With more advanced disease, deformities or fractures may occur. In early disease, standard radiographs may appear normal. At least 30% of total bone mass must be lost before abnormalities in density are

Table 36-1
Causes of Secondary Osteoporosis

Endocrine Diseases	Gastrointestinal Diseases
Hyperparathyroidism	Gastrectomy
Thyrotoxicosis	Malabsorption syndromes (sprue)
Hypogonadism	Chronic biliary obstruction
Hyperprolactinemia	
Glucocorticoid excess (Cushing's syndrome)	Genetic abnormalities of collagen synthesis
	Ehlers-Danlos syndrome
Malignant Diseases Myeloma Leukemia Lymphoma	Osteogenesis imperfecta Prolonged immobilization Bed rest Cast application to limb
Drugs Heparin Ethanol Glucocorticoids	

detectable by plain radiographs (Figure 36-4). Quantitative measurement of bone density is the primary means of diagnosing osteoporosis, using World Health Organization standards. The most widely used method for measuring bone mass is dual-energy x-ray absorptiometry, which uses x-ray beams of two different energy levels. Tissues of differing densities (bone and soft tissue) conduct the beams differently, allowing specific densities to be calculated. Quantitative bone density measurements are used to document the presence of osteopenia or osteoporosis and to predict the risk of fracture. A decline of one standard deviation below young normal bone density implies a doubling of fracture risk. The risk doubles again for each standard deviation decline.

Routine laboratory evaluation is limited and used to rule out causes of secondary osteoporosis. Serum creatinine, calcium, phosphorus, alkaline phosphatase, and TSH, as well as CBC, should be obtained in most patients. Patients with elevated serum calcium should have a measurement of serum PTH. Those at clinical risk for vita-

Figure 36-3

Clinical Manifestations of Osteoporosis

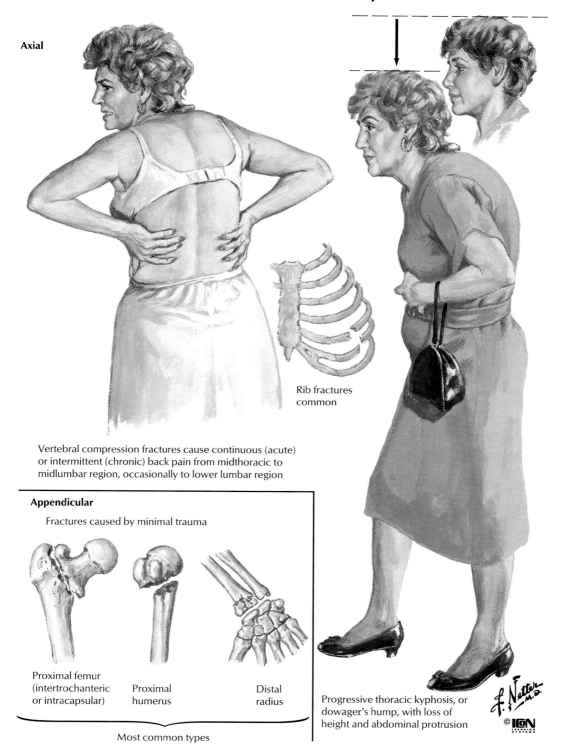

Axial

Rib fractures common

Vertebral compression fractures cause continuous (acute) or intermittent (chronic) back pain from midthoracic to midlumbar region, occasionally to lower lumbar region

Appendicular

Fractures caused by minimal trauma

Proximal femur (intertrochanteric or intracapsular)

Proximal humerus

Distal radius

Most common types

Progressive thoracic kyphosis, or dowager's hump, with loss of height and abdominal protrusion

Figure 36-4   Radiographic Findings in Axial Osteoporosis

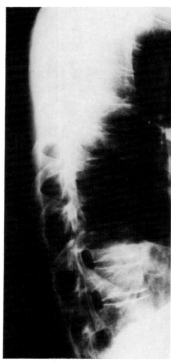

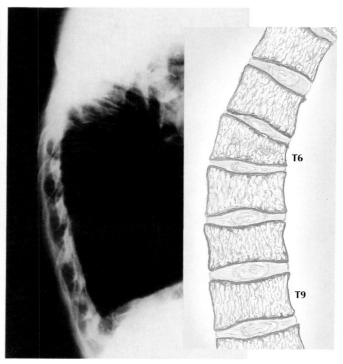

Mild osteopenia in post-
menopausal woman. Vertebrae
appear "washed-out"; no
kyphosis or vertebral collapse

Anterior wedge compression at T6 in same patient 16$^{1}/_{2}$ years later. Patient
has lymphoma, with multiple biconcave ("codfish") vertebral bodies and
kyphosis. Focal lesion at T6 suggests neoplasm

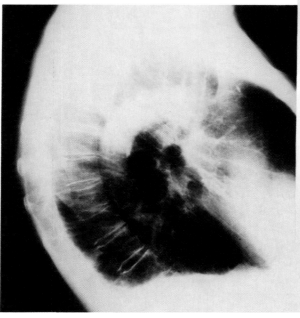

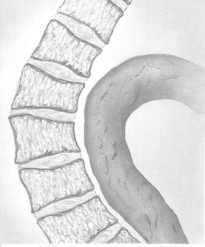

Severe kyphosis in postmenopausal
woman. Mild, multiple biconcavity and
wedging of vertebrae. Extensive
calcification of aorta

Table 36-2
Calcium Requirements for Optimal Bone Health

Children and Adolescents	Daily Calcium (mg)
1–3 years	500
4–8 years	800
9–18 years	1,300

Women and Men	
19–50 years	1,000
>50 years	1,200

Pregnant and Lactating Women	
15–18 years	1,300
19–50 years	1,000

min D deficiency, especially homebound or institutionalized individuals, should have a measurement of 25-hydroxyvitamin D.

MANAGEMENT AND THERAPY
Prevention

Osteoporosis is better prevented than cured. The health habits of individuals in early and middle life play a role in their risk of osteoporosis in later life. Adequate dietary intake of calcium and vitamin D, active physical exercise, and avoidance of excessive alcohol, tobacco, and drugs known to cause osteopenia are all useful measures for the prevention of osteoporosis.

The recommended daily allowance of vitamin D for most healthy individuals is 400 IU, but for the elderly, 800 IU is preferred. Recommended allowances for calcium are shown in Table 36-2.

Drug Therapy

The objectives of therapy include prevention of further excessive bone loss, promotion of bone formation, prevention of fractures, reduction or elimination of pain, and restoration of physical function. All of the agents listed below have been shown to improve bone density and to reduce the incidence of fractures in clinical trials. All are "anti-resorptive" agents, acting to reduce rates of bone resorption, rather than to stimulate bone formation. Estrogens are commonly used to relieve menopausal symptoms in postmeno-

pausal women, whether osteoporosis is present or not. With recent reports questioning routine hormone replacement therapy in postmenopausal women, the future role of estrogen therapy for prevention of osteoporosis will certainly need to be examined. Other anti-osteoporosis drugs are indicated for use in patients having either documented osteoporotic fractures or bone densities at least two standard deviations below normal young adult levels.

Estrogen replacement in postmenopausal women prevents the excessive bone loss due to estrogen deficiency. Estrogens should be given with a progestin in women who have an intact uterus to avoid the increased risk of endometrial cancer. Orally administered estrogens have a beneficial effect on the serum lipid profile and adversely affect the risk of venous blood clots in susceptible individuals. Clinical trials have shown that estradiol administered transdermally is also beneficial in postmenopausal osteoporosis.

Selective estrogen receptor modulators (SERMs) are synthetic analogs of estrogen that have some of the biological effects of natural estrogen, but lack other effects. Drugs in this class include tamoxifen, a drug used to treat breast cancer, and raloxifene, a drug approved for the treatment of osteoporosis. Raloxifene acts as an estrogen agonist with respect to bone and lipoprotein metabolism. It increases bone density and lowers serum cholesterol when given to postmenopausal women. Raloxifene does not stimulate the endometrium, and like tamoxifen it acts as an estrogen antagonist in breast tissue. Thus, raloxifene is a good choice as an anti–osteoporosis drug in women at high risk of breast cancer.

Bisphosphonates are a family of compounds that resemble pyrophosphate and are incorporated into the mineral structure of bone. There they inhibit bone resorption and promote increased bone mass. Clinical trials of several bisphosphonates, including etidronate, alendronate, and risedronate indicate that bone density is increased in postmenopausal women after 2 or more years of treatment. Further trials with alendronate, and risedronate provide strong evidence that these drugs can reduce fracture risk by 40% to 60% at various skeletal sites, including the spine and hip. These drugs are effective in men as well as women. Alendronate and risedronate are the only bisphosphonates currently approved in the United States for treatment of osteoporosis, but other drugs of this class are likely to be approved in the near future.

Calcitonin is a peptide hormone produced in small quantities by the parafollicular cells of the normal thyroid gland. The administration of synthetic human or salmon calcitonin in patients with osteoporosis causes a reduction in bone resorption and a modest increase in bone density. Clinical trials have found that intranasal calcitonin therapy reduces the occurrence of vertebral fractures in postmenopausal women. Large doses of calcitonin may have an analgesic effect through an independent action on the central nervous system.

FUTURE DIRECTIONS

Improved public knowledge about dietary and lifestyle issues affecting risk may offer the greatest promise for avoiding a growing epidemic of osteoporotic fractures. Wider availability of inexpensive and portable instruments for screening for low bone density should allow earlier recognition of high-risk individuals. Finally, new therapeutic strategies involving drugs that promote active bone formation are being developed. Among the agents being investigated are low-dose parathyroid hormone, growth hormone, and insulin-like growth factor 1. Large clinical trials with PTH, in particular, have shown impressive increases in bone density and a reduction in the incidence of fractures. The combination of anti-resorptive drugs, such as bisphosphonates, and bone-forming drugs, such as PTH, may provide even greater efficacy.

REFERENCES

Hochberg M. Preventing fractures in postmenopausal women with osteoporosis. A review of recent controlled trials of antiresorptive agents. *Drugs Aging.* 2000;17:317-330.

Raisz LG, Kream BE, Lorenzo JA. Metabolic bone disease. In: Larsen PR, Kronenberg HM, Melmed S, Polonsky KS, eds. *Williams Textbook of Endocrinology.* 10th ed. Philadelphia, Pa: WB Saunders Co; 2002.

Rodan GA, Martin TJ. Therapeutic approaches to bone diseases. *Science.* 2000;289:1508-1514.

Rosen CJ, Bilezikian JP. Clinical review 123: Anabolic therapy for osteoporosis. *J Clin Endocrinol Metab.* 2001; 86: 957-964.

Ross PD. Osteoporosis. Frequency, consequences, and risk factors. *Arch Intern Med.* 1996;156:1399-1411.

Shoback D, Marcus R, Bikle D, Strewler G. Mineral metabolism & metabolic bone diseases. In: Greenspan FS, Gardner DG, eds. *Basic & Clinical Endocrinology.* 6th ed. Los Altos, Calif: Lange Medical Publications; 2001:273-333.

Chapter 37

Paget's Disease of Bone

Sue A. Brown

Paget's disease of bone, also known as osteitis deformans, is a disorder of accelerated bone turnover. It is characterized by abnormal osteoclast activity which results in increased bone breakdown. Because bone formation and resorption are coupled, there is a concomitant increase in bone formation. However, the new bone that is laid down is abnormal in its organization. Bone biopsy specimens demonstrate loss of the usual lamellar structure that is important for bone strength. As a result, the bone is weakened with an abnormal bone remodeling surface.

The incidence of Paget's disease is difficult to estimate because the disease is largely asymptomatic. Autopsy and radiological series have found the incidence to be 3% to 3.7% of patients older than 55 years. Overall, it appears to be a disease of individuals of Anglo-Saxon descent and is much less common in Asian individuals. Nearly all individuals present at a later age, usually older than 40 years. Some series report a male predominance, while others suggest that males are equally as affected as females.

ETIOLOGY AND PATHOGENESIS

The exact etiology is unknown. Microscopically, osteoclasts are structurally abnormal, of increased size, and found in increased number. They have multinucleated structures with inclusion bodies similar to nucleocapsids found in paramyxoviruses such as measles, respiratory syncytial virus, and canine distemper virus. It has been postulated, but not definitively proven, that Paget's disease results from a viral infection. The involved osteoclasts appear to have an increased sensitivity to substances that alter osteoclast activity such as 1,25 dihydroxyvitamin D (calcitriol) and RANK-ligand, an important signaling protein secreted by osteoblasts to control osteoclast activity (Figure 37-1).

Paget's disease may also have a genetic predisposition. It has been reported that 12% to 25% of patients have an affected first-degree relative. The putative genetic abnormality has not been defined. A susceptibility gene on the long arm of chromosome 18 has recently been identified in at least one study. This was discovered after an abnormality at a different location on the same chromosome was identified in familial expansile osteolysis, a rare disorder in which osteoclasts also have paramyxoviral-like inclusions. Possibly, viral infection initiates abnormal osteoclast activity and the onset of Paget's disease in individuals with a genetic susceptibility.

CLINICAL PRESENTATION

Most individuals with Paget's disease of bone are asymptomatic. Often, it is incidentally diagnosed after serum alkaline phosphatase levels are obtained or plain radiographs are performed for unrelated reasons. It predominantly affects the calvarium and axial skeleton, most often involving vertebral bodies, pelvis, and long bones. It can occur in a monostotic form with a single site affected. However, the majority of individuals have polyostotic disease with multiple sites involved (Figure 37-2). Only 5% of individuals present with bone pain often described as a dull or persistent ache exacerbated by activity. However, pain is not a good indicator of extent of disease. In one study, only 30% of 863 sites of disease caused symptoms in 170 patients. Bone pain may result from irritation of the periosteum, increased vascularity in affected bone, or mechanical stress with microfractures. There may be warmth at the site of involvement with Paget's disease. Pain may be due to joint dysfunction rather than Pagetic involvement of the bone itself. Pain in or near a joint may reflect underlying osteoarthritic changes such as osteophyte formation due to the presence of Paget's disease in the adjoining long bone, which may deteriorate cartilage and alter the joint surface. Significant joint

Figure 37-1

Pathophysiology and Treatment of Paget's Disease of Bone

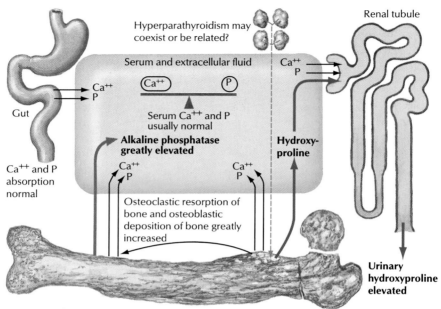

Hyperparathyroidism may coexist or be related?

Renal tubule

Serum and extracellular fluid

Ca^{++}
P

Ca^{++} ⬚ P ⬚

Serum Ca^{++} and P usually normal

Gut

Ca^{++}
P

Ca^{++} and P absorption normal

Alkaline phosphatase greatly elevated

Ca^{++}
P

Ca^{++}
P

Hydroxy-proline

Osteoclastic resorption of bone and osteoblastic deposition of bone greatly increased

Urinary hydroxyproline elevated

Abnormal bone structure, coarse trabeculation, thickening, bowing, pseudofractures, fractures, hypervascularity

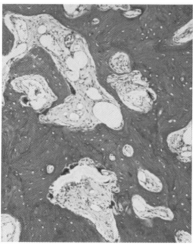

Section of bone shows intense osteoclastic and osteoblastic activity and mosaic of lamellar bone

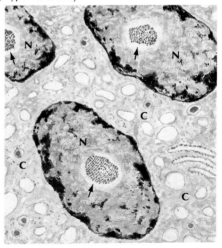

Electron-microscopic view of multinucleated osteoclast with nuclear inclusions that may be viruses (arrows). N = nuclei; C = cytoplasm

Figure 37-2

Paget's Disease of Bone

Manifestations of advanced, diffuse Paget's disease of bone (may occur singly or in combination)

Enlarged head, headache

Deafness due to compression of nerve in bony meatus

Increased cardiac output due to great bone vascularity (may progress to high-output failure)

Kyphosis

Bone pain, most commonly in back or hips; radicular pain with spine involvement

Bowing of limbs

Increased warmth and tenderness over bones; increased limb volume

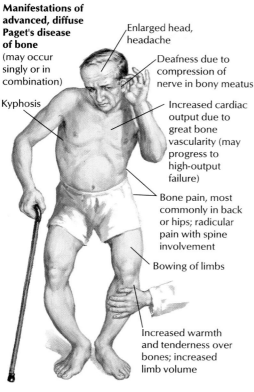

Mild cases often asymptomatic (may be discovered incidentally on radiographs taken for other reasons)

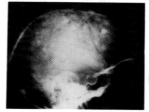

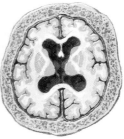

Lateral radiograph shows patchy density of skull, with areas of osteopenia (osteoporosis circumscripta cranii)

Extremely thickened skull bones, which may encroach on nerve foramina or brainstem and cause hydrocephalus (shown) by compressing cerebral aqueduct

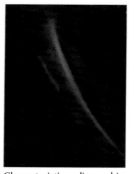

Characteristic radiographic findings in tibia include thickening, bowing, and coarse trabeculation, with advancing radiolucent wedge

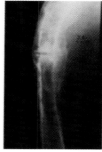

Healing chalk-stick fracture

deformities can occur with bowing of the lower extremities as well as abnormal facial structures such as frontal bossing. Fractures are a common complication in weight-bearing bones as a result of disorganized bone structure. Neurological compromise is a concerning complication. Involvement of the vertebral column can result in spinal cord or peripheral nerve root compression. Cranial nerves, particularly ocular and auditory nerves, can be affected due to skull deformities. Hearing loss has been reported in up to 37% of individuals and may also be due to acquired bony abnormalities in the cochlea. Rarely, hydrocephalus occurs due to deformities at the skull base. With active, widespread disease, high-output congestive heart failure may develop due to increased vascularity of the bone remodeling surface. A rare but dreaded complication is the development of osteosarcoma, which is estimated to occur in less than 1% of patients with long-standing disease.

DIFFERENTIAL DIAGNOSIS

Other conditions that can present with bone pain, lytic lesions, and elevated alkaline phosphatase levels include malignancies, primary or metastatic disease, and infiltrative diseases such as infections and sarcoidosis. With widespread involvement, it can be difficult to distinguish Paget's disease from an underlying malignancy. Usually, the underlying malignancy is more obvious on clinical examination and the bone metastases are a later complication. Paget's disease is much more likely if previous radiographs demonstrate relative stability of the lesions over time. A distinguishing radiological feature of Paget's disease is the increase in the diameter of affected bones, which remains unchanged in infiltrating or metastatic diseases. An isolated Pagetic focus in the vertebral body may resemble vertebral hemangiomas or compression fractures. Unfortunately, bone scans do not distinguish among these conditions. Biochemical findings, such as anemia, hypoalbuminemia, or hypercalcemia, may suggest other underlying disorders. Paget's disease may cause hypercalcemia but only with prolonged immobilization or recent fracture. Although characteristic radiographical features exist, the diagnosis of Paget's disease is not always clear, and a search for an underlying malignancy or other disorder may need to be pursued, including obtaining a bone biopsy specimen in some instances.

DIAGNOSTIC APPROACH

A diagnosis of Paget's disease is often made based on characteristic findings on plain radiographs. Early in the disease, lytic lesions predominate, reflecting increased areas of osteoclast resorption. They are characterized by flame or V-shaped resorption fronts on long bones, or isolated lytic lesions in the skull (also known as osteoporosis circumscripta). As the disease progresses, cortical thickening and sclerotic areas develop due to excessive bone formation from increased osteoblast activity. Bone scans demonstrate increased activity at the involved sites. The extent of the disease varies among individuals. Radiologic identification of sites of involvement is important to document the extent of the disease and to identify asymptomatic lesions located in fracture-prone sites that may require treatment. Although the disease may progress with advancing resorption fronts in a particular bone, there is usually not extensive spread to new bones after the initial diagnosis is made.

On laboratory examination, a significantly elevated alkaline phosphatase level occurs in approximately 95% of individuals. Baseline values are often greater than 3 times the upper limit of normal. However, monostotic or isolated Paget's disease may have a normal alkaline phosphatase level. The sensitivity of bone-specific alkaline phosphatase is slightly better than that of total alkaline phosphatase. The level of alkaline phosphatase usually correlates with disease activity if followed over time in a single individual. Serum levels of calcium, phosphate, parathyroid hormone, and vitamin D metabolites are usually normal. Hypercalcemia only occurs when the rates of bone formation decrease while the rate of bone resorption remains high, such as during prolonged immobilization or recent fracture. Bone turnover markers or collagen breakdown products, such as urinary N-telopeptides and deoxypyridinoline, are consistently elevated in active, extensive Paget's disease. However, these markers are not specific and have wide intrinsic variability, making their use difficult in treatment of patients. Other markers of osteoblast function, such as osteocalcin, are not helpful in the diagnosis or management of Paget's disease.

MANAGEMENT AND THERAPY

Treatment of Paget's disease has dramatically improved since the availability of potent oral bisphosphonates. Multiple studies have demonstrated an improvement in symptoms, notably bone pain, and a reduction in alkaline phosphatase and other bone turnover markers. Bisphosphonates have been shown to restore normal bone structure on bone biopsy specimens. However, there are no prospective long-term data that demonstrate prevention of future complications after treatment is initiated. Mild disease with isolated involvement in a location unlikely to cause complications, such as the scapula or pelvis, may not need to be treated. Short-term treatment with bisphosphonates or calcitonin may be indicated before orthopedic procedures to prevent excessive blood loss due to the hypervascularity of bone. The most common indications for therapy are bone pain, involvement of fracture-prone sites (weight-bearing bones, vertebral bodies), periarticular bone lesions, extensive skull involvement, prior orthopedic procedures, and prolonged immobilization.

Bisphosphonates are pyrophosphate analogs that decrease bone resorption rates by decreasing osteoclast activity and make the hydroxyapatite structure of the bone matrix less susceptible to resorption. Several preparations are available and are generally given in 3- to 6-month cycles every 1 to 2 years or 1 to 2 months before elective surgery. Etidronate, the initial drug available, is less potent than newer agents and has been associated with osteomalacia when used at higher doses. Alendronate and risedronate, potent oral bisphosphonates, are FDA approved for the treatment of Paget's disease (40 mg orally once daily and 30 mg orally once daily, respectively). One randomized controlled clinical trial of 89 patients comparing alendronate (40 mg once daily) and etidronate (400 mg once daily) for 6 months demonstrated a normalization of alkaline phosphatase in 63% of patients on alendronate compared to only 17% on etidronate. There were significant decreases in urinary bone turnover markers as well as improvements in pain and functional scores on alendronate. A follow-up extension study showed that 52% still had normal alkaline phosphatase levels 25 to 30 months after treatment ended. Radiographic evidence of improvement has varied with some studies demonstrating regression of bone resorption fronts while others have not shown a significant change. Similar improvements in bone turnover markers are seen with either risedronate or alendronate. Pamidronate is highly effective but must be given in IV form. Dosing has varied from 60 mg given as a single infusion for mild disease to 20 to 60 mg given IV every 3 to 6 months.

Calcitonin is FDA-approved in both salmon and human subcutaneous forms for the treatment of Paget's disease. However, bisphosphonates have superior efficacy in inducing and maintaining a remission, which has relegated calcitonin to second-line therapy if bisphosphonates are not tolerated. Calcitonin has a role in perioperative management because it is fast-acting and effective for decreasing blood loss during surgery. Other treatment options have included gallium and plicamycin, although they are rarely used today. Often, analgesics and joint replacement surgery need to be considered to treat the associated osteoarthritic changes.

The general goal of treatment is to normalize alkaline phosphatase levels and decrease pain. Serum levels are often measured every 4 to 6 months. An additional treatment course should be considered when the alkaline phosphatase level has increased more than 25% of that achieved after the initial treatment. Bone turnover markers, such as urinary N-telopeptides, may respond earlier than alkaline phosphatase to bisphosphonate therapy. A single 3- to 6-month course of a bisphosphonate can induce a remission for 1 to 2 years or longer. Plain radiographs show changes over time, but they do not always correlate with alkaline phosphatase levels or symptomatic improvement. Bone scans are more reliable for following changes, although radiation exposure and expense limit their use. Although uncontrolled studies suggest there are decreased fracture rates, there is no solid proof that treating individuals will prevent future complications.

FUTURE DIRECTIONS

Individuals can become less responsive to a single bisphosphonate after successive treatment courses. At least one study suggests, however, that these patients may retain responsiveness when changed to a different bisphosphonate. Combination therapy may prove to be a more effective strategy in the future. Newer, more potent bisphosphonates continue to be developed and may prove even more efficacious for the treatment of Paget's disease of bone.

REFERENCES

Delmas PD, Meunier PJ. The management of Paget's disease of bone. *N Engl J Med.* 1997;336:558-566.

Gutteridge DH, Ward LC, Stewart GO, et al. Paget's disease: acquired resistance to one aminobisphosphonate with retained response to another. *J Bone Miner Res.* 1999; 14(suppl 2):79-84.

Hosking D, Meunier PJ, Ringe JD, Reginster JY, Gennari C. Paget's disease of bone: diagnosis and management. BMJ. 1996;312:491-494.

Siris E, Weinstein RS, Altman R, et al. Comparative study of alendronate versus etidronate for the treatment of Paget's disease of bone. *J Clin Endocrinol Metab.* 1996;81:961-967.

Siris ES. Goals and treatment for Paget's disease of bone. *J Bone Miner Res.* 1999;14(suppl 2):49-52.

Chapter 38
Pituitary Diseases

David R. Clemmons

The anterior lobe of the pituitary gland produces six polypeptide hormones that regulate the function of other endocrine glands, such as the thyroid and the adrenal glands. The posterior lobe produces hormones that are involved in regulation of salt and water balance. Because of its strategic location, tumors that occur within the sella turcica, the cavernous sinuses, or in the hypothalamus can lead to disruption of pituitary hormonal function. From a functional perspective, diseases of the pituitary are grouped into those that destroy or impair hormone function and those that result in increased hormone secretion.

ETIOLOGY AND PATHOGENESIS
Normal Pituitary Anatomy and Physiology

The pituitary gland is encased within the sphenoid bone at the base of the brain and is connected directly to the hypothalamus. The hypothalamus contains specific neurons that, following electrochemical stimulation, release peptides termed releasing factors. The releasing factors that have been identified include growth hormone–releasing factor (GHRH); gonadotropin-releasing hormone (GRH), which stimulates both luteinizing hormone (LH) and follicle-stimulating hormone (FSH) secretion; thyrotropin-releasing hormone (TRH); and corticotropin-releasing factor (CRF). Prolactin secretion is negatively regulated by dopamine that is released from hypothalamic neurons. Following direct stimulation, hypothalamic neurons release these polypeptides into the hypophyseal portal vessels where they are transported to the anterior pituitary cells. Each releasing factor stimulates the synthesis and release of the appropriate trophic hormone by a specific pituitary cell type into the general circulation.

Each pituitary hormone acts at specific sites to produce its target effects. Growth hormone (GH) acts upon connective tissue cells to stimulate the synthesis of insulin-like growth factor-I (IGF-I). IGF-I stimulates trophic actions related to growth, including protein synthesis, inhibition of protein breakdown, and growth of connective tissue cell types such as bone, muscle, and cartilage. GH is necessary for normal statural growth, and for maintenance of normal muscle and bone mass in adults. GH has several important metabolic functions, including stimulation of lipolysis resulting in release of free fatty acids that are used as an energy source in maintaining normal glucose homeostasis and fat stores. GH also stimulates amino acid flux in muscle and contributes to the normal balance between bone formation and absorption. Prolactin acts primarily on the breast to stimulate milk production in the postpartum period. It antagonizes the effects of estrogen, and supraphysiologic concentrations impair normal fertility and estrogen action. Thyroid-stimulating hormone (TSH) acts directly upon the thyroid gland to increase the synthesis and secretion of both T3 and T4. Adrenocorticotropic hormone (ACTH) has a similar effect on the adrenal gland, stimulating the conversion of cholesterol to various adrenal steroids, the most important of which is cortisol. Both LH and FSH act in concert to stimulate gonadal function in males and females. FSH in males is primarily a stimulator of spermatogenesis and Sertoli cell function and LH functions primarily to stimulate testosterone biosynthesis by the Leydig cells. In females, FSH stimulates follicle maturation while LH is primarily responsible for stimulation of corpus luteal function.

Negative Feedback Regulation

All hormones produced by target cell types are secreted into the general circulation. They feed back on the normal pituitary gland and suppress trophic hormone secretion. For example, IGF-I feeds back directly on the somatotropes to inhibit GH release, T4 inhibits TSH production, cortisol inhibits ACTH secretion, and testosterone in men and estrogen in women inhibit LH and FSH release.

Regulation of posterior pituitary hormone secretion is quite different. The hypothalamus maintains direct neural connections to the posterior pituitary gland through axonal processes. Following their synthesis in the hypothalamic neurons, these small peptides are transported down axonal processes and stored in secretory granules within the posterior pituitary gland. Neural inputs regulate the release of vasopressin, which acts directly on the kidney to control free water clearance. Similarly, under the appropriate stimulus, the brain releases oxytocin, which stimulates uterine contractions. Suckling results in loss of dopaminergic inhibition of prolactin secretion with a direct reduction in dopamine levels. Lesions that sever the stalk while causing a major loss of stimulation of anterior pituitary hormone synthesis may not cause a complete ablation of posterior pituitary hormone synthesis because these hormones may be released by the severed neurons directly after hypothalamic stimulation. This type of lesion will increase prolactin secretion due to loss of dopamine inhibition.

A number of disease processes — tumors, other destructive lesions, vascular insults — interrupt the delicate balance of the hypothalamic/pituitary axis. A discussion of a selected group of disorders follows.

CLINICAL PRESENTATION, DIFFERENTIAL DIAGNOSIS, DIAGNOSTIC APPROACH, MANAGEMENT, AND THERAPY
Diseases of the Anterior Pituitary Gland

Most cases of anterior pituitary gland dysfunction are caused by tumors (Figure 38-1). Usually benign, these tumors disrupt normal pituitary gland function because of their anatomic location. Functionally, tumors are grouped into mass lesions that result in destruction of pituitary hormone secretion and those that result in adenomatous expansion of the specific cell type that produces a single hormone resulting in a hormonal overproduction syndrome.

Mass lesions that can result in pituitary cell destruction and hypofunction include cysts, such as Rathke cleft cyst, arachnoid, dermoid; tumors, such as craniopharyngioma, chordoma, glioma, sarcoma, hamartoma, dysgerminoma, metastases, hormone-secreting or nonfunctional pituitary adenomas; and miscellaneous causes, such as aneurysms, hypophysitis, sarcoidosis, histiocytosis-x, and Sheehan's syndrome.

Usually, tumors destroy multiple cell types. Mass lesions that result in pituitary dysfunction can be divided into three groups: those that arise within the sella turcica; those within the parasellar areas; and those within the hypothalamus. Hypothalamic tumors can cause anterior pituitary dysfunction by destroying hypothalamic-releasing factor production and usually not through expansion within the sella turcica. Chromophobe adenomas arise within the sella turcica, often secreting only the alpha subunit of the LH or FSH; therefore, they are hormonally silent. These tumors grow slowly and may destroy the entire anterior/pituitary gland by pressure necrosis. Extensive proliferation can lead to invasion into the cavernous sinus, or if they extend superiorly, they exert pressure on the optic chiasm leading to bitemporal heminopsia.

Other lesions that arise within the pituitary gland include cystic lesions that develop from partial infarction of preexisting pituitary tumors, and granulomatous diseases such as histiocytosis X or sarcoidosis. Hamartomas also occur within the region of the sella turcica, resulting in hypopituitarism. Sheehan's syndrome, a postpartum pituitary infarction due to massive blood loss at delivery that results in panhypopituitarism, is one of the most common circulatory diseases involving the pituitary gland. Carotid artery aneurysms can destroy the pituitary gland. Parasella and hypothalamic lesions that may produce hormonal dysfunction include meningiomas and craniopharyngiomas. These tumors, which often arise in the hypothalamus, result in disruption of hypothalamic hormone production. Dysgerminomas of the third ventricle can result in hypothalamic dysfunction.

Iatrogenic Causes of Hypopituitarism

Surgery for intrasellar or parasellar lesions can inadvertently result in destruction of the normal pituitary gland by damage to the hypothalamic neurons, stalk section, or direct damage to the anterior pituitary gland. Radiation treatment for pituitary tumors often results in destruction of the normal pituitary gland. Radiation for diseases such as gliomas, CNS leukemia or lymphoma, or for head and neck tumors can produce sufficient scatter radiation to destroy anterior pituitary gland function.

Figure 38-1 **Pituitary Anterior Lobe Deficiency in the Adult**

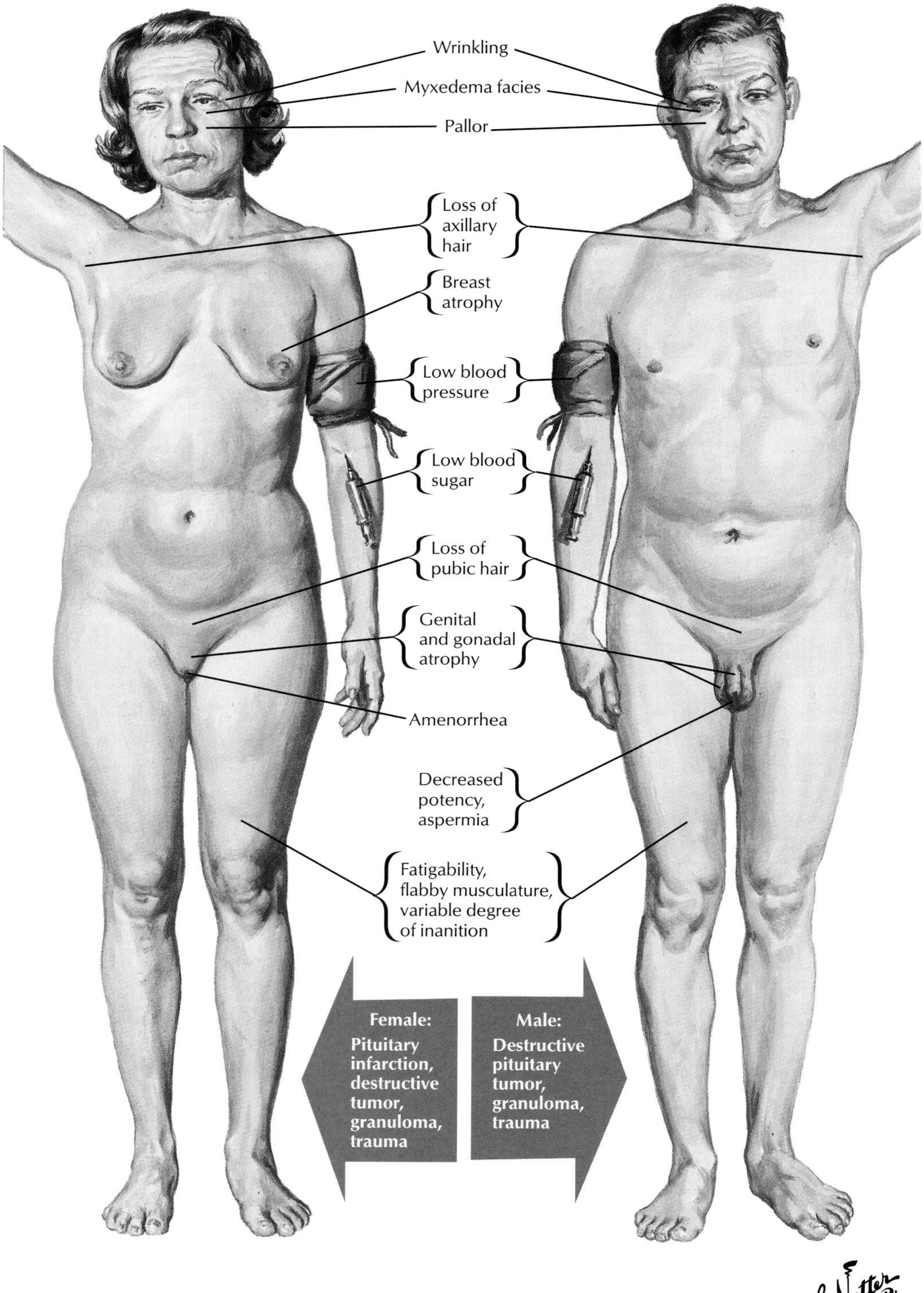
Wrinkling
Myxedema facies
Pallor
Loss of axillary hair
Breast atrophy
Low blood pressure
Low blood sugar
Loss of pubic hair
Genital and gonadal atrophy
Amenorrhea
Decreased potency, aspermia
Fatigability, flabby musculature, variable degree of inanition
Female: Pituitary infarction, destructive tumor, granuloma, trauma
Male: Destructive pituitary tumor, granuloma, trauma
F. Netter M.D.
© ICON LEARNING SYSTEMS

Consequences of Loss of Hormonal Function

Large mass lesions of the pituitary gland and/or hypothalamic region can result in complete anterior pituitary hormone destruction (Figure 38-1). Generally, the first hormone to be lost is GH followed by LH/FSH, followed by ACTH and TSH and, lastly, prolactin. Loss of normal GH secretion in children can result in significant growth failure and hypoglycemia as well as an increase in body fat and loss of normal muscle mass. In adults, GH deficiency is more likely to lead to changes in body composition with loss of muscle and bone mass. Hypoglycemia in adults is rare. Loss of gonadotrophin secretion in women results in anovulation first followed by amenorrhea and loss of secondary sexual characteristics. In men, loss of gonadotrophin secretion is associated with impotence, decreased testicular size, and a loss of male secondary sexual characteristics. Loss of TSH secretion results in secondary hypothyroidism. The symptoms, dry skin, constipation, cold intolerance, weight gain and loss of energy with increased fatigability, are similar to those of primary hypothyroidism. Loss of ACTH secretion leads to secondary hypoadrenalism with weight loss, loss of appetite, early satiety, nausea, extreme weakness and lassitude, and inability to mount a normal stress response with resulting circulatory collapse if the deficiency is severe. Unlike primary adrenal insufficiency, mineralocorticoid secretion remains nearly normal; therefore, severe disturbances of sodium and water balance are less common, although hyponatremia occurs due to the loss of direct effect of cortisol on free water clearance.

The loss of prolactin secretion due to diseases such as Sheehan's syndrome results in failure of postpartum lactation. Symptoms of antidiuretic hormone (ADH) deficiency include polyuria, polydipsia, postural hypotension, and hyperosmolarity. Patients with large tumors can present with symptoms due to the mass lesion, including visual field loss, diplopia, and headaches. The physical signs depend on which hormonal deficits have occurred. Patients with panhypopituitarism often present with dry thin skin, increased truncal fat, decreased muscle mass, loss of pubic and axillary hair, and deep tendon reflexes showing delayed relaxation phase. Ancillary laboratory abnormalities that may occur include anemia, hyponatremia (low cortisol), hypernatremia, hyposmolarity (ADH deficiency), and hypoglycemia (low GH). Usually the diagnosis of panhypopituitarism or of partial loss of pituitary hormone secretion is confirmed by stimulation tests (Table 38-1). When a hormonal deficit has been confirmed, an MRI of the sella turcica and parasellar region can determine if a mass lesion is present. Treatment usually includes removal of the tumor and institution of hormone replacement therapy. Thyroid hormone and cortisol are replaced orally, and gonadal steroids are replaced either orally (estrogen and progesterone), transdermally, or by injection. Growth hormone can be replaced only by injection. ADH is replaced orally or intranasally.

Pituitary Dysfunction Due to Hypersecretion of Specific Hormones

Adenoma formation with subsequent expansion of somatotropes, thyrotropes, gonadatropes, or lactrotropes results in hypersecretion of each of these hormones (Figures 38-2, 38-3, and 38-4). The most common disorder is prolactin hypersecretion, which accounts for more than 50% of pituitary adenomas followed by growth hormone and ACTH hypersecretion. TSH or gonadotropin hypersecretion are rare. The etiology of these tumors in most cases is unknown; however, they represent clonal expansion of a small group of cells. Mutations of oncogenes, such as PTTG that are cell growth activators, or mutations of tumor suppressor genes, such as G protein subunit alpha and menin, can result in the formation of pituitary tumors that overproduce hormones. To date, no specific mutation has been determined to be present for most patients that present with these symptoms. Menin gene mutations result in multiple endocrine neoplasia-1 (MEN-1) syndrome, which is accompanied not only by pituitary mass lesions but also by tumors of the parathyroid gland and pancreas.

Hyperprolactinemia

Overproduction of prolactin leads to different syndromes in men and women. Specifically, modest overproduction of prolactin by very small tumors (<1.0 cm) in women results first in anovulation and then leads to amenorrhea due to direct antagonism of gonadotrophin action in the ovary and attenuation of estrogen action in target tis-

Figure 38-2

Acromegaly

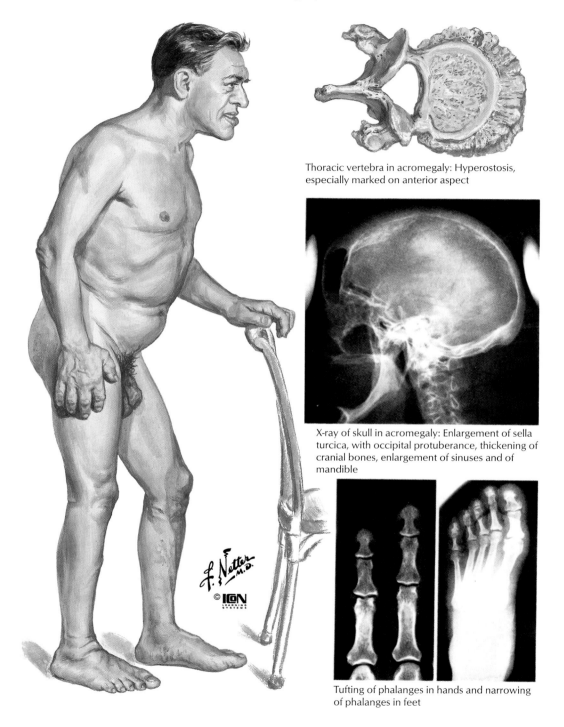

Thoracic vertebra in acromegaly: Hyperostosis, especially marked on anterior aspect

X-ray of skull in acromegaly: Enlargement of sella turcica, with occipital protuberance, thickening of cranial bones, enlargement of sinuses and of mandible

Tufting of phalanges in hands and narrowing of phalanges in feet

Figure 38-3

Acidophil Adenoma

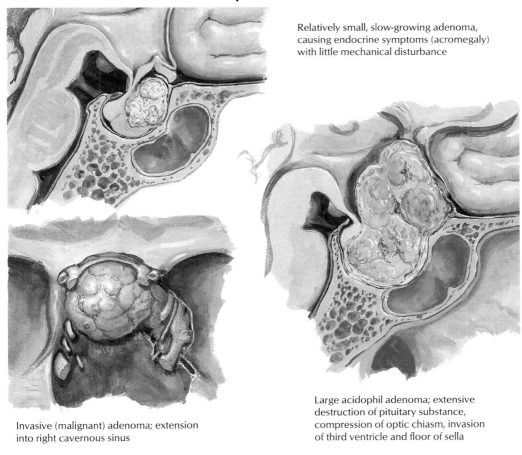

Relatively small, slow-growing adenoma, causing endocrine symptoms (acromegaly) with little mechanical disturbance

Large acidophil adenoma; extensive destruction of pituitary substance, compression of optic chiasm, invasion of third ventricle and floor of sella

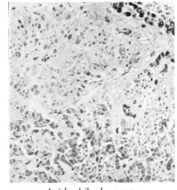

Invasive (malignant) adenoma; extension into right cavernous sinus

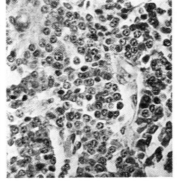

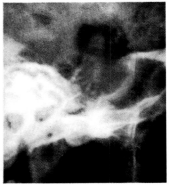

Acidophil adenoma (Mann stain, X 125

Mixed acidophil-chromophobe adenoma (Mann stain, X 250)

Enlarged sella turcica

Gigantism, acromegaly (may be asymptomatic if very small)

Figure 38-4

Basophil Adenoma

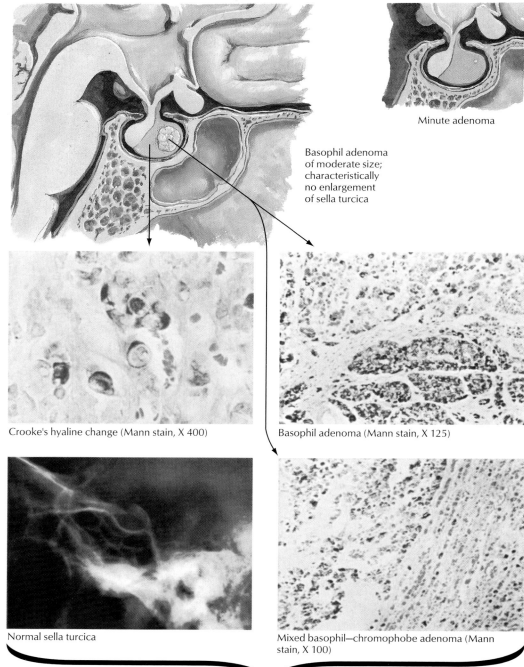

Minute adenoma

Basophil adenoma
of moderate size;
characteristically
no enlargement
of sella turcica

Crooke's hyaline change (Mann stain, X 400)

Basophil adenoma (Mann stain, X 125)

Normal sella turcica

Mixed basophil—chromophobe adenoma (Mann
stain, X 100)

May cause Cushing's syndrome
(may be symptom-free)

Table 38-1
Diagnostic Tests Used to Confirm Pituitary Hormone Deficiencies

Hormone	Screening Test	Stimulation Test	Peak Response
GH	IGF-I decreased in 57% of cases	Insulin tolerance test or Arginine infusion plus GHRH	<3 ng/mL <9 ng/mL
FSH/LH*	Testosterone plus LH (men) Estrogen plus FSH & LH (women)	GnRH	<10 IU/mL
TSH*	Free T4 and TSH	TRH	<5 uU/uL
ACTH	Urine cortisol	ACTH stimulation test	serum cortisol <18 ug/dL
ADH	Polyuria >3L/24 h with serum osmolarity >295 mOsm Urine osmolarity <300 mOsm	Water deprivation test	Correction of hyper osmolarity to <298mOsm after ADH administration

*Usually these deficiencies are confirmed with screening tests and stimulation testing is usually not required

sues such as the endometrium. Severe hyperprolactinemia results in major attenuation of estrogen action with breast and vaginal atrophy, hot flashes, and development of osteoporosis. Spontaneous lactation occurs in women who are producing sufficient estrogen to stimulate milk production. These patients often present with galactorrhea and amenorrhea. Laboratory diagnosis of hyperprolactinemia is confirmed by serum prolactin measurement greater than 25 ng/mL. Treatment depends on whether a microadenoma or a macroadenoma is present. Almost all tumors are reduced in response to dopaminergic agonists. Usually, dopaminergic agonist treatment is instituted first, then the decision as to whether surgery or radiation is made, depending on tumor responsiveness. If prolactin values are <100 ng/mL, other etiologies such as medications (e.g., phenothiazines) or hypothyroidism should be excluded. When prolactin values are greater than 150 ng/mL, they are almost always a result of pituitary tumors. Hypothalamic tumors that result in compression of the pituitary stalk (e.g., craniopharyngiomas) may cause an increase in prolactin.

Acromegaly

Over-production of GH leads to gigantism in children and acromegaly in adults (Figures 38-2 and 38-3). The physical features in adults are quite distinctive and are due to the fact that the long bones have undergone epiphyseal fusion but that there is overgrowth of the hands and feet, the supraorbital ridge, and mandible. Enlargement of soft tissues, including the tongue and skin, and visceromegaly are usually present. Symptoms include sweating, weakness, easy fatigability, and arthralgias. Laboratory abnormalities include fasting hyperglycemia, hyperinsulinemia, and hyperphosphatemia. Treatment includes surgery to remove the primary GH-producing lesion and, sometimes, follow-up radiation therapy. Medical therapy with dopaminergic antagonists, long-acting forms of somatostatin, and growth hormone receptor antagonists is an effective means for reducing the growth-promoting effects of GH. Left untreated, this disease is associated with increased mortality and morbidity, primarily from cardiovascular disease. Because of the increase in mortality, the treatment goals should be normalization of serum

IGF-I. The diagnosis of acromegaly is established either by obtaining an IGF-I value or by determining that growth hormone cannot be suppressed to less than 0.5 ng/mL following ingestion of 75 g of glucose.

Cushing's Disease

Overproduction of ACTH results in Cushing's syndrome, (see chapter 29, Figure 29-6), which presents with a distinct phenotypic appearance, including fat redistribution over the posterior cervical area (buffalo hump), supraclavicular fat pads, and truncal obesity. Connective tissue breakdown leads to the distinct appearance of striae over the abdomen, and easy bruisability is present due to capillary fragility. Other symptoms are hypertension due to increased sodium and water retention; hirsutism and amenorrhea (70% of females); weight gain (20 to 30 lb is common); proximal muscle weakness and poor wound healing; and, in most patients, a distinctive facial flush. Laboratory evaluation often reveals hypokalemia, decreased serum urea nitrogen, and decreased bone mineral density. The diagnosis is made by demonstrating that total urinary cortisol excretion over a 24-hour period is elevated (>120 mcg/day). If this test result is positive, one must distinguish between pituitary tumors and other causes of Cushing's syndrome. This is done by administering dexamethasome, 2.0 mg every 6 hours for 48 hours. Urinary cortisol will be suppressed by 50% or greater in patients with ACTH-producing pituitary tumors. Adequate treatment for Cushing's disease constitutes removal of the ACTH-producing tumor. If a surgical cure is not achieved, radiation treatment and consideration of adrenalectomy is given to alleviate the hormonal overproduction. If left untreated, Cushing's syndrome has a 50% 5-year mortality. Therefore, eliminating the hormonal abnormality is imperative.

FUTURE DIRECTIONS

Major advances have been made in the past decade regarding the quality of pituitary imaging and transphenoidal surgery. Progress in these areas is likely to accelerate. Specifically, surgery is now performed endoscopically and in many cases, this has been extremely successful with much less in-hospital and postoperative morbidity. Continuing improvement in radiation therapy, in terms of localizing the radiation to the pituitary mass that limits damage to surrounding structures, is also likely to be forthcoming. Molecular genetics is likely to continue to improve our ability to predict the development of pituitary tumors. Hormonal assays will improve in terms of sensitivity and specificity so that more reliable diagnostic testing can be performed more rapidly. Whether these tests will be sufficiently precise to obviate stimulation or suppression testing cannot be determined at this time.

REFERENCES

Black PM, Zervas NT, Candia G. Management of large pituitary adenomas by transsphenoidal surgery. *Surg Neurol.* 1988;29:443-447.

Greenman Y, Melmed S. Diagnosis and management of non-functioning pituitary tumors. *Annu Rev Med.* 1996;47:95-106.

Hurel SJ, Thompson CJ, Watson MJ, Harris MM, Baylis PH, Kendall-Taylor P. The short Synacthen and insulin stress tests in the assessment of the hypothalamic-pituitary-adrenal axis. *Clin Endocrinol (Oxf).* 1996;44:141-146.

Littley MD, Shalet SM, Beardwell CG, Ahmed SR, Applegate G, Sutton ML. Hypopituitarism following external radiotherapy for pituitary tumours in adults. *Q J Med.* 1989;70:145-160.

Maroldo TV, Dillon WP, Wilson CB. Advances in diagnostic techniques of pituitary tumors and prolactinomas. *Curr Opin Oncol.* 1992;4:105-115.

Melmed S, Ho K, Klibanski A, Reichlin S, Thorner M. Clinical review 75: recent advances in pathogenesis, diagnosis, and management of acromegaly. *J Clin Endocrinol Metab.* 1995;80:3395-3402.

Radovick S, Cohen LE, Wondisford FE. The molecular basis of hypopituitarism. Horm Res. 1998;49(suppl 1):30-36.

Vance ML. Hypopituitarism. *N Engl J Med.* 1994;330:1651-1662.

Section V

DISORDERS OF THE GASTROINTESTINAL TRACT

Chapter 39

Celiac Disease

William D. Heizer

Malabsorption syndrome results from disease or surgery of the small intestine or pancreas and is characterized by steatorrhea, weight loss, growth retardation in children, and nutrient deficiencies (Figure 39-1). As a result of early diagnosis and treatment, the full-blown syndrome is rarely seen today. In the absence of intestinal surgery, advanced celiac sprue is the most likely cause for malabsorption syndrome in the small bowel.

The prevalence of celiac sprue in whites is 1 in 200 to 1 in 400. However, only 10% to 20% of affected individuals are aware that they have the disease. It may be discovered unexpectedly during upper endoscopy for unrelated symptoms.

ETIOLOGY AND PATHOGENESIS

The etiology of celiac sprue which includes genetic and environmental factors, is complex and multifactorial. One genetic susceptibility locus is associated with the major histocompatibility complex (human leukocyte antigen [HLA] DQ2 and DQ8). In addition, there are probably one or more non-HLA susceptibility loci. Exposure to the wheat protein, gluten, or a similar prolamine present in rye and barley is the most important environmental factor. T-cell–mediated damage to the small intestinal mucosa is seen histologically with migration of lymphocytes to intraepithelial locations, shortening and thickening of the villi, and crypt hyperplasia. The enzyme, tissue transglutaminase, appears to play a role in T-cell damage by catalyzing the deamidation of glutamine side chains of gluten and also cross-linking of these residues to lysine in other proteins, including in the enzyme itself. Antibodies against tissue transglutaminase are recognized clinically as antiendomysial antibodies.

CLINICAL PRESENTATION

Patients with malabsorption syndrome present with diarrhea, weight loss or poor weight gain, and bulky, greasy, and unusually foul smelling stools (Figure 39-2). Signs of vitamin or mineral deficiencies may include glossitis (B vitamins and iron deficiency), osteomalacia (vitamin D and calcium deficiency), tetany (calcium and magnesium deficiency), and ecchymoses (vitamin K deficiency).

Edema results from hypoalbuminemia caused by decreased hepatic synthesis of albumin and protein-losing enteropathy. Endoscopic findings in the duodenum include notching of valvulae conniventes, pavement stone appearance of mucosa, and diminished (or absent) valvulae. Subtle presenting findings include anemia, osteopenia, glossitis, vomiting, muscle cramps, bleeding, infertility, seizures, paresthesias, abdominal distension, weakness, lassitude, growth retardation in children, or small bowel intussusception. Celiac sprue occurs with increased frequency in patients' relatives and in patients with type I diabetes, IgA deficiency, Down's syndrome, autoimmune thyroid disease, primary biliary cirrhosis, Sjögren's syndrome, and microscopic colitis. It is present in 100% of patients with dermatitis herpetiformis.

DIFFERENTIAL DIAGNOSIS

In addition to celiac sprue, the causes of malabsorption syndrome include tropical sprue, Whipple's disease, giardiasis, short bowel syndrome, immunoproliferative disease of the small intestine, intestinal lymphangiectasia, A-beta lipoproteinemia, pancreatic insufficiency, bacterial overgrowth syndrome (resulting from small bowel abnormalities including diverticula, short circuits, motility disorders, or strictures of the small bowel), HIV enteropathy, and radiation enteropathy. In the absence of small bowel resection, Crohn's disease and TB very rarely cause malabsorption.

DIAGNOSTIC APPROACH

If malabsorption syndrome is suspected, fat malabsorption should be documented by a semiquantitative test involving sudan staining of the stool or by quantitative analysis of stool collected

Figure 39-1

Malabsorption Syndrome: Pathophysiology

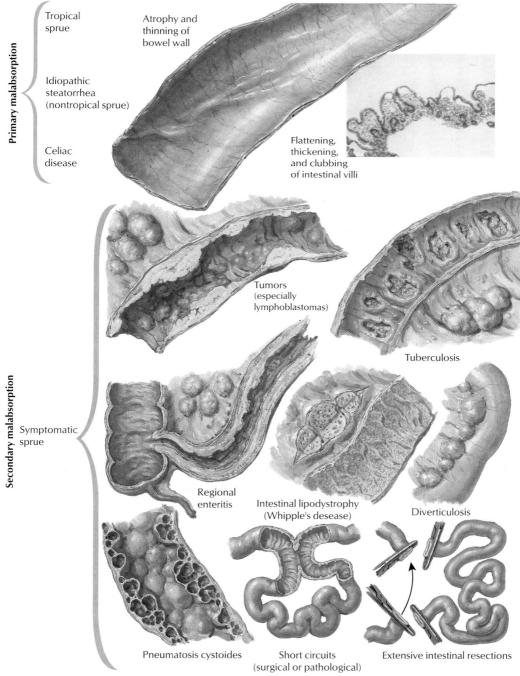

Primary malabsorption

Tropical sprue

Idiopathic steatorrhea (nontropical sprue)

Celiac disease

Atrophy and thinning of bowel wall

Flattening, thickening, and clubbing of intestinal villi

Secondary malabsorption

Symptomatic sprue

Tumors (especially lymphoblastomas)

Tuberculosis

Regional enteritis

Intestinal lipodystrophy (Whipple's desease)

Diverticulosis

Pneumatosis cystoides

Short circuits (surgical or pathological)

Extensive intestinal resections

Figure 39-2

Malabsorption Syndrome
Physical Findings

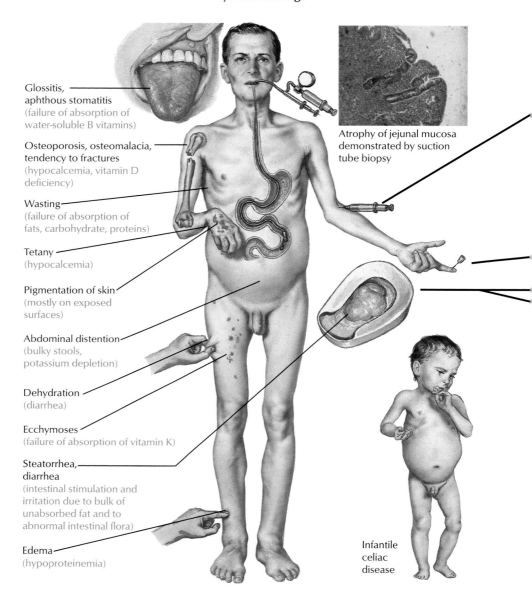

Glossitis, aphthous stomatitis
(failure of absorption of water-soluble B vitamins)

Osteoporosis, osteomalacia, tendency to fractures
(hypocalcemia, vitamin D deficiency)

Wasting
(failure of absorption of fats, carbohydrate, proteins)

Tetany
(hypocalcemia)

Pigmentation of skin
(mostly on exposed surfaces)

Abdominal distention
(bulky stools, potassium depletion)

Dehydration
(diarrhea)

Ecchymoses
(failure of absorption of vitamin K)

Steatorrhea, diarrhea
(intestinal stimulation and irritation due to bulk of unabsorbed fat and to abnormal intestinal flora)

Edema
(hypoproteinemia)

Atrophy of jejunal mucosa demonstrated by suction tube biopsy

Infantile celiac disease

Malabsorption Syndrome (continued)

Laboratory Findings

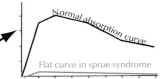

Absorption tests (with glucose, vitamin A, D–xylose, amino acids, radioactive triolein and oleic acids) yield flat curves

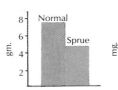

Low blood protein (failure to absorb protein)

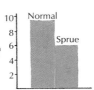

Low blood calcium (lack of Ca absorption plus loss of Ca in stool, plus formation of insoluble soaps with unabsorbed fatty acid)

Macrocytic, hyperchromic anemia (poor absorption of vitamin B_{12} and folic acid)

and/or

Microcytic, hypochromic anemia (poor absorption of iron and protein)

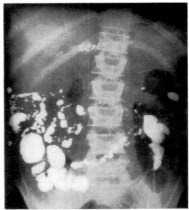

X-ray – typical "deficiency" pattern with breaking up and flocculation of barium column

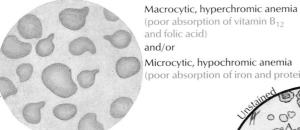

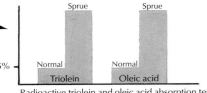

Radioactive triolein and oleic acid absorption tests (increased loss of both substances in feces)

Stool examination reveals abundance of:
A – neutral fats
B – fatty acid crystals
C – soaps

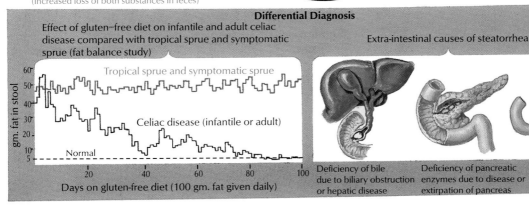

Differential Diagnosis

Effect of gluten–free diet on infantile and adult celiac disease compared with tropical sprue and symptomatic sprue (fat balance study)

Tropical sprue and symptomatic sprue

Celiac disease (infantile or adult)

Normal

Days on gluten-free diet (100 gm. fat given daily)

Extra-intestinal causes of steatorrhea

Deficiency of bile due to biliary obstruction or hepatic disease

Deficiency of pancreatic enzymes due to disease or extirpation of pancreas

Gastrectomy (partial or total)

over 72 hours (Figure 39-2). A stool osmotic gap (290 minus twice the sodium plus potassium concentration in stool water) >125 mosm/L and disappearance of diarrhea with fasting are consistent with diarrhea due to malabsorption.

A high index of suspicion is important for diagnosis of celiac sprue. Serologic tests are useful. Endomysial antibody positivity is approximately 95% sensitive and specific, similar to the presence of reticulin antibodies. Gliadin IgA antibody is at least 95% sensitive but somewhat less specific. Individuals with positive serologic tests and those with negative serologic tests suspected to have sprue should undergo small bowel biopsy. Four to 6 biopsy specimens from the mucosa of the duodenum wall beyond the bulb should be obtained endoscopically. Both the serologic tests and the biopsies can become normal after several months of a gluten-free diet. HLA typing is not routinely useful for diagnosis, but in equivocal cases or refractory cases where the diagnosis has become suspect, the absence of both DQ2 and DQ8 antigens should call the diagnosis into question. The d-xylose test is nonspecific and insensitive and is not indicated. Small-bowel radiographic changes may include dilatation, intussusception, and segmentation of barium but are neither specific nor sensitive for sprue. A trial of gluten withdrawal should not be used as a means to diagnose celiac sprue.

Blunting of villi and crypt hyperplasia are not specific for celiac sprue and occur in other diseases, including gastrinoma, giardiasis, and enteropathy-associated T-cell lymphoma. Intraepithelial lymphocytes may be the only visible changes on light microscopy in mild sprue. Whether there are patients with entirely normal small-bowel histologic appearances in whom symptoms (usually diarrhea) respond specifically to gluten withdrawal is questionable. A few cases have been reported. A thick band of collagen beneath the epithelial cells confirms the diagnosis of collagenous sprue, which is generally more refractory to treatment.

MANAGEMENT AND THERAPY

The mainstay of treatment for celiac sprue is lifelong avoidance of all wheat, rye, and barley. Some studies suggest that oats are not harmful, but until more studies are available, oats should be avoided until all symptoms have improved. Response usually occurs within 3 to 4 weeks of withdrawing gluten

from the diet but may be delayed for 1 year or more. Even entirely asymptomatic patients with biopsy-diagnosed sprue should avoid gluten to avoid complications, including osteopenia, anemia, and small-bowel malignancies.

Refractory symptoms should stimulate a careful review of the diet, including medications that may contain gluten. Patients unresponsive to gluten withdrawal often respond to treatment with steroids or other immunosuppressive agents, such as azathioprine or cyclosporin. All patients should take a multivitamin and mineral supplement daily until any symptoms have fully responded. Refractory or recurrent symptoms should prompt a search for complications or associated conditions including microscopic colitis, ulcerative jejunitis, small intestinal lymphoma or adenocarcinoma, and collagenous sprue.

FUTURE DIRECTIONS

Identification of the genes responsible for the disease should clarify pathogenesis and lead to tests that are more specific and sensitive. A potential therapeutic approach is to use oral proteolytic enzymes with meals to detoxify gluten similar to the use of lactose for lactose intolerance. Other possible therapeutic strategies may include inhibitors of tissue transglutaminase, treatment to produce immune tolerance to the toxic fractions of gluten, or development of wheat, rye, and barley that is genetically modified to be nontoxic to celiac patients. Even further study may clarify the prevalence, if any, of individuals with diarrhea or other symptoms and a normal small-bowel histologic appearance, who respond specifically (over and above placebo response) to withdrawal of gluten.

REFERENCES

Brasitus TA, Sitrin MD. Intestinal malabsorption syndromes. *Annu Rev Med.* 1990;41:339–347.

Ciclitira PJ, King AL, Fraser JS. AGA technical review on celiac sprue. American Gastroenterological Association. *Gastroenterology.* 2001;120:1526–1540.

Fasano A, Catassi C. Current approaches to diagnosis and treatment of celiac disease: an evolving spectrum. *Gastroenterology.* 2001;120:636–651.

Mulder CJ, Wahab PJ, Moshaver B, Meijer JW. Refractory coeliac disease: a window between coeliac disease and enteropathy associated T cell lymphoma. *Scand J Gastroenterol.* 2000;35(suppl 232):32–37.

Sollid LM. Molecular basis of celiac disease. *Annu Rev Immunol.* 2000;18:53–81.

Chapter 40
Cholelithiasis

Mark J. Koruda

The prevalence of gallstones in the United States is almost 10%. Cholecystectomy is the most common abdominal operation performed in this country with approximately 750,000 completed each year. The annual cost for the management of gallstones, their complications, and economic losses to society is close to $5 billion.

ETIOLOGY AND PATHOGENESIS

Gallstones are classified according to their composition. They vary in shape, number, size, and consistency; however these characteristics play little role in whether symptoms develop (Figure 40-1).

Cholesterol stones are the most common type of gallstone. Three factors are necessary for their formation: supersaturation of gallbladder bile with cholesterol, crystal nucleation, and gallbladder hypomotility (Figure 40-2). The solubility of cholesterol in bile depends on the incorporation of cholesterol in solubilizing bile acid–lecithin micelles. Alterations in the relative concentrations of cholesterol, bile acids, or lecithin can lead to cholesterol supersaturation. Mucin glycoprotein molecules act as nucleating agents to form gallstones. Cholesterol crystals in the mucin gel coupled with defective emptying of the gallbladder lead to the growth and development of stones.

Pigmented stones come in black or brown varieties. Black pigmented stones are composed of pure calcium bilirubinate or polymer-like complexes of calcium, copper, and large amounts of glycoproteins. These stones are most common in cirrhosis and chronic hemolytic states. Brown pigmented stones are usually associated with infection. Bacteria present in the biliary system hydrolyze glucuronic acid from conjugated bilirubin. Calcium salts of the now unconjugated bilirubin crystallize and form brown stones.

A majority of epidemiological series indicate the prevalence of gallstones in women varies from 5% to 20% between the ages of 20 and 55, and from 25% to 30% after age 50. The prevalence for men is approximately one half that of women at any age.

Risk Factors for Gallstone Development

- Older age
- Female
- Obesity
- Weight loss
- Total parenteral nutrition
- Pregnancy
- Genetic predisposition
- Diseases of the terminal ileum
- Hypertriglyceridemia

CLINICAL PRESENTATION

Gallstones cause symptoms by obstruction of the cystic duct, common bile duct, or erosion into neighboring organs (Figure 40-3). Seventy-five percent of gallstones do not cause symptoms; 20% cause intermittent pain or biliary colic; 10% result in acute cholecystitis; 5% pass into the common duct, causing bile duct obstruction or pancreatitis; and <0.1% are associated with fistulas or gallbladder cancer.

Biliary Colic and Chronic Cholecystitis

Approximately 75% of patients with cholelithiasis present with biliary colic. Pain results from the intermittent obstruction of the cystic duct by one or more stones. Inflammation is not present, so there are usually few, if any, systemic signs or symptoms. Biliary colic is a visceral pain that is poorly localized but typically felt in the epigastrium, right upper quadrant, or even the left upper quadrant. The pain is steady rather than intermittent or "colicky" and lasts from 1 to 6 hours. Pain lasting longer than 6 hours is more

---

Figure 40-1

Cholelithiasis
Pathologic Features, Choledocholithiasis

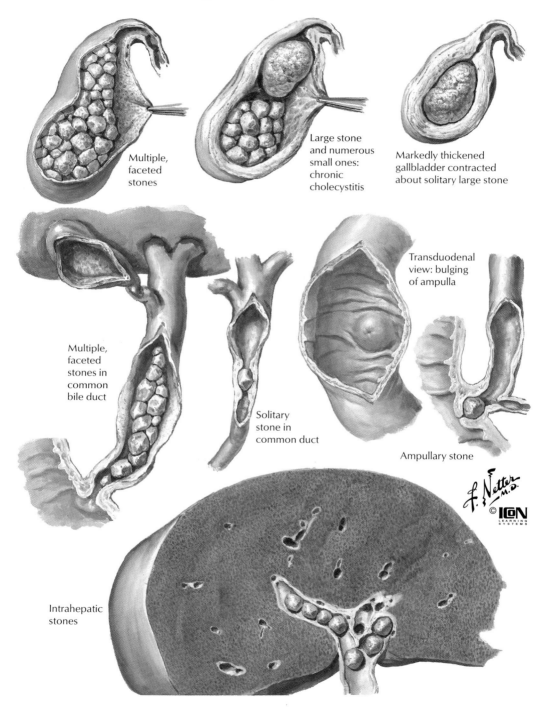

Multiple, faceted stones

Large stone and numerous small ones: chronic cholecystitis

Markedly thickened gallbladder contracted about solitary large stone

Multiple, faceted stones in common bile duct

Solitary stone in common duct

Transduodenal view: bulging of ampulla

Ampullary stone

Intrahepatic stones

Figure 40-2

Pathogenesis of Gallstones

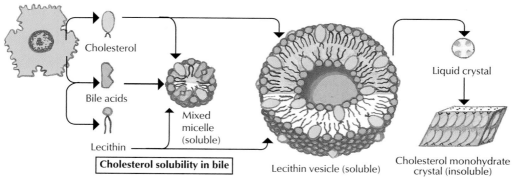

Cholesterol solubility in bile

Cholesterol

Bile acids

Lecithin

Mixed micelle (soluble)

Liquid crystal

Lecithin vesicle (soluble)

Cholesterol monohydrate crystal (insoluble)

Solubility of cholesterol in bile depends on incorporation of cholesterol in bile acid–lecithin micelles and lecithin vesicles. When bile becomes saturated with cholesterol, vesicles fuse to form liposomes, or liquid crystals, from which crystals of cholesterol monohydrate nucleate.

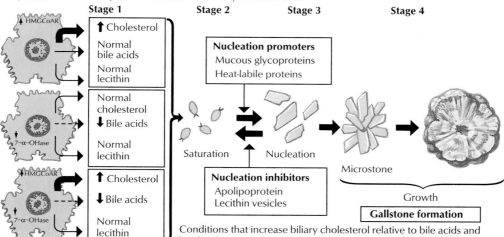

Stage 1

↓HMGCoAR

↑ Cholesterol
Normal bile acids
Normal lecithin

↓7–α–OHase

Normal cholesterol
↓ Bile acids
Normal lecithin

↑HMGCoAR
↓7–α–OHase

↑ Cholesterol
↓ Bile acids
Normal lecithin

Stage 2   **Stage 3**   **Stage 4**

Nucleation promoters
Mucous glycoproteins
Heat-labile proteins

Saturation   Nucleation

Nucleation inhibitors
Apolipoprotein
Lecithin vesicles

Microstone

Growth

Gallstone formation

Conditions that increase biliary cholesterol relative to bile acids and lecithin favor saturation of bile and formation of gallstones

Predisposing factors

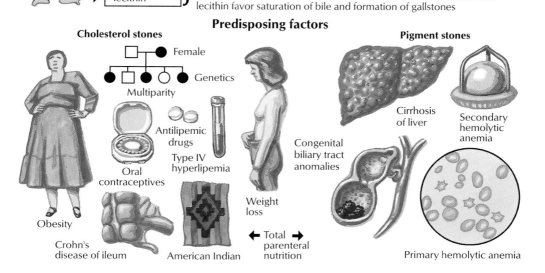

Cholesterol stones

Female
Genetics
Multiparity

Antilipemic drugs

Oral contraceptives

Type IV hyperlipemia

Obesity

Crohn's disease of ileum

American Indian

Congenital biliary tract anomalies

Weight loss

← Total parenteral nutrition →

Pigment stones

Cirrhosis of liver

Secondary hemolytic anemia

Primary hemolytic anemia

JOHN A. CRAIG—AD
© ICON

Figure 40-3

Mechanisms of Biliary Pain

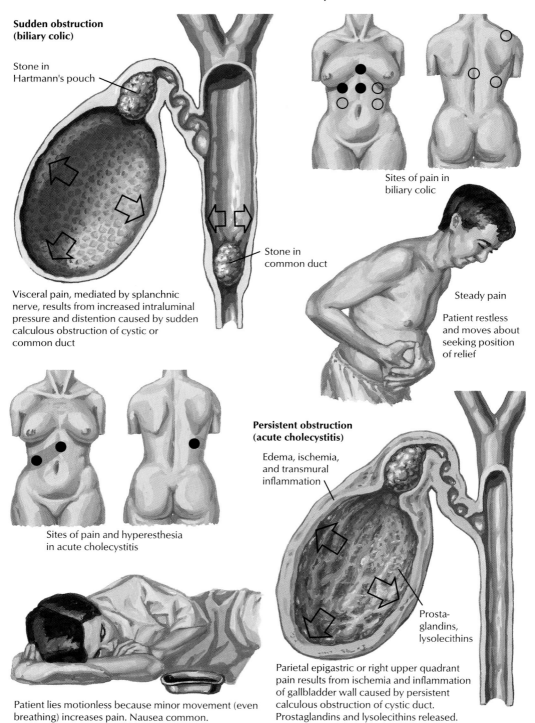

Sudden obstruction (biliary colic)

Stone in Hartmann's pouch

Stone in common duct

Visceral pain, mediated by splanchnic nerve, results from increased intraluminal pressure and distention caused by sudden calculous obstruction of cystic or common duct

Sites of pain in biliary colic

Steady pain

Patient restless and moves about seeking position of relief

Sites of pain and hyperesthesia in acute cholecystitis

Persistent obstruction (acute cholecystitis)

Edema, ischemia, and transmural inflammation

Prosta-glandins, lysolecithins

Patient lies motionless because minor movement (even breathing) increases pain. Nausea common.

Parietal epigastric or right upper quadrant pain results from ischemia and inflammation of gallbladder wall caused by persistent calculous obstruction of cystic duct. Prostaglandins and lysolecithins released.

JOHN A. CRAIG—AD
© ICON

commonly associated with the onset of inflammation and hence cholecystitis. Physical examination is typically normal, but mild tenderness in the right upper quadrant may be elicited. Laboratory tests are frequently unrevealing. Seventy percent of patients experience recurrent symptoms within 2 years of the initial attack. Recurrent episodes of biliary colic are referred to as chronic cholecystitis.

Acute Cholecystitis

Similar to biliary colic, acute cholecystitis is brought on by impaction of a gallstone or stones in the cystic duct or infundibulum. Prolonged obstruction of the cystic duct leads to stasis of bile within the gallbladder, damage to the gallbladder mucosa, and the consequent release of intracellular enzymes and activation of inflammatory mediators. As concentrations of inflammatory mediators rise within the gallbladder, ongoing inflammation produces increased protein and prostaglandin secretion, decreased water absorption, and white blood cell infiltration. Acute cholecystitis is initially a "chemically" mediated inflammatory process. Enteric bacteria may be cultured from the bile, but they are not responsible for the onset or activation of acute cholecystitis.

Symptoms persist and usually worsen. Over time, inflammation of the gallbladder ensues, and the pain becomes parietal in nature with localization to the right upper quadrant. Radiation of pain to the back or scapular area is common. Fever is fairly common, but the temperature is usually less than 102°F. Nausea and vomiting may occur. Jaundice is observed in approximately 20% of patients with bilirubin levels usually less than 4 mg/dL, and uniformly in those with higher bilirubin levels. Frequently, white blood cell counts are elevated. Abdominal examination often reveals right subcostal tenderness. A palpable gallbladder occurs in approximately one third of patients. "Murphy's sign," an insensitive but moderately specific finding, is described as inspiratory arrest during palpation of the right subcostal area during deep inspiration.

Choledocholithiasis, Cholangitis, and Gallstone Pancreatitis

Gallstones may pass from the gallbladder into the common bile duct and cause pain, obstructive jaundice, cholangitis, or pancreatitis (Figure 40-4). Five percent to 15% of patients with gallstones also have common duct stones. Stones within the common duct cause pain that is colicky, occurring in the epigastrium with radiation to the back. Jaundice is very common as bilirubin levels rise with the degree of obstruction. Elevations in alkaline phosphatase occur frequently.

Of all the complications of gallstones, *cholangitis* kills most quickly. The usual clinical presentation consists of pain, jaundice, and chills (i.e., Charcot's triad). Refractory sepsis characterized by altered mentation, hypotension, and Charcot's triad constitutes Reynold's pentad.

Gallstone pancreatitis occurs when a biliary stone causes a transient or sustained blockage of the ampulla of Vater. Most patients experience a mild, self-limited attack that resolves within several days, characterized by abdominal or back pain and elevated serum amylase and lipase levels. Abnormal serum biochemistries as well as clinical symptoms resolve slowly during this time. Severe pancreatitis develops in a finite number of patients, manifested by persistent retroperitoneal inflammation, pseudocyst formation, or pancreatic necrosis with or without peripancreatic sepsis.

Uncommon Complications of Gallstone Disease

Emphysematous cholecystitis occurs when gas-forming organisms infect the gallbladder secondary to acute cholecystitis. Gas pockets present within the gallbladder wall can be detected radiographically. Urgent cholecystectomy is recommended. *Cholecystenteric fistulas* occur when a stone erodes through the gallbladder wall into an adjacent viscus. The most common sites include the duodenum, the hepatic flexure of the colon, and the stomach.

DIFFERENTIAL DIAGNOSIS
Biliary Colic and Chronic Cholecystitis

Colic and chronic cholecystitis mimic episodic upper abdominal symptoms, including gastroesophageal reflux, peptic ulcer disease, pancreatitis, renal colic, diverticulitis, colon cancer, and angina pectoris. Complaints of gas, bloating, flatulence, and dyspepsia are frequent in patients with gallstones. These symptoms are nonspecific and should not be considered clinical manifesta-

Figure 40-4

Calculous Obstruction of Common Duct (Choledocholithiasis)

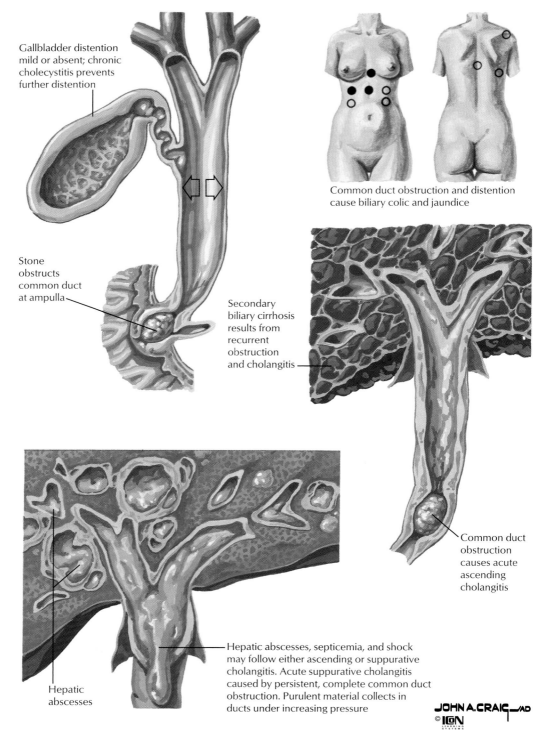

Gallbladder distention mild or absent; chronic cholecystitis prevents further distention

Common duct obstruction and distention cause biliary colic and jaundice

Stone obstructs common duct at ampulla

Secondary biliary cirrhosis results from recurrent obstruction and cholangitis

Common duct obstruction causes acute ascending cholangitis

Hepatic abscesses

Hepatic abscesses, septicemia, and shock may follow either ascending or suppurative cholangitis. Acute suppurative cholangitis caused by persistent, complete common duct obstruction. Purulent material collects in ducts under increasing pressure

JOHN A. CRAIG—AD
©IGN

tions of gallstone disease.

Acute Cholecystitis

The signs and symptoms of acute cholecystitis mimic those of acute appendicitis, acute pancreatitis, right kidney disease, pneumonia with pleurisy, acute hepatitis, hepatic abscesses, and gonococcal perihepatitis (Fitz-Hugh-Curtis syndrome).

Choledocholithiasis and Cholangitis

Because the symptoms associated with cystic and common duct obstruction are so similar, biliary colic and acute cholecystitis are always in the differential diagnosis. Malignant obstruction of the common bile duct, acute congestion of the liver associated with congestive heart failure, acute viral hepatitis, and acquired immunodeficiency cholangiopathy may also mimic choledocholithiasis.

DIAGNOSTIC APPROACH
Laboratory Tests

In uncomplicated biliary colic and chronic cholecystitis, there are usually no accompanying changes in hematologic and biochemical tests. In acute cholecystitis, leukocytosis is usually observed. Serum aminotransferase, alkaline phosphatase, bilirubin, and amylase levels may also be elevated.

Sonography

Ultrasonography is the modality of choice for examining the biliary tract. Ultrasound can detect stones as small as 2 mm in diameter within the gallbladder with sensitivity and specificity rates exceeding 95%.

Sonography is also valuable in the diagnosis of acute cholecystitis. Eliciting a sonographic Murphy's sign (focal gallbladder tenderness under the transducer) has a positive predictive value of >90% for diagnosis of acute cholecystitis when stones are seen. The presence of pericholecystic fluid in the absence of ascites and gallbladder wall thickening to >4 mm are nonspecific findings suggestive of acute cholecystitis.

Stones in the common bile duct are only seen with sonography in 50% of cases. Thus, sonography confirms, but does not exclude, common duct stones.

Hepatobiliary Scintigraphy

Hepatobiliary scintigraphy is most useful in evaluating patients with suspected acute cholecystitis. A normal hepatobiliary scan virtually rules out acute cholecystitis in patients who present with abdominal pain. The sensitivity of the test is approximately 95%, and the specificity is 90%. False-positive results occur primarily in fasting or critically ill patients.

Endoscopic Retrograde Cholangiopancreatography

Endoscopic retrograde cholangiopancreatography (ERCP) is the standard for evaluating common duct stones and pathology. Endoscopic therapeutic applications have revolutionized the treatment of common duct stones and other biliary tract disorders.

Computed Tomography and Magnetic Resonance Imaging

Although not well suited for the evaluation of uncomplicated stones, standard CT is an excellent test to detect complications such as abscess formation, perforation of the gallbladder or common bile duct, or pancreatitis. Spiral CT and MR cholangiography may prove useful as a noninvasive means of excluding common bile duct stones.

MANAGEMENT AND THERAPY

Cholecystectomy remains the mainstay of treatment of symptomatic gallstones.

Asymptomatic Cholelithiasis

Because up to 80% of all gallstones are asymptomatic and the risk for developing symptoms or complications is low, adult patients with silent or incidental gallstones should be observed and treated expectantly.

Biliary Colic and Chronic Cholecystitis

The natural history of biliary colic is such that recurrent biliary pain occurs in approximately 38% to 50% of patients per year. The risk of serious biliary complications is estimated at 1% to 2% per year. A reasonable approach is to offer cholecystectomy to those with recurring episodes of biliary colic. For asymptomatic patients not wanting to risk a future attack, a laparoscopic cholecystectomy is recommended. The laparoscopic approach to gallbladder removal is also the treatment of choice for symptomatic gallstones. Laparoscopy, unlike the traditional "open" operation, allows the surgery to be performed on an outpatient basis with a marked reduction in postoperative pain and a more rapid return to work and usual activities. Conversion to open cholecystectomy is uncommon, averaging <5% in most institutions. The incidence of bile duct injury associated with laparoscopic cholecystectomy has decreased to <0.5% and mortality rates are <0.1%.

Acute Cholecystitis

If acute cholecystitis is suspected, the patient should be hospitalized for evaluation and treatment. Antibiotics may be withheld in uncomplicated cases but are indicated in toxic-appearing patients or when complications such as perforation or emphysematous cholecystitis are suspected. Definitive therapy is cholecystectomy performed within 24 to 48 hours of the onset of symptoms. Delaying the procedure increases the difficulty in performing surgery and increases the complication rate and the need to convert to an open operation. Percutaneous cholecystostomy or transpapillary endoscopic cholecystostomy can be used to drain the inflamed gallbladder for patients deemed to be at high risk for surgery.

Choledocholithiasis

The optimal treatment for common duct stones depends on the level of local expertise in endoscopy and surgery. In general, the presence of obstructive jaundice with a dilated common bile duct should lead promptly to preoperative ERCP with sphincterotomy and stone extraction. Once the bile duct has been cleared, the patient can undergo a routine laparoscopic cholecystectomy within 1 or 2 days.

Cholangitis

The management of sepsis in cholangitis is of paramount importance. Drainage or decompression of the biliary system is definitive. ERCP with stone extraction or at least bile duct decompression with a stent is the treatment of choice. Alternatively, access to the obstructed biliary tract via percuta-

neous transhepatic cholangiography with drainage catheter placement can temporize by draining the infected obstructed bile duct. Once the patient has recuperated from the infectious insult, elective laparoscopic cholecystectomy can be undertaken.

Gallstone Pancreatitis

For more than three fourths of patients, gallstone pancreatitis is mild, self-limiting, and resolves with conservative management. Cholecystectomy should be performed during the initial admission when the pancreatitis has resolved. Delaying surgery increases the risk for recurrent symptoms and further complications. Prior to surgery, an evaluation of the biliary system for retained stones should be performed with either ERCP or intraoperative cholangiography. For patients with severe biliary pancreatitis, early ERCP with sphincterotomy, if indicated, is beneficial.

FUTURE DIRECTIONS

In light of the significant public health impact of gallstones, ongoing research continues to focus on finding the medical means to prevent gallstone formation. Further advances in nonsurgical therapy are expected. Perhaps the most exciting developments will occur in biliary tract imaging techniques with the application of improved resolution ultrasound, endoscopic ultrasound, magnetic resonance imaging, and cholangiography.

REFERENCES

NIH consensus conference. Gallstones and laparoscopic cholecystectomy. *JAMA.* 1993;269:1018–1024.

Acalovschi M. Cholesterol gallstones: from epidemiology to prevention. *Postgrad Med J.* 2001;77:221–229.

Ahmed A, Cheung RC, Keeffe EB. Management of gallstones and their complications. *Am Fam Physician.* 2000;61:1673–1680, 1687–1688.

Bilhartz LE, Horton JD. Gallstone disease and its complications. In: Feldman M, Friedman LS, Sleisenger MH, eds. *Sleisenger & Fordtran's Gastrointestinal and Liver Disease: Pathophysiology/Diagnosis/Management.* 7th ed. Philadelphia, Pa: WB Saunders Co; 2002.

Chapter 41
Cirrhosis

Roshan Shrestha

Cirrhosis of the liver is an irreversible alteration of hepatic architecture, characterized by diffuse fibrosis and areas of nodular regeneration. These nodules can be micronodular (less than 3 mm) or macronodular (more than 3 mm). Features of both micronodular and macronodular cirrhosis are frequently present in the same liver. Determining the etiology is often not possible from the gross and microscopic appearance of the cirrhotic liver and must therefore be based on results of history, physical examination, biochemical and serologic tests, and histochemical stains.

ETIOLOGY AND PATHOGENESIS

The relationship between alcohol abuse and cirrhosis is well established. Ethanol is a hepatotoxin that leads to the development of fatty liver, alcoholic hepatitis and, ultimately, cirrhosis (Figure 41-1). The pathogenesis may differ depending on the underlying causes of the liver disease. In general, there is ongoing chronic inflammation either due to toxins (alcohol and drugs), infections (hepatitis virus, parasites), autoimmune phenomenon (chronic active hepatitis, primary biliary cirrhosis [PBC]), or biliary obstruction (common bile duct stone, primary sclerosing cholangitis [PSC]), with the subsequent development of diffuse fibrosis and cirrhosis.

CLINICAL PRESENTATION

Patients may be entirely asymptomatic or may present with nonspecific constitutional symptoms, or symptoms of liver failure, complications of portal hypertension, or both.

Nonspecific symptoms include weakness, lethargy, anorexia, weight loss, abdominal pain, loss of libido, altered sleep-wake pattern, and nausea or vomiting. Specific symptoms due to hepatic synthetic dysfunction and portal hypertension include jaundice, pruritus, coagulopathy leading to easy bruising, fluid retention with ankle edema, ascites, gastroesophageal variceal bleeding leading to hematemesis or melena, and symptoms of hepatic encephalopathy ranging from mild confusion to coma.

On physical examination, patients may have stigmata of chronic liver disease such as Dupuytren's contractures, palmar erythema, spider angiomata, parotid enlargement, and bruising. Palpation of the

---

Causes of Cirrhosis

Infections: Hepatitis B, hepatitis C and possibly other viruses, schistosomiasis

Drugs and Toxins: Alcohol, methyldopa, methotrexate, isoniazid, amiodarone

Biliary Obstruction: Primary sclerosing cholangitis, cystic fibrosis, biliary atresia, common bile duct stones

Metabolic Disorders: Hereditary hemochromatosis, Wilson's disease, α1-antitrypsin deficiency, glycogen storage disease

Autoimmune Diseases: Chronic active hepatitis, primary biliary cirrhosis

Cardiovascular: Chronic right heart failure, Budd-Chiari syndrome, venoocclusive disease

Miscellaneous: Nonalcoholic steatohepatitis, sarcoidosis, jejunoileal bypass, neonatal hepatitis

---

abdomen may reveal an enlarged or shrunken liver, splenomegaly, ascites, or dilated superficial abdominal wall veins. Male patients may show signs of feminization (gynecomastia), testicular atrophy, and loss of body hair. Patients with hepatic encephalopathy may present with a "flapping tremor" or asterixis.

DIFFERENTIAL DIAGNOSIS

The new onset of ascites presenting with no history and stigmata of chronic liver disease may not be due to cirrhosis and portal hypertension. Other causes include portal vein occlusion, nephrotic syndrome, protein-losing enteropathy, severe malnutrition, myxedema, ovarian diseases (Meigs' syndrome, struma ovarii), pancreatic ascites, chylous ascites, nephrogenic ascites, tuberculous peritonitis, or secondary malignancy.

Figure 41-1

Septal Cirrhosis

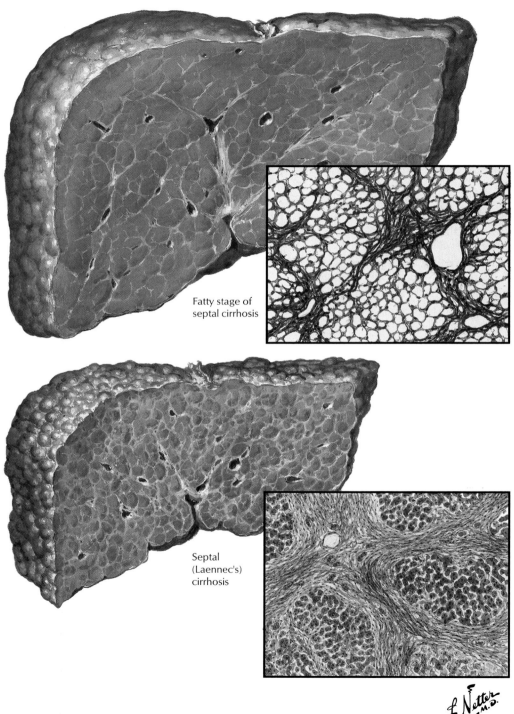

Fatty stage of septal cirrhosis

Septal (Laennec's) cirrhosis

Figure 41-2   **Endoscopic Appearance of Esophageal Varices**
with Evidence of Recent Hemorrhage

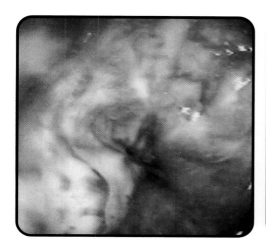 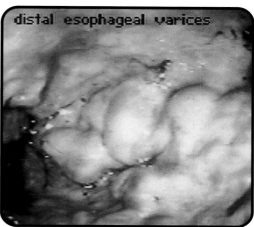

The differential diagnosis for hematemesis and melena includes duodenal ulcer, gastric ulcer, esophagitis, gastritis, Mallory-Weiss tear, hematobilia, anastomotic ulcer, and Ménétrier's disease.

DIAGNOSTIC APPROACH

After a thorough history and physical examination, complete laboratory data, radiologic examination, and histologic studies may be necessary to establish the diagnosis and possible cause of cirrhosis.

The complete blood cell count may show anemia, leukopenia, or thrombocytopenia. Hypersplenism causes both leukopenia and thrombocytopenia. Chronic blood loss and vitamin deficiency can cause anemia. The prothrombin time can be prolonged due to vitamin K deficiency or impaired clotting factor synthesis.

Serum biochemistry often shows elevated bilirubin level and a low albumin level. Some patients with established cirrhosis may have normal aspartate aminotransferase (AST) and alanine aminotransferase (ALT). Elevated AST and ALT levels are found in patients with autoimmune hepati-

tis, viral hepatitis, and alcoholic hepatitis. Patients with cholestatic liver disease usually have elevated alkaline phosphatase, gamma glutamyltransferase, and conjugated bilirubin levels.

Several other serologic tests are necessary to establish cause: viral serology for hepatitis B (HBsAg), C (anti-HCV Ab), and quantitative DNA and RNA levels for their activity status respectively; iron studies and HFE gene analysis for hereditary hemochromatosis; serum copper, ceruloplasmin level for Wilson's disease; α-1antitrypsin level and genotype for α-1 antitrypsin deficiency. Serum autoantibodies (antinuclear antibody, anti-smooth muscle antibody, anti-mitochondrial antibody) and quantitative serum immunoglobulins levels may help to diagnose autoimmune liver disease.

Radiologic studies (ultrasound with or without Doppler, CT, or MRI) provide additional diagnostic information. These studies are not always necessary, but they are indicated to screen for primary hepatocellular carcinoma, which is commonly associated with cirrhosis.

Histologic examination of the liver biopsy specimen is often key for diagnosis. Micronodules, fatty infiltration, and Mallory's hyaline usually accompany alcoholic cirrhosis. Primary biliary cirrhosis, primary sclerosing cholangitis, and autoimmune hepatitis have typical histologic findings. Special stains such as Prussian blue for iron and periodic acid-Schiff diastase for α-1 antitrypsin globules can confirm the diagnosis. Liver biopsy is necessary to stage the disease and may serve as a prognosticator in the natural history of the disease. This will then guide optimum therapy.

MANAGEMENT AND THERAPY

In general, management of cirrhosis includes:
- Withdrawal of the causative agent (e.g., alcohol, drugs).
- Treatment of specific underlying cause (e.g., antiviral therapy for viral hepatitis, prednisone or azathioprine for autoimmune hepatitis, phlebotomy for hemochromatosis, D-penicillamine or trientine for Wilson's disease).
- Treatment of decompensation of cirrhosis: ascites, infection, gastrointestinal hemorrhage, hepatic encephalopathy, and hepatorenal syndrome.
- Orthotopic liver transplantation for decompensated cirrhosis if the patient is a suitable candidate.

Ascites

Patients with cirrhosis in whom ascites develops need diagnostic (10 to 20 mL) abdominal paracentesis. Indications include new onset ascites, clinical deterioration with fever, abdominal pain, and change in mental status. The factors producing ascites in cirrhosis are a low serum albumin level, hepatic outflow block with overproduction of lymph, and portal venous hypertension. Ascites can be mild, moderate or severe on the basis of amount of fluid in the peritoneal cavity (Figures 41-3 and 41-4). The initial treatment involves restriction of dietary sodium intake and the use of oral diuretics. Approximately 20% of patients respond to sodium restriction alone. Sodium is usually limited to 2 g (90 mEq) per day. Diuretics include spironolactone and furosemide. More than 90% of patients respond to this combination therapy. The maximum spironolactone dose is 400 mg/day and for furosemide, the maximum dose that should be used is 160 mg/day. Amiloride, 10 to 20 mg/day, can be used in place of spironolactone if there are side effects such as tender gynecomastia.

Approximately 10% of patients with cirrhosis will have ascites refractory to routine medical treatment with sodium restriction and diuretic therapy. Large volume paracentesis (LVP) can be used before alternative therapies such as transjugular intrahepatic portosystemic shunt (TIPS) or peritoneovenous shunt. TIPS is a relatively safe nonsurgical procedure that is effective in reducing portal hypertension. It has gained wide popularity and provides a bridge to liver transplantation. Peritoneovenous shunt (LeVeen) can be used if the placement of a TIPS is contraindicated.

Gastrointestinal Hemorrhage

Gastroesophageal variceal bleeding is the most ominous complication of cirrhosis. Initial management of suspected variceal bleeding requires immediate hospitalization, volume resuscitation, and airway protection for massive bleeding. If the diagnosis is reasonably certain, pharmacologic therapy with somatostatin or octreotide can be initiated. If endoscopy confirms esophageal varices, endoscopic therapy with either variceal ligation or sclerotherapy can be performed. Endoscopic therapy controls acute variceal bleeding in 80% to 95% of patients, a success rate superior to pharmacologic agents or balloon tamponade. There is a 50% to 80% risk of recurrent variceal bleeding. Options to prevent recurrent variceal bleeding include endoscopic ligation or sclerotherapy, β-blockers (propranolol, nadolol), surgical shunts, TIPS, and liver transplantation.

TIPS is one of the most promising therapies for the control of acute variceal bleeding. The goal of TIPS is to achieve a hepatic venous gradient of <12 mm Hg and a reduction or loss of contrast opacification of varices. TIPS is reserved for those patients who are refractory to endoscopic therapy along with pharmacotherapy or acute bleeding from gastric varices. The technical success rate and control of acute variceal bleeding is >90%. (Figure 41-2)

Hepatic Encephalopathy

Hepatic encephalopathy represents a constellation of reversible neurologic signs and symptoms accompanying advanced, decompensated liver disease or extensive portosystemic shunting. The pathogenesis of hepatic encephalopathy remains unclear. It is partially attributable to toxic compounds that are derived from the metabolism of nitrogenous substrates in the gut that bypass the liver through an anatomical and functional shunt. The four stages of hepatic encephalopathy are based on mental state and neurologic findings.

Stage 1: Mild confusion and incoordination present.

Stage 2: Asterixis is consistently present and the patient has obvious personality changes.

Stage 3: The patient is somnolent, disoriented on arousal.

Stage 4: The patient is comatose.

Common precipitating factors include deterioration in hepatic function, gastrointestinal hemorrhage, excess protein intake, alcohol, sedatives or hypnotics, surgery, hepatoma, infection, dehydration, electrolyte imbalance (hypokalemia), constipation, and placement of a surgical shunt or TIPS. Management includes identification and correction of any precipitating factor, restriction of dietary protein (40 g/day) and administration of lactulose. Antibiotics to decontaminate the gut, such as neomycin, metronidazole, or amoxicillin, can be added if there is no response to dietary manipulation and lactulose. Patients with severe refractory hepatic encephalopathy need urgent liver transplantation.

Hepatorenal Syndrome

Hepatorenal syndrome is a distinct type of progressive acute renal failure that develops in a patient with cirrhosis in whom all other causes of renal dysfunction are excluded. It is a functional type of renal failure. If the liver disease improves, normal renal function returns. The pathogenesis of the hepatorenal syndrome is unknown. The probability of hepatorenal syndrome in cirrhosis is approximately 20% in 1 year and 40% in 5 years. Hyponatremia and azotemia characterize hepatorenal syndrome. The urinary sodium concentration is <10 mEq/L. The urinary sediment is unremarkable. The urine/plasma creatinine ratio is >30, and the urine/plasma osmolality ratio is >1.

In the management of hepatorenal syndrome, specific causes for renal failure should be excluded (i.e., acute tubular necrosis, pre-renal azotemia from intravascular volume depletion, drug-

induced nephrotoxicity, or preexisting chronic renal disease). Hemodialysis should be considered for patients who are potential candidates for liver transplantation. Experimental forms of therapy include prostaglandin E1, dopamine, peritoneovenous shunt, and TIPS.

Liver Transplantation

Cirrhosis is the seventh most frequent cause of death in the United States, and liver transplantation is the only successful therapy in decompensated advanced disease. Approximately 18,000 patients in the United States are on the United Network of Organ Sharing (UNOS) waiting list, and the number increases 25% per year. Only 4,500 cadaveric transplants are performed each year in the United States. Because there is an excess of potential recipients, careful identification and evaluation of transplant recipients is critical.

Liver transplantation is no longer experimental and is considered as standard of care for patients with advanced cirrhosis. With improved surgical technique and better immunosuppressive drugs, it has become a successful therapy for end-stage liver disease with long-term survivals approaching 90% and excellent quality of life. Unfortunately, the gap between the numbers of cadaveric donors and recipients continues to widen.

Living donor liver transplantation (LDLT) is used by many transplant centers worldwide. First used in a pediatric patient in 1989, LDLT has become a viable alternative for pediatric recipients. Over the past few years, LDLT has been used successfully in adult recipients with patient and graft survivals similar to those with cadaveric liver transplantation. In the future, with appropriate donor and recipient selection, further refinement in surgical technique, and increasing experience, LDLT may give superior results. It is predicted that approximately 10% to 30% of liver transplantation in the United States will be with living donors.

FUTURE DIRECTIONS

Major improvements in diagnostic techniques now allow the diagnosis of chronic liver diseases earlier in their course. Improvement in pharmacologic agents that include antiviral drugs (hepatitis B and C) will help to prevent progression to cirrhosis.

Liver transplantation is a highly effective option in the management of advanced cirrhosis. Hepa-

Figure 41-3

Ascites

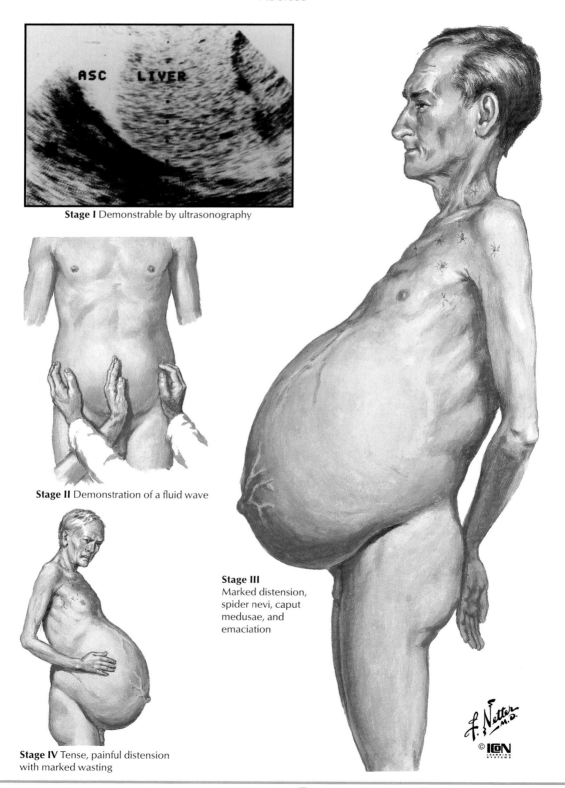

Stage I Demonstrable by ultrasonography

Stage II Demonstration of a fluid wave

Stage III
Marked distension,
spider nevi, caput
medusae, and
emaciation

Stage IV Tense, painful distension
with marked wasting

Figure 41-4

Pathophysiology of Ascites Formation

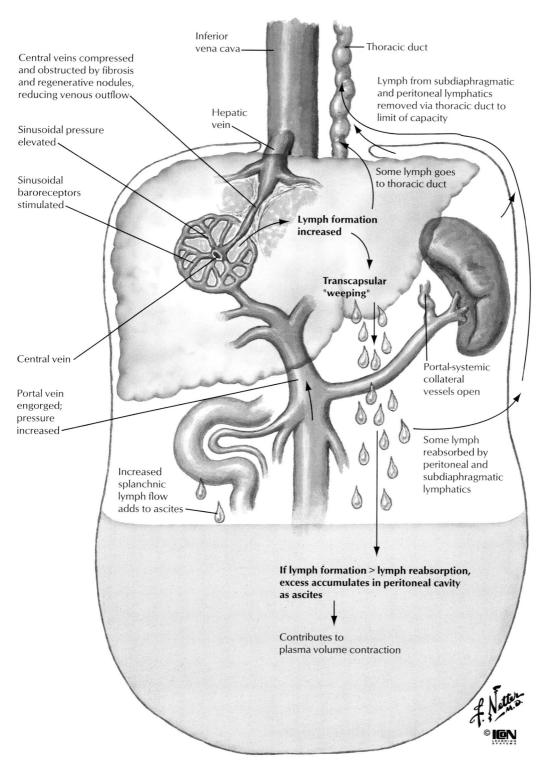

Central veins compressed and obstructed by fibrosis and regenerative nodules, reducing venous outflow

Sinusoidal pressure elevated

Sinusoidal baroreceptors stimulated

Central vein

Portal vein engorged; pressure increased

Inferior vena cava

Hepatic vein

Thoracic duct

Lymph from subdiaphragmatic and peritoneal lymphatics removed via thoracic duct to limit of capacity

Some lymph goes to thoracic duct

Lymph formation increased

Transcapsular "weeping"

Portal-systemic collateral vessels open

Some lymph reabsorbed by peritoneal and subdiaphragmatic lymphatics

Increased splanchnic lymph flow adds to ascites

If lymph formation > lymph reabsorption, excess accumulates in peritoneal cavity as ascites

Contributes to plasma volume contraction

tocyte, stem cell, and xenotransplantation may provide additional therapeutic options in the management of end-stage liver disease.

REFERENCES

Rector WG Jr. *Complications of Liver Disease.* St Louis, Mo: Mosby-Year Book Inc; 1992.

Rossle M, Haag K, Ochs A, et al. The transjugular intrahepatic portosystemic stent-shunt procedure for variceal bleeding. *N Engl J Med.* 1994;330:165–171.

Runyon BA. Care of patients with ascites. *N Engl J Med.* 1994; 330:337–342.

Starzl TE, Demetris AJ, Van Thiel D. Liver transplantation (1). *N Engl J Med.* 1989;321:1014–1022.

Starzl TE, Demetris AJ, Van Thiel D. Liver transplantation (2). *N Engl J Med.* 1989;321:1092–1099.

Stiegmann GV, Goff JS, Michaletz-Onody PA, et al. Endoscopic sclerotherapy as compared with endoscopic ligation for bleeding esophageal varices. *N Engl J Med.* 1992;326:1527–1532.

Chapter 42

Common Anorectal Disorders

Christopher C. Baker

Anorectal disorders, which often present as pain or defecation, are common and can be very serious for patients who present with them. The three most frequent causes of pain on defecation are thrombosed hemorrhoids, fissure in ano, and perirectal abscess. In evaluating these patients, it is important to obtain a thorough history concentrating on the events leading up to the problem and the aspects of defecation that are troublesome. General physical examination includes an anorectal examination concentrating on external inspection, digital examination, and anoscopy, which allows direct visualization of the anal canal. The pain is often too severe to allow a good anoscopic examination without anesthesia, and some patients may need a general anesthetic to facilitate the diagnosis.

THROMBOSED HEMORRHOID
Etiology and Pathogenesis

Hemorrhoids are protrusions of the submucosal veins into the anal canal. They tend to be caused by constipation with repeated straining to pass hard stool, leading to stretching of the anal mucosa, and prolapse. If prolapsed hemorrhoids remain out and are not reduced, then stasis leads to thrombosis of the hemorrhoids. The hemorrhoidal veins in most patients come from the internal hemorrhoids of the superior hemorrhoidal plexus.

Clinical Presentation

Patients usually present with bleeding followed by severe pain on defecation. A firm prolapsed thrombosed hemorrhoid that appears blue or purplish is seen on physical examination. Many patients have edematous tissue around the thrombosed hemorrhoid. The area is usually tender due to stretching of the anoderm.

Differential Diagnosis

Prolapsed hemorrhoids that are not thrombosed, anal condylomata, epidermal inclusion cysts, true rectal prolapse (with circumferential folds of rectal mucosa), or sentinel pile (associated with a fissure) should be considered. Other possibilities are pregnancy, which can cause increased venous pressure in the hemorrhoidal plexus, or the presence of cirrhosis with portal hypertension.

Diagnostic Approach

Generally, the diagnosis can be made by direct physical examination of the external anal canal. Occasionally, examination under local or general anesthesia may be necessary to evaluate the lesion. Anoscopy is rarely indicated.

Management and Therapy

Therapy is generally surgical. Incision and drainage of the clot may be adequate, but the excision of the thrombosed hemorrhoid itself is preferable because it allows the tissue to reduce and speeds recovery (Figure 42-1). Patients can have a local anesthetic with both procedures. Less severe cases can be treated with sitz baths, local steroid creams, and bulk-forming agents. Altering diet, stool consistency, and bowel habits are critical for the long-term treatment of these patients.

FISSURE IN ANO
Etiology and Pathogenesis

Fissure in ano is a superficial laceration or tear in the anoderm occurring just below the dentate line. The combination of constipation with hard stools and sphincter spasm causes the patient to strain against a spastic sphincter, and as a result causes the anoderm to give or tear. The skin in this area is richly innervated by sensory fibers, and the patient is enveloped in a cycle of pain, inflammation, spasm, and more pain. As the patient defecates, the area stretches again, leading to pain that can last several hours. Often, patients will resist having a bowel movement, making the subsequent passage of hard stool even more painful.

Figure 42-1

Thrombosed External Hemorrhoid

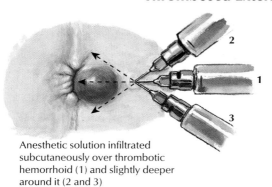

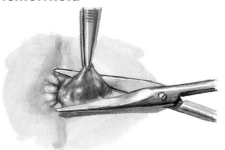

Anesthetic solution infiltrated subcutaneously over thrombotic hemorrhoid (1) and slightly deeper around it (2 and 3)

Skin over hemorrhoid drawn up by forceps and elliptical segment of skin excised

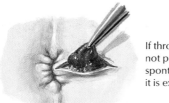

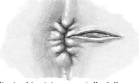

If thrombus does not pop out spontaneously, it is extracted

Elliptical incision partially falls together, ready for cotton dressing

Anal Fissure

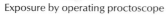

Area to be excised extending well beyond anal verge

Sentinel pile

Fissure

Hypertrophic papilla

Exposure by operating proctoscope

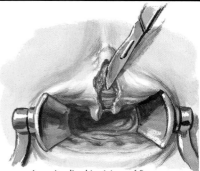

Longitudinal incision of fissure base, including papilla and sentinel pile but <u>not</u> sphincter

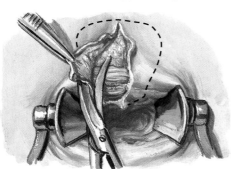

Excision of fissure and surrounding tissue

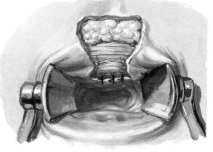

Suture of undermined mucosal margin to internal border of external sphincter

Clinical Presentation

The patient presents usually with an acute event or tear causing a cycle of pain and spasm. The physical finding that is pathognomonic in this entity is a sentinel pile or skin tag (Figures 42-1 and 42-2). This occurs in the posterior midline in 90% of adults. In children, 15% to 20% of lesions can be seen anteriorly. In general, having the patient lie in the lateral decubitus position and spreading the buttocks and asking the patient to strain allows the fissure to be seen. The anoderm will evert out, and the fissure can usually be seen underneath the sentinel pile. Digital examination should be avoided because the area is usually extremely tender. If the diagnosis is suspected and a fissure cannot actually be seen, it may be necessary to perform an examination with the patient under general anesthesia.

Differential Diagnosis

Some patients can sustain tears in this area from physical trauma. Patients with ulcerative colitis commonly have fissures. Various infectious lesions can cause fissures (e.g., amoebiasis and tuberculosis) but these are generally quite rare.

Diagnostic Approach

A good history and physical examination are essential to diagnosis. Occasionally, anoscopy with the patient under general anesthesia is necessary to make the diagnosis.

Management and Therapy

Occasionally, patients with mild fissures respond to local measures such as sitz baths, steroid cream (suppositories are contraindicated because they are so painful to administer), and bulk-forming agents. Using diazepam to decrease sphincter spasm is only occasionally successful. If the patient does not respond to conservative therapy by 3 to 7 days, consider an invasive approach. The gold standard treatment is a lateral anal sphincterotomy, performed by incising the inferior 1 cm of the internal anal sphincter with either an open or closed approach. Most patients require a general or spinal anesthetic for this procedure. Complications include bleeding, and rarely, abscess formation, and fistula. Incontinence, the most feared complication, occurs when the sphincterotomy performed is too large. This is avoidable with careful surgical

technique. Although patients often achieve prompt relief with this procedure, those with chronic fissures may take longer to heal and should be advised occasionally.

PERIRECTAL ABSCESS
Etiology and Pathogenesis

Perirectal abscesses occur in patients with constipation and usually start when inspissated stool gets caught in the anal crypts (Figure 42-3). This leads to crypt abscesses, which then perforate through the wall of the abdomen into the perirectal space. Abscesses can occur as perianal, intersphincteric, or supralevator. These abscesses are among the most feared infections, particularly in diabetics or immunocompromised patients, because they can proceed to necrotizing fasciitis of the perineum (Fournier's gangrene).

Clinical Presentation

Patients with perirectal abscesses tend to appear toxic and often have a fever. If symptoms include pain on defecation and induration in the perirectal tissues, a perirectal abscess should be suspected. The onset of pain is usually slower than a fissure and can be more diffuse. On physical examination, there may be edema or erythema overlying the abscess. Nonetheless, the hallmark of deep-seated soft tissue infection in these patients is induration. Because of the thick fascial bands around the anus, fluctuance is a relatively late sign. Digital examination may be rather painful. If the patient is able to tolerate it, the digital examination can show bogginess.

Differential Diagnosis

Very few entities are included in the differential diagnosis of perirectal abscess. Chronic abscesses with fistula formation can develop in patients with Crohn's disease. Rarely, patients with tuberculosis and actinomycosis can present with abscesses in these areas. The other entity that is sometimes confused with perirectal abscesses is a localized soft tissue infection from chronic bedsores as seen in paraplegic patients.

Diagnostic Approach

The diagnosis is usually made by careful physical examination, looking for induration and occasionally bogginess on the rectal examination (if the patient allows a digital examination). Some clinicians have

Figure 42-2

Anal Fissure

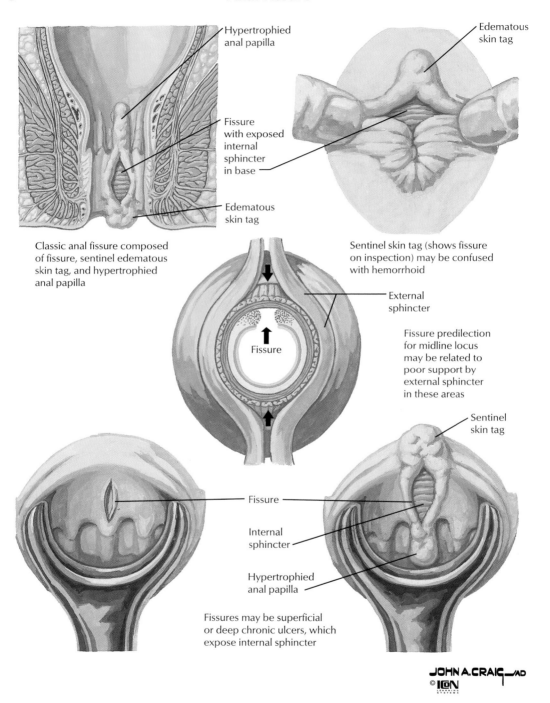

Hypertrophied anal papilla

Edematous skin tag

Fissure with exposed internal sphincter in base

Edematous skin tag

Classic anal fissure composed of fissure, sentinel edematous skin tag, and hypertrophied anal papilla

Sentinel skin tag (shows fissure on inspection) may be confused with hemorrhoid

External sphincter

Fissure

Fissure predilection for midline locus may be related to poor support by external sphincter in these areas

Sentinel skin tag

Fissure

Internal sphincter

Hypertrophied anal papilla

Fissures may be superficial or deep chronic ulcers, which expose internal sphincter

JOHN A. CRAIG—AD
© ICN

Figure 42-3

Surgical Management of Anorectal Abscess

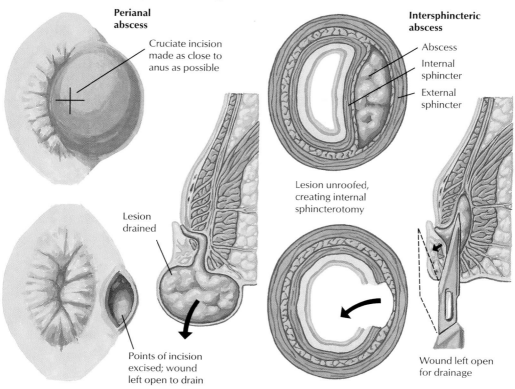

Perianal abscess

Cruciate incision made as close to anus as possible

Lesion drained

Points of incision excised; wound left open to drain

Intersphincteric abscess

Abscess
Internal sphincter
External sphincter

Lesion unroofed, creating internal sphincterotomy

Wound left open for drainage

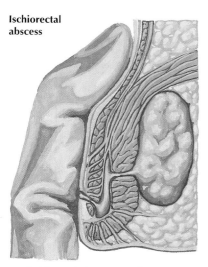

Ischiorectal abscess

Ischiorectal abscess may be palpated above anorectal ring, although located inferiorly

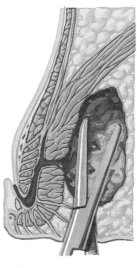

Abscess incised and loculations broken down

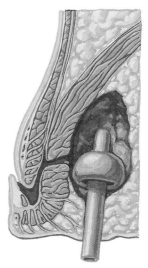

Mushroom catheter inserted to insure drainage

JOHN A. CRAIG—AD
© ICON

advocated a CT scan in difficult patients although this is usually not necessary. Examination with the patient under anesthesia, with aspiration of the suspected areas, may be necessary. In many cases, it is obvious where the perirectal abscess should be drained. Newer adjuncts such as endorectal ultrasound can be of value in selected patients, but generally are not necessary.

Management and Therapy

The critical approach to perirectal abscess is incision and drainage. Antibiotics are also important in treating these patients. Localized perianal abscesses may be drained under local anesthesia in the clinic or the emergency department. Patients with more complicated abscesses should be examined in the operating room under general or spinal anesthesia. Patients may be positioned either in lithotomy or in prone jackknife position, depending on the location of the abscess. Anoscopy should be performed to try to identify the offending crypt, and a generous incision of the entire infected/indurated area should be performed. A circumanal incision in the inner sphincteric groove is the safest incision to avoid damage to the sphincters (Figure 42-3). If the offending crypt can be identified, then a radial incision can be used to connect it in a submucosal fash-

ion to allow better drainage. Fistula in ano occurs in approximately 10% to 15% of cases, and these usually drain into the rectum into an area in which the offending crypt has not been identified. Patients with fistula in ano should be referred to a surgeon because of the complexity of management.

REFERENCES

Dennison AR, Whiston RJ, Rooney S, Morris DL. The management of hemorrhoids. *Am J Gastroenterol.* 1989;84:475–481.

Haas PA, Fox TA Jr, Haas GP. The pathogenesis of hemorrhoids. *Dis Colon Rectum.* 1984;27:442–450.

Johanson JF, Rimm A. Optimal nonsurgical treatment of hemorrhoids: a comparative analysis of infrared coagulation, rubber band ligation, and injection sclerotherapy. *Am J Gastroenterol.* 1992;87:1600–1606.

Lieberman DA. Common anorectal disorders. *Ann Intern Med.* 1984;101:837–846.

MacRae HM, McLeod RS. Comparison of hemorrhoidal treatments: a meta-analysis. *Can J Surg.* 1997;40:14–17.

Metcalf A. Anorectal disorders. Five common causes of pain, itching, and bleeding. *Postgrad Med.* 1995;98:81–84, 87–89, 92–94.

Pfenninger JL, Surrell J. Nonsurgical treatment options for internal hemorrhoids. *Am Fam Physician.* 1995;52:821–834, 839–841.

Shub HA, Salvati EP, Rubin RJ. Conservative treatment of anal fissure: an unselected, retrospective and continuous study. *Dis Colon Rectum.* 1978;21:582–583.

Chapter 43

Constipation

Yolanda V. Scarlett

Constipation refers to specific symptoms associated with impaired defecation, including abnormal stool frequency, straining with defecation, passage of hard stool, and a sense of incomplete evacuation. It is very common and affects persons of all ages, from children to the elderly. An individual with constipation may experience one or more of the symptoms. Millions of dollars are spent annually on over-the-counter laxatives, physician visits, and pharmacologic agents. The true prevalence is not known because many people do not seek medical care. Reported prevalence rates range from 2% to 20%. The Rome II consensus criteria for constipation include fewer than three bowel movements weekly, straining, hard or lumpy stools, sense of incomplete anorectal evacuation, or manual maneuvers to assist defecation with more than one fourth of the bowel movements. Functional constipation is described as having two or more of the outlined symptoms for at least 3 months of the year. It is important to define the patient's symptoms carefully to determine the most appropriate cost-effective diagnostic and therapeutic approach.

ETIOLOGY AND PATHOGENESIS

Most individuals are toilet-trained and able to control defecation by age 4. Successful continent evacuation requires that mental function be able to respond to cues indicating the need to evacuate, normal intestinal motility, proper internal and external anal sphincter function, and coordination of the puborectalis muscle. The rectum is a compliant reservoir with stretch or mechanoreceptors located in the rectal wall. The urge to defecate is experienced once stool is propelled from the distal sigmoid colon into the rectum and activates these mechanoreceptors. Defecation is initiated by sitting and straining, maneuvers that increase the intraabdominal pressure, decrease the resting tone of the internal anal sphincter, straighten the angle of the puborectalis muscle, relax the external anal sphincter, and allow expulsion of the fecal bolus. These maneuvers occur almost simultaneously, and an abnormality in any one of the steps can result in constipation.

The causes of constipation are broad and can be divided into metabolic, neurogenic, and idiopathic (Figure 43-1). In addition, numerous drugs are associated with constipation. Common metabolic and endocrine causes include hypothyroidism, diabetes mellitus, pregnancy, hypercalcemia, hypokalemia, uremia, glucagonoma, and porphyria. Neurogenic disorders include peripheral neuropathy, Hirschsprung's disease, autonomic neuropathy, neurofibromatosis, Chagas' disease, and intestinal pseudoobstruction. Central nervous system disorders include multiple sclerosis, Parkinson's disease, cerebrovascular accident, and spinal cord injury. Certain medications can cause constipation: narcotic analgesics, anticholinergic drugs, antidepressants, antihypertensives, diuretics, NSAIDs, antacids containing aluminum or calcium salts, antihistamines, and antiparkinson's agents. Long-term laxative use is also associated with constipation. Idiopathic causes include slow transit type constipation or colonic inertia, pelvic floor dyssynergia, constipation-predominant irritable bowel syndrome, megacolon, and megarectum.

CLINICAL PRESENTATION

Individuals who present with complaints of constipation may describe any of the following symptom complexes: infrequent bowel movements; excessive straining with defecation; inability to evacuate the rectum after experiencing an urge; a desire to have a bowel movement but with lack of an urge to defecate; evacuation of small, hard, or dry stools; digital manipulation to achieve evacuation; or a sense of incomplete evacuation. It is crucial to determine what the patient describes as constipation in order to guide the diagnostic approach.

Figure 43-1

Causes of Constipation

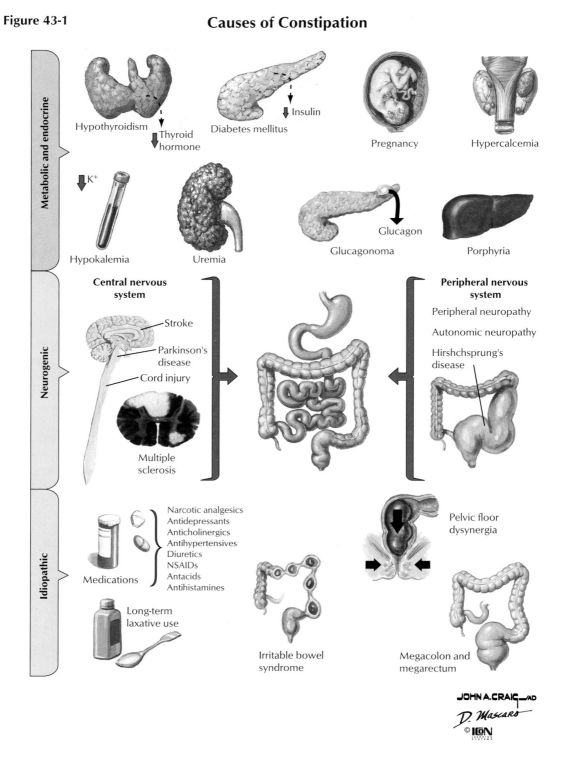

Metabolic and endocrine

Hypothyroidism → Thyroid hormone

Diabetes mellitus ↓ Insulin

Pregnancy

Hypercalcemia

↓K⁺

Hypokalemia

Uremia

Glucagonoma → Glucagon

Porphyria

Neurogenic

Central nervous system

Stroke
Parkinson's disease
Cord injury

Multiple sclerosis

Peripheral nervous system

Peripheral neuropathy

Autonomic neuropathy

Hirshchsprung's disease

Idiopathic

Medications
Narcotic analgesics
Antidepressants
Anticholinergics
Antihypertensives
Diuretics
NSAIDs
Antacids
Antihistamines

Long-term laxative use

Irritable bowel syndrome

Pelvic floor dysynergia

Megacolon and megarectum

JOHN A. CRAIG—AD
D. Mascaro
©ICN

Figure 43-2

Diagnosis and Management of Constipation

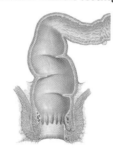

— Rectum

— Internal sphincter

— External sphincter

3 Balloon manometer inserted in rectum

Anorectal manometry

Normal   Hirshchsprung's disease

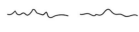
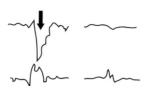

In normal circumstances, balloon distention should cause transient relaxation of internal sphincter

Balloon expulsion test

Normal   Abnormal (dysynergia)

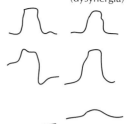

Expulsion should cause increase in rectal pressure and decrease in baseline pressure

Colonic transit testing

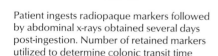

Radiopaque marker

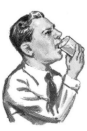

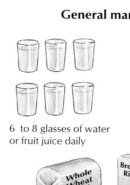

Radiopaque paste introduced into rectum. Fluoroscopic monitored digestion provides information on anorectal angle, pelvic floor descent, rectocele, intussusception and rectal prolapse.

Patient ingests radiopaque markers followed by abdominal x-rays obtained several days post-ingestion. Number of retained markers utilized to determine colonic transit time

General management measures

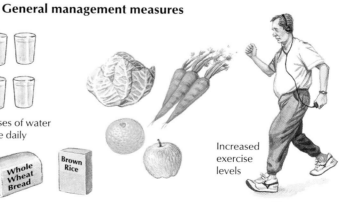

Increased fluid intake

6 to 8 glasses of water or fruit juice daily

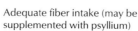

Whole Wheat Bread

Brown Rice

Adequate fiber intake (may be supplemented with psyllium)

Increased exercise levels

f. Netter M.D.

JOHN A. CRAIG—AD
© ICN

DIFFERENTIAL DIAGNOSIS

Most causes of constipation are not life-threatening and are of a functional rather than an organic nature. Functional causes of constipation include insufficient fluid and fiber intake as well as physical inactivity. Organic conditions to be considered include colorectal tumors, hernias, strictures, chronic intermittent volvulus, endometriosis, rectocele, rectal prolapse, and anal stricture.

DIAGNOSTIC APPROACH

A detailed history is critical when evaluating an individual with a complaint of constipation. Information obtained during the history guides selection of appropriate testing if testing is needed. The number of bowel movements in a 7-day period should be documented along with the appearance of the stool. Infrequent stools may reflect slow transit of fecal material through the colon. Small, hard, lumpy stool may indicate inadequate fiber and fluid intake. Long, small caliber or long, flat stools can be seen with inappropriate relaxation of the puborectalis muscle and external anal sphincter when attempting to evacuate. Small caliber stool can also be associated with tumors and necessitate colonoscopy to exclude malignancy.

Standard diagnostic testing includes the balloon expulsion test, colonic transit study, anorectal manometry, and defecography. Other studies such as pelvic floor electromyography, colonic motility testing, and pudendal nerve latency testing are not available at all testing centers, and adequate diagnostic information can usually be obtained without these studies.

The *balloon expulsion* study is a simple test that determines whether the patient can evacuate a 50-mL air or water-filled balloon. Some advocate balloon expulsion testing as a screening study for pelvic floor dysfunction. Inability to expel the balloon may reflect inability to appropriately relax the pelvic floor to allow defecation as seen with pelvic floor dyssynergia or paradoxical contraction of the pelvic floor in response to straining.

Colonic transit testing evaluates the time required for material to move through the colon. The most cost-effective method to determine the colonic transit time is ingestion of radiopaque makers in conjunction with having one or more abdominal radiographs obtained several days after ingestion. The number of retained radiopaque markers is used to determine the colonic transit time. There are several protocols for colonic transit marker studies, and the various protocols correlate well with each other. The colonic transit time can also be determined by radionuclide gamma scintigraphic studies that also quantitate the colon transit time. Radionuclide scintigraphic assessment of colon transit is not readily available, but it correlates well with determination of colon transit time when compared to radiopaque markers.

Anorectal manometry testing provides useful information about rectal sensation, internal anal sphincter relaxation, rectal compliance, and pelvic floor responses to straining. Testing is performed by placing pressure-recording catheters across the anal sphincters. Measurements are obtained by introducing increments of air into a balloon attached to the tip of the catheter. Balloon expulsion testing is often done in conjunction with anorectal manometry. Surface electromyography can be performed with skin pads or anal plugs and is often performed together with anorectal manometry to evaluate possible external anal sphincter and puborectalis dysfunction such as paradoxical pelvic floor motions that hinder evacuation. It is very helpful if there is a history of childhood constipation. Screening for Hirschsprung's disease is easily done with manometry. This diagnosis is excluded by demonstrating appropriate relaxation of the internal anal sphincter in response to balloon distention.

Defecography involves introducing soft barium paste into the rectum, then having the patient evacuate during fluoroscopic examination. It can provide information about the anorectal angle, pelvic floor descent, retentive rectoceles, intussusception, and rectal prolapse.

MANAGEMENT AND THERAPY

Initial management should include counseling regarding adequate fiber intake, sufficient fluid intake, and physical activity. Most Western diets do not provide the minimum recommended daily requirement of dietary fiber. If fiber intake is deficient, the patient should be instructed to gradually increase intake to 20 to 35 g daily. Psyllium supplements may provide a good source of fiber. Fiber intake should be increased over days to prevent abdominal bloating and increased flatulence. Fiber should be avoided if there is concern regarding colonic blockage or stricture because an impaction may occur proximal to the stricture. A minimum of 6 glasses of fluid, preferably water and fruit juices, should be taken daily. Physical limitations often restrict activity especially in older individuals, but the patient should be encouraged to remain physically active. Often with attention to fiber, water, and activity, the symptoms of constipation can be relieved. If there is still inadequate relief, the history should guide testing.

Patients with infrequent bowel movements without excessive straining may benefit from stool-softening agents such as docusate. Determination of the colonic transit time is indicated if there is inadequate symptom relief despite compliance with basic management. Documented slow colon transit or colonic inertia may be managed with laxatives. If chronic laxative use is required, bulk-forming agents (psyllium), hyperosmolar laxatives (polyethylene glycol, lactulose, and sorbitol), and saline laxatives (magnesium sulfate, magnesium citrate, and magnesium phosphate) are preferred to stimulant laxatives. Stimulant laxatives are not recommended for chronic use because they may cause degeneration of the nerve plexi in the gut, in turn causing more symptoms of constipation. Common stimulant laxatives include bisacodyl, senna, and cascara.

Anorectal manometry testing is indicated if there is concern about Hirschsprung's disease, sensory perception, or pelvic floor dysfunction. Balloon expulsion testing is often performed at the same time as anorectal manometry testing. If pelvic floor dysfunction is identified, pelvic floor retraining with biofeedback may be beneficial. Patients are taught to relax, instead of contract, the pelvic floor musculature when attempting to evacuate.

Subtotal colectomy with ileorectal anastomosis is reserved for individuals with constipation that does not respond to conservative measures and laxative therapy and who do not have pelvic floor dysfunction, including pelvic floor dyssynergia or outlet obstruction. These individuals should have demonstrated normal small bowel neuromuscular function because small bowel neuropathy and small bowel myopathy can contribute to constipation.

FUTURE DIRECTIONS

Current research includes clinical investigation of tegaserod, a medication that increases gut transit time in patients with constipation-predominant irritable bowel syndrome. Prucalopride is another agent that has been shown to decrease the colonic transit time in patients with constipation. Investigational agent RU-0211 is a bicyclic fatty acid that activates an intestinal chloride ion channel to secrete chloride and increase colonic fluid secretion. Preliminary data suggest that RU-0211 significantly increases the number of spontaneous bowel movements in patients with constipation.

REFERENCES

Barnes PR, Lennard-Jones JE. Balloon expulsion from the rectum in constipation of different types. *Gut.* 1985;26:1049–1052.

Bouras EP, Camilleri M, Burton DD, Thomforde G, McKinzie S, Zinsmeister AR. Prucalopride accelerates gastrointestinal and colonic transit in patients with constipation without a rectal evacuation disorder. *Gastroenterology.*2001;120:354–360.

Drossman DA, Corazziari E, Talley NJ, Thompson WG, Whitehead WE, and the Rome Multinational Working Teams, eds. *Rome II: Diagnostic Criteria for the Functional Gastrointestinal Disorders.* 2nd ed. McLean Va: Degnon Associates Inc; 2000:382–391.

Johanson JF, Gargano MA, Patchen ML, Ueno R. Efficacy and safety of a novel compound, RU-0211, for the treatment of constipation [abstract]. *Gastroenterology.*2002;122:A–315.

Metcalf AM, Phillips SF, Zinsmeister AR, MacCarty RL, Beart RW, Wolff BG. Simplified assessment of segmental colonic transit. *Gastroenterology.* 1987;92:40–47.

Prather CM, Camilleri M, Zinsmeister AR, McKinzie S, Thomforde G. Tegaserod accelerates orocecal transit in patients with constipation-predominant irritable bowel syndrome. *Gastroenterology.* 2000;118:463–468.

Wald A. Colonic and anorectal motility testing in clinical practice. *Am J Gastroenterol.* 1994;89:2109–2115.

Wald A, Caruana BJ, Freimanis MG, Bauman DH, Hinds JP. Contributions of evacuation proctography and anorectal manometry to evaluation of adults with constipation and defecatory difficulty. *Dig Dis Sci.* 1990;35:481–487.

Chapter 44

Diarrhea: Acute and Chronic

Yolanda V. Scarlett

Diarrhea is defined as increased stool output. The increased fecal output may represent increased frequency of stool, increased stool fluidity, or a combination of both. Objectively, diarrhea is defined as a stool weight in excess of 200 g in 24 hours and is classified as acute or chronic depending on the duration of symptoms. Acute diarrhea lasts no longer than 6 to 8 weeks with most cases resolving in 2 to 3 weeks. Cases lasting longer than 8 weeks are deemed chronic. Most cases of diarrhea in the United States are acute and self-limited. Still, diarrheal illnesses remain a major cause of morbidity and mortality worldwide.

ETIOLOGY AND PATHOGENESIS

Diarrhea develops secondary to abnormal fluid and electrolyte transport and altered intestinal motility. The major mechanisms of diarrhea include unusual amounts of poorly absorbable solute in osmotic diarrhea, abnormal ion absorption or ion secretion in secretory diarrhea, inflammatory processes, and abnormal intestinal motility.

In the normal state, in a 24-hour period, approximately 8 to 10 L of fluid enter the duodenum from a combination of dietary intake and gut secretions. Two thirds of the fluid is reabsorbed in the duodenum, and one third enters the proximal jejunum. Of the 10 L of fluid entering the small intestine, only 1,500 mL is presented to the colon. The small intestine has chloride (Cl^-) and bicarbonate (HCO_3^-) transport mechanisms that reduce the concentration of Cl^- and increase the concentration of HCO_3^- so that concentrations of these ions reflect the plasma concentrations. The colon absorbs the majority of the fluid with only 100 mL being excreted in a 24-hour period. The colon has active transport mechanisms that efficiently extract sodium (Na^+) and fluid and secrete potassium (K^+). Magnesium (Mg^{2+}) and calcium (Ca^{2+}) are poorly absorbed in the colon. The excreted stool product contains 3 mmol of Na^+, 8 mmol of K^+, and 2 mmol of Cl^-.

Osmotic diarrhea is the result of osmotically active, nonabsorbable solutes accumulating in the gut lumen, causing intraluminal salt and water retention. A classic feature of osmotic diarrhea is cessation of the diarrhea with fasting or if the individual stops ingestion of the osmotically active agent. In osmotic diarrhea, the electrolyte content of the excreted stool is normal and does not account for the total fecal osmolality. The difference between measured and calculated osmoles is termed the *osmotic gap*, and calculated by doubling the fecal sodium and potassium concentrations and subtracting the value from the plasma osmolality: Osmotic gap = 290 mosm/L − [2 x (fecal Na^+ + K^+)].

The normal stool osmotic gap is less than 125 mosm/dL and is usually less than 60. A fecal osmotic gap greater than 60 is suggestive of an osmotic diarrhea. In the setting of osmotic diarrhea, the osmotic gap it is usually greater than 125.

In contrast to osmotic diarrhea, secretory diarrhea does not abate during fasting. There may be a decrease in the stool volume and stool weight but not cessation of diarrhea as would be expected for osmotic diarrhea. In secretory diarrhea, there is a net luminal secretion of water and electrolytes into the gut, and the osmotic gap is less than 60.

Inflammatory diarrhea is characterized by the exudation of blood, mucus, pus, or serum proteins in the stool. This results in increased stool weight and diarrhea.

Abnormal intestinal motility may cause diarrhea secondary to rapid intestinal transit or by slow intestinal transit with stasis and resultant bacterial overgrowth.

CLINICAL PRESENTATION

Individuals presenting with diarrhea usually complain of frequent, loose, watery stools. They often seek medical attention because of accompanying dehydration, abdominal discomfort, fever, vomiting, gastrointestinal bleeding, pus in the stool, or chronicity of symptoms. It is crucial to characterize the patient's stool pattern and associated symptoms to guide the diagnostic approach.

DIFFERENTIAL DIAGNOSIS

The differential diagnosis for both acute and chronic diarrhea is extensive. Either may be caused by infectious agents. Pathogens commonly associated with acute infectious diarrhea include *Salmonella*, *Shigella*, enterohemorrhagic *Escherichia coli*, *Campylobacter*, rotaviruses, and Norwalk agent (Figure 44-2). *Vibrio cholera* and *Cyclospora* are less frequent causes of acute diarrhea. Microsporidia and Cryptosporidium can cause acute diarrhea and are more likely to affect immunocompromised individuals. *Clostridium difficile* is the agent most frequently associated with nosocomial diarrhea and antibiotic-associated diarrhea. Common causes of chronic infectious diarrhea include giardiasis, strongyloidiasis, and amebiasis.

Ischemic colitis is a noninfectious cause of acute diarrhea and occurs more frequently in the middle aged or elderly with significant peripheral vascular disease and/or atherosclerotic heart disease. Several medications, including nonsteroidal inflammatory agents, digitalis, vasopressin, and diuretics, have been associated with ischemic colitis.

Osmotic diarrhea with carbohydrate malabsorption from lactase deficiency is seen in lactose intolerance. An osmotic mechanism also underlies excessive sorbitol intake, lactulose use, fructose intake, ingestion of magnesium-containing compounds (laxatives, antacids, or supplements) and intestinal mucosal disease such as celiac sprue or gluten intolerance.

Enterotoxins identified as causes of secretory diarrhea include those produced by *E. coli* and *V. cholerae*. Senna-containing laxatives, and bisacodyl, vasoactive intestinal peptide, calcitonin, substance P, gastrin, serotonin, and prostaglandins also produce secretory diarrhea. Parasitic infection in giardiasis, strongyloidosis, and amebiasis can cause secretory diarrhea. Congenital chloridorrhea is due to a secretory stimulus secondary to a mucosal ion transport defect. Bile acid malabsorption, microscopic colitis, collagenous colitis, hyperthyroidism, medullary carcinoma of the thyroid gland, and collagen vascular diseases such as

systemic lupus erythematosus and scleroderma are additional causes of secretory diarrhea.

Inflammatory bowel disease (secondary to Crohn's disease, ulcerative colitis, or Behcet's disease) results in an exudative or inflammatory diarrhea (see Chapter 48, Figures 48-3 and 48-4). Inflammatory diarrhea also occurs as a complication of chemotherapeutic agents, radiation therapy, microscopic colitis, collagenous colitis, and graft-versus-host disease. Parasitic infections, viral agents, and bacterial pathogens may cause inflammatory diarrhea.

Abnormal intestinal motility underlies the functional diarrhea experienced with irritable bowel syndrome (IBS). Constipation may alternate with diarrhea in IBS. Typically, the diarrhea of IBS is associated with mucus production in the absence of inflammatory markers. The nocturnal diarrhea experienced by some patients with advanced diabetes mellitus is caused by deranged intestinal motility.

DIAGNOSTIC APPROACH

The initial evaluation of patients with both acute and chronic diarrhea should include a detailed history that includes the duration of symptoms, hydration status, severity of illness, travel history, exposure to potentially contaminated food or water, contact with ill individuals, recent use of antibiotics, medication use, and the immune status of the individual.

The physical examination should focus on findings usually observed in dehydration, such as orthostasis, dry mucous membranes, and poor skin turgor. The abdominal examination may demonstrate evidence of peritoneal inflammation, especially when the underlying cause is enteroinvasive infection. A rectal examination should be performed to assess for fistulas and abscesses.

The diagnostic evaluation of acute diarrhea should include stool examination for fecal leukocytes and fecal occult blood testing. Routine stool cultures are probably of little value in healthy individuals who lack fecal leukocytes and fecal occult blood. Similarly, stool cultures are of limited benefit in cases of nosocomial diarrhea. *C. difficile* is the most likely offending agent in the nosocomial setting and is effectively diagnosed with enzyme-linked immunosorbent assays for toxin A. Stool culture specimens should be obtained from immunocompromised individuals and from persons with

Figure 44-1

Diarrhea

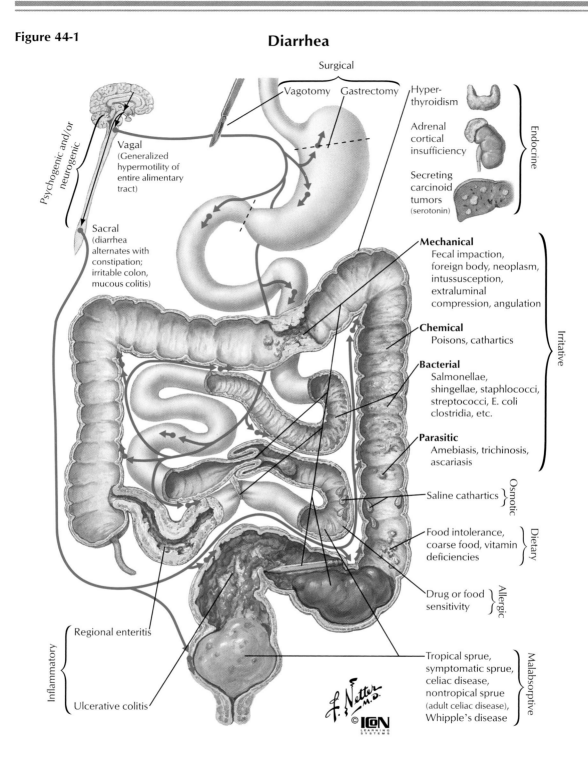

Surgical

Vagotomy Gastrectomy

Hyper-thyroidism

Adrenal cortical insufficiency

Secreting carcinoid tumors (serotonin)

Endocrine

Psychogenic and/or neurogenic

Vagal (Generalized hypermotility of entire alimentary tract)

Sacral (diarrhea alternates with constipation; irritable colon, mucous colitis)

Mechanical
Fecal impaction, foreign body, neoplasm, intussusception, extraluminal compression, angulation

Chemical
Poisons, cathartics

Bacterial
Salmonellae, shingellae, staphlococci, streptococci, E. coli clostridia, etc.

Parasitic
Amebiasis, trichinosis, ascariasis

Irritative

Saline cathartics — Osmotic

Food intolerance, coarse food, vitamin deficiencies — Dietary

Drug or food sensitivity — Allergic

Regional enteritis

Inflammatory

Ulcerative colitis

Tropical sprue, symptomatic sprue, celiac disease, nontropical sprue (adult celiac disease), Whipple's disease — Malabsorptive

Figure 44-2

Bacillary Dysentery

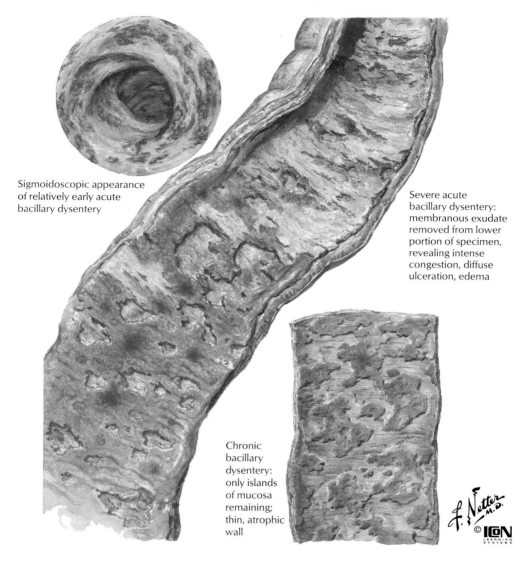

Sigmoidoscopic appearance
of relatively early acute
bacillary dysentery

Severe acute
bacillary dysentery:
membranous exudate
removed from lower
portion of specimen,
revealing intense
congestion, diffuse
ulceration, edema

Chronic
bacillary
dysentery:
only islands
of mucosa
remaining;
thin, atrophic
wall

known Crohn's disease or ulcerative colitis. Infectious agents can cause an acute exacerbation of diarrhea in patients with known inflammatory bowel disease. The role of endoscopy is usually limited in the evaluation of acute diarrhea; however, flexible sigmoidoscopy is helpful if ischemic colitis is suspected. The demonstration of pseudomembranes on endoscopic examination is diagnostic of C. difficile colitis and may be especially beneficial in patients who are clinically toxic.

Recommended laboratory testing for chronic diarrhea includes a complete blood cell count to evaluate for inflammation and serum electrolytes with blood urea nitrogen and creatinine to determine fluid status. Stool analysis for fecal leukocytes is helpful in differentiating inflammatory from noninflammatory diarrhea. Calculation of the stool osmotic gap helps to differentiate osmotic from secretory diarrhea. Fecal occult blood, when present, is suggestive of an inflammatory process. The determination of fecal fat helps to differentiate malabsorption. The Sudan fat stain provides a qualitative assessment and the 72-hour fecal fat level, a quantitative one. A fecal fat concentration greater than 7 g per 24 hours is consistent with a malabsorptive process. Measuring the stool pH may be beneficial in diagnosing carbohydrate malabsorption (pH of less than 5.6).

Endoscopy has a greater role in chronic diarrhea than in acute diarrhea. Lower endoscopy, flexible sigmoidoscopy, or colonscopy with biopsies can be helpful in the diagnosis of Crohn's disease, ulcerative colitis, microscopic colitis, and collagenous colitis. Esophogastroduodenoscopy, with biopsy specimens taken from the proximal duodenum, is the gold standard for confirming celiac disease or gluten intolerance. In the setting of chronic diarrhea, if the evaluation has been extensive and a diagnosis has not been established, factitious diarrhea should be considered and the stool should be analyzed for laxative use.

MANAGEMENT AND THERAPY

The management and therapy of diarrhea are based on the etiology of the disease. Most cases of acute diarrhea are self-limited and do not require therapy beyond supportive care with attention to fluid intake to prevent dehydration. Oral rehydration solutions consisting of sodium chloride, sodium bicarbonate, potassium chloride, and sucrose or glucose are designed to use the intestinal sodium-glucose transport system to promote water absorption and thereby decrease the risk of dehydration. Symptomatic therapy with loperamide or diphenoxylate can be considered for acute diarrhea if the stool is nonbloody and there is no fever. In general, empiric antibiotic therapy does not significantly alter the course of acute diarrhea. Empiric antibiotics are generally reserved for patients with bloody diarrhea, fever, and increased fecal leukocytes with associated dehydration. Such patients, who have often been symptomatic for 1 week or more, may require hospitalization. Antibiotic therapy should also be considered in immunocompromised hosts. Probiotic bacteria may be beneficial in reestablishing the intestinal flora with nonpathogenic organisms and in shortening the length of diarrhea in traveler's diarrhea and C. difficile infection.

The treatment of chronic diarrhea is guided by the etiology of the disease or disorder and the symptoms. Cases of chronic diarrhea of unknown etiology are often challenging. Loperamide can be used long term for symptomatic relief. Diphenoxylate, codeine, and tincture of opium should be used with caution because dependency may develop with the long-term use of these agents. Fiber supplementation or bulking agents such as polycarbophil can be beneficial for decreasing stool fluidity.

FUTURE DIRECTIONS

Current research includes the clinical investigation of serotonin 5-hydroxytryptamine 3 (5-HT3) antagonists for the management of diarrhea-predominant IBS. Alosetron is a highly selective 5-HT3 antagonist that was removed from the market in November 2000 due to potential serious side effects. Recently the FDA reapproved use of alosetron for diarrhea-predominant IBS when prescribed by practitioners knowledgeable of the side-effect profile and with close patient monitoring as recommended by the manufacturer.

Receptor antagonists of the M3 category, such as darifenacin and zamifenacin, are being investigated for possible clinical use in the management of diarrhea-predominant IBS.

Galanin is a neuropeptide with receptors expressed on colonic epithelial cells. Expression of galanin-1 receptors has been shown to be increased via activation of NF-kB in diarrhea caused by rotavirus. Rotavirus is the most frequent cause of severe diarrheal illness worldwide. Animal studies have confirmed the importance of galanin in the regulation of intestinal fluid secretion during rotavirus infection. Future research may provide crucial information for the control of viral diarrhea.

REFERENCES

American Gastroenterological Association medical position statement: guidelines for the evaluation and management of chronic diarrhea. *Gastroenterology.* 1999;116:1461–1463.

Camilleri M. Management of the irritable bowel syndrome. *Gastroenterology.* 2001;120:652–668.

DuPont HL. Guidelines on acute infectious diarrhea in adults. The Practice Parameters Committee of the American College of Gastroenterology. *Am J Gastroenterol.* 1997;92:1962–1975.

Eherer AJ, Fordtran JS. Fecal osmotic gap and pH in experimental diarrhea of various causes. *Gastroenterology.* 1992; 103:545–551.

Shaw R, Hempson S, Matkowsky J, Benya R. Galani-1 receptor expression contributes to rotavirus diarrhea [abstract 638]. *Gastroenterology.* 2002;122(suppl 1):A-76.

Chapter 45

Gastroesophageal Reflux Disease

Nicholas J. Shaheen and Melissa Rich

Gastroesophageal reflux disease (GERD) is one of the most common disorders encountered in medical practice. Almost half of Americans suffer heartburn symptoms at least once a month and greater than 10% experience heartburn weekly. Once considered a "nuisance problem," GERD is now associated with several serious conditions, including esophageal strictures, asthma, and esophageal adenocarcinoma. The toll of reflux on quality of life can be substantial. Patients with GERD sometimes rate their quality of life as worse than those with severe chronic diseases such as angina and mild heart failure. For these reasons, clinicians should be aggressive in the management of this disease.

ETIOLOGY AND PATHOGENESIS

The pathophysiology of GERD is complex and multifactorial. The body has developed an elegant system of defense mechanisms that allows it to keep gastric acid with a pH of 1 to 2 in proximity to sensitive esophageal tissues. Even minor perturbations of this defense may result in acid injury from reflux.

To a minor degree, reflux occurs in most individuals. However, small amounts of acid refluxate are usually neutralized by salivary secretions and propelled back into the stomach by peristalsis. In GERD, several deficiencies in this defense system are often present. Patients with severe GERD, on average, have *decreased lower esophageal sphincter (LES) pressure* compared with normal subjects, although there is much overlap between normal subjects and those with reflux. Perhaps more importantly, these subjects have an *increased number of transient lower esophageal relaxations*. Although these short periods of sphincter relaxation occur in normal individuals as well as in those with reflux, those with reflux appear to have them more commonly and also have a higher incidence of reflux during the relaxations than normal. *Hiatal hernia,* or displacement of the stomach through the hiatus so that part of the stomach is in the chest, occurs commonly in those with GERD, impairing the efficiency of the LES. Some patients demonstrate *impaired peristalsis,* decreasing their ability to propel the refluxate back into the stomach. Other mechanisms, such as differences in the potency and composition of the refluxate, are postulated but less well understood.

Some manifestations of GERD, including esophagitis, esophageal peptic strictures, and Barrett's esophagus, occur only in those with the most severe disease (Figure 45-1).

Esophagitis is the breakdown of mucosal tissue, so that erosions, exudates, and ulcers replace the normal squamous epithelium. Esophageal peptic stricture, or narrowing of the esophagus secondary to chronic acid exposure, sometimes requires endoscopic dilatation and, rarely, surgery. Barrett's esophagus is a metaplastic change of the lining of the esophagus so that it switches from its normal squamous epithelium to a columnar epithelium with goblet cells. It appears that chronic acid exposure is a necessary prerequisite in the pathogenesis. However, because many subjects with severe GERD never get Barrett's esophagus, other poorly understood host factors must also play a role.

CLINICAL PRESENTATION

Heartburn, or substernal chest burning, is the most common clinical presentation (Figure 45-2). This sensation is often worse when recumbent or after a large meal. Regurgitation of food, water brash (a filling of the mouth with saliva), dysphagia (difficulty swallowing), odynophagia (pain with swallowing), and chest pain are also common.

Recently, there has been an increased appreciation for the extra-esophageal manifestations of reflux. GERD may cause a variety of pulmonary and ear, nose, and throat conditions, including asthma, bronchitis, chronic cough, halitosis, hoarseness, pulmonary fibrosis, aspiration pneumonia, and erosion of the dental enamel.

Figure 45-1   ## Complications of Peptic Reflux (Esophagitis and Stricture)

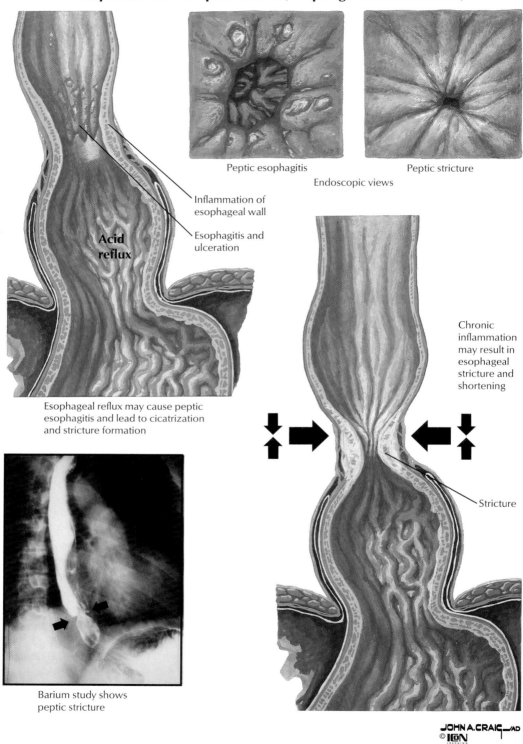

Peptic esophagitis

Peptic stricture

Endoscopic views

Inflammation of
esophageal wall

Esophagitis and
ulceration

**Acid
reflux**

Esophageal reflux may cause peptic
esophagitis and lead to cicatrization
and stricture formation

Chronic
inflammation
may result in
esophageal
stricture and
shortening

Stricture

Barium study shows
peptic stricture

JOHN A. CRAIG—AD
©ICN

Figure 45-2

Symptoms and Medical Management of Sliding Esophageal Hiatus Hernia

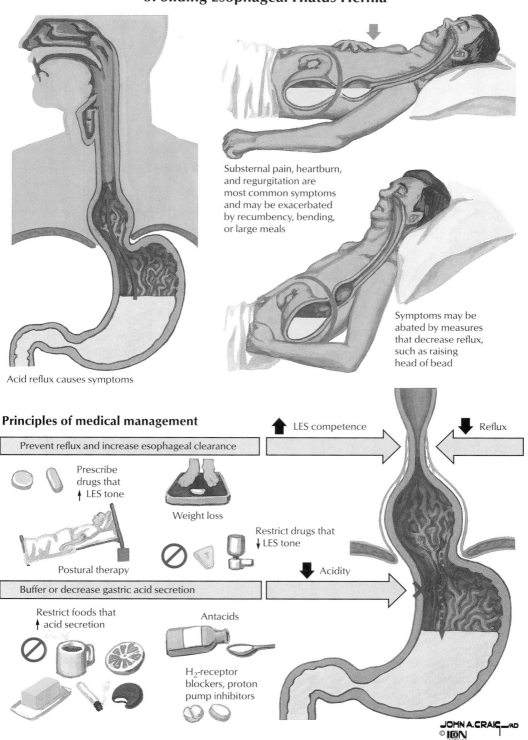

Substernal pain, heartburn, and regurgitation are most common symptoms and may be exacerbated by recumbency, bending, or large meals

Symptoms may be abated by measures that decrease reflux, such as raising head of bead

Acid reflux causes symptoms

Principles of medical management

Prevent reflux and increase esophageal clearance

Prescribe drugs that ↑ LES tone

Weight loss

Restrict drugs that ↓ LES tone

Postural therapy

Buffer or decrease gastric acid secretion

Restrict foods that ↑ acid secretion

Antacids

H_2-receptor blockers, proton pump inhibitors

LES competence

Reflux

Acidity

JOHN A. CRAIG—AD
© ICON

DIFFERENTIAL DIAGNOSIS

The presentation of GERD can be similar to many other conditions. Patients with heart disease may describe their chest pain as "burning." Among those complaining of chest pain, ruling out cardiac disease, especially in high-risk subgroups, is essential. Dysphagia is associated with esophageal cancer and esophageal strictures. The extra-esophageal symptoms of GERD may be especially hard to recognize. GERD-induced asthma is a commonly missed diagnosis and should be considered in patients who do not respond as expected to therapies directed at asthma.

DIAGNOSTIC APPROACH

Most individuals with classic reflux symptoms do not require further diagnostic workup beyond a good history and physical (Figure 45-2). In these patients, an empiric trial of anti-acid therapy may be used as both a diagnostic and therapeutic measure. Appropriate response to therapy confirms the diagnosis and obviates further workup.

Invasive workup in reflux disease is generally reserved for three categories of patients: those with "alarm symptoms" (dysphagia, weight loss, bleeding, and anemia); those with uncommon or unclear presentations, in whom the diagnosis is uncertain; and those who do not demonstrate the expected clinical response to therapy.

Several tests are available to evaluate symptoms (Figure 45-3). *Upper endoscopy* is a sensitive test for assessing mucosal damage and detecting strictures and cancers. Normal results of upper endoscopy do not rule out GERD, as many patients will have non-erosive reflux disease. The *24-hour pH probe* is a small tube placed through the nare into the esophagus. It continually monitors and electronically records esophageal acid exposures, allowing the clinician to note the extent of reflux, how high up the esophagus the reflux travels, and the relation of reflux episodes to other symptoms such as cough or wheezing. *Esophageal manometry* assesses the contractions of the esophagus and the function of the LES. Because many patients will have normal esophageal motility, it is not sensitive for reflux. *Barium radiographs* are excellent for identifying the presence and extent of esophageal strictures or cancer, but are not sensitive or specific for the presence of reflux. Other tests, such as the Bernstein acid perfusion test, scintigraphy, and esophageal impedance studies, either lack specificity or are not commonly available.

Some authorities advocate a once-in-a-lifetime upper endoscopy for those with chronic reflux symptoms, both to screen for adenocarcinoma and to identify those with Barrett's esophagus who might then be enrolled in endoscopic surveillance programs to identify any resultant cancer at an early and potentially curable stage. Neither the efficacy nor cost-effectiveness of such a screening endoscopy has been substantiated.

MANAGEMENT AND THERAPY

The goal of management is complete relief of symptoms. Given the armamentarium of medical and surgical therapies available, this goal is achievable in most patients.

Conservative Therapy

Some GERD patients may respond to simple dietary and lifestyle modifications (Figure 45-2). *Elevating the head of the bed*, preferably on blocks, is a simple measure that is especially effective in those with nighttime symptoms. *Weight loss* reduces intraabdominal pressure and may reduce symptoms. *Avoidance of late night meals* gives the stomach adequate time to empty before recumbency. Smoking decreases LES pressure, and *smoking cessation* may improve symptoms. *Caffeine, fatty foods*, and *alcohol may all decrease LES pressure*, and limited intake of these items is recommended.

Pharmacologic Therapy

For those with very occasional GERD symptoms precipitated by dietary indiscretion, self-medication with either antacids or over-the-counter H_2 receptor antagonists appears safe and is widely practiced. Patients with severe or frequent symptoms require more intensive therapy. Both *H_2 receptor antagonists,* such as cimetidine, ranitidine, famotidine, and nizatidine, and *proton pump inhibitors,* such as omeprazole, pantoprazole, rabeprazole, lansoprazole, and esomeprazole, may provide symptomatic relief. The proton pump inhibitors are more effective at decreasing acid production than the H_2 receptor antagonists, but are more expensive. Some authorities have advocated a "step-up" approach to therapy with these agents, whereby the clinician starts by treating with an H_2

Figure 45-3

Diagnostic Techniques

Esophagography

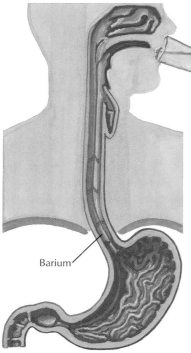

Barium

Barium esophagography demonstrates hernia, stricture, ulcer, or other complications in patients with symptomatic reflux

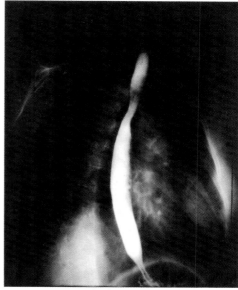

Barium contrast study shows normal esophagus and esophagogastric junction

Endoscopy

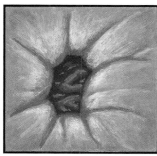

Normal esophagogastric junction

Sliding esophageal hiatus hernia

Endoscopic views

Endoscopy demonstrates esophagitis

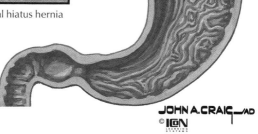

JOHN A. CRAIG—AD
© ICN

receptor antagonist and "steps up" therapy to a proton pump inhibitor only in patients unresponsive to the H$_2$ receptor antagonist. Others advocate a "step-down" approach so that therapy is initiated with a proton pump inhibitor to achieve symptom control, and then the patient is stepped down to the lowest level of acid inhibition that still provides good symptom control. No matter which strategy is adopted, it is important to assess symptom response shortly after the initiation of therapy and to adjust the medication regimen appropriately.

Rarely, patients will not achieve good symptom control with standard doses of proton pump inhibitors. In those situations, the dose of the proton pump inhibitor may be increased to twice a day. If the patient continues to be unresponsive, the clinician should question the diagnosis and consider further workup. If twice-a-day proton pump inhibitors do not control GERD, the addition of a nighttime H$_2$ receptor antagonist to the two doses of proton pump inhibitor or a third dose of proton pump inhibitor may help. Use of a *promotility agent* in addition to the anti-acid regimen is reasonable. Unfortunately, few agents are available. Metoclopramide use is limited. Cisapride is also effective, but safety concerns have curtailed its use and availability. Other promotility agents may soon be available. Sucralfate, a *mucosal coating agent,* may be used either alone or in combination with acid inhibition, but its frequent dosing interval and efficacy make it a less commonly used drug in reflux.

Duration of therapy is a commonly overlooked issue in reflux disease. GERD is a chronic condition often requiring chronic therapy. In the subgroup of patients with erosive esophagitis, the majority of those healed with medication will have recurrence of their esophagitis if taken off therapy. In these patients, symptom control after initial treatment may be maintained with less intensive therapy. For instance, a patient initially requiring proton pump inhibitors to heal erosive esophagitis may stay symptom- and disease-free on H$_2$ receptor antagonists.

Surgical Therapy

A surgical anti-reflux procedure for control of symptoms may be considered for patients requiring chronic pharmacologic therapy, especially high-dose proton pump inhibition. *Laparoscopic Nissen fundoplication* is the most common anti-reflux surgical procedure performed in the United States. The recovery time is short, and the procedure is generally well tolerated. Studies indicate that most patients obtain symptom relief and are not taking anti-reflux medications at 2 years. Long-term outcomes are less clear; data suggest that operator experience and appropriate patient selection are key to improving outcomes.

Recently, the FDA approved two devices for endoscopic manipulation of the LES area to relieve reflux symptoms. The first, an endoscopic sewing device, places a suture in the LES that tightens it, thereby decreasing reflux. It has demonstrated some promise in treating mild-to-moderate reflux. The second device delivers high radiofrequency waves into the LES, causing fibrosis and tightening of the LES, as well as destruction of nerves that mediate LES relaxation. This device has demonstrated short-term improvement in symptoms and decreased acid reflux as demonstrated by 24-hour pH probe data. It remains to be seen if either device will provide durable relief of reflux.

FUTURE DIRECTIONS

Several avenues hold promise for improving care of patients with reflux. Several new promotility agents are under development and are likely to be useful in GERD. Endoscopic alterations of the anatomy offer the chance to improve symptoms without subjecting the patient to surgery. Better treatments for the complications of reflux, such as strictures and Barrett's esophagus, may decrease the number of subjects who suffer the most severe manifestations of this disease. Finally, objective analysis of our practices in caring for the reflux patient should allow us to recognize the most cost-effective approaches to therapy.

REFERENCES

Kahrilas PJ. Gastroesophageal reflux disease. *JAMA.* 1996;276(12):983–988.

Katz PO. Treatment of gastroesophageal reflux disease: use of algorithms to aid in management. *Am J Gastroenterol.* 1999;94[11 Suppl]:S3–S10.

Nebel OT, Fornes MF, Castell DO. Symptomatic gastroesophageal reflux: Incidence and precipitating factors. *Am J Dig Dis.* 1976;21(11):953–956.

Pope CE. Acid-reflux disorders. *N Engl J Med.* 1994;331(10):656–660.

Szarka LA, DeVault KR, Murray JA. Diagnosing gastroesophageal reflux disease. *Mayo Clin Proc.* 2001;76(1):97–101.

Chapter 46

Giardiasis

Douglas R. Morgan

Giardia lamblia, the most common intestinal parasite worldwide, is a frequent cause of diarrhea and malabsorption. It is typically acquired through the ingestion of contaminated food and water, or person-to-person contact. Synonyms for *Giardia lamblia* include *G. intestinalis* and *G. duodenalis*.

Giardiasis occurs in sporadic, epidemic, and endemic forms. Sporadic infections are seen with international travel, rural camping, or person-to-person contact. Outbreaks have been reported with community water systems and in institutions such as day-care centers. Up to 35% of toddlers in day-care centers are infected, according to some studies. Giardiasis is endemic in the developing world. Studies based on stool specimens suggest that the prevalence is 2% to 5% in the developed world compared with 20% to 30% in the developing world. Infection occurs year-round, with a small peak in the spring in the United States. The annual incidence rate is approximately 10 per 100,000 population, based on Centers for Disease Control and Prevention surveillance data.

ETIOLOGY AND PATHOGENESIS

Phylogenetic analysis suggests that *G. lamblia* is a primitive eukaryote. This flagellated protozoan is an aerotolerant anaerobe. There are three species of giardia. *G. agilis* infects amphibians. *G. muris* infects birds and reptiles. *G. lamblia* infects many mammals in addition to humans, but it is unclear whether there are true animal reservoirs for the organism.

G. lamblia has two stages in its life cycle: cysts, the infectious form; and trophozoites, the replicating form.

The cyst form is inert and environmentally resistant, potentially viable for months outside the host. It is resistant to freezing and ultraviolet light. Water treatment, by filtration or boiling, prevents *G. lamblia* infections. The halogens (iodine, chlorine) also inactivate cysts under appropriate concentrations and exposure duration. The trophozoite is the motile form with four pairs of posteriorly directed flagellae. Trophozoites are adherent to the small bowel mucosa, possibly using the flagellae, or a

ventral surface adhesive disk. Replication occurs by binary fission within the intestine, with a doubling time of approximately 12 hours. Encystation occurs in the ileum, possibly triggered by exposure to bile, followed by cyst excretion in feces (Figure 46-1).

The pathogenesis of giardiasis remains ill-defined. Possible mechanisms include brush border disruption or villous blunting due to lymphocytic infiltration triggered by the infection. It is unlikely that pathogenesis is due to mucosal invasion or an associated enterotoxin. The humoral immune response is the primary mode of defense, and repeated exposure may induce partial immunity. Patients with hypogammaglobulinemia may have a more severe form of infection. Chronic infection may be related to strain differences, antigen variation, or limited antibody efficacy. Hypochlorhydria also predisposes to symptomatic infection. The disease course does not appear to be significantly altered in HIV infection.

CLINICAL PRESENTATION

G. lamblia, once thought to be commensal, is now known to be a definitive human pathogen. Transmission, primarily fecal-oral, occurs with contaminated water and food or via person-to-person contact. Contaminated surface water or shallow well water facilitates infection in the majority of patients. Such infections are manifest in the setting of community water system outbreaks, international travel, and camping. Deep wells provide adequate soil filtration. Spread via contaminated food is related to food handling and typically seen in restaurants, but also documented among office staff and at social events. Person-to-person transmission primarily occurs in day-care centers and among institutionalized patients. Infection may also occur via anal intercourse.

Figure 46-1   **Helminths and Protozoa Infesting the Human Intestine**

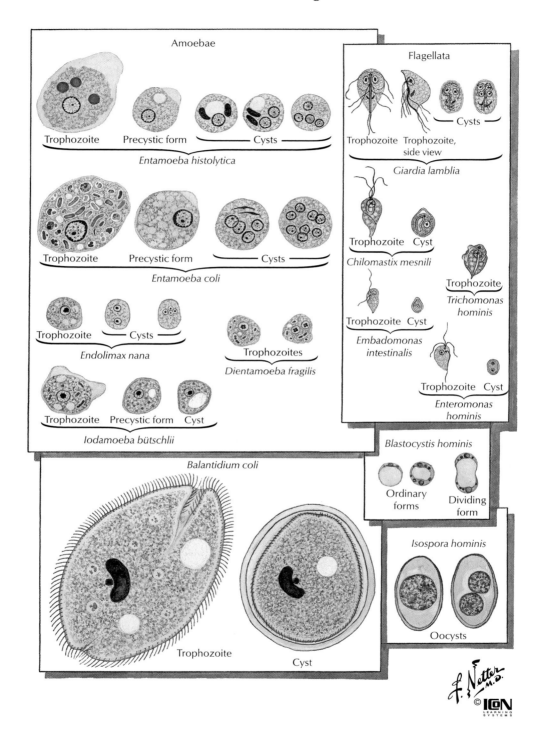

Determinants of disease severity remain an enigma. Infected patients are either asymptomatic (60%), have acute infection (40%), or have a chronic infection (40% of the acute infections). Approximately 10% of asymptomatic patients are cyst passers. A small percentage of chronically infected patients are initially without acute symptoms. Children and those with prior infection, particularly those from endemic areas, are more likely to have asymptomatic infection. The infectious inoculum may be as low as 10 to 25 cysts. The probability of symptomatic infection appears to be unrelated to the size of the innoculum. The incubation period is 1 to 2 weeks on average, with a range of 1 day to 6 weeks. Patients usually seek care following 1 to 2 weeks of symptoms, that is, 2 to 4 weeks following initial infection.

Protracted diarrhea is a central feature of giardiasis. Typically, stools are loose and foul-smelling and may contain mucus but not blood. Anorexia, nausea, abdominal cramping, bloating, and weight loss are common symptoms. Fever occurs in approximately 10% of patients. Lactose intolerance often persists for up to 4 weeks following eradication of the organism.

Patients chronically infected with *Giardia* typically have loose, but not watery stools, and associated malabsorption and weight loss. Malabsorption of vitamin B_{12}, folate, and protein may occur. For children in developing nations with chronic giardiasis, there are discordant studies regarding resultant growth and developmental delay. The extra-intestinal manifestations of giardiasis are rare and include urticaria, reactive arthritis, cholecystitis, cholangitis, and granulomatous hepatitis. Gastric infection has been documented in the setting of achlorhydria.

DIFFERENTIAL DIAGNOSIS

The primary focus in the evaluation of acute diarrhea is infectious agents. Important bacterial infections include *Salmonella, Shigella, Campylobacter, Yersinia,* and *Escherichia coli.* In the setting of antecedent antibiotic use, *Clostridium difficile* is a potential pathogen. Other parasitic infections include *Entamoeba histolytica* and *Cryptosporidium* (Figure 46-1). Viral enteritides are also common and include rotavirus and the Norwalk agent. Identification of high-risk groups such as institutionalized patients, international travelers, and patients with

HIV infection results in the highest yield from diagnostic studies. For acute diarrhea, dietary indiscretion, recent medication changes, and new-onset chronic diarrhea should be considered.

Chronic diarrhea has a broad differential diagnosis with a variety of classification schemes. Other infectious diseases may be considered, particularly for the returning international traveler. The differential diagnosis includes the inflammatory diarrheas (Crohn's disease), maldigestion (pancreatic insufficiency), and malabsorption (Whipple's disease, celiac sprue, bacterial overgrowth). Other considerations include systemic disease, lymphoma, medication side effects, and the rare tumor-related secretory diarrheas (gastrinoma, carcinoid tumor, vasoactive intestinal peptide-oma).

DIAGNOSTIC APPROACH

Examination of fecal specimens is the primary means for diagnosis. Many laboratories examine fresh fecal specimens with saline dilution for the identification of cyst and trophozoites. Diagnosis is usually made with the detection of cysts following specimen preservation and staining (trichrome, iron hematoxylin). Cyst passage in stool is sporadic, and 3 samples are recommended as sensitivity increases from 60% to 90% with examination of 1 to 3 specimens. The detection of fecal leukocytes or fecal fat varies. The presence of gross blood or hemoccult-positive stools typically implies another process.

Giardia antigen assays, using either immunofluorescent or ELISA technology, typically have single specimen sensitivities greater than 90%. Some laboratories now use antigen assays as the primary *Giardia* diagnostic test, but because of cost, their use is often limited to document infection clearance (in outbreak investigations) or screening within institutions. The submission of stool for ova and parasites also has the potential to detect other pathogens in the differential diagnosis.

In difficult cases, intestinal sampling or biopsy may be useful. Upper endoscopy with duodenal aspirate and mucosal biopsy is the alternative choice in difficult cases. While invasive, it is helpful for the evaluation of chronic diarrhea. Traditionally, the examination of stool specimens is more sensitive than upper endoscopy for giardiasis. A negative upper endoscopy result with aspirate and biopsy, in conjunction with three negative stool specimens, essentially rules out infection with *Giardia*.

Research and epidemiologic surveillance tools include serology, culture, and polymerase chain reaction techniques. These are not available clinically at present. Other laboratory testing or imaging studies are neither necessary nor useful. Of note, patients typically have neither leukocytosis nor eosinophilia.

MANAGEMENT AND THERAPY

Treatment is generally reserved for symptomatic patients or to prevent spread within institutions for asymptomatic patients (Table 46-1). Antibiotic susceptibility testing is not available, nor usually necessary. Metronidazole, although not approved by the US Food and Drug Administration, is currently the treatment of choice. Its side effects include nausea, headache, a metallic taste, and a disulfuram-like reaction. Tinidazole, also a nitroimidazole, is not available in the United States but is the most widely used antibiotic for giardiasis worldwide. It has the advantage of single-dose therapy. Furazolidone is often used for children because it is available in an elixir. Its efficacy is approximately 80%, and therefore a longer duration of therapy, up to 10 days, is recommended. The principal side effect is a mild hemolysis in patients with glucose-6-phosphatase deficiency. Other antibiotics, which have been evaluated in small studies, include albendazole and paromomycin. Quinacrine, which had been considered the drug of choice, is no longer available in the United States.

Treatment of giardiasis in pregnancy is difficult, and there are no consistent recommendations. For mild infection, treatment delay until the postpartum period is recommended. With significant symptomatic infection, paromomycin or metronidazole is often used. In giardiasis with persistent symptoms, lactose intolerance is the most likely etiology. For recurrent symptoms, infection relapse, other pathogens, or an alternative etiology should be considered.

The prevention of *Giardia* outbreaks in community water systems depends on adequate sedimentation, filtration, and possibly a higher chlorine concentration within the treated water. For individuals who have been camping or for international travelers, boiling (at least 10 minutes), filtration (pore size less than or equal to 2 μm), or halogens (chlorine,

Table 46-1
Treatment of Giardiasis

Medication	Dosage	Comments
Metronidazole	250 mg tid, 5 to 7 days	Recommended, not FDA approved
Furazolidone	100 mg qid, 5 to 10 days	Elixir available for children
Tinidazole	2 gm, single dose	Used worldwide, not available in US
Albendazole	400 mg bid, 5 days	Initial studies support efficacy
paromomycin	600 mg tid, 5 to 10 days	Consider in pregnancy

Note:
1) Quinacrine, previously considered the drug of choice, is no longer available in the US.
2) Preventive measures for water preparation for camping or international travel:
Filtration, 2 micron pore size or less; boiling, 10 minutes, minimum; halogenation, iodine or chlorine.

iodine) are recommended. Within day-care centers and other institutions, hand washing is important. In the absence of an outbreak, eradication is controversial. Breast-feeding is recommended because maternal IgA has been shown to be effective in preventing infection in infants.

FUTURE DIRECTIONS

Recent studies, which require validation, have suggested that specific *Giardia* genotypes predispose to acute and chronic diarrhea. Ongoing research will define the mechanisms of antimicrobial resistance as well as alternative therapies. A unified diagnostic pathway with a single stool specimen utilizing ELISA technology for the common parasitic pathogens will enhance evaluation efficiency.

REFERENCES

Farthing MJ. Giardiasis. *Gastroenterol Clin North Am.* 1996;25:493–515.
Hill DR. Giardia lamblia. In: Mandell GL, Bennett JE, Dolin R, eds. *Mandell, Douglas, and Bennett's Principles and Practice of Infectious Diseases.* 5th ed. Philadelphia, Pa: Churchill Livingstone; 2000.
Lengerich EJ, Addiss DG, Juranek DD. Severe giardiasis in the United States. *Clin Infect Dis.* 1994;18:760–763.
Ortega YR, Adam RD. Giardia: overview and update. *Clin Infect Dis.* 1997;25:545–549.

Chapter 47

Helicobacter Pylori Infection and Associated Disorders

Douglas R. Morgan

Helicobacter pylori, the most common chronic bacterial infection in the world, is associated with acute and chronic gastritis, peptic ulcer disease, gastric adenocarcinoma, and gastric lymphoma. Phylogenetic analysis suggests that the organism co-evolved with human beings, dating to the initial human migrations. After years of debate, Barry Marshall's pivotal work in the 1980s confirmed the presence of *H. pylori* in the stomach and its association with gastric disease.

Nearly half of the world's population is chronically infected with *H. pylori*. The infection is endemic in most of the developing world, affecting 50% of teenagers and 70% to 80% of adults, and in the developed world, 20% to 30% of adults. Childhood socioeconomic status is the strongest determinant of infection likelihood. Related risk factors include inadequate sanitation, crowded living conditions, and sibling infection. In the United States, there are significant racial differences with respect to infection (Table 47-1).

Person-to-person transmission, specifically, gastro-oral, is postulated as the mode of infection. Studies suggest that most infections are acquired by children younger than 5, with familial clustering. Viable organisms have also been isolated from feces and water supplies, suggesting that low-level sporadic transmission is possible. Adult infection in the developed world is uncommon, with an estimated rate of less than 1% per annum.

The decrease in *H. pylori* infections worldwide due to improved socioeconomic conditions has several implications. A phenomenon observed in both developing and developed nations is that older patients are more likely to be infected. This likely reflects childhood socioeconomic status rather than new adult infection. This explains, in part, the decrease in incidence in duodenal ulcers and gastric cancer in the developed world. Racial differences and decreasing prevalence support an individualized approach to dyspepsia.

ETIOLOGY AND PATHOGENESIS

H. pylori is a gram-negative spiral-shaped gastric organism. The bacteria inhabit the stomach mucosal surface without invasion. The usual organism burden in the stomach is 1 billion, with multiple quasi-species present within each individual. *H. pylori* infection triggers a robust host immune response, resulting in chronic active gastritis in the majority of infections. The organism uses a novel pH-dependent urea channel (UreI) and urease to generate ammonia and create a buffered microenvironment. The urease enzyme is produced at a higher level by *H. pylori* than by other bacteria and serves as the basis for many of the diagnostic tests.

The development of ulcer disease or cancer depends on the complex interaction at the gastric

H. Pylori Infection and Gastric Carcinogenesis
Host susceptible genotypes (e.g., Interleukin-1)
Childhood *H. pylori* infection
Interleukin-1-beta upregulation by *H. pylori*
Diffuse gastritis with achlorhydria
Atrophic gastritis
Environmental exposure (e.g., dietary, co-infections)
Microniche dysequilibrium: host, quasi-species
Intestinal metaplasia
Gastric dysplasia
Gastric adenocarcinoma

microniche level between host genetics, virulence factors, and the environment. Several virulence factors have been described for the organism, the most important of which is the cytotoxin-associated gene A (cagA), which increases the likelihood of both ulcer disease and cancer. There are several patterns of chronic active gastritis. Antral predominant gastritis is associated with peptic ulcers, and corpus gastritis with intestinal metaplasia and gastric adenocarcinoma (Figure 47-1).

CLINICAL PRESENTATION

The principal diseases associated with *H. pylori* infection are gastritis, acute and chronic; peptic ulcer disease; gastric adenocarcinoma; and low-grade B cell non-Hodgkin's lymphoma (mucosa-associated lymphoma [MALToma]).

Most infected persons have an asymptomatic chronic active gastritis. Dyspepsia is the hallmark of symptomatic infection. Initial infection with acute gastritis is self-limited, but may cause discomfort, halitosis, nausea, and vomiting. Transient achlorhydria often develops for 1 to 6 months.

H. pylori, the most important cause of peptic ulcer disease, is implicated in 75% of both duodenal and NSAID–negative gastric ulcers. The lifetime risk for an ulcer with infection is 5% to 20%. Active ulcer disease may cause epigastric pain, nausea, vomiting, and, if complicated, hemorrhage or obstruction. Eradication of *H. pylori* decreases the risk of ulcer recurrence, but less so than initially proposed. A meta-analysis of trials suggests that the duodenal ulcer recurrence rate with successful eradication is 20% at 6 months, versus 56% in untreated patients. Infection testing and treatment are strongly recommended for patients with past or current peptic ulcer disease.

The concept of antibiotic therapy for cancer prevention or cure is intriguing. Patients with *H. pylori*–related gastric cancer or MALToma usually have nonspecific symptoms until large tumors are present. While the etiology of gastric adenocarcinoma is multifactorial, *H. pylori* infection has a proven role, although neither necessary nor sufficient. Epidemiologic studies consistently suggest a relative risk increase of 3% to 9%, similar to the relation between tobacco and lung cancer. A definitive cancer prevention trial is difficult because 500,000 patient-years would be required. Cost effectiveness analyses recommend screening for high-risk patient populations: family history of gastric cancer and immigrants from high incidence regions (Asia, Latin America, Eastern Europe).

The majority of patients with gastric MALToma also have evidence of infection. Studies suggest that nearly 80% of patients with low-grade tumors attain remission with antibiotic therapy. Half of these patients demonstrate a persistent monoclonal B-cell clone, providing a cautionary note.

Controversial associations with *H. pylori* include nonulcer dyspepsia (NUD), gastroesophageal reflux (GERD), and synergistic effects with NSAIDs and proton pump inhibitors (PPIs). The majority of randomized controlled trials have failed to show benefit of eradication therapy for NUD, supporting the notion that it is a functional disease. This has important implications for the approach to uninvestigated dyspepsia. Some patients may derive benefit from antibiotic therapy, however, in general, eradication therapy cannot be recommended in NUD.

There may be an additive effect in peptic ulcer disease between *H. pylori* and NSAIDs. The current literature fails to provide a consensus regarding the benefit of testing and eradication before the initiation of chronic NSAID therapy. In the setting of a "dual" NSAID-*H. pylori* ulcer, eradication is indicated. Continued PPI therapy may be considered if ongoing NSAID use is needed. Similarly, subsequent studies have not substantiated the initial report of an increased risk of atrophic gastritis and, by inference, gastric cancer in infected patients treated with chronic PPI therapy. Currently, testing and treatment for *H. pylori* are not recommended before the initiation of chronic NSAID or PPI therapy.

Table 47-1
H. Pylori Seroprevalence in the US

RACE	ALL	AGE		
		20–30	*50–60*	*>70*
Whites	27	8	36	55
African American	51	38	54	73
Hispanic	58	49	63	74

Adapted from Everhart JE, Kruszon-Moran D, Perez-Perez GI, Tralka TS, McQuillan G. Seroprevalence and ethnic differences in Helicobacter pylori infection among adults in the United States. *J Infect Dis.* 2000;181:1359–1363.

Figure 47-1

Etiology and Pathogenesis of *Helicobacter Pylori*

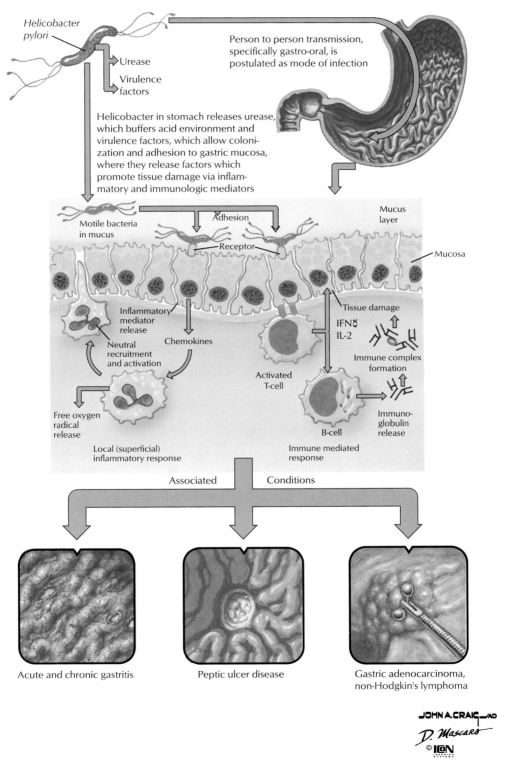

Helicobacter pylori

Urease

Virulence factors

Person to person transmission, specifically gastro-oral, is postulated as mode of infection

Helicobacter in stomach releases urease, which buffers acid environment and virulence factors, which allow colonization and adhesion to gastric mucosa, where they release factors which promote tissue damage via inflammatory and immunologic mediators

Motile bacteria in mucus

Adhesion

Mucus layer

Receptor

Mucosa

Inflammatory mediator release

Tissue damage

IFNɣ IL-2

Chemokines

Neutral recruitment and activation

Immune complex formation

Activated T-cell

Free oxygen radical release

B-cell

Immunoglobulin release

Local (superficial) inflammatory response

Immune mediated response

Associated   Conditions

Acute and chronic gastritis

Peptic ulcer disease

Gastric adenocarcinoma, non-Hodgkin's lymphoma

JOHN A. CRAIG—AD

D. Mascaro

© ICN

Figure 47-2 ### Diagnosis and Management of *Helicobacter Pylori*

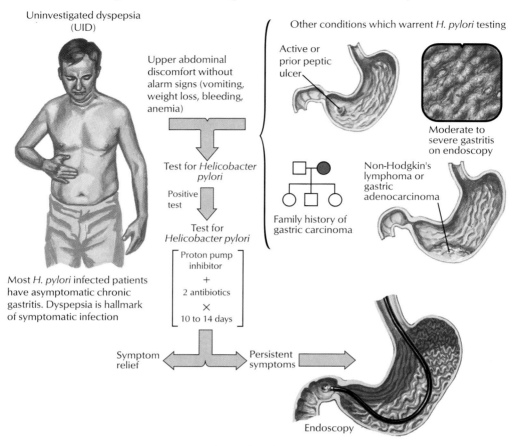

Uninvestigated dyspepsia
(UID)

Upper abdominal
discomfort without
alarm signs (vomiting,
weight loss, bleeding,
anemia)

Test for *Helicobacter
pylori*

Positive
test

Test for
Helicobacter pylori

Proton pump
inhibitor
+
2 antibiotics
×
10 to 14 days

Symptom
relief

Persistent
symptoms

Most *H. pylori* infected patients
have asymptomatic chronic
gastritis. Dyspepsia is hallmark
of symptomatic infection

Other conditions which warrent *H. pylori* testing

Active or
prior peptic
ulcer

Moderate to
severe gastritis
on endoscopy

Non-Hodgkin's
lymphoma or
gastric
adenocarcinoma

Family history of
gastric carcinoma

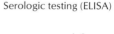

Endoscopy

Tests for *Helicobacter pylori*

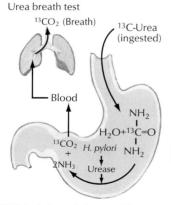

Urea breath test

$^{13}CO_2$ (Breath)

^{13}C-Urea
(ingested)

Blood

NH_2

$H_2O + ^{13}C=O$

$^{13}CO_2$ *H. pylori* NH_2
+
$2NH_3$ Urease

^{13}C-labeled urea is ingested if
H. pylori is present it provides
"urease" which splits off the
labeled CO_2 which is passed into
circulation and expired in breath
(active infection)

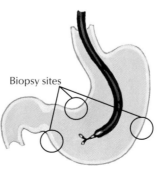

Endoscopy with biopsy

Biopsy sites

For patients undergoing upper
endoscopy, biopsy samples
submitted for histology or rapid
urea testing (RUT) histology is
gold standard (active infection)

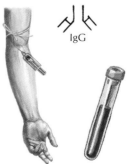

Serologic testing (ELISA)

IgG

Serology testing (ELISA) detects IgG
antibodies and documents past or
current infection, but not eradication

JOHN A. CRAIG—AD

D. Mascaro

© ICN
LEARNING SYSTEMS

Postulated extragastric manifestations of disease are more tenuous. Studies have yielded discordant results regarding the worsening of GERD and its complications in some patients following *H. pylori* treatment. In the moderate-to-severe GERD population, indications for initial testing should be clear, and patients with positive results, following discussion, should be offered treatment. Despite initial reports, there is little evidence for an association with coronary artery disease, stroke, iron deficiency anemia, rosacea, or growth delay.

DIFFERENTIAL DIAGNOSIS

Dyspepsia is broadly defined as the symptom of upper abdominal discomfort. The differential diagnosis includes peptic ulcer disease, gastric cancer, esophageal disease and GERD, myocardial ischemia, and hepatobiliary disease. *Nonulcer dyspepsia*, also known as functional or endoscopy negative dyspepsia, refers to pain in this region without alarm features, laboratory abnormalities, or findings on upper endoscopy. *Uninvestigated dyspepsia* (UID) refers to the initial presentation with epigastric pain or discomfort before evaluation. At upper endoscopy in patients with UID, approximately 15% each will have ulcer disease, esophageal disease, or gastritis, while the remaining 40% to 60% are negative, suggestive of nonulcer or self-limited dyspepsia.

The variety of approaches to UID include empiric acid suppression, immediate endoscopy, "test and treat," and "test and scope." The latter approaches refer to *H. pylori* testing with either treatment or endoscopy for positive results. The dominant strategy in the US is *test and treat*. Patients with new-onset dyspepsia, younger than 45 to 50, and without alarm signs or symptoms (vomiting, weight loss, bleeding, anemia) are tested for *H. pylori* infection and treated if results are positive. Persons with persistent symptoms are referred for endoscopy. Recent outcome studies support the efficacy of this approach. *Test and scope* is often used in Asia and Latin America where gastric cancer rather than ulcer disease is the main concern. Certain European centers use *immediate endoscopy* for UID. Small studies suggest that outcomes and patient satisfaction are slightly better with immediate endoscopy. If endoscopy costs in the US decrease, this may become a reasonable approach. *Empiric acid sup-*

pression for 1 to 2 months has returned to favor with the availability of PPIs. While the test-and-treat strategy is reasonable for most patients, the approach should be individualized with consideration of "test and scope" and immediate endoscopy based on symptoms, age, ethnicity, family history, and test availability.

DIAGNOSTIC APPROACH

Testing for *H. pylori* is suggested for those with active or prior peptic ulcer disease, UID, family history of gastric cancer, moderate-to-severe gastritis diagnosed on upper endoscopy, and gastric cancer or MALToma. All infected patients should be offered treatment.

Diagnostic tests include both noninvasive and invasive tests (Table 47-2). Serology (ELISA) detects IgG antibodies, documenting past or current infection, but not eradication. The urea breath tests (UBT) and stool antigen assay are "active tests," documenting operative infection. For patients undergoing upper endoscopy, gastric biopsy specimens may be submitted for either histologic studies or rapid urease testing (RUT). Histologic studies are the gold standard for testing. Both the UBT and RUT tests depend on the detection of bacterial urease activity. Culture of the organism remains difficult and is limited to the research setting.

In low prevalence populations, such as young whites in the US, the false-positive rate of serologic testing is unacceptable, and active testing is

Table 47-2
Diagnostic tests for *H. Pylori* Infection

Serology
ELISA, IgG Whole blood
Active tests

Urea breath tests
    ^{13}C, nonradioactive isotope
    ^{14}C, radioactive isotope
Stool antigen test

Endoscopy–based tests
Histopathology, gold standard Rapid urease tests

Table 47-3
Treatment Regimens

- PAC, bid

- PPI, clarithromycin (500 mg), amoxicillin (1g)

- PMC regimen, bid

- PPI, clarithromycin (250 to 500 mg), metronidazole (250 to 500mg)

- PBMT regimen, qid (bid PPI)

- PPI, metronidazole (250 mg), tetracycline (500 mg)

Note: PPI, proton pump inhibitor (omeprazole, esomeprazole, lansoprazole, pantoprazole, rabeprazole)

recommended, particularly the test-and-treat strategy for UID. Recent treatment (within 2 to 4 weeks) with any of the components of *H. pylori* treatment (PPIs, bismuth compounds, and antibiotics) decreases the sensitivity of all non-serologic tests.

In general, documentation of successful eradication is unnecessary. Confirmation of clearance is considered in patients with complicated peptic ulcer disease, gastric adenocarcinoma, MAL-Toma, persistent symptoms, and for those requesting such documentation. Active tests or endoscopy are used 6 weeks after treatment to avoid false-negative results in the immediate post-treatment period.

MANAGEMENT AND THERAPY

Optimal therapy for *H. pylori* infection requires a PPI with 2 antibiotics for 10 to14 days (Table 47-3). Offer treatment to all patients with positive diagnostic test results. The three principal regimens have similar efficacy of 80% to 85%.
- PAC regimen twice daily : PPI, clarithromycin (500 mg), amoxicillin (1 g).
- PMC regimen twice daily: PPI, clarithromycin (250 to 500 mg), metronidazole (250-500 mg).
- PBMT regimen qid (bid PPI): PPI, bismuth (525 mg), metronidazole (250 mg), tetracycline (500 mg).

The PAC regimen is the most common combination. The PMC combination is appropriate with penicillin allergy. The use of a PPI with the bismuth-based regimen significantly improves its efficacy. No significant difference is noted between PPIs. Prepackaged products may improve compliance. Use of other antibiotics such as rifabutin, furazolidone, and ciprofloxacin has been reported.

Eradication failure is usually due to patient non-compliance or antibiotic resistance. There is no significant resistance to either amoxicillin or tetracycline. Primary resistance rates with clarithromycin and metronidazole are 5% to 10% and 25% to 35%, respectively, with age, sex, racial, and regional differences. Higher resistance rates are noted in the elderly, females, and African Americans. Metronidazole resistance may be an in vitro effect and overcome with the use of bismuth or PPI. Clarithromycin resistance markedly decreases efficacy. PBMT is the principal retreatment regimen (Figure 47-2).

FUTURE DIRECTIONS

Ongoing research should provide insights into the mode of transmission, childhood infection, and immunology. New antibiotic regimens are expected. A combination pill that includes bismuth, metronidazole, and tetracycline is in clinical trials. A vaccine would provide the most cost-effective manner to prevent gastric cancer in high incidence regions of the developing world, but development has proved difficult due to the organism's genetic diversity. As *H. pylori* has co-evolved with humans, continued basic and clinical research will likely offer insights into the organism itself, other bacterial infections, and other human diseases.

REFERENCES

Howden CW, Hunt RH. Guidelines for the management of *Helicobacter pylori* infection. Ad Hoc Committee on Practice Parameters of the American College of Gastroenterology. *Am J Gastroenterol.* 1998;93:2330–2338.

Moran AP, ed. *Helicobacter 2001: Past, Present, and Future* [book on CD-ROM]. Englewood, NJ: Normed Verlag Inc; 2001.

Uemura N, Okamoto S, Yamamoto S, et al. *Helicobacter pylori* infection and the development of gastric cancer. *N Engl J Med.* 2001;345:784–789.

Veldhuyzen van Zanten SJ, Flook N, Chiba N, et al. An evidence-based approach to the management of uninvestigated dyspepsia in the era of *Helicobacter pylori.* Canadian Dyspepsia Working Group. *CMAJ.* 2000;162(suppl 12):S3–S23.

Chapter 48

Inflammatory Bowel Disease

Kim L. Isaacs

Inflammatory bowel disease (IBD) refers to idiopathic, chronic, relapsing inflammation of the gastrointestinal tract. IBD includes Crohn's disease and ulcerative colitis. The pathogenesis, clinical features, and treatments overlap.

Both ulcerative colitis and Crohn's disease are more common in individuals of Northern European origin with incidence rates from 5 to 12 per 100,000. The incidence of ulcerative colitis has remained fairly constant over the past 50 years. The incidence of Crohn's disease is increasing globally with the most marked changes from 1960 to 1987 with a recent plateau. The sex distribution is equal in ulcerative colitis; there is a slight female predominance in Crohn's disease. These diseases are more common in white, and Jewish, populations than in other groups. Both diseases show increased incidence in families, with 6% to 20% of patients having a positive family history of IBD. There is a high concordance of disease among monozygotic twins. As compared to a non-diseased population, those patients with Crohn's disease, have a higher prevalence of smokers while those with ulcerative colitis are more likely to be non-smokers. Environmental factors such as infections, toxin or drug exposure, and diet may play a permissive role in the development of disease. Specific agents such as NSAIDs and oral contraceptives have been implicated in Crohn's disease.

ETIOLOGY AND PATHOGENESIS

The etiology of ulcerative colitis and Crohn's disease is unknown. Studies indicate an interaction between genetic susceptibility, the host's immune response, and environmental influences. Once inflammation is initiated, there is a failure to down-regulate the immune response. Disordered immunoregulation is thought to occur in part through T cell responses. Bacteria and bacterial cell products have been implicated in pathogenesis. Recently, a *Nod2* gene mutation has been identified with increased frequency in patients with Crohn's disease. *Nod2* is responsible for immune system recognition and response to lipopolysaccharides in the outer membranes of certain bacteria.

Ulcerative colitis is a mucosal disease limited to the colon. It begins in the rectum and is contiguous throughout the bowel. There may be a sharp cutoff of normal and abnormal mucosa in the distal bowel, or the entire colon may be involved (pancolitis). The ileum is involved in 10% of patients with pancolitis (backwash ileitis). There are no skip lesions, although occasionally there will be a patch of inflammation in the cecum in patients with left-sided ulcerative colitis. Histologically, there is a neutrophilic infiltration with crypt abscess formation and crypt distortion. The inflammation is limited to the mucosal surface. There is foreshortening of the intestine and the development of pseudopolyps with healing.

In *Crohn's disease*, the inflammatory process may involve any part of the luminal GI tract from the mouth to the anus (Figure 48-1). The terminal ileum is affected in 70% to 80% of patients, either alone or in combination with colonic involvement. The inflammation is transmural and characterized by infiltration of the bowel wall with neutrophils, followed by mononuclear type cells and fibrous tissue. With chronicity, there is architectural distortion. In 60% of cases, non-caseating granulomas may be seen. Small aphthous ulcerations evolve into deep linear ulcerations and fissuring. Mucosal and submucosal fibrosis may lead to stricture formation. The disease is characterized by "skip lesions" with normal intervening mucosa. The serosa and mesentery exhibit reactive changes with thickening and fibrosis. Grossly "creeping fat" is noted along the serosal surface. The transmural nature of the disease along with the deep ulcerations and fissures lead to the complications of abscess and fistula formation.

CLINICAL PRESENTATION
Ulcerative Colitis

Patients typically present with bloody diarrhea and tenesmus. With rectal involvement, bleeding and constipation may be a presenting complaint. Other symptoms may include systemic symptoms, such as weight loss, fever, and anorexia; and localized abdominal cramping may occur with bowel movements. Steady constant pain in the absence of bowel movements suggests severe disease. In toxic dilatation, there are decreased bowel sounds and abdominal distension. Long-standing disease may present with a colonic malignancy. After 10 years of disease with pancolitis, the incidence of colon cancer increases at approximately 1% per year.

Crohn's Disease

The presentation of Crohn's disease depends on the affected location. In gastroduodenal disease, there are signs and symptoms that mimic peptic ulcer disease with mid-epigastric pain and nausea. In small bowel disease, pain is common; narrowing of the small bowel lumen may lead to obstructive symptoms with nausea, vomiting, abdominal distension, and pain. In ileal disease, non-bloody diarrhea occurs; patients with significant ileal disease may have vitamin B_{12} deficiency or bile salt diarrhea. Weight loss and nutrient malabsorption are common. Systemic symptoms include weight loss and fever; anemia and an elevated platelet count are more common than in ulcerative colitis. Growth retardation in children may be the presenting complaint.

Complications include abscess formation, enterocutaneous fistulas, and obstruction. Extraintestinal manifestations include axial or central and peripheral arthritis, pyoderma gangrenosum, erythema nodosum, iritis, episcleritis, sclerosing cholangitis, aphthous stomatitis, amyloidosis, gallstones, or kidney stones (Figures 48-2 and 48-3).

DIFFERENTIAL DIAGNOSIS

The differential diagnosis for ulcerative colitis includes infectious colitis from *Clostirdium difficile*, *Salmonella*, *Shigella*, *Campylobacter jejuni*, *Escherichia coli*, *Entamoeba histolytica*; radiation colitis; ischemic colitis; diverticulitis; Crohn's colitis; and lower GI bleeding from other causes such as hemorrhoids, malignancy, or polyps.

The differential diagnosis for Crohn's disease includes tuberculosis, appendicitis, lymphoma, pelvic inflammatory disease/tubo-ovarian abscess, ectopic pregnancy, *Yersinia entercolitica* infection, ulcerative jejunoileitis, Behçet's syndrome, chronic granulomatous disease, or sarcoidosis.

DIAGNOSTIC APPROACH

The clinical presentation dictates the types and timing of diagnostic testing. A stool specimen should be examined in patients presenting with a diarrheal illness. WBCs and blood are seen in ulcerative colitis and infectious colitis. Examination of stool culture specimens for bacterial pathogens, *C. difficile* toxin, and parasites will help rule out infectious etiologies. Comprehensive parasitic screening tests are required in anyone with a travel history or potential parasitic exposure. A qualitative stool fat helps identify a malabsorptive diarrhea.

Hematologic studies should include hemoglobin, white blood cell count, ESR, C-reactive protein, and albumin to help define the severity of disease. Serologic testing for antineutrophilic cytoplasmic antibody and anti-*Saccharomyces cerevisiae* antibody has limited diagnostic usefulness.

Sigmoidoscopy, colonoscopy, or both are useful in the diagnosis of colitis (Figure 48-4). Endoscopic evaluation can help determine the extent and severity of disease. Small bowel radiologic studies help with the diagnosis of small intestinal Crohn's disease with findings such as luminal narrowing, irregularity, and internal fistulous disease, as well as documenting the extent of small bowel involvement. In colitis, barium studies of the colon may show a shortened contracted bowel with a loss of bowel wall markings.

MANAGEMENT AND THERAPY
Principles of Therapy

The treatment of ulcerative colitis or Crohn's disease depends on disease location, extent of disease, and severity. Severe disease exacerbations may require inpatient hospitalization. Symptomatic and supportive treatment includes antidiarrheal agents, antispasmodic drugs, hydration, and nutritional support. The physical examination and clinical presentation should be targeted to determine whether signs and symptoms of toxicity and/or development of complications such

Figure 48-1

Regional Enteritis (Crohn's Disease)

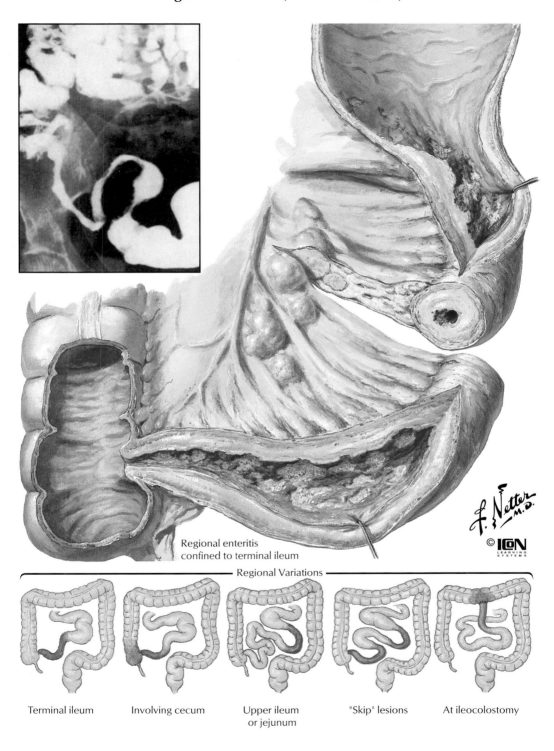

Regional enteritis
confined to terminal ileum

— Regional Variations —

| Terminal ileum | Involving cecum | Upper ileum or jejunum | "Skip" lesions | At ileocolostomy |

Figure 48-2

Regional Enteritis
(Crohn's Disease)

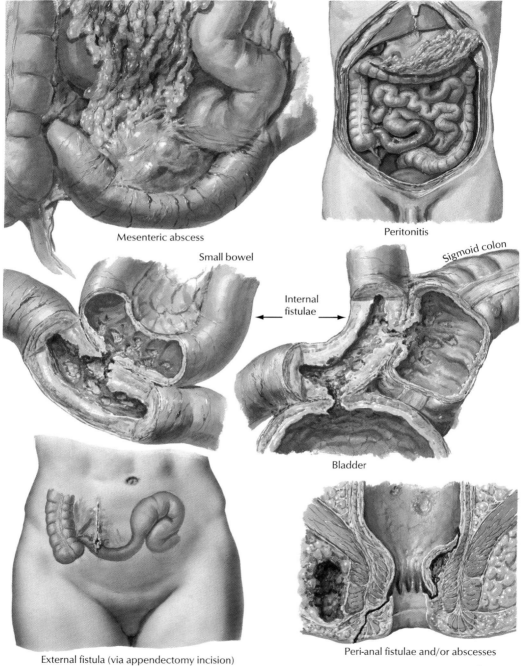

Mesenteric abscess

Peritonitis

Small bowel

Sigmoid colon

Internal fistulae

Bladder

External fistula (via appendectomy incision)

Peri-anal fistulae and/or abscesses

Figure 48-3

Extraintestinal Manifestations of Inflammatory Bowel Disease

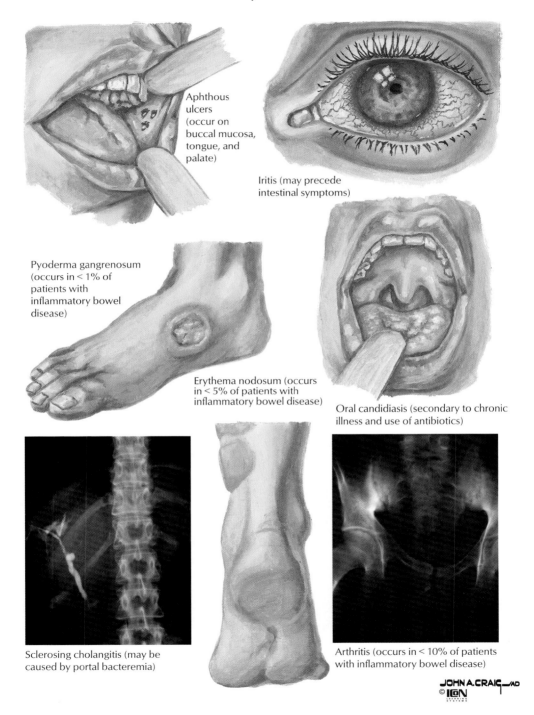

Aphthous ulcers (occur on buccal mucosa, tongue, and palate)

Iritis (may precede intestinal symptoms)

Pyoderma gangrenosum (occurs in < 1% of patients with inflammatory bowel disease)

Erythema nodosum (occurs in < 5% of patients with inflammatory bowel disease)

Oral candidiasis (secondary to chronic illness and use of antibiotics)

Sclerosing cholangitis (may be caused by portal bacteremia)

Arthritis (occurs in < 10% of patients with inflammatory bowel disease)

JOHN A. CRAIG—AD
© ICN

Figure 48-4

Inflammatory Bowel Disease: Colitis

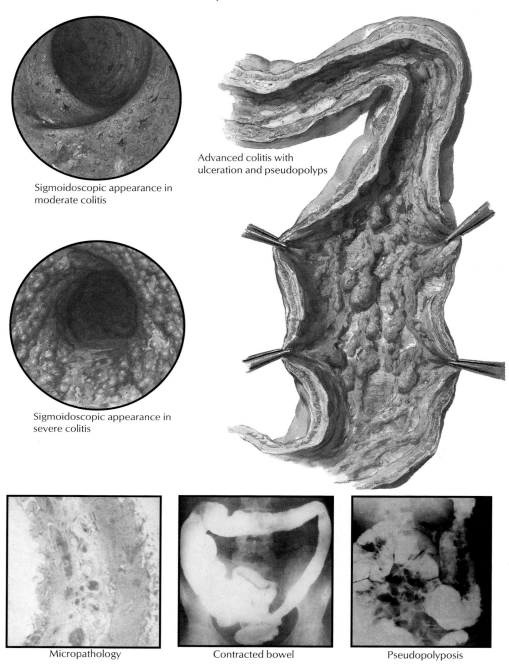

Sigmoidoscopic appearance in
moderate colitis

Advanced colitis with
ulceration and pseudopolyps

Sigmoidoscopic appearance in
severe colitis

Micropathology

Contracted bowel

Pseudopolyposis

as toxic dilatation, perforation, and abscess formation are present.

Specific Pharmacologic Therapy

In drug therapy, the goals are to use the least toxic drugs first, reduce long-term steroid use, and induce remission.

5-Aminosalicylates (5-ASAs), the first-line therapy in ulcerative colitis and Crohn's disease, are also useful in the maintenance of remission in ulcerative colitis. The 5-ASAs differ in the site and mechanism of release. Their activity is dose-dependent, and dosage escalation may enhance response to these agents.

Sulfasalazine is a 5-ASA bound to sulfapyridine by a diazo bond. Sulfapyridine is a carrier that prevents small bowel absorption. The diazo bond is broken down by bacteria in the colon, releasing 5-ASA and sulfapyridine. Side effects include nausea, vomiting, malaise, sun sensitivity, and rash, which may be caused by the sulfa component. Patients can be desensitized to some of these side effects. Male patients may experience a reduction in sperm count with decreased fertility. Agranulocytosis has also been described. Despite these potential problems, sulfasalazine is a very useful drug and may have benefit for arthritis in those patients with both bowel disease and arthritis.

Osalazine is a 5-ASA diamer in which the 5-ASAs are linked by a diazo bond, which is broken down by bacteria in the colon releasing the 5-ASAs. Up to 20% of patients may experience a secretory diarrhea, which limits its usefulness in treating colitis.

Oral mesalamine is available in a pH-dependent release form and a delayed release form. The delayed release form is delivered into the terminal ileum and colon. When the capsule opens in the ileum or colon, the drug is released. Standard dosing ranges from 2.4 to 4.8 g/day. The pH-dependent form relies on diffusion of water into an ethyl cellulose granule and displacement of the drug out of the granule. The drug is released in the duodenum. It can be used for disease involving the small bowel or the colon. Standard dosing is 4 g/day.

Topical mesalamine is available in enema and suppository forms. The suppositories (500 mg) are useful for the topical therapy of rectal disease. The enema form, dosed at 4 g, can be used for colonic disease to the splenic flexure; it does not require release from a carrier as with the oral agents.

Balsalazide is a 5-ASA with a diazo bond to an inert carrier, 4-aminobenzoyl-beta-alanine. Delivery to the colon is similar to that of sulfasalazine but without the sulfa side effects. Standard dosing is 6.75 g/day.

Steroids are used for more severe ulcerative colitis or Crohn's disease. Corticosteroids can be used topically, orally, or intravenously. Prednisone is the most commonly used oral steroid. Budesonide, an alternative steroid for the treatment of ileal Crohn's disease, has recently become available as an ileal release preparation. It has the advantage of a rapid first-pass metabolism and, theoretically, a lower steroid side-effect profile. Orally, the prednisone dosage range is typically 40 to 60 mg/day for 3 weeks with a variable slow taper if there is a response; there is no benefit to using doses higher than this. Intravenous steroids may be given as a bolus or a continuous infusion. There are anecdotal reports suggesting that continuous cortiosteriod infusion is better than bolus infusion. Short-term side effects include glucose intolerance, acne, mood swings, sleep disturbances, and weight gain. Long-term side effects include osteoporosis and cataracts. These agents have no maintenance benefit and should be used for acute disease therapy. Topical steroids are available in suppository, foam, and enema preparations. Foam and suppositories are used in rectal disease. Enemas may be used for left-sided colonic disease.

Antibiotics have been shown to have a role in colonic disease, perineal disease, small bowel bacterial overgrowth, and infectious complications such as abscess formation and pouchitis. Metronidazole at 10 to 20 mg/kg is the first-line antibiotic. Unfortunately, it is poorly tolerated by many patients due to nausea and taste disturbances. Peripheral neuropathy may occur with long-term use, and paresthesias are often an early sign of this side effect. Metronidazole should be discontinued if any paresthesias occur because neuropathy is progressive and can be irreversible. Other antibiotics that have been used with some success are ciprofloxacin and clarithromycin.

Immunosuppressive agents such as azathioprine or 6-mercaptopurine are used for medically refractory bowel disease, steroid-dependent disease, and perineal disease. These agents are most commonly used in Crohn's disease, but are increasingly used in ulcerative colitis. The wbc should be carefully monitored for evidence of bone marrow suppression. Measurement of metabolites may play a role in determining therapeutic efficacy and potential for toxicity. These agents have a delayed onset of action and should be used for 3 to 6 months before making decisions on lack of efficacy. Other side effects include pancreatitis and cholestasis. Long-term neoplasia risk is not clear.

Parenteral *methotrexate* has been shown to be of benefit in active Crohn's disease as well as for maintenance therapy. Dosages range from 15 to 25 mg intramuscularly or subcutaneously once per week. Signs of toxicity include liver abnormalities and pulmonary fibrosis. It is contraindicated in pregnancy, and caution should be used in women of childbearing age.

Cyclosporin is used in severe, acute colitis. It has a limited role in the treatment of Crohn's disease. In fulminant colitis, intravenous dosing has been shown to prevent or delay colectomy in patients treated with this drug. It has a narrow therapeutic window. Side effects include renal toxicity, hypertension, hirsutism, and seizures. A surgeon, watching for signs and symptoms that would lead to an urgent colectomy, should observe these patients.

Infliximab, a chimeric antibody to tumor necrosis factor-α, is very useful in the treatment of Crohn's fistulous disease as well as inducing remission and decreasing steroid requirements in patients with luminal disease. It is given as an IV infusion over 2 hours. The average duration of response is 8 weeks. Potential side effects include infusion reactions, infections, arthritis or arthralgias, and malignancy.

FUTURE DIRECTIONS

There has been an explosion of knowledge regarding important factors in the pathophysiology of inflammatory bowel disease. This is reflected in how we think and treat Crohn's disease and ulcerative colitis. As we move forward into a new era of treatment, clinical and genetic phenotyping of disease may allow for more specific therapeutic regimens. Advances are being made in terms of the use of biologics in the treatment of IBD, and we are likely to see drug regimens that include growth factors, antibodies to different components of immune active cells, and drugs that stimulate certain classes of white blood cells. The recognition that gut bacterial flora may play a role in disease activity will likely lead to increased manipulation of the gut flora with both probiotics and antibiotics. With these new therapies, attempts will be made to develop therapy regimens to avoid steroid exposure and allow for early intervention that may change the disease course.

REFERENCES

Hanauer SB, Dassopoulos T. Evolving treatment strategies for inflammatory bowel disease. *Annu Rev Med.* 2001;52:299–318.

Hanauer SB, Kane S. The pharmacology of anti-inflammatory drugs. In: Kirsner JB, ed. *Inflammatory Bowel Disease.* 5th ed. Philadelphia, Pa: WB Sanders Co; 2000:510–528.

Hanauer SB, Sandborn W, and The Practice Parameters Committee of the American College of Gastroenterology. Management of Crohn's disease in adults. *Am J Gastrolenterol.* 2001;96:635–643.

Lichtenstein GR. Inflammatory bowel disease. *Gastroenterol Clin North Am.* 1999;28:255–523.

Shanahan F. Inflammatory bowel disease: immunodiagnostics, immunotherapeutics, and ecotherapeutics. *Gastrolenterology.* 2001;120:622–635.

Chapter 49
Irritable Bowel Syndrome

Yehuda Ringel and Douglas A. Drossman

Irritable bowel syndrome (IBS), the most common functional gastrointestinal disorder, is defined as a combination of chronic or recurrent gastrointestinal symptoms, not explained by structural or biochemical abnormalities. Studies show that 8% to 23% of adults in the Western world have IBS of varying severity. It accounts for 12% of primary care and 28% of gastroenterological practice visits yearly.

IBS affects both genders and all ages and demographic groups. Prevalence is higher in females (female-to-male ratio 2:1) and decreases with age. IBS poses a considerable socioeconomic burden in terms of health-care utilization and costs. On average, patients with IBS miss 3 times more workdays, and have significantly more health care and physician visits annually than people without bowel symptoms. The cost of health services for patients with IBS is significantly higher than that for controls. The estimated annual direct cost in the United States is $1.6 billion, and the calculated indirect costs are as high as $20 billion.

ETIOLOGY AND PATHOGENESIS

There is no unique pathophysiologic mechanism that explains the symptoms of IBS. It is best understood as an integration of several contributing features. Patients may have exaggerated intestinal motor activity in response to intrinsic (e.g., meals, intraluminal balloon distention) or environmental (e.g., psychological stress) stimuli. However, while certain motility abnormalities have been described, they are not unique or well correlated with pain and the discomfort that characterize IBS. Patients can also exhibit lower pain thresholds to intestinal or rectal distention (i.e., visceral hypersensitivity and altered pain perception).

The pathophysiologic mechanisms by which visceral hypersensitivity and altered perception are induced or modulated are incompletely understood. Recent studies show that the autonomic nervous system, the neuroendocrine system, and the CNS have a major role in processing and modulating afferent visceral information from the gut and influencing the conscious experience of visceral sensations and pain via activation of 5-HT afferent receptors (Figure 49-1). Thus, the experience of IBS symptoms can result from dysfunction at the level of the gut (i.e., abnormal intestinal motor or sensory function) or from dysfunction at any level of neural control of the gut, including the autonomic nervous system, spinal pathways and the CNS (i.e., the brain-gut axis). Figure 49-2 describes the physiologic interactions between brain and gut (top) as well as the visceral pain modulation system (bottom).

Psychological factors, through their effects on the CNS (e.g., brain cognitive and affective centers) or through autonomic nervous system and neuroendocrine (e.g., hypothalamic-pituitary-adrenal axis) pathways also influence symptom perception as well as behavioral and emotional responses. Psychological distress affects intestinal motor function and reduces the intestinal sensation threshold, leading to increased gastrointestinal perception.

As both physiologic and psychological factors contribute to the patient's symptoms and illness, a *biopsychosocial model of illness and disease* is used for IBS (Figure 49-3). The *biopsychosocial model of illness and disease* integrates the physiological, psychological, behavioral, and environmental factors that contribute to clinical presentation, and outcome. Consistent with this model, all these factors interact simultaneously at multiple levels to define illness experience and outcome. The relative contribution and importance of each individual factor varies among patients and in an individual patient over time. Thus, the clinical presentation, the severity of the symptoms, and the outcome are determined by interaction of all these factors. This complexity carries important implications for establishing a comprehensive and effective diagnosis and treatment plan for patients with IBS.

CLINICAL PRESENTATION

Abdominal pain or discomfort is the most frequently reported symptom in IBS (Figure 49-4). It is often poorly localized, variable in nature, and usually relieved with defecation. Pain or discomfort is also associated with altered bowel habits (e.g., diarrhea, constipation, or combination of both at times) and with a change in the consistency or frequency of stools. Associated symptoms include bloating, urgency, and/or a feeling of incomplete evacuation. Although symptoms tend to occur in clusters, individual symptoms may also occur sequentially and they may vary in type, location, and severity over time. In addition, some patients may complain about other (i.e., non-colonic) GI symptoms (e.g., heartburn, nausea, early satiety) or non-GI (i.e., extraintestinal) symptoms including musculoskeletal symptoms (e.g., fibromyalgia), headache, genitourinary symptoms, sexual dysfunction, sleep disturbances, and chronic fatigue. Patients with more severe IBS are more likely to have an increased prevalence of co-morbid psychosocial disturbances (e.g., life stressors, a history of abuse). This is associated with an increase in symptom reporting, poorer health status, and poorer outcome.

IBS is classified as diarrhea-predominant, constipation-predominant, or mixed (combination of both), depending on the most prevalent bowel pattern. This subclassification is determined by stool frequency, form, and passage. However, because the predominant symptom often changes over time, it is not uncommon for a patient to alternate between these IBS subgroups or even between different functional disorders such as IBS and dyspepsia.

As noted, IBS symptoms are heterogeneous in their expression, may overlap other functional GI disorders (e.g., dyspepsia, functional heartburn), or may coexist with other disorders (e.g., ulcerative colitis, Crohn's disease). In these patients, treatment of both disorders is necessary for symptom control and prevention of long-term adverse outcomes. While symptoms may help direct diagnostic and treatment approaches, they are not sufficient to make a diagnosis.

DIFFERENTIAL DIAGNOSIS

The differential diagnosis is broad for IBS (Table 49-1). It includes lactase deficiency; bacterial overgrowth; GI malignancy (e.g. colon or rectal cancer); drugs such as use of laxative/cathartics, or antacids containing magnesium; infection due to *Salmonella* species, *Campylobacter jejuni, Yersinia enterocolitica, Clostridium difficile, Giardia lamblia, Entameba histolytica*; and opportunistic infections in an immunocompromised host. IBS can mimic inflammatory bowel disease (i.e., Crohn's disease, ulcerative colitis); chronic pancreatitis; celiac sprue; metabolic disorders such as diabetes mellitus, thyrotoxicosis; endocrine-producing tumors such as gastrinoma, carcinoid, and VIPoma; psychiatric illnesses including depression, somatization disorders; intestinal pseudoobstruction due to primary visceral myopathy/neuropathy, or secondary myopathy/neuropathy (e.g., scleroderma, diabetes mellitus). Other colonic diseases in the differential diagnosis include microscopic/collagenous colitis and villous adenoma.

DIAGNOSTIC APPROACH

Because there are no biological markers for IBS, it is diagnosed by identifying a cluster of clinical symptoms that are consistent with the disorder, excluding other conditions by looking for clinical alert signs, and performing limited diagnostic testing.

The use of symptom-based diagnostic criteria is standard for IBS. A widely accepted set of diagnostic criteria was developed by multinational working teams known as the "Rome Committees." By using the clinical diagnostic criteria, the physician can make a positive diagnosis of IBS,

---

Symptoms Suggestive of Diagnoses Other Than Functional Bowel Disease

- Anemia
- Fever
- Rectal bleeding
- Weight loss
- Nocturnal GI symptoms
- Family history of GI cancer, inflammatory bowel disease, or celiac disease
- New onset of symptoms after age 50

Figure 49-1

Irritable Bowel Syndrome

Serotonin (5-HT) Receptors on Sensory Afferent Nerves

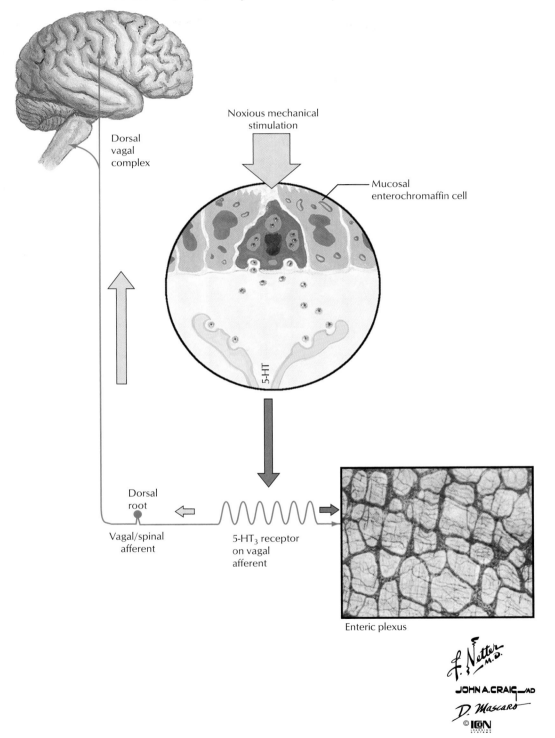

Enteric plexus

Figure 49-2

Irritable Bowel Syndrome
Pathophysiology

Input ➡️ Integration ↔️ Effect

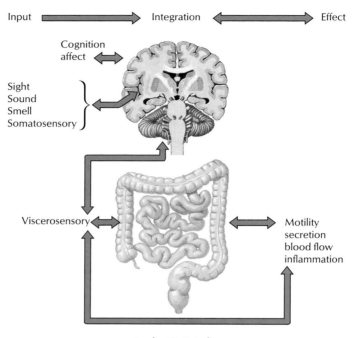

Cognition affect

Sight
Sound
Smell
Somatosensory

Viscerosensory

Motility
secretion
blood flow
inflammation

Brain-Gut Axis

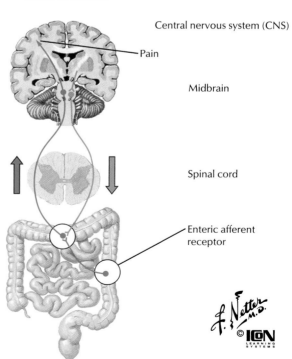

All gut functions (motor, sensory, and secretory) are controlled by intrinsic and extrinsic neural systems

Central nervous system (CNS)

Pain

Midbrain

Spinal cord

These systems interact in a bi-directional network between the brain and gut => brain-gut axis

Enteric afferent receptor

Figure 49-3

Conceptual (Biopsychosocial) Model for Irritable Bowel Syndrome

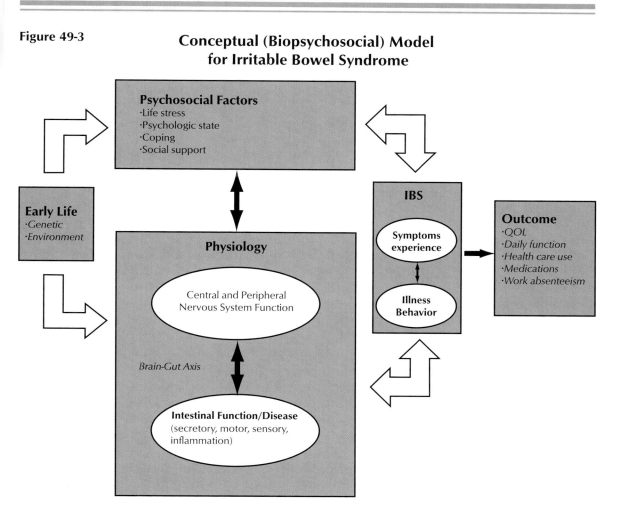

thereby reducing the need for excess diagnostic tests to exclude other conditions.

Abnormal stool symptoms include frequency (>3/day or <3/week); form (lumpy/hard or loose/ watery stool) in > 25% of the time. In addition, passage (straining, urgency, or feeling of incomplete evacuation) occurs > 1 of 4 defecations. Passage of mucus in > 25% of the time; and bloating or abdominal distension > are not essential, but when present, they increase diagnostic confidence and may be used to identify subgroups of IBS.

Obtaining the history of the patient's symptoms involves a careful inquiry about the pain or discomfort and its relation to bowel habits and stool characteristics. To meet the IBS criteria, the pain or discomfort must be associated with at least 2 of the 3 criteria linking pain to a change in bowel habit. Initial screening should include blood tests

(blood cell count, sedimentation rate, chemistries), stool tests (for ova, parasites, and blood), and sigmoidoscopy to rule out other potential diagnoses. To rule out other potential diagnoses, other studies such as colonoscopy, barium enema, ultrasound, or CT depend on the presence of "alarm" signs such as symptoms that awaken the patient from sleep, initial presentation at an older age; or evidence for GI bleeding, weight loss, fever, or a family history of colon cancer or IBD; an abnormal finding on physical examination on initial laboratory tests. More specific studies (e.g., lactose H2 breath test, thyroid-stimulating hormone, celiac sprue serology) should be considered depending on features in the history or from the screening studies that point to other diagnoses. If the initial screening is normal, further diagnostic studies should be withheld and

Figure 49-4

Irritable Bowel Syndrome

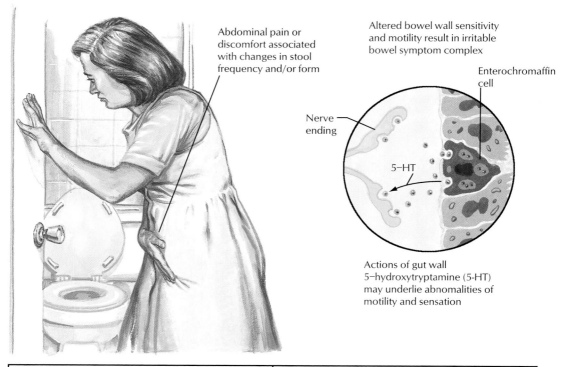

Abdominal pain or discomfort associated with changes in stool frequency and/or form

Altered bowel wall sensitivity and motility result in irritable bowel symptom complex

Enterochromaffin cell

Nerve ending

5-HT

Actions of gut wall 5-hydroxytryptamine (5-HT) may underlie abnormalities of motility and sensation

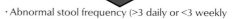

Rome II diagnostic criteria* for irritable bowel syndrome	Symptoms not essential for the diagnosis, but if present increase the confidence in the diagnosis and help to identify subgroups of IBS:
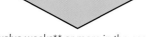	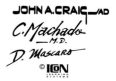

Twelve weeks** or more in the past twelve months of abdominal discomfort or pain that has two out of three features:
 	
  a. Relieved with defecation
  b. Onset associated with change in frequency of stool
  c. Onset associated with change in form (appearance) of stool
	· Abnormal stool frequency (>3 daily or <3 weekly
	· Abnormal stool form (lumpy/hard or loose/watery stool) >1/4 of defecations
	· Abnormal stool passage (straining, urgency, or feeling of incomplete evacuation) .1/4 of defecations
	· Passage of mucus .1/4 of defecations
	· Bloating or feeling of abdominal distension >1/4 of days

* In the absence of structural or metabolic abnormalities to explain the symptoms ** The twelve weeks need not be consecutive	

JOHN A. CRAIG—AD

C. Machado
—M.D.
D. Mascaro
© ICN

treatment can be started with a follow-up visit within 4 to 6 weeks. Any changes in the clinical status may lead to further investigation.

Because physiological and psychological factors influence the presentation of IBS, it is important to consider both in planning the diagnostic approach. Clinicians should evaluate patients for co-morbid disorders (e.g., anxiety, panic disorders,

DISORDERS OF THE GASTROINTESTINAL TRACT

Table 49-1
Differential Diagnosis of Irritable Bowel Syndrome

Lactase Deficiency

Drugs
    Laxative/cathartics
    Magnesium-containing antacids

Infection
    Bacterial infection
        Salmonella species
        Campylobacter jejuni
        Yersinia enterocolitica
        Clostridium difficile
    Parasitic infection
        Giardia lamblia
        Entameba ristolytica
    Opportunistic infections in immunocompromised
        host

Inflammatory Bowel Disease
    Crohn's disease
    Ulcerative colitis

Malabsorption
    Chronic pancreatitis
    Celiac sprue

Metabolic Disorders
    Diabetes mellitus

depressive disorders, post-traumatic stress disorder, and somatization disorders), personality disturbances, history of sexual or physical abuse, recent stressful life events, early life experiences, family dysfunction, and maladaptive coping strategies. Understanding the patient's psychosocial status helps to determine an appropriate diagnostic plan while minimizing investigative studies.

MANAGEMENT AND THERAPY

An effective physician-patient relationship is essential to any treatment plan. This includes appropriate reassurance and education about the condition, its natural history, and its consequences. The patient's understanding of the relevance of physiological and psychosocial factors to the symptoms, and the acceptance of the need to address both in diagnosis and treatment, is desired but not always achieved.

The specific treatment approach depends on the type of the symptoms and the severity of the disorder. Treatment for symptoms is determined by whether pain, diarrhea, or constipation is predominant. The severity of the symptoms is determined by their intensity, constancy, the degree of psychosocial difficulties, and the frequency of health-care utilization. Most subjects with IBS symptoms do not see physicians for their symptoms and are usually referred to as IBS nonpatients; the majority (approximately 70%) who do see physicians have mild and infrequent symptoms associated with little disability. These patients usually require only reassurance, education, recommendations for dietary and lifestyle changes, and encouragement for health-promoting behaviors. Short-term medication treatment can be prescribed during exacerbations. Another 25% of patients have moderate symptoms that occasionally interfere with daily activities (e.g., missing school, work, or social functions). These patients may require additional pharmacological or behavioral treatments. Only a small proportion of patients with IBS (approximately 5%) have severe symptoms that considerably affect their daily activities and quality of life. These patients usually require psychopharmacological (e.g., antidepressants) or psychological (e.g., cognitive-behavioral) treatments. In rare cases, referral to tertiary care centers may be needed.

Drug Therapy

Medications directed at the gut (e.g., anticholinergic agents for pain and diarrhea, or loperamide

---

Rome II Diagnostic Criteria* for IBS

Twelve weeks or more** in the past 12 months of abdominal discomfort or pain with at least 2 of 3 features:

· Relieved with defecation
· Onset associated with a change in frequency of stool
· Onset associated with a change in form (appearance) of stool

---

* In the absence of structural or metabolic abnormalities to explain the symptoms.

** The 12 weeks need not be consecutive.

for diarrhea, sorbitol or PEG solution for constipation, etc.) can relieve specific symptoms. Some new medications directed to reduce gut sensitivity and bowel dysfunction (e.g., 5-hydroxytryptamine 3 [5HT3] antagonists for diarrhea-predominant IBS, 5HT4 agonists for constipation-predominant IBS, and kappa opioid active agents for pain) have been recently approved for clinical use or are currently in clinical trials. Medications with central/psychotropic effects (e.g., antidepressants) can be used to treat co-morbid affective or psychiatric disorders (e.g., depression, anxiety). Low doses of antidepressants also have analgesic properties independent of their psychotropic effects. Tricyclic agents such as desipramine (50 to 150 mg) or amitriptyline (25 to 100 mg) appear to be effective in controlling IBS symptoms. However, serotonin reuptake inhibitors may be preferred in older patients or in those having constipation because they have little or no anticholinergic effect. Consistent with the biopsychosocial model, it is important to view medication therapy as part of a more comprehensive management plan.

Psychological Treatments

Several psychological treatment interventions are used for IBS including active psychotherapeutic treatments (e.g., cognitive-behavioral therapy, dynamic or interpersonal therapy) and more passive treatments (e.g., progressive muscle relaxation, hypnosis). Psychological treatments appear superior to conventional medical treatment in reducing psychological distress, improving coping, and reducing some bowel symptoms. However, no one specific treatment is found to be superior. Psychological treatments are recommended for patients with frequent or disabling symptoms, associated psychiatric disorders, history of abuse with maladjustment to the current illness, and somatization with multiple consultations across specialties.

FUTURE DIRECTIONS

Significant advances in our understanding of functional gastrointestinal disorders and IBS have occurred during the past decade; however, the diagnosis and management of these difficult yet common disorders are still a challenge in clinical practice. Hopefully, the growing interest and recent advances in the multidisciplinary research of these disorders will contribute to the development of novel and more effective diagnostic and treatment approaches.

REFERENCES

Drossman DA, Camilleri M, Mayer ER, Whitehead WE. AGA technical review on irritable bowel syndrome. *Gastroenterology*. 2002;123:2108–2131.

Ringel Y, Drossman DA. Irritable bowel syndrome. In: Humes HD, DuPont HL, Gardner LB, et al, eds. *Kelley's Textbook of Internal Medicine*. 4th ed. Philadelphia, Pa: Lippincott Williams & Wilkins; 2000:851–855.

Ringel Y, Drossman DA. Toward a positive and comprehensive diagnosis of irritable bowel syndrome. *MedGenMed* [serial online]. 2000;2(4). Available at: http://www.medscape.com/viewarticle/407962. Accessed February 12, 2003.

Ringel Y, Sperber AD, Drossman DA. Irritable bowel syndrome. *Ann Rev Med*. 2001;52:319–338.

Thompson WG, Longstreth G, Drossman DA, Heaton K, Irvine J, Muller-Lissner S. Functional bowel disorder and functional abdominal pain. In: Drossman DA, Corazziari E, Talley NJ, Thompson WG, Whitehead WE, and the Rome Multinational Working Teams, eds. *Rome II: Diagnostic Criteria for the Functional Gastrointestinal Disorders*. 2nd ed. McLean Va: Degnon Associates Inc; 2000:351–432.

Chapter 50

Pancreatitis

Ian S. Grimm

Pancreatitis is a general term that encompasses a broad spectrum of pathophysiologic disorders and clinical manifestations. Acute pancreatitis (AP) may range in severity from simple interstitial edema to extensive necrotizing pancreatitis with multisystem organ failure (Figure 50-1). Most episodes of AP are mild, with an excellent prognosis for complete recovery. However, pancreatic necrosis develops in approximately 20% of patients, which markedly increases the risk of severe complications and death. The mortality rate for patients with sterile necrosis is 10%, but mortality can exceed 25% in patients with infected pancreatic necrosis. Chronic pancreatitis (CP) refers to irreversible fibrosis and atrophy of the gland, often with a chronic inflammatory cell infiltrate, and progressive loss of exocrine and endocrine function (Figure 50-2).

ETIOLOGY AND PATHOGENESIS

The most common causes of pancreatitis in developed countries are gallstones (45%) and alcohol (35%). Approximately 10% of cases result from miscellaneous causes, while another 10% remain unexplained (Table 50-1).

CP can result from recurrent acute pancreatitis, however, it often develops insidiously. Most patients presenting with an initial attack of alcoholic pancreatitis, for instance, already have morphologic changes of chronic pancreatitis. Risk factors for chronic pancreatitis are listed in Table 50-2.

CLINICAL PRESENTATION

Acute pancreatitis presents with severe epigastric pain of sudden onset, frequently with radiation to the back, nausea, and vomiting (Figure 50-1). The pain typically reaches maximal intensity within 30 minutes, and persists for hours without relief. Fever, tachycardia, and leukocytosis may be present.

Chronic pancreatitis may initially present with an attack resembling acute pancreatitis, but it often progresses to a pattern of recurrent inflammatory flares or chronic persistent pain (Figure 50-2). Subsequently, malabsorption and diabetes mellitus may develop.

DIFFERENTIAL DIAGNOSIS

Acute pancreatitis can mimic many causes of an acute abdomen, such as biliary colic, perforated ulcer, mesenteric ischemia or infarction, bowel obstruction, inferior wall myocardial infarction, or ectopic pregnancy. Chronic pancreatitis can resemble ulcer disease, biliary disorders, gastrointestinal malignancies, malabsorption syndromes, or chronic functional abdominal pain.

DIAGNOSTIC APPROACH

Serum amylase or lipase elevations exceeding 3 times normal are characteristic of acute pancreatitis. Lesser elevations can occur in other conditions. Lipase values are slightly more accurate, especially when the presentation is delayed. Abdominal CT detects the presence or absence of pancreatitis in all but the mildest cases and is useful in excluding other conditions having a similar presentation.

The diagnosis of CP requires either evidence of characteristic morphologic abnormalities of the gland, or a combination of typical clinical features and abnormal pancreatic functional studies. Pancreatic calcifications on plain radiography or CT represent intraductal stones, which are pathognomonic for CP. Stones may also be seen on transabdominal ultrasonography. Endoscopic retrograde cholangiopancreatography (ERCP) and magnetic resonance cholangiopancreatography can provide fine detail of the ductal anatomy, such as irregular dilatation of the pancreatic duct, strictures, or ductal filling defects. Endoscopic ultrasonography is the most sensitive means for detecting subtle pancreatic parenchymal changes, although the clinical significance of such findings is uncertain.

The secretin test is the gold standard for docu-

Table 50-1
Causes of Acute Pancreatitis and Recurrent Acute Pancreatitis

Common
  Gallstones
    Microlithiasis
  Alcohol abuse
  Idiopathic causes

Uncommon
  ERCP*
  Metabolic
    Hypertriglyceridemia
    Hypercalcemia
  Obstructive
    Sphincter of Oddi dysfunction
    Pancreatic ductal lesions
      Tumor
      Stricture
    Duodenal or periampullary lesions
      Crohn's disease
      Blind loop
  Congenital
    Annular pancreas
    Pancreas divisum
  Trauma
  Medications
    e.g., azathioprine, 6-mercaptopurine,
    corticosteroids, DDI**, estrogens, furosemide,
    metronidazole, pentamidine, sulfonamides,
    tetracycline, thiazides, valproic acid
  Toxins
  Infections
    TB[†], CMV[††], mumps, coxsackie virus,
    mycoplasma, parasites
  Vascular
    e.g., vasculitis, embolism, hypotension
  Autoimmune
  Hereditary
    Hereditary pancreatitis
    Cystic fibrosis gene mutations

*ERCP, endoscopic retrograde cholangiopancreatography; **DDI, dideoxyinosine; [†]TB, tuberculosis; [††]CMV, cytomegalovirus. Adapted from Somogy L, Martin SP, Venkatsan T, Ulrich CD. Reccurrent acute pancreaitis: An algorithmic approach to identification and elimination of inciting factors. *Gastroenterology.* 2001;12:709, with permission from Elsevier.

Table 50-2
Risk Factors for Chronic Pancreatitis

Alcohol

Tobacco smoking

Chronic renal failure

Hypercalcemia

Hyperlipidemia (possible)

Obstructive
  Pancreas divisum
  Pancreatic ductal stricture
  Duodenal or ampullary lesions

Genetic
  Autosomal dominant hereditary pancreatitis
  Cationic trypsinogen mutations (codons 29, 122)
  Autosomal recessive
  Cystic fibrosis
  Cystic fibrosis gene (CFTR) mutations
  Secretory protease inhibitor (SPINK1) mutations
  Cationic trypsinogen mutations (codons 16, 22, 23)

Autoimmune
  Primary
  Associated with other diseases:
    Sjögren syndrome
    Inflammatory bowel disease
    Primary biliary cirrhosis

Recurrent acute pancreatitis

Necrotizing pancreatitis

Post-irradiation

Vascular diseases

Idiopathic
  Early onset
  Late onset
  Tropical

Adapted from Etemad B, Whitcomb C. Chronic pancreatitis: diagnosis, classification, and new genetic developments. *Gastroenterology.* 2001;120:691, with permission from Elsevier.

MANAGEMENT AND THERAPY
Acute Pancreatitis

Management of AP should focus on rapid treatment and early identification of patients at risk for severe AP. All patients should receive aggressive fluid replacement, pain management, and careful observation for signs of respiratory insufficiency

menting pancreatic insufficiency, but it is cumbersome and not widely available. The quantitative fecal fat stain is a simple test to document fat malabsorption, which, in a patient with suspected CP, implies loss of 90% of exocrine function.

Figure 50-1

Acute Pancreatitis

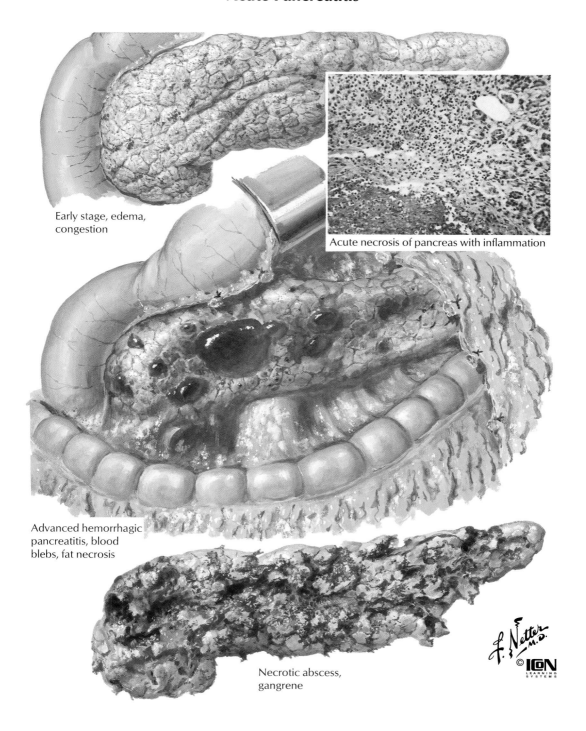

Early stage, edema,
congestion

Acute necrosis of pancreas with inflammation

Advanced hemorrhagic
pancreatitis, blood
blebs, fat necrosis

Necrotic abscess,
gangrene

Figure 50-2

Chronic (Relapsing) Pancreatitis

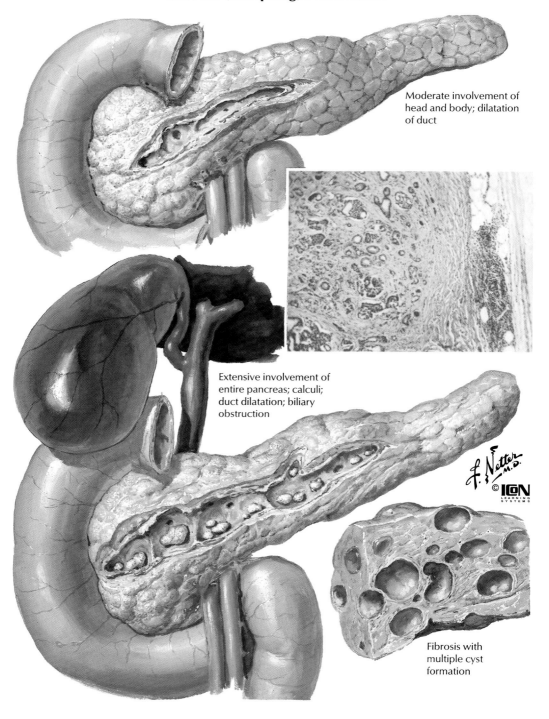

Moderate involvement of head and body; dilatation of duct

Extensive involvement of entire pancreas; calculi; duct dilatation; biliary obstruction

Fibrosis with multiple cyst formation

or significant third space fluid losses (hemoconcentration, oliguria, hypotension, tachycardia, or azotemia). To promptly identify individuals at risk for severe pancreatitis, the APACHE-II score should be calculated on the day of admission. Early predictors of severity include an APACHE-II score of 6 or above, obesity (body mass index >30), or pleural effusions. Severe AP is defined as an APACHE II score of 8 or more; a Ranson score of 3 or more; organ failure (shock, pulmonary insufficiency, renal failure, or gastrointestinal bleeding); or local complications, including necrosis, abscess, or pseudocyst. Abdominal ultrasound is indicated to screen for gallstones or biliary ductal dilatation. Patients with severe AP and suspected biliary obstruction should undergo urgent ERCP (within 72 hours) to remove bile duct stones. Patients with severe pancreatitis should be transferred to an intensive-care setting and undergo dynamic contrast-enhanced CT (ideally after 72 hours) to identify pancreatic necrosis. Oral intake is typically withheld while pain persists. Nasogastric suction is indicated for ileus or for refractory nausea and vomiting. In the absence of ileus, early jejunal feeding is safe and may reduce the risk of complications. Prophylactic antibiotics are recommended for severe pancreatitis (e.g., imipenem-cilastatin for 2 to 4 weeks). Patients with necrotizing pancreatitis and clinical deterioration or signs of infection should undergo guided, percutaneous fine-needle aspiration for bacteriology studies. Aggressive surgical debridement is the standard treatment for infected necrosis, which is otherwise uniformly fatal.

Chronic Pancreatitis

Therapy is directed at managing pain and fat malabsorption primarily. A low-fat diet, non-narcotic analgesics, and abstinence from alcohol are recommended. Narcotics may be required for severe pain. For persistent pain, high protease pancreatic enzyme replacement should be prescribed for at least 8 weeks. Microencapsulated enzyme preparations with high lipase content are useful for treatment of steatorrhea. Treatable problems should be sought, such as pseudocysts or stenosis of the duodenum or intrapancreatic common bile duct. Patients with refractory pain and pancreatic duct strictures or stones may benefit from endoscopic therapy. Those with intractable pain and a dilated main pancreatic duct often respond to surgical decompression (i.e., lateral pancreaticojejunostomy). Treatments of last resort for pain in patients with nondilated ducts include nerve blocks and pancreatic resection.

FUTURE DIRECTIONS

Newer diagnostic tests for pancreatitis (e.g., urinary trypsinogen-2) and biochemical markers of severity (e.g., urinary trypsinogen activation peptide, serum interleukins 6 and 8) may improve current practice. Novel therapies for severe AP will target inhibition of the systemic inflammatory response associated with this disease. The role of genetic factors in the development of pancreatic diseases will remain a major research focus.

REFERENCES

Banks PA. Practice guidelines in acute pancreatitis. *Am J Gastroenterol.* 1997;92:377–386.

Baron TH, Moran DE. Acute necrotizing pancreatitis. *N Engl J Med.* 1999;340:1412–1417.

Bradley EL III. A clinically based classification system for acute pancreatitis. Summary of the International Symposium on Acute Pancreatitis, Atlanta, Ga, September 11 through 12, 1992. *Arch Surg.* 1993;128:586–590.

Dervenis C, Johnson CD, Bassi C, et al. Diagnosis, objective assessment of severity, and management of acute pancreatitis. Santori consensus conference. *Int J Pancreatol.* 1999;25:195–210.

Etemad B, Whitcomb DC. Chronic pancreatitis: diagnosis, classification, and new genetic developments. *Gastroenterology.* 2001;120:682–707.

Somogyi L, Martin SP, Venkatesan T, Ulrich CD II. Recurrent acute pancreatitis: an algorithmic approach to identification and elimination of inciting factors. *Gastroenterology.* 2001;120:708–717.

Warshaw AL, Banks PA, Fernandez-Del Castillo C. AGA technical review: treatment of pain in chronic pancreatitis. *Gastroenterology.* 1998;115:765–776.

Chapter 51

Peptic Ulcer Disease

Melissa Rich and Nicholas J. Shaheen

Peptic ulcers are gastrointestinal mucosal defects that extend through the muscularis mucosa. Peptic ulcer disease (PUD) is associated with significant morbidity and expenditures related to work loss, hospitalizations, and outpatient care (excluding medications) of over $5 billion per year in the United States. Major advances have been made in the past three decades with the discovery and etiologic linkage of *Helicobacter pylori* (Hp) to peptic ulcer disease and the development of more effective medical therapies. However, despite advances in diagnosis and therapy, the prevalence of PUD remains unaltered, and the cumulative mortality rate in complicated ulcer disease remains at 10%.

The epidemiology of PUD mirrors that of Hp because this is the primary etiologic factor. As is the case for Hp, the prevalence of PUD varies with region and population. The worldwide lifetime prevalence of PUD is estimated at 5% to 10%. These estimates double in those harboring *H. pylori* infection.

The incidence of PUD increases with age. This is likely due to two major reasons. The first is that the incidence of Hp infection is decreasing in people younger than 30, primarily due to improved socioeconomic conditions. Second, use of nonsteroidal anti-inflammatory drugs (NSAIDs) is the number two leading cause of ulcer disease, and increasing age is an independent predictor of experiencing an NSAID–associated gastrointestinal complication.

ETIOLOGY AND PATHOGENESIS

H. pylori infection and NSAID use account for the majority of cases of PUD. Less common causes include hypersecretory states, stress ulcers, neoplasia, and idiopathic ulcers. Cigarette smoking can increase the risk of relapse and delay healing in ulcer disease. Corticosteroid use is a risk factor for PUD, but only when used in combination with NSAIDs.

In Europe and Australia, up to 95% of duodenal ulcers are attributed to Hp. Recent studies suggest that 75% of duodenal ulcers in the United States are associated with Hp. Infection with Hp universally results in antral gastritis. The infection inhibits somatostatin and subsequently increases gastrin release. These two hormonal alterations

cause parietal cells to increase secretion of acid in the gastric body. The increased acid secretion creates an increased duodenal acid load and gastric metaplasia—the conversion of the lining of the duodenum so that it resembles stomach epithelium. Hp then colonizes this gastric metaplasia in the duodenal bulb. This explains, in part, the paradoxical observation that Hp causes duodenal ulceration, but is generally not resident in normal duodenal epithelium.

NSAID use is the second most important etiologic factor in peptic ulcer disease in this country. Because of the "graying" of the American population and the ready availability of these agents over the counter, NSAID-induced gastrointestinal toxicity has risen in incidence over the past 3 decades. In the United States, more than 70 million prescription NSAIDs and more than 30 billion non-prescription NSAIDs are sold yearly. The FDA approximates the risk of a clinically significant gastrointestinal event, including perforations, ulcerations, or bleeding, to be 1% to 4% per year for the non-selective class of NSAIDs. The mechanisms by which NSAIDs cause ulceration involve both direct topical injury and systemic effects mediated by endogenous prostaglandins. NSAID use induces changes in the local mucosal blood flow of the stomach and duodenum. These changes impede repair of damaged mucosa. Additionally, traditional NSAIDs inhibit both the cyclooxygenase (COX-1 and COX-2) isoenzymes. While inhibition of the COX-2 isoenzyme leads to the antiinflammatory effects that provide the NSAIDs' beneficial effects, inhibition of the COX-1 isoenzyme causes an impaired response to mucosal damage. Because the COX-1 isoenzyme is involved in multiple "housekeeping" functions, such as hemostasis and protection of the gastric mucosa, inhibition of this enzyme is thought to be responsible for most of the mucosal toxicity of NSAIDs.

Nearly 100% of people infected with Hp will have gastritis, and likewise nearly 100% of people ingesting NSAIDs will have endoscopic evidence of erosions. However, symptoms of clinically important ulcers will develop in only a subset of these individuals (Figure 51-1). The inability to predict which individuals will develop PUD highlights our limited knowledge of the pathology of this disease.

CLINICAL PRESENTATION

The most common presenting complaint in patients with PUD is dyspepsia. Although classical teaching states that duodenal ulcers characteristically present with symptoms of a burning "hunger pain," occurring 2 to 3 hours after eating or awakening a patient from sleep, and relieved with antacids, it is now known that these symptoms lack sensitivity and specificity. The presence of symptoms does not reliably predict ulcers, nor does the absence of symptoms exclude disease. Occasionally, patients may present with symptoms of a complication of PUD, such as peritonitis from a free perforation, or gastric outlet obstruction from scarring or edema of the pyloric channel, leading to an inability to empty the stomach (Figures 51-2 and 51-3). Rarely, patients may present with syncope or angina secondary to previously undetected blood loss. Some subjects with PUD, especially those taking NSAIDs, may have no symptoms from the disease.

The clinical signs of PUD are often subtle. Vital signs are usually normal unless significant hemorrhage has occurred. Pain on palpation of the mid or right epigastrium is common, but not pathognomonic. Stool test results for fecal occult blood may be positive, but it is neither sensitive nor specific for PUD.

DIFFERENTIAL DIAGNOSIS

An accurate history is essential to discriminate between common and uncommon disorders that imitate peptic ulcer disease. With a detailed history and minimal testing, conditions such as gastroe-sophageal reflux, adenocarcinoma, biliary disease, or pancreatic disease can be excluded. Non-ulcer dyspepsia is the most common cause of epigastric pain in this country. This poorly understood entity likely represents several different pathologic processes, only some of which are peptic acid–related.

DIAGNOSTIC APPROACH

Older patients presenting with abdominal pain or any patient with alarm symptoms (anemia, weight loss, early satiety) should undergo endoscopy for exclusion of carcinoma. In patients younger than 45, a "test-and-treat" strategy may be pursued. To test and treat, one obtains a non-invasive measure of Hp infection such as a serum or breath test, and treats to eradicate the organism if it is present.

Endoscopy is the gold standard for the evaluation of PUD (Figure 51-4). It allows detection of ulcer disease with great accuracy and permits biopsy of lesions, to exclude carcinoma as well as confirm infection with Hp by histologic studies or rapid urease testing. Biopsy of all gastric ulcers should be performed to exclude malignancy.

Upper GI radiography is an acceptable substitute in areas where gastrointestinal endoscopy is not available. While certain radiographic features suggest benign or malignant disease, the test has insufficient accuracy to rule out malignancy as a cause of ulceration, especially in the case of gastric ulcers.

MANAGEMENT AND THERAPY

The goals of treatment are fourfold: to relieve symptoms, hasten healing, prevent complications, and decrease the risk of relapse of ulceration. The role of Hp in ulcer formation is indisputable. If infection is documented, eradication should be the initial management step for both duodenal and gastric ulcer. Follow-up testing is performed 4 weeks or more following therapy to ensure eradication in patients with complicated ulcer disease, such as bleeding ulcer or perforation. Repeat endoscopy has been advocated for gastric ulcer diseases to document healing and disprove malignancy; however, it is unclear whether this is necessary in all cases.

Multiple forms of therapy (histamine-2 receptor antagonists, proton pump inhibitors or misoprostol) are effective for healing an NSAID-associated

Figure 51-1   **Peptic Ulcer Disease: Acute Gastric Ulcers**

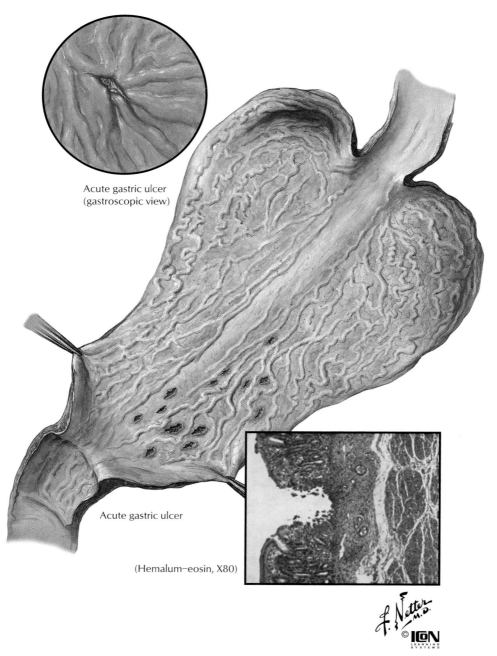

Acute gastric ulcer
(gastroscopic view)

Acute gastric ulcer

(Hemalum–eosin, X80)

ulcer if the agent is discontinued. If the patient must remain on the NSAID, proton pump inhibitors achieve superior healing rates. Treatment with COX-2 inhibitors appears to lessen the risk of gastrointestinal side effects in patients requiring chronic NSAID use, but the increased cost of these agents may be prohibitive for some patients. Surreptitious or inadvertent NSAID use is the most common reason for recurrent ulcer disease.

Although many chronic NSAID users are Hp-

Figure 51-2   **Peptic Ulcer Disease: Chronic Gastric Ulcers**

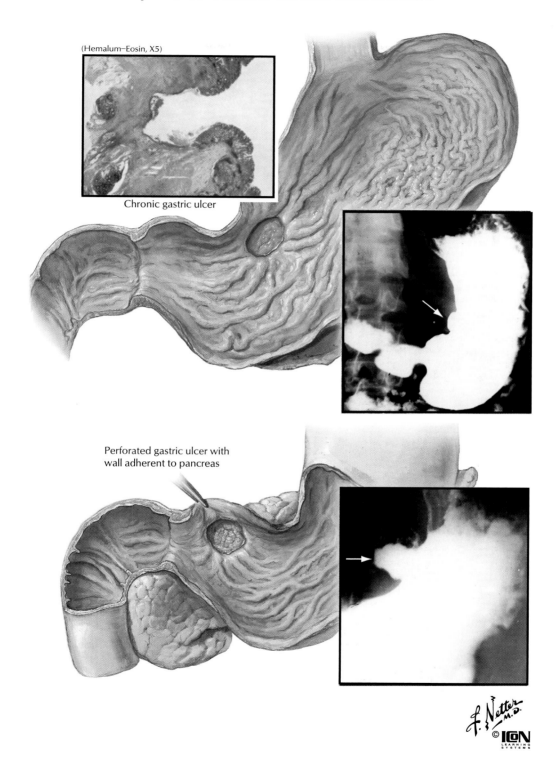

(Hemalum–Eosin, X5)

Chronic gastric ulcer

Perforated gastric ulcer with
wall adherent to pancreas

Figure 51-3

Peptic Ulcer Disease:
Complications of Gastric and Duodenal Ulcers

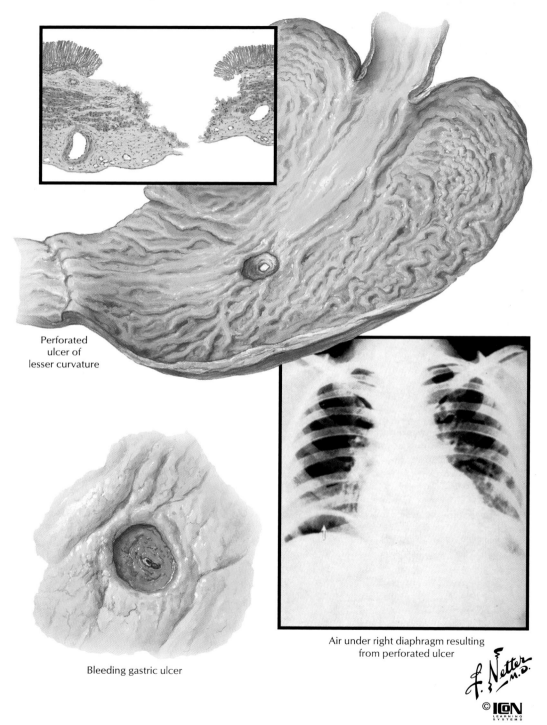

Perforated
ulcer of
lesser curvature

Air under right diaphragm resulting
from perforated ulcer

Bleeding gastric ulcer

Figure 51-4

Diagnostic Evaluation

Endoscopy

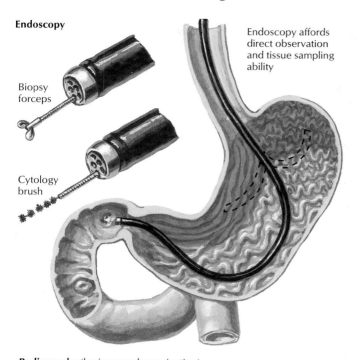

Biopsy forceps

Cytology brush

Endoscopy affords direct observation and tissue sampling ability

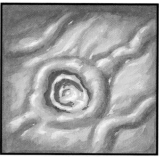

Duodenal ulcer

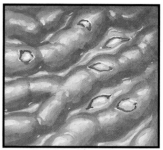

Gastritis with erosions

Radiography (barium meal examination)

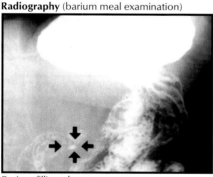

Barium-filling ulcer crater

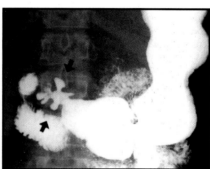

Deformed duodenal bulb

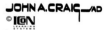

positive, the incremental benefit of eradicating the infection for all of those subjects who are *H. pylori* positive and require chronic NSAIDs remains controversial. Smoking cessation should be encouraged in any form of ulcer disease. Universal dietary modifications are not indicated.

Endoscopic therapy is the initial management step for complicated PUD (Figure 51-4). At the time of upper endoscopy, if either active bleeding or a non-bleeding, but visible, vessel is seen, hemostasis of bleeding can be accomplished with injection or thermal energy in the majority of cases. Successful endoscopic therapy can also lower the risk of recurrent bleeding for the following 72 hours, as well as the need for surgery. Upper endoscopy can be useful in gastric outlet obstruction secondary to chronic scarring from peptic ulcer disease, as endoscopic balloon dilatation may relieve the obstruction, obviating surgery. Generally, ulcers complicated by uncontrollable bleeding and ulcer perforation are managed surgically. Potent acid suppression and antimicrobial therapy have lessened the role of surgery in the management of chronic ulcers, and surgical intervention is rarely necessary.

FUTURE DIRECTIONS

While the relative risk of ulcer formation is increased in patients with Hp infection or NSAID ingestion, the absolute risk is low. Challenges facing investigators include identifying the subsets of these populations who are at higher risk. These high-risk patients could be targeted for *H. pylori* testing and eradication, or, in the case of those requiring chronic NSAID use, therapy with the COX-2 specific agents. The epidemiology of peptic ulcer disease is likely to change as infection with Hp, particularly in the United States, declines. As the prevalence of Hp decreases in the United States, the proportion of Hp-negative ulcers will rise. Thus, strategies to minimize NSAID–associated

ulcers are imperative. New medications, such as intravenous proton pump inhibitors, offer the promise of decreasing the acute mortality associated with ulcer hemorrhage.

REFERENCES

Ciociola AA, McSorley DJ, Turner K, Sykes D, Palmer JB. *Helicobacter pylori* infection rates in duodenal ulcer patients in the United States may be lower than previously estimated. *Am J Gastroenterol.* 1999;94:1834–1840.

Cryer B. Nonsteroidal anti-inflammatory drugs and GI disease. In: Feldman M, Friedman LS, Sleisenger MH, eds. *Sleisenger & Fordtran's Gastrointestinal and Liver Disease: Pathophysiology/Diagnosis/Management.* 7th ed. Philadelphia, Pa: WB Saunders Co; 2002.

Hawkey CJ, Karrasch JA, Szczepanski L, et al. Omeprazole compared with misoprostol for ulcers associated with nonsteroidal antiinflammatory drugs. Omeprazole versus Misoprostol for NSAID-induced Ulcer Management (OMNIUM) Study Group. *N Engl J Med.* 1998;338:727–734.

Kurata JH, Haile BM. Epidemiology of peptic ulcer disease. *Clin Gastroenterol.* 1984;13:289–307.

Sonnenberg A, Everhart JE. Health impact of peptic ulcer in the United States. *Am J Gastroenterol.* 1997;92:614–620.

Chapter 52

Viral Hepatitis:
Acute and Chronic Disease

Michael W. Fried

Viral hepatitis is a major public health concern worldwide. The most important etiologic agents are the five known hepatotropic viruses (Hepatitis A to E), whose predominant clinical manifestations are signs and symptoms of liver disease (Table 52-1). Infection with these viruses may result in a subclinical infection, acute, chronic, or acute and chronic hepatitis. A number of other viruses, such as cytomegalovirus, Epstein-Barr virus, and herpes simplex may also cause acute hepatitis, usually in the context of a systemic illness.

ACUTE HEPATITIS A
Clinical Presentation
and Diagnostic Approach

Symptoms of hepatitis A (HAV) are nonspecific and include malaise, anorexia, nausea and vomiting, low-grade fever, and mild right upper quadrant pain (Figure 52-1). Patients may note the onset of dark urine that usually accompanies jaundice in the icteric phase of acute hepatitis. Laboratory studies indicate acute hepatocellular injury with serum aminotransferases (alanine aminotransferase [ALT] and aspartate aminotransferase [AST]) greater than ten times the upper limit of normal. Serum bilirubin level will also be elevated but

usually below 10 mg/dL. Subclinical infections often occur in children who acquire hepatitis A in endemic areas. The likelihood of symptomatic acute icteric hepatitis A increases with age at acquisition. The definitive laboratory test for diagnosis of acute hepatitis A is HAV IgM in serum.

Management and Therapy

There are no specific interventions for treatment except for supportive care and monitoring for the development of fulminant liver failure, a rare sequela of HAV infection (Figures 52-2 and 52-3). The urgency of evaluation of hepatitis and considerations for hospital admission or referral

Table 52-1
Hepatotropic Viruses

	Mode of Transmission	Approximate Incubation	Endemic Areas	Potential for Chronicity
Hepatitis A	Fecal-Oral Food/waterborne outbreaks	1–6 wk	Developing countries	No
Hepatitis E	Fecal-Oral Food/waterborne outbreaks	1–6 wk	Mexico, SE Asia	No
Hepatitis B	Parenteral/Sexual/Perinatal	1–6 mo	Asia/Africa	Yes
Hepatitis D	Parenteral/Sexual	1–6 mo	Mediterranean	Yes
Hepatitis C	Parenteral	1–6 mo	Egypt	Yes

Figure 52-1

Viral Hepatitis
Acute Form

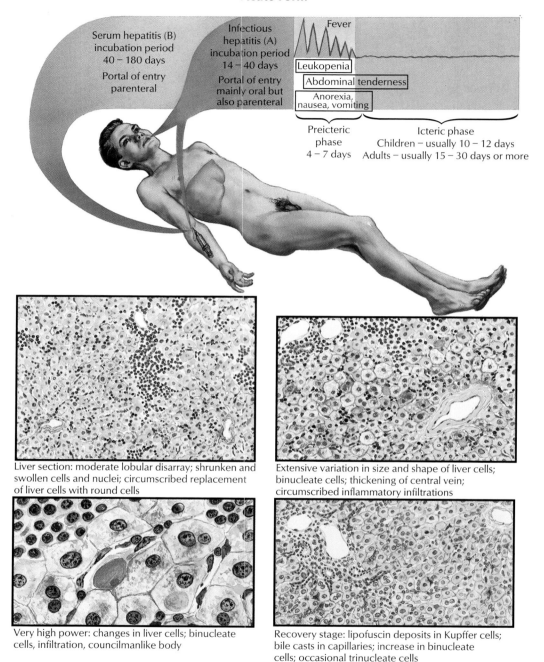

Serum hepatitis (B) incubation period 40 – 180 days

Portal of entry parenteral

Infectious hepatitis (A) incubation period 14 – 40 days

Portal of entry mainly oral but also parenteral

Fever

Leukopenia

Abdominal tenderness

Anorexia, nausea, vomiting

Preicteric phase 4 – 7 days

Icteric phase
Children – usually 10 – 12 days
Adults – usually 15 – 30 days or more

Liver section: moderate lobular disarray; shrunken and swollen cells and nuclei; circumscribed replacement of liver cells with round cells

Extensive variation in size and shape of liver cells; binucleate cells; thickening of central vein; circumscribed inflammatory infiltrations

Very high power: changes in liver cells; binucleate cells, infiltration, councilmanlike body

Recovery stage: lipofuscin deposits in Kupffer cells; bile casts in capillaries; increase in binucleate cells; occasional trinucleate cells

Figure 52-2

Viral Hepatitis
Fulminant Form
(Acute Massive Necrosis)

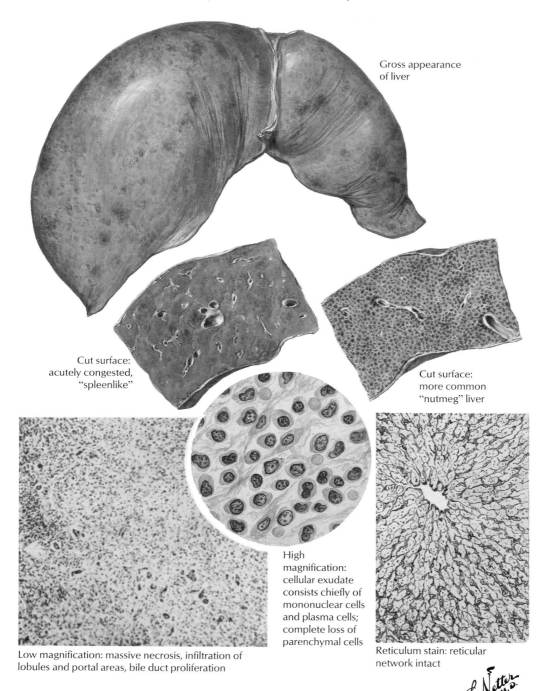

Gross appearance
of liver

Cut surface:
acutely congested,
"spleenlike"

Cut surface:
more common
"nutmeg" liver

High
magnification:
cellular exudate
consists chiefly of
mononuclear cells
and plasma cells;
complete loss of
parenchymal cells

Low magnification: massive necrosis, infiltration of
lobules and portal areas, bile duct proliferation

Reticulum stain: reticular
network intact

Table 52-2
Serologic Profile

	HBsAg	Anti-HBs	HbcAb	HBeAg	Anti-Hbe	HBV DNA	Serum ALT
Acute	+	–	+IgM	+/–	+/–	+/–	+++
Resolved	–	+	+ IgG	–	+	–	Normal
Chronic Hepatitis	+	–	+	+	–	+	++
Inactive Carrier	+	–	+	–	+	+/–	Normal
Vaccinated	–	+	–	–	–	–	Normal

Diagnosis of acute hepatitis B: HBsAg and HBc antibody I g.

to a liver specialist are based on the functional status of the patient, the tempo of changes in liver enzyme levels, and the presence of hepatic synthetic dysfunction. Patients with social support to monitor their status, who are sufficiently reliable to keep follow-up appointments, and who are able to maintain their oral intake do not require hospitalization. Patients who cannot remain hydrated or who have evidence of hepatic synthetic dysfunction (prolonged prothrombin time, altered mental status) should be hospitalized until clinical improvement is noted.

The index case is most infectious before the onset of jaundice, when fecal excretion of HAV is at its peak; thus, close personal and household contacts are at risk of acquiring hepatitis A from an index case. Cases should be reported to the local public health authorities who will monitor for clustering that may give clues about a common source outbreak. In addition, they will help trace potential contacts who are at risk of infection. Close contacts exposed to the index case within 2 weeks of the onset of jaundice should receive immune serum globulin, which may prevent infection.

Hepatitis A vaccine is now approved for use in the United States. Vaccination for hepatitis A is recommended for travelers to countries where HAV is endemic, men who have sex with men, intravenous drug users, residents and employees of institutionalized living facilities, and nursery/-day-care workers who may be exposed to HAV infection from fecal soiling. Patients with chronic liver disease who acquire hepatitis A may be at

risk for hepatic decompensation. Therefore, HAV vaccination is also recommended for this group.

HEPATITIS B

An estimated 45% of the world's population lives in an area where hepatitis B (HBV) is endemic. In the United States, approximately 200,000 new cases occur each year. Hepatitis B may be transmitted sexually, parenterally, or perinatally. Risk factors for acute hepatitis B in the United States are shown in Figure 52-4.

Persons who should be screened include those born in endemic areas, men who have sex with men, injecting drug users, hemodialysis patients, HIV-infected patients, pregnant women, and family/household and sexual contacts.

Clinical Presentation and Diagnostic Approach

Most adults who acquire acute hepatitis B resolve the acute infection and develop natural immunity; however, chronic infection develops in approximately 5% of adults. In neonates, who acquire hepatitis B through vertical transmission (highly endemic areas such as southeast Asia), the risk of chronicity approaches 90%. The potential clinical course of hepatitis B infection is shown in Figure 52-5.

The various clinical scenarios described above can be defined by specific serologic patterns (Table 52-2):

Extrahepatic manifestations include serum sickness or urticaria, membranous or membranoproliferative glomerulonephritis, and polyarteritis nodosa.

Figure 52-3

Viral Hepatitis
Subacute Fatal Form

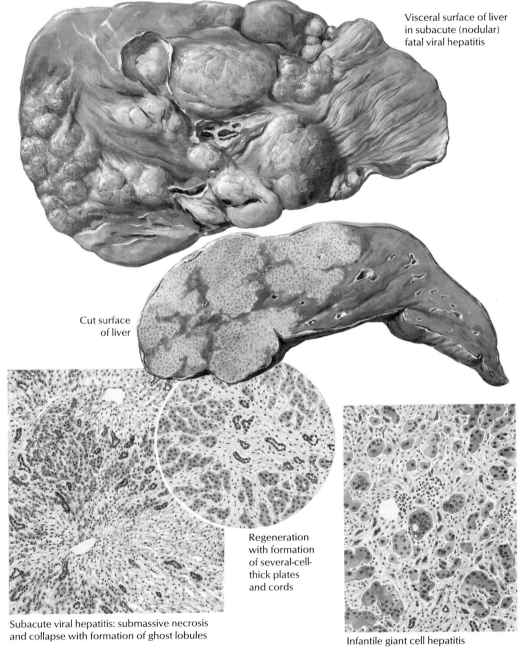

Visceral surface of liver
in subacute (nodular)
fatal viral hepatitis

Cut surface
of liver

Regeneration
with formation
of several-cell-
thick plates
and cords

Subacute viral hepatitis: submassive necrosis
and collapse with formation of ghost lobules

Infantile giant cell hepatitis

Figure 52-4

Acute Hepatitis B
Risk Factors

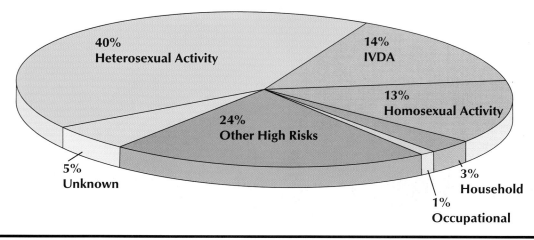

40%
Heterosexual Activity

14%
IVDA

13%
Homosexual Activity

24%
Other High Risks

5%
Unknown

3%
Household

1%
Occupational

Adapted from Epidemiology and Prevention of Viral Hepatitis. *Centers for Disease and Prevention* www.cdc.gov.

Management and Therapy

Acute hepatitis B does not require any treatment except supportive care and monitoring. Cases should be reported to local public health authorities. Sexual contacts within 2 weeks of presentation should be identified and receive hepatitis B immune globulin and hepatitis B vaccine. Repeat serologic testing for hepatitis B 6 months after the acute infection to verify resolution and absence of chronicity. Chronic hepatitis B may progress to cirrhosis, liver failure, and hepatocellular carcinoma. Patients may benefit from therapy with interferon or lamivudine, a nucleoside analogue. Both agents have demonstrated efficacy in resolving active viral replication and improving hepatic histological findings. Chronic hepatitis B carriers with clinical or histologic evidence of cirrhosis are at high risk for hepatocellular carcinoma and should be screened. Household and sexual contacts of carriers should receive hepatitis B vaccine to prevent inapparent parenteral exposure.

Prevention

Hepatitis B vaccine is highly immunogenic, and protective antibodies will develop in most people vaccinated for hepatitis B. Exceptions are patients who are immunocompromised and those with advanced liver disease. Universal vaccination is recommended for all newborns in the United States. With this aggressive strategy, it is likely that within 10 to 20 years, the incidence of acute hepatitis B will decrease significantly. In Taiwan, where hepatitis B is endemic and vertical transmission is the predominant mode of infection, aggressive vaccination of all newborns has dramatically reduced the incidence of hepatocellular carcinoma by preventing vertical transmission. Adolescents and adults born after mandatory vaccination for hepatitis B should be questioned about their vaccination status during routine visits to a health-care providers and every effort should be made to vaccinate them. Because hepatitis B is sexually transmitted, all unvaccinated individuals remain at risk for acquisition of this disease.

DELTA HEPATITIS (HEPATITIS D)

Hepatitis D (HDV) is a defective RNA virus that requires hepatitis B surface antigen to complete replication. Thus, delta infection is never seen in the absence of hepatitis B. It is most common in Mediterranean countries, particularly Italy and Turkey. HDV may be acquired at the time of acute HBV infection (co-infection) or after HBV has been established as a chronic infection (super-infection). Diagnosis can be made in HBsAg-positive individuals by testing for delta antibody in serum.

Figure 52-5

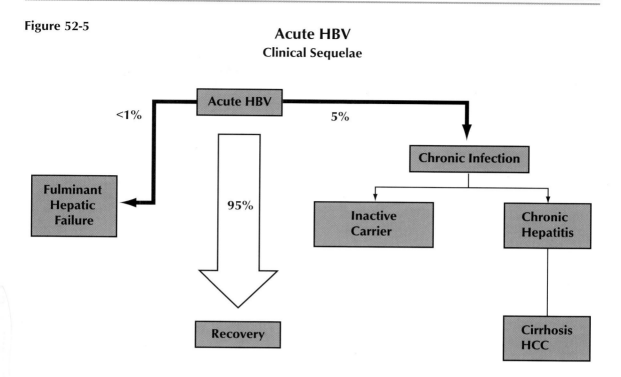

Acute HBV
Clinical Sequelae

HEPATITIS C

In the United States, it has been estimated that 1.8% of the population, or approximately 4 million people, are infected with hepatitis C virus (HCV). Hepatitis C virus is unique among hepatotropic viruses because of the high rate of chronicity. Chronic hepatitis C will develop in 50% to 85% of patients infected with hepatitis C, who will then be at risk for progressive liver disease. Most cases (75%) of acute hepatitis C are asymptomatic. Symptoms, most commonly fatigue, may develop in those who have chronic infection. In advanced cases, symptoms and signs of cirrhosis and portal hypertension may be present.

Hepatitis C is a single-stranded RNA virus. It is heterogeneous, with 6 major genotypes and multiple subtypes. The most common genotype in the United States is genotype 1 (70%), followed by genotypes 2 and 3 (30%). Genotype has no impact on disease progression. However, genotype 1 is strongly correlated with treatment resistance.

Clinical Presentation and Diagnostic Approach

Risk factors include intravenous drug use (70%), blood transfusion (6%), occupational exposure (3%), sexual exposure (~10%, although controversial), and unknown (~10%). The risks of tattoos, body piercing, and intranasal cocaine use are not well defined.

Screening

Because chronic hepatitis C is usually asymptomatic, diagnosis depends on ascertaining potential risk factors for infection during a thorough medical history. Screening for hepatitis C is recommended for all patients with the following: abnormal ALT, intravenous drug use (even on one occasion), blood transfusions before 1992 (before universal blood screening), hemophilia, organ transplant recipients before 1992, and patients on hemodialysis. In addition, health-care workers with documented exposure to HCV-infected blood and children born to HCV-positive mothers should be screened for hepatitis C.

Diagnosis

Anti-HCV antibody is the best screening test for anyone suspected of hepatitis C infection. It is very sensitive and specific in the setting of an identified risk factor and abnormal serum ALT. Supplemental assays, such as the recombinant immunoblot assay, are useful only for patients without risk factors to help resolve a possible false-positive anti-HCV antibody test result. HCV RNA in serum may be detected by using polymerase chain reaction (PCR) assays. It is the most sensitive and specific assay for the diagnosis of hepatitis C and denotes active infection. PCR tests are also used to monitor responses to therapy. Liver biopsy is a simple, generally safe, procedure that provides important information about the stage of liver disease. It is recommended for most patients with chronic hepatitis C.

The natural history of hepatitis C is somewhat controversial. Many patients will have stable disease; others will experience disease progression over 2 to 3 decades to cirrhosis, portal hypertension, and liver failure. No single characteristic or test accurately predicts the course of disease. Factors associated with more rapid disease progression include alcohol use, male gender, age at infection > age 40 years, and HIV coinfection.

Extrahepatic manifestations include cryoglobulinemia, glomerulonephritis, porphyria cutanea tarda, thyroid disease, and, possibly, diabetes mellitus, lichen planus, and B-cell lymphoma.

MANAGEMENT AND THERAPY

Acute hepatitis C is usually asymptomatic. Therefore, diagnosis of acute infection is uncommon. If identified early, therapy with interferon within 3 to 6 months of infection can prevent chronicity in 98% of patients.

Most patients are diagnosed with established chronic disease. Susceptible patients should receive the hepatitis A and B vaccines.

Treatment is indicated for those with evidence of significant inflammatory activity or fibrosis on liver biopsy specimen. Pegylated interferon, injected subcutaneously once per week, plus oral ribavirin, taken twice daily for 1 year results in sustained virological response in 56% of patients. Sustained virological response is defined as negative for HCV RNA in serum 6 months after stopping treatment. This is synonymous with "cure." Patients with genotype 1 have a lower sustained virologic response of 40% to 50%, while those with genotype 2 or 3 respond 75% to 80% of the time. Side effects include neutropenia, thrombocytopenia, hemolytic anemia, depression, and thyroid dysfunction. Treatment is contraindicated for those with significant depression, cardiac disease, or decompensated liver disease.

Prevention and Counseling

There is no risk of hepatitis C transmission by casual contact or hugging, kissing, or sharing food or eating utensils. It is important to avoid sharing objects with the potential for blood contamination, such as razors, toothbrushes, and nail clippers. The risk of sexual transmission is very low, but not zero. There are no recommendations to alter sexual practices when one partner has hepatitis C. The risk of vertical transmission of hepatitis C is very low. Women with hepatitis C are encouraged to have normal pregnancies and delivery, and there are no recommendations against breast-feeding or changing any birthing practices.

FUTURE DIRECTIONS

Extensive use of vaccinations will decrease the incidence of acute and chronic hepatitis B in the United States, although nonvaccinated immigrants from endemic countries remain at risk. For hepatitis C, the focus of future research will be to define host genetics and immune responses with the goal of better understanding the spectrum of disease severity and the development of progressive liver disease. Antiviral therapies for chronic hepatitis B and hepatitis C are likely to continue to improve. For hepatitis B therapy, the major emphasis will be on combination treatment with multiple nucleoside analogues hopefully preventing the development of resistance, as is regularly seen with a single agent, such as lamivudine. Understanding of the mechanism of hepatitis C replication has led to the development of novel agents that selectively inhibit enzymes crucial to HCV replication. These agents are in early phase clinical testing but will likely be useful in combination therapy for chronic hepatitis C within the next 3 to 5 years.

REFERENCES

Fried MW. Advances in therapy for chronic hepatitis C. *Clin Liver Dis.* 2001;5:1009–10023.

Fried MW. Diagnostic testing for hepatitis C: practical considerations. *Am J Med.* 1999;107:31S–35S.

Jonas MM. Viral hepatitis. From prevention to antivirals. *Clin Liver Dis.* 2000;4:849–877.

Lok AS, McMahon BJ, and the Practice Guidelines Committee, American Association for the Study of Liver Diseases. Chronic hepatitis B. *Hepatology.* 2001;34;1225–1241.

Regev A, Schiff ER. Viral hepatitis A, B, and C. *Clin Liver Dis.* 2000;4:47–71.

Section VI

DISORDERS OF COAGULATION AND THROMBOSIS

Chapter 53
Bleeding Disorders

Lee R. Berkowitz

The coagulation system is based on an intricate set of checks and balances between procoagulant and anticoagulant proteins, all interacting with platelets and the vascular endothelium. The end result is protection from bleeding and inhibition of excessive thrombosis. A great deal is known about many of the proteins in this system as well as the structure and function of platelets. This knowledge enables the internist to approach bleeding disorders with diagnostic and therapeutic sophistication.

ETIOLOGY AND PATHOGENESIS
Congenital Bleeding Disorders
von Willebrand Disease (vWD)

vWD is a common congenital bleeding diathesis. Both quantitative and qualitative abnormalities have been described in the von Willebrand protein, which allows platelet adherence to the endothelium and provides factor VIII stability. The most common variant of vWD is type I, which is autosomal dominant in inheritance. Patients have a quantitative decrease in vWD protein to 30% to 50% of normal. Type II variants are defined by qualitative differences in the multimeric structure of the von Willebrand protein. At least eight different type II variants have been described. They are labeled alphabetically as types IIa-IIh. Inheritance is either autosomal dominant or recessive.

Hemophilia A

Hemophilia A is the most common inherited bleeding disorder. The inheritance is X-linked, so this disorder is seen almost exclusively in males. Affected individuals have reduced factor VIII levels. Patients with severe hemophilia have no detectable factor VIII activity. Those with mild hemophilia have 1% to 5% factor VIII activity (Figure 53-1).

Acquired Bleeding Disorders

Disseminated intravascular coagulation (DIC) is a multisystem process resulting in bleeding and thrombosis in the microvasculature. Life-threatening disorders such as sepsis and massive trauma have the ability to overwhelm the clotting cascade, leading to excessive amounts of activated thrombin. This, in turn, causes fibrin deposition with activation of the lytic system and depletion of clotting factors (see Chapter 55, Figure 55-1).

Immune Thrombocytopenic Purpura (ITP)

ITP is an autoimmune process in which patients generate antibodies directed to surface proteins on platelets. The antibody-coated platelets are then prematurely destroyed in the reticuloendothelial system. ITP can occur spontaneously or can be a manifestation of an autoimmune disease or B-cell neoplasm.

Qualitative Disorders of Platelets

Platelet activation is dependent in part on cyclooxygenase-induced release of intracellular granules. Both aspirin and NSAIDs inhibit cyclooxygenase, causing impaired platelet function. This inhibition results in a mild bleeding tendency. Aspirin's effect is irreversible, whereas the NSAIDs cause reversible inhibition of cyclooxygenase.

Liver Disease

The liver is the site of synthesis of the majority of clotting proteins. In addition, activated factors are cleared from the circulation by the liver. Any disease causing impaired liver function will lead to decreased synthesis of clotting factors and a DIC-type picture due to a prolonged half-life of activated thrombin. The liver is also the site of vitamin K–dependent modulation of factors II, VII, IX, and X, a process that is also impaired with significant liver disease, resulting in decreased factor activity.

CLINICAL PRESENTATION AND DIFFERENTIAL DIAGNOSIS

Congenital bleeding disorders may present in childhood or in adults (Figure 53-2). Patients with hemophilia A have bleeding beginning in infancy. As these patients mature, spontaneous hemarthroses are common. Any trauma will result in local-

Figure 53-1

Hemophilia A and B

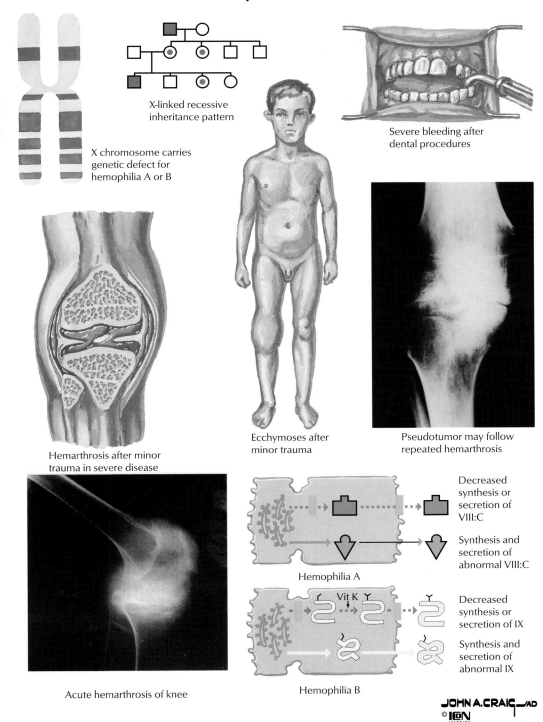

X-linked recessive
inheritance pattern

X chromosome carries
genetic defect for
hemophilia A or B

Severe bleeding after
dental procedures

Hemarthrosis after minor
trauma in severe disease

Ecchymoses after
minor trauma

Pseudotumor may follow
repeated hemarthrosis

Acute hemarthrosis of knee

Hemophilia A

Decreased
synthesis or
secretion of
VIII:C

Synthesis and
secretion of
abnormal VIII:C

Hemophilia B

Decreased
synthesis or
secretion of IX

Synthesis and
secretion of
abnormal IX

JOHN A. CRAIG—AD
© ICON
LEARNING
SYSTEMS

Figure 53-2   **Clinical Presentation of Patients with Bleeding Disorders**

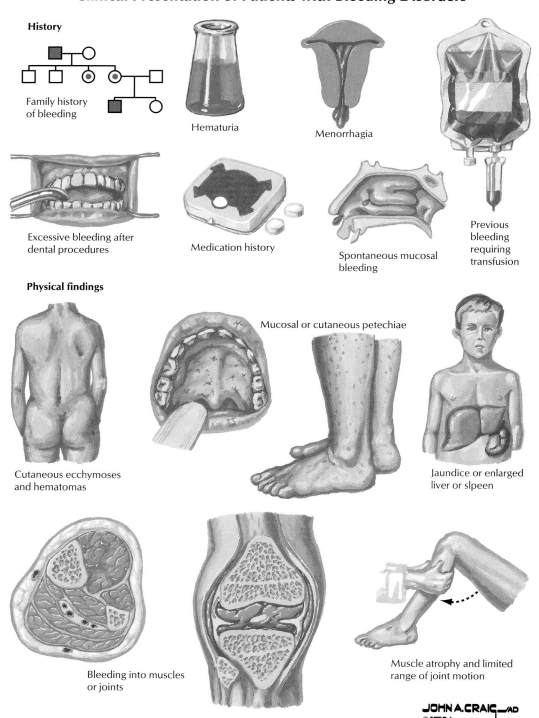

History

Family history of bleeding

Hematuria

Menorrhagia

Previous bleeding requiring transfusion

Excessive bleeding after dental procedures

Medication history

Spontaneous mucosal bleeding

Physical findings

Cutaneous ecchymoses and hematomas

Mucosal or cutaneous petechiae

Jaundice or enlarged liver or slpeen

Bleeding into muscles or joints

Muscle atrophy and limited range of joint motion

JOHN A. CRAIG—AD
©ICON
LEARNING
SYSTEMS

Table 53-1
Diagnostic Studies in Common Coagulations

Disorder	PT	aPTT	Platelet Count	Bleeding Time
Hemophilia A	nl	prolonged	nl	nl
vWD	nl	prolonged	nl	prolonged
DIC	prolonged	prolonged	decreased or nl	nl
ITP	nl	nl	decreased	nl
Qualitative platelet disorders	nl	nl	nl	prolonged
Liver disease	prolonged	prolonged	nl	nl

aPTT, Activated partial thromboplastin time; DIC, disseminated intravascular coagulation; ITP, immune thrombocytopenic purpura; nl, normal; PT, prothrombin time. vWD, von Willebrand's disease.

ized hemorrhage. Patients with vWD usually present later in life, and most often with easy bruisability, heavy menses, or significant bleeding secondary to dental work or surgery. Hemarthroses are rare.

With acquired bleeding disorders, there are several key findings. Patients with ITP or thrombocytopenia associated with DIC usually have petechiae on the lower extremities. The lesions are small para-follicular erythematous macules and are seen at platelet counts less than 50,000/μL. Oozing from any puncture site, such as from IVs, blood-drawing sites, and surgical scars, is common. Patients with qualitative platelet disorders or liver disease generally have an increased tendency to bruise.

With all bleeding problems, there is a great deal of overlap in findings, and none is pathognomonic for a particular disease process. With any of the above findings, the physician should have a low threshold to evaluate the coagulation system.

DIAGNOSTIC APPROACH

Several tests are readily available and will significantly narrow the diagnostic possibilities (Figure 53-3). The prothrombin time (PT) and activated partial thromboplastin time (aPTT) measure the activities of all clotting factors. Prolongations indicate significant factor deficiency, which is seen in hemophilia, vWD, DIC, and the coagulopathy of liver disease. The platelet count detects quantitative platelet problems (alterations in platelet num-

ber), and the bleeding time detects qualitative platelet problems (alterations in platelet function). Table 53-1 shows specific differences in these tests for the common coagulopathies.

Following the results of screening tests, more specific assays can be done. Tests are available for factor VIII and von Willebrand protein. Measurement of other factors and fibrinogen can be helpful for the diagnosis of DIC. The D-dimer assay, which measures lytic system activity, is often used in DIC. The diagnosis of ITP is usually a diagnosis of exclusion. Assays for platelet antibodies are available but have poor specificity (Figure 53-3).

MANAGEMENT AND THERAPY
Congenital Bleeding Disorders
von Willebrand Disease

Type I disease can be treated with desmopressin for mild bleeding and preoperative prophylaxis. The drug can be administered intravenously or subcutaneously and will increase levels of von Willebrand protein in several hours. For more significant bleeding, purified concentrates containing von Willebrand protein should be administered intravenously. Type II disease is treated similarly, except the IIb variant where DDAVP is contraindicated.

Hemophilia A

The treatment of choice for significant bleeding is administration of recombinant factor VIII intra-

BLEEDING DISORDERS

Figure 53-3

Hemostasis Tests

Platelet count

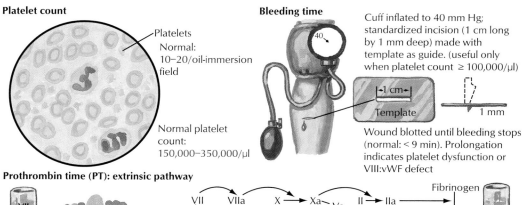

Platelets
Normal:
10–20/oil-immersion
field

Normal platelet
count:
150,000–350,000/μl

Bleeding time

Cuff inflated to 40 mm Hg;
standardized incision (1 cm long
by 1 mm deep) made with
template as guide. (useful only
when platelet count ≥ 100,000/μl)

|←1 cm→|
Template
1 mm

Wound blotted until bleeding stops
(normal: < 9 min). Prolongation
indicates platelet dysfunction or
VIII:vWF defect

Prothrombin time (PT): extrinsic pathway

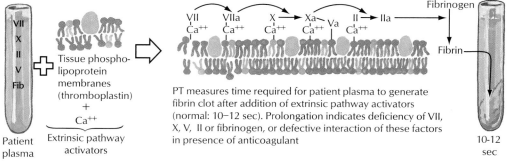

Patient
plasma

Tissue phospho-
lipoprotein
membranes
(thromboplastin)
+
Ca^{++}

Extrinsic pathway
activators

$VII \xrightarrow{} VIIa \xrightarrow{} X \xrightarrow{} Xa \xrightarrow{Va} II \xrightarrow{} IIa \xrightarrow{}$ Fibrinogen
$Ca^{++} \quad Ca^{++} \quad Ca^{++} \quad Ca^{++} \quad Ca^{++}$

Fibrin

PT measures time required for patient plasma to generate
fibrin clot after addition of extrinsic pathway activators
(normal: 10–12 sec). Prolongation indicates deficiency of VII,
X, V, II or fibrinogen, or defective interaction of these factors
in presence of anticoagulant

10-12
sec

Activated partial thromboplastin time (APTT): intrinsic pathway

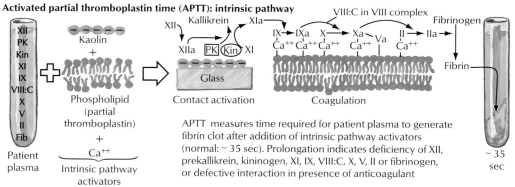

Patient
plasma

Kaolin
+
Phospholipid
(partial
thromboplastin)
+
Ca^{++}

Intrinsic pathway
activators

Contact activation

Coagulation

VIII:C in VIII complex

Kallikrein
XII, XIa
XIIa, PK Kin XI

$IX \xrightarrow{} IXa \quad X \xrightarrow{} Xa \xrightarrow{Va} II \xrightarrow{} IIa \xrightarrow{}$ Fibrinogen
$Ca^{++} Ca^{++} Ca^{++} \quad Ca^{++} \quad Ca^{++}$

Fibrin

APTT measures time required for patient plasma to generate
fibrin clot after addition of intrinsic pathway activators
(normal: ~ 35 sec). Prolongation indicates deficiency of XII,
prekallikrein, kininogen, XI, IX, VIII:C, X, V, II or fibrinogen,
or defective interaction in presence of anticoagulant

~ 35
sec

Mixing studies: prolonged PT or APTT

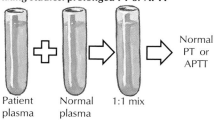

Patient
plasma

Normal
plasma

1:1 mix

Normal
PT or
APTT

Mixing factor-deficient patient plasma with
normal plasma in 1:1 ratio corrects prolonged
patient PT or APTT

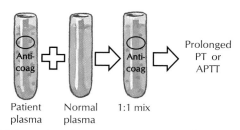

Patient
plasma

Normal
plasma

1:1 mix

Prolonged
PT or
APTT

Mixing patient plasma containing anticoagulant with
normal plasma in 1:1 ratio prolongs PT or APTT
of normal plasma

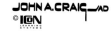

JOHN A.CRAIG—AD
© ICN

venously. The target factor VIII level depends on the severity of bleeding. For isolated hemarthroses, where the target level is 30% to 50%, patients can be taught to self-administer factor VIII.

With treatment, inhibitors to factor VIII develop in 10% to 15% of patients. A variety of approaches can be used in this situation, depending on the severity of the bleeding and the level of the inhibitor.

Acquired Bleeding Disorders
Disseminated Intravascular Coagulation

In patients with DIC, the primary focus should be to treat the underlying condition causing the coagulopathy. Until this is done, there will be no substantial improvement. This usually takes hours to several days. In the interim, fresh frozen plasma and cryoprecipitate can be given to replace clotting factors and fibrinogen. Platelets are also given if the platelet count is less than 50,000/µL with active bleeding. If there is no bleeding related to a surgical procedure, a lower platelet count can be tolerated without transfusion. The use of heparin is controversial because of its bleeding risk. In general, it is given if treatment of the underlying condition and replacement therapy do not appear to be working.

Immune Thrombocytopenic Purpura

At presentation, most patients are treated with prednisone (1 mg/kg body weight/day), which will normalize the platelet count in 3 to 7 days. The process is chronic, and an attempt at tapering steroids will often result in a decrease in the platelet count. Patients then must undergo splenectomy, which produces a complete response in 70% to 80% of cases. Intravenous immunoglobulin (IVIG) is an alternative to prednisone that improves the platelet count in days. Whether there is any advantage to IVIG is not clear, nor is it clear that the combination of prednisone and immunoglobulin is superior to either alone. For patients who continue with significant thrombocytopenia after splenectomy, there are a number of options including chemotherapy, high-dose pulse steroids, or chronic daily steroids. Responses are quite individualized.

Liver Disease

Because many patients have irreversible liver pathology, the coagulopathy is usually a chronic process. Repeated doses of vitamin K may be helpful. Otherwise, patients are treated for acute bleeding with fresh frozen plasma, which will transiently raise factor levels.

FUTURE DIRECTIONS

A considerable amount of effort has been made to initiate gene therapy in hemophilia, based on the observation that gene expression that produces a factor VIII level of a few percent would eliminate most of the bleeding. Clinical trials are currently in progress. Patients with hemophilia and inhibitors can also look forward to improved treatments. Recombinant factor VIIa is now available, and methods for development of immune tolerance are being improved. The treatment of patients with ITP refractory to prednisone and splenectomy is the target of a number of new agents, including thrombopoietin, rituximab, and mycophenolate mofetil.

REFERENCES

Bick RL. Disseminated intravascular coagulation: pathophysiological mechanisms and manifestations. *Semin Thromb Hemost.* 1998;24:3–18.

George JN, Woolf SH, Raskob GE, et al. Idiopathic thrombocytopenic purpura: a practice guideline developed by explicit methods for the American Society of Hematology. *Blood.* 1996;88:3–40.

Hedner U, Ginsburg D, Lusher JM, High KA. Congenital hemorrhagic disorders: new insights into the pathophysiology and treatment of hemophilia. *Hematology (Am Soc Hematol Educ Program).* 2000:241–265.

Chapter 54

Deep Venous Thrombosis and Pulmonary Embolism

Darren A. DeWalt and Marschall S. Runge

Deep venous thrombosis (DVT) and pulmonary embolism (PE) are the two most important clinical events that occur in individuals with venous thrombosis. Approximately 0.1% of the population will experience a DVT, and PE is the third leading cause of cardiovascular mortality. Early diagnosis and treatment of DVT and PE substantially reduce mortality and morbidity, but autopsy series find that DVT and PE are still underdiagnosed. The numerous publications of algorithms aimed at improving diagnostic accuracy and optimizing treatment illustrate the frequency with which both DVT and PE elude diagnosis. In this chapter, we will review the various presentations of these syndromes and provide an overview of the most promising modalities for early diagnosis and treatment.

ETIOLOGY AND PATHOGENESIS

Deep venous thromboses may occur anywhere in the venous system, but most begin in the lower extremities between the lower leg and the pelvis. Virchow's classic triad of vessel wall injury, stasis, and hypercoagulability is as relevant today as when proposed for understanding the pathogenesis and risk factors for thrombosis. Both stasis and vessel wall injury can lead to platelet aggregation, which triggers the clotting cascade, including cellular and protein components. This can result in an imbalance in the naturally occurring procoagulant and anticoagulant proteins, and formation of an intravascular thrombus. Chapter 56 describes this complex system in more detail.

Although pulmonary emboli usually result from thrombi in the venous system of the lower extremities or pelvis, one must also consider the inferior vena cava, renal or upper extremity veins, and even the right side of the heart as sources of pulmonary emboli (Figure 54-1). While thrombi can also form in smaller veins below the popliteal vein, these thrombi rarely embolize, and thus present a low risk.

Many of the classic risk factors for DVT or PE affect one aspect of Virchow's triad (Figure 54-2). Immobility from surgery, trauma, or paralysis can lead to stasis because venous flow in the lower extremities is partially dependent on muscular contraction. By entirely different mechanisms, surgery, trauma, or infection can cause vessel wall

injury. Additionally, the majority of malignancies are accompanied by some degree of hypercoagulability, a complication particularly well-documented in mucinous adenocarcinomas.

Another common cause of DVT involves pregnancy; the combination of a hypercoagulable state, local venous stasis (from the uterus compressing the inferior vena cava), and immobility (e.g., with travel) is a common setting for DVT in individuals who have none of the above risk factors. Indeed, other identified hypercoagulable states are increasing in number and are discussed in Chapter 56. Understanding the settings in which DVT and PE occur may offer the clinician a clue toward diagnosis. However, it is important to consider the clinical findings (Tables 54-1 and 54-2), particularly for patients with no known precipitants.

CLINICAL PRESENTATION

Patients with DVT or PE present with a spectrum of symptoms ranging from mild tenderness or swelling in the calf to acute dyspnea and syncope. A careful history may reveal one or more of the predisposing risk factors listed in Tables 54-1 and 54-2. The classic constellation of symptoms for an isolated DVT includes unilateral leg symptoms of swelling, tenderness, and dilated collateral veins. As previously noted, most patients do not present with this complete set of findings, making early diagnosis more challenging. Interestingly, approximately 40% of patients with iso-

Figure 54-1

Deep Venous Thrombosis

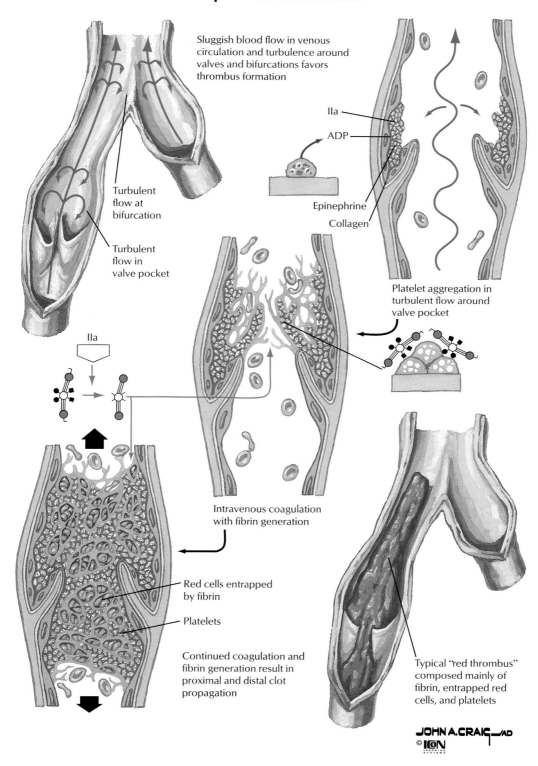

Sluggish blood flow in venous circulation and turbulence around valves and bifurcations favors thrombus formation

IIa

ADP

Epinephrine

Collagen

Turbulent flow at bifurcation

Turbulent flow in valve pocket

Platelet aggregation in turbulent flow around valve pocket

IIa

Intravenous coagulation with fibrin generation

Red cells entrapped by fibrin

Platelets

Continued coagulation and fibrin generation result in proximal and distal clot propagation

Typical "red thrombus" composed mainly of fibrin, entrapped red cells, and platelets

JOHN A. CRAIG—AD
© ICON

Figure 54-2   **Predisposing Factors for Pulmonary Embolism**

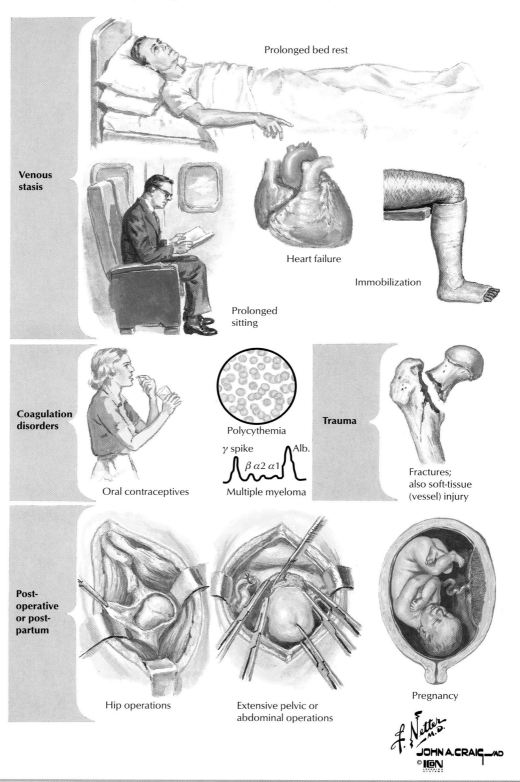

Prolonged bed rest

Venous stasis

Heart failure

Immobilization

Prolonged sitting

Coagulation disorders

Oral contraceptives

Polycythemia

γ spike   Alb.

β $\alpha 2$ $\alpha 1$

Multiple myeloma

Trauma

Fractures; also soft-tissue (vessel) injury

Post-operative or post-partum

Hip operations

Extensive pelvic or abdominal operations

Pregnancy

Table 54-1
Clinical Model for Predicting Pretest Probability for Deep Venous Thrombosis

Clinical Feature	Score
Active cancer (treatment ongoing or within previous 6 mo or palliative)	1
Paralysis, paresis, or recent plaster immobilization of the lower extremities	1
Recently bedridden >3 d or major surgery within 4 wk	1
Localized tenderness along the distribution of the deep venous system	1
Entire leg swollen	1
Calf swelling 3 cm > asymptomatic side (measured 10 cm below tibial tuberosity)	1
Pitting edema confined to the symptomatic leg	1
Collateral superficial veins (nonvaricose)	1
Alternative diagnosis as likely or greater than that of DVT	-2

In patients with symptoms in both legs, the more symptomatic leg is used. Pretest probability calculated as the total score: high ≥3; moderate 1 or 2; low ≤0.
Adapted from Wells PS, Anderson DR, Bormanis J, et al. Value of assessment of pretest probability of deep-vein thrombosis in clinical management. *Lancet.* 1997;350:1795–1798.

Table 54-2
Algorithm to Determine Pretest Probability of Pulmonary Embolism

Clinical Feature	Score
Clinical symptoms of DVT	3
Heart rate higher than 100 beats/min	1.5
Immobilization or surgery in the previous 4 wk	1.5
Previous objectively diagnosed DVT or PE	1.5
Hemoptysis	1
Malignancy	1
PE as likely as or more likely than an alternative diagnosis	3

Probability: High ≥6 pts, moderate 2–6 pts, low <2 pts.
Adapted from Wells PS, Anderson DR, Rodger M, et al. Excluding pulmonary embolism at the bedside without diagnostic imaging: management of patients with suspected pulmonary embolism presenting to the emergency department by using a simple clinical model and D-dimer. *Ann Intern Med.* 2001;135:98–107.

lated DVT will have asymptomatic PEs on ventilation/perfusion (V/Q) scans.

The more ominous presentation of PE may (but not invariably) include the symptoms of DVT and also reflect the effect of acute cessation of perfusion to parts of the lung. The sudden onset of dyspnea and tachycardia may be the initial clue (Figure 54-3). Other common symptoms and signs include chest pain (pleuritic or nonpleuritic), hemoptysis, pleural rub, hypoxemia, or fever (less than 38.9°C). A patient who also has syncope, hypotension, or signs of new-onset right-sided heart failure falls into the category of severe PE. At highest risk are those patients with PE who present with hemodynamic compromise. One should always include PE in the differential diagnosis for patients presenting in cardiogenic shock until another cause is proven.

DIFFERENTIAL DIAGNOSIS

Many processes can masquerade as a DVT or PE; keep them in mind while proceeding down the diagnostic algorithms. One of the most important factors in determining the probability of DVT or PE is the likelihood of a competing diagnosis. For DVT, the most common competing diagnoses are muscle strain or leg injury, venous insufficiency, lymphatic obstruction, popliteal cyst, drug-induced edema, and cellulitis. The differential diagnosis of dyspnea and tachycardia is also quite long and includes pneumonia, congestive heart failure, myocardial infarction, chronic obstructive pulmonary disease, pulmonary hemorrhage, and aspiration pneumonitis. One of the first steps in the diagnosis of DVT or PE is to assess the likelihood that one of the competing diagnoses accounts for the symptoms and physical examination findings.

DIAGNOSTIC APPROACH

The most accurate and cost-effective approach to the diagnosis of DVT and PE remains an active area of research and a challenge for clinicians. Currently, most authors recommend algorithms that combine the pretest probability with careful selection of diagnostic tests. Because DVT and PE are commonly missed, these diagnoses must be kept in mind until proven otherwise. This does not mandate comprehensive testing for a given patient, but the pretest probability for DVT and PE increases in circumstances when other leading diagnoses are excluded in the course of the initial assessment.

DEEP VENOUS THROMBOSIS

The diagnostic evaluation for suspected DVT should begin with an assessment of the pretest probability. Countless models have been proposed. The most widely used model was developed by Wells and associates (Table 54-1). Unfortunately, because of varied presentations, the clinical diagnosis of DVT is very inaccurate, leading to difficulty establishing an accurate pretest probability. This issue is presented in greater detail in Chapter 7. Pretest probability is extremely important, however, in interpreting the results of noninvasive tests, as described below.

The options for objective testing include D-dimer, compression venous ultrasonography (US), impedance plethysmography, and contrast venography. Contrast venography remains the gold standard for the diagnosis of DVT, and compression venous US has largely replaced impedance phethysmography as the noninvasive diagnostic test of choice. The accuracy of compression venous US has greatly reduced the need for contrast venography.

The D-dimer assays measure a degradation product of cross-linked fibrin and are commonly used in assessment of DVT. Theoretically, any patient with active coagulation should have an elevated D-dimer, suggesting the usefulness of a negative result to "rule-out" DVT. However, in clinical studies, the likelihood ratio of a negative D-dimer does not significantly lower the probability of disease. In practice, the D-dimer can sufficiently lower the probability of DVT in the low-risk group to avoid proceeding with ultrasonography. In the moderate- and high-risk groups, the false-negative rate of the D-dimer is too high to render it useful. Additionally, a positive result on a D-dimer test is woefully nonspecific and cannot be used to diagnose DVT. Certain patient groups are known to have especially high rates of false-positive results, including hospitalized patients and those who have had recent surgery or malignancy. We do not recommend routine use of D-dimer assays because they are, at best, useful only in the lowest-risk group that can still be adequately assessed noninvasively.

Compression venous US leads the list of noninvasive tests for the diagnosis of DVT. A positive test result occurs when the femoral or popliteal veins are noncompressible under ultrasound visualization. The ability to perform this test in a timely manner is the most difficult barrier because most studies must be done during normal working hours. The sensitivity and specificity of this test have been reported to be as high as 95% and 96%, respectively, for symptomatic, proximal DVT, although this clearly depends on the skill

Figure 54-3

Embolism of Lesser Degree Without Infarction

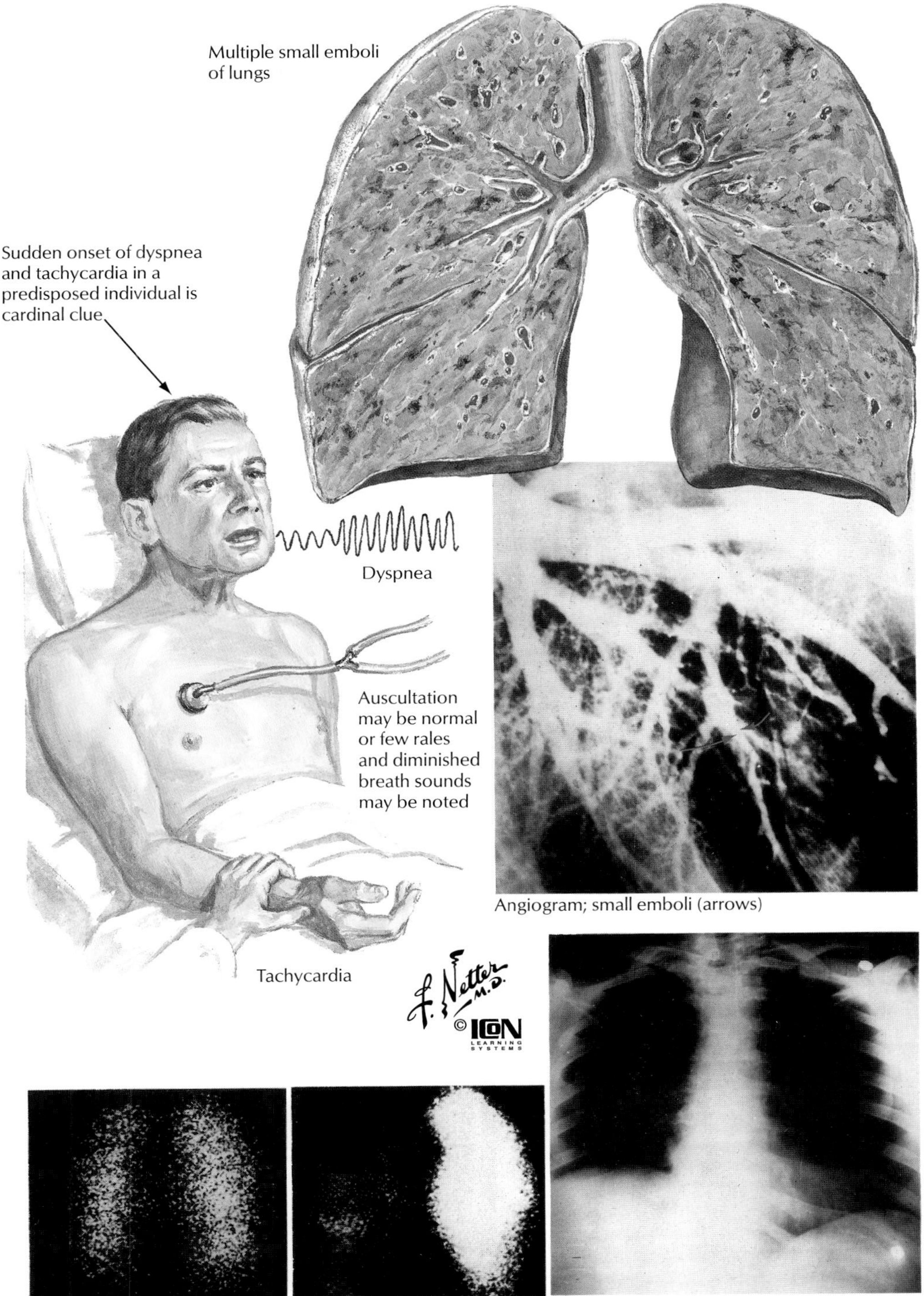

Multiple small emboli of lungs
Sudden onset of dyspnea and tachycardia in a predisposed individual is cardinal clue
Dyspnea
Auscultation may be normal or few rales and diminished breath sounds may be noted
Tachycardia
Angiogram; small emboli (arrows)
F. Netter M.D.
© ICON LEARNING SYSTEMS

Ventilation scan normal

Perfusion scan reveals defects in right lung. Emboli in left lung not visualized

X-ray film often normal.

and experience of the technologist and interpreting physician. For the diagnosis of isolated thrombosis in the calf vein, sensitivity and specificities are 60% to 70%, but as previously described, patients with only distal thromboses are at very low risk. When the US result confirms the clinical suspicion, one can stop further testing and proceed with therapy. Another test is required only if there is discord between the clinical suspicion and the US result.

Contrast venography is occasionally needed as the arbiter of discordant results between the clinical predictor model and the initial US. If a patient is thought to be at low risk, but has a positive US, venography is used to confirm the result. A negative venogram will abrogate long-term anticoagulation. Alternatively, if clinical suspicion is high but the US result is negative, most clinicians will consider venography to be certain that the US did not yield a false-negative result. The use of serial US examinations instead of venography has been proposed (Hirsch and Lee, 2002), but opinion varies. Certainly, this approach is preferable in individuals at risk of contrast dye nephropathy or with known dye allergy. Serial duplex examinations should be considered 7 days after the initial workup.

PULMONARY EMBOLISM

The diagnosis of PE begins in the same manner—with an assessment of the clinical probability of disease (Figure 54-3). Table 54-2 is a useful set of clinical criteria to determine pretest probability of pulmonary embolism. The last item is determined by the physician based on all available clinical data including history, physical examination, ECG, and chest radiography. In the initial study of this tool, patients in the high-risk group had an incidence of 41%; the moderate-risk group, 16%; and the low-risk group, 1.3%. This, again, illustrates the limitations of risk stratification and the difficulty of relying on clinical judgment alone for diagnosis.

The ECG does not reliably diagnose PE, but it may offer clues to its presence. The classic ECG finding of S1Q3T3 is infrequently present, and nonspecific ST or T wave changes appear more commonly (Figure 54-4). Evidence of new right ventricular strain or right axis deviation can be an early marker for massive PE. The ECG can also help determine whether other differential diagnoses, particularly myocardial infarction, are present.

The chest radiograph is mainly helpful in identifying other diagnoses and lessening the likelihood that the presentation is due to pulmonary embolism. The classic findings of pulmonary infarct that have been described (Hampton's hump or a dilated proximal pulmonary artery) are rarely seen.

The D-dimer test occupies the same place in the workup of PE as it does for DVT. In a patient in the lowest risk group, a negative D-dimer makes the presence of a PE unlikely. In any other group of patients, the D-dimer is not useful.

The imaging procedures for the determination of PE are ventilation-perfusion (V/Q) scan, helical CT scan, and pulmonary angiography. The V/Q scan remains the most time-tested and reliable noninvasive test for diagnosis of PE. The possible test results include normal, low probability, intermediate probability, and high probability. A normal V/Q scan will eliminate the possibility of PE, and a high probability scan will diagnose PE. Low or intermediate probability scans lack the accuracy to either dismiss the diagnosis of PE entirely or to begin therapy, and, depending on the clinical setting, may mandate further testing. Many other illnesses can complicate interpretation of the test, including neoplasm, infection, and heart failure; a normal baseline radiograph increases the chances that the V/Q scan will yield useful results. In our institution, many of our complicated patients, for whom knowing a diagnosis is essential, will be placed in the low or intermediate category and require further testing.

The *contrast-enhanced helical CT scan* has gained rapid acceptance in the diagnosis of PE and has decreased the use of V/Q scanning for some groups of patients. The CT has a high specificity and reasonable sensitivity for emboli in the proximal pulmonary arteries and the large branches. However, it is always limited in the diagnosis of subsegmental defects. Based on a number of studies, a positive CT result confirms the diagnosis of PE, but a negative CT result of the chest does not adequately rule out PE. CT can be used in settings where underlying lung pathology makes V/Q scanning difficult to interpret, and can often be used for assessing proximal PE concurrently with other suspected diagnoses. In some centers, CT scanning can be performed more rapidly and during off-hours when V/Q scanning is

Figure 54-4

Massive Embolization

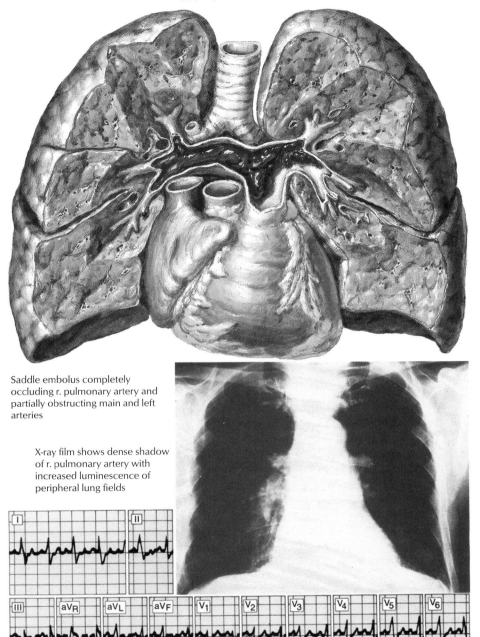

Saddle embolus completely occluding r. pulmonary artery and partially obstructing main and left arteries

X-ray film shows dense shadow of r. pulmonary artery with increased luminescence of peripheral lung fields

Characteristic electrocardiographic findings in acute pulmonary embolism. Deep S_1; prominent Q_3 with inversion of T_3; depression of S-T segment in lead II (often also in lead I) with staircase ascent of S-T_2; T_2 diphasic or inverted; r. axis deviation; tachycardia

not available. Besides the lack of sensitivity for distal PEs, CT scanning is limited in that it requires the administration of venous contrast material, which may be contraindicated in some groups of patients. Thus, CT scan offers an alternative for the V/Q scan, but neither is the perfect test and, unfortunately, the combination of the two tests does not carry the same diagnostic yield as a pulmonary angiogram.

As for DVT, angiography remains the gold standard for the diagnosis of PE. This invasive procedure requires passage of a catheter into the pulmonary arteries and injection of contrast under fluoroscopy. The risk of pulmonary angiography is less than 0.5% in skilled hands, and thus is far less than the complications of misdiagnosis of PE. Delaying anticoagulation in patients with thrombus can be disastrous, and chronic unnecessary anticoagulation should be avoided. Thus, any patient with a high clinical suspicion of PE but an ambiguous diagnosis should undergo pulmonary angiography.

In the stable patient, an often reasonable alternative is to perform lower-extremity venous US. Although not all PEs result from DVT, the presence of DVT offers confirmatory evidence that, in the presence of appropriate symptoms, the patient has had a PE.

MANAGEMENT AND THERAPY

The recommendations for therapy for DVT and PE are currently the same, except for very large PEs, or PEs in the presence of hemodynamic compromise. The efficacy of anticoagulation is clear, but controversies remain over the acute management of DVT and PE, and on the necessary length of long-term anticoagulation. Both of these are addressed in the American College of Chest Physicians (ACCP) guidelines (Hyers, 2001) in more detail.

Acute management of DVT and PE requires administration of heparin. Multiple studies have evaluated the effectiveness of continuous infusion unfractionated heparin (UH) and low-molecular-weight heparin (LMWH), both of which are indirect thrombin inhibitors (requiring the presence of antithrombin III). Most authorities consider both therapies effective for DVT and hemodynamically stable PE. Most hospitals have developed standard protocols for the administration of UH, and we strongly support this approach. At our hospital,

UH is started with a bolus dose of 80 IU/kg and a continuous infusion of 18 IU/kg/hr. The activated partial thromboplastin time (aPTT) should be checked 6 hours after initiation and the dose of heparin adjusted to reach an aPTT of 1.5 to 2.3 times normal. Many physicians prefer LMWH because of its ease of administration (subcutaneously once or twice daily) and because therapeutic monitoring is not usually required. However, the kidneys clear LMWH, and monitoring is needed if the creatinine clearance is less than 30 mL/min. To monitor LMWH, plasma anti-Xa activity is followed. In stable patients, LMWH can be given on an outpatient basis. Note that different preparations of LMWH vary in their relative antithrombin and anti-Xa activities, and they may not be readily interchangeable. Altogether, however, the only reason that LMWH is not the clear treatment of choice for patients with DVT and PE is its cost, which is much higher than that of UH.

Long-term anticoagulation is recommended for any patient with either DVT or PE, and, at this time, warfarin is the mainstay of this therapy. Warfarin exerts its effect by inhibiting the formation of vitamin K–dependent proteins, and thus does not achieve therapeutic anticoagulation until it has been administered for several days. It is currently recommended to start warfarin during the first 1 to 2 days of heparin therapy and continue the heparin until the International Normalized Ratio reaches the therapeutic range of 2.0 to 3.0 (approximately 1 week).

Duration of anticoagulation depends on the underlying cause of the thrombosis and is still a subject of much debate and research. The current ACCP guidelines are reasonable (Table 54-3), but these recommendations may change as we learn more about the causes of "idiopathic" venous thromboembolism.

Most patients can be treated according to the above guidelines. However, patients with either very large PEs or with PE and hemodynamic compromise may require a more aggressive approach. Thrombolytics have been studied in patients with massive PE, but have not been proven to decrease mortality, probably due to the comorbidities present in patients with massive PE. However, most experts agree that hemodynamically unstable patients should be considered for thrombolytic therapy. If thrombolytic therapy is considered, the potential for bleeding (particularly from an under-

Table 54-3
Duration of Anticoagulation for Deep Venous Thrombosis and Pulmonary Embolism

3–6 months	First event with reversible or time-limited risk factor
≥ 6 months	Idiopathic DVT and PE, first event
12 months or lifetime	First event with: Cancer, Anticardiolipin antibody, Antithrombin deficiency, Recurrent event, idiopathic or with thrombophilia

With permission from Hyers TM, Agnelli G, Hull RD, et al. Antithrombotic therapy for venous thromboembolic disease. *Chest* 2001; 119:184S

lying malignancy) must be carefully weighed. Surgical embolectomy should be considered for patients with massive PE and hemodynamic compromise with contraindications to thrombolytic therapy or who fail thrombolysis.

Another subset of patients who require special consideration are those with contraindications to anticoagulation or with repetitive DVT or PE. In individuals with contraindications to anticoagulation, an inferior vena cava (IVC) filter may be inserted to lessen the chance of further pulmonary emboli. Temporary filters that can be removed after the situation is resolved are now available. IVC filters can also be used with anticoagulation in patients with recurrent DVTs and PEs. Occasionally, long-term IVC filters will be used as a last option in patients with a contraindication to anticoagulation, although in this circumstance, complications can arise from local thrombosis at the site of the filter.

Prophylaxis

Prevention of DVT and PE has been well studied and proven effective in several instances.

Patients at high risk for DVT and PE include (in order of descending risk) those undergoing surgical procedures (especially orthopedic and neurosurgical); after ischemic stroke; and medical patients with cancer, heart failure, severe lung disease, or myocardial infarction. Those at highest risk clearly benefit from more aggressive measures to prevent clot. For instance, therapy with LMWH is clearly superior to other modalities for patients undergoing hip or knee replacements. For patients at lower risk (medical patients), the best therapy remains unclear. In practice, many centers give low-dose UH subcutaneously twice a day, but over time, LMWH will likely be shown to be more useful in preventing DVT and PE. Ultimately, DVT and PE prophylaxis should be instituted for any patients at risk. A detailed analysis of the vast research in this area can be found in the ACCP guidelines on prevention of venous thromboembolism (Geerts, 2001).

FUTURE DIRECTIONS

The diagnostic algorithms of DVT and PE will benefit from further refinement of the imaging modalities, but the most exciting developments will be in anticoagulants with fewer side effects and a broader therapeutic window.

REFERENCES

Geerts WH, Heit JA, Clagett GP, et al. Prevention of venous thromboembolism. *Chest.* 2001;119(suppl):132S–175S.

Hirsh J, Lee AY. How we diagnose and treat deep vein thrombosis. *Blood.* 2002;99:3102–3110.

Hyers TM, Agnelli G, Hull RD, et al. Antithrombotic therapy for venous thromboembolic disease. *Chest.* 2001;119(suppl): 176S–193S.

Rodger M, Wells PS. Diagnosis of pulmonary embolism. *Thromb Res.* 2001;103:V255–V238.

Wells PS, Anderson DR, Bormanis J, et al. Value of assessment of pretest probability of deep-vein thrombosis in clinical management. *Lancet.* 1997;350:1795–1798.

Wells PS, Anderson DR, Rodger M, et al. Excluding pulmonary embolism at the bedside without diagnostic imaging: management of patients with suspected pulmonary embolism presenting to the emergency department by using a simple clinical model and D-dimer. *Ann Intern Med.* 2001;135:98–107.

Chapter 55

Disseminated Intravascular Coagulation

Stephan Moll

Disseminated intravascular coagulation (DIC) is a complex coagulation disorder due to widespread activation of both the clotting system and the fibrinolytic system, with resultant thrombotic and hemorrhagic complications. DIC is not a disease, but a common pathologic pathway resulting from various triggering factors.

ETIOLOGY AND PATHOGENESIS

DIC is the result of inappropriate and excessive activation of the hemostatic process. The pathological activators of this process are only partially understood. Several mechanisms of activation are likely, including release of tissue factor into the systemic circulation (in extensive tissue trauma; abruptio placentae; retained dead fetus); production of tissue factor-like substances by malignant tumor cells; tissue factor-like activity of amniotic fluid; vessel wall endothelial injury leading to platelet activation, followed by activation of the hemostatic system (in endotoxin sepsis, extensive burns, hypothermia, hypoxemia and acidosis, extensive carcinomatosis); direct platelet activation by antigen-antibody complexes; and anaphylaxis (in amniotic fluid embolism).

The activation of the coagulation system leads to excessive thrombin, with subsequent fibrin formation. Fibrin is deposited in the vasculature of multiple organs, particularly the small caliber vessels. Thrombin and fibrin formation leads to activation of the fibrinolytic system, in which plasminogen gets activated to plasmin, which then breaks down fibrin. Procoagulant and fibrinolytic factors are thus consumed.

Thrombin also leads to platelet activation, which further enhances the prothrombotic state. The consumption of platelets leads to thrombocytopenia. When procoagulant activity dominates, thrombi form in the microvasculature, leading to multiorgan failure. If the fibrinolytic activity and the consumption of procoagulant factors dominate, bleeding results. Microangiopathic hemolytic anemia (MAHA) occurs when microthrombi narrow the lumen of the microvasculature, and erythrocytes, unable to pass through, become fragmented; hemolysis and circulation of fragmented red blood cells (helmet cells and schistocytes) result.

CLINICAL PRESENTATION

The clinical presentation of DIC varies (Figure 55-1). Low-grade DIC, often referred to as compensated DIC, is found most frequently in patients with malignant tumors and, rarely, in the

---

Clinical Conditions Associated with Disseminated Intravascular Coagulation

- Sepsis
- Trauma
- Cancer
- Obstetrical calamities
    Amniotic fluid embolism
    Preeclampsia, eclampsia, HELLP
    Abruptio placentae
- Endotoxin sepsis
- Retained dead fetus
- Vascular disorders
    Aortic aneurysm
    Hemangiomas
- Head injury
- Reactions to toxins
    Snake venom
- Drugs
- Allergic reactions
- Therapy with prothrombin complex concentrates

Figure 55-1

Disseminated Intravascular Coagulation (DIC)

Extensive exposure of subendothelium activates intrinsic pathway excessively

Large amounts of phospholipoprotein membranes entering the circulation activate extrinsic pathway excessively

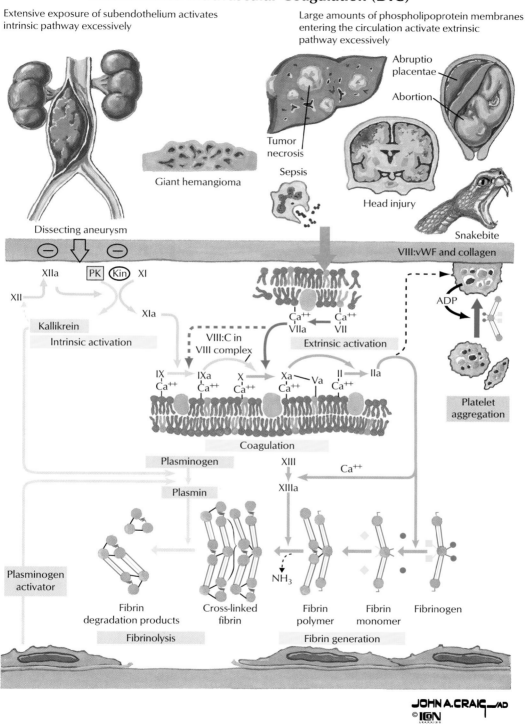

Abruptio placentae

Abortion

Tumor necrosis

Sepsis

Head injury

Giant hemangioma

Dissecting aneurysm

Snakebite

VIII:vWF and collagen

XIIa   PK Kin   XI

XII

XIa

Kallikrein

Intrinsic activation

VIII:C in VIII complex

Ca^{++} VIIa Ca^{++} VII

Extrinsic activation

ADP

IX Ca^{++} IXa Ca^{++} X Ca^{++} Xa Ca^{++} — Va   II Ca^{++} — IIa

Platelet aggregation

Coagulation

Plasminogen

XIII Ca^{++}

Plasmin

XIIIa

Plasminogen activator

NH_3

Fibrin degradation products

Cross-linked fibrin

Fibrin polymer

Fibrin monomer

Fibrinogen

Fibrinolysis

Fibrin generation

JOHN A. CRAIG—MD

© ICON

obstetrical patient with a retained dead fetus. Because liver synthetic function is able to replace the consumed coagulation proteins and a steady state is reached, the patient may be asymptomatic, and DIC is detected only by laboratory testing. More severe DIC leads to subacute or acute systemic bleeding, sometimes in conjunction with end-organ failure. The hemorrhagic diathesis may present as easy bruising, microscopic or macroscopic hematuria, or bleeding from venipuncture, intravenous catheter sites, surgical wounds, or endotracheal tubes. At the most extreme end is fulminant DIC, presenting as massive and diffuse bleeding, unmanageable by blood product transfusions.

DIC in the obstetrical patient can present in several different ways. Amniotic fluid embolism occurs in 1:20,000 to 1:30,000 deliveries, carries a 26% to 86 % maternal mortality, and is responsible for approximately 10% of maternal deaths. It occurs during labor or caesarean section, or within 30 minutes postpartum. Fulminant, diffuse hemorrhage develops due to the consumption of coagulation factors, or acute hypotension, hypoxemia, and cardiopulmonary arrest due to widespread microthrombi. Previous pregnancy, carrying a male fetus, and a history of allergies and atopy are risk factors, but prolonged labor or the use of oxytocin are not. A less severe DIC, ranging from mild vaginal bleeding to maternal hemorrhagic shock, may occur in abruptio placentae. The extent of DIC in septic abortion, intra-amniotic infection, and postpartum endometritis varies (Figure 55-1).

DIFFERENTIAL DIAGNOSIS

Often the presentation is such that DIC cannot be diagnosed with absolute certainty. Many of the patients in whom the diagnosis of DIC is entertained are in the intensive care unit and have multiple medical problems. The coagulopathy and thrombocytopenia in these patients are often multifactorial. A diagnosis of "probable component of DIC" is the best conclusion to which even the hematologist and coagulationist can commit.

The differential diagnosis includes coagulopathy due to liver synthetic dysfunction in chronic or acute liver failure; thrombocytopenia due to hypersplenism; vitamin K deficiency in the postsurgical or ICU patient; dilutional coagulopathy and thrombocytopenia after multiple red blood cell transfusions; drug- or heparin-induced thrombocytopenia; thrombotic thrombocytopenic purpura (TTP); hemolytic-uremic syndrome (HUS); other microangiopathic hemolytic anemias; immune-mediated thrombocytopenia (ITP) triggered by infection; or a defective heart valve in infective endocarditis.

In the pregnant or postpartum patient, the differential diagnosis includes preeclampsia, eclampsia, HELPP syndrome, and TTP/HUS.

DIAGNOSTIC APPROACH

A diagnosis of DIC is best made by verifying that the patient has an underlying disease that can be associated with DIC, and by obtaining a combination of coagulation tests (e.g., PT, aPTT, fibrinogen, antithrombin III, D-dimer, factor VII, factor V) and a platelet count that are consistant with DIC; a review of the peripheral blood smear should be done as well. In addtion, it is important to exclude other disease entities that could cause a similar picture and to use factor VIII activity levels to differentiate between severe DIC and severe liver synthetic dysfunction. The activity of the vitamin K–dependent factors (II, VII, IX, X) should be compared with non-vitamin K–dependent factors (fibrinogen, ATIII, V, VIII, XI, XII) to differentiate between vitamin K deficiency and DIC. Finally, coagulation tests (e.g., antithrombin III , fibrinogen, platelet count, possibly factor VII and factor V) should be followed over time to assess for progression, stabilization, or improvement of DIC.

MANAGEMENT AND THERAPY

Management of DIC centers around treatment of the underlying disorder that triggered DIC, blood product support in the bleeding patient, and consideration of the use of low-dose heparin, antithrombin III concentrate, or activated protein C concentrate (Drotrecogin alfa).

The literature on DIC is full of reviews and opinions on the treatment, but there are very few clinical treatment studies; therefore, therapy is mostly empirical. The bleeding patient clearly needs blood product support. In the non-bleeding patient with DIC who is at increased risk for bleeding (postsurgical, postpartum, intubated, etc.), blood products are often indicated. In other non-bleeding patients with DIC, blood product transfusions are probably not indicated. However, no randomized trials on the use of fresh frozen plasma

(FFP) and platelets in DIC have been published. The theory that blood product transfusions, such as plasma and platelets, may "fuel the fire" and worsen DIC, has never been proven. However, avoidance of transfusion products in DIC patients not at risk for bleeding appears prudent. The clinician should not focus on treating laboratory abnormalities. The clinical picture should guide management.

Blood Products

Fresh frozen plasma (FFP) contains all coagulation factors, but none in concentrated form. A bleeding patient with severe DIC should receive as much FFP as possible, but fluid overload is a limitation. To avoid a dilutional coagulopathy in the patient who receives multiple packed red blood cell transfusions, use one bag of FFP for every 4 units of packed red blood cells.

Cryoprecipitate contains mainly fibrinogen, von Willebrand factor, and fibronectin. In the patient who is bleeding or who is at high risk of bleeding, fibrinogen levels should be kept above 100 mg/dL, possibly above 150 mg/dL. In some countries, purified fibrinogen products are available. In the United States, cryoprecipitate is the product of choice. One dose of cryoprecipitate (derived from 10 donors) increases the fibrinogen plasma level by 100 mg/dL in a non-DIC patient, less in a patient with ongoing DIC.

Platelet counts should be kept at or above 50,000/μL in the bleeding patient. One bag of platelets, typically one apheresis unit from a single donor, leads to an anticipated increase in platelet count of 30,000 to 60,000 /μL in the non-DIC patient, less in the DIC patient.

Packed red blood cells (PRBCs) should be transfused as needed.

Antithrombin III concentrate (ATIII) indications are not clear-cut. ATIII has been shown to have a beneficial effect on DIC severity score, on improvement of organ function, and on the duration of DIC. It is unclear which type of patient derives benefits from ATIII concentrate. Several studies have shown a modest, but not statistically significant, reduction in mortality. It has therefore remained unclear who should be treated with ATIII concentrate. The appropriate dose of ATIII concentrate in the treatment of DIC is also unclear. Several different ATIII dosing regimens have been studied, but not directly compared.

Other Treatments

Basic research suggests that *heparin* by inactivating thrombin and thus blocking the coagulation process would be beneficial in the treatment of DIC, but the role of heparin is also unproven due to a lack of good clinical studies. Heparin use is based on personal opinions and preferences. Some authorities recommend low doses of heparin (300 to 500 U/hour), particularly in patients with clinically overt thromboembolism or extensive deposition of fibrin, as occurs with purpura fulminans or acral ischemia. Others rarely use heparin in the treatment of DIC, unless larger vessel arterial or venous thrombosis or multiorgan failure due to presumed microthrombi dominates the clinical picture.

Drotrecogin alfa (recombinant activated protein C concentrate) is a new intravenous anticoagulant that interrupts the coagulation process by inactivating coagulation factors Va and VIIIa. It has been shown to decrease mortality in patients with severe sepsis and was approved by the FDA for this indication in 2001. The benefit of the drug in non-infectious DIC has not been examined yet.

FUTURE DIRECTIONS

The role of established and new anticoagulants in the treatment of DIC will be further examined: a multicenter phase III trial on use of antithrombin III concentrate is presently awaiting publication; drotrecogin alfa will be examined in non-sepsis–related DIC and recombinant thrombomodulin and other new anticoagulants in phase II and III studies. FDA approval of fibrinogen concentrate for bleeding patients with DIC is desirable, as is a clinical study of recombinant factor VIIa.

REFERENCES

Bernard GR, Vincent JL, Laterre PF, et al, and the Recombinant human protein C Worldwide Evaluation in Severe Sepsis (PROWESS) study group. Efficacy and safety of recombinant human activated protein C for severe sepsis. *N Engl J Med.* 2001;344:699–709.

Eisele B, Lamy M, Thijs LG, et al. Antithrombin III in patients with severe sepsis. A randomized, placebo-controlled, double-blind, multicenter trial plus a meta-analysis on all randomized, placebo-controlled, double-blind trails with antithrombin III in severe sepsis. *Intensive Care Med.* 1998;24:663–672.

Feinstein DI. Diagnosis and management of disseminated intravascular coagulation: the role of heparin therapy. *Blood.* 1982;60:284–287.

Levi M, Ten Cate H. Disseminated intravascular coagulation. *N Engl J Med.* 1999;341:586-592.

Chapter 56
Hypercoagulable States

Stephan Moll

Conditions that predispose to thrombosis are referred to as hypercoagulable states. They can be inherited or acquired. Thrombophilia is the tendency to form thromboses. Formerly, "idiopathic thrombosis" applied to thromboses in which the underlying hypercoagulable state could not be identified. The term is best avoided because most "idiopathic" thrombosis can be attributed to one or more of the recently discovered thrombophilic abnormalities. Thromboses can be separated into those associated with transient risk factors and those not associated with transient risk factors.

ETIOLOGY AND PATHOGENESIS

In hypercoagulable states, an unbalance in the procoagulant and fibrinolytic mechanisms leads to unphysiologic thrombosis. Several disturbances of plasmatic coagulation are known that result predominantly in venous thromboembolism. Relatively little is known about disturbances in blood vessel wall and platelet function that lead to hypercoagulability. Of patients with venous thromboembolism without transient risk factors, 50% have a detectable thrombophilic abnormality (Table 56-1). In arterial thromboembolism, a hypercoagulable abnormality cannot usually be identified.

CLINICAL PRESENTATION

Factor V Leiden is a point mutation in the coagulation factor V gene discovered in 1994 and named for the city of Leiden, The Netherlands. The mutation results in a factor V protein (Arg506Gln) that cannot be normally inactivated by its physiologic inactivator, activated protein C (APC), thus causing APC resistance. It is the most common inherited risk factor for venous thromboembolism (Figure 56-1). The heterozygous state is a mild risk factor for venous thrombosis (risk increased 3-fold to 8-fold); the homozygous state is a stronger one (risk increased 80-fold). Factor V Leiden is not a risk factor for arterial events, except in young women who smoke cigarettes. Found primarily in whites (approximately 5% of Americans are heterozygous), the mutation does not occur in native Africans or Asians. However, due to the mixture of races in the United States, 1.2% of the African-American population is heterozygous for factor V Leiden.

Hypercoagulable States Predisposing to Venous Thromboembolism

Acquired
- Surgery, trauma, prolonged immobilization
- Older age
- Obesity, smoking
- Hormones (oral contraceptives, pregnancy, hormone replacement therapy)
- Malignancy, chemotherapy
- Previous venous thromboembolism
- Inflammatory disorders (Crohn's disease, ulcerative colitis)
- Myeloproliferative disorders
- Hyperhomocysteinemia (inherited or acquired)
- Antiphospholipid antibodies
    Anticardiolipin antibodies
    Lupus anticoagulant
- Paroxysmal nocturnal hemoglobinuria

Inherited
- Factor V Leiden (G1691A mutation)
- Prothrombin G20210A mutation
- Protein C deficiency
- Protein S deficiency
- Antithrombin III deficiency
- Rare causes (dysfibrinogenemia, elevated PAI1 levels, etc.)
- Elevated levels of factor VIII, factor IX, factor XI, or fibrinogen (inherited or acquired)
- Factor XIII Val34 Leu polymorphism (protective effect against venous thromboembolism)

Table 56-1
Prevalences of Hypercoagulable States in Venous Thromboembolism

Hypercoagulable State	Prevalence in Unselected Patients with Venous Thromboembolism	Prevalence in Patients with Venous Thromboembolism Without Transient Risk Factors*
Protein C deficiency	3%	1%–9%
Protein S deficiency	1%–2%	1%–13%
Antithrombin III deficiency	1%	0.5%–7 %
Factor V Leiden	12%–21%	52%
Prothrombin 20210 mutation	6%	16%–19%
Hyperhomocysteinemia	10%–4%	18.8%
Antiphospholipid antibodies	8.5%–14%	No reliable studies available

*Transient risk factors: surgery, trauma, and immobilization.

Prothrombin 20210 mutation, a point mutation in the non-coding sequence of the prothrombin gene (G20210A), is associated with elevated prothrombin (factor II) levels. Discovered in 1996, it is the second most common risk factor for venous thromboembolism (Table 56-1). It is a mild risk factor for venous thromboembolism (risk of heterozygotes increased 2-fold to 4.8-fold compared to individuals without this mutation), but is not a risk factor for arterial thrombosis. The mutation is found in the same population as the factor V Leiden mutation; 2.3% of the overall US population and 0.5% of the African-American population is heterozygous for the mutation.

Protein C deficiency, a moderate risk factor for venous thromboembolism (risk is 7 to 15 times increased compared to a control population), is caused by a multitude of mutations. However, clinical penetrance is variable, and selected families are at greater risk. Arterial thrombotic problems are less common in individuals with protein C deficiency.

Protein S deficiency is a mild risk factor for venous thromboembolism. There is a 2-fold increased risk of venous thromboembolism compared to a control group. The clinical picture is variable between families.

Antithrombin III (ATIII) deficiency is associated with venous thromboembolism and has variable clinical penetrance. Selected families are at high risk; 50% of individuals in these families have thromboses before the age of 25 years. Overall, ATIII deficiency appears to be a moderate to strong risk factor for venous thromboembolic disease, but accurate risk estimates are not available because the disorder is uncommon.

Homocysteinuria is a rare homocysteine metabolism disturbance in children, leading to extremely high serum homocysteine levels. Fifty percent of these patients have arterial or venous thromboses before the age of 30. Homocysteinemia is a disorder of mildly to moderately increased serum homocysteine levels, associated with an increased risk of venous thromboembolism, arteriosclerosis, and arterial thromboembolism. Elevated levels are also found in patients with a homozygous mutation in the methylene-tetrahydrofolate reductase gene (thermolabile C677T MTHFR), but this mutation is not a risk factor for arterial thromboembolic disease by itself. The data on the association of the MTHFR polymorphism with venous thromboembolism are inconsistent.

Elevated homocysteine levels can be decreased in approximately 60% of patients with folate, 0.4 mg per day. If after 2 months the levels are still elevated, folate can be increased to 2 to 5 mg per day. If after 2 months homocysteine levels are still elevated, 25 to 50 mg of vitamin B6 and 0.4 to 1 mg vitamin B_{12} per day can be added.

Antiphospholipid antibody syndrome (APLA) is defined as the occurrence of thrombosis (arterial or venous) or recurrent pregnancy loss in patients with repeatedly positive antiphospholipid antibody tests (lupus anticoagulant and/or at least moderately elevated IgG or IgM anticardiolipin antibodies). It occurs as the primary APLA syndrome not associated with any other diseases, or as secondary APLA syndrome, associated with autoimmune diseases, malignancy, or drugs. Patients in whom thrombosis develops are at high risk for recurrence, and indefinite anticoagulation is usually recommended after one episode of venous or arterial thromboembolism. The optional International Normalized Ratio (INR) for oral anticoagulation is a matter of debate. In some patients, the INR is invalid because of a lupus anticoagulant effect, and alternative tests to measure the oral anticoagulant effect are indicated (factor II or X activity, chromogenic factor II or X). Individual INR treatment decisions are best made with the help of a thrombophilia specialist. Recurrent pregnancy loss associated with APLA syndrome can be treated successfully with unfractionated heparin (5,000 U every 12 hours) plus 75 mg aspirin every day. Low-molecular-weight heparins can likely be used instead of unfractionated heparin, but have not been well studied in this disorder.

Thorough exclusion of all causes for arterial thromboembolism (arteriosclerosis, intracardiac thrombus, cardiomyopathy, atrial fibrillation, patent foramen ovale, etc.) and for venous thromboembolism (especially malignancy) is essential.

DIAGNOSTIC APPROACH

Opinions vary as to what constitutes an appropriate workup. The extent of the workup needs to be tailored to the individual patient.

In venous thromboembolism not associated with surgery, trauma, or prolonged immobilization, the following tests may be helpful: factor V Leiden; prothrombin 20210 mutation; protein C activity; protein S activity; antithrombin III activity; homocysteine level; antiphospholipid antibodies (lupus anticoagulant plus anticardiolipin IgG and IgM antibodies).

Hypercoagulable States Predisposing to Arterial Thromboembolism

Acquired
- Arteriosclerosis
- Vasculitis
- Heparin-induced thrombocytopenia
- Thrombotic thrombocytopenic purpura (acquired or inherited)
- Hemolytic-uremic syndrome (usually acquired)
- Hyperhomocysteinemia (acquired or inherited)
- Antiphospholipid antibodies
  Lupus anticoagulant
  Anticardiolipin antibodies

Inherited
- Deficiency of protein C, protein S, antithrombin III
- Rare causes (dysfibrinogenemia)
- Elevated levels of fibrinogen, factor VIII, and von Willebrand factor (inherited or acquired)
- Factor XIII Val34 Leu polymorphism (protective effect against arterial thromboembolism)

In unexplained arterial thromboembolic events, thrombophilia tests include lipid profile (LDL cholesterol, triglycerides, lipoprotein-a), protein C activity, protein S activity, antithrombin III activity, and antiphospholipid antibodies (lupus anticoagulant plus anticardiolipin IgG and IgM antibodies), and homocysteine.

The diagnosis of factor V Leiden is made by either genetic (polymerase chain reaction), or coagulation (activated protein C resistance) testing. APC resistance and factor V Leiden are not synonyms because 5% to 10 % of patients with APC resistance do not have factor V Leiden, but another abnormality such as a lupus anticoagulant that interferes with the APC-resistance assay. An abnormal APC-resistance test needs to be followed by the genetic test for factor V Leiden.

The diagnosis of prothrombin 20210 mutation is made by genetic testing (PCR). Factor II activity levels are not helpful.

For evaluation of protein C deficiency, protein C activity levels should be measured. Protein C antigen levels are not helpful because normal levels do not exclude a dysfunctional protein that causes functional protein C deficiency. Protein C activity levels are low in patients taking vitamin K antago-

Figure 56-1   **Factor V Leiden, Prothrombin 20210 Mutation**

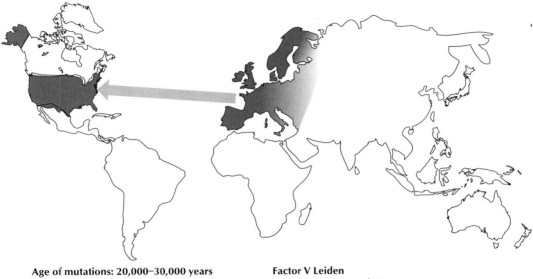

Age of mutations: 20,000–30,000 years
Origin: Europe

Factor V Leiden
· 5% Caucasian population
· 1.2% in African Americans

Prothrombin 20210 mutation
· 2% Caucasian population
· 0.5% in African Americans

nists (warfarin, phenprocoumon, etc.). Levels take up to 2 weeks to normalize after discontinuation of warfarin. They are also low in liver disease.

Protein S circulates in the plasma in 2 forms: bound to the transport protein C4b-binding protein, and unbound, as free protein S. Only the free protein is enzymatically active. Tests include protein S activity, free protein S antigen, and total protein S antigen. Obtaining only free or total protein S antigen levels is insufficient to rule out protein S deficiency because a patient may have normal amounts of protein S antigen, but a functional deficiency due to a dysfunctional protein S molecule. Protein S activity levels can be low in the patient on oral contraceptives or hormone replacement, during pregnancy, with oral anticoagulant treatment, and with liver synthetic dysfunction. Congenital protein S deficiency cannot be diagnosed under these circumstances. Levels take up to 2 weeks to normalize after discontinuation of oral anticoagulants.

ATIII activity can be low in the acute setting of a venous thromboembolism, during heparin ther-

apy, with synthetic liver dysfunction, and in nephrotic syndrome. Low levels in these circumstances do not necessarily indicate congenital ATIII deficiency.

Plasma homocysteine levels increase after a protein-rich diet and when the blood sample is left uncentrifuged at room temperature for more than 60 minutes after phlebotomy. Levels should be checked in the fasting patient, and the iced sample should be sent to the laboratory at once.

Antiphospholipid antibodies (APLA) are a heterogenous group of antibodies (Figure 56-2) that can be detected in the laboratory by either a functional coagulation assay (then termed lupus anticoagulant), or by enzyme-linked immunoabsorbent assay (ELISA). Because phospholipids are needed in the test tube for coagulation to take place, binding of phospholipids by the antibodies leads to a prolongation of coagulation tests, such as the activated partial thromboplastin time (aPTT), prothrombin time (PT), dilute Russel viper venom time (dRVVT), or Kaolin clotting time (KCT). A lupus anticoagulant is diagnosed when

Figure 56-2

Antiphospholipid Antibodies

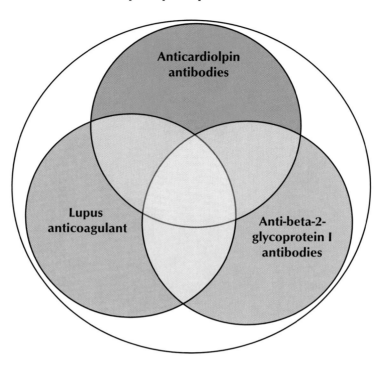

Anticardiolpin antibodies

Lupus anticoagulant

Anti-beta-2-glycoprotein I antibodies

excess phospholipids added to the test tube lead to normalization of the clotting time ("hexagonal phospholipid confirm," "dRVVT confirm," "platelet neutralization procedure"). A complete workup for APLA includes testing for a lupus anticoagulant by 2 coagulation methods (for example, aPTT and dRVVT), and measurement of IgG and IgM anticardiolipin antibodies. The clinical significance of other antiphospholipid antibodies (IgA anti-cardiolipin, anti-β2-glycoprotein I, anti-phosphatidylserine, anti-phosphatidylethanolamine, anti-phosphatidylinositol) has not been defined, and testing for these antibodies for clinical decision making is not indicated. Plasma of patients on warfarin can be reliably tested for lupus anticoagulant. In the patient taking heparin, the test may produce false-negative results. APLA can interfere with the determination of individual coagulation factor activity levels, leading to falsely low factor levels.

Testing for rare causes of thrombophilia, such as dysfibrinogenemia, plasminogen deficiency, paroxysmal nocturnal hemoglobinemia, and others is preferably done only after consultation with a thrombophilia specialist.

MANAGEMENT AND THERAPY

The presence or absence of certain thrombophilic risk factors has bearing on the length of anticoagulant treatment after venous thromboembolism, on the intensity of anticoagulation (in the case of the presence of antiphospholipid antibodies), and may have implications for other family members. Management and therapy of various arterial and venous thromboembolic problems are discussed in the other chapters of this book. Referral for evaluation in a specialized thrombophilia center should be considered in any patient with thrombosis and in asymptomatic individuals with known thrombophilia.

FUTURE DIRECTIONS

Significant developments in thrombophilia include the identification of new genetic polymorphisms and haplotypes that predispose carriers to venous or arterial thromboembolism, and performance of clinical studies that assess the risk of recurrent thrombosis in patients with various thrombophilias and determine the best length and intensity of oral anticoagulant treatment.

Patients will also benefit from the formation of comprehensive thrombophilia centers and active patient interest groups.

REFERENCES

American Thrombosis Association Web site. Available at: http://www.bloodclot.org. Accessed February 23, 2003.

Hirsh J, Bates SM. Clinical trials that have influenced the treatment of venous thromboembolism: a historical perspective. *Ann Intern Med.* 2001;134:409–417.

Lane DA, Grant PJ. Role of hemostatic gene polymorphisms in venous and arterial thrombotic disease. *Blood.* 2000;95: 1517–1532.

Reiner AP, Siscovick DS, Rosendaal FR. Hemostatic risk factors and arterial thrombotic disease. *Thromb Haemost.* 2001;85:584–595.

Seligsohn U, Lubetsky A. Genetic susceptibility to venous thrombosis. *N Engl J Med.* 2001;344:1222–1231.

University of Southern Indiana School of Nursing and Health Professions Web site. Anticoagulation therapy management certificate program. Available at: http://health1.usi.edu/anticoag. Accessed February 26, 2003.

Wilson WA, Gharavi AE, Koike T, et al. International consensus statement on preliminary classification criteria for definite antiphospholipid syndrome: report of an international workshop. *Arthritis Rheum.* 1999;42:1309–1311.

Section VII

HEMATOLOGIC DISORDERS

Chapter 57

Anemias

Lee R. Berkowitz

Anemia, a hemoglobin below the normal range for a standard complete blood count (CBC), is a common finding in internal medicine patients. Most anemias have a specific etiology. Defining the cause is critical for determining therapy and for uncovering other significant associated disease processes. Although these anemias are familiar to most clinicians, understanding them continues to be a dynamic process because new information is always emerging.

ETIOLOGY AND PATHOGENESIS
Iron Deficiency

This common anemia should be considered in any patient presenting with a microcytic anemia and a low or normal reticulocyte count. Because adults have several grams of iron in circulating red blood cells and another gram in storage iron, the diagnosis of iron deficiency requires searching for a source of blood loss. The sequence of findings in iron deficiency is loss of storage iron, followed by development of anemia, and finally development of microcytosis.

Thalassemia

This disorder is a common anemia in certain areas of the world, including the Mediterranean, India, Southeast Asia, and Africa. A high prevalence has also been observed in Western countries in individuals descended from those regions where thalassemia is common. At a molecular level, there are hundreds of globin abnormalities leading to either *alpha chain underproduction (alpha thalassemia)* or *beta chain underproduction (beta thalassemia)*. The phenotype is similar. The underproduction of either alpha or beta chains results in a microcytic red blood cell. There is also hemolysis because the imbalance results in excess globin chains, which are oxidized and precipitate on the surface of the red blood cell, resulting in premature red blood cell removal in the spleen. The bone marrow partially compensates by increasing the number of reticulocytes.

Vitamin B_{12}/Folate Deficiency

The folate metabolic pathway results in thymidine synthesis. Thymidine is then incorporated into DNA. Vitamin B_{12} is a cofactor in this pathway. Vegetables and fruits are rich in folates, but vitamin B_{12} is only found in foods from animals. The absorption of folate occurs in a straightforward pathway in the jejunum. Vitamin B_{12} absorption is more complex, requiring intrinsic factor production in the stomach, pancreatic secretion, and then passage through the mucosa of the terminal ileum.

The hematologic findings in folate and vitamin B_{12} deficiency are identical. Because nuclear maturation is arrested, red blood cells are macrocytic. Reticulocytes are low or normal. The folate/B_{12} pathway is also present in neutrophils and platelets, so deficiencies can result in reductions in all 3 cell lines. Neutrophils are often hypersegmented.

Vitamin B_{12} deficiency can also lead to neurologic findings as a consequence of demyelination. These include peripheral neuropathy, decreased proprioception, optic atrophy, and dementia. These abnormalities may precede hematologic changes and improve after by B_{12} replacement if recognized late.

Anemia of Chronic Disease

A *normocytic anemia* with a suboptimal reticulocyte response may develop in patients with a variety of chronic inflammatory diseases, infections, or neoplastic diseases. Because a precise cause has not been found, this anemia is called the anemia of chronic disease and is the most common cause of anemia in hospitalized patients. One theory is that elevated levels of cytokines induce blockage of the release of storage iron into circulating iron. Another theory is that elevated levels of cytokines result in

Figure 57-1

Anemia

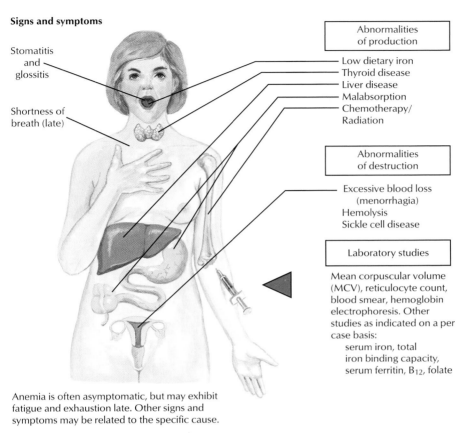

Signs and symptoms

Stomatitis and glossitis

Shortness of breath (late)

Abnormalities of production
- Low dietary iron
- Thyroid disease
- Liver disease
- Malabsorption
- Chemotherapy/Radiation

Abnormalities of destruction
- Excessive blood loss (menorrhagia)
- Hemolysis
- Sickle cell disease

Laboratory studies

Mean corpuscular volume (MCV), reticulocyte count, blood smear, hemoglobin electrophoresis. Other studies as indicated on a per case basis:
 serum iron, total iron binding capacity, serum ferritin, B_{12}, folate

Anemia is often asymptomatic, but may exhibit fatigue and exhaustion late. Other signs and symptoms may be related to the specific cause.

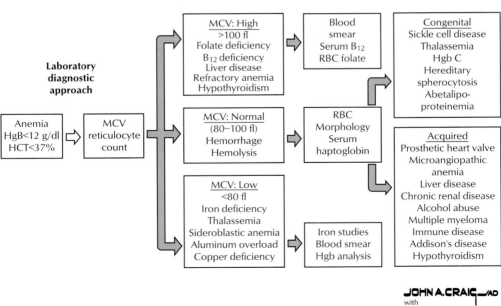

Laboratory diagnostic approach

Anemia HgB<12 g/dl HCT<37%

MCV reticulocyte count

MCV: High >100 fl
Folate deficiency
B_{12} deficiency
Liver disease
Refractory anemia
Hypothyroidism

Blood smear
Serum B_{12}
RBC folate

Congenital
Sickle cell disease
Thalassemia
Hgb C
Hereditary spherocytosis
Abetalipo-proteinemia

MCV: Normal (80–100 fl)
Hemorrhage
Hemolysis

RBC Morphology
Serum haptoglobin

MCV: Low <80 fl
Iron deficiency
Thalassemia
Sideroblastic anemia
Aluminum overload
Copper deficiency

Iron studies
Blood smear
Hgb analysis

Acquired
Prosthetic heart valve
Microangiopathic anemia
Liver disease
Chronic renal disease
Alcohol abuse
Multiple myeloma
Immune disease
Addison's disease
Hypothyroidism

JOHN A. CRAIG—AD
with
E. Hatton
© ICN

Figure 57-2 **Categorizing Anemia Based on Reticulocyte Count**

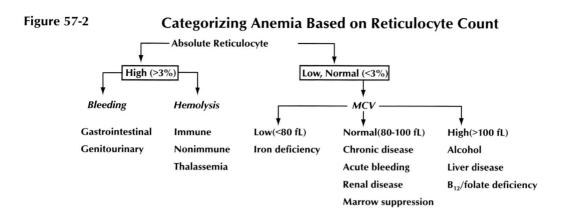

decreased endogenous erythropoietin levels. There are no specific diagnostic tests, so the diagnosis is made by clinical observation.

CLINICAL PRESENTATION

Patients with anemia may or may not be symptomatic (Figure 57-1). Key factors include the degree of anemia and how rapidly it develops. In general, symptoms develop at a hemoglobin level of 8.0 to 9.0 g/dL, when the anemia develops over hours to a few days. A slower evolving process will allow the patient to compensate hemodynamically, so patients with hemoglobin values below 7.0 g/dL may have few symptoms. All patients will have symptoms at a hemoglobin level of 5.0 to 6.0 g/dL.

Early symptoms of anemia include fatigue and dyspnea on exertion. As the anemia worsens, patients will experience organ ischemia, often presenting with angina pectoris or focal neurologic findings. Shock is common with acute blood loss. With ischemic symptoms or shock, patients should undergo an emergency transfusion before a cause for the anemia is investigated.

DIAGNOSTIC APPROACH

Because there are many causes of anemia, a selective diagnostic approach is recommended. A prudent place to begin is to categorize the anemia based on the mean cell volume (MCV) of the patient's red blood cells and the reticulocyte count (Figures 57-1 and 57-2). Dividing the red blood cells into microcytic, MCV less than 80 fL; normocytic, 80 to 100 fL; or macrocytic, greater than 100 fL will greatly narrow the diagnostic possibilities. The reticulocyte count gives additional information regarding the status of the bone mar-

row. If the bone marrow's red blood cell productive mechanism is intact, anemia will result in an increased production of reticulocytes. A low or even normal reticulocyte count in the anemic patient (3% or less) indicates the marrow is not responding appropriately, and a search for a marrow abnormality will define the cause of the anemia. A word of caution about interpreting reticulocyte counts is warranted. They are usually reported as a percent of the red blood cells, a relative value. To convert this to an absolute value, the patient's percent reticulocytes should be multiplied by the ratio of the patient's hematocrit, divided by a normal hematocrit value.

Figure 57-2 illustrates how the MCV and reticulocyte count can be utilized to categorize anemias. Once the anemia has been categorized by MCV and the reticulocyte count, more specific tests can be done.

Iron Deficiency

A number of diagnostic tests are useful for diagnosing iron deficiency. Serum markers include serum iron, total iron binding capacity, and ferritin. A low serum ferritin (<18 ug/L) has a positive likelihood ratio over 40, and a serum ferritin of 19 to 45 ug/L has a positive likelihood ratio of about 3. A transferrin saturation (fe/tibc) of 0.05 has a positive likelihood ratio of 16.5. However, a transferrin saturation of 0.06 to 0.08 only has a positive likelihood ratio of 1.43. The gold standard for iron deficiency is a Prussian blue stain of the bone marrow, indicating the presence or absence of iron. Since bone marrow aspiration is an invasive procedure, the morbidity must be considered on an individual basis. Finally, a trial of iron can be diagnostic. The response will take weeks, and patient compliance is necessary. The diagnostic approach, whether serologic markers, bone marrow aspiration, or a trial of iron, depends on the severity of illness.

Thalassemia

Because the erythrocytes underproduce hemoglobin in individuals with thalassemia, microcytsis is universally present. This underproduction also results in hemolysis. The combination of microcytosis and increased reticulocytes seen in thalassemia is unique, and thus can be used to make the diagnosis. Further information can be obtained from a hemoglobin electrophoresis, which in beta thalassemia shows increased hemoglobin A2 and increased hemoglobin F.

B$_{12}$/Folate Deficiency

The diagnosis of folate deficiency is made when there is a macrocytic anemia with or without pancytopenia in clinical settings that could lead to folate deficiency. These include pregnancy, poor nutrition, hemolysis, and malabsorption. A serum folate assay may be helpful, but it should be noted that levels increase quickly with proper diet. A red blood cell folate assay that does not change with refeeding may confirm the diagnosis. The diagnosis of vitamin B$_{12}$ deficiency is usually made by measuring serum vitamin B$_{12}$. Current assays have high sensitivity but are only moderately specific. Assays of homocysteine and methylmalonic acid are helpful in that both increase with vitamin B$_{12}$ deficiency. The Schilling test, in which a patient ingests radiolabeled vitamin B$_{12}$ with or without intrinsic factor, is rarely done because of the difficulty in obtaining an adequate urine collection and the reduced sensitivity of the test in early vitamin B$_{12}$ deficiency.

MANAGEMENT AND THERAPY
Iron Deficiency

A diagnosis of iron deficiency in an adult requires that a source of blood loss be found. In premenopausal females, menstruation is the most likely cause. In postmenopausal females and men, a bleeding site in the gastrointestinal tract should be thoroughly evaluated. Once the cause is found, patients need supplemental iron to restore iron in erythrocytes as well as storage iron. The standard treatment is ferrous sulfate 325 mg orally 3 times a day for 6 months. Other iron preparations are also available and equally efficacious with the exception of enteric-coated products. These reduce gastrointestinal toxicity but have poor absorption. Iron can also be given intravenously if a patient cannot tolerate oral iron. A single total replacement dose is given. This carries a small risk of anaphylaxis. Transfusions also provide intravenous iron, 250 mg per unit of packed red blood cells.

Thalassemia

Patients with heterozygous alpha or beta thalassemia have a mild *hemolytic anemia*. Folic acid daily (1 mg orally) will more than meet the increased demands resulting from the increased red blood cell turnover. A severe anemia develops in patients with homozygous thalassemia, which requires transfusions, usually beginning in childhood.

Vitamin B$_{12}$/Folate Deficiency

The most common cause of vitamin B$_{12}$ deficiency is *pernicious anemia*, where loss of intrinsic factor does not allow vitamin B$_{12}$ absorption; vitamin B$_{12}$ must be given intramuscularly. At diagnosis, 1 mg of vitamin B$_{12}$ is given weekly for 4 weeks followed by monthly injections. The same treatment is applicable for other causes of vitamin B$_{12}$ deficiency such as gastric achlorhydria from protein-pump inhibitors and diseases of the terminal ileum. The treatment for all causes of folate deficiency is daily oral folate, 1 mg. If the patient cannot take oral folate, it can be given intravenously.

Anemia of Chronic Disease

If improvement of the underlying condition occurs, an improvement in the anemia will follow. This is not always the case in conditions that are chronic. Measurement of the endogenous erythropoietin level is recommended. If the level is less than 500 mu/mL, patients are candidates for recombinant human erythropoietin, given weekly by subcutaneous injection. An increase in the hemoglobin is usually seen in 4 to 8 weeks. Administration is maintained as long as the chronic condition is present.

FUTURE DIRECTIONS

A significant number of new proteins that are involved in iron metabolism have been identified. One, the soluble fragment of the transferrin receptor, may be useful in the detection of iron deficiency as well as in distinguishing iron deficiency from the anemia of chronic disease.

For beta thalassemia, allogenic bone marrow transplantation has been done in more than 1,000 patients. A subgroup analysis shows high mortality in older patients (ages 17 to 35 years). Safer variants of transplantation such as mini-allografts are being investigated.

Patients with vitamin B_{12} deficiency from gastric achlorhydria or pernicious anemia may respond to high doses of oral vitamin B_{12} (2 mg/day). Large studies are needed to see if early reports of the efficacy of oral vitamin B_{12} are generally applicable to these two groups of patients.

REFERENCES

Brittenham GM, Weiss G, Brissot P, et al. Clinical consequences of new insights in the pathophysiology of disorders of iron and heme metabolism. *Hematology* (Am Soc Hematol Educ Program). 2000:39-50.

Goodnough LT, Brecher ME, Kanter MH, AuBuchon JP. Transfusion medicine. First of two parts—blood transfusion. *N Engl J Med.* 1999;340:438-447.

Guyatt GH, Patterson C, Ali M, et al. Diagnosis of iron-deficiency anemia in the elderly. *Am J Med.* 1990;88:205-209.

Chapter 58
Blood Component Therapy

Mark E. Brecher

The transfusion of blood was the first successful transplant of living tissue in humans. Today, transfusion of blood components is so common and safe that it is rarely thought of as a transplant. In 1999, for allogeneic transfusions within the United States alone, it is estimated that 12,022,000 units of whole blood/red blood cells, 3,036,000 units of whole blood–derived platelets, 1,003,000 units of apheresis platelets, and 3,319,000 units of plasma were administered. For red blood cell–containing products alone, this equates to 1 unit transfused every 2.6 seconds. A basic understanding of compatibility, indications, and the risks of blood component therapy are essential for both optimal patient care and for providing patients within formation for a truly informed decision.

BASIC IMMUNOHEMATOLOGY

Pre-transfusion testing confirms compatibility between the blood component and the recipient, and detects unexpected but clinically significant antibodies that might harm the recipient or compromise the survival of the transfused cells. *Red blood cell serological testing* depends on in-vitro hemolysis or agglutination resulting from red blood cell antigen-antibody interaction. *ABO typing* involves testing of the recipient's red blood cells with potent anti-A and anti-B typing reagent ("forward" typing) and reaction of the recipient's plasma or serum with A_1 (the major subtype of group A) and B red blood cells ("reverse" typing). Typically ABO antibodies are IgM antibodies and are reactive at room temperature. Rh typing tests the recipient's red blood cells with a chemically modified IgG anti-D antibody that is reactive at room temperature.

Antibody screening for unexpected red blood cell antibodies requires testing of serum or plasma with group O reagent red blood cells selected to express all commonly occurring clinically significant antigens. Clinically significant antibodies present in serum or plasma are detected after 37° C incubation or after the addition of anti-human globulin (an indirect anti-human globulin test or indirect Coombs' test). If an unexpected antibody is detected, further serological testing to identify the antigen specificity of the antigen is performed. A *non-reactive antibody screen* allows for the rapid selection of red blood cells that require only a confirmation of ABO compatibility. The presence of unexpected antibodies requires the more time-consuming identification of antigen-negative units and a full cross-match. A full cross-match requires testing of the recipient's serum or plasma with red cells from the units to be transfused, incubation at 37° C, and testing with anti-human globulin.

With the exception of infants, the lack of expression of either the A or B antigen results in the formation of anti-B or anti-A, respectively. A group O individual lacks both the A and the B antigens and thus forms both anti-A and anti-B. The ABO antigens, their antibodies, and compatibility of red blood cell and plasma components are summarized in Table 58-1.

Table 58-1
ABO Types and Compatibility of Red Cells and Plasma

ABO Type (antigens expressed)	Percent of Population	ABO RBC* Compatibility	Plasma Compatibility
O	46	O	O, A, B, AB
A	41	A, O	A, AB
B	9	B, O	B, AB
AB	4	AB, A, B, AB	AB

*RBC, red blood cell.

Platelets can be thought of as bags of plasma, and ideally one would transfuse platelets with the compatibility of plasma. However, because of the short shelf life of platelets (5 days), platelets are frequently transfused across ABO compatibility barriers. Cryoprecipitate due to the limited volume transfused is also frequently transfused across ABO plasma compatibility barriers. Group O is a universal red blood cell unit. Group AB is a universal plasma unit.

Rh-negative (D-negative) red blood cells and platelets (which account for only 15% of the donor base) are reserved principally for female recipients of childbearing potential, and thus at risk for hemolytic disease of the newborn with pregnancy. To preserve an inventory of Rh-negative units, trauma cases involving males, in which the type is not initially known, are frequently transfused with Rh-positive red blood cells.

BLOOD COMPONENTS AND INDICATIONS FOR TRANSFUSION

Individual institutions must have guidelines for the transfusion of blood components. These guidelines are based on the scientific literature and local practice and serve as the basis for the focused review of transfusion practices. Although guidelines represent institution consensus, they cannot substitute for clinical judgment and the need for flexibility in practice, and should not be considered a mandate to transfuse or not to transfuse.

Before the administration of blood or blood components, the indications, risks, and benefits of a blood transfusion and possible alternatives must be discussed with the patient and documented in the medical record. Transfusions should be documented in the patient's record, including both indications and outcome. Specific notations should be made when exceptions to the institutional guidelines exist.

Red Blood Cells

The purpose of red blood cell transfusion is to provide oxygen-carrying capacity and to maintain tissue oxygenation when the intravascular volume and cardiac function are adequate for perfusion. One unit of red blood cells should increase the patient's hemoglobin level by 1 g/dL or the hematocrit by 3% in a 70-kg recipient. Red blood cell transfusion should only be used when time or underlying pathophysiology precludes other management (e.g., iron, erythropoietin, folate).

Criteria: (1) Hemoglobin (Hgb) <8 g/dL in an otherwise healthy patient; (2) Hgb <11 g/dL in cases of increased risk of ischemia (pulmonary disease, coronary artery disease, cerebral vascular disease etc.); (3) acute blood loss resulting in blood loss ≥15% of total blood volume (750 mL in 70-kg male) or with evidence of inadequate oxygen delivery (e.g., electrocardiographic signs of cardiac ischemia, tachycardia, cyanosis); (4) symptomatic anemia in a normovolemic patient (e.g., tachycardia, mental status changes, electrocardiographic signs of cardiac ischemia, angina, shortness of breath, lightheadedness or dizziness with mild exertion); or (5) regular predetermined therapeutic program for severe hypoplastic/aplastic anemia or for bone marrow suppression for hemoglobinopathies. The post-transfusion Hgb should not exceed 11.5 g/dL (12.5 g/dL in those cases of increased risk of organ/tissue ischemia).

It is not acceptable to use red blood cell transfusions to increase wound healing or merely to take advantage of readily available predonated autologous blood without an acceptable medical indication.

Platelets

Platelets are used for patients suffering from or at significant risk of hemorrhage due to thrombocytopenia or platelet dysfunction. One unit of whole blood–derived platelets (a "random" unit) should increase the platelet count by 7 to 10 × 10^9/L in a 70-kg recipient. Dosing is generally a pool of 4 to 6 U. A single donor apheresis platelet transfusion should increase the platelet count by 40 to 60 × 10^9/L in a 70-kg recipient.

Criteria: (1) platelet count ≤10 × 10^9/L (for prophylaxis in stable, non-febrile patient), or ≤20 × 10^9/L for prophylaxis with fever or instability; (2) platelet count ≤50 × 10^9/L in a patient with documented hemorrhage or rapidly decreasing platelet count or planned invasive or surgical procedure; (3) diffuse microvascular bleeding in a patient with disseminated intravascular coagulation or following a massive blood loss (>1 blood volume) with a platelet count not yet available; or (4) bleeding in a patient with platelet dysfunction.

Unacceptable indications for platelet transfusion include patients with the following syndromes, but no evidence of bleeding or coagulopathy: thrombotic thrombocytopenic purpura (TTP), hemolytic-uremic syndrome (HUS), or idiopathic thrombocytopenic purpura (ITP); empiric use during massive transfusion in which the patient does not exhibit a clinical coagulopathy; and extrinsic platelet dysfunction, such as in renal failure, hyperproteinemia, or von Willebrand's disease.

Fresh Frozen Plasma

This component contains adequate levels of all soluble coagulation factors. Fresh frozen plasma (FFP) is indicated for the correction of multiple or specific coagulation factor deficiencies, or for the empiric treatment of thrombotic thrombocytopene purpura (TTP) or hemolytic uremic syndrome (HUS). One unit contains approximately 220 mL, and the usual starting dose is 5 to 15 mL/kg (2 to 4 units in a 70-kg recipient).

Criteria for transfusion include treatment or prophylaxis of multiple or specific coagulation factor deficiencies (PT and/or PTT > 1.5 times the mean normal value). Congenital deficiencies (antithrombin III; factors II, V, VII, IX, X, XI; plasminogen; or antiplasmin) or acquired deficiencies related to warfarin therapy, vitamin K deficiency, liver disease, massive transfusion (>1 blood volume in 24 hours), and disseminated intravascular coagulation are acceptable indications for the transfusion of FFP. FFP is also indicated in patients with a suspected coagulation deficiency (PT/PTT pending) who are bleeding, or at risk of bleeding, from an invasive procedure. Unacceptable criteria are empiric use during massive transfusion in which patient does not exhibit clinical coagulopathy, nutritional supplementation, or volume replacement.

Cryoprecipitate

Cryoprecipitate is a cold insoluble fraction of FFP; each bag contains approximately 80 to 100 U of factor VIII and 150 to 250 mg of fibrinogen. It also contains factor XIII and von Willebrand's factor. The usual starting dose is one concentrate per 7 to 10 kg. In a 70-kg male, 10 U would be expected to raise the fibrinogen 40 mg/dL. Cryoprecipitate may also be applied topically, with an equal volume of bovine thrombin, taking advantage of its adhesive and hemostatic/sealant properties. Single units are appropriate as a fibrin sealant or glue.

Appropriate indications for cryoprecipitate use include treatment or prevention of bleeding associated with certain known or suspected clotting factor deficiencies (factor VIII, von Willebrand's, factor XIII, or factor I) and of a prolonged bleeding time or fibrinogen <150 mg/dL or other specific coagulation factor assay–documented deficiency. Cryoprecipitate may also be used for the treatment of surface oozing and the maintenance of tissues in tight apposition to each other or the sealing of leaking spaces (fibrin glue). The use of desmopressin acetate may frequently be a preferred or acceptable alternative to use of cryoprecipitate for patients with type I von Willebrand's disease, mild hemophilia A (factor VIII deficiency), or certain platelet dysfunctional disorders.

Other Blood-Derived Products

Other blood-derived products, such as intravenous immunoglobulin preparations, normal serum albumin, and coagulation factor concentrates, are beyond the scope of this chapter. Their use is covered in other relevant chapters.

INFECTIOUS DISEASE RISK OF BLOOD PRODUCTS

Although blood products today are considered "safer than ever," a truly zero-risk blood supply is probably unattainable. Currently, blood donations in developed countries are screened for human immunodeficiency virus I/II (anti-HIV I/II, HIV p-24 Ag), hepatitis C (anti-HCV), hepatitis B (HbsAg, anti-HBc), and syphilis (RPR or VDRL). Recently, many countries have begun testing for hepatitis C and HIV with nucleic amplification testing (NAT). Knowledge of the current risk of disease transmission (summarized below) is a prerequisite for proper informed consent for transfusion (Table 58-2).

NON-INFECTIOUS DISEASE RISK OF BLOOD PRODUCTS

The greatest risk of transfusion involves non-infectious complications. The most common non-infectious cause for death is the transfusion of ABO-incompatible allogeneic red blood cells (with the administration of ABO-incompatible red

Table 58-2
Risk of Infectious Disease

Infectious Agent	Estimated Risk/Unit	Estimated Risk/Unit with NAT* Testing
Virus		
HIV 1 and 2	1:1,326,399	1:1,900,000
HTLV I/II	1:641,000	N/A
Hepatitis B	1:63,000	N/A
Hepatitis C	1:233,000	1:1,600,000
Bacteria		
Red blood cells	<1:1,000,000	N/A
Platelets[†]	1:2,000	N/A
Parasites		
Malaria, Babesia	<1:1,000,000	N/A

* NAT, nucleic amplification testing.

[†] The high risk of bacterial contamination of platelets is due to the required storage at 20 to 24° C, 1:2,500 per pool of 6 or 1:13,400 single donor apheresis platelets result in clinical sepsis. The related mortality is approximately 1:17,000 for random donor pools and 1:16,000 for single donor apheresis platelets.
Modified from Brecher ME, ed. *Technical Manual*, 14th ed. Bethesda, MD: *American Association of Blood Banks*, 2002: 622.

blood cells at a rate of 1:38,000 units and a fatality rate 1:1,300,000 units transfused). These events are invariably due to human error, classically, the misidentification of a patient or sample. It is because of the recognition of this avoidable source of error that blood banks and transfusion services have very stringent policies regarding patient and sample identification. Non-infectious complications of transfusion can be divided into acute (within 24 hours of transfusion) and delayed (greater than 24 after transfusion) (Table 58-3).

FUTURE DIRECTIONS

Future directions for blood component therapy include additional initiatives to reduce the risk of infectious disease such as wider application of NAT testing, use of viral and bacterial inactivation technologies, or both. Alternatively, routine bacterial detection in platelets may allow for extended storage that would impact platelet availability. Red blood cell "substitutes" made from polymerized hemoglobin are currently in clinical trials. Such products with a prolonged shelf life will not require compatibility testing and may provide transient (24 to 48 hours) oxygen-carrying capacity in patients for whom transfusion of red blood

Table 58-3
Non-infectious Complications of Transfusion

Type	Rate
Acute (within 24 hours of transfusion)	
Immunologic	
Hemolytic	1:38,000−1:70,000
Febrile/chill non-hemolytic	1:100−1:200
Transfusion-related acute lung injury	1:10,000
Allergic (mild)	1:33−1:100
Anaphylactic	1:20,000−1:50,000
ACE* inhibitor−mediated hypotension	Variable
Nonimmunologic	
Fluid overload	<1%
Air embolism	Rare
Citrate toxicity (hypocalcemia)	Variable
Pseudohemolytic	Unknown
Delayed (greater then 24 hours after transfusion)	
Immunologic	
Delayed hemolytic	1:5000-1:11,000
Graft-versus-host disease	Rare
Post-transfusion purpura	Rare
Nonimmunologic	
Iron overload	after > 100 units of RBCs[†]

*ACE, angiotensin-converting enzyme; [†]RBCs, red blood cells.
Modified from Brecher ME, ed. *Technical Manual*, 14th ed. Bethesda, MD: American Association of Blood Banks, 2002: 586-589.

cells is not an option (e.g., trauma patients in the field) or allow extensive acute normovolemic hemodilution in the operative setting.

REFERENCES

Brecher ME, ed. *Technical Manual*. 14th ed. Bethesda, Md: American Association of Blood Banks; 2002.

Goodnough LT, Brecher ME, Kanter MH, AuBuchon JP. Transfusion medicine. First of two parts—blood transfusion. *N Engl J Med*. 1999;340:438-447.

Goodnough LT, Brecher ME, Kanter MH, AuBuchon JP. Transfusion medicine. Second of two parts—blood conservation. *N Engl J Med*. 1999;340:525-533.

Stehling L, Luban NL, Anderson KC, et al. Guidelines for blood utilization review. *Transfusion*. 1994;34:438-448.

Chapter 59
Bone Marrow Failure States

Maria Q. Baggstrom and Thomas C. Shea

Bone marrow failure refers to any condition in which the peripheral blood cell count is low because of a failure of the marrow to produce adequate numbers of circulating cells. Marrow failure is due to many different causes and is usually classified according to either the morphological and clinical picture or etiology. The following classification system is based on bone marrow morphology: aplastic anemia (fatty bone marrow), myelodysplasia (disordered hematopoiesis), and agnogenic myeloid metaplasia and myelofibrosis (fibrosis).

APLASTIC ANEMIAS
Etiology and Pathogenesis

Aplastic anemia is a disorder that can be further subdivided into conditions with multi-lineage or single lineage cytopenias. Both types can be acquired or inherited.

While the majority of cases of aplastic anemias are thought of as idiopathic, certain associated factors should be considered as potentially causative, including radiation, chemicals, drugs, infections, and immunologic diseases (Table 59-1).

Clinical Presentation

Usually, the patient presents with a history of infection, bleeding, or symptomatic anemia (Figure 59-1). Upon examination, there are signs of petechiae, ecchymoses, pallor, and infection. Aplastic anemia has a bimodal age distribution, with one peak at about 20 years of age and a second peak in the fifth decade.

Differential Diagnosis

The differential diagnosis is very broad because many diseases can cause cytopenias. If the cytopenias are particularly severe, diseases such as alcoholic cirrhosis, cancer, systemic lupus erythematosus, and tuberculosis should be considered.

Diagnostic Approach

The diagnosis of aplastic anemia lies primarily in the examination of the peripheral blood smear and the bone marrow biopsy specimen. The *peripheral blood smear* shows few abnormalities except a decrease in the overall number of white blood cells, red blood cells, and platelets. *Microscopic examination* of the bone marrow biopsy specimen reveals that the bone marrow is replaced by fat. Other diagnostic tests include *cytogenetic analysis*, which is usually normal in these patients, flow cytometry of blood or marrow to look for the co-expression of the CD55/59 antigens (diagnostic of paroxysmal nocturnal hemoglobinuria), and/or antibodies for parvovirus. If thymoma is suspected, a CT scan of the neck and chest is indicated.

Management and Therapy

Management involves a combination of supportive care and immunosuppressive therapy and, for selected individuals, bone marrow transplantation. Patients commonly need medical support with antibiotics and transfusions of platelets and red blood cells. Red blood cell and platelet transfusions should be depleted of white blood cells before infusion to reduce the risk of alloimmunization. Use of cytokines such as G-CSF, GM-CSF, and erythropoietin, are frequently helpful with recurrent infections or profound anemia. *Immunosuppressive therapy* includes the use of antithymocyte globulin (ATG), cyclosporine, cyclophosphamide, and steroids. Response to immunosuppressive therapy affects long-term survival (Table 59-2). The frequency of durable remission is higher in children, but secondary malignancies including myelodysplasia and acute leukemia may occur as often as 15%.

Table 59-1
Classification of Aplastic Anemias and Single Cytopenias

Aplastic Anemia
Acquired
 Radiation
 Drugs and chemicals
  ·Regular effects—cytotoxic agents, benzene
  ·Idiosyncratic reactions—chloramphenicol,
   nonsteroidal antiinflammatory drugs, antiepileptic
   drugs, gold, other drugs and chemicals

 Viruses
  ·Epstein-Barr virus (infectious mononucleosis)
  ·Hepatitis (non-A, non-B, non-C hepatitis)
  ·Human immunodeficiency virus (HIV)
  ·Parvovirus

 Immune diseases
  ·Eosinophilic fasciitis
  ·Hypoimmunoglobulinemia
  ·Thymoma and thymic carcinoma
  ·Graft-versus-host disease in immunodeficiency

 Paroxysmal nocturnal hemoglobinuria
 Pregnancy
 Idiopathic—the most frequent diagnosis

Inherited
  ·Fanconi's anemia
  ·Dyskeratosis congenita
  ·Schwachman-Diamond syndrome
  ·Reticular dysgenesis
  ·Amegakaryocytic thrombocytopenia
  ·Familial aplastic anemias

·Non-hematological syndromes (Down, Dubovitz,
 Seckel)

Cytopenias
Acquired
 Anemias
  ·Pure red blood cell aplasia
  ·Transient erythroblastopenia of childhood

 Neutropenias
  ·Idiopathic
  ·Drugs, toxins

 Thrombocytopenias
  ·Drugs, toxins
  ·Inherited

Inherited
 Anemias
  ·Congenital pure red blood cell aplasia

 Neutropenias
  ·Kostmann's syndrome
  ·Schwachman-Diamond syndrome

 Reticular dysgenesis

 Thrombocytopenias
  ·Thrombocytopenia with absence of radii
  ·Idiopathic amegakaryocytic thrombocytopenia

Reprinted from *Hematology: Basic Principles and Practice*, Hoffman R, Benz EJ Jr, Shatttil SJ, et al, Aplastic Anemia, 298, 2000, with permission from Elsevier

Allogeneic transplantation is generally used for patients younger than 40 or after failure of immunosuppressive therapy. Transplant-related mortality and morbidity are significant, however.

Certain clonal hematologic diseases appear to arise from aplastic anemia. *Paroxysmal nocturnal hemoglobinuria* develops early, generally with hematologic recovery after ATG treatment for the aplastic anemia. *Myelodysplasia* develops later, after months or years of unsuccessful immunosuppressive therapy and can progress to acute myeloid leukemia. These clonal diseases develop in up to 15% to 20% of patients within 10 years after treatment with immunosuppressive therapy but are rare after allogeneic transplantation.

One proposed algorithm is to offer transplantation as first-line therapy to patients younger than 40 with a matched sibling donor. For all patients over age 40 or those without a matched sibling donor, immunosuppression should be the first-line therapy.

Future Directions

Future directions for the therapy of aplastic anemias include non-ablative bone marrow transplantation, the use of growth factors (interleukin 11, stem cell factors, other cytokines), high-dose cyclophosphamide, recombinant humanized anti-IL-2 receptor antibody–directed therapy, and gene therapy for identifiable lesions such as Fanconi's anemia.

Figure 59-1

Bone Marrow Failure

Clinical Presentation

Symptoms of anemia (pallor, dyspnea, and tiredness) are common to **aplastic anemias**, **myelodysplasia** (when it affects the red cell line), **agnogenic myeloid metaplasia**, and **myelofibrosis**.

Examination of peripheral blood smear:

Aplastic anemia: Decrease in overall number of platelets, white and red cells

Myelodysplasia: Anisocytosis is common with both microcytic and macrocytic red blood cells present in the majority of cases

Agnogenic myeloid metaplasia and **myelofibrosis:** Immature granulocytes, nucleated red cells, and teardrop-shaped red cells

Hepatomegaly routinely present in the **agnogenic myeloid metaplasia syndromes**

Replacement of the bone marrow by fatty tissue is seen in **aplastic anemia. Myelofibrosis** is characterized by the presence of diffuse fibrotic tissue replacing the bone marrow

Peripheral edema is another sign seen in patients with **agnogenic myeloid metaplasia** and **myelofibrosis**.

Patients with **agnogenic myeloid metaplasia** present night sweats; low-grade fever; digestive symptoms such as early satiety and diarrhea; marked splenomegaly

Ecchymoses and petechiae are common findings in those conditions that affect platelet production, such as **aplastic anemia**, and **myelodysplasia**

Examination of the bone marrow smear:

Myelodysplasia: Most marrow biopsies are hypercellular and abnormal cytogenetics are important prognostic markers found in 50% of these patients

Agnogenic myeloid metaplasia and **myelofibrosis:** Fibroblasts, reactive myelofibrosis, dysplastic-megakaryocyte hyperplasia, osteosclerosis, and dilation of marrow sinusoids with intravascular hematopoiesis

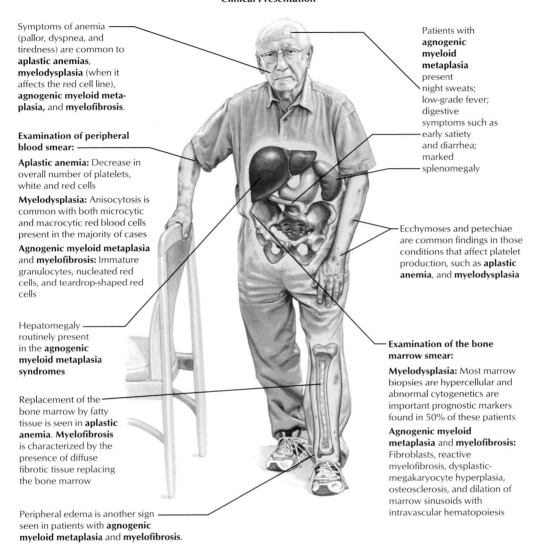

Histopathology of normal and abnormal marrow states

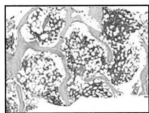

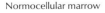

Normocellular marrow

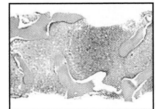

Hypercellular marrow

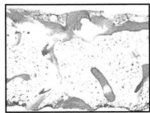

Hypocellular marrow

C. Machado
—M.D.

© **ICN**
LEARNING
SYSTEMS

Table 59-2
Aplastic Anemia and Therapies

Therapy	Response Rate (%)	Relapse Rate (%)
Antithymocyte Globulin (ATG)	20–85	35
Cyclosporine A (CsA)	16–57	40–63
ATG/CsA	65–80	3–36
Cyclophosphamide	70	40
Bone marrow transplantation	66–90	10–36

With permission from Ball SE. The modern management of severe aplastic anemia. *Br J Haematol* 2000;110:41–53.

MYELODYSPLASIA
Etiology and Pathogenesis

Myelodysplasia is a clonal disorder of hematopoietic progenitor cells, which results in ineffective hematopoiesis. Usually, the marrow cavity is hypercellular but unable to differentiate into mature cells that leave the marrow cavity and function normally in the peripheral blood. Myelodysplastic syndromes are classified into five categories (Table 59-3).

Myelodysplasia is generally an idiopathic acquired process, but it has been associated with exposure to chemicals (e.g., solvents, pesticides), chemotherapy, and radiation therapy. It causes bone marrow failure through ineffective hematopoiesis. There are intrinsic defects in the neoplastic clone causing impaired cellular maturation. The rate of cell division and growth is actually higher than normal; however, apoptosis is also increased.

Clinical Presentation

Presentation depends on which cell line is primarily affected (Figure 59-1). If the red blood cell line is affected, there can be symptoms of anemia: fatigue, dyspnea on exertion, and pallor. If the white blood cell line is affected, there can be signs of infection. If the platelets are affected, there can be signs of petechiae, ecchymosis, and bleeding. However, there is usually progressive pancytopenia. The abnormalities are often found on a routine blood cell count in an otherwise asymptomatic patient.

Table 59-3
Myelodysplastic Syndromes Classification

Refractory Anemia
Findings encompass cytopenia of at least one lineage in the peripheral blood (usually anemia) with normal or hypercellular bone marrow with dysplastic changes. Less than 1% blasts in the peripheral blood and less than 5% blasts in the bone marrow.

Refractory Anemia with Ringed Sideroblasts
This disorder presents with cytopenia (almost always anemia), dysplastic changes, and the same percentages of blood and bone marrow blasts as in refractory anemia. Ringed sideroblasts account for more than 15% of all nucleated cells in the bone marrow.

Refractory Anemia with Excess Blasts
This type of anemia shows cytopenia of 2 or more lineages in the peripheral blood. Dysplastic changes are present in all 3 lineages. Less than 5% blasts in the peripheral blood and between 5% and 20% blasts in the bone marrow.

Chronic Myelomonocytic Leukemia
Findings include peripheral-blood monocytosis (monocyte count $>1 \times 10^9$ per liter). Less than 5% blasts in the peripheral blood and up to 20% blasts in the bone marrow.

Refractory Anemia with Excess Blasts in Transformation
The hematologic features are similar to those of refractory anemia with excess blasts. More than 5% blasts in the peripheral blood or between 21% and 30% blasts in the bone marrow, or the presence of Auer rods in the blasts.

With permission from Heaney ML, Golde DW. Myelodysplasia. *N Engl J Med.* 1999;340(21):1650–1651.

Differential Diagnosis

The differential diagnosis of the pancytopenia in MDS patients can include congenital causes, hypersplenism, paroxysmal nocturnal hemoglobinuria, viral marrow suppression, marrow infiltration, and anemia of chronic disease. Dysplastic changes in the bone marrow can also be caused by vitamin deficiency (B_{12} and folate), drugs (antibiotics, chemotherapeutic agents), ethanol, benzene, lead, and viral infections such as infection with HIV.

Table 59-4
International Prognostic Scoring System for Myelodysplastic Syndromes

Prognostic Variable	Survival and AML Evolution Score Value				
	0	0.5	1.0	1.5	2.0
Marrow blasts (%)	<5	5–10	—	11–20	21–30
Karyotype	Good	Inter-mediate	—	Poor	—
Cytopenias	0–1	2–3	—	—	—

Karyotypes: good = normal, -Y, del(5q), del(20q); poor = complex (>3 abnormalities) or chromosome 7 anomalies; intermediate = other abnormalities.
Cytopenias: neutrophils <1800/uL, platelets <100,000/uL, hemoglobin <10g/dL.
Reprinted from *Hematology: Basic Principles and Practice*, Hoffman R, Benz EJ Jr, Shatttil SJ, et al, Aplastic Anemia, 298, 2000, with permission from Elsevier

Table 59-5
Survival by IPSS Score

Risk Category	Combined Score	Median Survival(yrs)
Low	0	5.7
Intermediate 1	0.5–1.0	3.5
2	1.5–2.0	1.2
High	>2.5	0.4

Note: Median age at diagnosis is seventh decade with a 3:2 proportion favoring men. Many patients progress to acute myeloid leukemia (AML). This can range from 5% transformation in refractory anemia with ringed sideroblasts (median survival 73 months) to 40% to 50% in refractory anemia with excess blasts (median survival 12 months) and refractory anemia with excess blasts in transformation (median survival 5 months), respectively. AML following evolution of myelodysplastic syndrome (MDS) is an especially aggressive form of leukemia that is difficult to treat and is fatal in 90% of the one third to one half of MDS patients in whom it develops.
With permission from Heaney ML, Golde DW. Myelodysplasia. *N Engl J Med.* 1999;340:1651.

Diagnostic Approach

Diagnosis requires examination of the peripheral blood smear and the bone marrow biopsy specimen. The peripheral blood smear may show macrocytic red blood cells, hypogranular granulocytes (pseudo-Pelger-Huet anomaly), and giant platelets. Bone marrow evaluation shows normal or frequently increased cellularity, megaloblastic red-blood-cell precursors, ringed sideroblasts, immature myeloid cells, asynchronous maturation of the nucleus and cytoplasm in granulocytic precursors, the pseudo-Pelger-Huet anomaly, micro-megakaryocytes, nuclear and cytoplasmic blebs, karyorrhexis, misshapen nuclei, and often an increase in myeloblasts. Cytogenetic analysis is important for determining the biology and prognosis of the disease. Half of all cases of myelodysplasia will have a cytogenetic abnormality. Abnormalities of chromosome 7 and complex abnormalities of chromosome 5 are associated with a particularly aggressive course and rapid progression to acute leukemia. However, those with an isolated deletion of chromosome 5 (5q- syndrome) have a more benign course; the median survival is longer than 5 years, and only 25% experience progression to acute leukemia (Tables 59-4 and 59-5).

Management and Therapy

Supportive care includes the administration of hematopoietic cytokines and growth factors, especially the combination of erythropoietin and G-CSF. Patients with <20% blasts in their marrow can be given a trial of agents such as 5-azacytidine or decitabine to induce differentiation and maturation of the abnormal cells. Further management includes chemotherapy and stem cell transplant. Patients in whom acute leukemia evolves and who have blast counts greater than 20% are frequently treated with standard induction regimens for acute leukemia. Results have been disappointing with a remission rate of 50% to 60% and a relapse rate of 90% for anthracycline/cytarabine combinations. Immunomodulation may be promising. In a pilot study of 25 patients, 11 patients became transfusion-independent after treatment with ATG. While bone marrow transplantation is the only curative therapy for such patients and should be undertaken when feasible, these patients often fare poorly due to their advanced age and more resistant disease.

Future Directions

Future directions include nonablative bone marrow transplant, immunomodulation, and molecular genetic approaches.

AGNOGENIC MYELOID METAPLASIA AND MYELOFIBROSIS
Etiology and Pathogenesis

Fibrosis of the bone marrow (myelofibrosis) is divided into primary and secondary (myelophthisis) processes. Myelofibrosis can be caused by infiltration of the bone marrow by a neoplastic process, granulomatous infections, and metabolic abnormalities.

Nonmalignant conditions associated with myelofibrosis include tuberculosis, histoplasmosis, renal osteodystrophy, vitamin D deficiency, hypoparathyroidism, hyperparathyroidism, gray platelet syndrome, systemic lupus erythematosus, scleroderma, radiation exposure, osteopetrosis, Paget's disease, benzene exposure, thorotrast exposure, and Gaucher disease.

Malignant disorders associated with myelofibrosis include agnogenic myeloid metaplasia, other myeloproliferative disorders, polycythemia vera, chronic myeloid leukemia, primary thrombocythemia, acute myelofibrosis, acute myeloid leukemia, acute lymphocytic leukemia, hairy cell leukemia, acute myelodysplasia with myelofibrosis, multiple myeloma, systemic mastocytosis, non-Hodgkin's lymphoma, and carcinoma, including breast, lung, prostate, and stomach.

Clinical Presentation

Patients present with marked splenomegaly, progressive anemia, and constitutional symptoms including fatigue, weight loss, night sweats, low-grade fever, early satiety, diarrhea, and peripheral edema (Figure 59-1). Upon examination, they have pancytopenia, extramedullary hematopoiesis, leftward shift in the granulocyte count, and increased levels of lactate dehydrogenase. Complications can include portal hypertension, splenic infarction, and other sites of hematopoiesis causing lymphadenopathy (enlarged lymph nodes), pleural effusions, ascites (serosal surfaces), pneumonia-like process (lung), hematuria (urogenital system), and compression of the spinal cord and nerve roots (paraspinal and epidural spaces). Median age at diagnosis is 65 with no definitive gender distribution.

Differential Diagnosis

The differential diagnosis includes other hematological malignancies such as chronic myeloge- nous leukemia, lymphoma, multiple myeloma, Hodgkin's disease, hairy cell leukemia, and myelodysplastic syndromes. Solid tumors such as metastatic breast, prostate, or lung cancer can also cause this syndrome.

Diagnostic Approach

The diagnosis is made through examination of the peripheral blood smear and the bone marrow. The peripheral blood smear shows immature granulocytes, nucleated red cells (leukoerythroblastosis), and teardrop-shaped red blood cells. Biopsy of the bone marrow shows fibroblasts in the marrow space with reactive myelofibrosis along with dysplastic-megakaryocyte hyperplasia, osteosclerosis, and dilatation of marrow sinusoids accompanied by intravascular hematopoiesis. Cytogenetic studies are useful only for excluding chronic myelogenous leukemia. The criteria for the diagnosis of myelofibrosis with myeloid metaplasia (MMM) include the following:

Necessary criteria: (a) diffuse bone marrow fibrosis, and (b) absence of Philadelphia chromosome or BCR-ABL rearrangement in peripheral-blood cells.

Optional criteria: splenomegaly of any grade; anisopoikilocytosis with teardrop erythrocytes; circulating immature myeloid cells; circulating erythroblasts; clusters of megakaryoblasts and anomalous megakaryocytes in bone marrow sections; myeloid metaplasia.

The diagnosis of MMM can be made if the following combinations are present: the 2 necessary criteria plus any 2 optional criteria when splenomegaly is present, or the 2 necessary criteria plus any 4 optional criteria when splenomegaly is absent.

Management and Therapy

Median survival is between 3 and 6 years (Table 59-6). Causes of death include leukemic transformation, infection, thrombohemorrhagic events, and heart failure. Prognostic factors associated with shortened survival include advanced age, anemia, hypercatabolic symptoms, leukocytosis, leukopenia, circulating blasts, increased numbers of granulocyte precursors, thrombocytopenia, and abnormalities in karyotype.

Management and therapy of myelofibrosis are largely palliative. Androgen preparations and cor-

Table 59-6
Lille Scoring System for Predicting Survival in Myelofibrosis with Myeloid Metaplasia

No. of Adverse Prognostic Factors	Risk Group	Median Survival (mo)
0	Low	93
1	Intermediate	26
2	High	13

Note: Adverse prognostic factors were hemoglobin count less than 10 g/dL and WBC count less than 4 or greater than $30 \times 10^9/_L$.
With permission from Barosi G. Myelofibrosis with myeloid metaplasia: Diagnostic definition and prognostic classification for clinical studies and treatment guidelines. *J Clin Oncol.* 1999;17(9):2961.

ticosteroids are used to alleviate anemia. Hydroxyurea is used to control leukocytosis, thrombocytosis, and organomegaly. Alternative treatments include interferon-alpha and cladribine. Splenectomy is recommended for patients with hydroxyurea-resistant symptomatic splenomegaly, overt portal hypertension, and progressive anemia requiring transfusion. For patients with contraindications to surgery, splenic irradiation can be done. Allogenic stem cell transplantation is an option in young patients.

Future Directions

Future directions for therapy include antifibrotic and antiangiogenic therapy, cytokine-directed approaches, and safer and more effective methods of allogeneic transplantation.

REFERENCES

Ball SE. The modern management of severe aplastic anaemia. *Br J Haematol.* 2000;110:41-53.

Barosi G. Myelofibrosis with myeloid metaplasia: diagnostic definition and prognostic classification for clinical studies and treatment guidelines. *J Clin Oncol.* 1999;17:2954-2970.

Greenberg PL. Myelodysplastic syndrome. In: Hoffman R, Benz EJ Jr, Shattil SJ, et al, eds. *Hematology: Basic Principles and Practice.* 3rd ed. New York, NY: Churchill Livingstone; 2000:1106-1129.

Heaney ML, Golde DW. Myelodysoplasia. *N Engl J Med.* 1999;340:1649-1660.

Hoffman R. Agnogenic myeloid metaplasia. In: Hoffman R, Benz EJ Jr, Shattil SJ, et al, eds. *Hematology: Basic Principles and Practice.* 3rd ed. New York, NY: Churchill Livingstone; 2000:1172-1188.

Tefferi A. Myelofibrosis with myeloid metaplasia. *N Engl J Med.* 2000;342:1255-1265.

Young NS, Maciejewski JP. Aplastic anemia. In: Hoffman R, Benz EJ Jr, Shattil SJ, et al, eds. *Hematology: Basic Principles and Practice.* 3rd ed. New York, NY: Churchill Livingstone; 2000:297-331.

Chapter 60

Hematopoietic Stem Cell Transplantation

John Powderly and Thomas Shea

Over the past 3 decades, hematopoietic stem cell transplantation has been established as curative therapy for hematopoietic malignancies, marrow failure syndromes, primary immunodeficiencies, and genetic disorders. Current efforts are designed to improve the efficacy of transplantation in these patients as well as expanding the role of transplantation for the treatment of other disorders such as solid tumors and autoimmune diseases.

Underlying the use of bone marrow or stem cell transplantation is the principle of dose response in regard to tumor cell kill (i.e., increasing dose overcomes drug resistance and eradicates more malignant cells). The ensuing hematopoietic deficiency is abrogated by the infusion of the stem cells from an autologous (a patient's own stem cells) or allogeneic (histocompatible donor) source (Figure 60-1). In the autologous setting, tumors that are still sensitive to the effects of standard doses of chemotherapy (chemosensitive disease) respond even better to the dose escalation used in transplantation. An additional therapeutic component of allogeneic transplantation is the graft-versus-tumor (GVT) immune effect mediated by donor lymphoid cells against residual host cancer cells. Advances in the fields of immunology, infectious disease, and transfusion medicine have all contributed to the encouraging results listed in Table 60-1.

AUTOLOGOUS STEM CELL TRANSPLANTS

While responses have been achieved in breast cancer and other solid tumors, these responses have not been confirmed or shown to be superior to conventional therapy in randomized trials. Such trials have identified a disease-free survival (DFS) and overall survival (OS) benefit for autologous transplants over conventional therapy in relapsed Hodgkin's and non-Hodgkin's lymphoma, acute myeloid leukemia in first complete response (CR), and in multiple myeloma. Because of more rapid hematopoietic recovery, fewer infections, and shorter hospital stays, the vast majority of these transplants are now undertaken with peripheral blood stem cells (PBSC) rather than bone marrow. While autologous transplantation is tolerated better than allogeneic transplantation, it is not feasible in patients with disease in the marrow and is generally unsuccessful in disease that is resistant to conventional doses of chemotherapy. Whether the increased risk of relapse associated with reinfusion of tumor cells that may be present in the autologous graft can be improved by more effective techniques for their removal is unknown, but currently being studied in randomized clinical trials.

ALLOGENEIC TRANSPLANTS

If a suitable donor is available, the decision to undergo an allogeneic transplant depends on the underlying disease and the existing comorbidities of the patient. The decreased leukemia relapse rate in allogeneic transplants compared to that in identical twin (syngeneic) or autologous transplants exemplifies the advantage of an alloimmune GVT response. Clinically favorable mild chronic graph-versus-host-disease (GVHD) enhances GVT in diseases such as chronic myelogenous leukemia (CML) and is associated with a decreased relapse rate. This immune effect is also the basis for treating recurrent disease after transplant with infusions of lymphocytes collected from the donor (donor lymphocyte infusions) and the development of nonmyeloablative transplants.

Usually, allogeneic transplantation is preferable for relapsed leukemias and patients with refractory lymphomas or multiple myeloma because of the

Table 60-1
Diseases Responsive to Hematopoietic Stem Cell Transplantation

Disease	Type of Transplant	Timing	Clinical Results
AML	Allogeneic	First CR	OS 40%–50%
ALL (children)	Allogeneic	Second CR	OS 40%–65%
ALL (high risk)	Allogeneic	First CR	OS 50%
Chronic phase CML	Allogeneic	Chronic Phase (CP)	OS 50%–80%
Accelerated phase CML	Allogeneic	Individualized	OS 30%–40%
Blast phase CML	Allogeneic	Second CP	OS 15%–25%
Myelodysplastic syndrome	Allogeneic	Age < 60	OS 40%
Aplastic anemia	Allogeneic	Individualized	OS 70%–90%
CLL	Allogeneic or Autologous	Participation in clinical trial	Small series of patients with durable CR. Nonablative transplants under investigation
Intermediate-grade NHL	Autologous	Chemosensitive relapse	OS 40%–50%
High-risk NHL	Autologous	First CR	OS 50%–60%
Low-grade NHL	Allogeneic or Autologous	Chemosensitive relapse	DFS 25%–50% at 5 yr
Mantle cell lymphoma	Allogeneic or Autologous Clinical trial	First CR	Small series with durable CR rates of 25%–50%
Lymphoblastic lymphoma	Allogeneic or Autologous Clinical trial	Chemosensitive relapse or first CR	Small series with durable CR
NHL or Hodgkin's disease	Allogeneic Clinical trial	Advanced Refractory Disease	15%–25% DFS
Multiple myeloma	Autologous	Chemosensitive relapse or first CR	5-yr OS 50%; DFS of 20%
High-risk breast, testicular or ovarian cancer	Autologous Clinical trial	Chemosensitive disease	Improved survival over historical controls not confirmed in randomized trials
Renal cell carcinoma	Nonablative Allogeneic	Clinical trial	Small series with durable CR
Thalassemia	Allogeneic	Clinical trial	OS 75% for patients without cirrhosis
Sickle cell anemia	Allogeneic	Clinical trial	OS 75%
Autoimmune disorders	Allogeneic	Clinical trial	Small series of remissions

CR, Complete response; DFS, disease-free survival; OS, overall survival; AML, acute myelogenous leukemia; CML, chronic myelogenous leukemia; ALL, acute lyphocytic leukemia; CP, chronic phase, NHL, non-Hodgkin's lymphoma.

immune effect of the donor cells against residual tumor and the lack of contaminating tumor cells in the infusion product. Some cases may favor early transplantation. Early identification and transplantation of patients with high-risk features who are destined to do poorly with standard therapies provides the best chance for cure in such settings.

HISTOCOMPATIBILITY

Major histocompatibility (MHC) *class I* (HLA; A, B, C) and *class II* (HLA-D; DR, DQ, DO, DN, DP, DR) antigens are the human leukocyte antigens (HLA) used to determine patient/donor compatibility. Six alleles from 3 HLA antigens (A, B, and DR) are used for routine typing of siblings. A 6 of 6 match is considered to be an HLA identical full match. Additional alleles can be evaluated for unrelated donor transplants.

DONOR AVAILABILITY

Matched sibling donors are available for approximately 30% of patients and are preferred over unmatched donors due to the decreased risk of graft rejection and GVHD. The National Marrow Donor Program includes a registry with more than 3.5 million volunteer donors that can provide a match for approximately 65% of Caucasians but only 30% to 40% of African American and other minority patients. Transplants using cells from unrelated donors who are mismatched at one or more alleles, or umbilical cord blood cells are available for certain patients at a limited number of centers. Virtually all patients have a haplotype or 3-antigen mismatched donor, provided they have a living first-degree relative. Infusion of large numbers of stem cells along with depletion of T cells from the donor product and aggressive immunosuppression may overcome the high risk of acute graft rejection and severe GVHD in these transplants.

SOURCES OF HEMATOPOIETIC STEM CELLS
Bone Marrow

Marrow harvesting usually requires general anesthesia for multiple aspirations from the iliac crest. Typically, 15 to 20 mL/kg recipient body weight yielding a minimum of 2×10^8 cells/kg is adequate for engraftment. Donors usually go home the same day and seldom require more than oral analgesics for 1 to 2 days postoperatively.

Peripheral Blood

Low numbers of CD34+ stem cells exist in peripheral blood under normal circumstances. This number can be markedly increased, allowing for collection by a process called pheresis following treatment with granulocyte–colony-stimulating factor (G-CSF) alone, or, for autologous transplant patients, in combination with chemotherapy. Advantages over bone marrow collection include a more rapid hematopoietic recovery and a decreased transplant-related mortality. This process results in infusion of 10 times more donor T cells in allogeneic transplants, leading to an increased risk of GVHD. This complication appears to be offset by earlier graft recovery and a lower risk of both infection and relapse.

Umbilical Cord Blood

An increased concentration of hematopoietic stem cells is present in umbilical cord blood, which can be collected from the placenta after delivery. Because neonatal lymphocytes remain immunologically naïve, they are less likely to result in GVHD and can be used in partially matched patient/donor pairs. The ability to undertake transplants with mismatched donors and the rapid availability of these frozen and stored cord blood products are the major advantages of this approach. Disadvantages include the low number of stem cells resulting in delayed engraftment and an increased risk of infection. Currently, umbilical cord transplants are used primarily for children, but research on expanding cord stem cells in vitro may provide sources for adults.

TRANSPLANT-RELATED THERAPY
Conditioning Regimens

Preparative regimens given before stem cell or bone marrow infusion are designed to eradicate the underlying disease and permit engraftment of donor stem cells without rejection. Full myeloablation of the hematopoietic system may be accomplished by total body irradiation (TBI) or high dose busulfan. In addition to marrow aplasia and infection, major toxicities include infertility, lung and liver toxicity, and severe mucositis. Each of these ablative modalities is generally administered with high-dose cyclophosphamide and/or etoposide to augment both the immunosuppressive and anti-tumor effect of the treatment. In the

Figure 60-1

Hematopoietic Stem Cell Transplantation

Autologous and allogeneic stem cell transplantation

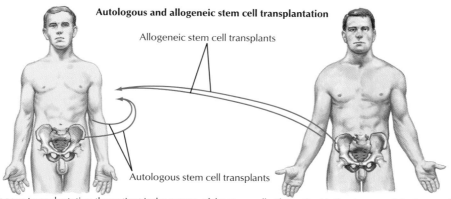

Allogeneic stem cell transplants

Autologous stem cell transplants

In autologous transplantation the patient is the source of the stem cells (the patient is the donor and the host at the same time). When the stem cells come from another person who is a histocompatible donor, this is called allogeneic transplantation

Sources of hematopoietic stem cells

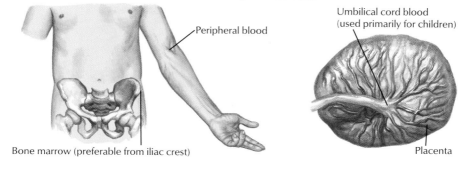

Peripheral blood

Umbilical cord blood (used primarily for children)

Bone marrow (preferable from iliac crest)

Placenta

Transplant complications

Graft versus host disease (graft rejection)

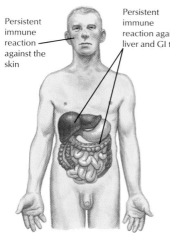

Persistent immune reaction against the skin

Persistent immune reaction against liver and GI tract

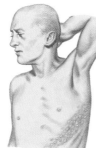

Reactivation of Varicella Zoster

Infections

Invasive pulmonary infections: **Fungi:** nocardiosis, aspergillosis, pneumocystis, bacteria: **Gram+:** Staphylococcal, pneumococcal infections. **Gram−:** E. coli, klebsiella, pseudomonas aeruginosa: **Viral:** CMV, herpes simplex, influenza infections.

Encephalitis: viruses: herpes simplex. Protozoa: toxoplaplasmosis fungi: aspergillosis

Sinus infections: fungal: mucormycosis

Bacteremias and catheter infections: Staphylococcal, streptococcal, Gram-negative infections

Hepatic infections: Fungal: Aspergillosis. Viral: CMV

GU tract infections: Adenoviruses CMV, bk

GI tract infections: CMV and adenoviral infections

C. Machado
M.D.

© ICON
LEARNING
SYSTEMS

autologous setting, a variety of combination regimens have used additional drugs including carmustine, thiotepa, and melphalan.

Nonmyeloablative regimens with immunosuppressive drugs such as fludarabine and cyclophosphamide or low dose TBI have been used to establish a mixed-chimera (both donor and host cells) hematopoietic state. In less aggressive tumors such as chronic leukemias or indolent lymphomas, the advantages of this approach include less toxicity and shorter duration of pancytopenia while maintaining a GVT effect. This cell-mediated response has been shown to evoke complete responses in both hematologic malignancies and solid tumors such as renal cell cancer. Although still preliminary, these less toxic transplants may be ideal for older patients or those with underlying organ compromise.

Immunosuppression

The main factor allowing allogeneic transplantation is the use of medications that dampen the T cell response. Initial treatment with agents such as methotrexate, corticosteroids, and either cyclosporin or tacrolimus is used to prevent graft rejection and subsequent GVHD during the initial period after transplant. Additional agents such as anti-thymocyte globulin (ATG) or mycophenolate have also been used to prevent rejection.

Transfusion Therapy

Transfusions for immunosuppressed patients require removal of leukocytes from infused blood products to lower the risk of alloimmunization and CMV reactivation or transmission. Blood products must also be irradiated after transplantation to reduce the risk of transfusion-associated GVHD. These measures should be continued as long as patients are receiving immunosuppressive medication or have evidence of GVHD.

TRANSPLANT COMPLICATIONS
Treatment-Related Morbidity and Mortality

Weighing the potential for cure with transplantation against the complications, quality of life, and risk of relapse of the underlying malignancy are paramount considerations for both the transplant team and patient (Table 60-2). Overall mortality rates with allogeneic transplants range from 15%

Table 60-2
Comparison of Complications Between Autologous, Allogeneic and Nonablative Transplants

Complication	Autologous	Allogeneic	Nonablative
Bacterial infection	3+	4+	2+
Viral infections	1+	4+	4+
Fungal infections	1+	4+	4+
Graft vs host	—	3+	3+
Graft rejection	Slow recovery 1+	2%–5%	5%–10%
Graft vs tumor	—	2+	3+
Veno-occlusive disease	1%–3%	10%	Rare
Relapse	4+	2+	3+
Secondary MDS* or AML[†]	5%–15%	—	—
Treatment-related mortality	5%	20%–40%	15%–25%

*MDS, myelodysplastic syndrome; [†]AML, Acute myelogenous leukemia.

to 50% in the first 1 to 2 years, depending on patient age, organ function, and quality of the donor-patient match. Treatment-related mortality rates vary from 2% to 10% for autologous transplants, depending primarily on the type and stage of malignancy and physiological status of the patient. While complications are more common following allogeneic transplants than autologous transplants, the risk of relapse is substantially higher for most autologous transplant patients. This leads to a complicated decision process regarding the optimal type of transplant for an individual patient that is based on the availability of a match, organ function, performance status, age, and disease status. Such decisions are best made by an informed patient at an experienced center where multiple options are available.

Graft-Versus-Host Disease

The degree of HLA disparity is directly associated with severity of GVHD. Acute GVHD occurs before day 100 and develops in 10% to 70% of matched sibling transplants. More severe GVHD is associated with matched unrelated or mismatched donor transplants. This can be reduced by T cell depletion of the donor product before infusion, but such maneuvers also lead to higher rates of relapse and graft rejection. Chronic GVHD that occurs beyond day 100 manifests as a persistent autoimmune reaction against the host's skin, gut, and liver. While mild GVHD is associated with an enhanced GVT effect and decreased relapse rate, severe GVHD is an unrelenting process that conveys a poor quality of life and higher risk of treatment-related mortality.

Infection

Bacterial infections occur early after transplantation during the period of neutropenia and mucosal injury. Infection with CMV and other viral pathogens such as adenovirus usually occur 30 to 100 days after transplantation. Risk of bacterial, fungal, and viral infection continues with prolonged immunosuppression and can present months to years later as unexplained fevers (Figure 60-1). Patients requiring prolonged immunosuppression for GVHD are at risk for rapidly fatal bacterial infections with encapsulated organisms such as streptococcus and pneumococcus. Fevers in these patients must be treated aggressively with broad-spectrum antibiotics while the underlying cause is being investigated. Reactivation of varicella zoster occurs in 30% to 40% of patients, typically within 12 months of transplant. Life-threatening dissemination may occur if not recognized and treated early with medications such as acyclovir. Late fungal infections with invasive organisms such as aspergillus or mucormycosis can also be seen in patients on long-term immunosuppressive therapy.

FUTURE DIRECTIONS

Continued improvements in supportive care and expansion of the donor transplant pool through the use of cord blood cells, mismatched, and matched unrelated donors will continue to increase the number of transplant candidates in upcoming years. Combining new vaccine and other immunotherapy approaches with either autologous or allogeneic transplants will be used to eliminate tumor cells and the risk of relapse in the future.

REFERENCES

Childs R, Chernoff A, Contentin N, et al. Regression of metastatic renal-cell carcinoma after nonmyeloablative allogeneic peripheral-blood stem-cell transplantation. N Engl J Med. 2000;343:750-758.

Childs R, Clave E, Contentin N, et al. Engraftment kinetics after nonmyeloablative allogeneic peripheral blood stem cell transplantation: full donor T-cell chimerism precedes alloimmune responses. Blood. 1999;94:3234-3241.

Negrin RS, Blume KG. Allogeneic autologous hematopoietic cell transplantation. In: Beutler E, Lichtman MA, Coller BS, Kipps TJ, Seligsohn U, eds. Williams Hematology. 6th ed. New York, NY: McGraw-Hill; 2001:209-247.

Thomas ED, Blume KG, Forman SJ, eds. Hematopoietic Cell Transplantation. 2nd ed. Malden, Mass: Blackwell Science Inc; 1998.

Chapter 61

Leukemias

Beverly S. Mitchell

The leukemias are a group of disorders characterized by neoplastic transformation of hematopoietic cells, with resultant accumulation of these cells in the bone marrow and commonly, although not universally, in the peripheral blood. Leukemias may arise from lymphoid or from myeloid cells and are generally classified as acute if the cells are arrested early in differentiation (blasts or early progenitors), or as chronic if the cells are mature. Most leukemias are characterized by chromosomal or cytogenetic abnormalities that contribute to the assessment of overall prognosis. Risk factors for leukemia include exposure to ionizing radiation, previous chemotherapy, and increasing age.

ACUTE MYELOID LEUKEMIA
Etiology and Pathogenesis

Acute myeloid leukemia (AML) arises in a stem cell capable of giving rise to granulocytes, monocytes, red blood cells, and platelets. Malignant transformation occurs at different stages of differentiation, giving rise to subtypes that can be distinguished by morphology, histochemistry, and specific surface markers using a panel of monoclonal antibodies (flow cytometry). The subtypes of AML have been codified in a French-American-British (FAB) classification system that divides the leukemias into 7 groups (M1–7) based on the myeloid phenotype. Because cells accumulate at a very immature stage of development, they replace the bone marrow and cause anemia and thrombocytopenia. Many cytogenetic abnormalities have been described that lead to the production of specific proteins that cause the leukemias. Of these, the translocation of a portion of chromosome 17 onto the long arm of chromosome 15 in acute progranulocytic or M3 leukemia is the best understood. The resulting aberrant gene product contains a portion of the nuclear retinoic acid receptor, and clinical remissions in this disorder can be achieved with pharmacological doses of all-*trans*-retinoic acid. This vitamin A derivative binds to the receptor and overcomes the block in differentiation, allowing maturation of the leukemic cells into neutrophils.

Clinical Presentation

Patients present with symptoms related to anemia (fatigue, pallor, dyspnea), neutropenia (infection), or thrombocytopenia (petechiae, bleeding).

Different subtypes may have specific manifestations. Acute *progranulocytic leukemia* (M3) may present with disseminated intravascular coagulation and bleeding or purpura. Leukemias derived from monocytes (M4 and M5) may present with skin, gum, or lung infiltration. AML may also develop from preexisting myelodysplasia that is characterized by a period of low blood counts, frequently requiring blood product support.

Differential Diagnosis

Patients presenting with high white blood counts consisting predominantly of blasts are easily diagnosed based on examination of the peripheral blood smear (Figure 61-1). Patients with pancytopenia may have acute leukemia on the basis of blasts in the bone marrow only. The differential diagnosis includes aplastic anemia, myelodysplasia, marrow infiltration with fibrosis or tumor, or, rarely, hypersplenism.

Diagnostic Approach

Examination of the peripheral blood smear is always warranted. A bone marrow aspiration and biopsy should be performed with requests for flow cytometry and cytogenetics. Bone marrow specimens are generally hypercellular, and a blast count of greater than 30% is diagnostic of acute leukemia.

Management and Therapy

Patients with AML are treated with combination chemotherapy in an attempt to empty the bone marrow of malignant cells and allow normal progenitors to repopulate the marrow. Patients are generally hospitalized for 3 to 4 weeks and require intensive blood product and antibiotic support. Following the induction of remission (less than 5% blasts in the marrow), patients are treated with several cycles of high-dose chemotherapy as consolidation of the remission. Patients with cytogenetic abnormalities portending a poor prognosis or who relapse are candidates for bone marrow transplantation. The overall survival rate is 30% to 40% at 3 to 5 years, with most deaths due to relapse of the disease.

ACUTE LYMPHOBLASTIC LEUKEMIA
Etiology and Pathogenesis

The acute lymphoblastic leukemias (ALLs) are associated with cytogenetic abnormalities and translocations. Most frequently they occur in immunoglobulin or T cell receptor loci that undergo recombination in the normal course of lymphoid maturation and are regions of active transcription. These diseases may also be subcategorized as of pre-T, T, pre-B, or B cell origin based on their surface markers. The presence of a Philadelphia chromosome (a translocation between chromosomes 9 and 22) occurs in some patients with ALL and has a poor prognosis.

Clinical Presentation

As with AML, ALL presents with anemia and thrombocytopenia. The white blood cell count may be elevated or low, and blasts have a lymphoid morphology. In contrast to AML, patients with ALL more frequently have lymphadenopathy and splenomegaly. The disease may also involve the central nervous system and present with cranial nerve abnormalities and/or headache. Lumbar puncture is indicated to make a diagnosis of leukemic meningitis in such cases.

Differential Diagnosis

Toxoplasmosis or acute viral infections such as cytomegalovirus and infectious mononucleosis may present with a *reactive lymphocytosis* that is difficult to distinguish from an acute leukemia. Appropriate antibody titers in conjunction with suspicion of an infectious etiology should establish the appropriate diagnosis. The leukemic phase of certain lymphomas and the occasional lymphoid blast crisis of chronic myelogenous leukemia are also in the differential diagnosis.

Diagnostic Approach

Examination of the peripheral blood and bone marrow by morphology, cytogenetics, and flow cytometry should establish the diagnosis (Figure 61-1). Specific T and B cell surface markers identify the subset of leukemia. Monoclonality is indicative of an acute leukemia, as opposed to a reactive lymphocytosis and can be determined by finding identical rearrangements of the immunoglobulin or T cell receptor loci in all cells.

Management and Therapy

The treatment of ALL consists of intensive induction chemotherapy with multiple drugs and consolidation treatment that is carried out over 1 to 2 years. The regimens are very intensive and include prophylactic intrathecal administration of chemotherapy drugs such as methotrexate and cytosine arabinoside. Although most patients enter remission, patients may relapse years following treatment, and the overall cure rate with chemotherapy alone in adults is roughly 20%, with a worse prognosis for individuals over 50. Childhood ALL has a far better prognosis, with an overall cure rate of more than 80%.

CHRONIC MYELOGENOUS LEUKEMIA
Etiology and Pathogenesis

The hallmark of *chronic myelogenous leukemia* (CML) is the presence of the Philadelphia chromosome (Ph'), involving a reciprocal translocation between chromosomes 9 and 22. This leads to the formation of a fusion protein between the *bcr* region of chromosome 22 and the *c-abl* tyrosine kinase on chromosome 9. The fusion protein has increased kinase activity and is sufficient to cause the disease in transgenic mice. The disease frequently undergoes progression to a blast crisis form by a progression of genetic change(s) that have not been well characterized.

Clinical Presentation

CML presents with a high white blood count that may be detected on routine complete blood cell count and splenomegaly in 90% of cases. Patients may complain of generalized fatigue or abdominal discomfort and early satiety. Occasionally, patients present with hypermetabolic symptoms of fever and weight loss. Hepatomegaly is also common. The peripheral blood smear shows mature neutrophils with occasional earlier myeloid forms and an occasional blast (Figure 61-1). The platelet count is frequently elevated, and platelets may appear somewhat large and dysmorphic on peripheral smear. An accelerated phase of the disorder is a harbinger of blast crisis and is characterized by progressive splenomegaly and elevation of the WBC count with basophils and an increasing percentage of blasts. Blast crisis occurs in untreated patients at a mean of 3 to 4 years from diagnosis and is characterized by more than 30% blasts in the bone marrow of either myeloid or lymphoid type.

Differential Diagnosis

Reactive leukocytosis, resulting most commonly from infection, malignancy, or drug reaction, is the most common entity to be differentiated from CML. Other myeloproliferative disorders, including polycythemia vera and myelofibrosis, also present with elevated WBC counts and splenomegaly. The blast crisis of CML must be distinguished from de novo forms of AML and ALL.

Diagnostic Approach

The Ph', generally obtained from a bone marrow examination, definitively distinguishes CML from both infectious causes of a high WBC count and from other myeloproliferative diseases. ALL may also be associated with a Ph'. A leukocyte alkaline phosphatase score may be obtained on peripheral WBCs and is generally high in reactive leukocytosis and low in CML.

Management and Therapy

Patients presenting with a very high WBC count may require initial therapy with hydroxyurea, which controls the blood counts but does not prolong overall survival. Until recently, the optimal treatment of CML included bone marrow transplantation for younger patients (<40 years) with a donor and the combined use of alpha interferon and cytosine arabinoside for all other patients. The relatively small percentage of patients who lost the Ph' with this regimen had a decrease in the incidence of blast crisis and prolongation of survival. However, a drug that specifically inhibits the tyrosine kinase activity of the bcr-abl fusion protein (imatinib) has recently been approved. Imatinib is both highly effective and less toxic than prior therapy. Imatinib results in hematological remissions in more than 90% of patients and is the first chemotherapy drug that specifically targets an oncogenic protein. Although it is not yet known what its overall effect on survival will be, it offers the least toxicity and highest response rate of any therapy developed to date.

CHRONIC LYMPHOCYTIC LEUKEMIA
Etiology and Pathogenesis

CLL is the most common type of leukemia, frequently occurring in patients older than 50. This disorder involves the accumulation of slowly dividing mature B, or rarely T, lymphocytes in the peripheral blood and bone marrow. The molecular basis for this disorder remains obscure, although a number of different cytogenetic abnormalities have been described. It appears to be associated with an increase in the anti-apoptotic or anti-cell death proteins, such as bcl-2, that characterize the indolent lymphomas.

Clinical Presentation

Patients most commonly present with an elevated WBC count on routine CBC. The majority of cells are mature lymphocytes (Figure 61-1). Other less common presentations include lymph node enlargement, recurrent infections due to associated hypogammaglobulinemia, or immune-mediated hemolytic anemia or thrombocytopenia. A simple Rai staging classification, which has prognostic import, defines the stage of the disease:

Stage	Features	Median Survival (yr)
0	Lymphocytosis only (>5x10^9/L)	>15
I	Lymphocytosis and lymphadenopathy	8
II	Lymphocytosis and splenomegaly	6
III	Lymphocytosis and anemia (Hgb <11 g/dL)	3
IV	Lymphocytosis and thrombocytopenia (platelets <100x10^9/L)	2

The anemia and thrombocytopenia in this classification results from decreased production due to bone marrow involvement. More recent studies

Figure 61-1

Leukemias

Clinical Presentation of Leukemias

Acute myeloid leukemia (AML), acute lymphoblastic leukemia (ALL), chronic myelogenous leukemia (CML), and chronic lymphocytic leukemia (CLL)

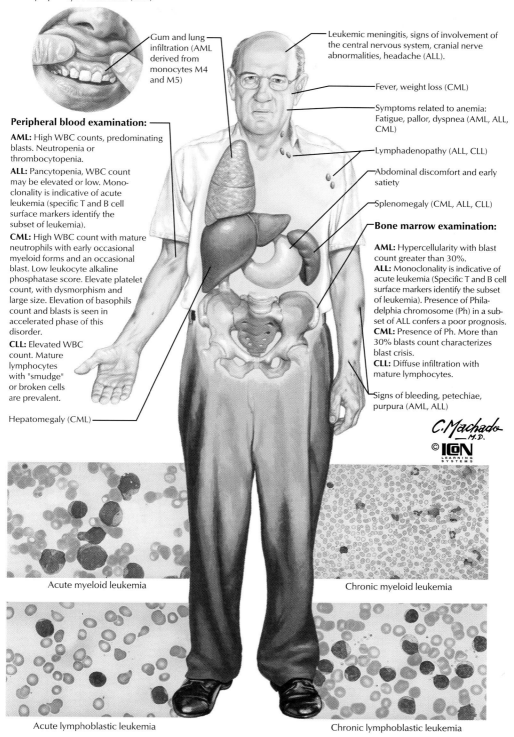

Gum and lung infiltration (AML derived from monocytes M4 and M5)

Leukemic meningitis, signs of involvement of the central nervous system, cranial nerve abnormalities, headache (ALL).

Fever, weight loss (CML)

Symptoms related to anemia: Fatigue, pallor, dyspnea (AML, ALL, CML)

Lymphadenopathy (ALL, CLL)

Abdominal discomfort and early satiety

Splenomegaly (CML, ALL, CLL)

Peripheral blood examination:

AML: High WBC counts, predominating blasts. Neutropenia or thrombocytopenia.

ALL: Pancytopenia, WBC count may be elevated or low. Mono-clonality is indicative of acute leukemia (specific T and B cell surface markers identify the subset of leukemia).

CML: High WBC count with mature neutrophils with early occasional myeloid forms and an occasional blast. Low leukocyte alkaline phosphatase score. Elevate platelet count, with dysmorphism and large size. Elevation of basophils count and blasts is seen in accelerated phase of this disorder.

CLL: Elevated WBC count. Mature lymphocytes with "smudge" or broken cells are prevalent.

Hepatomegaly (CML)

Bone marrow examination:

AML: Hypercellularity with blast count greater than 30%.
ALL: Monoclonality is indicative of acute leukemia (Specific T and B cell surface markers identify the subset of leukemia). Presence of Phila-delphia chromosome (Ph) in a sub-set of ALL confers a poor prognosis.
CML: Presence of Ph. More than 30% blasts count characterizes blast crisis.
CLL: Diffuse infiltration with mature lymphocytes.

Signs of bleeding, petechiae, purpura (AML, ALL)

C. Machado
— M.D.

© ICON
LEARNING SYSTEMS

Acute myeloid leukemia

Chronic myeloid leukemia

Acute lymphoblastic leukemia

Chronic lymphoblastic leukemia

on gene expression in CLL have been useful in its classification and in defining prognosis.

Differential Diagnosis

Viral infections, the leukemic phase of non-Hodgkin's lymphoma, and hairy cell leukemia, an unusual lymphoproliferative disease characterized by pancytopenia, splenomegaly, and a distinctive surface marker phenotype, are in the differential diagnosis.

Diagnostic Approach

Examination of the peripheral blood reveals mature lymphocytes, frequently with "smudge" or broken cells characteristic of lymphoproliferative diseases. Bone marrow transplantation may be indicated in patients presenting with cytopenias. Flow cytometry is a useful diagnostic tool in difficult cases. A serum protein electrophoresis and Coombs' test with reticulocyte count are indicated in patients with recurrent infections and anemia, respectively.

Management and Therapy

Patients with stage 0, I, or II disease can be observed at 3- to 6-month intervals with physical examination and CBC to assess disease progression. Patients with stable disease can be observed annually. Initial therapy for patients with stage III or IV disease is either intermittent treatment with an alkylating agent and prednisone or therapy with fludarabine, a nucleoside analog. Although fludarabine results in a higher remission rate and longer disease-free intervals, overall survival is similar with the 2 regimens. Fludarabine results in prolonged immunosuppression, and patients should be monitored for opportunistic infections. Patients with more aggressive CLL or who have failed primary therapy are candidates for combination chemother-

apy. Richter's syndrome represents a transformation of the disease into a more aggressive lymphoma and confers a poor prognosis. Patients with recurrent infections and hypogammaglobulinemia should receive intravenous immunoglobulin. Immune-mediated hemolysis or thrombocytopenia requires treatment of the underlying disease for a good response.

FUTURE DIRECTIONS

Progress in treating the acute leukemias has been slow. New approaches include the combined use of monoclonal antibodies with chemotherapeutic drugs and stimulation of the host immune system to leukemia-associated antigens. As new molecular mechanisms of oncogenesis are discovered, they will be become subjects for specific targeting by pharmacologic agents. CML has opened a new era of tumor-specific therapies that should revolutionize the current approaches to leukemia treatment.

REFERENCES

Druker BJ, Talpaz M, Resta DJ, et al. Efficacy and safety of a specific inhibitor of the BCR-ABL tyrosine kinase in chronic myeloid leukemia. *N Engl J Med.* 2001;344:1031-1037.

Hoelzer D, Gokbuget N. New approaches to acute lymphoblastic leukemia in adults: where do we go? *Semin Oncol.* 2000;27:540-559.

Keating MJ, O'Brien S, Lerner S, et al. Long-term follow-up of patients with chronic lymphocytic leukemia (CLL) receiving fludarabine regimens as initial therapy. *Blood.* 1998;92:1165-1171.

Laport GF, Larson RA. Treatment of adult acute lymphoblastic leukemia. *Semin Oncol.* 1997;24:70-82.

Savage DG, Szydlo RM, Goldman JM. Clinical features at diagnosis in 430 patients with chronic myeloid leukaemia seen at a referral centre over a 16-year period. *Br J Haematol.* 1997;96:111-116.

Schiffer CA, Dodge R, Larson RA. Long-term follow-up of Cancer and Leukemia Group B studies in acute myeloid leukemia. *Cancer.* 1997;80(suppl):2210-2214.

Chapter 62
Malignant Lymphomas

Robert Z. Orlowski

Lymphomas arise from a malignant transformation of lymphoid tissue and are classified as *Hodgkin's disease* (HD) or *non-Hodgkin's lymphoma* (NHL). HD is divided into 5 subtypes that share many characteristics, according to the Revised European-American Lymphoma (REAL) classification. NHL, however, comprises a heterogeneous group of more than 20 malignancies that are distinct not only from HD, but in many cases from one another.

First described by Dr. Thomas Hodgkin, the term Hodgkin's disease was coined later by Sir Samuel Wilks. In developed areas, its incidence is approximately 3/100,000 population, but in the developing world it is <1/100,000. A bimodal age distribution is seen, with one peak at 20 to 30 years of age and a second peak in incidence after age 50. The median age at diagnosis is approximately 33 years of age. HD afflicts men more frequently than women, although in the 20- to 30-year-old age group there is a slight female preponderance. HD incidence and mortality have been decreasing, and it is an example of the success of radiation therapy and chemotherapy.

NHL is also more frequent in the developed world and in men, but has an approximate 4-fold higher incidence than HD, and represents about 4% of all new cancer diagnoses in the United States. It is one of the few malignancies with a rising incidence, at approximately 3% to 4% per year. From 1973 to 1996, the incidence of NHL has increased by 81%. This is due in part to HIV, and is contributed to by an aging population because the incidence of NHL rises with age (median age of diagnosis is approximately 65), although certain subtypes, such as some aggressive lymphomas, afflict younger populations.

ETIOLOGY AND PATHOGENESIS

The etiology of HD remains unknown, although several factors support a possible role for an infectious agent. Some notable associations include Epstein-Barr virus (EBV) infection (especially recent infectious mononucleosis, but EBV is not found in all tumors), HIV infection, and a genetic predisposition (approximately 1% of patients have a family history of HD, with first-degree relatives and monozygotic compared with dizygotic twins at increased risk).

Whereas in HD the most common karyotype is normal, in NHL non-random translocations play important roles in the pathogenesis of certain subtypes: t(8;14), t(2;8), or t(8;22)—*c-myc* drives proliferation in Burkitt's lymphoma (BL); t(14;18)—anti-apoptotic *bcl-2*, seen in 85% of follicular and some higher-grade NHLs; and t(11;14)—cyclin-D1 cell-cycle control protein in mantle cell lymphoma.

Several risk factors for NHL have been identified. *Primary immunodeficiency syndromes*: ataxia-telangiectasia, and Wiskott-Aldrich.

Viral infection: EBV, associated with African BL; hepatitis C virus (HCV); HIV and intermediate/high-grade NHL; and human T-cell leukemia virus-I (HTLV-I) and adult T-cell leukemia/lymphoma.

Helicobacter pylori infection: associated with some gastric lymphomas, as are celiac sprue and inflammatory bowel diseases.

Secondary immunodeficiency: particularly as a result of immune suppression in organ transplant recipients.

Autoimmune disorders: rheumatoid arthritis, Felty's syndrome, Sjögren's disease.

Occupational exposures: pesticides, hair dyes, radiation.

CLINICAL PRESENTATION

Patients with HD typically have asymptomatic adenopathy that is firm, non-tender, and mobile, although nodes can be matted together. Supradiaphragmatic presentations involving the neck, supraclavicular fossa, or axilla are most common, as is mediastinal involvement, but disease limited to areas below the diaphragm is less frequent, as is epitrochlear or Waldeyer's ring involvement. Systemic symptoms can include fever, night sweats, weight loss, fatigue, and pruritus. Rare manifestations include pain in affected nodes after drinking alcohol and Pel-Ebstein fever, which builds to a peak over several days, lasts several weeks, wanes, and then begins anew.

Asymptomatic progressive adenopathy is also common in NHL, although the sites of involvement are more varied, and extranodal disease is more frequent. Patients with indolent NHL may have had several years of waxing/waning adenopathy and tend not to have systemic symptoms or primary extranodal involvement until disease is more advanced. With intermediate- and high-grade lymphomas, constitutional findings and early extranodal involvement, such as of the gastrointestinal tract, bone marrow, or central nervous system, can occur even in early-stage disease.

DIFFERENTIAL DIAGNOSIS

Adenopathy with or without systemic symptoms should prompt consideration of infectious etiologies, including mononucleosis, histoplasmosis, toxoplasmosis, and tuberculosis; autoimmune processes, including rheumatoid arthritis, systemic lupus erythematosus, and Wegener's granulomatosis; hypersensitivity reactions, such as to drugs or vaccinations and serum sickness; benign disorders, such as hyperthyroidism or amyloidosis, and Kawasaki's or Whipple's disease; and other malignancies, including metastatic breast, renal cell, prostate gland, and lung cancer. With mediastinal masses, one should consider sarcoidosis, thymoma, germ cell tumors, and HD versus NHL, especially lymphoblastic, peripheral T-cell, and large cell lymphomas. Pathologically, it may be difficult to distinguish certain HD cases from large cell lymphoma, T-cell–rich B-cell lymphoma, or Ki-1+ anaplastic large cell lymphoma.

DIAGNOSTIC APPROACH

For patients with asymptomatic adenopathy, watchful waiting for a few weeks, possibly with a course of antibiotics, is usually reasonable. Steroids should be avoided because they are lympholytic. Regression of adenopathy does not rule out a malignant process because nodes may wax and wane. Patients with persistent or progressive adenopathy should be referred for a biopsy. Patients with unex-plained constitutional symptoms, abnormal screening laboratory studies including anemia, elevations of the ESR or LFTs or lactate dehydrogenase (LDH), abnormal chest radiographs, or at high HIV risk should be considered for prompt referral.

An incisional or excisional biopsy is required to diagnose lymphoma. The most accessible node is generally targeted. If there is concern for transformation of an indolent lymphoma into an aggressive one, the most symptomatic node should be removed. Standard hematoxylin-and-eosin staining is supplemented with flow cytometry or immunohistochemistry for antigens such as CD30 and CD15 in HD, and to identify clonal populations and lymphocyte lineage markers such as CD19/20 for B-cell NHL and CD3/5 for T-cell NHL. Cytogenetics should be performed for NHL because certain karyotypic abnormalities are helpful diagnostically. Needle aspiration is not adequate because the neoplastic Reed-Sternberg cells in HD can make up 1% or less of the total cell population, and the nodal architecture used in histologic classification of lymphomas is lost. Reed-Sternberg cells must be present to diagnose HD, but are rarely seen in other hematological malignancies.

HISTOLOGY

The REAL classification recognizes 4 "classic" Hodgkin's diseases and a fifth subtype, nodular lymphocyte-predominant (NLPHD):

Nodular sclerosis (NS) (40% to 80% of cases): Typically young adults, especially women; with early stage supradiaphragmatic disease.

Mixed cellularity (MC) (15% to 40%): Often in men with generalized lymphadenopathy or extranodal disease and systemic symptoms.

NLPHD (5% to 6%): Considered by some an NHL, patients generally have early stage disease with mediastinal sparing; late relapses and other cancers are more common.

Classic lymphocyte predominant (<1% to 2%): Approximately one third of LPHD cases, similar to MC HD.

Lymphocyte depleted (<1% to 2%): Common in elderly patients with advanced, extranodal disease and abdominal adenopathy, or with MC HD associated with EBV/HIV.

REAL characterizes non-Hodgkin's lymphoma based on a T- or B-cell origin, and on its stage of differentiation as either a precursor- or peripheral-

Figure 62-1

Malignant Lymphomas – Staging

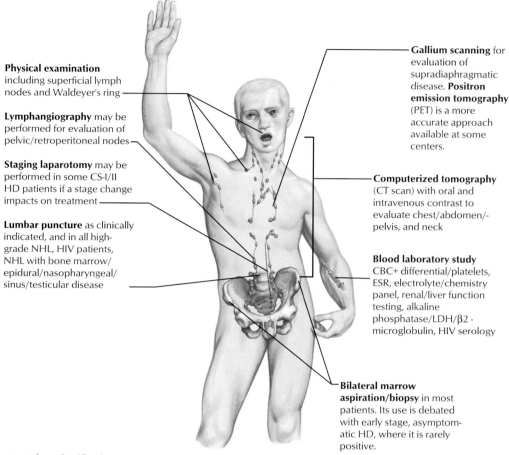

Physical examination including superficial lymph nodes and Waldeyer's ring

Lymphangiography may be performed for evaluation of pelvic/retroperitoneal nodes

Staging laparotomy may be performed in some CS-I/II HD patients if a stage change impacts on treatment

Lumbar puncture as clinically indicated, and in all high-grade NHL, HIV patients, NHL with bone marrow/epidural/nasopharyngeal/sinus/testicular disease

Gallium scanning for evaluation of supradiaphragmatic disease. **Positron emission tomography** (PET) is a more accurate approach available at some centers.

Computerized tomography (CT scan) with oral and intravenous contrast to evaluate chest/abdomen/-pelvis, and neck

Blood laboratory study CBC+ differential/platelets, ESR, electrolyte/chemistry panel, renal/liver function testing, alkaline phosphatase/LDH/β2 - microglobulin, HIV serology

Bilateral marrow aspiration/biopsy in most patients. Its use is debated with early stage, asymptomatic HD, where it is rarely positive.

C.Machado —M.D.

© **ICON** LEARNING SYSTEMS

Ann Arbor Classification

Stage I
Involvement of a single lymph node region (I) or of a single extralymphatic organ or site (IE)

Stage II
Involvement of two or more lymph node regions on the same side of the diaphragm (II) or localized involvement of extralymphatic organ or site and of one or more lymph node regions on the same side of the diaphragm (IIE)

Stage III
Involvement of lymph node regions on both sides of the diaphragm (III) which may also be accompanied by localized involvement of extralymphatic organ or site (IIIE) or by involvement of the spleen (IIIS) or both (IIISE)

Stage IV
Diffuse or disseminated involvement of one or more extralymphatic organs or tissues with or without associated lymph node enlargement

Certain symptoms are commonly associated with lymphoma:

* Night sweats
* Fever >38.5°C
* Weight loss >10%

These are called "B" symptoms, and are included in the stage designated to a patient. For instance, a patient with involved lymph nodes in the neck and under the arms only, and without any of the "B" symptoms, has stage IIA disease. The same patient with night sweats has stage IIB disease

neoplasm, and is undergoing clinical validation. The Working Formulation is still in use and divides NHL based on its nodal/cytologic morphology and biological aggressiveness, although it doesn't consider cell origin and excludes many newer lymphomas. Low-grade lymphomas include small lymphocytic/follicular-small, -mixed, and -small cleaved and large cell; intermediate grade includes follicular large cell, diffuse small cleaved, mixed small and large, and diffuse large cell; and high-grade includes large-cell immunoblastic, lymphoblastic, and diffuse small noncleaved cell. The diffuse large B-cell and follicular lymphomas are most commonly diagnosed.

STAGING OF HODGKIN'S DISEASE AND NON-HODGKIN'S LYMPHOMA

Management of HD and NHL depends upon accurate staging (Figure 62-1). Staging depends on complete history and physical examination as well as a number of diagnostic techniques. The goal is to classify the extent of disease according to a standard classification system.

The most commonly used classification system is the Ann Arbor Classification, which synthesizes information into a stage designation for HD and NHL, although HD has a greater tendency for anatomical spread. NHL is more likely to skip adjacent node groups and shows a greater tendency for extranodal involvement.

MANAGEMENT AND THERAPY FOR HODGKIN'S DISEASE

HD is treated with radiation therapy, chemotherapy, or both, applied according to stage.

Early, stage I/II classic HD: Patients with supradiaphragmatic, laparotomy-staged disease receive primary radiation therapy. Subtotal lymphoid irradiation, including the mantle/para-aortic fields, yields a 75% to 85% relapse-free survival and a 90% 20-year survival rate because many relapsed patients are salvaged. Patients without laparotomy present a greater challenge, and several risk stratifications have been developed. One recommendation for patients with an unfavorable presentation (≥1 B symptom, or age >50, or high ESR, or large mass, or ≥4 sites involved) is to receive combined modality chemotherapy-radiation therapy, while others receive radiation alone. Combined modality therapy previously included a full course of chemotherapy, but increasing evidence supports the use of 4 chemotherapy cycles instead of 6, followed by involved field radiation therapy (IFRT).

Advanced, stage III/IV classic HD: Although there has been some controversy about IIIA patients, most stage III/IV patients receive combination chemotherapy, administered as 6 to 8 cycles, each over 1 month. Freedom from relapse in stage IIIB/IV disease can be up to 70%, with overall survival >80%. The most common regimens include ABVD (adriamycin/bleomycin/vinblastine/dacarbazine) or MOPP (mechlorethamine/oncovin/procarbazine/prednisone). ABVD is generally preferred because it avoids alkylating agents that can induce myelodysplasia or secondary leukemia, is better tolerated, and improves the chance of preserving fertility.

NLPHD: Most patients have early stage disease, and radiation therapy, sometimes with more limited fields, is a consideration given their good prognosis.

Relapsed HD: Most patients who received primary radiation undergo combination chemotherapy. For those who underwent chemotherapy and had a long remission, repeat chemotherapy is reasonable, but after a brief or no remission, patients are candidates for bone marrow or stem cell transplantation.

Late toxicities are seen years after therapy and include hypothyroidism, accelerated atherosclerosis, avascular bony necrosis, and secondary malignancies, including lung/breast/head and neck/skin cancers/sarcomas/myelodysplasia/leukemia and NHL.

THERAPY FOR NON-HODGKIN'S LYMPHOMA

The histologic type and stage are taken into account in making treatment recommendations. General guidelines for follicular and diffuse large cell lymphomas, the most common NHLs, are presented below.

Indolent, Follicular Lymphomas

Early, stage I/II disease: Indolent lymphomas are incurable with standard chemotherapy, and there is no evidence that early treatment prolongs survival. A watchful waiting approach is reasonable for asymptomatic patients. Patients with locally symptomatic disease are candidates for IFRT, which may be curative in a subset. For many with systemic symptoms, chemotherapy can decrease tumor burden and symptoms, although relapse is inevitable.

Advanced, stage III/IV disease: Watchful waiting is still appropriate for some asymptomatic patients, especially those with stage III disease because up to 75% are alive at 5 years. Most, however, especially those with stage IV disease, will shortly become symptomatic and require treatment. Symptomatic patients are candidates for systemic chemotherapy. Options include chlorambucil or cyclophosphamide, alone or with prednisone (these are oral regimens, but expose patients to alkylators that risk myelodysplasia/secondary leukemia); fludarabine, alone or in combination with mitoxantrone and dexamethasone, or cyclophosphamide (higher response rates, more immunosuppressive); rituximab monoclonal anti-CD20 antibody alone or especially with drugs, such as CHOP (cyclophosphamide/doxorubicin/-oncovin/prednisone) or combination regimens CHOP or CVP (CHOP without doxorubicin). Interferon addition improves disease-free survival in some studies.

Relapsed disease: When patients experience relapse, they can be treated with another of the available chemotherapeutic modalities. Transplantation is investigational.

Diffuse Large Cell/Intermediate and Immunoblastic Lymphomas

Early, stage I/II disease: CHOP for 3 cycles followed by IFRT: 70% to 80% progression-free and overall survival at 5 years.

Advanced, stage-III/IV disease: CHOP for 6 to 8 cycles: complete response rates up to 60%, but therapy is curative in <50%. Addition of Rituxan to CHOP, especially in patients >60, but probably in younger patients as well, appears to be superior to CHOP alone. The IPI index, an independent predictor of survival, provides a useful therapeutic guide. Factors include age (≤60 vs. >60), LDH (normal vs. abnormal), performance status (ECOG 0-1 vs. 2-4), stage (I/II vs. III/IV), and extranodal sites (≤1 vs. >1). Patients in the high-intermediate or high-risk groups (three to five poor risk factors) may be candidates for dose-intense treatments.

Relapsed disease: When patients experience relapse, they receive salvage chemotherapy, followed in some cases by bone marrow or stem-cell transplantation.

FUTURE DIRECTIONS

Future HD therapy will likely involve shortened dose-intense regimens, such as the 12-week Stanford-V protocol, followed by radiation to involved sites that were 5 cm or larger. In NHL, rituximab/chemotherapy combinations have improved remission rates for indolent and more aggressive B-cell NHL. Some patients with follicular lymphoma achieve molecular remissions with clearance of *bcl-2*-positive cells, raising the possibility that a proportion might be cured.

REFERENCES

The Leukemia & Lymphoma Society Web site. Available at: http://www.leukemia.org. Accessed February 27, 2003.

National Cancer Institute Web site. Cancer information. Available at: http://cancer.gov/cancerinformation. Accessed February 27, 2003.

National Cancer Institute Web site. Clinical trials. Available at: http://cancer.gov/clinicaltrials. Accessed February 27, 2003.

Section VIII
ONCOLOGIC DISORDERS

Chapter 63

Breast Cancer

Lisa A. Carey

Breast cancer was diagnosed in nearly 200,000 US women in the year 2000, making it the most common malignancy in women. The lifetime risk of the development of breast cancer for an American woman is approximately 1 in 10, with advancing age as the strongest risk factor. Two thirds of cases occur in postmenopausal women; the disease is extremely rare in women under the age of 30. Incidence increased 40% from 1973 to 1998 while breast cancer mortality within the entire population decreased 20% during this same period. Most of that decrease in mortality occurred after 1995, and likely reflects improved screening and early detection as well as more effective treatment.

ETIOLOGY AND PATHOGENESIS

Age is the strongest risk factor for breast cancer. Women older than 65 have a risk several-fold higher than a 40-year-old woman. At any age, a history of breast or ovarian cancer increases the risk of subsequent breast cancer. Family history is an important, but smaller contributor to risk (approximately twofold to fivefold increased risk for first-degree relatives); except in those families with an inherited form of breast cancer, in whom the risk is very large. Inherited breast cancer, which is rare and primarily due to mutations in the genes *BRCA1* or *BRCA2*, is inherited in an autosomal dominant fashion with a 60% to 80% lifetime risk and an increased risk of premenopausal and bilateral disease. Only 5% to 10% of all breast cancers are due to inherited mutations. Identification of families with inherited breast cancer patterns is crucial because genetic testing can identify carriers of a mutation, and there are effective prevention strategies.

Hormonal risk factors may be broadly grouped as factors that increase the number of normal menstrual cycles in a lifetime, especially if the cycles occur before a first full-term pregnancy. They include early age of menarche, late menopause, and nulliparity or age at first pregnancy older than 30. There are several other variables that have been associated with breast cancer risk, possibly by increasing hormone levels. For example, obesity, a high fat diet, and alcohol can all cause higher circulating estrogen levels. Certain benign breast diseases confer increased risk of breast cancer. Atypical hyperplasia is asso-

ciated with an up to 1% yearly risk of invasive breast cancer. Despite the name, lobular carcinoma in situ (LCIS) is not a neoplastic or preneoplastic lesion, but is a marker of increased breast cancer risk in any quadrant of either breast. This risk can approach 1.5% per year for invasive breast cancer.

CLINICAL PRESENTATION

There are two major forms of primary breast cancer: invasive and noninvasive. Noninvasive breast cancer includes ductal carcinoma in situ (DCIS), which is truly a preneoplastic lesion in that up to 30% of inadequately treated DCIS recur or progress to invasive cancer. Most DCIS are detected by mammography; only 10% are palpable. Paget's disease is a rare variant of DCIS with or without invasive disease. It appears as eczematous changes of the nipple that represent extension of the DCIS component of the cancer into the main ducts.

Invasive breast cancer usually presents as a painless mass or mammographically detected calcifications, architectural distortion, or asymmetrical density. Clinical or self-breast examination may also detect a tumor by overlying dimpling or retraction of the skin or asymmetry of the breasts (Figure 63-1). Occasionally, breast cancer will be associated with nipple inversion or discharge. Suspicion of malignancy should be higher if the discharge is guaiac positive. Rarely, breast cancers will present with inflammatory changes in the skin of the breast. Since the advent of screening, more breast cancers present at an early curable stage, with disease limited to the breast only or breast and local lymph nodes. Fewer than 10% of patients with breast cancer present with distant metastases.

Most invasive primary breast cancers are adenocarcinomas of ductal, lobular, or a mixed pattern. Less than 5% are pure tubular, colloid, mucinous, or medullary type, which are considered to have a better prognosis. Clinical oncologists use several features of the patient and the tumor to gauge likelihood of recurrence. The "TNM" system, although imperfect, is used most commonly. T refers to tumor size or fixation to local structures, with larger sizes or fixed status conferring worse prognosis. N refers to regional lymph node metastasis; the presence of involved axillary, mammary, supraclavicular or infraclavicular lymph nodes connotes poorer prognosis. M refers to distant metastasis, which is generally considered incurable. There are several prognostically relevant features of the patient or the tumor that are not included in the TNM system. Some studies suggest that high-grade tumors carry a worse prognosis. The presence of the nuclear hormone receptors for estrogen (ER) and progesterone (PR) suggests slightly better prognosis and later recurrence, if it occurs, and predicts success of treatment with hormonal agents and approaches. In several studies, younger age at diagnosis appears to carry a worse prognosis; however, this may be due to the larger, more nodally involved tumors often found in young patients. Overexpression of the cell-surface receptor tyrosine kinase HER-2/neu found in 20% to 30% of breast cancers may portend a worse prognosis; however, this phenomenon may not be wholly independent of other prognostic variables. As with the ER and targeted hormonal agents, such as tamoxifen, HER-2/neu predicts success of treatment with the targeted anti-HER-2 antibody trastuzumab.

Most patients present with early stage nonmetastatic breast cancer, at a time when prompt multimodality therapy can reduce breast cancer recurrence and death. Breast cancer recurrence as metastatic disease can occur at any time; however, the risk is highest within the first 5 to 10 years after diagnosis. There are multiple tumor and host factors that affect a tumor's ability to exit the breast, survive in the blood and lymphatics, arrest and extravasate in a new site, and finally

survive and grow in that site to become clinically evident metastatic disease (Figure 63-2). The most common sites of recurrence are local (including conserved breast or chest wall), bone, lymph nodes, lung, and liver. CNS recurrences, rare before the era of aggressive systemic therapy, appear to be increasing, probably because the drugs used to prevent systemic relapse do not penetrate the CNS adequately. Local recurrence, particularly in a conserved breast, is curable with surgery and radiation therapy; however, it is a poor prognostic factor. Metastatic breast cancer is considered incurable and has a median survival after relapse of 24 months, although a small percentage of patients live longer than 10 years.

DIFFERENTIAL DIAGNOSIS

Several nonmalignant conditions can mimic breast cancer. Cysts and fibroadenomas often present with palpable masses. These may be distinguished from malignancy on clinical or radiographic grounds, such as the tenderness, cyclic changes, and sonographic appearance of cysts, and the characteristic mammographic density and circumscribed feel and appearance of fibroadenomas. Papillomas or mammary duct ectasia can produce nipple discharge. Mastitis or cellulitis of the breast is very difficult to distinguish clinically from inflammatory breast cancer. Breast malignancies other than primary breast cancer are rare. These include sarcomas (cystosarcoma phyllodes among others), lymphomas, and chloromas as well as metastases from melanomas or other carcinomas. Breast cancer metastasis to the contralateral breast is rare. A woman with a history of breast cancer is at increased risk of developing breast cancer in the contralateral breast. In general, these represent second primary tumors.

DIAGNOSTIC APPROACH

Approximately 20% to 30% of invasive and 80% of noninvasive breast cancers are not palpable; 10% of invasive cancers are not visible on mammograms. For this reason, physical examination and radiology are considered complementary (Figure 63-3). Ultrasound may provide valuable information in evaluating palpable masses. The American Cancer Society guidelines for breast cancer screening are that women older than 20

Figure 63-1

Palpation of the Breasts

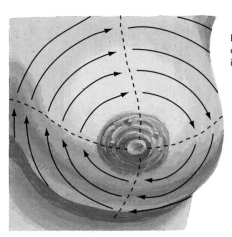

Breast is palpated systematically, either quadrant by quadrant or in increasing or decreasing circles

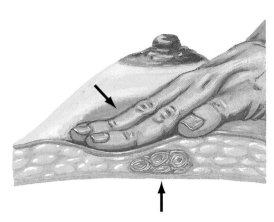

Flat parts of the fingers are used to gently compress breast tissue against chest wall to reveal breast masses

Nipple is squeezed gently to detect bleeding or discharge

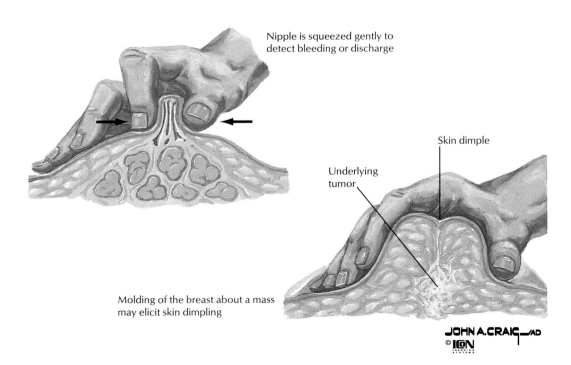

Skin dimple

Underlying tumor

Molding of the breast about a mass may elicit skin dimpling

JOHN A.CRAIG—AD
© ICON

Figure 63-2

Pathways of Tumor Dissemination

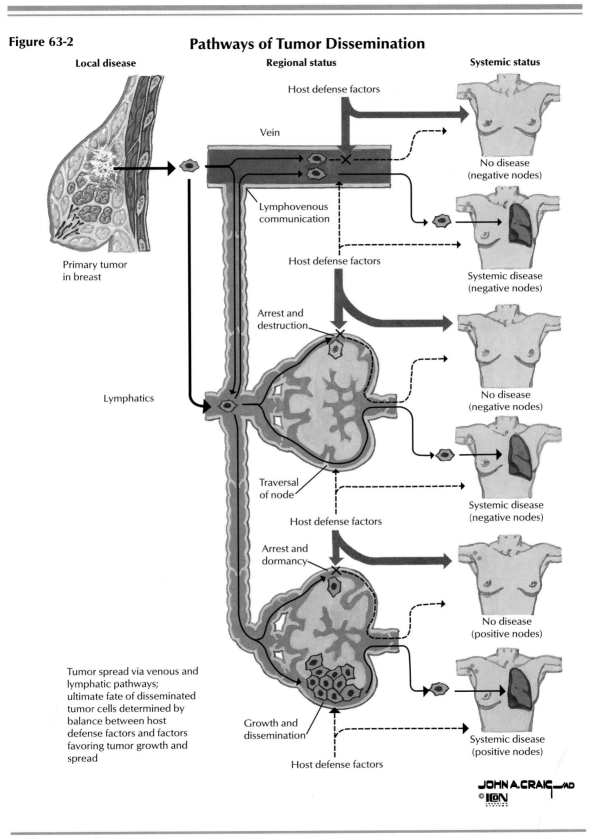

Local disease

Primary tumor
in breast

Regional status

Host defense factors

Vein

Lymphovenous
communication

Host defense factors

Arrest and
destruction

Lymphatics

Traversal
of node

Host defense factors

Arrest and
dormancy

Growth and
dissemination

Host defense factors

Systemic status

No disease
(negative nodes)

Systemic disease
(negative nodes)

No disease
(negative nodes)

Systemic disease
(negative nodes)

No disease
(positive nodes)

Systemic disease
(positive nodes)

Tumor spread via venous and
lymphatic pathways;
ultimate fate of disseminated
tumor cells determined by
balance between host
defense factors and factors
favoring tumor growth and
spread

JOHN A. CRAIG—MD
©ICN

Figure 63-3   ## Mammograms

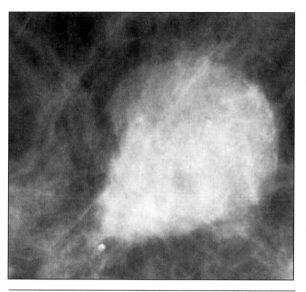

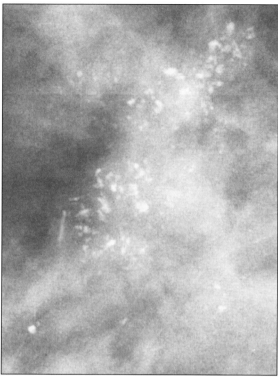

Mammogram depicting a partially lobulated, partially indistinct mass that proved to be infiltrating ductal carcinoma.

Mammogram depicting branching, casting, pleomorphic calcifications that proved to be ductal carcinoma in situ. (Mammograms courtesy of Etta Pisano, M.D.)

should perform breast self-examination every month; women should have clinical breast examination by a health professional every 3 years from ages 20 to 39 and yearly thereafter; and that women 40 and older should undergo annual mammography. Mammography in women between 40 and 50 has been controversial, although emerging data suggest a smaller but real benefit in this age group. The benefit is smaller in younger women because breast cancer is less prevalent and mammograms are technically limited in more glandular and dense premenopausal breasts.

Diagnosis of a palpable lesion can be made by fine needle aspiration, core needle biopsy, or open surgical biopsy. Lesions seen by mammography and/or ultrasound only can be biopsied by stereotactic core needle biopsy, by ultrasound-guided needle biopsy, or by needle localized open biopsy. A complete history and physical examination is the best screening test for systemic spread of cancer. Chest radiography, complete blood cell count, and screening liver chemistries

are often performed to screen for metastatic disease; however, these tests are unlikely to be abnormal in early stage tumors. More aggressive evaluations such as bone scans and CT scans are generally reserved for symptomatic patients or those with more locally advanced or metastatic disease.

MANAGEMENT AND THERAPY
Prevention

There are both medical and surgical strategies for breast cancer prevention. In women at moderate to high risk, the selective estrogen receptor modulator tamoxifen has been shown to reduce the risk of noninvasive and invasive breast cancer by 49%. As expected, tamoxifen decreases the incidence of ER-positive breast cancer, and does not appear to affect the development of ER-negative breast cancer. Toxicity includes increased endometrial cancer risk, venous thrombosis, menopausal symptoms, and a small increase in cataract progression. Surgical strategies used primarily in very high-risk patients include prophylactic mastectomy and prophylactic oophorectomy in premenopausal women. Prophylactic mastectomy reduces the risk of breast cancer by at least 90% in high-risk patients treated by skilled surgeons. Prophylactic oophorectomy has been evaluated only in BRCA1 mutation carriers, in whom it reduces breast cancer by 50%.

Local/Regional Therapy

Surgical options include breast conservation, which is local excision of the tumor with dissection of the level I and II axillary lymph nodes followed by radiation therapy to the breast. Breast conservation is standard of care, and offers comparable 5-year survival to modified radical mastectomy. Some tumors are too large or poorly placed for conservation; for those patients mastectomy is standard. Dissection of the ipsilateral axillary lymph nodes allows tumor debulking and prognostication. Sentinel lymphadenectomy, a recently developed technique, allows surgeons to selectively identify the first draining lymph node or nodes (the "sentinel" node) from a tumor region using vital blue dye and/or radiolabeled colloid. In experienced hands, if this first draining lymph node does not contain tumor, the remainder of the axilla is also free of tumor and does not require dissection. Radiation therapy is required for patients who have breast conservation; otherwise, the local recurrence rate may exceed 30% with long-term follow-up. Local recurrance in conserved and radiated breasts is under 10%. Radiation is also given to the chest wall and local lymph node groups remaining after surgery for large tumors or for some tumors with involved axillary lymph nodes.

Systemic Therapy

Systemic therapy refers to chemotherapy, hormone therapy, bisphosphonates, or biotherapy given to patients to prevent or treat metastatic disease throughout the body. Adjuvant therapy is given as an adjunct to local therapy to decrease the chance of recurrence. Neoadjuvant, or preoperative, therapy is a newer approach that involves the same drugs as in adjuvant therapy given before the surgery to decrease the tumor size and allow breast conservation. The use of adjuvant therapy, primarily chemotherapy or hormone therapy, is determined by the patient's general health,

age, ER status of the tumor, and the probability of recurrence based on stage and other prognostic variables. Chemotherapy includes several non-cross-resistant drugs, called polychemotherapy. Overall, adjuvant chemotherapy decreases the risk of recurrence by 24% and the risk of death by 15%. Hormone therapy is useful only in preventing recurrence of tumors that express the ER; it is not effective in ER-negative cancer. The selective estrogen receptor modulator tamoxifen decreases the risk of recurrence by 47% and risk of death by 26%. In premenopausal patients with ER-positive tumors, oophorectomy may be a useful adjunct to tamoxifen, particularly in high-risk patients who cannot or will not take chemotherapy. Combination chemohormonal therapy is more effective than either strategy alone.

Metastatic therapy is given to women with systemic relapse. The goals of metastatic therapy are to palliate symptoms and prolong life; however, given the incurable nature of the disease at this stage, quality of life considerations become very important in choosing therapy. This therapy may include chemotherapy, either with one of the many single agents with documented effectivness or polychemotherapy; hormone therapy such as tamoxifen or other antiestrogen; aromatase inhibitors (postmenopausal), or ovarian ablation (premanopausal); if ER-positive, bisphosphonates for lytic bone metastases, or targeted biotherapy such as the anti-HER-2 monoclonal antibody trastuzumab. Surgery and radiation are also sometimes used for treatment of local complications. A number of clinical trials are evaluating the best combinations of chemotherapy and other drugs for adjuvant treatment and newer drugs and compounds for metastatic therapy.

FUTURE DIRECTIONS

Since 1990, breast cancer mortality in the United States has markedly decreased, largely because of aggressive efforts to detect and treat the disease at early stages. A significant additional strategy has been to develop effective preventive treatments for those at high risk. Certain groups, such as African Americans and the medically underserved populations in the United States and many populations in undeveloped countries, have not seen these improvements in outcome. An important accomplishment will be to provide better screening and prevention efforts to these groups. Improved imaging techniques such as digital mammography and breast MRI are currently under evaluation. New strategies are at hand to determine the metastatic potential of the tumor and to refine selection of adjuvant therapy. These include examination of bone marrow or blood for evidence of micrometastases, definition of individual tumor biology through tumor markers, and classification of tumor subtypes through gene expression array analysis. Bisphosphonates, new hormonal approaches other than tamoxifen, and targeted molecular therapies such as trastuzumab are being tested in the adjuvant setting to try to improve the cure rate in early breast cancer. The success and low toxicity of tamoxifen and trastuzumab suggest that the future of breast cancer therapy is likely to involve other targeted therapies, with treatment determined by the molecular profile of the particular tumor.

REFERENCES

Early Breast Cancer Trialists' Collaborative Group. Polychemotherapy for early breast cancer: an overview of the randomized trials. *Lancet.* 1998;352:930-942.

Early Breast Cancer Trialists' Collaborative Group. Tamoxifen for early breast cancer: an overview of the randomized trials. *Lancet.* 1998;351:1451-1467.

Fisher B, Constantino JP, Wickerham DL, et al. Tamoxifen for the prevention of breast cancer: report of the National Surgical Adjuvant Breast and Bowel Project P-1 Study. *J Natl Cancer Inst.* 1998;90:1371-1388.

Chapter 64

Cancer of the Oral Cavity and Oropharynx

David R. White and William W. Shockley

The oral cavity and oropharynx are among the most common sites for head and neck cancer. In the United States, there are 30,000 new cases of cancer arising in these sites, accounting for 8,000 deaths per year. In developing nations, these numbers are much higher, with oral cavity cancer being the third most common malignancy after cervical and gastric cancers. Squamous cell carcinoma (SCC) accounts for greater than 90% of oral cavity and oropharyngeal malignancies followed by minor salivary gland malignancies in the oral cavity and lymphoma in the oropharynx. Discussion in this chapter will be limited to SCC of the oral cavity and oropharynx.

ETIOLOGY AND PATHOGENESIS

The oral cavity is defined as the region beginning at the vermilion border of the lip extending posteriorly to the end of the hard palate superiorly and the circumvallate papillae inferiorly. Subsites of the oral cavity are the lips, buccal mucosa, gingiva and alveolar ridge, hard palate, floor of the mouth, retromolar trigone, and the anterior two thirds of the tongue. The oropharynx begins at the posterior border of the oral cavity and extends posteriorly to the posterior pharyngeal wall, inferiorly to the epiglottis, and superiorly to the soft palate. Subsites of the oropharynx are the base of the tongue (posterior one third), lateral and posterior pharyngeal walls, tonsillar area (including pharyngeal tonsils, tonsillar pillars, and tonsillar fossae), and soft palate. Together, the oral cavity and oropharynx have important roles in airway protection, deglutition, and communication. Loss or compromise of these functions increases with tumor extent, and preservation of these functions is an important principle in treatment.

RISK FACTORS AND PREMALIGNANT LESIONS

Alcohol consumption and cigarette use are the primary risk factors in the development of SCC of the oral cavity and oropharynx. Other forms of tobacco use, including cigar smoking, pipe smoking, and smokeless tobacco, are also associated with these lesions. While alcohol consumption and tobacco use are accepted independent risk

factors for SCC, their concurrent use results in a synergistic effect with an even greater propensity for malignancy. Betel nut chewing, popular in India and Southeast Asia, is also a known risk factor. Although it is included in discussion of oral cavity carcinoma, SCC of the lip differs from other oral cavity SCCs in that ultraviolet radiation exposure is the primary risk factor. Other risk factors include Plummer-Vinson syndrome and tertiary syphilis.

The concept of "field cancerization," where widespread epithelial dysplasia occurs in high-risk individuals, applies to SCC of the upper aerodigestive tract. The presence of SCC of the upper aerodigestive tract increases the chance that a second primary SCC is present by up to 15%.

Premalignant lesions should be recognized and followed closely because early identification of asymptomatic lesions is associated with much lower morbidity and mortality. Erythroplasia is the most important premalignant lesion of the oral cavity and oropharynx. Generally seen as a red, slightly raised lesion or a smooth, atrophic red lesion, erythroplasia is associated with up to 90% presence of dysplasia, carcinoma in situ, or SCC at the time of presentation. Erythroplasia may also represent an inflammatory lesion of the mucosa, and management includes removal of irritating factors and treatment of infection with follow-up in 10 to 14 days. If the lesion has not resolved, incisional biopsy of the periphery of the lesion is recommended to rule out carcinoma.

Leukoplakia (Figure 64-1), defined as a white patch of mucosa not associated with any other disease, is associated with less than 5% malignant transformation. Management of leukoplakia involves serial examination by the clinician. Biopsy is necessary only for lesions that undergo rapid growth, become symptomatic, or are otherwise clinically suspicious. Lichen planus (LP) is associated with malignancy rarely (3%–5%), and observation is adequate for most cases. Erosive LP occasionally merits biopsy for diagnosis. Like leukoplakia, suspicious areas of LP should be biopsied.

CLINICAL PRESENTATION
Oral Cavity

The lip is a common site for SCC of the oral cavity, comprising 25% to 30% of all oral cavity malignancies. SCC of the lip (Figure 64-1) presents as a nonhealing, crusting, ulcerative lesion or a scaly, hyperkeratotic lesion of the vermilion; approximately 90% occur on the lower lip due to increased sun exposure.

In the remainder of the oral cavity, SCC is likely to present as a nonhealing ulcer, an exophytic lesion, or an indurated infiltrating mass. The most common sites are the anterolateral tongue and anterior floor of the mouth (Figure 64-2). These tumors are often asymptomatic until advanced stages, when they present with pain, bleeding, dysphagia, loose teeth, or difficulty with articulation.

A palpable neck mass representative of metastasis to a cervical lymph node is present on initial evaluation in 15% to 30% of patients with oral cavity SCC (Figure 64-3). Submental and submandibular lymph nodes are the first-echelon drainage for most of the oral cavity, and these regions are most likely to be involved when metastasis is present. The upper deep jugular lymph nodes are also often involved. Because of the rich lymphatic drainage and near midline position of many oral cavity SCCs, bilateral or contralateral cervical metastases are relatively common.

Oropharynx

Oropharyngeal tumors typically appear as ulcerative or infiltrating mucosal lesions. SCC of the base of tongue (Figure 64-3) is often not visible during routine physical examination and is noticeable only upon palpation. The most common sites for oropharyngeal SCC are the tonsil and the anterior tonsillar pillar. To a greater extent than its counterpart in the oral cavity, SCC of the oropharynx remains asymptomatic until the disease is advanced. The most common presenting symptoms are pain and dysphagia. In more advanced cases, these symptoms can be accompanied by dysarthria, referred otalgia, weight loss, hemoptysis, hoarseness, and stridor. Cervical metastases are identifiable upon presentation in up to 60% of patients and are most commonly seen in the deep jugular nodes.

DIFFERENTIAL DIAGNOSIS

Differential diagnosis includes inflammatory processes and benign lesions (see Chapter 1 Aphthous Ulcers and Other Common Oral Lesions), salivary gland neoplasms, lymphoma (primarily with tonsillar involvement), and sinonasal malignancies, which may erode into the oral cavity and oropharynx.

DIAGNOSTIC APPROACH

A thorough history and physical examination is the most important step in diagnosis of lesions of the oral cavity and oropharynx. Early diagnosis is of paramount importance because small, asymptomatic lesions may be treated with a high rate of cure, with minimal morbidity. Once lesions become symptomatic, the cure rate drops and the morbidity of treatment modalities increases dramatically.

A history of cigarette smoking or alcohol use should alert the clinician that the patient is at high risk for SCC of the oral cavity and oropharynx. The patient may present with an unusual appearing lesion or simply with persistent mouth or throat symptoms. Thorough physical examination should incorporate the use of headlights and dental mirrors to facilitate examination of all mucosal surfaces in the oral cavity and oropharynx. Lesions of the retromolar trigone and anterior floor of mouth are missed most often during cursory examination because of their location behind the teeth. A tongue blade is instrumental in examining these "hidden" lesions. After examination of all mucosal surfaces, palpation of the floor of the mouth, tongue, base of the tongue, and tonsillar region should be performed. Palpable masses, areas of induration, ulceration, and tenderness should alert the clinician to the possibility of malignancy. Cranial nerve function should be documented with particular attention

Figure 64-1

Leukoplakia

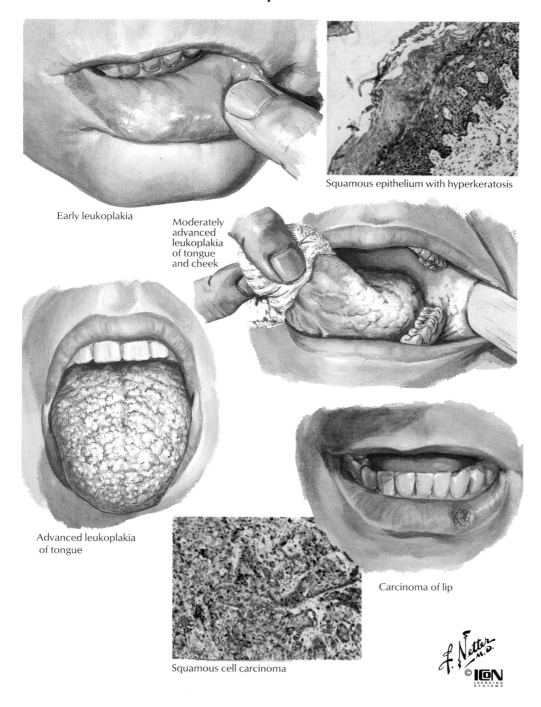

Early leukoplakia

Squamous epithelium with hyperkeratosis

Moderately advanced leukoplakia of tongue and cheek

Advanced leukoplakia of tongue

Carcinoma of lip

Squamous cell carcinoma

Figure 64-2

Malignant Tumors of Oral Cavity

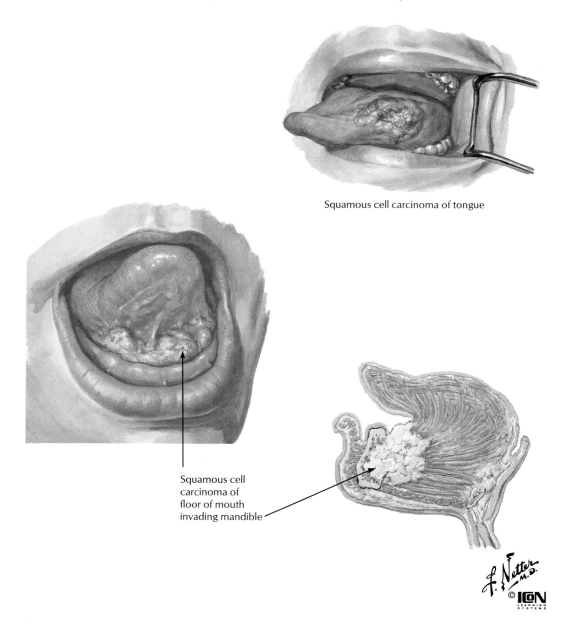

Squamous cell carcinoma of tongue

Squamous cell
carcinoma of
floor of mouth
invading mandible

to the hypoglossal nerve as well as the mandibular and lingual branches of the trigeminal nerve. Trismus may indicate invasion of the muscles of mastication. Examination of the neck for lymphadenopathy should always be performed.

After treatment for 10 to 14 days and removal of irritants, the lesion should be re-evaluated. If substantial improvement has not occurred, biop-

sy is merited. Sore throat unresponsive to medical treatment, otalgia without evidence of ear disease, and unexplained dysphagia should receive further workup. Biopsy of suspicious lesions may be performed under local anesthesia if the lesion is easily accessible. Biopsy should not be excisional and should include a section of the lesion as well as a small portion of adjacent

Table 64-1
AJCC Staging of Oral Cavity and Oropharyngeal Cancer

Primary Tumor	Oropharyngeal Cancer
TX: primary tumor cannot be assessed T0: No evidience of primary tumor Tis: Carcinoma *in situ* T1: 2 cm or less T3: More than 4 cm T2: Tumor more than 2 cm but not more than 4 cm T4(lip): Tumor invades adjacent structures (e.g., through cortical bone, inferior alveolar nerve, floor of mouth, skin of face) T4(oral cavity): Tumor invades adjacent structures (e.g., through cortical bone, into deep (extrinsic) muscle of tongue, maxillary sinus, skin. Superficial erosion alone of bone/tooth socket by gingival primary is not sufficient to classify as T4)	T1: Tumor diameter ≤2 cm in greatest dimension T2: Tumor diameter ≥2 cm, but not ≥4 T3: Tumor diameter ≥4 cm T4: Tumor invades adjacent structures (e.g., pterygoid muscle(s), mandible, hard palate, deep muscle of tongue, larynx)
Regional Lymph Nodes (N)	Distant Metastases

NX: Regional lymph nodes cannot be assessed
N0: No regional lymph node metastasis
N1: Metastasis in a single ipsilateral lymph node, <3 cm in greatest dimension
N2: Metastasis in a single ipsilateral lymph node, ≥3 cm but not ≥6 cm in greatest dimension; or in multiple ipsilateral lymph nodes, none ≥6 cm in greatest dimension; or in bilateral or contralateral lymph nodes, none more than 6 cm in greatest dimension
  N2a: Metastasis in a single ipsilateral lymph node, ≥3 cm but not ≥6 cm in greatest dimension
  N2b: Metastasis in multiple ipsilateral lymph nodes, none ≥ 6 cm in greatest dimension
  N2c: Metastasis in bilateral or contralateral lymph nodes, none ≥ 6 cm in greatest dimension
N3: Metastasis in a lymph node, ≥ 6 cm in greatest dimension
	MX: Distant metastasis cannot be assessed
	M0: No distant metastases
	M1: Distant metastases present

Used with permission of the American Joint Committee on Cancer (AJCC®), Chicago, Illinois. The original source of material is in the *AJCC® Manual for staging cancer,* 5th edition (1997) published by Lippincott-Raven Publishers, Phila.

"normal" appearing mucosa. Biopsy of oropharyngeal lesions may be difficult to perform without general anesthesia.

MANAGEMENT AND THERAPY
Management

If the lesion is a superficial early SCC of the oral cavity, excision without extended workup may be appropriate. Otherwise, once the diagnosis is confirmed or strongly suspected, the patient should undergo panendoscopy (laryngoscopy, bronchoscopy, and esophagoscopy) to rule out a second primary SCC of the upper aerodigestive tract. As previously noted, a second primary will occur in as many as 15% of patients with SCC of the oral cav-

ity or oropharynx. Preoperative studies include a chest radiograph and liver function tests to rule out distant metastasis or synchronous lung cancer. Radiographic evaluation of the mandible with a dental x-ray is indicated in some oral cavity cancers. CT or MRI may be indicated to better define the location and extent of the tumor and cervical metastases. Generally, contrast-enhanced CT of the neck (from skull base to clavicles) is most useful and expedient. Exceptions include base of tongue cancers or suspicion of perineural invasion, when tissue planes are better imaged with MRI. On occasion, these imaging studies will identify pathological lymph nodes not palpable on physical examination.

Tumor staging is the most reliable predictor of

Figure 64-3

Malignant Tumors of Oropharynx

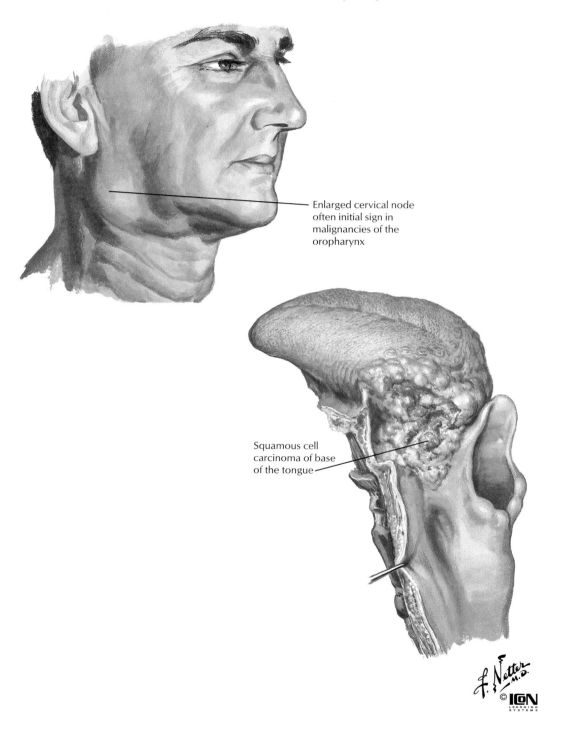

Enlarged cervical node often initial sign in malignancies of the oropharynx

Squamous cell carcinoma of base of the tongue

prognosis. Staging is performed according to the guidelines of the American Joint Committee on Cancer (Table 64-1). T1 and early T2 lesions have an associated 60% to 95% 5-year survival rate when no cervical metastases are present. The presence of cervical metastasis results in a worse prognosis with only 25% to 40% 5-year survival. More advanced disease (T3 and T4 lesions) carry 5-year survival rates of 11% to 40%. In general, oropharyngeal cancers have a worse prognosis than oral cavity tumors.

Other considerations in prognosis include tumor thickness and patient age. Tumor thickness has recently been shown to affect prognosis of oral cavity SCCs, with lesions ≥5 mm thick associated with significantly lower 5-year survival rates. Presence of SCC in young patients (<35 years old) is generally a poor prognostic indicator, with the majority of these tumors representing aggressive disease.

Treatment

Treatment is comprised of surgical excision, radiation therapy, and combined modalities. Chemotherapy alone has not been shown to have curative potential in SCC of the head and neck, but does have a role in palliation of advanced disease.

Early lesions (T1 and early T2) are generally amenable to single-modality treatment. Surgical resection with wide margin (1–2 cm) of excision is the treatment of choice for most of these lesions. Radiation provides an alternative for patients in poor health or in whom surgical morbidity is deemed too great. Advanced lesions (infiltrative T2, and all T3 and T4) require combined modality treatment. In the oral cavity, resection is accompanied by postoperative radiation treatment. Advanced oropharyngeal SCC is treated with resection and adjuvant radiation therapy traditionally, but recent studies show increasing effectiveness of combined radiation and chemotherapy. Tonsillar and base of tongue tumors appear to be particularly amenable to combined chemoradiation as the primary treatment.

Treatment depends on the size of the primary tumor and the presence of nodal disease. Patients with early lesions and no clinical evidence of lymphatic spread may be followed closely without specific therapy directed to the cervical lymph nodes. For more advanced disease, neck dissection with removal of lymph nodes at risk or radia-

tion of the neck is required, even in the absence of clinically evident cervical metastasis. Presence of enlarged cervical lymph nodes requires neck dissection and adjuvant radiation treatment.

Treatment for advanced cancer of the oral cavity and oropharynx often results in functional loss. Despite continued improvement in reconstructive techniques, dysphagia, dysarthria, and aspiration may occur following treatment. Patients often require tracheostomy and feeding tubes in the immediate postoperative period, and some require one or both for an extended period. Xerostomia, mucositis, woody edema, and dysphagia are common side effects of radiation treatment.

FUTURE DIRECTIONS

Several new chemotherapeutic agents such as epidermal growth factor-receptor inhibitors show promise as adjuvant therapies for head and neck cancer. Other areas of promise include the use of intraoperative radiation therapy and genetically engineered adenoviruses, which target tumor markers to specifically lyse cancer cells while sparing healthy cells. In the surgical realm, sentinel node biopsy is being evaluated as an alternative to neck dissection in patients with larger primary lesions and no evidence of nodal spread.

While many new therapeutic options may soon be available, the role of tobacco and alcohol use in the development of oral and oropharyngeal cancer cannot be overemphasized. Avoidance of these risk factors is the most effective measure in reducing the incidence of head and neck cancer, and the clinician should take the responsibility of patient education as seriously as diagnosis and treatment.

REFERENCES

Genden EM, Thawley SE, O'Leary MJ. Malignant neoplasms of the oropharynx. In: Cummings CW, Fredrickson JM, Harker LA, et al, eds. *Otolaryngology – Head and Neck Surgery*. 3rd ed. St Louis, Mo: Mosby-Year Book Inc; 1998:1463-1511.

Mashberg A, Samit A. Early diagnosis of asymptomatic oral and oropharyngeal squamous cancers. *CA Cancer J Clin*. 1995;45:328-351.

Prince S, Bailey BM. Squamous carcinoma of the tongue: review. *Br J Oral Maxillofac Surg*. 1999;37:164-174.

Sharma PK, Schuller DE, Baker SR. Malignant neoplasms of the oral cavity. In: Cummings CW, Fredrickson JM, Harker LA, et al, eds. *Otolaryngology – Head and Neck Surgery*. 3rd ed. St Louis, Mo: Mosby-Year Book Inc; 1998:1418-1462.

Summerlin DJ. Precancerous and cancerous lesions of the oral cavity. *Dermatol Clin*. 1996;14:205-223.

Chapter 65

Colorectal Cancer

Robert S. Wehbie

Deaths due to colorectal cancer (CRC) are second only to lung cancer in site-specific mortality and comprise approximately 11% of the cancer-related deaths in the United States. Over the past decade, advances have been made in our understanding of CRC genetics, screening, surgical techniques, adjuvant therapies, and treatment of the patient with metastatic disease. Despite these advances, the etiology of most CRC remains ill defined, metastatic disease develops in a number of patients with localized disease at diagnosis despite adjuvant therapy, and, metastatic CRC, with a few exceptions, remains fatal.

ETIOLOGY AND PATHOGENESIS

Usually, CRC is a disease of the elderly, with incidence not rising appreciably until the fifth decade of life (Figure 65-1). Incidence varies around the world with rates higher in Western industrialized nations. Migrating populations tend to assume the relative risk of the region into which they move; thus, environmental factors have long been suspected to play a role in CRC development. Epidemiologic data suggest an association between dietary constituents such as fats and risk; however, identification of the specific dietary or other environmental factor(s) involved in CRC development has been elusive.

A family history of CRC is a strong predictor of development with up to 20% of patients reporting a family history of the disease. Having an affected first-degree relative increases the lifetime risk to approximately 10%. However, defined genetic syndromes account for approximately 5% of CRC.

The sequence of molecular events leading to carcinogenesis is better described for CRC than for any other solid tumor. This is mostly due to insights offered by the inherited CRC syndromes: familial adenomatous polyposis (FAP) and hereditary nonpolyposis colorectal cancer (HNPCC).

FAP accounts for less than 1% of CRC. It is caused by an inherited defect in one of 2 adenomatous polyposis coli (APC) genes. Affected individuals lose their only functional APC copy in certain somatic cells (such as colonocytes) through random deletion and develop hundreds to thousands of colorectal adenomas during adolescence. CRC develops in nearly all of these patients by age 40. Spontaneous loss of both APC copies is thought to be a key event in the development of colorectal adenomas in most patients with sporadic CRC.

HNPCC accounts for 2% to 4% of CRC. It is due to an inherited defect in one of a family of DNA mismatch repair (MMR) genes and leads to an accumulation of genetic errors. CRC develops in more than 60% of affected individuals by age 50. Approximately 15% of sporadic CRC have identified microsatellite instability, the genetic manifestation of MMR mutation.

It is believed that almost all CRC develops from adenomatous polyps. The current hypothesis of colorectal carcinogenesis suggests that CRC is caused by an accumulation of mutations. While there is probably an order to these defects, it is the overall accumulation of abnormalities that is most important. More than 90% of cancers have 2 or more defects. In general, genetic changes accumulate with an initial mutation in the 5q chromosome (APC gene mutations) noted in polyps and followed by changes in chromosome 12 (K-ras oncogene) as the polyps become more dysplastic. Deletions are then noted in a chromosome 18 gene (deleted in colon cancer —[DCC]). Finally, p53 (chromosome 17p) mutations appear and mark the transition from benign adenoma to malignant carcinoma.

Chronic inflammatory bowel diseases such as ulcerative colitis and Crohn's disease may lead to CRC development in up to 10% of affected individuals. Other conditions associated with an increased risk include Gardner's syndrome, Turcot's syndrome, and juvenile polyposis. Together,

Figure 65-1

Risk Factors

Heredity

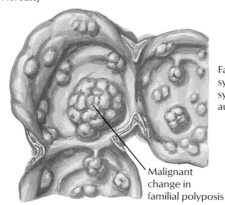

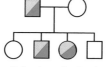

Familial polyposis, Gardner's syndrome, and cancer family syndrome inherited via autosomal dominant pattern

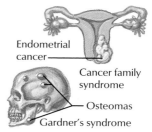

Endometrial cancer

Cancer family syndrome

Osteomas

Gardner's syndrome

Malignant change in familial polyposis

CNS tumor

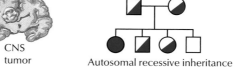

Autosomal recessive inheritance in Turcot's syndrome

Multiple polyposis syndromes. Colon polyps often associated with other systemic abnormalities show definite inheritance patterns and indicate significant increased incidence of colorectal cancer.

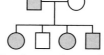

First-degree relatives of patients with colorectal cancer show increased incidence of cancer

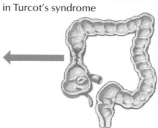

Diet

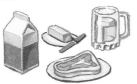

Diets high in animal fat seem to increase incidence of colorectal cancer; high-fiber diets are associated with lower incidence

Age

Incidence of colorectal cancer increases with age

Colorectal polyps

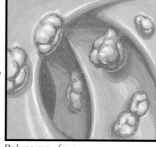

Polyps may favor cancer formation

Inflammatory bowel disease

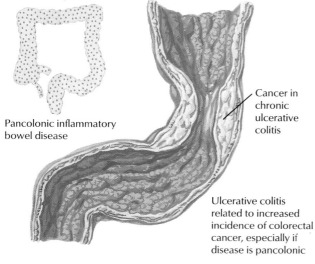

Pancolonic inflammatory bowel disease

Cancer in chronic ulcerative colitis

Ulcerative colitis related to increased incidence of colorectal cancer, especially if disease is pancolonic

Other predisposing conditions

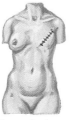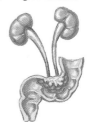

Gynecologic or breast cancer

Uretero-sigmoidostomy

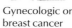

JOHN A. CRAIG—AD
© ICON

Table 65-1
American Cancer Society Colorectal Cancer Screening Guidelines

Average - or standard - risk patients, defined as the absence of any high-risk factors, should be screened annually beginning at age 40:

· An annual digital rectal examination after age 40

Starting at age 50, both men and women should have:

· Yearly fecal occult blood test (FOBT) and flexible sigmoidoscopy every 5 years; or
· FOBT yearly (acceptable but not preferred); or
· Flexible sigmoidoscopy every 5 years; and
· Double contrast barium enema every 5 years; or
· Colonoscopy every 10 years

High-risk patients should begin colorectal cancer screening earlier and/or more often. Some high-risk populations include:

· A strong family history of colorectal cancer or polyps (cancer or polyps in a first-degree relative younger than 60 or in 2 first-degree relatives of any age)
· A known family history of hereditary colorectal cancer syndromes (familial adenomatous polyposis and hereditary non-polyposis colon cancer)
· A personal history of colorectal cancer or adenomatous polyps
· A personal history of chronic inflammatory bowel disease

Note: Flexible sigmoidoscopy together with FOBT is preferred when compared to FOBT or flexible sigmoidoscopy alone. All positive tests should be followed up with colonoscopy. Polyps discovered on flexible sigmoidoscopy mandate total colon evaluation by either high-quality barium enema or colonoscopy.
Adapted from ASC Guidelines on Screening and Surveillance for the Early Detection of Adenomatous Polyps and Colorectal Cancer. Update 2001:8, 11.

these conditions account for approximately 1% of CRC cases.

CLINICAL PRESENTATION

Symptoms depend on the size and location of the tumor (Figure 65-2). Typical presenting symptoms include abdominal pain, changes in bowel habits, and rectal bleeding. Colon cancers on the right side tend to be large and present with occult bleeding resulting in anemia (fatigue, heart failure). Left-sided cancers tend to present with symptoms of bowel obstruction (e.g., cramping, change in bowel habits). Blood mixed with the stool is the most frequent symptom of rectal cancer. Other symptoms include mucous discharge, changes in bowel habit, unsatisfied defecation, rectal discomfort, abdominal pain, and the symptoms (or signs) of anemia. Not uncommonly, patients present with signs or symptoms of metastatic disease. The liver is the most common site of CRC metastasis, but other sites can be involved.

DIFFERENTIAL DIAGNOSIS

Most CRC are adenocarcinomas; other histologic varieties account for less than 5% of cases

and include carcinoid tumors, sarcomas, lymphomas, melanomas, and, in patients with HIV, Kaposi's sarcoma. Locally advanced tumors from other pelvic structures can involve the rectum and present with rectal cancer–like symptoms. Because symptoms of CRC are nonspecific, malignancy should be included in the differential diagnosis of nearly any chronic gastrointestinal or abdominal illness. Never dismiss the possibility of CRC because of a patient's age.

DIAGNOSTIC APPROACH
Screening

Fecal occult blood testing and sigmoidoscopy screening have been shown to decrease CRC-related mortality (Table 65-1). The concept that most cases of CRC follow the adenoma to carcinoma pathway has led to the important application of colonoscopy and polypectomy, because more than 90% of polyps can be removed via colonoscopy. Adenoma removal has been shown to decrease the incidence of CRC by 70% to 90%. With increasing use of screening technologies, more CRC are asymptomatic. Most cancers that present today are symptomatic because screening is still not uniformly practiced (Figure 65-3).

Figure 65-2

Clinical Manifestations of Colorectal Cancer

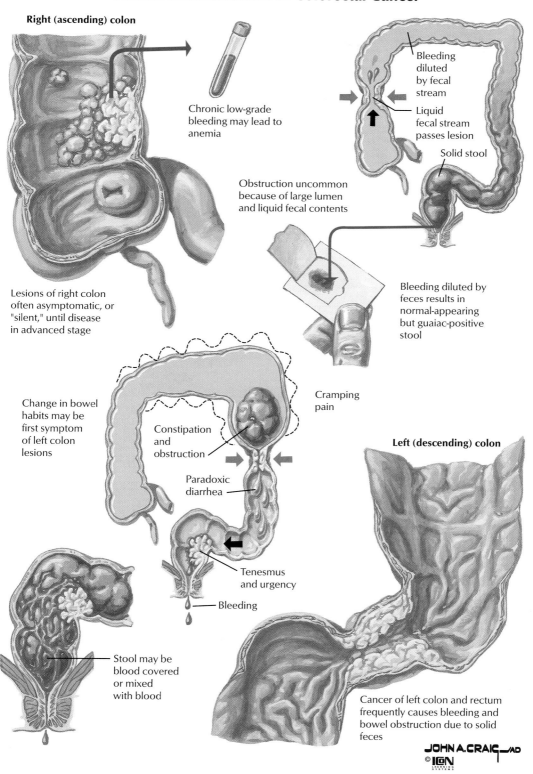

Right (ascending) colon

Chronic low-grade bleeding may lead to anemia

Lesions of right colon often asymptomatic, or "silent," until disease in advanced stage

Obstruction uncommon because of large lumen and liquid fecal contents

Bleeding diluted by fecal stream

Liquid fecal stream passes lesion

Solid stool

Bleeding diluted by feces results in normal-appearing but guaiac-positive stool

Change in bowel habits may be first symptom of left colon lesions

Constipation and obstruction

Paradoxic diarrhea

Cramping pain

Left (descending) colon

Tenesmus and urgency

Bleeding

Stool may be blood covered or mixed with blood

Cancer of left colon and rectum frequently causes bleeding and bowel obstruction due to solid feces

JOHN A.CRAIG—AD
© ICON

Figure 65-3

Screening Techniques

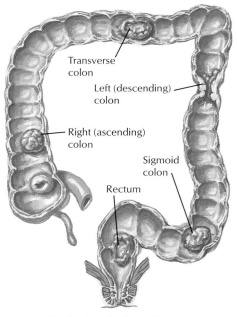

Transverse colon

Left (descending) colon

Right (ascending) colon

Sigmoid colon

Rectum

Distribution of colorectal cancer

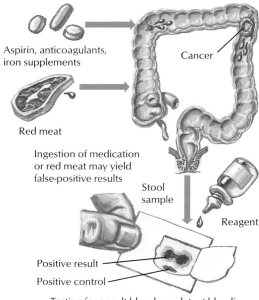

Aspirin, anticoagulants, iron supplements

Red meat

Cancer

Ingestion of medication or red meat may yield false-positive results

Stool sample

Reagent

Positive result

Positive control

Testing for occult blood can detect bleeding in entire bowel but results are inaccurate

Direct screening techniques are most reliable

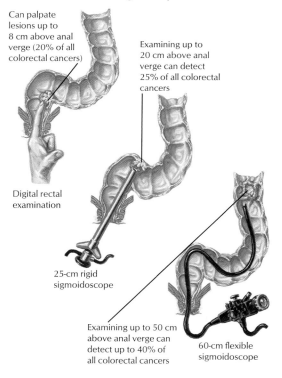

Can palpate lesions up to 8 cm above anal verge (20% of all colorectal cancers)

Examining up to 20 cm above anal verge can detect 25% of all colorectal cancers

Digital rectal examination

25-cm rigid sigmoidoscope

Examining up to 50 cm above anal verge can detect up to 40% of all colorectal cancers

60-cm flexible sigmoidoscope

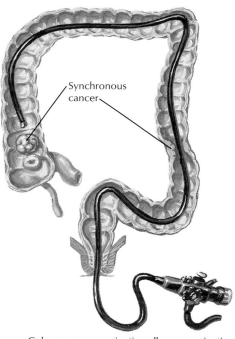

Synchronous cancer

Colonoscope examination allows examination of complete colon

JOHN A. CRAIG—MD
© ICON

Endoscopy

A rigid sigmoidoscope facilitates reliable examination of the rectum, but frequently the rectosigmoid junction cannot be negotiated; therefore, the sigmoid colon may not be visualized. Flexible sigmoidoscopy allows visualization of only the distal third of the colon. Colonoscopy provides a view of the entire colon and is more sensitive for both early CRC and colorectal adenomas than double-contrast barium enema. Synchronous lesions are present in up to 15% of patients; thus, the entire colon should be assessed whenever possible (Figure 65-3).

Staging

The TNM classification for rectal cancer has replaced the Dukes staging system (Table 65-2). Tumor stage, determined by the depth of tumor penetration into the bowel wall, the number of regional lymph nodes involved, and the presence or absence of distant metastases, is an important prognostic indicator of survival.

Imaging Studies

Most patients with CRC do not require preoperative studies beyond a chest radiograph. There is little evidence to support the use of CT to detect liver metastases as compared with careful clinical examination at surgery; intraoperative evaluation will accurately evaluate the extent of disease. Preoperative staging with CT scanning may be helpful in avoiding unnecessary laparotomy in patients with a relatively asymptomatic primary tumor and clinical evidence of metastases (Figure 65-4). Transrectal ultrasound can determine the depth of tumor invasion and the presence of pelvic lymph node metastases. It is an important rectal cancer staging tool at many institutions, particularly those where preoperative chemoradiation therapy is employed.

Laboratory Studies

Routine preoperative laboratory studies including a complete blood cell count and blood chemistry studies with liver-related tests usually suffice. A preoperative carcinoembryonic antigen (CEA) may be helpful in the postoperative follow-up of patients.

MANAGEMENT AND THERAPY
Surgery

Tumor resection is the cornerstone of CRC management. The goal of surgery is the removal of all macroscopic tumor. Most colon cancers can be treated with a one-stage resection and anastomosis. The rectum is divided into equal thirds. Tumors arising in the upper third are handled most satisfactorily by low anterior resection. A proportion of low rectal cancers and cancers of the anal canal are best managed by abdominoperineal resection of the rectum together with the anal canal, and subsequent permanent colostomy. Some low mobile cancers, especially in poor operative candidates, may be best treated by transanal local excision.

Adjuvant and Neoadjuvant Therapy

Adjuvant chemotherapy with 5-fluorouracil (5-FU) and leucovorin (LV) for 6 months improves survival for patients with T3NxM0 or TxN1M0 CRC. There is increasing evidence that there may also be a survival advantage with adjuvant chemotherapy in some patients with T2N0M0 disease. Rectal cancers (tumors arising below the peritoneal reflection) present an additional challenge. Nearly 40% of patients will have local recurrence if the tumor extends through the bowel wall (T3 disease) or if there are positive lymph nodes. Postoperative adjuvant pelvic radiation therapy is effective in controlling these local recurrences. Standard practice now is to augment this radiation therapy with the protracted infusion of 5-FU.

Over the past few years there has been an evolution in rectal cancer management with the delivery of chemoradiation therapy preoperatively. Although the value of this neoadjuvant therapy is not proven in clinical trials, many oncologists prefer this approach and emphasize the smaller volume of irradiated tissue, the potential decreased risk of tumor seeding at surgery, less acute effects of radiation, and the potential that tumor downstaging will permit more sphincter-sparing surgeries. Because a number of cases are pathologically downstaged with preoperative chemoradiation therapy, all patients treated in this manner should be considered for completion of their 6-month adjuvant chemotherapy course with additional chemotherapy postoperatively, regardless of the pathologic stage at surgery.

Follow-up includes colonoscopy 12 months postoperatively and then at 2- to 3-year intervals. Patients should be seen every 6 to 12 months for 5 years. There is no evidence to support routine imaging studies in the follow-up period.

Figure 65-4

Metastasis in Colorectal Cancer

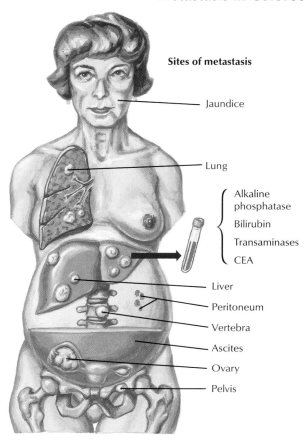

Sites of metastasis

Jaundice

Lung

Alkaline phosphatase

Bilirubin

Transaminases

CEA

Liver

Peritoneum

Vertebra

Ascites

Ovary

Pelvis

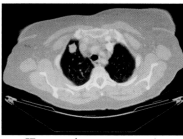

CT scan: pulmonary metastasis

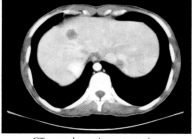

CT scan: hepatic metastasis

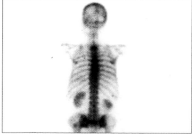

Bone scan: bony metastasis

Surgical management of colorectal metastasis

Local excision
Single lesion near margin confined to single lobe

Lobectomy
Single or multiple lesions confined to single lobe

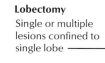

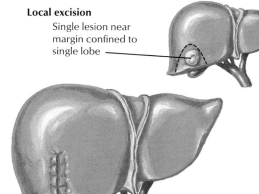

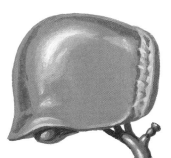

Solitary or multiple hepatic or pulmonary metastases restricted to single lobe potentially curable with surgery

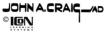

JOHN A. CRAIG—AD
© ICON

Table 65-2
Stage Grouping

AJCC/UICC				Dukes
Stage 0	Tis*	N0	M0	
Stage I	T1	N0	M0	A
	T2	N0	M0	
Stage II	T3	N0	M0	B
	T4	N0	M0	
Stage III	Any T	N1	M0	C
	Any T	N2†	M0	
	Any T	N3	M0	
Stage IV	Any T	Any N	M1	

*Carcinoma *in situ*.
†Metastasis in 4 or more regional nodes.
Note: Dukes B is a composite of better (T3, N0, M0) and worse (T4, N0, M0) prognostic groups, as is Dukes C (Any T, N1, M0 and Any T, N2, N3, M0).
Used with permission of the American Joint Committee on Cancer (AJCC®), Chicago, Ill. The originial source for this material is the AJCC® Cancer Staging Manual, 4th edition (1992) published by Lippincott–Raven Publishers, Philadelphia, Pa.

Management of Metastatic Disease

Recurrent CRC is frequently localized to resectable organs. The most common organ is the liver with the lung second. When confined to a resectable segment, long-term survival is 25% to 40%. In selected patients, unresectable liver lesions may be directly ablated by freezing, ethanol injection, or radiofrequency thermal ablation. Hepatic artery infusion of floxuridine has not been shown to be superior to systemic chemotherapy for liver metastasis, but may be an adjuvant modality in those patients rendered free of disease by either hepatic surgery or ablative therapies.

Patients with unresectable or widespread metastatic disease may benefit from systemic chemotherapy. Combination chemotherapy regimens appear more effective than the core regimen of 5FU/LV. The past several years have seen the addition of irinotecan to 5-FU/LV regimens with enhanced tumor response, albeit with increased toxicities. Roughly one half of patients fail to respond to first-line chemotherapy and progressive disease essentially develops in all that do.

FUTURE DIRECTIONS

The future for advances in all aspects of CRC management is bright. Increasing knowledge of CRC molecular biology and genetics is pivotal in these developments. Identification of molecular targets and lesions will allow the rational design of strategies for CRC prevention, screening, and treatment.

Better identification of environmental factors will have obvious ramifications for CRC prevention. Current clinical studies are focusing on several types of agents in the chemoprevention of CRC. NSAIDs are one such group; inhibition of cyclooxygenase-2 by the NSAID celecoxib in patients with familial adenomatous polyposis leads to a significant reduction in the number of colorectal polyps. This approach may have broader application and CRC chemoprevention trials with NSAIDs' are underway. New screening modalities promise both increased sensitivity and specificity by analyzing for genetic anomalies linked to CRC (such as K-ras) in stool samples.

CT and colonography may provide noninvasive means of detecting polyps and CRC. *Positron emission tomography* (PET) has already made its way into some centers as a means of detecting metastatic disease; however, some tumors including mucinous adenocarcinomas may escape detection.

Advances in adjuvant therapies will consist of both more effective regimens and improved patient selection for these treatments. New treatment strategies showing efficacy in metastatic CRC are expected to make their way into the adjuvant setting. Molecular analysis of nodes may permit more accurate staging and decrease the

Figure 65-5

Prognostic Indicators in Colorectal Cancer

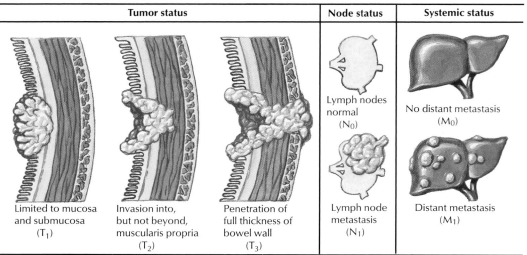

Tumor status			Node status	Systemic status

Limited to mucosa and submucosa (T₁)

Invasion into, but not beyond, muscularis propria (T₂)

Penetration of full thickness of bowel wall (T₃)

Lymph nodes normal (N₀)

Lymph node metastasis (N₁)

No distant metastasis (M₀)

Distant metastasis (M₁)

Tumor staging assesses depth of invasion (T) into or through bowel wall, presence or absence of lymph node (N) and distant organ metastasis (M)

Histology

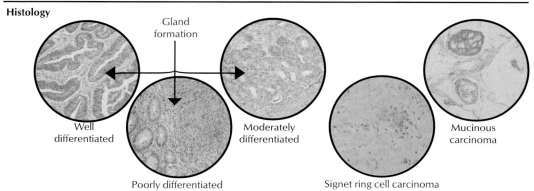

Gland formation

Well differentiated

Poorly differentiated

Moderately differentiated

Signet ring cell carcinoma

Mucinous carcinoma

Well-differentiated tumors have better outcome than poorly differentiated tumors; intracellular or extracellular mucin indicates poor prognosis

Flow cytometry

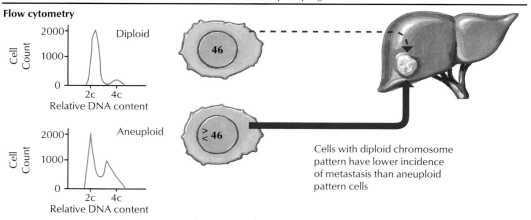

Cells with diploid chromosome pattern have lower incidence of metastasis than aneuploid pattern cells

Flow cytometry shows DNA chromosome pattern of tumor cells

JOHN A. CRAIG—AD
© ICN

false-negative rate of nodal examination. Evidence suggests that analysis for CEA expression in nodes can detect micrometastasis in what would otherwise have been scored nonmetastatic on routine pathologic studies.

An increased understanding of CRC biology and markers of treatment responses will likely permit a more patient-directed approach to treatment (Figure 65-5). As examples, CRC with high-level thymidylate synthase expression may have a poorer response to 5-FU. A host of other molecular markers also have prognostic importance. In stage III colon cancer patients, retention of 18q alleles (the DCC gene region) in microsatellite-stable colon cancers and mutation of the gene for the type II receptor of T-cell growth factor-ß1 in those cancers with microsatellite instability predicts an improved survival with 5-FU–based adjuvant chemotherapy.

New agents and regimens are needed for the treatment of metastatic CRC. As with irinotecan, oxaliplatin-containing combinations have been shown to increase efficacy over the 5-FU/LV core. Oral forms of 5-FU (such as capecitabine) may replace parenteral 5-FU/LV. More effective future therapies for metastatic CRC will likely wed biologic agents with conventional chemotherapy. Recently, a chimeric monoclonal antibody (cetuximab) that binds selectively to the epidermal growth factor receptor (EGFR) was shown in combination with irinotecan to produce major objective responses in patients with EGFR-positive, irinotecan-refractory CRC.

REFERENCES

Harms BA, Grochow L, Neiderhuber JE, Ritter MA. Chapter 62 – Colon and Rectum. pp 1611-1660. In: Abeloff MD, Armitage JO, Lichter AS, Niederhuber JE, eds. *Clinical Oncology. 2nd ed.* New York, NY: Churchill Livingstone; 2000.

Leichman CG, Gallinger S, Sinicrope F. Integration of molecular biology in the diagnosis and treatment of colorectal cancer. In: Program and abstracts at the 37th Annual Meeting of the American Society of Clinical Oncology; May 12-15, 2001; San Francisco, Calif.

Saltz L, Rubin M, Hochster H, et al. Cetuximab (IMC-C225) plus irinotecan (CPT-11) is active in CPT-11-refractory colorectal cancer (CRC) that expresses epidermal growth factor receptor (EGFR). In: Program and abstracts of the 37th Annual Meeting of the American Society of Clinical Oncology; May 12-15, 2001; San Francisco, Calif. Abstract 7.

Watanabe T, Wu TT, Catalano PJ, et al. Molecular predictors of survival after adjuvant chemotherapy for colon cancer. *N Engl J Med.* 2001;344:1196-1206.

Chapter 66

Lung Cancer

Mark A. Socinski

Lung cancer is diagnosed in approximately 169,000 people annually in the United States. It is the second most common cancer in men (after prostate gland cancer) and in women (after breast cancer), accounting for 14% of all cancers in men and 13% in women. It is the most common cause of cancer-related death with approximately 160,000 deaths annually. In men, the number of lung cancer deaths has been decreasing since the late 1980s, but it still accounts for 31% of all cancer deaths. In women, lung cancer deaths surpassed breast cancer deaths in 1986 and now accounts for 25% of all cancer deaths. The number of deaths from lung cancer exceeds the number of deaths from colon, breast, prostate gland, and pancreatic cancer combined.

ETIOLOGY AND PATHOGENESIS

Smoking is the major risk factor for lung cancer. Although 85% to 90% of all patients have a history of direct exposure to tobacco, it is likely that the cause of lung cancer is multifactorial because cancer does not develop in the vast majority of lifetime smokers. A dose-response relationship exists between the number of cigarettes smoked and lung cancer risk. Once smoking cessation occurs, risk decreases but remains above the risk of lifetime nonsmokers for at least 18 years. More than half of all lung cancers are diagnosed in current nonsmokers.

Lung cancer is classified into 2 major categories: small cell lung cancer (SCLC) and non-small cell lung cancer (NSCLC). NSCLC includes squamous cell, adenocarcinoma (including the bronchoalveolar subtype), and large cell carcinoma. Each category and subtype of lung cancer has variations in the histology and degree of differentiation. Approximately 1% to 4% of lung cancers have mixed histology consisting of both small cell and non-small cell. The differentiation by pathologists between SCLC and NSCLC is good (above 90%). However, it is not 100% and careful attention to the clinical presentation is necessary.

CLINICAL PRESENTATION

The clinical presentation of lung cancer is generally related to symptoms referable to the disease in the chest or to metastatic disease. The most common chest symptoms are cough, dyspnea, chest pain, and hemoptysis. Other symptoms may occur from invasion into or obstruction of vital thoracic structures including superior vena cava syndrome, pleural/pericardial effusion, post-obstructive pneumonia, and Pancoast's syndrome.

Metastatic disease may occur anywhere, but the most common sites include the liver, adrenal glands, bone, brain, and lymph nodes. Patients often present with symptoms referable to sites of metastases including bone pain, seizures, hemiplegia, or hepatomegaly. Generalized symptoms such as weight loss, fatigue, malaise, and anorexia are very common and occur more often with advanced disease.

Several paraneoplastic syndromes are associated with lung cancers including the syndrome of inappropriate antidiuretic hormone (SIADH), hypercalcemia, gynecomastia, Cushing's syndrome, and several neurological syndromes including Eaton-Lambert syndrome, and other conditions such as cerebellar degeneration, peripheral neuropathy, and dementia.

DIAGNOSTIC APPROACH

Histologic or cytologic confirmation is required to make the diagnosis of lung cancer. Options include:

Sputum cytology: least invasive but accuracy depends on rigorous sample collection and optimal preservation. The sensitivity is approximately 65% and highly dependent on tumor size and location (large central tumors have the highest sensitivity rates). There is a 2% false-positive rate and a 10% false-negative rate.

Table 66-1
Stage Groupings

Stage	T	N	M	Approx % of cases*
IA	1	0	0	Stage I – 36%
IB	2	0	0	
IIA	1	1	0	Stage II – 7%
IIB	2	1	0	
	3	0	0	
IIIA	1-3	2	0	Stage IIIA – 10%
IIIB	1-4	3	0	Stage IIIB – 20%
	4	0-3	0	
IV	any	any	1	Stage IV – 27%

*Clinical stage.
Adapted from Mountain, CF. Revisions in the International System for Staging Lung Cancer. *Chest.* 1997;111:1712.

Bronchoscopy: the overall sensitivity is 80% to 85% in central tumors and 60% to 65% in more peripheral lesions. In tumors less than 2 cm, the sensitivity is 33%.

Transthoracic fine needle aspiration: the overall sensitivity is 88%, specificity 97%, and a false-positive rate of 1%. It carries a 27% false-negative rate; so, lesions highly suspicious for lung cancer should still be considered malignant even with a negative transthoracic fine needle aspiration.

Cervical mediastinoscopy or anterior mediastinotomy: Mediastinal lymph node sampling is often the method of diagnosing lung cancer. A cervical mediastinoscopy involves an incision in the sternal notch and sampling lymph nodes with the mediastinoscope in the paratracheal (R2, R4, L2, and L4 positions) and subcarinal (station 7) spaces. In tumors arising in the left upper lobe, it is necessary to sample nodes in the aortopulmonary window via an anterior mediastinotomy. This procedure involves an incision in the left second intercostal space and direct visualization on the AP window (station 10).

Biopsy or fine needle aspiration of a metastatic site: Biopsy of extra thoracic sites is a strategy that can accomplish both diagnosis and staging. For example, biopsies of the liver, bones, adrenal glands, or a brain lesion will provide the diagnosis and the stage (IV). Each patient suspected of having a lung cancer should have multidisciplinary input into the optimal approach to making the diagnosis.

DIFFERENTIAL DIAGNOSIS AND STAGING

Lung cancer should be suspected when the appropriate signs and symptoms suggest this diagnosis, particularly in a patient with a history of smoking. Radiographic abnormalities often suggest the diagnosis but new abnormalities need to be differentiated from benign pulmonary lesions including infectious, inflammatory, granulomatous, vascular abnormalities, hamartomas, and metastatic lesions.

Staging is the most important determinant of a patient's treatment plan and prognosis. All patients must be carefully staged at the time of initial presentation. Staging is done with use of the TNM system briefly summarized in the table below and illustrated in Table 66-1, Figures 66-1 and 66-2.

> **TNM Staging System**
> **T Status**
> T0 – primary cannot be defined
> Tis – in situ carcinoma
> T1 – lesions less than 3 cm and surrounded by lung
> T2 – lesions greater than 3 cm or invading the visceral pleura
> T3 – lesions in a structure that can potentially be resected (chest wall or pericardium)
> T4 – a lesion that invades a vital structure that cannot be resected (aorta or heart) or a malignant pleural or pericardial effusion
>
> (continued on page 446)

Figure 66-1

Lung Cancer

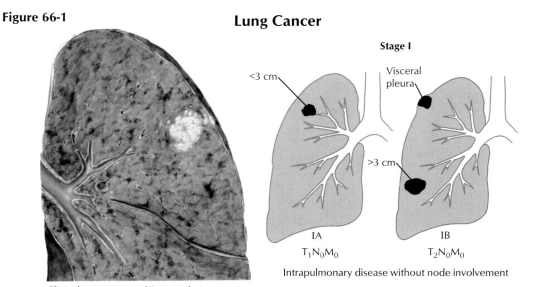

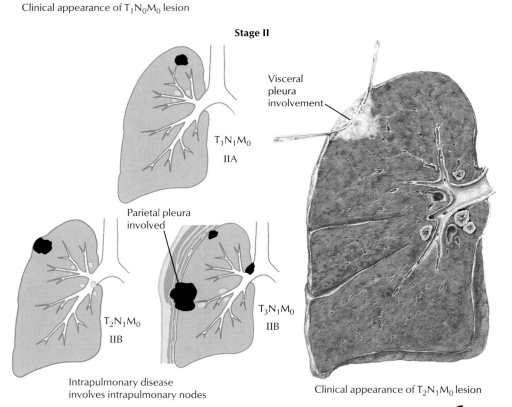

Clinical appearance of $T_1N_0M_0$ lesion

Stage I

<3 cm

Visceral pleura

>3 cm

IA
$T_1N_0M_0$

IB
$T_2N_0M_0$

Intrapulmonary disease without node involvement

Stage II

$T_1N_1M_0$
IIA

$T_2N_1M_0$
IIB

Parietal pleura involved

$T_3N_1M_0$
IIB

Intrapulmonary disease involves intrapulmonary nodes

Visceral pleura involvement

Clinical appearance of $T_2N_1M_0$ lesion

F. Netter M.D.
with
E. Hatton
© ICON
LEARNING SYSTEMS

Figure 66-2

Lung Cancer
Stage IIIA

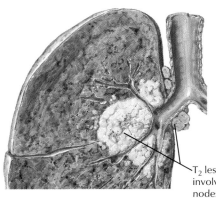

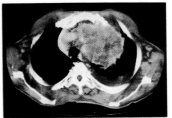

CT scan. Chest wall extension (T_3)

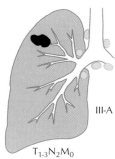

III-A

$T_{1-3}N_2M_0$

Ipsilateral
mediastinal lymph
nodes involved (N_2)

T_2 lesion with N_2 (ipsilateral)
involvement of mediastinal
nodes (III-A)

Stage IIIB

T_4 N_3

III-B
$T_4N_{1-3}M_0$
$T_{1-4}N_3M_0$

Regional extension of
extrapulmonary disease

T_4 invasion of mediastinum
with compression of
superior vena cava (III-B)

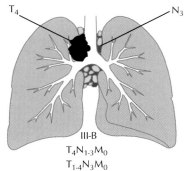

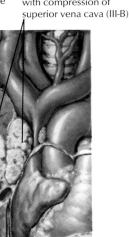

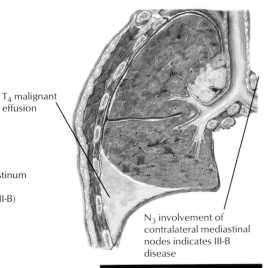

T_4 malignant
effusion

N_3 involvement of
contralateral mediastinal
nodes indicates III-B
disease

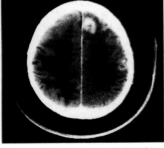

CT scan. Distant metastasis (M_1) in
brain indicates stage IV

with
E. Hatton
© ICON

TNM Staging System (cont'd)

N Status

N0 – no lymph nodes involved

N1 – lymph nodes within the lung only (peri-bronchial or hilar)

N2 – ipsilateral mediastinal nodes

N3 – contralateral mediastinal or supraclavicular nodes

M Status

M0 – no metastatic disease

M1 – metastatic disease

Clinical staging (CS) relies on physical examination and radiographic studies. Pathologic surgical staging (PSS) confirms the findings of radiographic studies with biopsies of suspected areas of pathologic involvement. In general, PSS is more accurate than CS staging because noninvasive radiologic tests are not sufficiently accurate at defining the presence of cancer.

All patients require a complete history and physical examination, chest radiograph, and a staging chest CT (a chest CT extending all the way through the liver and adrenal glands). Additional testing may include a head CT or MRI, radionuclide bone scan, and a PET scan. PSS may include mediastinoscopy, thoracoscopy, or biopsy of suspected metastatic lesions.

Although the TNM system should also be used for SCLC, a more simplified system, limited or extensive stage disease, has historically been used: Limited stage disease is defined as disease limited to a "reasonable" thoracic radiation port. This typically includes the primary tumor and N1 to N3 nodes. Areas of controversy include the contralateral hilar and supraclavicular nodes. Disease beyond this definition is classified as extensive stage SCLC and includes patients with malignant pleural/pericardial effusions.

MANAGEMENT AND THERAPY

Accurate staging is essential because treatment depends on histology and stage of the disease.

Non-Small Cell Lung Cancer
Stage I

The standard of care is complete surgical resection via lobectomy or more if needed. Systematic

sampling or complete mediastinal node dissection is performed on all patients at resection. The expected cure rates or 5-year survival rates range from 70% to 80% for stage IA to 50% to 65% for stage IB. Routine postoperative radiation therapy or postoperative adjuvant chemotherapy is not indicated.

Stage II

Complete surgical resection via lobectomy is the standard of care. Systematic sampling or complete mediastinal node dissection is performed on all patients at resection. The expected cure rates or 5-year survival rates range from 30% to 50% in stage II NSCLC. If a complete surgical resection is accomplished, postoperative radiation therapy or chemotherapy is not indicated.

Stage IIIA/B

Stage IIIA includes two groups: those with bulky mediastinal disease and those with non-bulky mediastinal disease. In patients with non-bulky disease, surgical resection may be entertained. Survival with surgery alone has been poor with a 5-year survival rate of 9% to 30%. Several small phase III studies suggest that preoperative chemotherapy improves the 5-year survival rate. Postoperative chemotherapy (with or without thoracic radiation) does not improve long-term survival. In resected stage IIIA patients, postoperative thoracic radiation therapy reduces local recurrences but does not improve survival. In this resectable population of patients, the 5-year survival rate is approximately 20% to 35% for these patients.

In patients with unresectable stage IIIA/B NSCLC with a good performance status (PS), combined chemotherapy and thoracic radiation therapy is the standard of care. When concurrent approaches have been directly compared to sequential therapy in phase III trials, concurrent chemotherapy and radiation therapy has yielded superior survival results. In this population of patients, the 5-year survival rate is approximately 10% to 20%.

Stage IV

Combination platinum-based chemotherapy improves survival and palliates disease-related symptoms in the majority of patients with a good PS. Studies comparing platinum-based chemotherapy versus best supportive care (BSC) have shown improvement in survival as a result of the chemotherapy. The 1-year survival rate with BSC alone is approximately 10%; with platinum-based chemotherapy, the 1-year survival rate is approximately 20% to 25%. Recently developed cytotoxic agents (paclitaxel, docetaxel, gemcitabine, vinorelbine, irinotecan) when used with the platinums have improved the survival outcomes in stage IV NSCLC. These new agents are associated with a 1-year survival rate of 30% to 40%.

Best supportive care is the standard for patients with a poor PS because these patients suffer more treatment-related morbidity and mortality and show no improvement in survival as a result of treatment.

Small Cell Lung Cancer

Limited stage small cell lung cancer (LS SCLC) comprises one third of all cases of SCLC. The optimal therapeutic approach is combined chemotherapy and radiation therapy. Cisplatin/etoposide is the standard regimen and radiation therapy is given concurrently with chemotherapy early in the course. Because brain relapse is so common in patients achieving remission, prophylactic cranial irradiation (PCI) is recommended.

Extensive stage small cell lung cancer (ES SCLC) is a treatable but incurable disease. Although response rates to combination chemotherapy range from 60% to 80%, the 2-year survival rate is 10%. The median survival is 8 to 12 months. The standard regimen is either cisplatin or carboplatin in combination with etoposide.

FUTURE DIRECTIONS

Several targeted agents are being tested in advanced NSCLC. These new drugs are targeted at novel pathways including angiogenesis, signal transduction, apoptosis, and matrix metalloproteinases. They will likely lead to further improvements in survival and be incorporated into treatment in earlier stages of NSCLC. New radiation therapy techniques including 3-dimensional treatment planning, intensity-modulated approaches, stereotactic radiation therapy, and the use of protective agents to ameliorate the toxicity of radiation will likely improve the therapeutic index of radiation therapy. Current studies of adjuvant and neoadjuvant systemic therapy in early stage operable NSCLC will help define which of these approaches is appropriate as an adjunct to surgery. Chemopreventive strategies in early stage disease are under study and may lead to a reduction in the risk of second primary tumors. Rapid spiral CT scanning has brought about a resurgence of interest in screening for lung cancer, although the role of screening remains controversial. Lastly, reduction in the number of smokers would dramatically decrease the incidence of lung cancer. Strategies directed at prevention of smoking and more effective smoking cessation therapies should be high priorities.

REFERENCES

Detterbeck FC, Rivera MP, Socinski MA, Rosenman JG, eds. *Diagnosis and Treatment of Lung Cancer: An Evidence Based Guide for the Practicing Clinician.* Philadelphia, Pa: WB Saunders Co; 2001.

Mountain CF. Revisions in the International System for Staging Lung Cancer. *Chest.* 1997;111:1710-1717.

Reif MS, Socinski MA, Rivera MP. Evidence-based medicine in the treatment of non-small-cell lung cancer. *Clin Chest Med.* 2000;21:107-120, ix.

Chapter 67

Palliative Care for Patients With Advanced Cancer

Thomas E. Stinchcombe and Stephen A. Bernard

Palliative care focuses on care of patients whose disease is no longer responsive to curative treatment. The goal of interventions is to provide the best quality of life possible for the patient and his or her family. These interventions have been used in patients with the advanced stages of cancer; however, they are increasingly being used in patients with a variety of diseases such as end-stage heart disease, end-stage pulmonary diseases, and a variety of neurological conditions. The focus of any medical intervention is to provide optimal relief from distressing symptoms such as pain, constipation, nausea, and vomiting. The social, psychological, and spiritual aspects of the patient's illness must also be carefully considered and addressed. This interdisciplinary approach often involves the patient, family members, physicians, nurses, social workers, home health aids, and spiritual advisors to treat the multiple aspects of the patient's illness.

PAIN

The chronic pain seen in this setting is divided into nonmalignant and malignant categories based on the concept that the pathophysiology and the patient populations in the 2 conditions are different; therefore, the treatment approaches and goals should be different. Approximately 70% of patients with cancer report pain when the disease is in advanced stages, and approximately 35% have pain severe enough to impair their ability to function.

There is great variability in a patient's perception of pain; a careful history of its location, character, and severity provides the most accurate assessment. Perception of pain may be altered by other symptoms (eg, fatigue, weakness, nausea, constipation, dyspnea, coughing); or psychological factors (eg, depression, anxiety, and feelings of hopelessness or anger). The impact that the pain has on a patient's daily activities and psychosocial functioning varies greatly. The physiological processes that cause or modify pain character, intensity, and frequency change in response to the patient's clinical course and treatment. Pain should be reevaluated on a regular basis, and modifications in the treatment made when indicated. Treatment of symptoms contributing to the pain should also be implemented.

Pathophysiology of Pain

The afferent pathways of the nervous system have nociceptors, specialized receptors that respond to noxious physical or chemical stimuli widely distributed throughout the body except in the brain. These pain afferent fibers enter the spinal cord via the dorsal root, and synapse in the dorsal horn and then ascend to the brain. The efferent pathways, which modulate nociceptive transmission, originate in the central nervous system and travel down the lateral posterior column into the peripheral nerves. The efferent pathways are activated by endogenous endorphins and can be activated centrally by opioids that mimic the activity of endogenous endorphins. The neurotransmitter serotonin is also believed to be important in some of these descending pathways, and this may account for the action of antidepressants in the treatment of pain.

Classification of Pain

Nociceptive pain arises from direct stimulation of the nociceptors by physical or chemical stimulation of the nerve endings due to tissue damage; it is often divided into somatic and visceral pain. Somatic pain is described as aching pain that is often well localized. Visceral pain is poorly localized and described as squeezing or a pressure sensation; it may be referred to distant cutaneous sites. It is caused by infiltration, compression, or distention of thoracic or abdominal viscera that are innervated by the sympathetic nervous system. Neuropathic pain is burning or tingling with intermittent lancinating pain that results from tumor infiltration or compression of a peripheral nerve or the spinal cord. This type of pain is seen in diabetic neuropathy or postherpetic neuralgia.

Treatment of Pain

Often, analgesic therapy is initiated for the treatment of the pain at the start of treatment for the underlying malignancy. If the disease is responsive, treatment of the underlying condition can provide significant pain relief. Pain related to bone metastases or to spinal cord compression can be significantly alleviated by the initiation of localized radiation therapy to the symptomatic lesion. Orthopedic surgery plays an important role in the management of lytic lesions because the stabilization of the lesions can reduce incident pain as well as prevent pathological fractures. In breast cancer or multiple myeloma, pamidronate, a bisphosphonate, reduces the pain associated with bone lesions and may reduce the development of new bone lesions. Systemic chemotherapy or hormonal therapy can provide pain relief in treatment-responsive tumors. Treatment of pain with opioid and non-narcotic medications is usually the mainstay of cancer pain treatment.

ANOREXIA AND CACHEXIA

Anorexia is defined as the decline in food intake to the point that caloric intake does not provide enough energy for the amount of caloric expenditure. In advanced cancer the presence of this symptom is due to several causes. Specific tumor types may play a role in the degree of anorexia, and certain treatments may exacerbate the symptom by causing persistent nausea, worsening gastroparesis, or altering the patient's sense of taste or smell. Inadequately controlled pain may also contribute to this problem.

Cancer cachexia refers to the weight loss, and particularly loss of muscle mass and adipose tissue commonly associated with advanced cancer. It was originally thought to be a form of starvation as a result of the consumption of calories by a highly metabolic tumor creating a "calorie deficit" for the body. Recent research indicates cachexia develops as a result of a fundamental alteration in the body's metabolism by the tumor mediated by the release of cytokines such as tumor necrosis factor (TNF), interleukin-6 (IL-6), and interleukin-1 (IL-1). The 2 syndromes often occur simultaneously and symptoms can be very disturbing to the patient's family or caretakers; however, they do not always cause the patient any discomfort. Patient and family education is very important.

Clinical Management

The initial treatment involves encouraging increased oral intake or the use of high calorie nutritional supplements; however, as the patient becomes more ill, these measures may not be sufficient. Treating symptoms that may be contributing to the syndrome is an important aspect of managing anorexia and cachexia.

Pharmacologic approaches may result in an increased appetite or sense of well-being for the patient; less frequently they result in improvement in objective parameters such as weight gain or lean muscle mass. Potential adverse effects must be balanced against the relatively modest benefits. Often, decisions are made based on the patient's and the family's preferences and the level of anxiety and discomfort created by the anorexia and cachexia.

Corticosteroids, usually dexamethasone or methylprednisolone, are used most often. Trials have shown an improvement in appetite and performance status, but they have been associated with adverse events such as gastrointestinal hemorrhage, cushingoid body features, and myopathy. These relatively inexpensive medications are also beneficial in the treatment of chronic nausea and pain, and may be beneficial in the treatment of cancer-associated fatigue. The proper dose and duration of treatment have not yet been definitively determined.

The progestational agent, megestrol acetate, is often used in this situation. Several studies have documented its effectiveness in increasing appetite and food intake in a significant percentage of patients. The dose used has varied from 480 to 1600 mg daily. Side effects include fluid retention, edema, and erectile dysfunction in men. There is some concern about a possible increased risk of deep vein thrombosis. The high cost of megestrol acetate, especially in comparison to corticosteroids, must be considered with the use of this agent.

Emerging Therapies

Dronabinol, a derivative of marijuana, has shown some activity as an appetite stimulant and in the treatment of chronic nausea, benefits that have resulted in interest in its use in the treatment of cancer cachexia and anorexia. As expected, there are associated mood effects, somnolence, and confusion. Thalidomide is believed to alter levels of TNF, a cytokine that may be responsible for anorexia and cachexia. A preliminary study revealed some therapeutic efficacy. Thalidomide may be of benefit in the treatment of coexisting insomnia also. It is a teratogen and has been associated with adverse events such as dry mouth, somnolence, and peripheral neuropathy. Melatonin is believed to alter TNF levels and is relatively well tolerated. A preliminary study revealed some efficacy in preventing weight loss in patients with metastatic cancer. Anabolic steroids have been considered as a possible treatment for these symptoms, although a recent randomized controlled trial showed that they were inferior to dexamethasone or megestrol acetate.

HYDRATION

Often patients with advanced cancer have a decline in their oral intake due to cancer fatigue, persistent nausea and vomiting, and cancer anorexia and cachexia. Family members and members of the medical staff will often raise the issue of the palliative benefits of intravenous hydration. Many family members have concerns that if intravenous fluids (IVF) are not initiated, the patient will "die of thirst," and this fear is often compounded if the patient has dry mucous membranes or the appearance of dehydration. The family may perceive the decision to discontinue intravenous hydration as "letting him or her die" and they must be educated before any discussion or decision to forgo or discontinue hydration.

The risks and benefits of IVF are debated in the palliative care community because many studies evaluating its use have been done in very heterogeneous patient populations. The symptoms, clinical outcomes evaluated, and the evaluation methods used have varied among studies making direct comparison difficult. The argument in favor of the use of IVF is that the patient may have less delirium related to dehydration, and a lower frequency of adverse events from altered drug metabolism due to renal insufficiency. There is no evidence that the use of IVF in this setting prolongs life to any significant degree The argument against the use of IVF is that there is the risk of fluid overload, and some experts argue that there is a palliative benefit to fluid deficiency. Some purported benefits include decreased pulmonary and gastrointestinal secretions with less nausea and vomiting and decreased urine production with fewer episodes of incontinence and a decreased need for use of urinary catheters.

Many patients complain of thirst or dry mouth while in the terminal phases of their illness, and this can cause significant discomfort for the patient and the patient's family. A study by McCann et al. found that 66% of patients admitted to a palliative care unit complained of thirst or dry mouth on admission, but with the use of small amounts of oral fluids, ice chips, and routine mouth care, these symptoms were relieved for several hours in most patients. This study supports the use of these simple measures initially to address a patient's complaint of thirst or dry mouth before considering the initiation of IVF.

Given the relative paucity of data on the risks and benefits of intravenous hydration and the relative risks and benefits of fluid deficiency in the palliative setting, it is impossible to give definitive recommendations on this subject. Often the decision will have to be made based on the condition and wishes of the individual patient, and his or her family and the opinion of the physician and medical staff caring for the patient.

FUTURE DIRECTIONS

There are increasing numbers of palliative care specialists throughout the world. In the United States, there is a certification process for physicians and nurses interested in this area. Hospital-based units have been formed at community and academic centers. The success of these programs is dependent on the system for reimbursement of medical care in the United States. Currently, this system imposes restraints on the services that can be provided. Whether changes can be made in the reimbursement for these types of services is not clear, but an increasing demand has been seen in many areas of the United States.

REFERENCES

Bruera E, Neumann CM, Pituskin E, Calder K, Ball G, Hanson J. Thalidomide in patients with cachexia due to terminal cancer: preliminary report. *Ann Oncol.* 1999;10:857–859.

Cleeland CS, Gonin R, Hatfield AK, et al. Pain and its treatment in outpatients with metastatic cancer. *N Engl J Med.* 1994;330:592–596.

Fainsinger R, Bruera E. The management of dehydration in terminally ill patients. *J Palliat Care.* 1994;10:55–59.

Lissoni P, Paolorossi F, Tancini G, et al. Is there a role for melatonin in the treatment of neoplastic cachexia? *Eur J Cancer.* 1996;32A:1340–1343.

Loprinzi CL, Kuglet JW, Slaon JA, et al. Randomized comparison of megestrol acetate versus dexamethasone versus fluoxymesterone for the treatment of cancer anorexia/cachexia. *J Clin Oncol.* 1999;17:3299–3306.

McCann RM, Hall WJ, Groth-Juncker A. Comfort care for terminally ill patients. The appropriate use of nutrition and hydration. *JAMA.* 1994;272:1263–1266.

Chapter 68

Prostate Cancer

Young E. Whang and Paul A. Godley

Prostate cancer is the most commonly diagnosed visceral malignancy in males, comprising 30% of diagnosed cancers. An estimated 189,000 new cases are anticipated in the United States in 2002. These figures represent a sharp decline from the 1997 estimates of 334,500 new cases, a trend consistent with an effect from the recent adoption of prostate-specific antigen (PSA) screening for prostate cancer. Prostate cancer is the second leading cause of male cancer deaths, with 30,200 deaths anticipated in 2002. Mortality rates from prostate cancer as well as several other cancers also decreased in 1998, although a relationship of this decrease to current screening efforts has not been established.

The incidence rates among African American men surpass those of other racial and ethnic groups and are twice as high as those of white Americans. The mortality rate of African Americans is also more than twice that of whites. Risk increases sharply as men age, and men with a strong family history of prostate cancer may have several times the risk of prostate cancer as men without such a history.

ETIOLOGY AND PATHOGENESIS

Research on men who migrate from areas of low prostate cancer mortality to areas of high mortality provides compelling evidence for unidentified environmental causes. Japanese males ages 65 to 74 who migrated to the United States had age-specific prostate cancer mortality rates (40.2/100,000/year) intermediate between the high rate of US whites (92.6/100,000/year) and Japan's lower rate (11.2/100,000/year). These studies imply that immigrants are exposed to environmental or lifestyle factors that place them at higher risk for prostate cancer. Reviews of prostate cancer risk factors have not demonstrated consistent environmental, behavioral, or dietary risk factors amenable to primary prevention measures, although some studies have suggested that dietary saturated fat consumption may increase risk.

CLINICAL PRESENTATION

Prostate cancer in the earlier stages is often asymptomatic. Symptoms referable to the prostate gland may be due to benign prostatic hyperplasia, which is not related to prostate cancer. Locally advanced prostate cancer may present with symptoms of bladder outlet obstruction or hematuria, and patients with metastatic disease may present with bone pain and, less commonly, spinal cord compression or obstructive uropathy (Figure 68-1).

DIAGNOSTIC APPROACH

Screening remains a controversial issue. The lack of consensus on PSA screening is reflected in the diversity of recommendations from public health and physician organizations. The American Cancer Society, the American Urological Association and others recommend annual screening with PSA and digital rectal examination (DRE) starting at age 50, while the *National Cancer Institute* (NCI), the US *Preventive Services Task Force*, the *Canadian Task Force on the Periodic Health Exam*, the Office of Technology Assessment, and the American College of Physicians have either abstained from a recommendation, recommended that screening be discussed with patients, or recommended explicitly against screening.

Of the screening tests for early prostate cancer, only the PSA blood test stands out as both convenient to administer and potentially sensitive enough to detect cancer while it is localized to the prostate gland. DRE is not a reliable screening test, having failed to demonstrate effectiveness in preventing metastatic prostate cancer or death from prostate cancer in a case-control study and a quasi-cohort study. DRE, however, does detect some prostate cancers that are missed by PSA testing.

Uncertainty about the natural history of prostate cancer and the wisdom of detecting and treating asymptomatic patients is reflected in the extraordinarily high prevalence of *unsuspected prostate cancers* in unselected series of autopsies. Several large autopsy studies of unselected men from various countries and without a diagnosis of prostate cancer document the large proportion of men (20%–30%) with unsuspected prostate cancers.

Pathology and Staging

Tissues obtained from transurethral resection of the prostate may be incidentally found to be involved with cancer. Patients with an elevated PSA level or a palpable nodule on DRE should undergo a needle biopsy of the prostate gland. Almost all the prostate carcinomas are adenocarcinomas. In the Gleason grading system, the glandular differentiation patterns of the primary and secondary tumors are each scored from 1 (well-differentiated) to 5 (poorly differentiated) and then added together to give a number from 2 to 10 (Figure 68-1). The Gleason score also provides prognostic information. High-grade tumors are more likely to spread outside of the prostate gland and relapse following therapy.

Staging using the TNM system classifies T1 and T2 tumors as nonpalpable and palpable tumors confined to the prostate gland. Stage T1c describes nonpalpable tumors detected by random prostate biopsies after an elevated PSA test. Stage T3 tumors extend beyond the gland and T4 tumors invade adjacent organs. N1 and M1 denote the presence of positive lymph nodes and metastatic disease, respectively.

MANAGEMENT AND THERAPY
Localized Disease

Treatment of localized prostate cancer is controversial in the absence of randomized prospective trials directly comparing surgery and radiation. Radical prostatectomy is the most frequently chosen treatment (Figure 68-2). With a retropubic approach, the procedure is frequently preceded by a regional pelvic lymph node dissection. Over one third of patients with clinically localized disease are upstaged with capsular penetration, positive surgical margins, or involvement of the seminal vesicles or lymph nodes. The risk of finding positive lymph nodes increases with the stage and Gleason grade. A frozen section can be obtained intraoperatively

and the prostatectomy aborted if the results are positive for metastatic nodal disease. If a perineal approach is used, the lymph nodes cannot be simultaneously sampled. The major side effects associated with radical prostatectomy include erectile dysfunction and urinary incontinence.

Radiation therapy can be delivered by external beam or by brachytherapy using iodine or palladium prostatic interstitial implants. External beam radiation is given to a dose of approximately 70 to 78 Gy in daily fractions over 7 to 8 weeks. Androgen deprivation therapy may be administered for several weeks preceding radiation therapy. Seed implants permanently placed during an outpatient procedure may be used in combination with external beam radiation. Temporary high-dose-rate brachytherapy devices, inserted into the prostate gland for less than an hour and removed, remain investigational. Radiation therapy is associated with erectile dysfunction and rectal damage (radiation proctitis) frequently and urinary symptoms less commonly.

The third option is no treatment, also termed watchful waiting, expectant management, or observation. It involves treating patients when symptoms develop, but not initially attempting to eradicate the disease. The advantage is the lack of early complications associated with aggressive therapy. The trade-off is late complications from locally advanced or metastatic prostate cancer, and death from prostate cancer—a possibility also faced by men who choose more aggressive treatment. Patients who choose watchful waiting should not experience prostate cancer–specific mortality for 10 years or more, so this may be an option that those with low-grade disease, or a less than 10-year life expectancy should consider. The treatment of locally advanced disease (T3 or T4) consists of radiation and androgen deprivation, either alone or in combination. Radiation plus androgen deprivation may be more effective in terms of survival than radiation alone.

Metastatic Disease

Metastatic prostate cancer is incurable. Patients are treated palliatively with androgen deprivation because prostate cancer cells initially require circulating testosterone for viability and proliferation (Figure 68-3). Advantages of surgical castration with bilateral orchiectomy include immediate efficacy,

Figure 68-1

Prostate Cancer

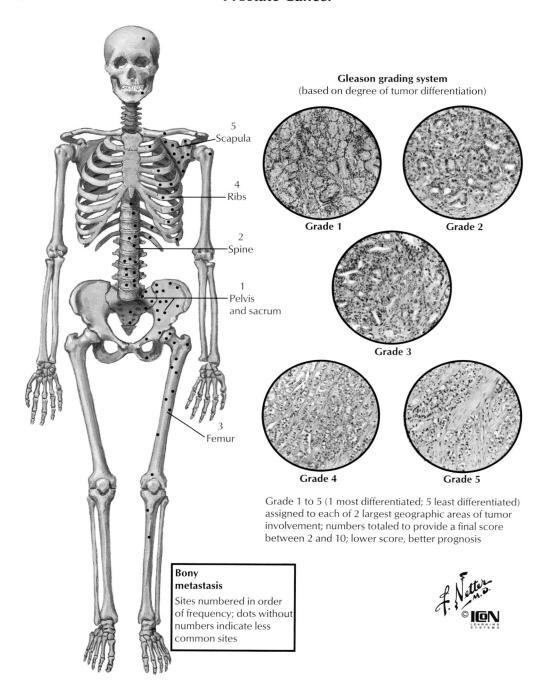

Gleason grading system
(based on degree of tumor differentiation)

Grade 1

Grade 2

Grade 3

Grade 4

Grade 5

Grade 1 to 5 (1 most differentiated; 5 least differentiated)
assigned to each of 2 largest geographic areas of tumor
involvement; numbers totaled to provide a final score
between 2 and 10; lower score, better prognosis

5
Scapula

4
Ribs

2
Spine

1
Pelvis
and sacrum

3
Femur

**Bony
metastasis**

Sites numbered in order
of frequency; dots without
numbers indicate less
common sites

Figure 68-2

Radical Prostatectomy

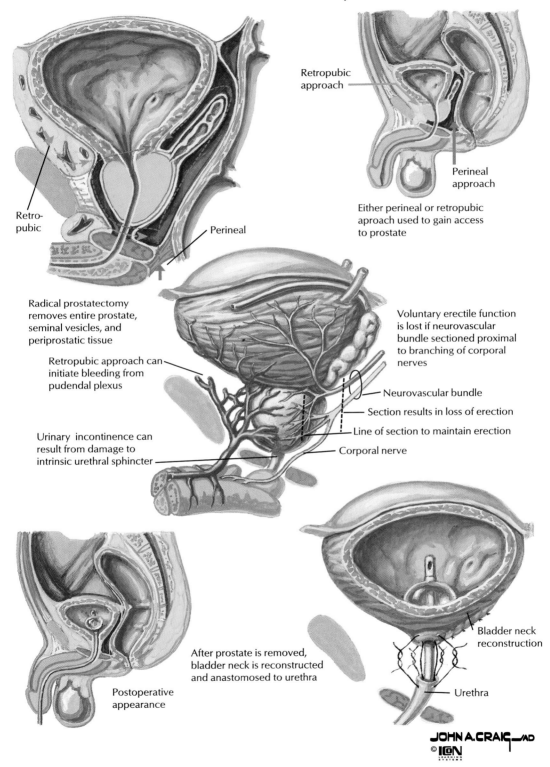

Retropubic approach

Perineal approach

Either perineal or retropubic aproach used to gain access to prostate

Retro-pubic

Perineal

Radical prostatectomy removes entire prostate, seminal vesicles, and periprostatic tissue

Retropubic approach can initiate bleeding from pudendal plexus

Urinary incontinence can result from damage to intrinsic urethral sphincter

Voluntary erectile function is lost if neurovascular bundle sectioned proximal to branching of corporal nerves

Neurovascular bundle

Section results in loss of erection

Line of section to maintain erection

Corporal nerve

After prostate is removed, bladder neck is reconstructed and anastomosed to urethra

Postoperative appearance

Bladder neck reconstruction

Urethra

JOHN A. CRAIG AD
© ICON
LEARNING SYSTEMS

Figure 68-3

Androgen Deprivation in Metastatic Disease

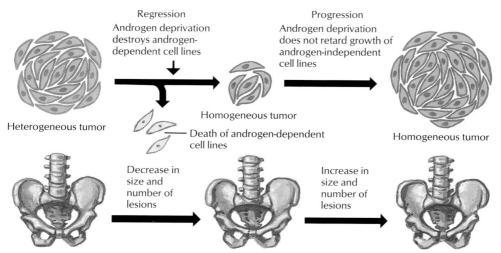

Feedback inhibition

Androgen receptor

LHRH

Androgen-receptor blockade

DES and other sex hormones

LHRH-receptor complex

LH

LH-receptor complex

LHRH-receptor blockade

LHRH analogues

Ketoconazole

Blockade of testosterone synthesis

Testosterone

Cytoplasmic androgen-receptor blockade

Bicalutamide

Flutamide

Orchiectomy removes primary androgen source

Tumor growth

5α-reductase

5-DHT dihydrotestosterone

Protein synthesis cell division

mRNA

DHT-receptor complex

Androgen-dependent tumor cell

Blockade of specific receptors in hypothalamic-pituitary-testicular axis and at cellular level can produce androgen deprivation of androgen-dependent prostate tumor cells

"Escape" phenomenon in metastatic disease

Regression
Androgen deprivation destroys androgen-dependent cell lines

Progression
Androgen deprivation does not retard growth of androgen-independent cell lines

Heterogeneous tumor

Homogeneous tumor

Death of androgen-dependent cell lines

Homogeneous tumor

Decrease in size and number of lesions

Increase in size and number of lesions

Tumor contains heterogeneous population of androgen-dependent and androgen-independent cell lines. Androgen-deprivation therapy has no direct influence on androgen-independent cell lines

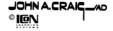

compliance, and low cost. Medical castration utilizing the long-acting preparations of a luteinizing hormone–releasing hormone (LH-RH) agonist (leuprolide or goserelin) is used more commonly possibly because of the psychological trauma associated with orchiectomy (Figure 68-3). The LH-RH agonist initially causes a transient surge in the testosterone level decreases due to the stimulation of the pituitary LH-RH receptor before the testosterone level to the castrate level over 3 weeks ("flare" phenomenon). Short-term use of an anti-androgen agent such as flutamide or bicalutamide, which acts as a competitive inhibitor of the androgen receptor, is indicated for the first several weeks after administration of the LH-RH agonist. The major common side effects of androgen deprivation therapy (both surgical and medical) include loss of libido, erectile dysfunction, gynecomastia, hot flashes, loss of muscle mass, osteoporosis, anemia, and fatigue.

Androgen deprivation is effective only temporarily because progressive disease will develop again after a median of 18 to 24 months (Figure 68-3). In this setting, second-line endocrine manipulations involving anti-androgens, low-dose steroids, or ketoconazole are often attempted. For patients who have been on long-term anti-androgen therapy, its discontinuation leads to reduction in PSA in 15% to 20% of cases; however, responses to second-line hormonal treatment tend to be infrequent and short-lived.

The traditional view of prostate cancer as resistant to chemotherapy is changing to the extent that many patients with hormone-refractory prostate cancer may benefit from a referral to medical oncologists. Mitoxantrone improved pain control and the quality of life in 2 randomized clinical trials. Estramustine has synergistic activity with several cytotoxic agents including taxanes (docetaxel or paclitaxel), vinblastine, and etoposide. A combination of estramustine and taxanes is currently regarded as one of the most active regimens in this setting. Zoledronic acid, a new potent bisphosphonate, decreases skeletal complications such as bone pain, fracture, and spinal cord compression in patients with bone metastases. In addition to chemotherapy, palliation of pain associated with bone metastases may be achieved by external beam radiation or systemic administration of bone-seeking radioactive isotopes (strontium-89 or samarium-153).

Medical Emergencies in Prostate Cancer Management

The metastatic sites frequently involved by prostate cancer are bones and lymph nodes in the pelvis and retroperitoneum. Spinal cord compression, a common oncologic emergency, arises from epidural metastasis in the vertebral bodies and usually presents with midline accelerating back pain. Loss of ambulation due to weakness, and bowel/bladder incontinence are late symptoms that are usually irreversible despite treatment. The diagnosis can be made with computed tomography myelography or noninvasively with MRI. Treatment consists of corticosteroids and radiation therapy. Use of the LH-RH agonist by itself is not recommended in this setting due to concerns about the flare phenomenon.

Obstructive uropathy may result from primary prostate cancer locally invading into the urethra and the bladder or extrinsic compressive obstruction of ureters by soft tissue nodal masses in the pelvis or retroperitoneum. It may progress to complete renal failure. Renal function can be preserved by relief of obstruction through percutaneous nephrostomy tube or internal stent placement.

FUTURE DIRECTIONS

Availability of the human genome sequence and advances in molecular profiling of tumors hold great promise for developing better prognostic and predictive markers and therapeutic agents specifically targeting cancer cells (e.g. drugs inhibiting kinases). Approaches to improve the treatment outcome of those patients unlikely to be cured by local treatment alone (e.g. high Gleason score, T3 or T4 stage, etc.) will be explored. Treatment approaches to hormone-refractory prostate cancer will continue to be refined with available chemotherapeutic agents and novel molecularly targeted agents.

Several prostate cancer prevention strategies are under investigation. The Prostate Cancer Prevention Trial examined chemoprevention of prostate cancer using finasteride, an inhibitor of 5-alpha reductase. The results from this large randomized trial should be available before 2010. The Prostate, Lung, Colorectal, and Ovarian Cancer Screening Trial, should also be completed around 2010. SELECT, a large randomized, controlled trial of selenium and vitamin E as nutritional cancer prevention agents, began in 2002.

REFERENCES

American Cancer Society Web site. Available at: http://www.cancer.org. Accessed February 10, 2003.

National Cancer Institute Web site. PDQ® cancer information summaries. Available at: http://www.nci.nih.gov/cancer info/pdq. Accessed February 10, 2003.

National Cancer Institute Web site. About SEER. Available at: http://seer.cancer.gov/about. Accessed February 10, 2003.

US TOO! International, Inc Web site. Available at: http://www.ustoo.com. Accessed February 10, 2003.

Chapter 69
Skin Cancer

Robert S. Tomsick

Skin cancer is a major health problem in the United States with 1.3 million new nonmelanoma skin cancers and 51,000 new melanomas diagnosed annually. Nonmelanoma and melanoma skin cancers together account for 40% of all malignancies. The annual cost to treat nonmelanoma skin cancers in the United States approaches $650 million. The incidence of both nonmelanoma and melanoma skin cancers has been steadily increasing. Early detection and treatment can have a significant impact on morbidity and mortality.

BASAL CELL CARCINOMA
Etiology and Pathogenesis

Basal cell carcinoma (BCC) is the most common skin cancer. It accounts for more than 75% of all nonmelanoma skin cancers. There are 750,000 to 900,000 new cases in the United States each year. Most of these cancers are located on sun-exposed areas, 85% of them on the head and neck. Incidence increases with age; it is uncommon in those under age 50 and rare in young adults. Persons with light skin, blue eyes, and blonde hair are at greater risk because of their relative lack of natural photoprotection with melanin pigment. The patient is often unaware of these painless tumors because of their very slow growth rate. Frequently slight bleeding after minor trauma (e.g., face washing) brings the patient to the physician.

Clinical Presentation

The most common clinical appearance of a BCC is a discrete, smooth, pink papule or nodule with a translucent or "pearly" sheen and telangiectasias, often with a central erosion or ulceration; however, the appearance may vary considerably. Superficial BCC may present as a thin, scaly, red plaque easily confused with eczema or tinea. Morpheaform BCC may appear similar to a yellow-white scar. Pigmented BCC has sufficient melanin to appear as a black nodule. The diagnosis is an easy one once a biopsy is performed.

Differential Diagnosis

The common, nodular type of BCC has a distinctive appearance that is seldom missed because of its "pearly" sheen and central dell or ulceration (Figure 69-1). At times, nodular BCC may resemble sebaceous adenoma or other appendage tumors. Superficial BCC is often mistaken for actinic keratosis, tinea, or eczema. Morpheaform BCC may resemble scar tissue, morphea, or chronic radiodermatitis.

Management and Therapy

Basal cell carcinomas are slow-growing tumors, and treatment is usually not urgent. Metastasis is rare, but the tumor is capable of unrestricted growth causing local destruction; hence, complete ablation of the tumor is indicated. BCCs with morpheaform, infiltrating, or micronodular histopathologic patterns are more difficult to cure. Tumors in certain facial sites are more

Figure 69-1   Nodular Basal Cell Carcinoma

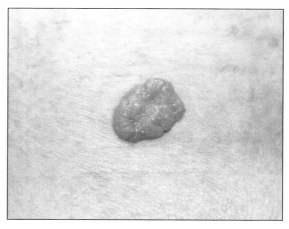

resistant to ablation regardless of the method used. High-risk areas include the medial canthus, nasolabial fold, alar crease, postauricular sulcus, and concha. Treatment type requires consideration of several factors: the size and location of the tumor, its histologic subtype, ready access to and cost of the treatment, time frame available for treatment, skill of the physician, patient age, and intervening medical conditions. Guidelines for use of different modalities:

Curettage and electrofulguration: small tumors (<1 cm), sites not prone to high recurrence rates, nonaggressive histologic patterns, speed and ease of treatment, when secondary intention healing is adequate, to minimize cost.

Cryosurgery: indications similar to those for curettage and electrofulguration.

Radiation therapy: larger tumors, older patients, tissue conservation, to avoid disfiguring scars.

Topical chemotherapy: for superficial tumors only (in the epidermis and at the dermal-epidermal junction), to avoid or minimize scarring.

Surgical excision: any size tumor, any location or histopathologic pattern, rapid healing.

Mohs' chemosurgery (micrographic surgery): any size tumor, aggressive histopathologic patterns, sites prone to high recurrence rates, recurrent tumors, tissue conservation.

The prognosis for BCC is excellent. Overall, the 5-year cure rate for small, primary (i.e., previously untreated) BCCs is approximately 95%, regardless of the treatment used. Larger tumors, tumors in select sites, and tumors with certain histopathologic patterns will not have as high a cure rate.

SQUAMOUS CELL CARCINOMA
Etiology and Pathogenesis

Squamous cell carcinoma (SCC) is the second most common cutaneous malignancy with an incidence of 7 to 12 per 100,000 in the white population of the United States. It is a sun-associated tumor, and more likely to develop in those with blue eyes, blonde hair, and fair skin. Persons with outdoor occupations, heavy recreational sun exposure, and those living in semitropical or tropical regions are at greatest risk. Most SCCs probably arise from an antecedent lesion, the actinic keratosis, a premalignant focus of intraepidermal dysplasia brought about by chronic sun exposure. It is an erythematous, scaly lesion from a few millimeters

Figure 69-2   Bowen's Disease

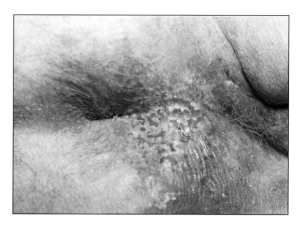

to several centimeters in size. The scale may be so thick as to form a cutaneous horn. SCC in situ is referred to as Bowen's disease (Figure 69-2).

Factors other than sunlight that can play a significant role in the pathogenesis include certain strains of human papillomavirus (HPV), especially in the periungual and genital regions, topical agents (tar, creosote, nitrogen mustard), and some ingested chemicals (arsenic). Any chronic inflammatory focus on the skin can lead to SCC, but usually the inflammation is present for years before the cancer forms; chronic discoid lupus erythematosus lesions or vascular ulcers are examples of cancer-inciting lesions. Old thermal burn scars and sites of therapeutic x-ray exposure are well known to cause SCC decades after the initial injury or treatment.

Clinical Presentation

SCC presents as papules, nodules, or plaques, which are erythematous and hyperkeratotic (Figure 69-3). Bowen's disease is a thin, pink scaly plaque, which may mimic a superficial fungal infection or dermatitis; the scale may be thin or compact, yellow, and thick. Although the tumor begins in the epidermis and may remain superficial for a long time, ultimately it invades into the dermis, and even subcutaneous tissues, forming a deep nodular mass. Erosion of the epidermis or deeper ulceration may occur early or late. The growth rate is variable. It may grow slowly or may double in size in a matter of weeks. In an early, superficial phase, it may be indistinguishable from an actinic keratosis or eczema. Later, its malignant

Figure 69-3   Squamous Cell Carcinoma

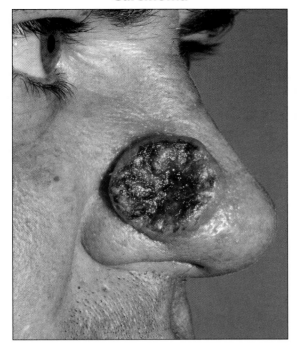

nature is more obvious when a deeper, ulcerated nodule develops. The clinical appearance of even the advanced SCC may not be sufficiently distinct from other, less common cutaneous malignancies; however, its localization in an area of sun-damaged skin or in an area of old burn injury or radiation dermatitis leads one to suspect the diagnosis.

Differential Diagnosis

SCC that is in situ can resemble actinic keratosis, eczema, dermatophytosis or, in the perineum, extramammary Paget's disease. Invasive SCC must be differentiated from actinic keratosis, keratoacanthoma, granulomas, and a wide variety of benign and malignant, primary and metastatic, cutaneous tumors.

Management and Therapy

The modalities and the criteria for selection used in the treatment of BCC are also used for SCC. The prognosis for SCC of the skin is good. Five-year cures are greater than 90% overall, although rates for larger and more deeply invasive tumors are lower. Metastases are not rare, approaching 3% to 4%. Tumors on the ears and lips, and those that develop in thermal burn or radiation treatment sites are particularly likely to metastasize.

MELANOMAS
Etiology and Pathogenesis

Melanomas develop in fair-skinned people most frequently; they are unusual in dark-skinned people. In 1% to 6% of cases, there is a familial history. Patients with large numbers of nevocellular nevi may have an increased risk, especially if some of those nevi are dysplastic). Melanomas develop in normal-appearing skin most often, but may evolve from a preexisting nevus of either the congenital or acquired type. History of perceptible change in any pigmented lesion is of paramount importance. Although there is an association between melanomas and sun exposure, it is quite common for melanomas to develop on relatively sun-protected sites; head and neck, torso, and upper and lower extremities are all common sites. Usually, they first appear as nonpalpable, pigmented lesions. Their innocuous appearance and small size cause them to be overlooked or thought of as a "mole" or "age spot." They expand laterally at the dermal-epidermal junction, and increasing diameter or perimeter irregularities prompt the patient or the physician to be suspicious. Eventually they change from macular, nonpalpable, lesions to nodular lesions.

Clinical Presentation

On examination, one usually sees a pigmented lesion with color that may vary from light brown to black, but areas of red or white are not rare (Figure

Figure 69-4   Melanoma

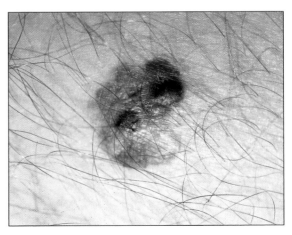

69-4). The size of the lesion can vary from a few millimeters to several centimeters and borders are usually irregular and indistinct. Ulceration is a late change. The natural variation in the appearance of benign, nevocellular nevi makes the diagnosis difficult.

Several tools have been developed recently to more precisely define melanomas. Epiluminescence is the use of an illuminated magnifying lens to examine lesions for subtle variations in pigment pattern, which might indicate malignancy. Digital epiluminescence microscopy is available to store and compare images of suspicious lesions. Ultimately, the diagnosis is made histopathologically after a biopsy specimen is taken. Incisional biopsy of a portion of a melanoma does not predispose to metastasis or worsen prognosis; however, it is important to get a representative specimen to make a diagnosis and aid in prognosis. A "shave biopsy" should not be done for it may not provide the opportunity to assess the depth of invasion of the melanoma. The dermatopathologist will make the diagnosis of melanoma and assess a level of invasion. A number of subclassifications exist, with corresponding histopathologic and clinical features: lentigo maligna melanoma, nodular melanoma, superficial spreading melanoma, acral lentiginous melanoma, and desmoplastic melanoma. These classifications are less important than the level of invasion in planning treatment and making a prognosis.

Differential Diagnosis

Melanoma most often must be differentiated from benign, congenital, or dysplastic nevi; seborrheic keratosis; tattoo; foreign body; or in the case of amelanotic melanoma, pyogenic granuloma.

Management and Therapy

The treatment of melanomas is surgical. The extent of surgery depends on the location, size, and depth of invasion of the melanoma. A microstaging is done at biopsy to determine the histopathologic level of invasion, measured in millimeters (Breslow levels). The Breslow level is the single most important predictor of survival for patients with melanoma. Patients with tumors less than 0.76 mm thick have a 96% 5-year survival rate, while patients with tumors greater than 4 mm have a 47% chance of 5-year survival. Larger melanomas, deeper melanomas, and melanomas on the head, neck, hands and feet require wider margins of excision. The Breslow level determines the margin of excision: in general, tumors with levels less than 2 mm are excised with 1.0 to 1.5 cm margins of clinically normal skin; tumors with levels of 2 to 4 mm are excised with 2.0 to 2.5 cm margins. Elective lymph node dissection for patients with melanoma confined to the skin has not been shown to improve survival. It may improve survival if there are clinically involved regional lymph nodes. Sentinel lymph node biopsy uses lymphoscintigraphy to determine the first ("sentinel") node in a regional basin with subsequent biopsy of that node to search for metastatic foci. This may be a useful staging procedure but imparts no survival benefit for the patient and is not the standard of care. Interferon-alfa-2b for patients with metastatic disease has been approved by the FDA, although no statistically significant benefit has been demonstrated in prospective trials. Numerous tumor vaccine therapy trials are ongoing.

Follow-Up Care

Patients who have had a BCC or an SCC should be observed for 5 years with routine skin examinations and palpation for lymph nodes to check for recurrence of the tumors as well as surveillance for the development of new, primary cutaneous malignancies. Approximately 30% to 50% of patients with skin cancer experience another, separate skin cancer within a few years. The frequency of the follow-up examinations varies depending on the character of the initial tumor and the level of sun damage, and precancerous change.

Patients who have had a melanoma should undergo lifelong follow-up to check for recurrence or the development of second primary melanomas, which may occur in as many as 5% of patients. Initially check-up visits should be no longer than every 6 months, extending to 12 months in later postoperative years. Patients with a family history of melanoma and dysplastic nevi should be observed more closely. Screening for occult metastases from early melanomas is generally not warranted.

All patients should be educated about the risks of sun exposure, and the use of sunscreens that have sun protection factor of 15 or higher and provide ultraviolet A and ultraviolet B protection. Instruction in self-examination should also be a routine part of follow-up care.

FUTURE DIRECTIONS

While the principal treatment for all skin cancers remains surgical ablation, several new treatment modalities are under investigation. Photodynamic therapy uses a systemic or topical application of a photosensitizing chemical followed by intense or laser light to the area to bring about a more or less selective destruction of the tumor tissue with relative sparing of adjacent tissue. Immunomodulators are currently under investigation. Imidazoquinolin, a heterocyclic amine, has shown potent antiviral and antitumor action both experimentally and in recent clinical trials.

REFERENCES

Balch CM, Soong SJ, Bartolucci AA, et al. Efficacy of an elective regional lymph node dissection of 1 to 4 mm thick melanomas for patients 60 years of age and younger. *Ann Surg.* 1996;224:255-266.

Buzaid AC, Ross MI, Balch CM, et al. Critical analysis of the current American Joint Committee on Cancer staging system for cutaneous melanoma and proposal of a new staging system. *J Clin Oncol.* 1997;15:1039-1051.

National Institutes of Health Consensus Development Conference Statement on Diagnosis and Treatment of Early Melanoma, January 27-29, 1992. *Am J Dermatopathol.* 1993;15:34-43.

Kanzler MH, Mraz-Gernhard S. Treatment of primary cutaneous melanoma. *JAMA.* 2001;285:1819-1821.

MEDLINEplus Health Information Web site. Skin cancer. 2002. Available at: http://www.nlm.nih.gov/medlineplus/skincancer.html. Accessed December 14, 2002.

Randle HW. Basal cell carcinoma. Identification and treatment of the high-risk patient. *Dermatol Surg.* 1996;22:255-261.

The Skin Cancer Foundation Web site. Available at: http://www.skincancer.org. Accessed December 15, 2002.

Szepietowski JC, Salomon J. Typical and atypical locations of basal cell carcinoma: relationship with clinical and histological types. *Skin Cancer.* 2000;15:193-198.

Chapter 70

Upper Gastrointestinal Tract Cancer

Mark Taylor and Robert S. Webhie

Cancer of the stomach is second only to lung carcinoma in incidence, with over 750,000 new cases diagnosed worldwide each year. Incidence is highest in the Russian Federation and Japan. In the US, there were an estimated 21,900 new cases and 13,500 deaths in 1999. This represents a dramatic decline in the past 7 decades.

Tumors of the esophagus account for 4% of malignancies and 3% of cancer deaths worldwide. Prevalence is highest in South Africa, China, Southern Asia, Iran, and France. In the United States, it accounts for 5.5% of malignancies and 3% of cancer deaths and is more common in metropolitan areas such as New York; Washington, DC; and Los Angeles. There has been a decline in proximal squamous cell carcinoma (SCC) of the esophagus and distal adenocarcinoma of the stomach, whereas incidence of distal esophageal adenocarcinoma and proximal gastric carcinoma has increased. Upper gastrointestinal cancers are 2 to 3 times more common in men than in women. SCC of the esophagus is 4 to 5 times more common in African Americans; adenocarcinoma is more prevalent in the white population.

ETIOLOGY AND PATHOGENESIS

Most (95%) gastric carcinomas are either intestinal or diffuse type adenocarcinomas (Figure 70-1). Diffuse type has a poorer prognosis. Gastric adenocarcinomas are further classified by macroscopic appearance as fungating, ulcerated, ulcerated with infiltration, diffusely infiltrating (linitis plastica) (Figure 70-1), or unclassifiable. SCC is located most frequently in the upper two thirds of the esophagus (Figure 70-2) adenocarcinoma in the distal third (Figure 70-3). Until recently, SCC was the most common pathology in the United States, but there has been an increase in adenocarcinoma, making it the most common histological subtype since 1994. SCC remains the most common histological type worldwide.

Environmental and genetic factors both play a role in development (Table 70-1). Migrants from high-risk areas who move to low-risk areas have an intermediate risk for development of cancer, as do their subsequent generations. *Helicobacter pylori* infection is associated with a three- to six-fold increase in the risk of developing distal intestinal type adenocarcinoma, although its exact role in the development of carcinoma is unknown. For SCC of the esophagus, the most significant risk factors are alcohol consumption and tobacco use, which act independently as well as synergistically. Patients with upper aerodigestive tract tumors have a 4% to 7% risk per year of esophageal cancer, suggesting a field effect of the aforementioned agents. Risk factors for adenocarcinoma are not as well defined, however. The presence of Barrett's esophagus is associated with a 30- to 40-fold increase in risk.

PROGNOSIS

The most important prognostic factor is stage at presentation. Tumor staging is based on the depth of invasion, lymph node involvement, and presence of metastasis. In gastric cancer, both depth of invasion and the number of lymph nodes involved significantly alter prognosis (Table 70-2). Adverse prognostic factors include advancing age, linitis plastica type, aneuploidy, and tumors of the gastric cardia or the gastroesophageal junction. Metastatic disease is essentially incurable; the median survival time for both gastric and esophageal cancer is less than 1 year.

The prognosis for esophageal cancer is poor regardless of stage. There appears to be no difference in prognosis between adenocarcinoma and SCC; however, 5-year survival rates are approaching 40% because of improvements in surgical techniques and combined modality therapy. Several factors may account for the poor prognosis

Figure 70-1

Carcinoma of the Stomach

Polypoid Adenocarcinoma

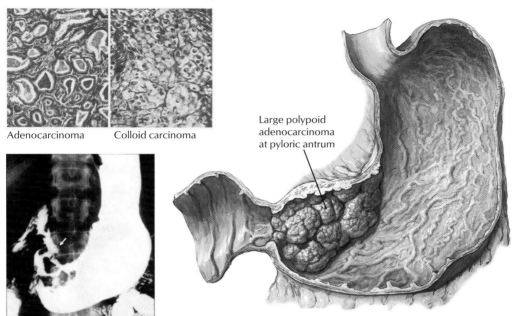

Adenocarcinoma   Colloid carcinoma

Radiographic appearance of
polypoid adenocarcinoma

Large polypoid
adenocarcinoma
at pyloric antrum

Scirrhous Carcinoma

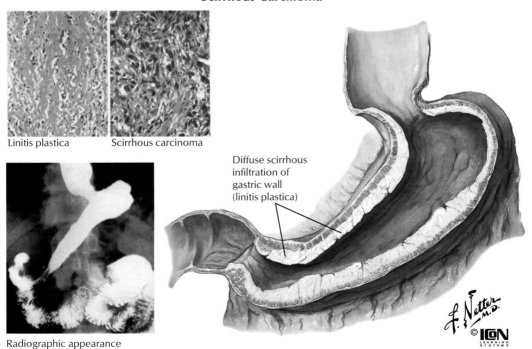

Linitis plastica   Scirrhous carcinoma

Diffuse scirrhous
infiltration of
gastric wall
(linitis plastica)

Radiographic appearance
of linitis plastica

Figure 70-2 **Carcinoma of the Upper Part of Esophagus**

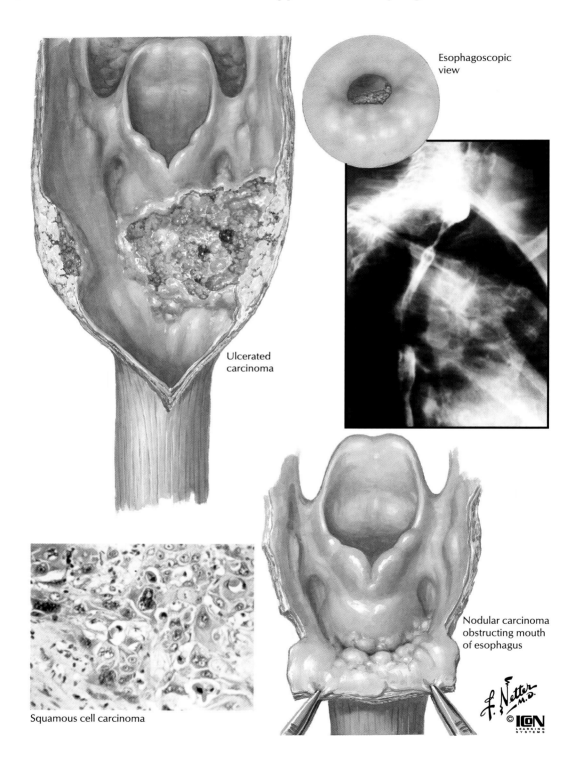

Esophagoscopic view

Ulcerated carcinoma

Nodular carcinoma obstructing mouth of esophagus

Squamous cell carcinoma

Figure 70-3

Malignant Tumors of Midportion of Esophagus

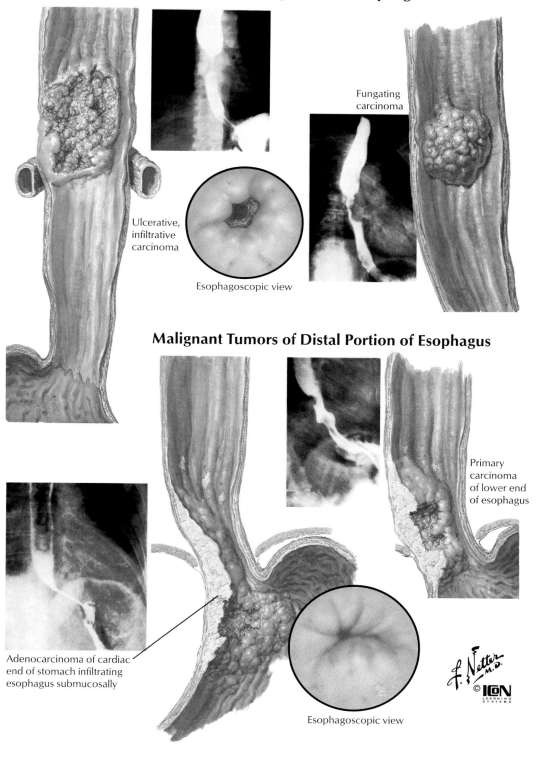

Fungating carcinoma

Ulcerative, infiltrative carcinoma

Esophagoscopic view

Malignant Tumors of Distal Portion of Esophagus

Primary carcinoma of lower end of esophagus

Adenocarcinoma of cardiac end of stomach infiltrating esophagus submucosally

Esophagoscopic view

Table 70-1
Risk Factors

Gastric Cancer	Esophageal Cancer (SCC)
Nutritional Factors	
High salt consumption	Alcohol
High nitrate consumption	
Low dietary vitamin A and C	
Lack of refrigeration	
Exposure	
Rubber workers	Smoking
Coal workers	Lye ingestion
Helicobacter pylori infection	Human papilloma virus infection
Epstein-Barr virus infection	
Radiation exposure	
Prior gastric surgery for benign disease	
Genetic Factors	
Type A blood	Tylosis Autosomal dominant condition manifest by hyperkeratosis of palms and soles
Pernicious anemia	Plummer-Vinson syndrome Esophageal webs and iron deficiency anemia
Hereditary nonpolyposis colon cancer	
Li-Fraumeni syndrome	
Autosomal dominant syndrome involving p53 tumor suppressor gene mutation associated with soft tissue sarcoma, breast, osteosarcoma, brain tumors, adrenal cortical tumors, acute leukemia	
Family history	
Preexisting Conditions	
Adenomatous gastric polyps	Achalasia
Chronic atrophic gastritis	Celiac sprue
Dysplasia	Other aerodigestive cancer
Intestinal metaplasia	Barrett's esophagus (adenocarcinoma)
Ménétrier's disease Poorly outlined disease, diagnosed in patients with giant gastric folds, dyspeptic symptoms, and hypoalbuminemia due to gastrointestinal protein loss; the etiology is unknown	
Gastric ulcers	

Adapted from Karpeh M, Kelsen DP, et al as in DeVita VT, Hellman S, et al. *Cancer Principles and Practice of Oncology*, 6th ed. Philadelphia, Pa: Lippincott, Williams & Wilkins, 2001:1092–1126.

Table 70-2
Five-Year Survival Rates in Gastric Cancer

	% 5-year Survival Rates			
T Stage	Invading lamina propria/submucosa	Invading muscularis propria	Invading adventitia	Invading adjacent structures
	85% – 95%	50% – 80%	25% – 40%	5% – 25%
N Stage	No regional lymph node metastasis	1-6 positive nodes	7-15 positive nodes	>15 positive nodes
	80% – 85%	50% – 60%	25% – 30%	10%

Adapted from Karpeh M, Kelsen DP, et al as in DeVita VT, Hellman S, et al. *Cancer Principles and Practice of Oncology*, 6th ed. Philadelphia, Pa: Lippincott, Williams & Wilkins, 2001:1092–1126.

of esophageal cancer. Most importantly, the esophagus is a distensible organ, allowing for primary tumors to grow quite large before causing symptoms. The average patient has symptoms for 3 to 6 months before presentation. This delay results in approximately 50% of patients presenting with locally advanced or metastatic disease. Anatomy also plays a role. The esophagus has an exceptionally rich lymphatic and venous drainage system leading to a high rate of distant failure, even in disease initially thought to be curable. The size of the tumor correlates with risk for distant disease; tumors <5 cm are localized 65% of the time whereas tumors >5 cm are localized only 25% of the time.

CLINICAL PRESENTATION

Gastric carcinoma presents most commonly with vague abdominal symptoms (anorexia, abdominal discomfort, nausea and vomiting, melena, and weakness) that are not clearly attributable to carcinoma; therefore, most gastric cancers are not diagnosed until the disease is advanced. Early satiety, a classic but not usually observed (20%), is the symptom [most common] associated with diffusely infiltrating carcinoma (Figure 70-1). Weight loss, seen in more than 80% of patients, is associated with poorer survival. Often, symptoms attributable to metastatic disease including jaundice from biliary obstruction, abdominal swelling from ascites, abdominal pain from metastatic disease, or direct extension into adjacent organs are found at presentation (Figure 70-4).

In carcinoma of the esophagus, progressive dysphagia is present in 90% of patients. Dysphagia for solids precedes that for liquids. Typically, patients give a history of symptoms for 3 to 6 months before seeking medical attention. Weight loss is common and symptoms can include cough or pneumonia from tracheoesophageal fistulas, chest pain from invasion of mediastinal structures, hoarseness from recurrent laryngeal nerve palsy, odynophagia, and hematemesis from tumor bleeding.

DIFFERENTIAL DIAGNOSIS

Other histological types of cancers include small cell carcinoma, melanoma, lymphoma, and sarcomas. Gastrointestinal stromal tumors (GIST) are seen in the stomach as well. Metastatic disease to the esophagus is unusual but can be seen with breast, lung, or ovarian carcinoma; lymphoma; and melanoma. More commonly, the esophagus is involved by direct extension of the tumor originating in adjacent organs. The symptoms of upper gastrointestinal cancers can be nonspecific, so cancer should be suspected with dysphagia or abdominal pain, especially when associated with weight loss.

DIAGNOSTIC APPROACH

The diagnosis and staging of gastric and esophageal carcinoma are similar. Until recently, double-contrast barium swallow followed by endoscopy for pathologic confirmation was the mainstay of diagnosis. Many patients are now diagnosed via initial endoscopy. For esophageal cancer, CT of the chest and upper abdomen is performed to evaluate for metastatic disease and gross invasion of local structures that may preclude surgery. Gastric cancer is evaluated by abdominal CT and a chest

Figure 70-4

Carcinoma of Stomach

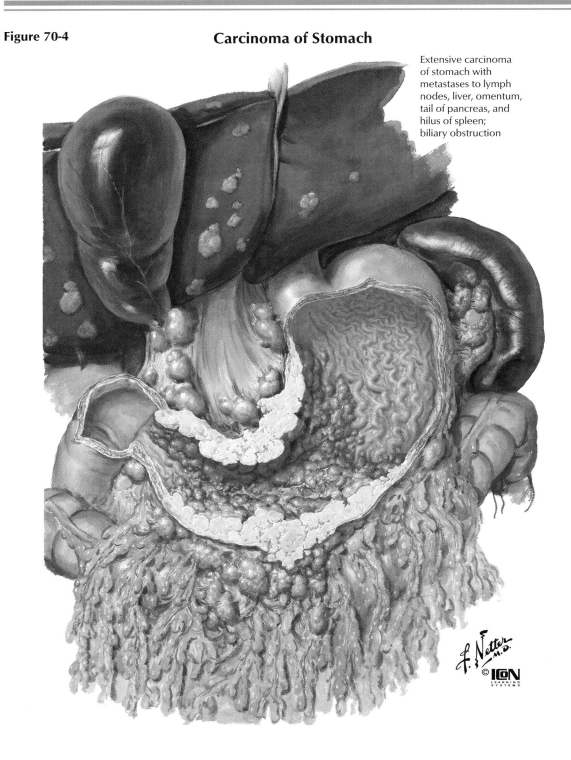

Extensive carcinoma
of stomach with
metastases to lymph
nodes, liver, omentum,
tail of pancreas, and
hilus of spleen;
biliary obstruction

radiograph. A CT of the chest should be obtained for tumors in the gastric cardia or those extending into the esophagus. CT is insensitive for evaluation of lymph node involvement. There is enthusiasm for using endoscopic ultrasound to evaluate the depth of tumor invasion and lymph node involvement to provide more accurate staging. Diagnostic laparoscopy at surgery is used to evaluate for disease commonly missed by CT (serosal liver metastasis and peritoneal disease) and for more accurate assessment of gross invasion by the primary tumor. For tumors of the upper and mid esophagus, a bronchoscopy is performed before surgery to evaluate for tracheobronchial fistula and for concurrent bronchial lesions.

MANAGEMENT AND THERAPY
Surgery
Gastric Cancer

Localized gastric cancer is treated with the intent to cure with a partial gastrectomy for distal tumors. A total gastrectomy is the standard for proximal gastric tumors or tumors of the gastroesophageal junction. There is controversy as to the extent of lymph node dissection required at the time of surgery. In Japan, a more extensive nodal dissection is performed with reports of better overall survival rates. In the United States and Europe, a more limited dissection is performed, as it is thought more extensive operations only add to morbidity. The difference in mortality rates has been attributed to more accurate staging with the Japanese procedure. Operative mortality is approximately 5% and long-term sequelae include dumping, heartburn, and reduced appetite. Gastric cancer can recur at the site of the initial tumor, local lymph nodes, in the peritoneal cavity, or distantly (usually to the liver or lungs).

Esophageal Cancer

Surgery should be considered in localized or regional spread disease that has not invaded essential structures. Patients must be fit enough to withstand the thoracotomy. Even with lymphatic spread, prolonged survival and relief of symptoms are best achieved if surgery is included in the therapy. The decision on surgical approach is based on location of the tumor and the surgeon's preference. Right thoracoabdominal (Ivor-Lewis), left thoracoabdominal, and transhiatal approaches are most common; morbidity and mortality rates are similar. Prognosis is related to tumor stage, not type of procedure performed. Long-term survival after surgical resection ranges from 10% to 30% in most series. Most recurrences occur at the site of the initial tumor, but metastatic recurrence is seen most commonly in the liver and lungs.

Radiation Therapy and Chemotherapy

As primary treatments, radiation therapy and chemotherapy are inferior to surgical resection or chemoradiation therapy. Chemotherapy or radiation therapy alone given before (neoadjuvant) or after (adjuvant) surgery has not shown a survival advantage. Use of these modalities in this setting should be reserved for clinical trials.

In esophageal cancer, the combination of cisplatin and 5-fluorouracil (5-FU) in conjunction with radiation given before surgery has improved local failure rates, median survival, and 5-year survival rates. The benefit of combined modality treatment comes at the expense of significantly increased toxicity. It is unknown whether chemoradiation therapy alone is equivalent to surgery in esophageal cancer. Combination therapy is an appropriate alternative that provides a chance for long-term disease-free survival for patients who are not deemed surgical candidates.

Recent consideration has been given for treating carcinomas of the cardia as adenocarcinoma of the esophagus. The rationale is the similarity in epidemiology, genetic abnormalities, prognosis of these malignancies, and the frequency at which gastric carcinoma invades submucosally into the distal esophagus. Chemoradiation therapy may provide a survival benefit after surgical resection in patients with close surgical margins, gross residual disease, or node positive disease.

Palliative Treatment

Dysphagia is the main symptom requiring palliation in esophageal carcinoma. Intubation with stents, laser ablation, photodynamic therapy, or alcohol injection can be effective. Obstruction or major bleeding can occur in both gastric and esophageal carcinoma and may necessitate palliative resection or radiation.

Agents that have activity against gastric carcinoma include 5-FU, doxorubicin, cisplatin, methotrexate, mitomycin C, and nitrosourea. In western countries, most regimens include 5-FU and most have failed to show any survival benefit. Cisplatin or 5-FU based regimens have been the basis for treatment in the United States. In Japan, mitomycin C is used more frequently and may provide a small survival benefit in that population.

Combination chemotherapy may enhance survival and improve quality of life in patients with systemic disease, although the median survival time remains at 8 months. Cisplatin-based regimens usually in combination with 5-FU are the mainstay of therapy in esophageal carcinoma.

In both gastric and esophageal cancer, management of pain is a significant issue that may benefit from analgesics or radiation therapy. Attention to nutritional support must not be overlooked and can include supplements, or placement of a gastric or an enteral feeding tube.

Screening and Follow-up

In the United States, routine screening with upper endoscopy is not advocated for upper gastrointestinal tract cancer. In high-risk regions of the world, such as Japan, screening programs have resulted in the diagnosis of earlier stage cancers, which has translated into reduced gastric cancer mortality rates. It is currently recommended that those with Barrett's metaplasia undergo screening endoscopy with biopsy every 2 years. If high-grade dysplasia is found, management is controversial. Some advocate immediate esophagectomy because it is believed that this condition invariably progresses to adenocarcinoma; however, the time of progression is unknown. Others advocate delaying surgery in favor of frequent screening until adenocarcinoma is detected. There is no evidence that treatment of gastroesophageal reflux disease reduces the incidence of adenocarcinoma.

After initial treatment of gastric cancer, current guidelines recommend follow-up every 3 months for the first year and then every 6 months until 5 years. Complete blood count, liver chemistries, and chest radiographs are often obtained every 6 months for 3 years; further imaging is based on symptoms. Monthly vitamin B12 injections are needed if a total gastrectomy was performed. Follow-up evaluations of esophageal cancer should be monthly for the first year, biannually for the following 2 years, and then annually. Recommended radiographic and blood work evaluations are similar to those for gastric cancer.

FUTURE DIRECTIONS

Despite improvements in survival over the past few decades, the prognosis of upper GI tract malignancies remains poor. New agents under investigation include paclitaxel, docetaxel, capecitabine, vinorelbine, and irinotecan. Optimum timing of radiation, chemotherapy, and surgery has yet to be fully answered and await results of clinical trials. For gastric cancer, chemotherapy delivered directly into the peritoneal cavity holds promise. To date, there has been a reduction in peritoneal relapse but no survival advantage to this approach; clinical trials are ongoing.

Identifying patients who may benefit from treatment remains a challenging task. More accurate means of staging are being evaluated. The role of newer imaging modalities, such as positron emission tomography, is being investigated. Molecular genetics may provide prognostic information as well as potential targets for new biologic agents. The need for improvement in current therapies for upper gastrointestinal tract cancers stresses the importance of enrolling patients in clinical trials.

REFERENCES

Gunderson LL, Donohue JH, Burch PA. Chapter 60 - Stomach. pp 1545-1585. In: Abeloff MD, Armitage JO, Lichter AS, Niederhuber JE, eds. *Clinical Oncology*. 2nd ed. New York, NY: Churchill Livingstone; 2000.

Hietmiller RF, Forastiere AA, Kleinberg LR. Chapter 59 - Esophagus. pp 1517-1544. In: Abeloff MD, Armitage JO, Lichter AS, Niederhuber JE, eds. *Clinical Oncology*. 2nd ed. New York, NY: Churchill Livingstone; 2000.

Karpeh M, Kelsen DP, Tepper JE. Chapter 33.3 - Cancer of the stomach. pp 1092-1126. In: DeVita VT Jr, Hellman S, Rosenberg SA, eds. *Cancer Principles & Practice of Oncology*. 6th ed. Philadelphia, Pa: Lippincott Williams & Wilkins; 2001.

Landis SH, Murray T. Bolden S, Wingo PA. Cancer statistics, 1999. *CA Cancer J Clin*. 1999;49:8-31.

Shrump DS, Altorki NK, Forastiere AA, Minsky BD. Chapter 33.2 - Cancer of the esophagus. pp 1051-1091. In: DeVita VT Jr, Hellman S, Rosenberg SA, eds. *Cancer Principles & Practice of Oncology*. 6th ed. Philadelphia, Pa: Lippincott Williams & Wilkins; 2001.

Section IX
INFECTIOUS DISEASES

Chapter 71
Endocarditis

Kristine B. Patterson, Cam Patterson, and Meera K. Kelley

Infective endocarditis (IE) is an infection of the endocardial surface of the heart and implies the presence of microorganisms in the lesion. Despite advances in antimicrobial therapy, IE continues to be associated with high morbidity and mortality. Early diagnosis, prompt and appropriate antimicrobial therapy, and timely surgical intervention are cornerstones of successful management. Annually, 10,000 to 15,000 new cases of IE are diagnosed. Congenital heart disease underlies 6% to 24% of the cases. The mitral valve is most commonly involved, followed by the aortic valve. Degenerative aortic valve disease and mitral valve prolapse with regurgitation are the leading predisposing factors. The tricuspid and pulmonic valves are rarely involved, except in injection drug users. In addition, increasing numbers of hospital-acquired infections due to central venous catheter use, pacemakers, and other forms of parenteral access have resulted in an increased incidence of IE in susceptible individuals. (Figure 71-1)

ETIOLOGY AND PATHOGENESIS

Typically, IE occurs in the setting of a previously damaged valve surface, which provides a suitable site for bacterial colonization. Bacteria then reach the site, adhering to the lesion. After colonizing the valve, bacteria replicate to a critical mass, in turn allowing a mature infected vegetation to form.

IE stimulates humoral and cellular immune responses, as manifested by hypergammaglobulinemia, splenomegaly, and monocytosis. Circulating immune complexes, found in virtually all patients, may cause extravalvular manifestations and hypocomplementemia. Glomerulonephritis and peripheral manifestations, such as Osler's nodes may develop, as can rheumatoid factor and antinuclear antibodies.

CLINICAL PRESENTATION

Any organ system can be involved in patients with IE, and thus the clinical presentation is highly variable. Four processes contribute to the clinical manifestations of IE: 1) the infectious process on the valve, including local intracardiac complications (Figure 71-2); 2) embolization to any organ; 3) bacteremic seeding of remote sites; and 4) circulating immune complexes. Fever is the most common sign and symptom. Heart murmurs are present in over 85% of patients, but may be absent, particularly in right-sided disease. The classic changing murmur is uncommon. Valve destruction or rupture of chordae tendineae may alter auscultatory findings and result in congestive heart failure (CHF). Peripheral manifestations, including Roth's spots, Janeway lesions, Osler's nodes, splinter hemorrhages, petechiae, and clubbing, are found in 50% of cases and are associated with untreated IE of long duration. Splenomegaly is common. Musculoskeletal manifestations include low back pain, arthralgias, arthritis, and diffuse myalgias. Clinical findings of systemic emboli are unique to the organ involved. Central nervous system injury occurs in 20% to 40% of patients and is associated with increased mortality. Although embolic stroke is most common, other CNS complications include rupture of mycotic aneurysm, seizures, cranial nerve palsies, cerebritis, and microabscesses (Figure 71-3).

DIAGNOSTIC APPROACH

The diagnosis of IE is based on microbiological and echocardiographic findings. Several nonspecific laboratory studies may be suggestive of IE. These include: anemia, thrombocytopenia, leukocytosis, an elevated sedimentation rate, hypergammaglobulinemia, positive rheumatoid factor, hypocomplementemia, false-positive Venereal Disease Research Laboratory (VDRL) test results, and false-positive Lyme disease serology. Blood cultures are the most important laboratory test. At least 3 sets of blood cultures should be obtained during the first 24 hours of observation. More cultures may be necessary if the patient has received antibiotics in the preceding weeks. Almost 50% of culture-negative IE can be attributed to antibiotic

Figure 71-1 ## Common Portals of Bacterial Entry in Bacterial Endocarditis

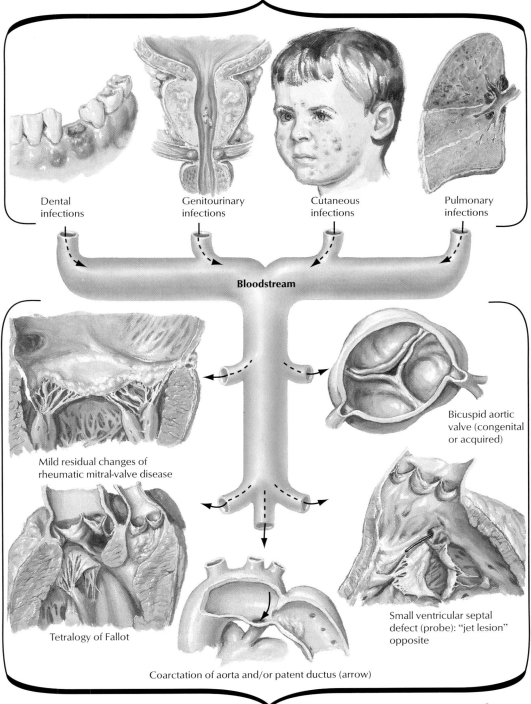

Dental
infections

Genitourinary
infections

Cutaneous
infections

Pulmonary
infections

Bloodstream

Mild residual changes of
rheumatic mitral-valve disease

Bicuspid aortic
valve (congenital
or acquired)

Tetralogy of Fallot

Small ventricular septal
defect (probe): "jet lesion"
opposite

Coarctation of aorta and/or patent ductus (arrow)

Common Predisposing Lesions

use before obtaining cultures. Organisms, such as the HACEK group and *Brucella*, are slow growing and require extended incubation of cultures (4 weeks). Special culture techniques or media may be required for some organisms (e.g., *Legionella*). Blood culture results are negative in more than 50% of fungal endocarditis cases. Serological studies are necessary to diagnose Q fever, brucellosis, legionellosis, and psittacosis.

Echocardiography should be performed in all patients. Transthoracic echocardiography (TTE) is rapid, noninvasive, and has excellent specificity for vegetations (98%); however, sensitivity is less than 60%. Transesophageal echocardiography (TEE) allows imaging of very small vegetations and is the procedure of choice for assessing the pulmonic valve, prosthetic valves and the perivalvular areas for abscesses. TEE has a substantially higher sensitivity (76% to 100%) and specificity (94%) than TTE for perivalvular extension of infection. If clinical suspicion of IE persists after an initially negative TEE, a repeat study is warranted within 7 to 10 days. The combination of a negative TEE and a negative TTE confers a 95% negative predictive value.

Streptococcal Endocarditis

Streptococci are the most common causative agents of IE, with the viridans streptococci the most common subgroup. The cure rate of nonenterococcal streptococcal IE exceeds 90%, but complications are seen in approximately 30% of cases.

Enterococcal endocarditis usually affects older men after genitourinary tract manipulation or younger women after an obstetrical procedure. Treatment is difficult because classic peripheral manifestations are uncommon.

Streptococcus pneumoniae IE is rare, however it frequently has a fulminant course and is often associated with perivalvular abscess and pericarditis as well as concurrent meningitis. The aortic valve is typically involved. Patients frequently have a history of alcohol abuse.

IE due to nutritionally variant streptococci typically is indolent in onset and associated with previous heart disease. Therapy is difficult because of systemic embolization and frequent relapse.

Staphylococcal Endocarditis

Staphylococci are the second most common cause of IE. *Staphylococcus aureus* is the most common cause of native valve IE, and may also affect prosthetic valves. The course is typically fulminant with widespread metastatic infection. Myocardial and valve-ring abscesses and peripheral foci of suppuration are common. Thirty percent of patients experience neurologic manifestations. IE caused by methicillin-resistant *S. aureus* is particularly common in injection drug users or patients with nosocomial infection. Coagulase-negative staphylococci are an important cause of prosthetic valve endocarditis (PVE), and are less common but recognized to cause native valve endocarditis.

Gram-negative Endocarditis

Persons addicted to narcotics, prosthetic valve recipients, and patients with cirrhosis are at increased risk for gram negative bacillary endocarditis.

Salmonella species are associated with valvular destruction, atrial thrombi, myocarditis, and pericarditis.

Pseudomonas species are usually seen in injection drug users and often affect normal valves. Embolic phenomena, inability to sterilize valves, neurological complications, ring and annular abscesses, splenic abscesses, bacteremic relapses, and progressive heart failure are common.

Neisseria gonorrhoeae occasionally causes IE and typically follows an indolent course, with aortic valve involvement, large vegetations, valve-ring abscesses, CHF, and nephritis.

HACEK Endocarditis

The HACEK group of organisms includes *Haemophilus* species, *Actinobacillus actinomycetemcomitans*, *Cardiobacterium hominis*, *Eikenella corrodens*, and *Kingella* species. All are fastidious and may require 2 to 3 weeks for primary isolation. HACEK endocarditis is more common in patients who have dental infections or injection drug users who contaminate the injection with saliva.

Fungal Endocarditis

Candida parapsilosis and *Candida tropicalis* predominate in injection drug users. *Aspergillus* species and *Candida albicans* predominate in non-injection drug users. Blood culture results are usually negative in *Aspergillus* IE. Prognosis is poor and surgical intervention is usually required.

Table 71-1
Antimicrobial Therapy for Infective Endocarditis*

Etiology	Antimicrobial Therapy
Viridans Streptococci and Streptococcus bovis penicillin-susceptible (MIC < 0.2 ug/mL):	Penicillin G 12–18 million U/24 hrs IV in 6 doses** for 4 wks OR Ceftriaxone 2 g IV once daily for 4 wks. OR Penicillin G 12–18 million U/24 hrs IV in 6 doses** for 2 wks WITH gentamicin 1mg/kg IV every 8 hrs for 2 wks.†† OR Vancomycin 30mg/kg/24 hrs IV in two divided doses for 4 wks. (Recommended only for patients allergic to β-lactams.)
Viridans Streptococci and Streptococcus bovis relatively resistant to penicillin (MIC 0.1–0.5 µg/mL):	Penicillin G 18 million U/24 hrs IV continuously or 6 doses for 4 wks WITH Gentamicin 1mg/kg IV every 8 hrs for 2 wks. (First-generation cephalosporins may be substituted for penicillin in patients with penicillin hypersensitivity not of the immediate type.) OR Vancomycin 30 mg/kg/24 hrs IV in two divided doses for 4 wks. (Only recommended for patients allergic to β-lactams.)
Enterococci (and viridans streptococci with penicillin MIC > 0.5 ug/mL, nutrient variant viridans streptococci):	Penicillin G 12-18 million U/24 hrs IV in 6 doses WITH gentamicin 1mg/kg IV every 8 hrs for 4–6 wks. OR Ampicillin 12 g/24 hrs in six doses WITH gentamicin 1 mg/kg IV every 8 hrs for 4–6 wks. OR Vancomycin 30mg/kg/24 hr IV in two divided doses for 4–6 wks WITH gentamicin 1 mg/kg IV every 8 hrs†† for 4–6 wks. (Only recommended for patients allergic to β-lactams; cephalosporins are not acceptable alternatives for patients allergic to penicillins.)†
Staphylococci (penicillin-susceptible):	Penicillin G 20 million U/24 hrs IV in six doses for 4–6 wks.**
Staphylococci (methicillin-susceptible, penicillin-resistant):	Nafcillin (or oxacillin) 2 g IV every 4 hrs** for 4-6 wks WITH gentamicin 1 mg/kg IV†† every 8 hr for 3–5 d.** OR Cefazolin (or other first generation cephalosporin) 2 g IV every 8 hr for 4–6 wks WITH gentamicin 1 mg/kg IV every 8 hrs** for 3–5 d.
Staphylococci (methicillin-resistant):	Vancomycin 30 mg/kg/24 hr IV in two divided doses for 4–6 wks.
HACEK microorganisms:	Ceftriaxone 2 g once daily IV for 4 wks. OR Ampicillin 2 g every 4 hrs or 12 g/24hrs I0V continuously WITH gentamicin 1 mg/kg IV every 8 hrs for 4 wks.

* Antibiotic dosages for adults patients with normal renal and hepatic function.

† Test infecting strain of Enterococcus for resistance to aminoglycosides. High-level resistance means loss of synergy and thus aminoglycosides should not be used in these instances. Therapy should be prolonged to 8–12 wk.

** Dosing of penicillin, nafcillin, and oxacillin is quite frequent and often problematic for home therapy patients. Because these drugs are stable for 24 hr at room temperature, they may be given via a pump that remains with patient, requiring adjustment only once every 24 hr.

†† Aminoglycosides are used for synergy for gram-positive infections. Requires continuous therapy.

Figure 71-2

Bacterial Endocarditis

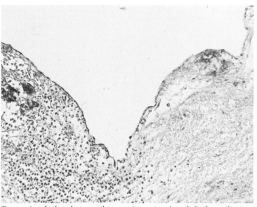

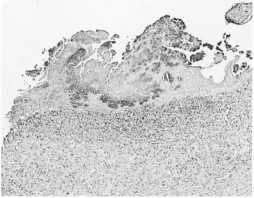

Deposit of platelets and organisms (stained dark), edema, and leukocytic infiltration in very early bacterial endocarditis of aortic valve

Development of vegetations containing clumps of bacteria on tricuspid valve

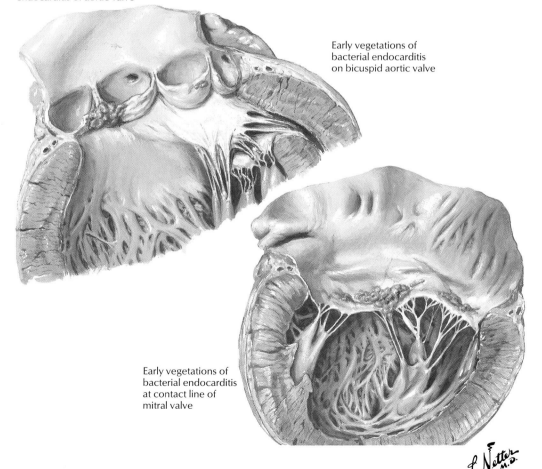

Early vegetations of bacterial endocarditis on bicuspid aortic valve

Early vegetations of bacterial endocarditis at contact line of mitral valve

Figure 71-3

Bacterial Endocarditis: Remote Embolic Effects

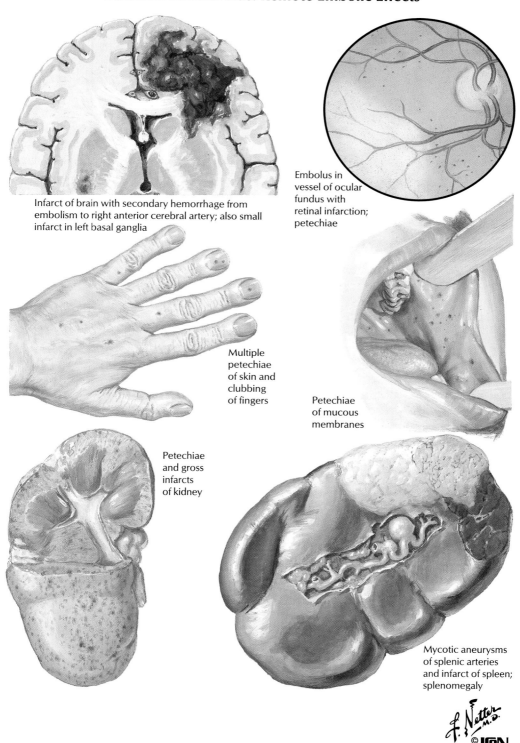

Infarct of brain with secondary hemorrhage from embolism to right anterior cerebral artery; also small infarct in left basal ganglia

Embolus in vessel of ocular fundus with retinal infarction; petechiae

Multiple petechiae of skin and clubbing of fingers

Petechiae of mucous membranes

Petechiae and gross infarcts of kidney

Mycotic aneurysms of splenic arteries and infarct of spleen; splenomegaly

Culture-negative Endocarditis

Culture-negative IE is common. Causes include recent administration of antimicrobial agents; slow growth of fastidious organisms, such as the HACEK group; fungal endocarditis; intracellular parasites, such as *Bartonella* or *Chlamydia* species; and noninfectious endocarditis.

MANAGEMENT AND THERAPY
Antimicrobial Therapy

After initial empiric therapy, antimicrobial agents should be selected based on susceptibility testing of the isolated causative microbe (Table 71-1). Prolonged administration of antimicrobial agents is required, almost always via the parenteral route. Bactericidal agents or antibiotic combinations that produce synergistic, rapidly bactericidal effects are the agents of choice. Serum concentrations must be closely monitored when using aminoglycosides. Blood culture specimens should be obtained early in therapy to ensure eradication of the bacteremia, and throughout therapy when persistent or recurrent fever is present. Patients with IE complicated by cardiac arrhythmias and CHF require close observation in an intensive care unit. Anticoagulation is contraindicated in patients with native valve IE.

Cardiac Surgery

Indications for surgery during active IE include:
- Refractory CHF
- More than 1 serious systemic embolic episode
- Uncontrolled infection
- Hemodynamically significant valve dysfunction
- Ineffective antimicrobial therapy
- Resection of mycotic aneurysms
- PVE caused by antibiotic-resistant pathogens
- Local suppurative complications including perivalvular or myocardial abscesses

Prosthetic Valve Endocarditis

PVE occurs in up to 10% of patients during the lifetime of the prosthesis. Early PVE (within 60 days after implantation) usually results from valve contamination during the perioperative period. Late PVE (after 60 days) results from transient bacteremia. Clinical manifestations are similar to those of native valve IE, however, new or changing murmurs are more common. Persistently positive blood culture results are the hallmark. TEE is recommended for diagnosis and assessment of complications such as perivalvular abscess, regurgitation, etc. Coagulase-negative staphylococci are the dominant cause of PVE in the first year. After 1 year, the causative organisms are similar to those of native valve IE. Therapy is, by necessity, aggressive. Rifampin and gentamicin can be added to nafcillin for methicillin-sensitive *S. aureus* or to vancomycin for methicillin-resistant *S. aureus*. For culture-negative PVE, use vancomycin and gentamicin provide broad bactericidal coverage.

Prophylaxis

Antimicrobial prophylaxis is recommended for patients with increased risk of endocarditis due to underlying cardiac conditions undergoing invasive procedures likely to generate bacteremia. Detailed prophylaxis recommendations are available at the American Heart Association Web site.

FUTURE DIRECTIONS

Some clinicians believe that the size of the vegetation and other echocardiographic characteristics predict who is at risk for poor outcome and needs early surgery. At the present time specific echocardiographic criteria have not been demonstrated. Future studies will help to determine whether echocardiographic findings other than perivalvular or myocardial abscesses are added to the current list of indications for surgery.

REFERENCES

Bayer AS, Bolger AF, Taubert KA, et al. Diagnosis and management of infective endocarditis and its complications. *Circulation*. 1998;98:2936–2948.

Berbari EF, Cockerill FR III, Steckelberg JM. Infective endocarditis due to unusual or fastidious microorganisms. *Mayo Clin Proc*. 1997;72:532–542.

Dajani AS, Taubert KA, Wilson W, et al. Prevention of bacterial endocarditis. Recommendations by the American Heart Association. *JAMA*. 1997;277:1794–1801.

Ellis M. Fungal endocarditis. *J Infect*. 1997;35:99-103.

Mandell GL, Bennett JE, Dolin R, eds. *Mandell, Douglas, and Bennett's Principles and Practice of Infectious Diseases*. 5th ed. New York, NY: Churchill Livingstone; 2000.

Root RK, Waldvogel F, Corey L, Stamm WE. *Clinical Infectious Disease – A Practical Approach*. New York, NY: Oxford University Press; 1999.

Schlant RC, Alexander RW, O'Rourke RA, Roberts R, Sonnenblick EH, eds. *Hurst's The Heart*. 10th ed. New York, NY: McGraw-Hill Inc; 2001.

Chapter 72

Fever of Unknown Origin

William C. Miller

Fever is common with many acute illnesses and usually resolves spontaneously or with treatment. However, persistent fever develops in certain patients without clear cause, posing a diagnostic challenge for their physicians.

Petersdorf and Beeson established the classic definition of fever of unknown origin (FUO). They defined FUO as: 1) illness of more than 3 weeks' duration, 2) fever of 38.3°C (101°F) on several occasions, and 3) diagnosis uncertain after 1 week of study in hospital. Although this definition of FUO has been very useful, changes in the practice of medicine have significantly altered the approach to patients with persistent fever. Suggested changes to the definition include the substitution of 3 outpatient visits or 3 hospital days for the third criterion. Alternatively, the third criterion can be replaced with uncertain diagnosis after 1 week of evaluation.

ETIOLOGY AND PATHOGENESIS

The 5 primary categories of FUO are infection, 30% to 50% of cases; malignancy, 20% to 30%; rheumatologic/connective tissue disease, 10% to 20%; miscellaneous, 15% to 25%; and undiagnosed, 5% to 15% (Figure 72-1). The frequencies vary geographically, with infections more common in developing countries and tropical regions.

The most commonly identified infections are abscesses, tuberculosis, and viral infections. Subacute bacterial endocarditis (SBE), osteomyelitis, sinusitis, and urinary tract infections also cause FUO.

Abscesses, predominantly intraabdominal, have remained a leading cause of FUO over the past 3 decades. Hepatic, subhepatic, and subdiaphragmatic abscesses are common. Other locations include the retroperitoneal, splenic, appendiceal, pericolonic, perinephric, and pelvic areas.

Tuberculosis associated with FUO is often miliary or extrapulmonary. Viral infections have been increasingly recognized due to the availability of serologic markers for cytomegalovirus (CMV) and Epstein-Barr virus (EBV). HIV infection, either with primary disease or with previously undiagnosed disease, and a concurrent opportunistic infection is also in the differential diagnosis. Many other infections are associated with FUO, including cat-scratch disease (*Bartonella* infection), brucellosis, histoplasmosis, leishmaniasis, malaria, psittacosis, relapsing fever, and leptospirosis.

SBE is a less common cause of FUO than in the past due to improvements in blood culture methods and echocardiography. However, true culture-negative cases still constitute 3% to 5% of large series. Fastidious organisms are often missed in routine culture.

Several neoplastic diseases cause fever and present as FUO. Hematologic malignancies are most common including Hodgkin's and non-Hodgkin's lymphomas. Leukemia is also in this list, but less commonly presents as FUO.

Solid tumors cause FUO less commonly than lymphomas and leukemias. Renal cell carcinoma is typically listed as a cause of FUO, although only 2.5% of cases present with FUO. Other solid tumors occasionally associated with FUO include colon carcinoma, hepatocellular carcinoma, gastric carcinoma, pancreatic carcinoma, mesothelioma, and leiomyosarcoma.

Still's disease and giant cell arteritis are the most common rheumatologic diseases associated with FUO. Still's disease occurs in young adults and is associated with episodic fever, arthralgias, arthritis and, commonly, a rash. Giant cell arteritis is an important cause of FUO in older patients. Other rheumatologic diseases causing FUO include polyarteritis nodosa, systemic lupus erythematosus (SLE), polymyositis, and rheumatoid arthritis.

Many other disorders fall under the miscellaneous category. Drug fever is one of the most common. Factitious fever, most often identified in

Figure 72-1

Potential Causes of Fever of Unknown Origin

Infectious origin (30% to 50%)

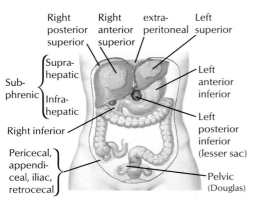

Right posterior superior

Right anterior superior

extra-peritoneal

Left superior

Supra-hepatic

Sub-phrenic

Infra-hepatic

Right inferior

Left anterior inferior

Left posterior inferior (lesser sac)

Pericecal, appendi-ceal, iliac, retrocecal

Pelvic (Douglas)

Abdominal and pelvic abscesses often cause of FUO

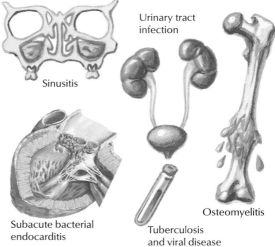

Sinusitis

Urinary tract infection

Osteomyelitis

Subacute bacterial endocarditis

Tuberculosis and viral disease

Malignancy (20% to 30%)

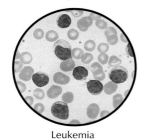

Leukemia

Hematologic malignancy (lymphoma, leukemias) frequent cause of FUO - solid tumors less so

Rheumatologic and connective tissue disorders (10% to 20%)

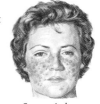

Still's disease

Polyarteritis nodosa, giant cell arteritis

Systemic lupus erythematosus

Miscellaneous causes (15% to 20%)

Drug fever

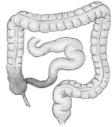

Crohn's disease

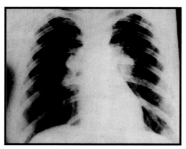

Sarcoid

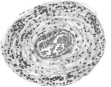

Wegener's granulomatosis

Undiagnosed (5% to 15%)

????

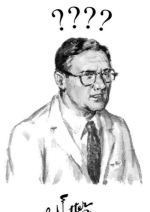

JOHN A. CRAIG—MD

C. Machado—M.D.

©ICN

Figure 72-2   ## Diagnostic Considerations in Fever of Unknown Origin

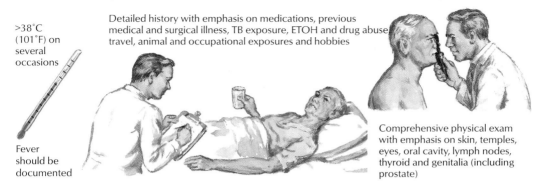

>38°C
(101°F) on
several
occasions

Detailed history with emphasis on medications, previous
medical and surgical illness, TB exposure, ETOH and drug abuse,
travel, animal and occupational exposures and hobbies

Fever
should be
documented

Comprehensive physical exam
with emphasis on skin, temples,
eyes, oral cavity, lymph nodes,
thyroid and genitalia (including
prostate)

Laboratory Studies
(many have been completed to establish criteria for FUO)

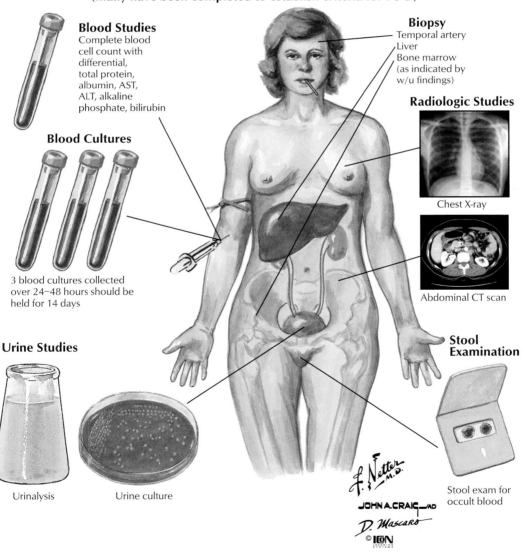

Blood Studies
Complete blood
cell count with
differential,
total protein,
albumin, AST,
ALT, alkaline
phosphate, bilirubin

Blood Cultures

3 blood cultures collected
over 24–48 hours should be
held for 14 days

Urine Studies

Urinalysis

Urine culture

Biopsy
Temporal artery
Liver
Bone marrow
(as indicated by
w/u findings)

Radiologic Studies

Chest X-ray

Abdominal CT scan

**Stool
Examination**

Stool exam for
occult blood

young persons who are associated with the medical profession, is surprisingly common. Granulomatous diseases associated with fever at presentation include Crohn's disease, Wegener's granulomatosis, sarcoidosis, and granulomatous hepatitis. Alcoholic hepatitis is associated with persistent fever and appears to be common in the community setting. Other conditions to consider include recurrent pulmonary emboli, thyroid disease, atrial myxoma, and familial Mediterranean fever.

Despite adequate diagnostic evaluation, a significant proportion of patients with FUO will remain without a confirmed diagnosis. Many will recover spontaneously without sequelae. In others, manifestations of the underlying illness will develop over time, leading to a definitive diagnosis.

CLINICAL PRESENTATION

By definition, the clinical presentation of FUO includes fever. The fever may be high or low, relatively constant or intermittent. Generally, the more prolonged the fever, the less likely that an infection is the cause. Other symptoms and signs may or may not be present. If present, they may provide important clues to the diagnosis. Relatively minor findings should not be overlooked or dismissed.

DIFFERENTIAL DIAGNOSIS

A wide variety of diseases can cause FUO. Evidence of particular organ system involvement should lead to a narrowing of the differential diagnosis. For example, lymph node involvement suggests lymphoma, CMV, EBV, tuberculosis, toxoplasmosis, or *Bartonella* infection (cat-scratch disease), among others.

DIAGNOSTIC APPROACH

The clinician should first document the fever—a critical but commonly overlooked step in evaluation. If fever is not demonstrated, the patient should document it with a reliable thermometer. Documentation and evaluation of fever patterns, however, rarely leads to the diagnosis. (Figure 72-2)

An extremely thorough history and physical examination are essential. Frequently, the bedside evaluation provides the critical clues to the selection of additional tests. The history should include detailed questions about medications, previous medical and surgical illnesses, tuberculosis expo-

sure, prior evaluations with purified protein derivative, alcohol and illicit drug use, travel, animal and occupational exposures, and hobbies. Careful questioning about all body systems is essential to detect minor symptoms that might prove important to the diagnosis (Figure 72-2).

The examination should be comprehensive with special attention paid to the skin, temples, eyes, oral cavity, lymph nodes, thyroid, and genitalia. In men, the prostate examination is very important. A careful pelvic examination is essential in women. Positive results on physical examination should lead to a targeted investigation and early diagnosis. However, subtle physical findings may be overlooked, especially in older patients. Findings may change over time, necessitating repeated examinations.

Many common laboratory tests are likely to have been completed before a patient satisfies the criteria for FUO. Initial laboratory testing includes routine studies, such as complete blood cell count with differential, total protein, albumin, aspartate aminotransferase, alanine aminotransferase, alkaline phosphatase, bilirubin, urinalysis, and urine culture.

Typically, 3 blood cultures spaced over a 24- to 48-hour period are sufficient. False-negative blood culture results can occur during antibiotic therapy, necessitating repeat cultures if empirical therapy was initiated before collection. With the satisfaction of FUO criteria, blood cultures for rare pathogens are often necessary. Blood culture specimens should be observed for up to 14 days. Consider a culture using alternative techniques, such as lysis centrifugation procedure, to enhance detection of fastidious organisms. It is important to communicate with the microbiology laboratory to identify preferred procedures for isolating rare or fastidious organisms.

The patient should have a chest radiograph and a tuberculin skin test early in the evaluation. Stool is examined for occult blood at least 3 times to provide clues to underlying gastrointestinal diseases, such as Crohn's disease or carcinoma of the colon.

The erythrocyte sedimentation rate (ESR) often provides useful information. An ESR greater than 100 mm/hour suggests the presence of a major systemic disease, such as giant cell arteritis, a neoplastic process, or tuberculosis. Slightly or moderately elevated ESRs (20–40 mm/hr) are common in FUO, and can be difficult to interpret, especially in elderly patients. A normal ESR argues against connective tissue diseases.

An abdominal and pelvic CT should be obtained early in the evaluation to identify occult abscesses, one of the most common causes of FUO. Detection of an abnormality with CT may be followed by a CT-guided biopsy to establish the definitive diagnosis. CT of the chest occasionally provides evidence of lung disease not readily apparent by radiography.

Several radionuclide scanning techniques are helpful in the evaluation of FUO. The most commonly used are gallium-67 scans and indium-labeled leukocyte scans. Bone scans are useful in the diagnosis of occult osteomyelitis or metastatic neoplastic disease. Positron emission tomography (PET) with ^{18}F-fluoro-deoxyglucose has also been used. Generally, these tests do not provide a specific diagnosis, but may yield a focus for further evaluation. Physicians should not rely heavily on these studies and should interpret the results very cautiously.

In younger patients, serologic studies can play a role in the diagnostic evaluation. Generally, serum samples should be obtained during the initial evaluation and frozen for later testing. Indiscriminate use of serologic studies is not cost effective and leads to false positive results. The clinician should select serological tests only in response to diagnostic clues in the history, physical examination, and routine laboratory tests. An important exception is serologic tests for systemic lupus erythematosus. Antinuclear antibody and anti–double-stranded DNA are key in the evaluation of most young patients with persistent fever.

Patients with lymphadenopathy and persistent fever may be evaluated with serologic titers for CMV, EBV, and HIV. Antibody titers for CMV and EBV require cautious interpretation. Repeat serologic tests for HIV after 2 to 3 months to identify seroconversion. Polymerase chain reaction assay for HIV also helps to assess for primary HIV infection.

Biopsy procedures, particularly of the bone marrow and liver, are important diagnostic tools. Bone marrow biopsy is helpful in identifying hematologic malignancies and miliary tuberculosis. Culture testing for mycobacteria, as well as bacteria and fungi, should be performed on all biopsy specimens. Bone marrow aspiration alone is probably not adequate in the evaluation of FUO. Liver biopsy can yield the diagnosis if abnormalities are detected on routine studies of liver function.

Temporal artery biopsy is indicated early in the evaluation of the elderly patient with FUO and elevated ESR. Signs and symptoms of giant cell arteritis may be minimal, or limited to persistent fever alone. The surgeon should obtain a generous length (2-3 cm) of temporal artery at biopsy. Bilateral specimens may be necessary.

In older patients, colonoscopy to search for colon carcinoma is reasonable. Echocardiography, both transthoracic and transesophageal, is essential to evaluate for valvular lesions consistent with endocarditis, especially if blood cultures may have been obscured by previous antibiotic therapy.

Laparoscopy is occasionally necessary when other evaluations fail to yield a diagnosis. CT scans identify most intraabdominal processes and facilitate percutaneous biopsies. Generally, if the imaging study results are negative, invasive exploration of the abdomen is not indicated.

Many patients with FUO will have no diagnosis at the end of an intensive evaluation. If no diagnosis has been established after a thorough investigation and the patient is stable, a period of observation is indicated. It may lead to new findings that point to the diagnosis or the symptoms may resolve spontaneously.

MANAGEMENT AND THERAPY

The appropriate management depends primarily on the identification of the underlying etiology. However, the clinician should follow certain general rules of management.

Early in the evaluation, especially in older patients, discontinue all nonessential medications, including those that have been used long term. Long-term use of certain medications can cause drug fevers, and a costly investigation can be avoided if fever resolves after discontinuation.

Avoid empirical therapeutic trials if possible. Given the frequent spontaneous resolution of the FUO, "cure" cannot be ascribed to the treatment with certainty. Use of therapeutic agents, especially antibiotics, can obscure findings or tests that might lead to a definitive diagnosis.

FUTURE DIRECTIONS

FUO is likely to become increasingly uncommon, but more difficult to diagnose. The advances in imaging and diagnostic tests have led to more rapid diagnosis of persistent fever. Those cases that remain undiagnosed present a substantial challenge to the physician.

REFERENCES

Durack DT, Street AC. Fever of unknown origin—reexamined and redefined. *Curr Clin Top Infect Dis.* 1991;11:35–51.

Hirschmann JV. Fever of unknown origin in adults. *Clin Infect Dis.* 1997;24:291–302.

Mackowiak PA, Durack DT. Fever of unknown origin. In: Mandell GL, Bennett JE, Dolin R, eds. *Principles and Practice of Infectious Diseases.* 5th ed. Philadelphia: Churchill Livingstone; 2000:622–633.

Petersdorf RG. Fever of unknown origin. An old friend revisited. *Arch Intern Med.* 1992;152:21–22.

Petersdorf RG, Beeson PB. Fever of unexplained origin: Report of 100 cases. *Medicine.* 1961;40:1–30.

Chapter 73

Herpes Simplex Virus Infections

Peter A. Leone

Genital and oral infections due to herpes simplex virus (HSV) are endemic in the United States. Genital herpes infection is caused by HSV-2 and less frequently by HSV-1. Genital HSV infection causes vesicular and ulcerative disease in adults and severe systemic disease in neonates and immunocompromised individuals. HSV-2 transmission is almost always sexual, while HSV-1 is usually transmitted through nonsexual human contact. The incidence of new HSV-2 infections is estimated at greater than 1.5 million cases annually. HSV-2 seroprevalence, which is extremely rare under the age of 12, rises sharply with the onset of sexual activity, and peaks by the early 40s. The seroprevalence of HSV-2 infection rose 30% between 1978 to 1991 to 21.7%. The majority of individuals with genital HSV infection have undiagnosed initial infections and unrecognized recurrent outbreaks. Orolabial HSV-2 infection is rare, and is almost always associated with genital infection. HSV-1 infection frequently occurs in childhood with seropositivity in approximately 20% of children under the age of 5 years. The seroprevalence of HSV-1 rises almost linearly with increasing age to approximately 50%. HSV-1 is increasingly common, with an estimated 50% of incident genital infection attributable to it.

ETIOLOGY AND PATHOGENESIS

Primary HSV infection occurs at the mucosal site of inoculation with retrograde infection of sensory nerve ganglia. Following resolution of primary infection, HSV enters a latent state in the sensory nerve ganglia and can reactivate to cause active infection at any mucosal site innervated by the infected ganglia.

During primary HSV infection, natural killer (NK) cells are important effectors of immunity. NK cell activation depends on the production of several cytokines that have direct and indirect effects important in limiting viral replication. As the immune response matures, clearance of HSV from infected tissues is T cell mediated and involves cytokine-mediated effector mechanisms and direct cytolysis of virus-infected cells. Both CD4+ and CD8+ T cells are important in resolution of infection.

The efficiency of the immune response appears to influence the quantity of virus-established latency in the ganglia. The elements that contribute to this control are not completely known, but interferon gamma is likely to be important. Initial evidence suggests that immune response may play a supplemental role in maintaining latency of HSV but this remains to be confirmed.

CLINICAL PRESENTATION

Genital infection with HSV is classified into five categories.

The *primary first episode* refers to infection with either HSV-1 or HSV-2 in an individual who has never been infected with a herpes simplex virus. In immunocompetent hosts, this event usually goes unrecognized. After an incubation period of 1 to 14 days (average, 4 days), a papule appears that evolves into a vesicle within 24 hours (Figure 74-1). These vesicles can be clear or pustular and rapidly evolve into shallow, nonindurated, painful ulcers. Clinical associations include dysuria, inguinal lymphadenitis, vaginal discharge, and cervicitis. Systemic symptoms, including myalgias, malaise, fever, and other "flu-like" symptoms, may also develop. Crops of lesions occur over 1 to 2 weeks. Crusting and healing require an additional 1 to 2 weeks.

A *nonprimary first episode* is an infection in an individual who has had a previous infection with either HSV type, typically a previous orolabial infection with HSV-1, in whom a genital HSV-2 infection develops. Generally, it is less severe than the primary first episode due to a partial humoral and cellular immune response. There are fewer lesions, less pain, fewer systemic symptoms, and more rapid resolution of lesions (usually 5 to 7 days). This episode is clinically similar to that of recurrent disease and can be mistaken for recurrent infection.

A *First recognized episode* is an initial infection whether it is a first episode or recurrent infection.

Figure 73-1

Lesions of Herpes Simplex

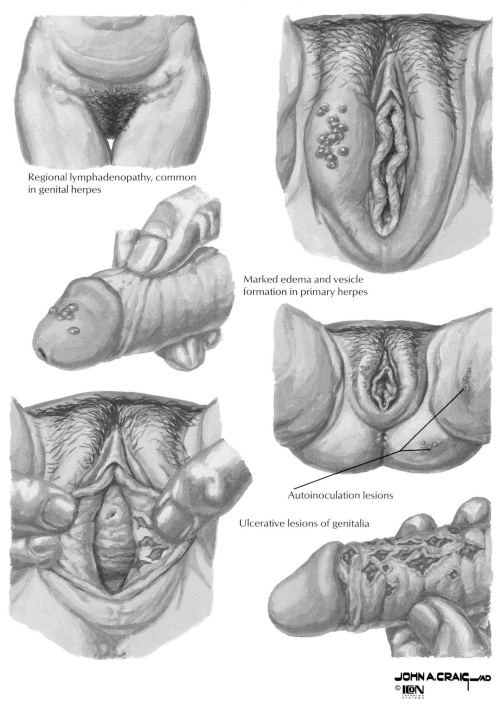

Regional lymphadenopathy, common
in genital herpes

Marked edema and vesicle
formation in primary herpes

Autoinoculation lesions

Ulcerative lesions of genitalia

JOHN A.CRAIG—AD
©ICN

A *Recurrent episode* is the second or subsequent episode of genital herpes with the same virus type. HSV-2 accounts for more than 90% of recurrent genital herpes. The median number of recurrences is 4 with 38% of individuals having 6 or more recurrences annually. Recurrent outbreaks are usually not associated with systemic symptoms, and are fairly mild and often go unrecognized, but may be preceded by a prodrome of paresthesia or dysesthesia. A cluster of localized vesiculopustular or ulcerative lesions develops and tends to lateralize to one side of the midline. "Atypical" lesions are common and may be mistaken for excoriation or irritation. Predominant locations of lesions are the glans or shaft of the penis in men, the vaginal introitus or labia in women, and the buttocks and anal area in both sexes. A neuropathic prodrome may occur 6 to 24 hours before the appearance of lesions.

Subclinical shedding refers to the detection of virus in the absence of visible lesions. Our understanding of genital herpes has shifted from that of intermittent outbreaks to one of low grade shedding of virus that can be detected by viral culture of the genitals and anus 5% to 7% of days and 15% to 20% of days by polymerase chain reaction (PCR). The frequency of subclinical shedding is greatest the first 6 to 12 months after acquiring genital herpes. It is less common in HSV-1. In HSV-2, subclinical shedding occurs in almost all individuals but is more common in women and diminishes in frequency over time. Many episodes are temporarily associated around clinically recognized outbreaks, with virus detected one to several days preceding or following resolution of lesions. Patients who are counseled about the mild signs and symptoms of recurrent outbreaks may learn to recognize some periods when they are at risk of transmitting HSV to partners.

DIFFERENTIAL DIAGNOSIS

Discrete genital or anal ulcers in sexually active young adults have a relatively narrow differential diagnosis. Chancroid is rare in the United States, and syphilis is at an historic low and highly concentrated in certain geographic areas.

The differential diagnosis should include the following infectious etiologies: genital herpes, syphilis, chancroid, primary HIV, lymphogranuloma venereum, and donovanosis.

Primary syphilis may be distinguished from other ulcers by the presence of a nontender, indurated, nonpurulant ulcer. Other ulcer characteristics are not helpful in distinguishing infectious etiologies, but are more likely to be due to herpes. Diagnostic testing is critical to prevent a missed diagnosis of genital herpes for any genital ulcer.

DIAGNOSTIC APPROACH

Viral culture is the "gold standard" for the diagnosis. It allows a definitive diagnosis for a genital ulcer and permits distinction of HSV-1 from HSV-2, an important consideration for prognosis and counseling. Cultures are most sensitive while lesions are in the vesicular-pustular stage. Sensitivity rapidly declines as lesions ulcerate and crust. PCR is a more sensitive assay and although offered by many reference laboratories, it is not commercially available. Direct immunofluorescent antibody testing is more rapid (4 to 6 hours) than culture, but does not differentiate HSV-1 and HSV-2.

Enzyme-linked immunosorbent assay (ELISA) testing for HSV antigens in clinical specimens is a rapid alternative to culture (results in 3 to 4 hours), but its use is generally confined to large laboratories and teaching institutions. Microscopy of Papanicolaou smears or Giemsa staining (Tzanck test) is insensitive and nonspecific. A type-specific antibody test based on HSV glycoprotein G is the most important and reliable diagnostic tool for HSV infection. Antibody tests based on complement fixation, indirect immunofluorescence, or neutralization technologies do not distinguish antibodies to HSV-1 from HSV-2. A negative antibody test result is reassuring in that it excludes the diagnosis in a patient who has symptoms suggestive of recurrent herpes. A positive test result that is not HSV glycoprotein G based is of little diagnostic value because it does not distinguish reliably between type 1 and type 2 infections. Because more then one-half of US adults are HSV-1 seropositive, a positive test result is useless in the evaluation of genital ulcer disease. IgM antibody is often present with recurrent HSV outbreaks and does not indicate recent infection.

The new type-specific serological assays have specificities of over 98% for the detection of HSV-2 antibody and sensitivities of higher than 90%,

Table 73-1
Drug and Dose for a Specific Type of HSV-2 Infection

Type of Infection or Therapy	Acyclovir	Famciclovir	Valacyclovir
Initial	200 mg po q4h, 5× d for 10 days	250 mg po tid for 10 days	1 g po bid for 10 days
Recurrent	200 mg po q4h, 5× d for 5 days	125 mg po bid for 5 days	500 mg po bid for 3 days

depending on the population studied. A rapid, office-based assay that can be run on serum or fingersticks and provide results in less than 10 minutes is available. It is imperative to specify a glycoprotein G-based test when ordering an HSV serologic test.

The following are the current FDA-approved type-specific assays: Western blot; ELISA; immunoblot; and rapid assay.

MANAGEMENT AND THERAPY

There is an undeserved stigma attached to genital herpes, and most patients require reassurance and appropriate counseling. This can be given only if one has full access to the facts and myths surrounding this condition.

Pharmacologic and Other Treatment

Antiviral therapy for initial genital herpes prevents new lesion formation and rapidly reduces viral shedding, infectivity, and the risk of autoinfection. However, it has no effect on preventing subsequent recurrences. When taken continuously, it effectively suppresses HSV recurrences and reduces subclinical shedding. Episodic treatment shortens the course of recurrences. The current recommended antiviral regimens for genital herpes cause few adverse effects but serum levels can become elevated when renal function is impaired (requiring a reduction in dosage) (Table 73-1). Acyclovir, famciclovir, and valacyclovir, are not approved for use during pregnancy. Some experts recommend the use of suppressive acyclovir therapy during the last month of pregnancy for women with symptomatic recurrent herpes to prevent unnecessary cesarean sections by reducing the likelihood of an outbreak near term.

Topical lidocaine jelly 2% is a useful adjunct to oral antiviral drugs in managing severe first episodes in women. It should be applied frequently, and especially before voiding, but for no longer than 24 to 36 hours. There is a theoretical risk of sensitization, but this is very rarely seen in practice. Antifungal or antibacterial agents may be needed to treat secondary infections.

There is no evidence that salt baths, topical antiseptics, lysine, vitamins, or other nonmainstream remedies are more effective than placebo in the treatment or prevention of genital herpes.

Optimum Treatments
First Episodes

After diagnosis, assess the need for further immediate tests if there is clinical suspicion of syphilis, chancroid, primary HIV, or other infection. Tests include darkfield examination, serum for rapid plasma reagin (RPR), HIV p24 antigen, or antibody testing.

Use of an oral antiviral for 7 to 10 days should be considered. Symptoms usually resolve in 3 to 4 days. If this is not the case, consider the possibility of secondary infection. Lesions persisting for longer than 14 days should prompt consideration of HIV coinfection and one should consider repeat serologic testing for syphilis and examination for other genital infections at 2 to 4 weeks. If the initial HSV virologic test results were negative, HSV type-specific serology should be obtained at 6 weeks and again at 3 months after presentation.

Recurrent Episodes

Virologic specimens should be obtained from active lesions if the diagnosis has not yet been confirmed. Consider obtaining type-specific serology in patients with atypical lesions, negative virologic tests, or lesions that cannot be tested for the presence of HSV.

HIV testing should be strongly encouraged for those who have not been recently tested.

Other important considerations include: episodic treatment with oral antiviral agents; and counselling of patients on treatment options, including continued episodic therapy that may be started at the first signs or symptoms of an outbreak, or suppressive therapy to prevent recurrences.

Counseling

First and most importantly, accurate information about all aspects of the disease should be provided. New diagnoses of genital herpes can be emotionally devastating and may make comprehension and retention of information difficult. Important information to cover at the first visit includes:

- The availability of effective therapy for primary infection
- The availability of effective therapy for recurrences
- Recurrent episodes tend to be milder than the initial episode.
- Transmission of herpes usually occurs from a partner who was not aware of his or her infection or did not believe he or she was infectious when exposure occurred.

Time should be taken at follow-up visits to address the patient's concerns and to provide appropriate counseling. Patients may be given written information and referred to Internet web sites and telephone hotlines.

Prevention

The majority of patients, once educated on the mild signs and symptoms of outbreaks, will recognize symptomatic outbreaks. The following steps can help prevent the acquisition and transmission of genital herpes:

- Abstinence during outbreaks
- Condoms can reduce transmission, especially during the first 6 to 12 months after initial infection.
- Choosing partners with like serologic status
- Chronic suppressive therapy: although no data are available demonstrating reduction in HSV transmission while on suppressive therapy, it is reasonable to believe that the reduction in recurrences of outbreaks and subclinical shedding decreases the risk of transmission.

FUTURE DIRECTIONS

Preventive and therapeutic vaccines are currently in Phase 2 and Phase 3 clinical trials. Clinical efficacy data on these vaccines will be available in four years. Even with an effective vaccine, questions concerning the acceptability of an STD vaccine for the general public and whether the target population should be preteens or young adults will need to be addressed. The development of vaginal microbicides will offer women protection against HSV and a broad array of other STD's.

REFERENCES

Ashley RL, Wald A. Genital herpes: review of the epidemic and potential use of type-specific serology. *Clin Microbiol Rev.* 1999;12:1–8.

Ebel C., Wald A. *Managing Herpes: How to Live and Love with a Chronic STD.* Research Triangle Park, NC: American Social Health Association; 2002.

Fleming DT, McQuillan GM, Johnson RE, et al. Herpes simplex virus type 2 in the United States, 1976 to 1994. *N Engl J Med.* 1997;337:1105–1111.

Handsfield HH. *Genital Herpes.* New York, NY: McGraw-Hill; 2001.

Wald A. New therapies and prevention strategies for genital herpes. *Clin Infect Dis.* 1999;28(suppl 1):S4–S13.

Chapter 74

Herpes Simplex Encephalitis

Joseph J. Eron

Acute encephalitis, the most common form of fatal sporadic encephalitis in developed countries, is a frightening and potentially devastating manifestation of Herpes simplex virus (HSV) infection. Estimated incidence is between 2 to 4 cases per million individuals per year. HSV encephalitis occurs throughout the year and in patients of all ages, although it may be more common in adolescents and young adults, and in individuals older than 50.

ETIOLOGY AND PATHOGENESIS

Most HSV encephalitis is caused by HSV-1. Like all herpesviruses, HSV-1 and HSV-2 have a lytic phase and a latent phase. For HSV this latent phase occurs in neuronal cells in nerve root ganglia. The virus enters through mucosal or cutaneous surfaces with initial local, sometimes subclinical infection, which then leads to infection of autonomic or sensory nerve endings with subsequent transport to the nerve cell bodies in the ganglia. In initial infection, HSV replication occurs in the ganglia and surrounding neural tissue before the establishment of latency. In children and some young adults, HSV encephalitis may result from oral/labial infection and neurotropic extension via the olfactory bulb. In many adults, the presence of serological or historical evidence of HSV-1 infection at the time of HSV encephalitis presentation suggests that the encephalitis is a manifestation of reactivation of latent infection in the ganglion with extension to the central nervous system (CNS). HSV DNA has also been identified with polymerase chain reaction (PCR) in brain tissue from individuals dying of non-neurological causes; therefore, reactivation of latent infection within the CNS itself may be possible. The temporal lobe is the characteristic site of infection early in the course of encephalitis, which suggests a common mode of entry into the CNS when HSV-1 causes encephalitis, for example from reactivation in the trigeminal ganglia and entry into the brain via the rami meningeals of the trigeminal nerve. In some cases, the HSV-1 variant associated with encephalitis differs from the variant isolated from a patient's oropharynx, suggesting that encephalitis may result from a second HSV infection. The encephalitis is caused by lytic HSV infection of neuronal and astroglial cells resulting in necrosis of brain tissue. The infection may extend from the temporal lobe to other areas of the brain

CLINICAL PRESENTATION

The clinical presentation of HSV encephalitis is typically the acute onset of fever, mental status and/or behavior changes, with or without focal findings, which if present, localize to the temporal lobe (Figure 74-1). Dysphasia may be one localizing finding on presentation, and behaviors may be bizarre. Seizure activity is common, and patients usually present within a week of initial symptoms.

DIFFERENTIAL DIAGNOSIS

The differential diagnosis is broad, although other causes with specific therapeutic interventions are more limited. Bacterial meningitides, brain abscesses, and meningoencephalitis (e.g., *Listeria*) should be excluded and may require empiric therapy until the appropriate diagnostic tests have been completed. Additional viral infections include enteroviral and vector-borne viral encephalitides (eastern equine, St. Louis, and West Nile encephalitis, among others). Less common sporadic viral encephalitides such as those related directly or indirectly to adenoviruses, other herpesviruses, influenza, mumps, measles, and acute HIV infection should be considered. Additional infectious causes are suggested by medical/travel history and/or physical, laboratory, or radiological examinations and include Rocky Mountain spotted fever, syphilis, Lyme disease, tuberculosis, and opportunistic CNS pathogens

Figure 74-1

HSV - Encephalitis

Possible Route of Transmission in Herpes Simplex Encephalitis

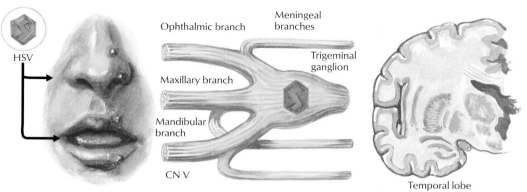

HSV

Ophthalmic branch

Meningeal branches

Trigeminal ganglion

Maxillary branch

Mandibular branch

CN V

Temporal lobe

Primary Infection	Latent Phase	Reactivation (Lytic Phase)
Virus enters via cutaneous or mucosal surfaces to infect sensory or autonomic nerve endings with transport to cell bodies in ganglia	Virus replicates in ganglia before establishing latent phase	Reactivation of HSV in trigeminal ganglion can result in spread to brain (temporal lobe) via meningeal branches of CN V

Clinical Features of HSV Encephalitis

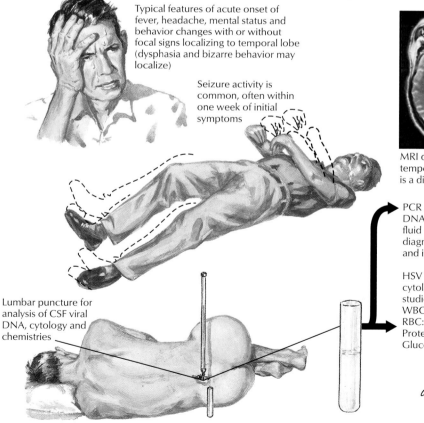

Typical features of acute onset of fever, headache, mental status and behavior changes with or without focal signs localizing to temporal lobe (dysphasia and bizarre behavior may localize)

Seizure activity is common, often within one week of initial symptoms

Lumbar puncture for analysis of CSF viral DNA, cytology and chemistries

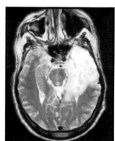

MRI demonstrating temporal lobe involvement is a diagnostic cornerstone

PCR amplification of HSV DNA from cerebrospinal fluid provides major diagnostic information and is very sensitive

HSV encephalitis CSF cytology and chemical studies typically show:
WBC: moderate
RBC: +/−
Protein: moderate
Glucose: normal

F. Netter M.D.

JOHN A. CRAIG—AD

D. Mascaro

© ICN

such as *Cryptococcus neoformans* or *Toxoplasma gondii* in undiagnosed advanced HIV infection. Noninfectious causes include intracranial hemorrhage, CNS autoimmune diseases with or without systemic manifestations such as systemic lupus erythematosus, Wegener's granulomatosis, or primary CNS vasculitis. Thyrotoxicosis, neuroleptic malignant syndrome, and exposure to certain toxins or drugs should also be considered.

DIAGNOSTIC APPROACH

Currently, MRI and PCR amplification of HSV DNA from cerebrospinal fluid (CSF) are the cornerstones of diagnosis. Typically, the MRI will have abnormalities ranging from localized edema with increased signal on T2-weighted images to large areas with radiographic evidence of frank necrosis and hemorrhage. However, only minimal abnormalities may be seen early in the disease (Figure 74-1). The CSF usually has a moderate number of WBCs (10 to 250 cells/mm^3) and usually, but not always, some RBCs (0 to 150 cells/mm^3), the number of which remains stable when CSF samples obtained at the beginning and at the end of a lumbar puncture are compared. The CSF protein level may be modestly elevated, while glucose levels are typically normal. PCR detection of HSV DNA in CSF is very sensitive. Specificity has been reported to be 100%, although false-positive results from either error in the assay (such as contamination) or detection of HSV DNA in the absence of HSV-mediated encephalitis are possible. CSF HSV antibody levels can also be used to diagnose HSV encephalitis if initial diagnostic procedures were not performed or were inconclusive.

MANAGEMENT AND THERAPY

The therapy of choice is intravenous acyclovir, administered as soon as the diagnosis is entertained. Administration of acyclovir should not be delayed for diagnostic certainty. Acyclovir is initially phosphorylated by the herpes simplex enzyme thymidine kinase and then cellular enzymes to produce the diphosphorylated and triphosphorylated forms, the latter of which inhibits the synthesis of viral DNA by competing with 2'-deoxyguanosine triphosphate as a substrate for HSV DNA polymerase. Acyclovir terminates viral DNA synthesis and cannot be removed by viral exonucleases resulting in inactivation of the polymerase. Acyclovir has poor oral bioavailability and must be given at high doses (10 to 15 mg/kg) intravenously every 8 hours for 10 to 21 days to ensure adequate levels in the CNS. In the initial comparative study with vidarabine, acyclovir reduced mortality by 50% (from 54% to 28%). Therefore, despite the fact that HSV-1 is very sensitive to inhibition by acyclovir, death or serious sequelae related to HSV encephalitis remain common, especially if therapy is initiated when the patient is near coma or comatose. In one study, none of the patients who began acyclovir when their Glasgow Coma Scale was above 10 died while 42% of the patients presenting with similar mental status who received vidarabine died. Supportive care is an important part of management and may include airway intubation, sedation, and mechanical ventilation when mental status is significantly compromised. The potential for rapid deterioration requires that even patients with minimal alteration in sensorium be carefully observed.

Mechanism-based toxicity of acyclovir is typically limited, because acyclovir is poorly phosphorylated in uninfected cells and its affinity for human DNA polymerases is low. Crystallization in the renal tubules with obstructive uropathy is the most frequent serious toxicity but is uncommon especially with adequate hydration.

Foscarnet is the alternative therapy of patients who do not tolerate acyclovir. Foscarnet is the drug of choice in encephalitis caused by HSV resistant to acyclovir, a problem that has been described in immunocompromised patients.

Sequelae of HSV encephalitis are common. Even with acyclovir therapy, only 38% of patients with confirmed HSV encephalitis were considered to be functioning normally 6 months following infection, although only 9% were considered to have moderate debility. Long-term cognitive and memory impairments are not uncommon.

FUTURE DIRECTIONS

The single most important area to be addressed for HSV encephalitis is consideration of its diagnosis early and institution of therapy coupled with enhancing the speed of definitive diagnosis. Microchip electrophoresis of PCR products reduces the time from when a CSF sample is obtained and the PCR result is available. However rapid institution of acyclovir therapy as soon as the diagnosis is suspected remains the key to therapeutic success in this potentially devastating illness.

REFERENCES

Baringer JR, Pisani P. Herpes simplex virus genomes in human nervous system tissue analyzed by polymerase chain reaction. *Ann Neurol.* 1994;36:823–829.

Hofgartner WT, Huhmer AF, Landers JP, Kant JA. Rapid diagnosis of herpes simplex encephalitis using microchip electrophoresis of PCR products. *Clin Chem.* 1999;45:2120–2128.

Schmutzhard E. Viral infections of the CNS with special emphasis on herpes simplex infections. *J Neurol.* 2001;248:469–477.

Studahl M, Rosengren L, Gunther G, Hagberg L. Difference in pathogenesis between herpes simplex virus type 1 encephalitis and tick-borne encephalitis demonstrated by means of cerebrospinal fluid markers of glial and neuronal destruction. *J Neurol.* 2000;247:636–642.

Whitley RJ, Alford CA, Hirsch MS, et al. Vidarabine versus acyclovir therapy in herpes simplex encephalitis. *N Engl J Med.* 1986;314:144–149.

Whitley RJ, Cobbs CG, Alford CA Jr, et al. Diseases that mimic herpes simplex encephalitis. Diagnosis, presentation, and outcome. NIAD Collaborative Antiviral Study Group. *JAMA.* 1989;262:234–239.

Zunt JR, Marra CM. Cerebrospinal fluid testing for the diagnosis of central nervous system infection. *Neurol Clin.* 1999;17:675–689.

Chapter 75

Infectious Diseases in Travelers

David J. Weber, David A. Wohl, and William A. Rutala

Each year, more than 25 million Americans travel to overseas destinations. During international travel, 1% to 5% of travelers seek medical attention, 0.01% to 0.1% require emergency medical evaluation, and 1 in 100,000 dies. This chapter will review the medical hazards faced by travelers, methods of reducing the risks associated with travel, and evaluation of fever in the traveler returning from lesser-developed countries. The focus is on prevention and management of infectious diseases.

PREVENTION OF TRAVEL-ASSOCIATED ILLNESSES

Healthcare providers should counsel travelers to lesser-developed countries on travel-related risks and methods to prevent illness. An accurate risk assessment requires information regarding the patient's medical condition (i.e., age, immunization history, underlying medical disorders, pregnancy status, allergies, and host defense abnormalities) and exact travel itinerary (i.e., locations to be visited including exact length of stay, urban versus rural locales, and level of accommodations and activities such as freshwater exposure, contact with animals, and sexual relations). Special efforts should be made to identify and counsel travelers who are at high risk, such as those traveling to physically unsafe locations, persons planning a prolonged stay, those traveling off the usual tourist routes, and immunocompromised persons. Current information regarding prevention of travel-associated diseases is available on the Web site maintained by the Centers for Disease Control and Prevention.

General risk counseling includes advice on how to avoid the following: 1) accidents, trauma, and injuries; 2) transportation-related injuries; 3) altitude illness; 4) heat-, humidity-, and sun-related illnesses; and 5) water-related illnesses. Counseling on avoiding infections includes the following categories of infectious diseases: 1) traveler's diarrhea, 2) respiratory tract infections, 3) arthropod-borne illnesses (especially malaria, dengue, yellow fever, and Japanese B encephalitis), 4) sexually transmitted diseases, 5) blood-borne illnesses (especially HIV), and 6) animal bites (especially rabies) and envenomations.

All patients should have their immunization status reviewed and, if deficiencies are noted in universally recommended vaccines (e.g., measles, mumps, rubella, diphtheria tetanus), the vaccinations should be provided. Travelers should be offered vaccines available to prevent travel-associated illnesses based on an individual risk assessment. Physicians prescribing vaccines should be familiar with indications, contraindications, and administration guidelines. Although immunoglobulin can be used to protect against hepatitis A, hepatitis vaccine is preferred provided there is time for immunity to develop before travel.

ETIOLOGY AND PATHOGENESIS
Causes of Fever After Travel to Tropical Countries

Only limited data are available regarding the causes of fever in returning travelers. A recent series of patients (1998 to 1999) noted the following diagnoses: malaria 27%, respiratory tract infections 24%, gastroenteritis 14%, dengue 8%, typhoid fever 3%, hepatitis A 3%, rickettsiae 2%, tropical ulcers 2%, connective tissue disease 2%; all other causes were 1% or less. Only 9% of patients in this series had a febrile illness without a confirmed diagnosis.

DIAGNOSTIC APPROACH
Fever in Returning Travelers

In evaluating fever in the returning traveler, checking the vital signs to assess whether the patient is medically stable is the first step. If cardiorespiratory distress is present, initial therapy should be targeted towards stabilizing the patient. Next, one should assess whether the patient has a potentially communicable disease and determine the need for isolation and personal protective equipment. Treat all patients using standard precautions including the

Figure 75-1

Amebiasis

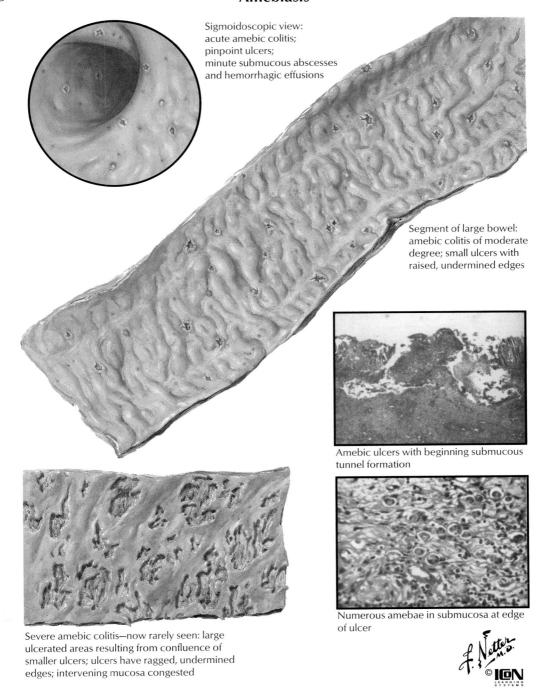

Sigmoidoscopic view:
acute amebic colitis;
pinpoint ulcers;
minute submucous abscesses
and hemorrhagic effusions

Segment of large bowel:
amebic colitis of moderate
degree; small ulcers with
raised, undermined edges

Amebic ulcers with beginning submucous
tunnel formation

Numerous amebae in submucosa at edge
of ulcer

Severe amebic colitis—now rarely seen: large
ulcerated areas resulting from confluence of
smaller ulcers; ulcers have ragged, undermined
edges; intervening mucosa congested

Figure 75-2

Typhoid Fever
Paratyphoid Fever, Enteric Fever

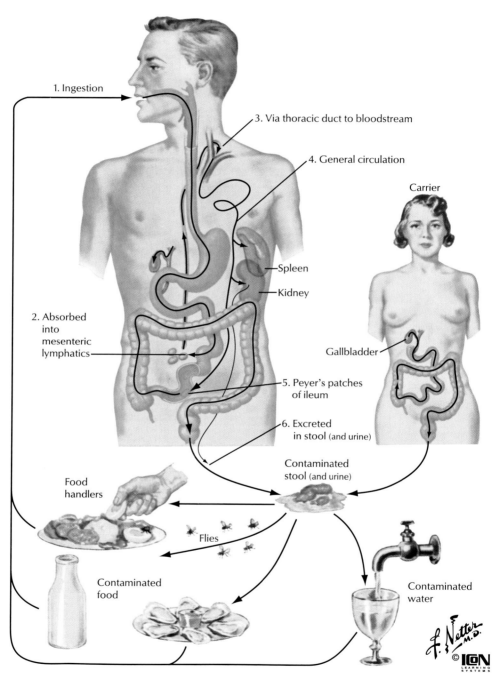

1. Ingestion

3. Via thoracic duct to bloodstream

4. General circulation

Carrier

Spleen

Kidney

2. Absorbed into mesenteric lymphatics

Gallbladder

5. Peyer's patches of ileum

6. Excreted in stool (and urine)

Contaminated stool (and urine)

Food handlers

Flies

Contaminated food

Contaminated water

Table 75-1
Possible Physical Findings in Selected Tropical Infections

Physical Finding	Infection or Disease
Rash	Acute HIV seroconversion disease, brucellosis, Ebola virus, CMV, dengue fever, EBV, gonorrhea, measles, syphilis, typhoid, typhus
Eschar	Anthrax, *Borrelia*, Congo-Crimean fever, South African tick-bite fever, scrub typhus, tick typhus
Jaundice	CMV, leptospirosis, malaria, relapsing fever, viral hepatitis, yellow fever
Lymphadenopathy	Acute HIV seroconversion disease, brucellosis, dengue fever, Lassa fever, visceral leishmaniasis
Hepatomegaly	Amebiasis, leptospirosis, malaria, typhoid, viral hepatitis
Splenomegaly	Acute American trypanosomiasis, African trypanosomiasis, brucellosis, CMV, dengue fever, EBV, malaria, relapsing fever, trypanosomiasis, typhoid, visceral leishmaniasis
Hemorrhage	Congo-Crimean fever, dengue hemorrhagic fever, Ebola viruses, epidemic louse-borne typhus, Lassa fever, Marburg virus, meningococcemia, Rift Valley fever, Rocky Mountain spotted-fever, yellow fever, CMV, EBV, HIV

CMV, cytomegalovirus; EBV, Epstein-Barr virus; HIV, human immunodeficiency virus.

use of gloves when in contact with body secretions or excretions (except sweat). Wear a surgical mask if the patient may have a droplet- (e.g., meningococcemia) or airborne-transmitted (e.g., varicella) disease. An N-95 respirator should be worn if pulmonary tuberculosis is suspected.

Clinicians may find use of an algorithm helpful in evaluating fever in returning travelers. First, assess the patient for the presence of hemorrhagic manifestations. If present, consider viral hemorrhagic fevers (e.g., Ebola, Lassa, Marburg, Congo-Crimean, yellow fever), meningococcemia, gram-negative sepsis, and rickettsial infections. If viral hemorrhagic fever is possible based on history, clinical presentation, and incubation period, institute appropriate isolation precautions, seek expert consultation and consider ribavirin therapy. Second, consider the diagnosis of malaria. If *Plasmodium falciparum* is possible and the patient is acutely ill with signs of severe malaria, begin empiric therapy. If the patient is not acutely ill, obtain serial thick and thin blood smears and treat based on laboratory results. Finally, perform a complete his-

tory and physical examination, and perform preliminary laboratory tests. If localized findings are present, pursue the appropriate differential diagnosis (Table 75-1). If no localizing findings are present, consider enteric fever, dengue, rickettsial infections, leptospirosis, schistosomiasis, brucellosis, and noninfectious causes of disease.

Key historical questions include exact itinerary, immunization history, and prophylaxis. Physical examination should focus on a thorough dermatologic examination; inspection of the eyes for scleral icterus, conjunctival suffusion, or conjunctival petechiae; and assessment for lymphadenopathy, splenomegaly, and hepatomegaly. Initial laboratory examination includes a complete blood cell count, serum chemistries, liver profile, and a urinalysis. Additional tests are obtained as directed by the results of the history, physical examination, and preliminary laboratory results.

Caveats for the evaluation of fever in the returning traveler are:
- Evaluate thoroughly for all causes of febrile illnesses, both travel- and nontravel-related (e.g., pneu-

Table 75-2
Differential Diagnosis of Fever in the Returning Traveler

Short Incubation (<10 days)

- Arboviral infection (including dengue fever)
- Enteric bacterial infections
- Influenza
- Paratyphoid
- Plague
- Relapsing fever (*Borrelia* spp.)
- Typhus (louse-borne, flea-borne)
- Viral hemorrhagic fever (Ebola, Lassa, Marburg)

Medium Incubation (10 to 21 days)

- African trypanosomiasis
- Brucellosis
- Leptospirosis
- Malaria
- Measles
- Q fever
- Scrub typhus
- Typhoid fever
- Typhus
- Viral hemorrhagic fever (Ebola, Lassa, Marburg)

Long Incubaton (>21 days)

- Amebic liver abscess
- Brucellosis
- Filariasis
- Hepatitis A, B, C
- HIV
- Malaria
- Melioidosis
- Schistosomiasis (Katayama fever)
- Tuberculosis
- Visceral leishmaniasis

monia, urinary tract infections, etc.) infections
- The most common tropical infections are malaria, viral hepatitis, infectious gastroenteritis, dengue, and enteric fever
- Malaria is potentially fatal and may progress rapidly; it should be excluded as rapidly as possible in all febrile patients with epidemiologic exposure
- Useful diagnostic points include travel history, travel itinerary, immunization and prophylaxis history, an assessment of incubation period (Table 75-2), and specific exposure history

EVALUATION AND MANAGEMENT OF 2 SPECIFIC DISEASE SYNDROMES
Traveler's Diarrhea
Clinical Presentation

Traveler's diarrhea (TD) is characterized by a twofold or greater increase in the frequency of unformed bowel movements. Symptoms often include abdominal cramps, nausea, vomiting (approximately 15%), bloating, urgency, fever, and malaise. Episodes usually begin abruptly and are generally self-limited. The most important determinant of risk is the destination of the traveler; high-risk destinations include Latin America, Africa, the Middle East, and Asia. TD is acquired via ingestion of fecally contaminated food or water. TD typically causes 4 to 5 loose or watery stools per day. The average duration of diarrhea is 3 to 4 days, but approximately 10% of cases persist longer than 1 week. Fever or bloody stools occur in 2% to 10% of cases. A causative pathogen is demonstrated in 50% to 75% of patients. The most common bacterial causes of TD are enterotoxigenic *Escherichia coli*, *Salmonella*, *Shigellae*, *Campylobacter jejuni*, and *Vibrio parahaemolyticus*. Viral etiologies include rotaviruses and Norwalk-like viruses. While less common, parasitic enteric pathogens including *Giardia*, *Entamoeba histolytica* (Figure 75-1), *Cryptosporidium parvum*, and *Cyclylospora cayetanensis* may cause TD.

Management and Therapy

Prevention of TD rests on 3 approaches: counseling regarding food and beverage consumption, use of nonantimicrobial medications, and use of prophylactic antibiotics. Bismuth subsalicylate decreases the incidence of diarrhea by approximately 60% but may result in temporary blackening of the tongue and stools, occasional nausea and constipation, and rarely tinnitus. Bismuth subsalicylate should be avoided in infants and young children, persons with aspirin allergies, and persons taking anticoagulants, probenecid, or methotrexate. Several antibiotics (sulfamethoxazole & trimethoprim, doxycycline, trimethoprim alone, and fluoroquinolones) decrease the incidence of TD by 50% to 95%. However, their efficacy depends on local antibiotic resistance patterns. Antimicrobial prophylaxis is not recommended because of potential side effects. Prophylaxis is reasonable in travelers who are immunosuppressed, although no data directly support this practice.

Figure 75-3

Typhoid Fever
Paratyphoid Fever, Enteric Fever

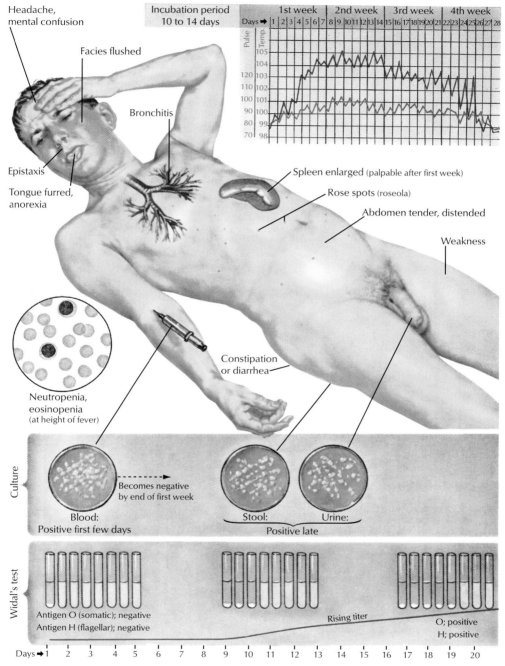

Headache, mental confusion

Facies flushed

Bronchitis

Epistaxis

Tongue furred, anorexia

Incubation period 10 to 14 days

Spleen enlarged (palpable after first week)

Rose spots (roseola)

Abdomen tender, distended

Weakness

Neutropenia, eosinopenia (at height of fever)

Constipation or diarrhea

Culture

Becomes negative by end of first week

Blood: Positive first few days

Stool:

Urine:

Positive late

Widal's test

Antigen O (somatic); negative
Antigen H (flagellar); negative

Rising titer

O; positive
H; positive

Initial treatment of TD includes fluid replacement (oral or intravenous), bismuth subsalicylate, and antimotility agents (e.g., tincture of opium, diphenoxylate, loperamide). Avoid antimotility agents in persons with fever or bloody stools. Furthermore, antimotility agents should be discontinued if symptoms persist longer than 48 hours. Consider antibiotic therapy with a fluoroquinolone in patients with prolonged TD, severe TD, bloody stools, or fever. Workup should include stool culture, stool for ova and parasites, and rotavirus.

Typhoid Fever
Clinical Presentation

Typhoid fever is an acute, life-threatening febrile illness caused by *Salmonella typhi*, although a similar syndrome may result from other *Salmonella* species (paratyphoid disease) (Figures 75-2 and 75-3). Clinical manifestations include fever, headache, malaise, anorexia, splenomegaly, and a relative bradycardia. Infection may result in mild symptoms.

Management and Therapy

Preventive measures include careful selection of food and drink and immunization. Immunization is recommended for travelers to high-risk destinations (e.g., Indian subcontinent and lesser developed countries in Asia, Africa, and Central and South America).

Typhoid fever should be considered in any returned traveler with high fever and systemic disease. The diagnosis is confirmed by cultures of stool and blood. Treatment should be initiated with intravenous antibiotics, usually a third-generation cephalosporin or a quinolone. Because *S. typhi* may demonstrate antimicrobial resistance, susceptibility tests should be performed on all isolates.

FUTURE DIRECTIONS

The events of September 11, 2001, have raised the specter of bioterrorism. Although the ultimate impact remains to be seen, physicians must remain ever vigilant of this new threat. Because many of the potential agents of bioterrorism (with the exception of smallpox) represent potential infections in travelers, clinicians providing care to travelers should be familiar with these agents including anthrax, plague, Q fever, tularemia, and botulism.

The most active research area that will affect travelers to less developed countries is the worldwide effort to develop safe and effective vaccines for pandemic diseases including HIV, malaria, and tuberculosis. It is likely that such vaccines will become available within the next 10 years.

REFERENCES

Centers for Disease Control and Prevention. *Health Information for International Travel 2001–2002*. Atlanta Ga: US Department of Health and Human Services; 2001.

Doherty JF, Grant AD, Bryceson AD. Fever as the presenting complaint of travelers returning from the tropics. *QJM*. 1995;88:277–281.

Humar A, Keystone J. Evaluating fever in travellers returning from tropical countries. *BMJ*. 1996;312:953–956.

MacLean JD, Lalonde RG, Ward B. Fever from the tropics. *Travel Med Advisor*. 1994;5:1–27.

Magill AJ. Fever in the returned traveler. *Infect Dis Clin North Am*. 1998;12:445–469.

O'Brien D, Tobin S, Brown GV, Torresi J. Fever in returned travelers: review of hospital admissions for a 3-year period. *Clin Infect Dis*. 2001;33:603–609.

Ryan ET, Kain KC. Health advice and immunizations for travelers. *N Engl J Med*. 2000;342:1716–1725.

Strickland GT. Fever in the returned traveler. *Med Clin North Am*. 1992;76:1375–1392.

Virk A. Medical advice for international travelers. *Mayo Clin Proc*. 2001;76:831–840.

Chapter 76

Infectious Mononucleosis

Bruce F. Israel and Shannon C. Kenney

Infectious mononucleosis (IM) is a clinical syndrome characterized by fever, pharyngitis, lymphadenopathy, and mononuclear lymphocytosis. Primary infection with the Epstein-Barr virus (EBV) causes the vast majority (90%) of cases, while a wide variety of other agents constitute the remainder. Classic IM is commonly a disease of adolescents and young adults, although occasionally it occurs in young children and older adults. The symptoms of primary EBV infection tend to be less severe in young children (many are asymptomatic), whereas first-time infection in the elderly often results in severe, atypical illness. Although IM is an often severe, but self-limited, disease in the healthy young adult, EBV infection can be fatal in immunosuppressed individuals.

EBV is endemic throughout the world as evidenced by 90% to 95% seropositivity in adults. There is some variance in different populations in the age of initial infection. With intimate contact and saliva exchange as the mode of transmission, primary EBV infection often occurs during the early years, and appears to be a less serious illness when acquired early. Earlier infection is more common in groups of lower socioeconomic status. Only 50% of children in the United States and United Kingdom are EBV positive by age 5, while 80% to 100% of children in developing nations are seropositive by age 4. In countries where infection is often delayed until adolescence or later, the IM syndrome ("the kissing disease") is much more common.

ETIOLOGY AND PATHOGENESIS

EBV is a herpesvirus that primarily infects B cells and epithelial cells. Viral infection most commonly occurs after contact with saliva from asymptomatically infected individuals. The virus initially infects B cells (and possibly epithelial cells) in the tonsils, followed by a systemic infection of circulating B cells. IM is characterized by an extremely vigorous T-cell response, and it is the host immune response that is thought to be responsible for many of its symptoms. The atypical lymphocytes that are the hallmark of IM are due to the T cells responding to the EBV-infected B cells.

EBV, like other herpesviruses, infects cells in both a latent and cytolytic (active) form. During primary infection, the virus uses the cytolytic form

of infection, which results in cell killing and allows the virus to be replicated and spread from cell to cell. In the immunocompetent host, cells infected with this form of EBV are eventually eliminated by T cells. Only cells containing a latent form of EBV infection evade the immune response. The latently infected B cells persist for the life of the host. From this reservoir, virus is periodically reactivated and shed into the saliva (allowing infection of a new host). In the immunocompetent individual, the latent form of EBV infection, while never completely eliminated, generally causes no illness. In contrast to infection with the latent forms of other herpesviruses (such as herpes simplex and cytomegalovirus [CMV]), latent EBV infection in cells is associated with expression of virally encoded transforming proteins. In individuals with insufficient T-cell function (such as transplant recipients and patients with AIDS), the latent EBV infection sometimes leads to lymphoproliferative B cell malignances. EBV is also commonly found in certain types of cancers in immunocompetent hosts (including African Burkitt's lymphoma, nasopharyngeal carcinoma, and Hodgkin's disease), although in these conditions the etiologic relationship between the virus and malignancy is less clear.

The host-immune response plays a critical role in the pathogenesis of primary EBV infection. A very vigorous adaptive cytotoxic T lymphocyte (CTL) response to EBV-infected B cells (such as occurs in the IM syndrome) results in the characteristic lymphocytosis with large "atypical lymphocytes"—representing the highly activated

Table 76-1
Clinical Findings in Infectious Mononucleosis

Common*	Uncommon*	Very Rarely Reported*
Fever	Cholestatic jaundice	Hemolytic anemia
Pharyngitis	Airway compromise	Thrombocytopenia
Cervical lymphadenopathy	Splenic rupture	Aplastic anemia
Hepatitis		Neutropenia
Splenomegaly		Meningitis/Encephalitis
Transient periorbital edema		Cranial nerve palsy/neuritis
Lymphocytosis		Guillain-Barré syndrome
Atypical lymphocytes		Hemophagocytic syndrome

*Acute infection in preadolescent children and adults older than 35 may lack common features, and are more likely to have the atypical features.

CTLs. EBV infection of B cells in the IM syndrome is commonly associated with a polyclonal B-cell activation and the production of multiple antibody species. Many of the serious consequences of acute IM (including hepatitis, thrombocytopenia, and hemolytic anemia) are thought to be secondary to the T-cell response and the production of autoantibodies. An effective immune response is required for eventual control of the infection. For example, individuals with the rare inherited genetic syndrome X-linked lymphoproliferative disease, are unable to control the primary EBV infection and fatal IM commonly develops. Primary EBV infection in children after bone marrow transplant also commonly results in lymphoproliferative disease.

CLINICAL PRESENTATION

Age is associated with distinct patterns in the presentation of primary EBV infection. Classic IM is most common in the adolescent and young adult, and is characterized by fever, pharyngitis, lymphadenopathy, and atypical lymphocytosis (Table 76-1). The pharynx is usually erythematous and may have an exudate. The adenopathy is commonly bilateral and involves the anterior (and sometimes posterior) cervical nodes. Enlarged nodes in other regions are less common. Splenomegaly is observed in up to one half of cases and up to one third of patients have periorbital edema early in the disease. A diffuse morbilliform rash is often observed in patients who have received beta-lactam antibiotics.

The most common laboratory abnormality is an atypical lymphocytosis (Figure 76-1). Liver function tests, especially transaminase levels, are elevated, although a severe increase in liver function tests (over tenfold normal) should prompt a search for an alternative diagnosis.

Primary EBV infection in young children is thought to be often asymptomatic, although the lack of sensitivity of the heterophile antibody tests in this age group, and the relative infrequency of atypical lymphocytosis, may compromise diagnosis. Children who present with a more classic IM picture seem more prone than adolescents to significant pharyngeal inflammation and even airway obstruction from reactive lymphoid tissue and edema.

Primary EBV infection in the elderly, although rare, is associated with a more severe, and atypical, clinical syndrome. Pharyngitis, lymphadenopathy, and atypical lymphocytosis are frequently absent. However, cholestatic liver disease, including fulminant liver failure, is much more common.

Complications

Symptoms in the adolescent usually resolve after several weeks, although more severe cases may require months for a full recovery. Complications involve almost every organ system and include airway compromise due to severe inflammation, hepatitis, cholestatic jaundice (particularly in the elderly), thrombocytopenia, hemolytic anemia, and rupture of an enlarged spleen. Cranial neuritis, encephalitis, meningitis, transverse myelitis, Guillain-Barré syndrome, neutropenia, and aplastic anemia/bone marrow suppression

Figure 76-1

Infectious Mononucleosis

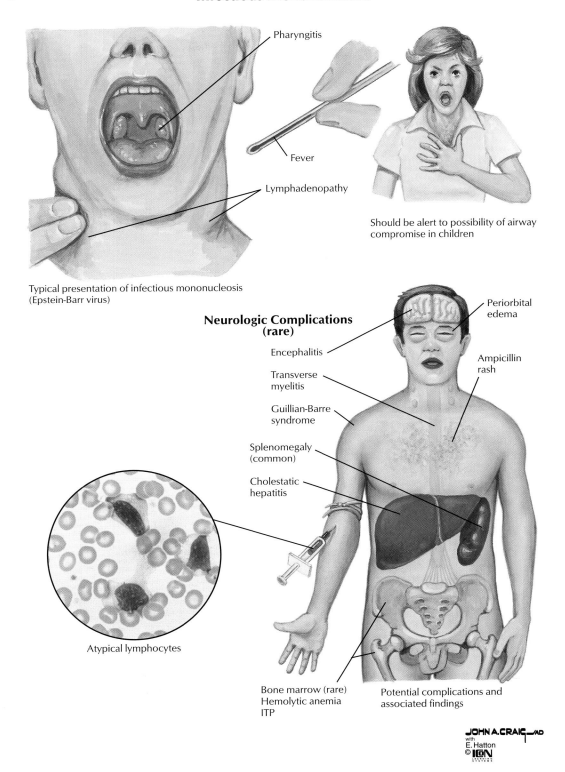

Pharyngitis

Fever

Lymphadenopathy

Should be alert to possibility of airway compromise in children

Typical presentation of infectious mononucleosis (Epstein-Barr virus)

Neurologic Complications (rare)

Periorbital edema

Encephalitis

Ampicillin rash

Transverse myelitis

Guillian-Barre syndrome

Splenomegaly (common)

Cholestatic hepatitis

Atypical lymphocytes

Bone marrow (rare)
Hemolytic anemia
ITP

Potential complications and associated findings

JOHN A. CRAIG—AD
with
E. Hatton
© ICON

are less common. In the rare familial X-linked lymphoproliferative syndrome (XLP), primary EBV infection results in either immediate, fulminant, and usually fatal IM, or subsequent hypogammaglobulinemia or B cell lymphoma. Very rarely, primary EBV infection is followed by a severe hemophagocytic syndrome, in which histiocytes attack the bone marrow, engulfing red blood cells. This syndrome appears to be associated with EBV-infected T cells. There is increasing evidence that, in rare cases, "chronic active EBV infection" develops, characterized by persistent infection with the cytolytic form of EBV infection, multiple organ involvement, and eventual death. Diagnosis of these fulminant processes is best accomplished using PCR–based assays that can quantitate the characteristic high viral load. These very rare syndromes should not be confused with chronic fatigue syndrome, which has not been shown to have an etiologic link with EBV. Periodically, immunosuppressed patients may suffer from a chronically active localized EBV infection in epithelial cells along the side of the tongue (oral hairy leukoplakia).

DIFFERENTIAL DIAGNOSIS

The differential diagnosis of IM-like syndrome in patients with negative EBV serology includes the other human herpesviruses (especially CMV, human herpesvirus-6 [HHV-6], and HHV-7), primary HIV infection, toxoplasmosis, and hepatitis viruses. In cases that do not resolve in a timely manner, malignancy is possible.

DIAGNOSTIC APPROACH
Heterophile Antibody

Patients with acute EBV infection commonly have polyclonal B-cell activation that generates nonadaptive, nonspecific IgM antibody species. The polyclonal IgM specificities usually include antibodies (the heterophile antibodies) that can bind sheep or horse red blood cells. Thus, acute phase sera agglutinate equine red blood cells, while convalescent sera lose this ability. Heterophile antibody is positive in more than 90% of adolescent IM cases. False-positive heterophile antibody test results, although rare, can be caused by lymphoma and hepatitis. The heterophile antibody test is insensitive in the diagnosis of primary EBV infection in children (less than 33%), and in patients older than 40.

Table 76-2
Interpretation of EBV-Specific Serology

Serology	No Prior EBV Infection	Acute IM	Past Infection
VCA IgM	−	+	−
VCA IgG	−	+/−	+
EBNA1 IgG	−	−	+

EBNA1, Epstein-Barr nuclear antigen 1; VCA, viral capsid antigen.

Specific Epstein-Barr Virus Serology

When the diagnosis needs confirmation, specific serology should be used (Table 76-2). The most useful antibody test is the IgM antibody to viral capsid antigen (VCA), as this is usually present at the time of presentation and disappears following the acute illness. In contrast, the IgG antibody to VCA, although often present at onset of symptoms, remains positive for life and cannot distinguish between acute versus past infection. Antibodies to the Epstein-Barr nuclear antigen 1 (EBNA1) do not develop until months following infection, and remain positive throughout a person's life. A definitive diagnosis of IM in a symptomatic patient can be made by positive IgM- or IgG-VCA antibody titer in the absence of EBNA1 titer, while positive VCA and EBNA1 titers together indicate past infection, and other causes for a patient's symptoms should be considered. Antibodies to the viral early antigens (EA-D and EA-R) are seen in both primary and reactivated (asymptomatic) infection, and are not particularly useful in diagnosing IM.

Quantification of Epstein-Barr Virus Load

Semiquantitative EBV PCR technology allows reproducible quantitation of EBV viral load from blood, although commercial facilities vary in reliability. Patients with IM often have a significantly higher burden of EBV present than can be found in chronically infected normal carriers. However, in most cases this assay is not required to make the diagnosis of IM.

MANAGEMENT AND THERAPY

The treatment of IM is primarily supportive. Beta-lactam antibiotics should be avoided (to prevent rash), and contact sports prohibited for several weeks due to the small risk of splenic rupture. A variety of antiviral agents (including acyclovir, ganciclovir, and foscarnet) inhibit the cytolytic form of EBV infection in tissue culture, although they have no effect in treating latent EBV infection. Because B cells are infected with both cytolytic and latent EBV during IM, it was anticipated that drugs such as acyclovir would be useful for this syndrome. To date, clinical trials have demonstrated no significant benefit in using acyclovir for IM, although the amount of oropharyngeal viral shedding is decreased. The failure to note a clinical benefit with acyclovir in these trials likely reflects the fact that many of the symptoms of IM are due to the immune response, rather than the virus, and immunocompetent individuals generally recover quickly from EBV without specific therapy. A subset of patients (particularly immunosuppressed individuals) may benefit from acyclovir during primary EBV infection. It is not surprising that antiviral drugs such as acyclovir are not useful in controlling the latent type of EBV infection involved in lymphoproliferative disease, because the virus replicates using the host cell DNA polymerase during this form of infection.

The addition of a short course of high-dose steroids may be useful in a few specific circumstances where an overactive immune response plays a role, including severe obstructive pharyngitis, hemolytic anemia, thrombocytopenia, and possibly CNS complications. The indiscriminate use of steroids may increase the risk of virally associated complications.

FUTURE DIRECTIONS

The development of commercially available tests for rapid quantification of EBV load may prove useful for observing patients with IM who have an unusually protracted or severe course, or who are at increased risk for the subsequent development of lymphoproliferative disease. Future studies will hopefully determine if acyclovir, although not proven to have significant clinical benefit in healthy patients with IM, has any role for treating patients who are at special risk for developing more severe disease. Recently, it has been shown that administration of exogenous EBV-specific cytotoxic T cells is useful for certain EBV-induced lymphoproliferative diseases in immunocompromised hosts. It is important to determine if EBV-specific cytotoxic T cells are also useful for treating severe IM in individuals at particularly high risk for complications (for example, patients with XLP). The development of drugs directed against the latent form of EBV infection will be an important advance in the treatment of EBV-induced lymphoproliferative disease.

REFERENCES

Auwerter PG. Infectious mononucleosis in middle age. *JAMA*. 1999;281:454–459.

Jenson HB. Acute complications of Epstein-Barr virus infectious mononucleosis. *Curr Opin Pediatr*. 2000;12:263–268.

Linde A. Diagnosis of Epstein-Barr virus-related diseases. *Scand J Infect Dis Suppl*. 1996;100:83–88.

Ohga S, Nomura A, Takada H, et al. Epstein-Barr virus (EBV) load and cytokine gene expression in activated T cells of chronic and active EBV infection. *J Infect Dis*. 2001;183:1–7.

Torre D, Tambini R. Ancyclovir for treatment of infectious mononucleosis: a meta-analysis. *Scand J Infect Dis*. 1999; 31:543–547.

Chapter 77

Influenza

Adaora A. Adimora

Influenza is an acute respiratory illness characterized by fever, cough, myalgias, and malaise due to influenza type A or B virus that occurs in epidemics each winter. Influenza's public health importance is largely due to the magnitude of its annual global epidemics and associated morbidity and mortality.

ETIOLOGY AND PATHOGENESIS

Influenza viruses are RNA viruses classified as type A, B, or C on the basis of antigenic differences. All belong to the family *Orthomyxoviridae*. Influenza C causes only mild illness and does not occur in epidemics, so its public health importance is substantially less than that of types A and B. Influenza A viruses are further subtyped based on two structural proteins: hemagglutinin and neuraminidase. Hemagglutinin binds the virus to cell receptors; neuraminidase may be involved in release of virus from infected cells following replication (Figure 77-1). At least nine neuraminidases and 15 hemagglutinins have been identified in influenza A viruses. Antibodies to these antigens are important determinants of the immune response to influenza virus. The ability of influenza A to cause epidemics is largely due to the propensity of its hemagglutinin and neuraminidase antigens to undergo major antigenic variation, known as antigenic shifts and minor variations, known as antigenic drift. Influenza B only undergoes antigenic drift. As a result of these periodic antigenic variations in circulating influenza virus strains, a large proportion of the population lacks immunity and is left vulnerable to infection.

Transmission occurs predominantly through droplet and airborne transmission produced by coughs and sneezes and by other mechanisms, such as hand contact. The virus infects the respiratory epithelium, where it replicates within infected cells, causes degenerative changes and cell death, and is then released to infect other cells. Illness severity appears to be related to the amount of viral replication and host defenses. Extrapulmonary viral infection is rare. The host immune response is complex and involves an array of defenses including cell-mediated immunity, local and systemic antibody, and interferon production. Constitutional symptoms, such as myalgias, fever, and headache, may be due to cytokine production because viremia is rare.

CLINICAL PRESENTATION

The illness usually begins abruptly after an incubation period of 24 to 72 hours. Fever, chills, headache, malaise, and myalgias are the predominant symptoms. Respiratory symptoms, such as cough, clear nasal discharge, and sore throat, are typically present but less prominent than the systemic manifestations. The presentation varies widely, from the classic presentation described above to minimal or no symptoms. The elderly may present with only fever, confusion, and weakness. Typically, the physical examination is notable for a toxic-appearing patient with pharyngeal erythema but no exudate and tender cervical lymphadenopathy. Fever and systemic symptoms usually last about 3 days, but convalescence is often marked by malaise and weakness. Complete recovery may require several weeks.

A variety of respiratory tract conditions can complicate influenza, such as tracheobronchitis, croup, and exacerbation of chronic pulmonary disease. Primary influenza viral pneumonia is associated with fever, cough, dyspnea, and respiratory compromise with minimal evidence of bacteria on sputum Gram stain (Figure 77-2). Sputum culture specimens show growth of only normal oral flora. A common complication, secondary bacterial pneumonia, is usually due to *Streptococcus pneumoniae*, *Haemophilus influenzae*, or less commonly *Staphylococcus aureus*, and is usually seen among the elderly or those with chronic lung, heart, or renal disease, or in dia-

Figure 77-1

Influenza Virus and its Epidemiology

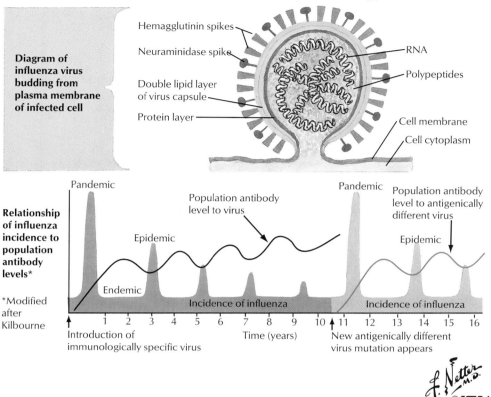

Diagram of influenza virus budding from plasma membrane of infected cell

Hemagglutinin spikes

Neuraminidase spike

Double lipid layer of virus capsule

Protein layer

RNA

Polypeptides

Cell membrane

Cell cytoplasm

Relationship of influenza incidence to population antibody levels*

*Modified after Kilbourne

Pandemic

Epidemic

Endemic

Population antibody level to virus

Incidence of influenza

Pandemic

Population antibody level to antigenically different virus

Epidemic

Incidence of influenza

1 2 3 4 5 6 7 8 9 10 11 12 13 14 15 16

Time (years)

Introduction of immunologically specific virus

New antigenically different virus mutation appears

betes mellitus. It tends to occur approximately 7 days after onset of influenza, usually after the patient appears to be recovering.

Non-pulmonary complications are relatively uncommon but include myositis, myocarditis, pericarditis, Guillain-Barré syndrome, encephalopathy, and toxic shock syndrome. Reye's syndrome is now a rare complication of influenza since recognition of aspirin as a risk factor in children and recommendations to avoid aspirin use in children with influenza.

DIFFERENTIAL DIAGNOSIS

Because a variety of infectious diseases are associated with abrupt onset of fever, headache, malaise, and myalgias, the differential diagnosis is generally based on epidemiological evidence of an illness characteristic of influenza occurring during a confirmed outbreak. The differential diagnosis includes adenoviruses, respiratory syncytial

virus, *Mycoplasma pneumoniae*, Legionella, and *Chlamydia psittaci*.

DIAGNOSTIC APPROACH

The most useful laboratory techniques for diagnosis of influenza in the setting of acute illness involve either virus isolation or detection of viral antigen in respiratory secretions. Nasal swabs or washes, throat swabs, or sputum samples provide acceptable specimens. Virus can be detected in culture within 3 to 7 days by cytopathic effect or hemadsorption. The time for diagnosis can be decreased to 1 or 2 days by centrifuging specimens onto cells in shell vials and using either immunofluorescence or ELISA to detect antigen. Some assays yield results within a few hours with comparable sensitivity and specificity to culture results.

Serological testing of acute and convalescent sera via complement fixation or hemagglutination

Figure 77-2

Influenzal Pneumonia

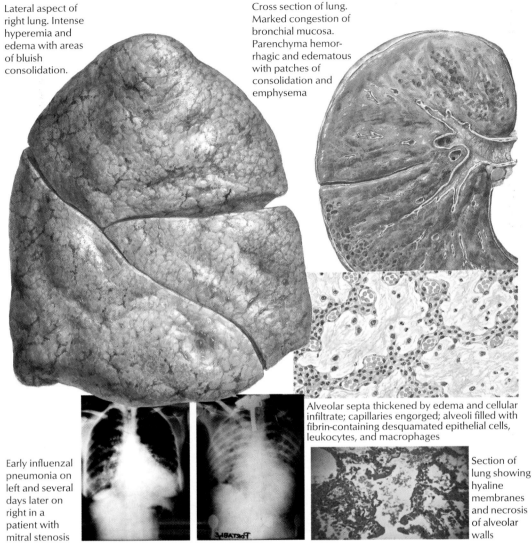

Lateral aspect of right lung. Intense hyperemia and edema with areas of bluish consolidation.

Cross section of lung. Marked congestion of bronchial mucosa. Parenchyma hemorrhagic and edematous with patches of consolidation and emphysema

Alveolar septa thickened by edema and cellular infiltrate; capillaries engorged; alveoli filled with fibrin-containing desquamated epithelial cells, leukocytes, and macrophages

Early influenzal pneumonia on left and several days later on right in a patient with mitral stenosis

Section of lung showing hyaline membranes and necrosis of alveolar walls

assays is sensitive and specific but is not useful in treating acute illness.

MANAGEMENT AND THERAPY

Uncomplicated cases of influenza usually require only supportive care and therapy for relief of symptoms. Appropriate recommendations include rest, maintenance of adequate hydration, and if needed, use of acetaminophen for relief of fever and headache. Children should not receive aspirin because of its association with Reye's syndrome.

Antiviral therapy is available for treatment of influenza. Amantadine and rimantadine are active against influenza A, and the neuraminidase inhibitors, zanamivir and oseltamivir, have activity against both influenza A and B. None of the available agents have demonstrated efficacy in preventing pneumonia, exacerbations of chronic pulmonary disease, or other serious complications of influenza. Their efficacy for treatment of patients at high risk for influenza-related complications is unclear.

Amantadine or rimantadine, when given within 48 hours of the onset of illness, can decrease the duration of influenza A symptoms by approximately 1 day. The most common adverse effects are related to the CNS and include nausea, nervousness, insomnia, and difficulty concentrating. These side effects resolve upon discontinuation of the medication. Amantadine is associated with a higher incidence of side effects than rimantadine. Both amantadine and rimantadine can be given in doses of 100 mg twice daily. Elderly patients and those with renal insufficiency should receive only 100 mg daily, because both drugs are renally excreted. To decrease risk of emergence of drug-resistant viruses, therapy should be discontinued within 24 to 48 hours of resolution of symptoms or after 3 to 5 days.

When given to otherwise healthy adults within 2 days of the start of illness, zanamivir and oseltamivir can decrease the duration of uncomplicated influenza A or B by about 24 hours. Zanamivir is given as an inhaled powder at doses of 10 mg twice daily for 5 days. Because zanamivir inhalation can exacerbate bronchospasm among patients with asthma or chronic obstructive pulmonary disease, it is not recommended for persons with underlying airway disease. Oseltamivir is given in doses of 75 mg orally twice daily. Its most common adverse effects are nausea and vomiting, which may be reduced by taking the drug with food.

PREVENTION

The primary method for preventing influenza is annual administration of influenza vaccine. Influenza vaccine is prepared from influenza A and B strains isolated during the previous influenza season and therefore likely to circulate in the United States in the upcoming winter. Immunization is recommended for people at high risk for complications from influenza infection, including persons older than 50; and those of any age who have chronic diseases of the heart, lung, or kidneys; diabetes mellitus; immunosuppression; or hemoglobinopathies. Also recommended for vaccination are residents of nursing homes and other facilities that house persons with chronic medical conditions; children and teenagers who receive chronic aspirin therapy and might therefore be at risk for Reye's syndrome; and women who will be beyond the first trimester of pregnancy during influenza season. Vaccination of health-care workers and household members of persons in high-risk groups is also recommended to decrease risk of influenza transmission. People known to have anaphylactic hypersensitivity to eggs or other vaccine components should not receive influenza vaccine. The optimal time for vaccine administration in the United States is from the beginning of October through mid-November.

Influenza vaccine efficacy depends on the vaccine recipient's age and immunocompetence as well as the degree of similarity between the vaccine virus strains and strains in circulation during influenza season. When vaccine and circulating virus strains are well matched, efficacy in healthy adults younger than 65 is 70% to 90%. Although the vaccine is less effective among elderly persons living in nursing homes (30%–40%), its efficacy is approximately 50% to 60% in preventing pneumonia and 80% in preventing death.

Although the primary method of influenza prevention is vaccination, antiviral agents are important adjuncts. Amantadine and rimantadine do not prevent influenza B infection but are 70% to 90% effective in preventing influenza A and have been used extensively in nursing home and other populations for this purpose. However, resistance may rapidly develop in such situations. There is substantially less experience with zanamivir and oseltamivir for prophylaxis against influenza, and neither drug is FDA-approved for this purpose. Recent studies suggest that both drugs are approximately 82% to 84% effective for prevention of influenza infection, although experience is limited in patients with chronic medical conditions or in those who reside in nursing homes. If, during the course of an influenza outbreak, patients at high risk for influenza-related complications are unvaccinated, they should receive the vaccination immediately followed by rimantadine for approximately 4 weeks while awaiting development of protective antibody titers.

FUTURE DIRECTIONS

Influenza remains one of the most common and important infectious diseases. Recent threats of potentially more virulent strains in Asia will galvanize both vaccine and treatment strategies. Improved vaccines with mucosal delivery are in advanced stages of development; their implementation should improve vaccine distribution and may also increase duration of immunity. New therapies directed against influenza are expected to play an important role in both endemic and epidemic situations.

REFERENCES

Centers for Disease Control and Prevention. Prevention and control of influenza: recommendations of the Advisory Committee on Immunization Practices (ACIP). *MMWR Morb Mortal Wkly Rep.* 2002;51:1–38.

Dolin R. Influenza. In: Braunwald E, Fauci AS, Kasper DL, Hauser SL, Longo DL, Jameson JL, eds. *Harrison's Principles of Internal Medicine.* 15th ed. New York, NY: McGraw-Hill; 2001:1125–1130.

Smith C. Influenza viruses. In: Gorbach SL, Bartlett JG, Blacklow NR, eds. *Infectious Diseases.* 2nd ed. Philadelphia, Pa: WB Saunders Co; 1998:2120–2124.

Treanor J. Influenza virus. In: Mandell GL, Bennett JE, Dolin R, eds. *Mandell, Douglas, and Bennett's Principles and Practice of Infectious Diseases.* 5th ed. Philadelphia, Pa: Churchill Livingstone; 2000:1823–1849.

Chapter 78

Malaria

William C. Miller

Malaria is a common and important infectious disease globally (Figure 78-1). An estimated 300 to 500 million cases of malaria occur worldwide each year, with over one million deaths, primarily in Africa, Asia, and South and Central America. Although once common in parts of the United States, most of the approximately 1200 cases reported each year are travelers to endemic regions.

ETIOLOGY AND PATHOGENESIS

One of four species causes malaria: *Plasmodium falciparum*, *Plasmodium vivax*, *Plasmodium ovale*, and *Plasmodium malariae*. The species are morphologically distinct, providing the basis for specific diagnosis.

The life cycles of the four species are similar except for a few important differences (Figure 78-2). Infection of humans begins with the inoculation of sporozoites from the salivary glands of an infected female *Anopheles* mosquito. The sporozoites rapidly invade hepatocytes and are largely cleared from the blood within 30 minutes of inoculation. In the liver, the parasite undergoes asexual multiplication to from hepatic or tissue schizonts. After a variable period of development, merozoites emerge from the liver cells into the bloodstream. The duration of the liver stage is typically 1 to 3 weeks, but it is 2 to 4 weeks for *P. malariae*.

A critical difference between species is the existence of persistent liver forms, or hypnozoites, in *P. ovale* and *P. vivax* infections. The hypnozoites remain dormant for months or years before becoming active and causing relapse. Neither *P. falciparum* nor *P. malariae* have persistent liver forms. However, persistent, low-grade infections in the blood with *P. falciparum* or *P. malariae* may cause recrudescence of clinical disease.

The merozoites released from the liver attach to and invade erythrocytes. In the erythrocyte, ring forms with a small nucleus and a ring of pale cytoplasm develop. The parasite then develops into a trophozoite and finally into an erythrocytic schizont. Rupture of the schizont releases merozoites into the bloodstream, leading to another asexual development cycle in fresh erythrocytes.

The parasite also undergoes a sexual cycle, which requires both humans and mosquitoes. In the erythrocyte, some merozoites develop into male and female gametocytes. These gametocytes are taken up during a blood meal by the female *Anopheles* mosquito. In the mosquito stomach, gametes form. Macrogametes are fertilized by microgametes forming zygotes, which then develop into ookinetes. The ookinetes invade the gut wall, form oocysts, and sporozoites develop within the oocysts. The sporozoites migrate to the salivary gland of the mosquito and await inoculation into the human host.

The cycle within the human host is affected by several host and parasite factors. *P. malariae* invades mature erythrocytes. *P. vivax* and *P. ovale* invade young erythrocytes. *P. falciparum* is capable of invading erythrocytes of any age. Thus, parasitemia is limited in *P. malariae*, *P. vivax*, and *P. ovale* infections, but can reach extremely high levels in *P. falciparum* infections.

Persons with high levels of hemoglobin F and hemoglobin S have increased resistance to falciparum malaria due to reduced survival of the parasite in the erythrocytes. Persons with the heterozygous state of hemoglobin AS have a survival advantage and experience less severe falciparum malaria. Persons with glucose-6-phosphate dehydrogenase deficiency also appear to have increased resistance to falciparum malaria.

Persons lacking the Duffy group antigens on erythrocytes are resistant to infection with *P. vivax*. This trait, common throughout much of Africa, accounts for the low incidence of vivax malaria in Africa.

The symptoms, signs, and complications of malaria are due to the intraerythrocytic cycle. Fever occurs with schizont rupture (Figure 78-3). Anemia is common in all forms of malaria and is

Figure 78-1

Geographic Distribution of Malaria

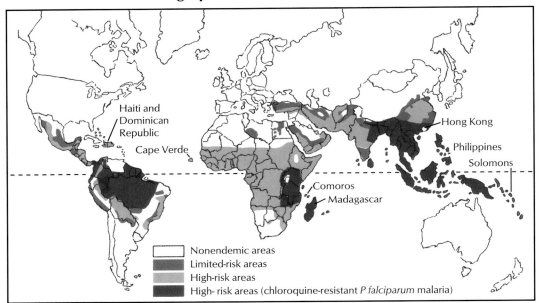

Haiti and
Dominican
Republic

Cape Verde

Hong Kong

Philippines

Solomons

Comoros

Madagascar

☐ Nonendemic areas
■ Limited-risk areas
■ High-risk areas
■ High-risk areas (chloroquine-resistant *P falciparum* malaria)

due primarily to destruction and phagocytosis of infected erythrocytes.

CLINICAL PRESENTATION

Many patients with malaria experience a prodrome with headache, decreased appetite, malaise, myalgias, and, in some cases, low-grade fever lasting 2 to 3 days or longer in persons with partial immunity or incomplete suppression due to prophylaxis.

Fever is the classic manifestation of malaria. The onset of a paroxysm of fever begins with abrupt onset of chills, often with teeth chattering and shivering. The subsequent fever, as high as 40° C to 41° C in falciparum malaria, typically lasts 2 to 4 hours and is followed by diaphoresis. The duration of the entire paroxysm is 8 to 12 hours. Between paroxysms, the persons may feel well.

The paroxysms are intermittent and may have periodicity (Figure 78-3). Paroxysms associated with *P. vivax* and *P. ovale* infections occur every 48 hours, whereas with *P. malariae* the interval between episodes is 72 hours. The paroxysms of

fever with these species are more common during the daylight hours. Fever is often irregular during the first few days of the illness. Periodicity is often absent in falciparum malaria, but may occur with an interval of about 48 hours. Malaria cannot be excluded on the basis of the lack of periodicity.

Other symptoms, in addition to fever, include headache, backache, and myalgias. Nausea and vomiting commonly occur during the febrile paroxysm, and diarrhea may develop. Lightheadedness and postural hypotension are due to volume depletion. Confusion and delirium may complicate the paroxysm of fever.

Physical findings in patients with malaria include fever, tachycardia, and orthostatic hypotension. Splenomegaly is typical, and tender hepatomegaly is often present. Jaundice and crackles in the lungs are also observed.

Cerebral malaria is the most severe complication of falciparum malaria. Typically, it occurs after several days of illness, but may develop early in the course. Common manifestations include confusion and hallucinations, but coma

Figure 78-2

Life Cycle of Malaria Parasites (*P. vivax*)

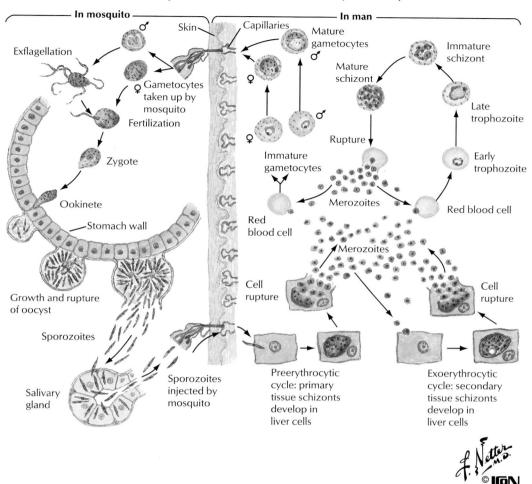

is required for a definitive diagnosis. Physical examination may be non-focal or exhibit focal findings including dysconjugate gaze, increased muscle tone, hemiparesis, and meningismus.

Splenic rupture may occur spontaneously or in association with minor trauma. Abdominal pain, possibly with radiation to the left shoulder, is typical. Hypotension and tachycardia may complicate the rapid fall in blood volume. Rapid surgical intervention is essential.

Patients often have a normocytic, normochromic anemia, usually with evidence of hemolysis. Thrombocytopenia is also common. Other laboratory findings include hyponatremia, elevated blood urea nitrogen, bilirubinemia, and mildly elevated liver transaminase levels. Elevation of the serum creatinine suggests acute renal failure due to hypovolemia or acute tubular necrosis.

The clinical presentation of malaria in adults from endemic regions is usually milder, manifested primarily by fever, headache, and gastrointestinal symptoms. The mild form of the illness is due to the acquisition of partial immunity. This immunity is not permanent and may wane after a prolonged period without exposure. In fact, natives to endemic regions represent one of the most common groups of travelers with imported malaria in the United States. Use of prophylaxis is uncommon among persons who have previously lived in malarious regions and are returning after staying overseas.

Figure 78-3

Malaria: Clinical Course and Diagnosis

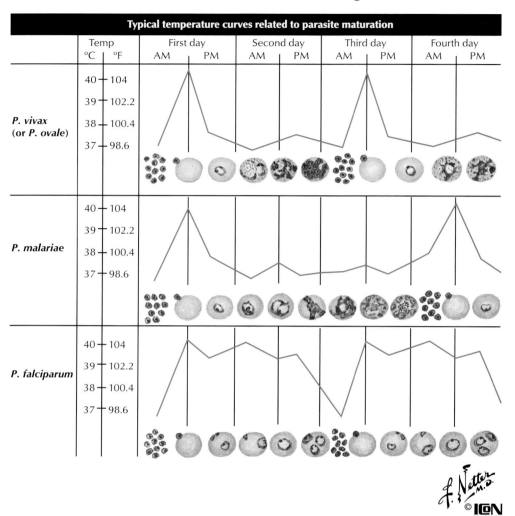

Malaria during pregnancy is often more severe than in other adults. Infection is associated with stillbirth, premature delivery, low birthweight, and an increased mortality. Anemia is worse in malaria during pregnancy. Hypoglycemia is common in malaria during pregnancy and may be exacerbated by treatment with quinine or quinidine.

DIFFERENTIAL DIAGNOSIS

The clinical manifestations of malaria are nonspecific and may be present in a variety of other febrile illnesses. Common infections in the United States, such as influenza, bacteremia, viral gastroenteritis, viral hepatitis, viral encephalitis, and viral or bacteri-

al meningitis may present similarly. Other febrile illnesses associated with travel include typhoid fever, relapsing fevers, yellow fever, leptospirosis, brucellosis, and traveler's diarrhea. Non-infectious causes of fever such as drug-induced fever with hemolysis should also be considered.

DIAGNOSTIC APPROACH

Malaria should be suspected in any person with fever and a history of travel to an endemic area. A carefully elicited travel history will assist in making the diagnosis and eliminating several of the other possible infectious causes. The travel history will provide insight into the likely species of *Plasmodi-*

Figure 78-4

Malaria: Clinical Course and Diagnosis

Thick blood smear (*P. falciparum*)   Thin blood smear (heavy *P. falciparum* infestation)

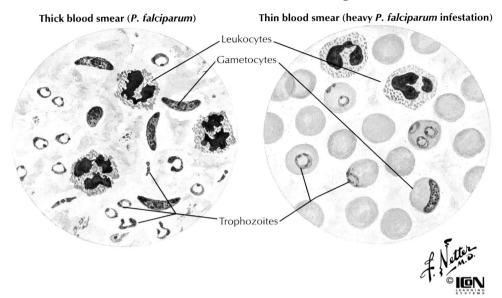

Leukocytes

Gametocytes

Trophozoites

um and guide treatment choices. *P. falciparum* occurs throughout the malarious regions of the world, but predominates in Africa, Haiti, and New Guinea. It is common in India, Southeast Asia, Oceania, and South America. *P. ovale* occurs primarily in Africa. *P. vivax* occurs in Central and South America, western Asia, and North Africa. *P. vivax* is rarely found in sub-Saharan Africa. *P. malariae* is widespread throughout the malarious regions of the world.

The primary diagnostic methods include the thick and thin blood films (Figure 78-4).

Thick films are prepared by placing a fresh drop of blood, preferably from a finger stick, on a microscope slide. After drying, the cells are lysed with distilled water and the slide is stained with Giemsa or Wright-Giemsa stain. Thin films are prepared in the same manner as slides for examination of erythrocyte morphology. Preparation of thin films may be made from tubes of blood with anticoagulant, although the anticoagulant may distort parasite morphology. Thick films are more sensitive than thin films, but thin films are necessary for species identification. Speciation is critical for determining the appropriate therapy.

Thick and thin films may be falsely negative. Collection of specimens repeatedly is essential to confirm the diagnosis. Specimens taken at various times of day increase the likelihood of detecting the parasite. An experienced laboratory technologist should review the smears.

MANAGEMENT AND THERAPY

The treatment decisions for malaria depend on the species and the severity of the illness. Severe falciparum malaria requires parenteral therapy with quinine or quinidine. Because intravenous quinine is not routinely available in the United States, quinidine is the drug of choice. In cases with high parasitemia (greater than 5% of erythrocytes infected), exchange transfusion can be considered as an adjunct to quinidine.

In uncomplicated falciparum malaria, treatment is guided by the location of acquisition of the infection. In most of the areas with endemic malaria, chloroquine resistance is common. Persons with travel history to these areas should receive one of several alternatives: oral quinine and doxycycline, oral quinine and pyrimethamine-sulfadoxine, mefloquine, or atovaquone and proguanil.

P. falciparum in Central America, Haiti, the Dominican Republic, and the Middle East remains sensitive to chloroquine. For falciparum malaria from these areas, as well as infections due to *P. vivax*, *P. ovale*, and *P. malariae*, chloroquine is the drug of choice. Chloroquine does not treat the liver forms of *P. vivax* and *P. ovale*. Persons with these infections by *P. vivax* and *P. ovale* must also receive primaquine to prevent relapse.

Cases of chloroquine-resistant *P. vivax* have been reported in Indonesia and Papua, New Guinea. Treatment of persons with *P. vivax* acquired in these regions should consist of oral quinine and doxycycline, oral quinine and pyrimethamine-sulfadoxine, or mefloquine.

Prophylaxis is a critical component of prevention of malaria for travelers to endemic regions. Mefloquine, administered once weekly, is effective prophylaxis. Alternatives include atovaquone and proguanil or doxycycline. Chloroquine is effective for travel to areas with chloroquine-sensitive *P. falciparum* and the other species of *Plasmodium*.

FUTURE DIRECTIONS

Malaria is likely to remain a problem worldwide for the foreseeable future. New antimalarial agents are needed to limit the impact of resistance to available therapeutic agents. Side-effect profiles for prophylaxis must also be improved. Given that malaria is relatively uncommon in the United States and the diagnosis requires an experienced laboratory technologist, the ongoing development of rapid, alternative diagnostic techniques may be beneficial.

REFERENCES

Bradley D, Newbold CI, Warrell DA. Malaria. In: Weatherall DJ, Ledingham JGG, Warrell DA, eds. *Oxford Textbook of Medicine*. 3rd ed. Oxford, United Kingdom: Oxford University Press; 1996:835–863.

Centers for Disease Control and Prevention Web site. National Center for Infectious Diseases: traveler's health. Information for health care providers: prescription drugs for preventing malaria. 2001. Available at: http://www.cdc.gov/travel/malariadrugs2.htm. Accessed January 2, 2003.

Miller KD, Greenberg AE, Campbell CC. Treatment of severe malaria in the United States with a continuous infusion of quinidine gluconate and exchange transfusion. *N Engl J Med*. 1989;321:65–70.

Wyler DJ. Plasmodium and babesia. In: Gorbach SL, Bartlett JG, Blacklow NR, eds. *Infectious Diseases*. 2nd ed. Philadelphia, Pa: WB Saunders Co; 1998:1969–1978.

Chapter 79

Meningitis

Shannon Galvin and Meera K. Kelley

Meningitis is an inflammation of the meninges, characterized by cellular pleocytosis in the cerebrospinal fluid. It usually manifests as headache, fever, meningismus (painful stiff neck) as well as seizures, focal neurological deficits, and disturbances of consciousness. The most common acute presentations result from bacterial and aseptic meningitis. Aseptic meningitis is associated with viral etiologies most commonly. Other causes include drug reactions and vasculitis. A subacute picture, where CSF pleocytosis persists for longer than 4 weeks, is more likely to be associated with fungal or tuberculous meningitis.

ETIOLOGY AND PATHOGENESIS

The most common cause of bacterial meningitis in adults is *Streptococcus pneumoniae*, which accounts for 38% of community-acquired cases. Other causes include *Neisseria meningitidis*, 14%; *Haemophilus influenzae*, 4%; and *Listeria monocytogenes*, 11%. Rarely, bacterial meningitis is associated with other bacteria, including gram negative bacilli, other streptococci, *Staphylococcus aureus*, anaerobes, and diphtheroids. The elderly or immunocompromised are more likely than others to develop infection due to *Listeria monocytogenes* and gram-negative bacilli. Patients with prior neurosurgery are more likely to develop infection with skin organisms: *Staphylococcus aureus*, and *Staphylococcus epidermis*, as well as *Pseudomonas aeruginosa* and other gram-negative bacilli.

Viral meningitis is most commonly caused by coxsackie and echoviruses. HIV, arboviruses, herpes simplex types 1 and 2, adenovirus, cytomegalovirus, varicella zoster, Epstein-Barr virus, lymphocytic choriomeningitis virus, and influenza are less common causes. Viral meningitis is often less severe, shows a lymphocytic pleocytosis, and has a self-limited course of 5 to 7 days. Other infectious causes include cryptococcosis, tuberculosis, leptospirosis, syphilis, Lyme disease, and amebic meningoencephalitis.

Aseptic meningitis can be caused by a number of drugs and can also be a manifestation of certain systemic disorders (Table 79-1). Carcinomatous meningitis is frequently seen in hematological malignancies and in some adenocarcinomas. The presentation is usually subacute and a large volume (10 cc) of CSF should be sent for cytological analysis when aseptic meningitis is suspected.

CLINICAL PRESENTATION

Headache, fever, and neck stiffness are the hallmarks of meningitis. The headache is usually severe and frontal and can be accompanied by photophobia and vomiting. In bacterial meningitis, the temperature usually exceeds 37.7°C but can be low grade in viral meningitis, and absent in immunocompromised patients. Neck stiffness is a more specific sign and has a sensitivity of approximately 70%. Mental status changes occur in bacterial meningitis in 44% of cases, but are found in only 3% of viral meningitis cases. Seizures occur up to 23% of the time, and focal findings such as cranial nerve deficits occur in as many as 28% of cases of bacterial meningitis.

Meningeal signs, most commonly meningismus, are present in approximately 88% of cases of bacterial meningitis. Other classical signs are Kernig and Brudzinski signs (Figure 79-1). The Kernig sign is pain in the back upon passive extension of one leg at the knee and the thigh. The Brudzinski sign is flexion of the legs at the thighs when the patient's neck is flexed. Jolt accentuation of headache is a very sensitive finding for meningitis. This is elicited by having the patient turn the head rapidly horizontally a number of times per second to assess for worsening of the headache.

A thorough neurological examination should be performed with attention to accurate assessment of the level of consciousness, the presence or absence of cranial nerve deficits, assessment for papilledema, and documentation of any

Figure 79-1

Kernig's Sign and Brudzinski's Neck Sign

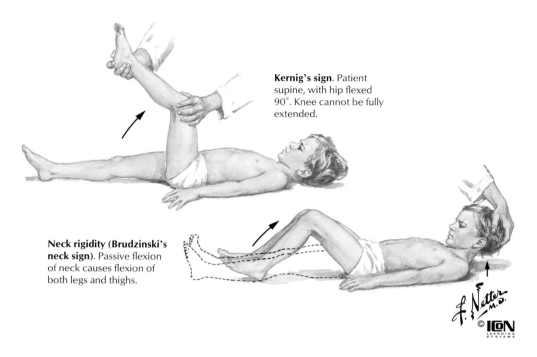

Kernig's sign. Patient supine, with hip flexed 90°. Knee cannot be fully extended.

Neck rigidity (Brudzinski's neck sign). Passive flexion of neck causes flexion of both legs and thighs.

Table 79-1
Etiology of Aseptic Meningitis

Viral	echovirus, coxsackievirus, arboviruses, Herpes simplex type 2, HIV, lymphocytic choriomeningitis, adenovirus, mumps, influenza, parainfluenza, CMV, Epstein-Barr, varicella zoster, others
Drugs	NSAIDs, trimethoprim-sulfamethoxazole, isoniazid, penicillin, ciprofloxacin, OKT3, azathioprine, immunoglobulin, carbamazepine, cytosine arabinoside, others
Systemic	sarcoidosis, Behcet's syndrome, systemic lupus erythematosus, CNS vasculitis, Vogt-Koyanagi-Harada syndrome, Wegener's granulomatosis, carcinomatous meningitis, others
Other infectious syndromes where CSF cultures can be negative	Rocky Mountain spotted fever, typhus, human ehrlichiosis, endocarditis, amebiasis, others

CMV, cytomegalovirus; CNS, central nervous system; CSF, cerebrospinal fluid; HIV, human immunodeficiency virus; NSAIDs, nonsteroidal anti-inflammatory drugs.

focal motor or sensory defects. Examine the skin for rashes. Purpura strongly suggests meningococcal disease. Petechiae are almost as frequently seen as purpura in meningococcal meningitis and can occur in rickettsial diseases and sometimes in pneumococcal meningitis.

Embolic phenomena such as splinter hemorrhages, Janeway lesions, and Roth spots suggest endocarditis, both a cause and a mimic of meningitis. A note should be made of cerebrospinal fluid shunts, prior neurosurgical procedures, or head trauma.

Figure 79-2

Bacterial Meningitis

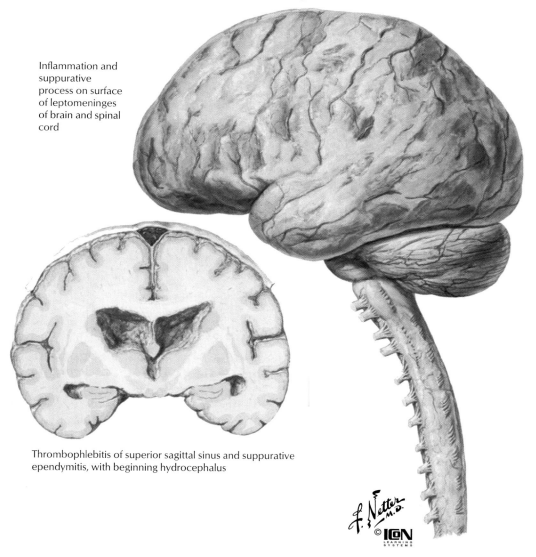

Inflammation and suppurative process on surface of leptomeninges of brain and spinal cord

Thrombophlebitis of superior sagittal sinus and suppurative ependymitis, with beginning hydrocephalus

The meningitis of leptospirosis is associated with jaundice and renal dysfunction in a patient with a history of exposure to rodent, dog, or livestock urine. Both syphilis and Lyme disease present with the clinical picture of aseptic meningitis during their secondary phases. Amebic disease secondary to *Naegleria fowleri* and *Acanthamoeba* is much more fulminant.

Patients can also present with evidence of infections associated with bacterial meningitis such as sinusitis, otitis media, and mastoiditis; as well as complications of meningitis such as cav-ernous sinus thrombosis and thrombophlebitis of the cranial sinuses (Figure 79-2).

DIAGNOSTIC APPROACH

The diagnosis is made by lumbar puncture (Figure 79-3). It is important to document the opening pressure and appearance of the CSF. CSF should be sent for cell count and differential, glucose, protein, Gram stain, and culture in all cases (Table 79-2). The addition of a VDRL and a cryptococcal antigen is helpful where an immunocompromised state is possible or in a subacute presentation.

Figure 79-3

Bacterial Meningitis

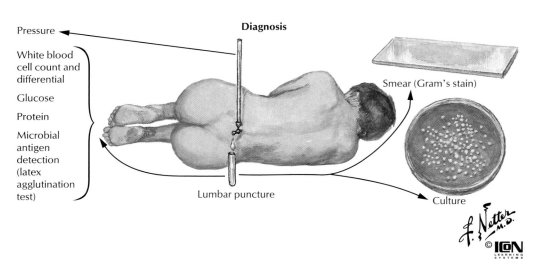

Diagnosis

Pressure

White blood cell count and differential

Glucose

Protein

Microbial antigen detection (latex agglutination test)

Lumbar puncture

Smear (Gram's stain)

Culture

Other important tests include latex agglutination for *Haemophilus influenzae* type b, *Streptococcus pneumoniae, Streptococcus agalatiae, Neisseria meningitidis* serogroups; viral PCR for herpes family viruses; examination for acid-fast organisms and tuberculosis PCR; and CSF cell cytology.

Some controversy surrounds the appropriate use of imaging studies and the timing of antibiotics. Meningitis is an infectious diseases emergency and, if lumbar puncture is to be delayed at all, empiric antibiotics should be started immediately. CSF cultures are often sterile for bacterial pathogens if taken after antibiotics have been given. CSF cell count and makeup are not affected to any great degree if taken within the first 24 hours of treatment. The risk of causing herniation in a patient by performing a lumbar puncture is no more than 6% and probably only happens when the intracranial pressure is not evenly distributed due to mass effect. Papilledema is a contraindication to lumbar puncture, but it occurs rarely in meningitis. The current recommendation is to obtain a CT scan before doing lumbar puncture on all comatose patients, those with focal deficits or papilledema, and in HIV-positive patients.

Culture is the gold standard for making a diagnosis of bacterial meningitis. In those patients who received antibiotics before lumbar puncture, latex agglutination tests can be helpful. Currently, tests are available for *Haemophilus influenza* type

b; *Neisseria meningitidis* serogroups A, C, Y, and W135; *Streptococcus agalactiae*; and *Streptococcus pneumoniae*.

Neurosyphilis is associated with a mild CSF pleocytosis, and the CSF VDRL test result is positive in only 60% of cases. The diagnosis of leptospirosis is made by serology, as is that of Lyme disease. PCR testing has recently become available for Lyme disease. The diagnosis of amebic disease requires CSF examination for motile amoebas.

DIFFERENTIAL DIAGNOSIS

The differential diagnosis for patients presenting with fever, headache, and altered mental status includes encephalitis, focal brain lesion, and systemic infections including endocarditis and rickettsial infections. Encephalitis is classically distinguished from meningitis by the absence of meningeal symptoms and the presence of diffuse neurological deficits such as altered mentation, confusion, and seizures. A brain lesion may be more likely to present with focal neurological complaints and be detected by CT imaging. Blood cultures to detect systemic bacteremia and consideration of rickettsial diseases are always warranted.

MANAGEMENT AND THERAPY

Treatment has been adjusted in the past several years due to the problem of antibiotic resistance

Table 79-2
Typical CSF Findings in Meningitis

	Normal	Bacterial	Viral	Fungal	TB	Other
WBC count	0–5/mm³	100–10,000/mm³	5–3000/mm³	5–500/mm³	5–500/mm³	
WBC makeup		>50% PMNs	>50% lymphocytes	>50% lymphocytes	>50% lymphocytes	Carcinomatous can have monoclonal population and cellular atypia
Protein	50–80 mg/dL	>200 mg/dL	Normal or slightly high	Normal or slightly high	Elevated	Protein can be elevated in any illness that disrupts blood brain barrier
Glucose	70–80 mg/dL or >60% of serum glucose	<40 mg/dL or <60% of serum glucose	Normal	Normal	<40 mg/dL may be normal in 20% of cases	Can be low in carcinomatous meningitis
Gram stain	Negative	60% positive	Negative	India ink positive 50% for cryptococcus	Acid fast stain positive 25%–37%	
Pressure	75–200 mm Hg	Elevated	Normal	Elevated	Normal or elevated	

Note: Exceptions to these values can occur and clinical findings should be taken into account when making a diagnosis.

among pneumococci, *Haemophilus influenzae*, and meningococcus. The current recommendation is to use a third-generation cephalosporin such as ceftriaxone 2 g IV every 12 hours. Vancomycin should be added in areas of high resistance (>10%), when *S. pneumoniae* has been isolated and sensitivity is pending in an ill patient, or if an isolate with an minimum inhibitory concentration greater than 0.5 ug/mL to ceftriaxone or cefotaxime has been identified. *Listeria monocytogenes* is not optimally treated with ceftriaxone. At-risk patients and any ill patient with meningitis not responding to therapy should receive ampicillin 2 g IV every 4 hours in addition to empiric therapy while awaiting cultures. Doxycycline should be added at 100 mg twice daily to any patient with meningitis and an illness consistent with Rocky Mountain spotted fever in an endemic area. Vancomycin 1 g IV every 12 hours is warranted in patients after neurosurgery or with recent head trauma. This can be switched to nafcillin or oxacillin if the organism is sensitive. Tuberculous meningitis is treated with 4 drugs with consideration of adding steroids. Cryptococcal disease requires amphotericin B therapy. At present, the only treatment for viral meningitis is supportive.

Prevention

Vaccination with *H. influenzae* type b should be part of the routine immunization schedule for children. Vaccination with pneumococcal vaccine protects against invasive disease and is helpful in reducing cases of pneumococcal meningitis in at-risk populations. It should be given to all adults older than 65, persons with chronic diseases, and people with asplenia. In January 2001, the Centers for Disease Control recommended administering the recently licensed heptavalent pneumococcal polysaccharide protein conjugate vaccine to children as part of the routine childhood immunization schedule.

A polysaccharide vaccine against *Neisseria meningitidis* serogroup A, C, Y, and W-135 is available and is currently recommended for use in disease outbreaks and in persons with complement deficiencies and functional asplenia as well as travelers to endemic areas of sub-Saharan Africa.

Prophylaxis

Close contacts of persons with meningococcal meningitis should receive one dose of ciprofloxacin 500 mg orally or four doses of rifampin 600 mg orally every 12 hours to eradicate colonization of the pharynx. Close contacts refer to household contacts, or those with other significant or prolonged contact.

FUTURE DIRECTIONS

Agents that mediate the inflammatory cytokines formed during meningitis are under investigation. Studies have looked at using antagonists of TNF, IL-1, and prostaglandins or giving IL-10. Ongoing assessment of local, national, and worldwide resistance patterns will be essential in guiding future therapy.

REFERENCES

Archer BD. Computed tomography before lumbar puncture in acute meningitis: a review of the risks and benefits. *CMAJ*. 1993;148:961–965.

Attia J, Hatala R. Cook DJ, Wong JG. The rational clinical examination. Does this adult patient have acute meningitis? *JAMA*. 1999;282:175–181.

Centers for Disease Control and Prevention. Prevention and control of meningococcal disease. Recommendations of the Advisory Committee on Immunization Practices (ACIP). *MMWR Recomm Rep*. 2000;49:1–10.

Centers for Disease Control and Prevention. Meningococcal disease and college students. Recommendations of the Advisory Committee on Immunization Practices (ACIP). *MMWR Recomm Rep*. 2000;49:13–20.

Centers for Disease Control and Prevention. Recommended childhood immunization schedule–United States, 2002. *MMWR Morb Mortal Wkly Rep*. 2002;50:7–10.

Centers for Disease Control and Prevention Web site. Available at: http://www.cdc.org. Accessed January 4, 2002.

Durand ML, Calderwood SB, Weber DJ, et al. Acute bacterial meningitis in adults. A review of 493 episodes. *N Eng J Med*. 1993;328:21–28.

Grimwood K, Collignon PJ, Currie BJ, et al. Antibiotic management of pneumococcal infections in an era of increased resistance. *J Paediatr Child Health*. 1997;33:287–295.

Hoban DJ, Witwicki W, Hammond GW. Bacterial antigen detection in cerebrospinal fluid of patients with meningitis. *Diagn Microbiol Infect Dis*. 1985;3:373–379.

Lambert HP. Meningitis. *J Neurol Neurosurg Psychiatry*. 1994; 57:405–415.

Meningitis Foundation of America Web site. Available at: http://www.musa.org. Accessed January 4, 2002.

Meningitis Research Foundation Web site. Available at: http://www.meningitis.org. Accessed January 4, 2002.

Pruitt AA. Infections of the nervous system. *Neurol Clin*. 1998;16:419–447.

Tunkel AR, Scheld WM. Acute meningitis. In: Mandell GL, Bennett JE, Dolin R, eds. *Mandell, Douglas, and Bennett's Principles and Practice of Infectious Diseases*. 5th ed. Philadelphia, Pa: Churchill Livingstone; 2000:959–997.

Chapter 80
Parasitic Infections

Mina C. Hosseinipour and Meera K. Kelley

Enteric parasitic infections remain an important cause of morbidity in developing countries. With the constant influx of immigrants, the growing number of travelers to developing countries, and immunosuppression related to HIV, transplantation, and chemotherapy; knowledge of parasitic diseases is of increasing importance. Parasitic diseases can be largely defined into two categories, those due to helminths and those due to protozoa.

NEMATODES: ROUNDWORMS

Nematodes are categorized according to where the adult form of the worm resides. Intestinal nematodes are the most prevalent. While intestinal nematode infections occur worldwide, the majority of cases occur in tropical or subtropical countries and disproportionately afflict children. Poor sanitation plays a major role because maturation of eggs within the environment must occur to maintain the worm life cycle and human infections. Symptoms are highly dependent on worm burden; light infections are generally asymptomatic while heavy infections result in more severe symptoms and complications. Eosinophilia generally occurs with the tissue migration phase of the immature worm and may be absent when the adult worm resides in the intestine. Co-infections with the intestinal worms are common.

Enterobiasis (Pinworm)
Etiology and Pathogenesis

Pinworm infection is caused by *Enterobius vermicularis* (Figure 80-1). When infectious eggs are ingested, larvae mature within the intestine, and adult female worms lay eggs on the perianal skin. Immature eggs must mature in the environment to become infectious. Because the maturation of *Enterobius* eggs occurs within hours, re-infection of the child and infection of family members and close contacts is common.

Clinical Presentation

Nocturnal pruritus ani is the predominant symptom, particularly among children. Pruritus vulvae and genitourinary symptoms may occur in girls.

Diagnostic Approach

The "scotch-tape" test is the best diagnostic method. Cellophane tape pressed on the perianal skin in the morning will reveal eggs and possibly female worms. Fecal smear for ova and parasites is frequently negative.

Management and Therapy

Single dose therapy with mebendazole 100 mg, pyrantel pamoate 11 mg/kg, or albendazone 400 mg is effective. Clothing and bedding should be washed to eradicate infectious eggs in the environment. The entire family should be treated simultaneously and retreatment of all family members should occur in approximately 2 weeks.

Trichuriasis (Whipworm)
Etiology and Pathogenesis

Whipworm infection is caused by *Trichuris trichiura*. This infection is also maintained via a direct life cycle. However, trichuris eggs require weeks to months to mature, therefore autoinfection (repeated infection of oneself) generally does not occur.

Clinical Presentation

Most infections are asymptomatic. Heavy infections in malnourished infants may result in diarrhea and rectal prolapse.

Diagnostic Approach

A fecal smear for ova and parasites is the best diagnostic method.

Management and Therapy

Either mebendazole 100 mg twice daily for 3

Figure 80-1

Parasitic Diseases
Enterobiasis

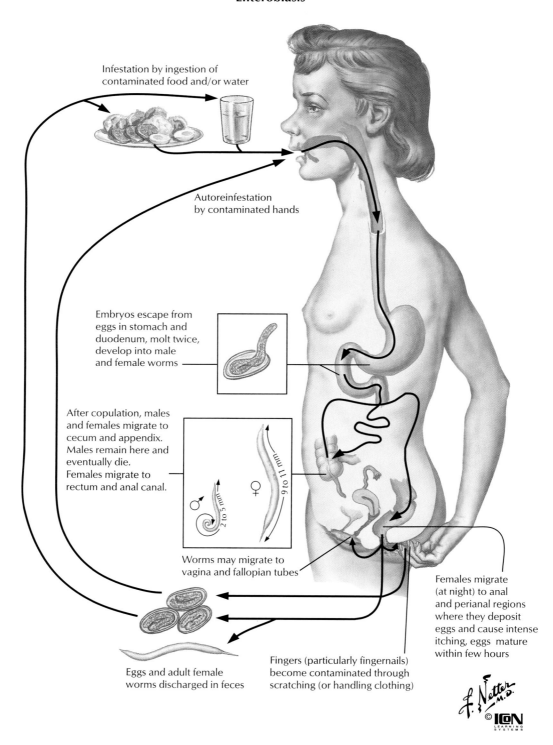

Infestation by ingestion of contaminated food and/or water

Autoreinfestation by contaminated hands

Embryos escape from eggs in stomach and duodenum, molt twice, develop into male and female worms

After copulation, males and females migrate to cecum and appendix. Males remain here and eventually die. Females migrate to rectum and anal canal.

2 to 5 mm

9 to 11 mm

Worms may migrate to vagina and fallopian tubes

Females migrate (at night) to anal and perianal regions where they deposit eggs and cause intense itching, eggs mature within few hours

Eggs and adult female worms discharged in feces

Fingers (particularly fingernails) become contaminated through scratching (or handling clothing)

days, mebendazole 500 mg single dose, or albendazole 400 mg once daily for 3 days is effective.

Ascariasis
Etiology and Pathogenesis

Ascaris lumbricoides infection occurs via a complex life cycle (Figure 80-2). After ingestion of infectious eggs, the immature larvae migrate through the lungs before reaching the adult stage in the intestine.

Clinical Presentation

Pulmonary symptoms, such as cough, dyspnea, and wheezing with infiltrates and eosinophilia may occur during the lung migration phase. Low levels of infection are largely asymptomatic while high worm burdens may cause gastrointestinal symptoms of abdominal pain, nausea, and small bowel obstruction. Rarely, ascarids may migrate into the biliary tract or pancreatic duct, causing symptoms consistent with biliary colic or pancreatitis. Occasionally, patients present with fecal passage of a large adult worm.

Diagnostic Approach

A fecal smear for ova and parasites is generally positive due to the high egg output of this parasite.

Management and Therapy

Either mebendazole 100 mg twice daily for 3 days, mebendazole 500 mg single dose, albendazole 400 mg single dose, or pyrantel pamoate 11 mg/kg single dose is effective.

Hookworm Infections
Etiology and Pathogenesis

Hookworm infections are caused by either *Necator americanus* or *Ancylostoma duodenale* (Figure 80-3). Their life cycle begins with the percutaneous penetration of the infectious filariform larvae, usually through bare feet. The larvae migrate from the skin to the lung and eventually transit to the small intestine where the adult worm resides and releases eggs into the feces. The eggs must embryonate into rhabditiform larvae, then to filariform larvae before they are infectious again. The repetitive release and reattachment of the adult worm to intestinal mucosa may result in low grade bleeding and anemia.

Clinical Presentation

A pruritic maculopapular rash may result after the penetration of the filariform larvae. Migration of the larvae through the lung is associated with cough, wheezing, pulmonary infiltrates, and eosinophilia. Abdominal symptoms include abdominal pain, diarrhea, and nausea and vomiting. Symptoms of iron deficiency anemia such as fatigue, dyspnea, or pica may develop with chronic infection. Hypoproteinemia and growth retardation occur in children who have chronic infection.

Diagnostic Approach

A fecal smear for ova and parasites is diagnostic.

Management and Therapy

Either mebendazole 100 mg twice daily for 3 days, mebendazole 500 mg single dose, albendazole 400 mg single dose, or pyrantel pamoate 11 mg/kg once daily for 3 days is effective. Iron supplementation may be necessary to correct the iron deficiency anemia.

Strongyloidiasis
Etiology and Pathogenesis

Strongyloides stercoralis penetrates intact skin, transits the lung, and then resides in the small intestine as an adult. It is capable of maintaining an autoinfective cycle where rhabditiform larvae transform into the infectious filariform larvae within the host allowing reinfection and persistence of the cycle for years. Autoinfection in an immunocompromised host can result in life-threatening disseminated illness known as hyperinfection. In the southern United States, strongyloidiasis occurs at an estimated prevalence of 0.4% to 4%.

Clinical Presentation

Larva currens, a recurrent serpiginous urticarial rash usually around the buttocks, is consistent with autoinfection. During the pulmonary transit phase, the patient may experience cough, wheezing, and pulmonary infiltrates. Abdominal symptoms include pain, diarrhea, nausea, and vomiting. Malabsorption and weight loss occurs with heavier infections. Hyperinfection results in ileus, pneumonia, meningitis, polymicrobial gram-negative bacteremia, and multi-organ failure. Eosinophilia may be absent in hyperinfection.

Figure 80-2

Parasitic Diseases
Ascariasis

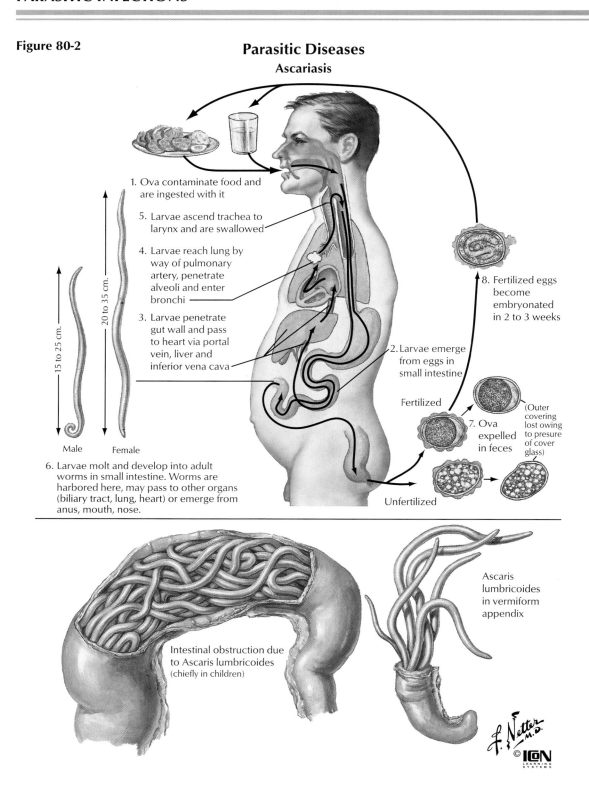

1. Ova contaminate food and are ingested with it

5. Larvae ascend trachea to larynx and are swallowed

4. Larvae reach lung by way of pulmonary artery, penetrate alveoli and enter bronchi

3. Larvae penetrate gut wall and pass to heart via portal vein, liver and inferior vena cava

8. Fertilized eggs become embryonated in 2 to 3 weeks

2. Larvae emerge from eggs in small intestine

Fertilized

7. Ova expelled in feces

(Outer covering lost owing to presure of cover glass)

Male

Female

15 to 25 cm.

20 to 35 cm.

6. Larvae molt and develop into adult worms in small intestine. Worms are harbored here, may pass to other organs (biliary tract, lung, heart) or emerge from anus, mouth, nose.

Unfertilized

Intestinal obstruction due to Ascaris lumbricoides (chiefly in children)

Ascaris lumbricoides in vermiform appendix

Figure 80-3

Parasitic Diseases
Necatoriasis and Ancylostomiasis

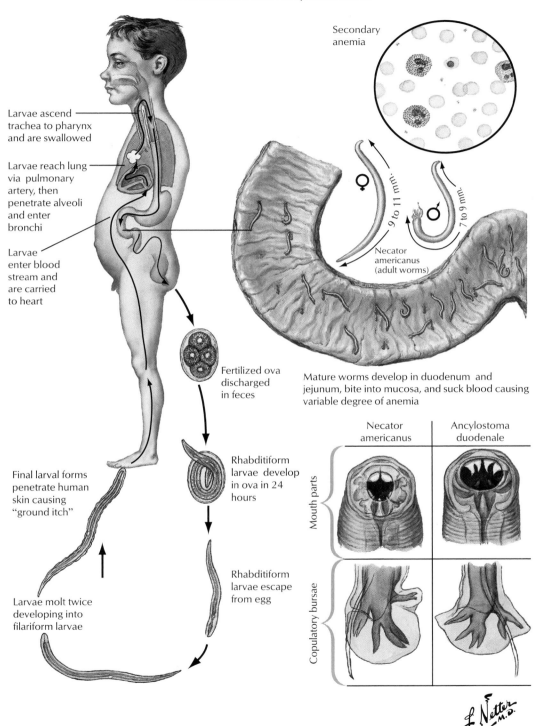

Secondary anemia

Larvae ascend trachea to pharynx and are swallowed

Larvae reach lung via pulmonary artery, then penetrate alveoli and enter bronchi

Larvae enter blood stream and are carried to heart

9 to 11 mm.

7 to 9 mm.

Necator americanus (adult worms)

Fertilized ova discharged in feces

Mature worms develop in duodenum and jejunum, bite into mucosa, and suck blood causing variable degree of anemia

Final larval forms penetrate human skin causing "ground itch"

Rhabditiform larvae develop in ova in 24 hours

Larvae molt twice developing into filariform larvae

Rhabditiform larvae escape from egg

	Necator americanus	Ancylostoma duodenale
Mouth parts		
Copulatory bursae		

Diagnostic Approach

A fecal smear is often negative and multiple stool specimens using concentration techniques may be required for diagnosis. Duodenal aspirate specimens from endoscopy or a "string test" may be necessary. In hyperinfection, sputum examination may reveal larvae. Patients from endemic areas planning immunosuppressive treatment such as chemotherapy or organ transplantation should have serologic testing.

Management and Therapy

Ivermectin 200 µg/kg/day for 1 to 2 days is highly efficacious and nontoxic for uncomplicated disease. Albendazole 400 mg per day for 3 days or thiabendazole 25 mg/kg twice daily for 2 days is also effective. In hyperinfection, ivermectin has not been well studied and thiabendazole should be used for up to 10 days.

Cestodes (Tapeworm)
Etiology and Pathogenesis

Tapeworm infection results in humans when uncooked or undercooked infected meat is ingested (Figure 80-4). The infection transmitted depends on the meat consumed: beef, *Taenia saginata*; pork, *Taenia solium*; and fish, *Diphyllobothrium latum*.

Clinical Presentation

Infection is often asymptomatic or individuals may sense the movement of the proglottids through the anus. Infection with *D. latum* may result in megaloblastic anemia secondary to vitamin B_{12} deficiency.

Diagnostic Approach

Fecal demonstration of proglottids or eggs is diagnostic.

Management and Therapy

Praziquantel 10 mg/kg single dose or niclosamide 2 g single dose is effective.

Cysticercosis
Etiology and Pathogenesis

The tapeworm, *T. solium* has the potential to cause cysticercosis (Figure 80-4). When the egg of *T. solium* is ingested either directly through fecal contamination or auto-infestation by reverse peristalsis, the larval form of the disease, cysticercus cellulosae, develops and tissue cysts (cysticerci) may develop in subcutaneous tissues, muscle, and the brain.

Clinical Presentation

Subcutaneous nodules may be palpable. Neurologic symptoms vary widely according to the location and number of cysts, stage of the infection, and the host response. Asymptomatic disease is common, particularly in the first years after infection. Seizure is the most common presenting symptom; headache, increased intracranial pressure, altered mental status, and focal neurologic findings occur less frequently.

Diagnostic Approach

CT scan and MRI are the primary methods to diagnose neurocysticercosis. MRI is more sensitive in the diagnosis of extraparenchymal cysts and inflammatory reactions to cysts. The enzyme-linked immunotransfer blot assay (serum titer) is highly specific for *T. solium* and highly sensitive in patients with multiple active cysts.

Management and Therapy

Treatment with antiparasitic agents should be individualized according to the location and activity of the cysts. Albendazole 400 mg twice daily, for 8 to 30 days or praziquantel 33 mg/kg thrice daily for 30 days with concomitant corticosteroids may be effective if therapy is indicated. Consultation with an infectious disease physician is recommended.

INTESTINAL PROTOZOA

While several species of protozoa may be found in the human intestinal tract, many are regarded as non-pathogenic commensals. *Giardia lamblia* and *Entamoeba histolytica* cause the majority of enteric protozoal disease among immunocompetent individuals in the United States. Cryptosporidium, Cyclospora, Microsporidia, and Isospora are important enteric protozoal diseases in patients with AIDS and are discussed elsewhere.

Giardiasis
Etiology and Pathogenesis

Giardia lamblia is a protozoal infection of the intestinal tract that develops after ingestion of

Figure 80-4

Parasitic Diseases
Taeniasis Solium (Cysticercosis Cellulosae)

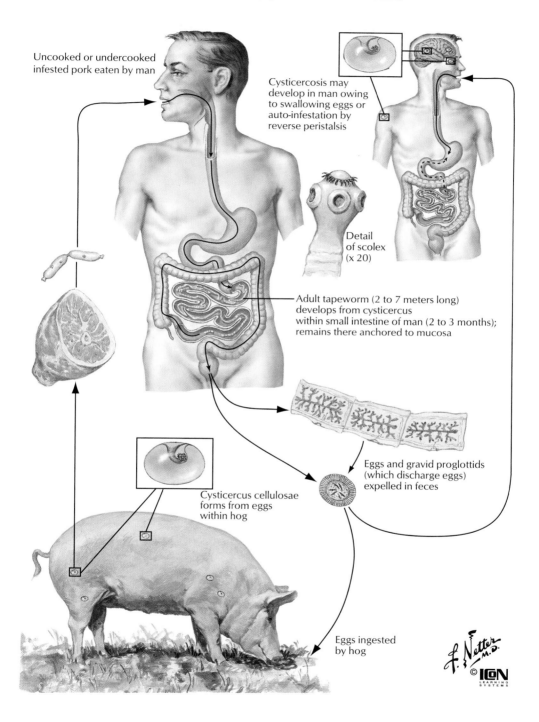

Uncooked or undercooked infested pork eaten by man

Cysticercosis may develop in man owing to swallowing eggs or auto-infestation by reverse peristalsis

Detail of scolex (x 20)

Adult tapeworm (2 to 7 meters long) develops from cysticercus within small intestine of man (2 to 3 months); remains there anchored to mucosa

Eggs and gravid proglottids (which discharge eggs) expelled in feces

Cysticercus cellulosae forms from eggs within hog

Eggs ingested by hog

Figure 80-5

Giardiasis

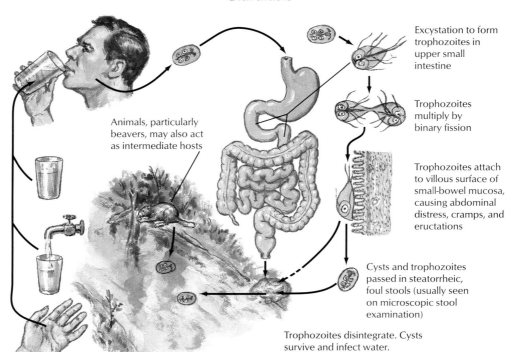

Excystation to form trophozoites in upper small intestine

Trophozoites multiply by binary fission

Trophozoites attach to villous surface of small-bowel mucosa, causing abdominal distress, cramps, and eructations

Animals, particularly beavers, may also act as intermediate hosts

Cysts and trophozoites passed in steatorrheic, foul stools (usually seen on microscopic stool examination)

Trophozoites disintegrate. Cysts survive and infect water.

Cysts ingested in contaminated, untreated stream water; in inadequately treated tap water; or via infected food handlers

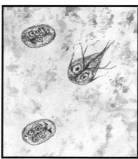

Cysts and trophozoite in stool

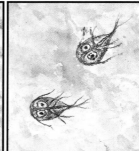

Giardia trophozoites in duodenal mucus

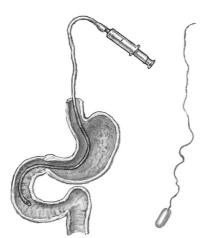

When infection is suspected but stool examination results are negative, duodenal or jejunal fluid (obtained by aspiration or gelatin capsule with string) should be examined

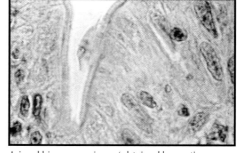

Jejunal biopsy specimen (obtained by suction or endoscopically) shows trophozoite on villous surface of mucosa

Figure 80-6

Amebiasis

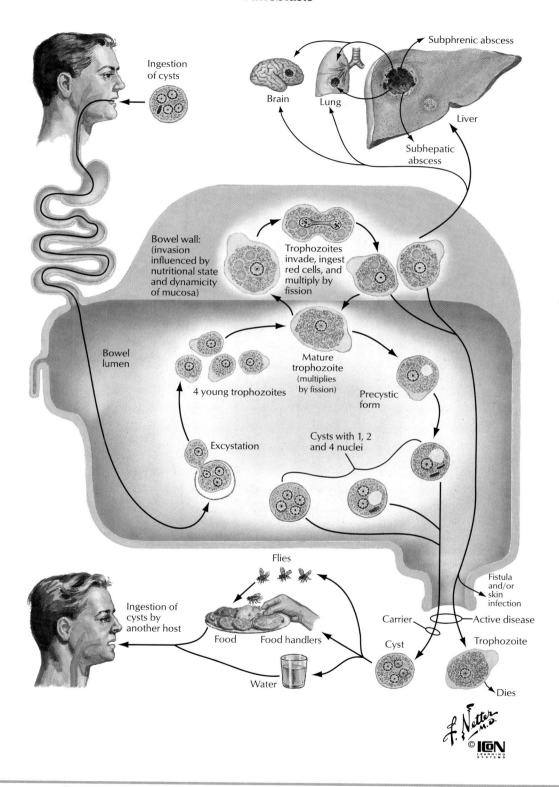

Ingestion of cysts

Subphrenic abscess

Brain

Lung

Liver

Subhepatic abscess

Bowel wall: (invasion influenced by nutritional state and dynamicity of mucosa)

Trophozoites invade, ingest red cells, and multiply by fission

Bowel lumen

Mature trophozoite (multiplies by fission)

Precystic form

4 young trophozoites

Excystation

Cysts with 1, 2 and 4 nuclei

Flies

Ingestion of cysts by another host

Food

Food handlers

Water

Carrier

Cyst

Fistula and/or skin infection

Active disease

Trophozoite

Dies

infective cysts via fecally contaminated water or food (Figure 80-5). Both wild and domestic animals may serve as a reservoir for the infection.

Clinical Presentation

Newly infected patients present with acute diarrhea, abdominal bloating, flatulence, steatorrhea, and weight loss. If untreated, chronic diarrhea may persist with associated malabsorption.

Diagnostic Approach

Microscopy of feces or duodenal aspirate specimens confirms the diagnosis. Stool testing for *Giardia* antigen is also diagnostic.

Management and Therapy

Metronidazole 250 mg orally thrice daily for 5 days; tinidazole is also effective but not available in the United States.

Amoebiasis
Etiology and Pathogenesis

E. histolytica infection is spread by fecal-oral contamination with infectious cysts (Figure 80-6). Symptoms develop if the cysts become trophozoites capable of invading the colonic mucosa. *E. histolytica* cysts are morphologically indistinguishable from the non-pathogenic *Entamoeba dispar*.

Clinical Presentation

The majority of infected individuals with *Entamoeba* cysts in the stool are asymptomatic because most are actually infected with *E. dispar*. Symptomatic disease will develop in only 10% of *E. histolytica* cyst carriers. Among symptomatic patients, diarrhea with blood and mucus, and abdominal pain developing over 1 to 2 weeks are the predominant complaints. Rarely, patients present with a localized painful abdominal mass secondary to amoeboma formation. Chronic amebic colitis presents with recurrent episodes of bloody diarrhea over years and may be confused with inflammatory bowel disease. Extraintestinal

manifestations include abscess formation of the liver, lung, brain, or pericardium, with liver abscess the most common. Most patients with amebic liver abscess present with fever, right upper quadrant pain, and tenderness of the liver; others may present solely with fever.

Diagnostic Approach

The finding of *Entamoeba* cysts and hematophagous trophozoites in a fresh stool wet mount is diagnostic of *E. histolytica*. In asymptomatic cyst passers, *E. histolytica* may be differentiated from *E. dispar* by the presence of positive amebic serology. Liver ultrasound, CT, and MRI are useful in the diagnosis of liver abscess.

Biopsy of colonic tissue revealing trophozoites is diagnostic of amebic colitis.

Management and Therapy

Asymptomatic *E. dispar* cyst carriers do not require treatment. Treat asymptomatic *E. histolytica* cyst carriers with either iodoquinol 650 mg thrice daily for 20 days or paromomycin 12 mg/kg orally thrice daily for 7 days. Amebic colitis and extraintestinal amebic disease are treated with metronidazole 750 mg thrice daily for 10 days followed with treatment with iodoquinol or paromomycin.

FUTURE DIRECTIONS

Efforts toward improving waste sanitation, food handling processes, animal husbandry processes, and ensuring quality control of water purification can virtually eliminate these enteric infections. Focused treatment of high-risk individuals, such as children, in developing countries, in conjunction with improved sanitation should be a global health priority.

REFERENCES

Centers for Disease Control and Prevention Web site. Available at: http://www.cdc.org. Accessed January 4, 2002.

Guerrant RL, Walker DH, Weller PF, eds. *Tropical Infectious Diseases: Principles, Pathogens, & Practice.* Philadelphia, Pa: Churchill Livingstone; 1999.

Chapter 81

Pulmonary Tuberculosis

David J. Weber, Peter A. Leone, and William A. Rutala

Tuberculosis remains a major scourge of mankind with an estimated one-third of the world's population currently infected. Each year more than 8 million persons are infected by *Mycobacterium tuberculosis*, leading to an estimated 2.6 million deaths. In the United States, 16,377 cases (5.8 cases/100,000 population) were reported in 2000, the lowest rate ever recorded. Overall, an estimated 15 million Americans are infected with *M. tuberculosis*. The incidence of tuberculosis in the United States varies independently by age, gender, and race/ethnicity with higher rates reported among older persons, men, non-white individuals, and foreign-born persons.

ETIOLOGY AND PATHOGENESIS

Human tuberculosis is caused by three closely related mycobacteria grouped in the *Mycobacterium tuberculosis*-complex: *M. tuberculosis*, *M. bovis*, and *M. africanum*. They are aerobic, non-spore-forming, non-motile, slightly curved or straight bacilli, 0.2 to 0.6 by 1.0 to 10 μm in size. Their cell walls have a high lipid content that render them impermeable to Gram staining (termed acid-fastness). Most laboratories use a fluorochrome stain that allows visualization of the mycobacteria using a fluorescent microscope (Figure 81-1).

In the United States, *M. tuberculosis* is the only important human pathogen in the *M. tuberculosis*-complex. It is found worldwide, and humans are the only known reservoir. *M. bovis*, an important pathogen in lesser developed countries, is most commonly acquired from cattle by ingestion of contaminated milk. The disease produced in humans by *M. bovis* is virtually indistinguishable from that caused by *M. tuberculosis* and is treated similarly. The bacillus of Calmette-Guerin (BCG), an attenuated strain of *M. bovis*, is used in many parts of the world as a vaccine to prevent tuberculosis. Although there is evidence that BCG vaccine protects against disseminated tuberculosis and meningitis in children, the efficacy of BCG to protect against pulmonary disease has not been proven.

Tuberculosis is spread from person-to-person through the air by droplet nuclei, particles 1 to 5 μm in diameter that contain *M. tuberculosis* (Figure 81-2). Droplet nuclei are produced when persons with pulmonary or laryngeal tuberculosis cough, sneeze, speak, or sing. *M. tuberculosis* infection occurs if after inhalation of infective droplet nuclei, viable bacilli survive the initial host defenses. The organisms grow for 2 to 12 weeks at which time they elicit a cellular immune response that can be detected by a reaction to the tuberculin skin test (TST). Before development of cellular immunity, tubercle bacilli spread via the lymphatics to the hilar lymph nodes and then through the bloodstream to distant sites. Tuberculosis will develop at some time in approximately 10% of individuals who acquire tuberculous infection and are not given preventive therapy.

CLINICAL PRESENTATION

Primary tuberculosis is generally a self-limited, mild pneumonic illness that often goes undiagnosed. Primary infection may result in granulomas visible on chest radiography. Most pulmonary tuberculosis infections are inapparent radiographically. A positive TST result is the only indication that infection has occurred.

The symptoms of tuberculosis are protean and nonspecific and can be classified as either systemic or organ-specific. Classic systemic symptoms include fever (present in approximately 35%–85%), night sweats, weight loss, anorexia, and fatigue. Laboratory findings may include an increased peripheral blood leukocyte count (~10%), anemia (~10%), and, occasionally, increased monocyte or eosinophil count. The lung is the most common site involved, accounting for 80% of cases reported to the Centers for Disease Control and Prevention (Figure 81-3). Organ-specific symptoms in pulmonary tuberculosis include

Figure 81-1

Tuberculosis: Sputum Examination
(Stained Smear)

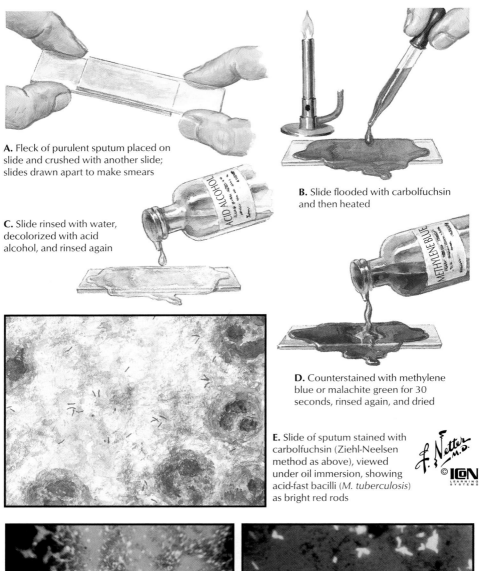

A. Fleck of purulent sputum placed on slide and crushed with another slide; slides drawn apart to make smears

B. Slide flooded with carbolfuchsin and then heated

C. Slide rinsed with water, decolorized with acid alcohol, and rinsed again

D. Counterstained with methylene blue or malachite green for 30 seconds, rinsed again, and dried

E. Slide of sputum stained with carbolfuchsin (Ziehl-Neelsen method as above), viewed under oil immersion, showing acid-fast bacilli (*M. tuberculosis*) as bright red rods

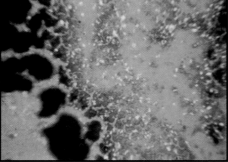

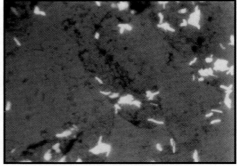

F. *M. tuberculosis* stained with auramine O which causes acid-fast bacilli to fluoresce (x 200)

G. Auramine O stain of *M. kansasii* (acid-fast "atypical" mycobacteria) which are much larger than *M. tuberculosis* (x 200)

Figure 81-2

Dissemination of Tuberculosis

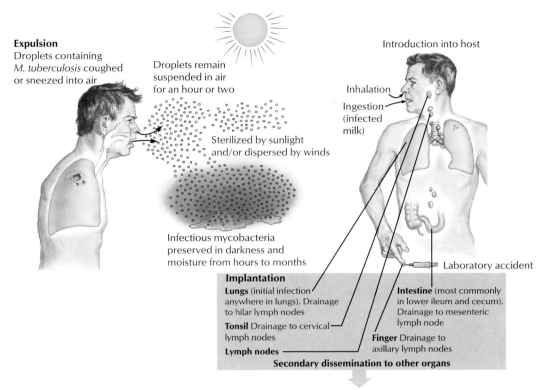

Expulsion
Droplets containing *M. tuberculosis* coughed or sneezed into air

Droplets remain suspended in air for an hour or two

Sterilized by sunlight and/or dispersed by winds

Infectious mycobacteria preserved in darkness and moisture from hours to months

Introduction into host

Inhalation

Ingestion (infected milk)

Laboratory accident

Implantation
Lungs (initial infection anywhere in lungs). Drainage to hilar lymph nodes

Tonsil Drainage to cervical lymph nodes

Lymph nodes

Intestine (most commonly in lower ileum and cecum). Drainage to mesenteric lymph node

Finger Drainage to axillary lymph nodes

Secondary dissemination to other organs

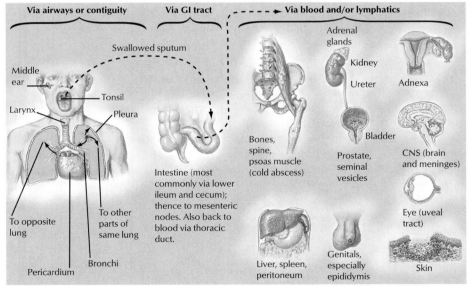

Via airways or contiguity   **Via GI tract**   **Via blood and/or lymphatics**

Swallowed sputum

Middle ear

Tonsil

Larynx

Pleura

To opposite lung

To other parts of same lung

Pericardium

Bronchi

Intestine (most commonly via lower ileum and cecum); thence to mesenteric nodes. Also back to blood via thoracic duct.

Adrenal glands

Kidney

Ureter

Adnexa

Bones, spine, psoas muscle (cold abscess)

Bladder

Prostate, seminal vesicles

CNS (brain and meninges)

Liver, spleen, peritoneum

Genitals, especially epididymis

Eye (uveal tract)

Skin

---

cough, pleuritic chest pain, and hemoptysis. In primary tuberculosis, chest radiographs often show infiltrates in the middle or lower lung zones, with ipsilateral hilar adenopathy (Figure 81-3). In reactivation tuberculosis, classic radiographic findings include upper lobe infiltrates, frequently with cavitation. In patients infected with HIV with <200 CD4 cells/mm³, the radiographic findings frequently are atypical; cavitation is uncommon, lower lung zone or diffuse infiltrates and mediastinal adenopathy are frequent, and extrapulmonary disease occurs in ~50% of cases.

Extrapulmonary tuberculosis may involve the pleura, lymphatics, bone or joints, genitourinary system, meninges, peritoneal cavity, or other sites. It often presents a diagnostic challenge with varied symptoms and signs depending on the organ system involved. Signs and symptoms of disseminated tuberculosis are generally nonspecific and include fever, weight loss, night sweats, anorexia, and weakness. A productive cough is common because most patients with disseminated disease also have pulmonary tuberculosis. Physical findings are variable but often include fever, wasting, hepatomegaly, pulmonary findings, lymphadenopathy, and splenomegaly. Small, 1- to 2-mm granulomas, are visible on chest radiography in approximately 85% of patients. These lesions that look like "millet seeds" have led to disseminated disease being termed "miliary" tuberculosis.

DIFFERENTIAL DIAGNOSIS

Patients with pulmonary tuberculosis may present with acute or chronic disease. The differential diagnosis of acute infection includes the common viral and bacterial causes of pneumonia such as *Streptococcus pneumoniae, Haemophilus influenzae, Mycoplasma spp*, and respiratory viruses. Chronic infection may be confused with noninfectious causes of pulmonary disease including sarcoidosis, collagen-vascular diseases, autoimmune diseases, and cancer. It may also be confused with other causes of chronic pulmonary infection, especially endemic fungi (blastomycosis, cryptococcosis, histoplasmosis, coccidioidomycosis) and nontuberculous mycobacteria.

Tuberculosis must be considered in the diagnosis of fever of unknown origin. Mycobacterial cultures of blood, bone marrow, and/or liver may sometimes establish the diagnosis. Biopsy speci-

mens of organs with evidence of dysfunction or abnormalities on radiographic scans should also include culture testing for mycobacteria.

Mycobacterial infection should be considered in many cases in chronic organ system disorders including meningitis, peritonitis, epididymitis, pericarditis, pleuritis, and osteomyelitis. The finding of granulomas on biopsy should always raise the suspicion of tuberculosis, although they may also be found in histoplasmosis, coccidioidomycosis, blastomycosis, and sarcoidosis.

DIAGNOSTIC APPROACH

Latent tuberculosis infection (LTBI) is detected by a TST using purified protein derivative (PPD) (Figure 81-4). This test is subject to both false-positive and false-negative results (Table 1) that can be minimized by careful attention to proper placement and interpretation of the test. In most persons, PPD skin test sensitivity persists throughout life; however, the size of the skin test may decrease and disappear over time. If PPD is administered to infected persons whose skin tests have waned, an initial test may be small or absent but a subsequent test (2–4 weeks later) may demonstrate an accentuated response. This "booster effect" should not be misinterpreted as skin test conversion but rather the second test should be considered as reflecting the individual's true exposure to *M. tuberculosis*. Two-step testing is recommended in people who are likely to undergo repeated tuberculin testing (i.e., healthcare workers) or for whom immunity is likely to have waned (i.e., the elderly), and who have not had a TST within the previous 12 months. The criteria used for classifying a TST result as positive are based on the size of induration, and epidemiological and clinical characteristics of the patient (Table 2). The sensitivity of the TST to detect active tuberculosis is in the range of 75% to 80% but may be lower is some groups such as the elderly and HIV-infected persons. The specificity of the TST is approximately 99% in populations that have no other mycobacterial exposure or BCG vaccination, but decreases to approximately 95% in populations where cross-reactivity with other mycobacteria is common (e.g., Southeast United States). Routine testing is recommended only for high-prevalence and high-risk groups (Table 2). Prior receipt of BCG vaccination does not alter

Figure 81-3

Initial (Primary) Tuberculous Complex

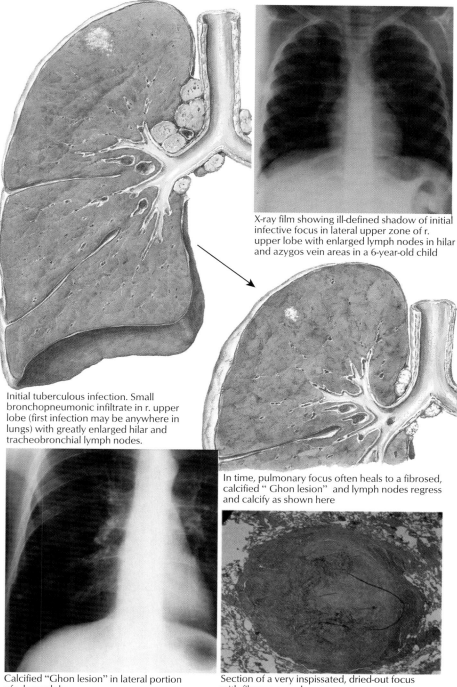

X-ray film showing ill-defined shadow of initial infective focus in lateral upper zone of r. upper lobe with enlarged lymph nodes in hilar and azygos vein areas in a 6-year-old child

Initial tuberculous infection. Small bronchopneumonic infiltrate in r. upper lobe (first infection may be anywhere in lungs) with greatly enlarged hilar and tracheobronchial lymph nodes.

In time, pulmonary focus often heals to a fibrosed, calcified " Ghon lesion" and lymph nodes regress and calcify as shown here

Calcified "Ghon lesion" in lateral portion of r. lower lobe

Section of a very inspissated, dried-out focus with fibrous capsule

Figure 81-4

Tuberculin Testing

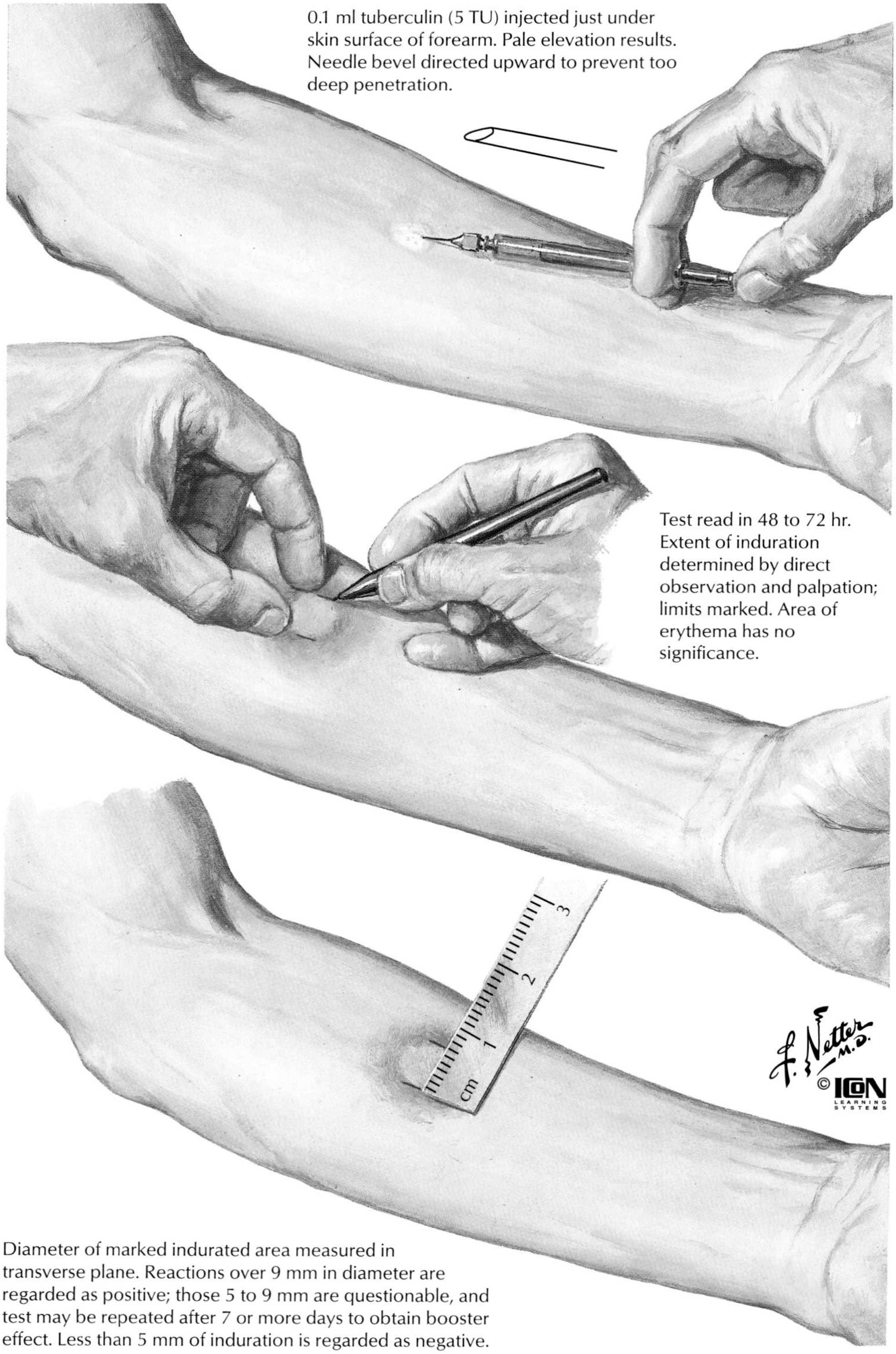
0.1 ml tuberculin (5 TU) injected just under skin surface of forearm. Pale elevation results. Needle bevel directed upward to prevent too deep penetration.
Test read in 48 to 72 hr. Extent of induration determined by direct observation and palpation; limits marked. Area of erythema has no significance.
cm
1
2
3
F. Netter M.D.
© ICON LEARNING SYSTEMS
Diameter of marked indurated area measured in transverse plane. Reactions over 9 mm in diameter are regarded as positive; those 5 to 9 mm are questionable, and test may be repeated after 7 or more days to obtain booster effect. Less than 5 mm of induration is regarded as negative.

Table 81-1
Potential Causes of False-positive and False-negative Tuberculin Reactions

Causes of False-Positive Reactions	Causes of False-Negative Reactions
Mistaking erythema for induration	Anergy due to overwhelming tuberculous infection
Infection with nontuberculous mycobacteria	Recent infection with *M. tuberculosis* (<12 weeks)
Receipt of BCG vaccine	Drugs (steroids, immunosuppressive agents)
Early reading of skin test with reaction due to immunoglobulins rather than cell-mediated immunity	Metabolic derangements (e.g., chronic liver or renal disease)
Use of incorrect strength of PPD (i.e., 250 TU)	Immune suppressive diseases (e.g., HIV, hematologic malignancies, or lymphoma)
Poorly standardized antigen	Malnourishment
	Recent receipt of live virus vaccine (e.g., measles)
	Newborns, elderly population
	Improper storage or dilution of PPD
	Inappropriate administration (e.g., too little antigen, or subcutaneous administration)
	Errors in reading or recording TST

Adapted with permission from Diagnostic Standards and Classification of Tuberculosis in Adults and children. *Am J Respir Crit Care Med.* 2000; 161:1390

the interpretation of TST reactivity. Pregnancy is not a contraindication to TST.

For suspected active tuberculosis, all patients should be evaluated with a reactive TST. A careful history should attempt to elicit the nonspecific symptoms of tuberculosis and organ-specific symptoms, especially of pulmonary disease. Physical examination is of limited utility in the diagnosis but may aid in detecting specific organ infection requiring further investigation. All patients with a positive TST result or symptoms of tuberculosis should have a chest radiograph to aid in the diagnosis of pulmonary tuberculosis and to determine the extent of disease.

A presumptive diagnosis of pulmonary tuberculosis can often be made using the chest radiograph. Demonstration of *M. tuberculosis* in cultured sputum specimens is the key to definitive diagnosis. Sputum should be obtained in early morning on 3 consecutive days. Induction of sputum with hypertonic saline may increase the yield of obtaining adequate sputum specimens, especially in HIV-infected patients. A CT scan may be useful in assessing whether an abnormal chest radiograph is consistent with tuberculosis. Aspiration of gastric fluid for culture may be useful in young children unable to produce sputum. Fiberoptic bronchoscopy can be used to obtain specimens from the respiratory tract in patients unable to produce sputum.

The diagnosis of extrapulmonary tuberculosis usually requires an invasive procedure to obtain fluid (e.g., CSF) for smear or culture, and biopsy to obtain tissue for culture. A first morning-voided midstream urine specimen should be cultured to establish the diagnosis of genitourinary tuberculosis. Blood for mycobacterial culture should be anticoagulated with heparin and processed by a lysis-centrifugation system or inoculated into broth media designed for mycobacterial blood cultures. The diagnosis of central nervous system tuberculosis may be established by culture of the CSF; a

Table 81-2
Criteria for Tuberculin Positivity, by Risk Group

Induration ≥5 mm	Induration ≥10 mm	Induration ≥15 mm
HIV-positive persons	Recent arrivals (<5 years) from high-prevalence countries*	Persons with no risk factors for TB
Recent contacts of TB cases*	Injection drug users	
Fibrotic changes on chest radiograph consistent with old tuberculosis	Mycobacterial laboratory personnel*	
Patients with organ transplants and other immunosuppressed patients (receiving the equivalent of ≥15 mg/d prednisone for ≥1 mo)	Residents and employees of high-risk congregate settings: prisons and jails, nursing homes and other healthcare facilities, residential facilities for AIDS patients, and homeless shelters*	
	Persons with clinical conditions that make them high risk[††, **]	
	Children <4 years of age or infants, children, and adolescents exposed to adults in high-risk categories[†, ††]	

* Epidemiologic criteria used in classifying the TST skin reaction.
[†] Clinical conditions used in classifying the TST skin reaction.
[††] "High-risk" medical conditions include silicosis, diabetes mellitus, chronic renal failure, leukemia, Hodgkin's disease, immunosuppressive therapy, and malnutrition.
With permission from Targeted tuberculin testing and treatment of latent tuberculosis infection. A joint statement of the American Thoracic Society and the Centers for Disease Control and Prevention. *Am J Respir Crit Care Med.* 2000;161:2345 Table 7; and adapted from Centers for Disease Control and Prevention. Screening for tuberculosis and tuberculosis infection in high-risk populations. Recommendations of the Advisory Council for the Elimination of Tuberculosis. *MMWR Recomm Rep.* 1995;44:19–34.

minimum of 5 mL of fluid should be submitted to the laboratory in a sterile container for culture. Invasive procedures to obtain specimens from the lung, pericardium, lymph nodes, bones and joints, bowel, salpinges, and epididymis should be considered when noninvasive techniques do not provide a diagnosis. Antimicrobial susceptibility testing should be obtained on all cultures that yield *M. tuberculosis*.

MANAGEMENT AND THERAPY

All patients with known or suspected tuberculosis should be placed on airborne precautions (≥6–12 air exchanges per hour, negative pressure, and air directly exhausted to the outside) when receiving care within a health-care facility. Healthcare personnel should don an N-95 respirator before entering a room where a patient with potentially communicable tuberculosis is housed. Patients should be maintained on airborne isolation until they have received at least 2 weeks of appropriate chemotherapy, demonstrated clinical improvement, and have three consecutive negative sputum smears obtained on different days. Patients with known or suspected multidrug-resistant *M. tuberculosis* should remain isolated until culture results are negative. Close contacts of persons with active pulmonary tuberculosis should be evaluated for tuberculosis, because active disease is already present in 2% to 3% and latent infection in 5% to 15%.

All persons with a reactive TST (Table 81-2) should consider therapy of LTBI (Table 81-3) after excluding active tuberculosis with history, physical examination, chest radiography, and bacteriologic studies (when indicated). Patients should receive follow-up evaluations at least monthly if receiving isoniazid or rifampin alone and at 2, 4, and 8 weeks if receiving rifampin and pyrazinamide. Follow-up evaluations should include questioning about adverse drug reactions and a brief physical assessment for signs of hepatitis. Baseline testing of liver function (i.e., alanine transaminase/aspartate transaminase and biliru-

Table 81-3
Recommended Therapy for Latent Tuberculous Infection

Drugs	Duration (mo)	Interval	Rating* (Evidence)[†] HIV Negative	HIV Positive
Isoniazid	9	Daily	A (II)	A (II)
		Twice weekly	B (II)	B (II)
Isoniazid	6	Daily	B (I)	C (I)
		Twice weekly	B (II)	C (I)
Rifampin-pyrazinamide[††]	2	Daily	B (II)	A (I)
	2–3	Twice weekly	C (II)	C (I)
Rifampin	4	Daily	B (II)	B (III)

* A = preferred; B = acceptable alternative; C = offer when A and B cannot be given.
[†] I = randomized clinical trial data; II = data from clinical trials that are not randomized or were conducted in other populations; III = expert opinion
[††] Recently has been shown to be associated with fulminant liver failure; use with caution.
With permission from targeted tuberculin testing and treatment of latent tuberculosis infection. A joint statement of the American Thoracic Society and the Centers for Disease Control and Prevention. *Am J Respir Crit Care Med.* 2000;161:S221–S247.

bin) is recommended only for persons at high risk for liver dysfunction, including patients with HIV infection, persons with a history of chronic liver disease (e.g., hepatitis C), pregnant women, postpartum women within 3 months of delivery, and persons who use alcohol regularly. Active hepatitis and end-stage liver disease are relative contraindications to the use of isoniazid or pyrazinamide. Routine monitoring during treatment of LTBI is indicated for persons whose baseline liver function test results are abnormal and persons at risk for hepatic disease. Such tests should also be performed on persons with signs or symptoms of hepatitis. Isoniazid therapy should be stopped if transaminase levels exceed three times the upper limit of normal if associated with symptoms, and five times the upper limit of normal if the patient is asymptomatic.

Patients with active tuberculosis require therapy with multiple drugs to prevent the development of resistance, enhance tuberculocidal therapy, and properly treat if their strain of *M. tuberculosis* is resistant to one or more drugs. The preferred regimen for patients with fully susceptible bacilli is a 6-month course consisting of isoniazid, rifampin, and pyrazinamide, given for 2 months, followed by isoniazid and rifampin for 4 months. Include ethambutol (or streptomycin in children too

young to be monitored for visual acuity) until the results of drug susceptibility studies are available. If there is evidence of a slow or suboptimal response, therapy should be given for a total of 9 months, or for 4 months after culture results become negative. Consider treating all patients with directly observed therapy (DOT) to ensure compliance. Extrapulmonary tuberculosis should be managed in a manner similar to that for pulmonary tuberculosis, except for children who have miliary tuberculosis, bone/joint tuberculosis, or tuberculous meningitis, all of whom should receive a minimum of 12 months of therapy. Expert consultation is usually needed when treating tuberculosis in HIV-infected persons because treatment is more difficult due to the possibility of malabsorption of antituberculous medications and because of drug interactions between rifampin and protease inhibitors.

Physicians should be familiar with the administration, adverse reactions, and contraindications of the first-line antituberculous medications. In pulmonary tuberculosis, the response to therapy should be monitored by obtaining follow-up sputa for culture. Reevaluate therapy if sputum culture results have not become negative after 2 months. In this case, drug susceptibility testing should be repeated, and DOT therapy continued or initiated. Patient education with regard to compliance, symptoms of drug toxicity, and drug interactions is critical to ensure proper therapy.

Drug resistance to first-line antituberculous therapy is a growing problem worldwide. In the United States, resistance is more common in persons who are foreign born, remain culture positive or whose symptoms do not resolve after 3 months of therapy. All patients with drug-resistant *M. tuberculosis* should receive DOT and be managed by persons familiar with use of second-line medications such as amikacin, capreomycin, quinolones, ethionamide, aminosalicylic acid, and cycloserine.

FUTURE DIRECTIONS

The major challenges of tuberculosis are the increasing proportion of drug-resistant strains, and the prevention and treatment of tuberculosis in HIV-infected persons. Progress against tuberculosis is being made on several fronts. New diagnostic tests for rapid detection of *M. tuberculosis* (e.g., PCR) in sputum or tissue samples are being studied. Rapid methods to identify drug-resistant tuberculosis, a new blood test for latent tuberculosis based on the detection of gamma-interferon, and serodiagnosis based on a combination of purified mycobacterial antigens are under investigation. New drugs may become available soon for the therapy of tuberculosis. The efficacy of quinolones still needs to be demonstrated in clinical trials. Two novel classes of drugs, the oxazo-lidinones (e.g., linezolid) and the nitroimidazopy-rans, are promising agents for the treatment of tuberculosis. Finally, a major research effort is being direct toward developing new tuberculosis vaccines. Several candidate vaccines should be ready for human testing within a few years.

REFERENCES

Diagnostic Standards and Classification of Tuberculosis in Adults and Children. Official statement of the American Thoracic Society and the Centers for Disease Control and Prevention. *Am J Respir Crit Care Med.* 2000;161:1376– 1395.

Targeted tuberculin testing and treatment of latent tuberculosis infection. A joint statement of the American Thoracic Society and the Centers for Disease Control and Prevention. *Am J Respir Crit Care Med.* 2000;161:S221–S247.

Bass JB Jr, Farer LS, Hopewell PC, et al. Treatment of tuberculosis and tuberculosis infection in adults and children. American Thoracic Society and The Centers for Disease Control and Prevention. *Am J Respir Crit Care Med.* 1994;149:1359–1374.

Centers for Disease Control and Prevention. Screening for tuberculosis and tuberculosis infection in high-risk populations. Recommendations of the Advisory Council for the Elimination of Tuberculosis. *MMWR Recomm Rep.* 1995;44:19–34.

Havlir DV, Barnes PF. Tuberculosis in patients with human immunodeficiency virus infection. *N Engl J Med.* 1999;340: 367–373.

Iseman MD. Treatment of multidrug-resistant tuberculosis. *N Engl J Med.* 1993;329:784–791.

Murthy NK, Dutt AK. Tuberculin skin testing: present status. *Semin Respir Infect.* 1994;9:78–83.

Small PM, Fujiwara PI. Management of tuberculosis in the United States. *N Engl J Med.* 2001;345:189–200.

Chapter 82
Septicemia

Joseph J. Eron

The clinical condition characterized by fever, tachycardia, hypotension, and metabolic acidosis in the presence of demonstrated or suspected infection has been labeled with various terms such as septicemia, sepsis, sepsis syndrome, and septic shock. These terms are used interchangeably by some clinicians, but experts in this area have worked to develop more precise definitions so that clinicians and clinical research scientists will have a common understanding to serve as a basis for their observations and treatments.

Sepsis is defined as infection (organisms in a normally sterile site) with clinical evidence of a systemic response with alterations in body temperature (>38° C or <36° C), tachycardia, metabolic acidosis, usually accompanied by compensatory respiratory alkalosis and tachypnea, and an elevated or depressed white blood cell count. *Sepsis syndrome* implies evidence of decreased organ perfusion such as decreased renal function, hypoxemia, or altered mental status. *Septic shock* is the presence of hypotension accompanied by organ hypoperfusion despite fluid resuscitation.

Sepsis and septic shock are common clinical conditions that are extremely challenging to manage successfully. Often, the microbiologic diagnosis is obscured due to antimicrobial therapy given before the patients arrive at the treating facility or during acute resuscitation before diagnostic cultures are obtained. Frequently, patients have underlying severe illness such as immune deficiency or immune suppression, hematologic or other malignancies, or disruption of host defenses such as severe burns. Patients may present with altered mental status so that medical history is unobtainable or unreliable. The rapid progression to multi-organ failure may make identification of the initial pathogenic process (e.g., pneumonia, pyelonephritis, or intra-abdominal infection) difficult. Erythroderma associated with gram-positive bacterial sepsis may mimic or mask cellulitis, thereby confusing the primary cause of the infection.

Sepsis is the tenth leading cause of death in the United States, but it may be the immediate cause of death in other common, independently categorized causes of mortality such as cancer and pneumonia. Depending on the type of hospital, sepsis or septicemia may be listed as a diagnosis in 1% to 2% of hospital discharges. Severe sepsis and septic shock are associated with substantial utilization of health care resources. There are an estimated 751,000 cases (3.0 cases per 1000 individuals) of sepsis or septic shock yearly in the United States, which may result in as many deaths as are caused by acute myocardial infarction (215,000, or 9.3% of all deaths). The incidence and severity of sepsis and septic shock are greater in the elderly. Therefore, the number of cases of sepsis will increase as the U.S. population continues to age.

ETIOLOGY AND PATHOGENESIS

For consistency in this chapter, sepsis and septic shock will be considered to be caused by a microbiologic organism with or without documented bloodstream infection. Other conditions can cause clinical syndromes indistinguishable from sepsis-related infection, although the exact mechanisms leading to the clinical presentation in those conditions are less clearly defined.

In the past, gram-negative bacilli were most commonly associated with bacteremia and sepsis in the United States. Over the last 15 to 20 years, gram-positive bacteria, in particular cocci such as *Staphylococcus aureus,* have become more common, especially as a cause of nosocomial bloodstream infections. However, almost any overwhelming microbiologic infection can lead to sepsis syndrome and septic shock. Possible etiologic agents include rickettsia and rickettsia-like organisms; fungi, such as candida, aspergillus and cryptococcus; parasites such as those that cause malaria; acute toxoplasmosis in the immunocompromised host; and even some viral infections. The lung, abdomen, and urinary tract are common sites of infection, but in up to one third of cases, the primary organ of involvement is not identified. Blood culture specimen results are positive in only approximately 30% of cases. Culture of other sites such as sputum, urine, CSF, or pleural fluid may reveal a specific etiology but areas of localized infection that trigger the process may not be accessible to culture.

The pathogenesis and clinical manifestations of sepsis and septic shock are the result of the systemic inflammatory response to bacteremia, endotoxemia, fungemia, or more localized severe infection designed to protect the host (Figure 82-1). In sepsis and septic shock, the inflammatory responses are pushed to a point at which the cascade is no longer appropriately regulated and the release of inflammatory mediators proceeds unchecked. Host cytokines play a key role in this process. Tumor necrosis factor-α (TNF-α) and interleukin-1 (IL-1) are stimulated by foreign antigens such as endotoxin. These cytokines produce leukocyte-endothelial adhesion and then release of proteases; platelet-activating factor; IL-8; arachidonic acid metabolites, such as thromboxane A$_2$, prostacyclin, and prostaglandin E2; and clotting factors, which contribute to the generation of fever, tachycardia, tachypnea, ventilation-perfusion abnormalities, lactic acidosis, and disseminated intravascular coagulation. TNF-α, although not the sole mediator of sepsis syndrome, may be the most potent mediator of the sepsis inflammatory response and levels of TNF-α are associated with mortality in human gram-negative infections.

CLINICAL PRESENTATION

The initial presentation of sepsis may be subtle, but the rapid progression of this syndrome usually makes the general diagnosis obvious although the specific infectious agent may remain obscure. Minor mental status changes or confusion may be very early signs of sepsis. Hyperventilation has been noted as an early sign in closely monitored patients who are found subsequently to be septic. Most patients are either hyperthermic or hypothermic and complain of chills or have rigors. Some debilitated and elderly patients may have minimal symptoms other than confusion, and minimal signs other than orthostasis or frank hypotension. Neutrophil counts may be high but neutropenia is also a common manifestation.

Although the line between primary clinical manifestations and subsequent complications is arbitrary, the complications of sepsis, manifestations of organ hypoperfusion, coagulopathy, and endothelial damage, represent a continuum into the sepsis syndrome and septic shock. Patients frequently present with evidence of organ hypoperfusion such as hypotension, oliguria, hypoxemia, acidosis, and liver function abnormalities and may also have signs of a consumptive coagulopathy with thrombocytopenia and bleeding and evidence of depressed myocardial function. Adult respiratory distress syndrome (ARDS) or diffuse pulmonary capillary leak syndrome may be a somewhat later finding. Due to the very rapid progression of sepsis, some patients may present with evidence of ARDS.

DIFFERENTIAL DIAGNOSIS

Other processes or stimuli may cause systemic inflammatory responses resulting in a clinical syndrome that is indistinguishable from sepsis. Burns and pancreatitis are the most common non-infectious causes. Other causes of severe tissue injury may also result in a sepsis-like appearance.

DIAGNOSTIC APPROACH

Diagnostic signs of septic shock syndrome may be subtle during the very early manifestations, but they are usually obvious once the process has evolved. Determining the source of the infection and the specific microbial agent is the main issue in diagnosis. Medical history including predisposing disorders, recent antimicrobial therapy, diet, travel, and exposure information is important. If possible, one should obtain a history of symptoms from the patient to help localize the infection or pinpoint the etiology. Cultures of blood and other fluids are essential. Stool culture and screening for *Clostridium difficile* toxin are sometimes overlooked.

MANAGEMENT AND THERAPY

Therapy is divided into several categories

Table 82-1
Empiric Antibiotic Therapy

Clinical Setting	Possible Therapies
Outpatient admission	Third-generation cephalosporin (e.g., ceftriaxone, cefotaxime) or piperacillin/tazobactam, or imipenem (or meropenem) each with an aminoglycoside
Intra-abdominal	Piperacillin/tazobactam or imipenem (or meropenem) each with an aminoglycoside
Possible MRSA	Add vancomycin
Hospitalized patient*	Imipenem (or meropenem) or piperacillin/tazobactam (at doses to cover *Pseudomonas aeruginosa*) plus aminoglycoside; ceftazidime, cefepime, and ciprofloxacin are alternatives
Neutropenic patient	Imipenem (or meropenem), cefepime, ceftazidime alone or with an aminoglycoside; piperacillin/tazobactam (at doses to cover *Pseudomonas aeruginosa*) is an alternative; vancomycin if fevers persist or likelihood of MRSA is high
Possible tick exposure	Add doxycycline

MRSA, methicillin-resistant *Staphylococcus aureus*.
*Local epidemiology of nosocomial infection and antibiotic resistance patterns should be used to guide therapy.

including antimicrobial, hemodynamic support, tissue oxygenation goal-directed therapy, and specific interruption of the inflammatory cascade. Ideally, antimicrobial therapy is directed at a specific pathogen; however, early in the course of septic shock the precise pathogen is usually not known and it may remain obscure after extensive investigation. In general, the severity of the illness dictates broad antimicrobial coverage unless there is a high degree of certainty as to the likely pathogen. Table 82-1 presents suggested empiric antibiotic therapy for patients with sepsis or septic shock in a variety of settings.

Despite advances in antimicrobial therapy over the past half-century, dramatic improvements in mortality from severe sepsis syndrome have not occurred. Imbalance between oxygen demand and oxygen supply resulting in total tissue and organ hypoxia is the result of the many physiologic abnormalities that are the hallmark of sepsis and septic shock such as peripheral vasodilatation, decreased cardiac function, intravascular volume loss, and increased metabolic demand. Recently, therapeutic interventions based on optimization of tissue oxygen delivery as measured by mixed venous oxygen saturation, pH, or arterial lactate levels have demonstrated improved outcomes compared to standard therapy based predominantly on fluid resuscitation and maintenance of blood pressure.

This "goal-oriented therapy" is predominantly used during early resuscitation of patients who present with severe sepsis syndrome. Physiologic goals include maintaining central venous pressure greater than 8 to 12 mm Hg, mean arterial pressure between 65 and 90 mm Hg, and central venous oxygen saturation at or above 70% (using transfusion, inotropic agents, and supplemental oxygen with or without mechanical ventilation).

Over the past decade, attempts to disrupt the inflammatory cascade that is responsible for the dysregulation of hemodynamics and coagulation in early sepsis, and leads to organ hypoperfusion, morbidity, and mortality have been disappointing. Glucocorticoids, agents to neutralize endotoxin, and interventions to inhibit the activity of TNF-α and IL-1 including IL-receptor antagonists, monoclonal antibodies to TNF-α and soluble TNF receptors, have in some small or uncontrolled studies offered preliminary evidence of activity. However, large comparative trials have essentially been negative for each of these agents. Studies

Figure 82-1

Septicemia

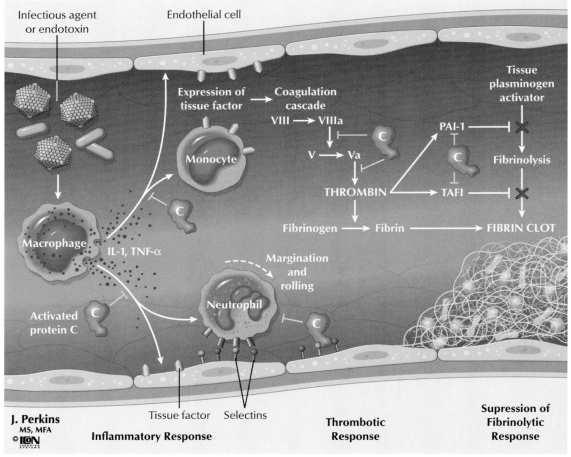

J. Perkins
MS, MFA
© ICON

Inflammatory Response

Thrombotic Response

Supression of Fibrinolytic Response

Indicates inactivation or inhibition

of inhibitors of platelet-activating factor, bradykinins, and cyclooxygenase (e.g., ibuprofen) have also been disappointing.

Recently, recombinant human activated protein C, which promotes fibrinolysis and inhibits thrombosis and inflammation, has been shown to improve mortality in severe sepsis. This protein has been postulated as an important counter-regulatory factor of the severe inflammation and coagulation of septic shock. In a randomized trial of patients with systemic inflammation, organ failure, and acute infection, recombinant human activated protein C (drotrecogin alpha) or placebo was administered by IV infusion within 48 hours of first evidence of organ dysfunction. Infusion was maintained for 96 hours. Mortality over 28 days was reduced from 30.8% to 24.7% in the patients

who received drotrecogin. Not surprisingly, serious bleeding was higher in the treated group. This agent is now available for treatment of severe sepsis when there is evidence of organ dysfunction. Many health-care institutions are limiting its use because of the very narrow window of activity defined by one large clinical study, the risk of significant bleeding, and the high cost of the drug.

FUTURE DIRECTIONS

Septicemia is an extremely common clinical syndrome with a high mortality rate (30% to 50%) despite modern interventions. Given the increasing number of elderly and immune-suppressed patients and the increasing prevalence of antibiotic resistance, the number of cases of sepsis is likely to continue to increase and antibiotic therapy alone is unlikely to improve mortality. After many failed attempts at disrupting the inflammatory and coagulation cascade in early sepsis, recent evidence that a fibrinolytic agent that is an inhibitor of thrombosis improves mortality in severe sepsis should spur continued interest in this treatment strategy. Decreases achieved with recombinant activated protein C were significant but modest (overall 6.1% decrease) and further definition of the window of activity of this agent is needed. Whether this agent can be used in earlier stages of sepsis needs to be understood. Additional inhibitors of the inflammatory and coagulation cascade are in development and need to be further studied. Combinations of agents that target more than one step in the cascade may prove more effective than a single agent. Supportive care and assessment of supportive therapy targeted to achieve specific physiologic goals will likely continue. Refinement of target physiologic parameters and elucidation of the specific interventions most effective at achieving them should result in increased use of the strategy in a wider array of clinical settings and increase the numbers of patients who survive this syndrome.

REFERENCES

Angus DC, Linde-Zwirble WT, Lidicker J, Clermont G, Carcillo J,Pinsky MR. Epidemiology of severe sepsis in the United States: analysis of incidence, outcome, and associated costs of care. *Crit Care Med*. 2001;29:1303–1310.

Bernard GR, Vincent JL, Laterre PF, et al, for the Recombinant human protein C Worldwide Evaluation in Severe Sepsis (PROWESS) study group. Efficacy and safety of recombinant human activated protein C for severe sepsis. *N Engl J Med*. 2001;344:699–709.

Bone RC, Balk RA, Cerra FB, et al. Definitions for sepsis and organ failure and guidelines for the use of innovative therapies in sepsis. The ACCP/SCCM Consensus Conference Committee. American College of Chest Physicians/Society of Critical Care Medicine. *Chest*. 1992;101:1644–1655.

Matthay MA. Severe sepsis—a new treatment with both anticoagulant and antiinflammatory properties. *N Engl J Med*. 2001;344:759–762.

Rivers E, Nguyen B, Havstad S, et al. Early goal-directed therapy in the treatment of severe sepsis and septic shock. *N Engl J Med*. 2001;345:1368–1377.

Wheeler AP, Bernard GR. Treating patients with severe sepsis. *N Engl J Med*. 1999;340:207–210.

Young, L. Sepsis syndrome. In: Mandell GL, Bennett JE, Dolin R, eds. *Mandell, Douglas, and Bennett's Principles and Practice of Infectious Diseases*. 5th ed. Philadelphia, Pa: Churchill Livingstone; 2000:806–819.

Chapter 83
Staphylococcal Infections

Andrew H. Kaplan

Staphylococcus aureus is an important bacterial pathogen. It is a major cause of serious nosocomial as well as community-acquired infections including skin and soft tissue infections, septicemia, endovascular infections, and infections of indwelling catheters. Resistance to many of the available classes of antibiotics is widespread and represents a serious challenge for clinicians. The mainstays of treatment are appropriate antibiotics, removal of infected tissues or foreign objects, and surgical drainage of infected fluid collections.

Asymptomatic carriers of *S. aureus* are relatively common—between 20% and 40% of adults are colonized with the organism at any one time and studies suggest that 50% of adults will be colonized at some time during their life. In adult carriers, the organism is most commonly recovered from the anterior nares and *S. aureus* is more commonly recovered from the nasopharynx of health-care workers than those who work outside of hospitals. Cross-sectional studies in high-risk patients have demonstrated carriage rates as high as 90%. Those at higher risk include patients with diabetes mellitus or chronic exfoliative skin conditions, and those receiving chronic hemodialysis. Users of intravenous drugs are also at greater risk for colonization. The clinical relevance of asymptomatic carriage is underlined by several studies that demonstrated both an increased risk for infection in colonized patients and for the transfer of strains from colonized health-care workers to patients.

The nosocomial spread of *S. aureus* has significant impact on both clinical outcomes and health-care costs. *S. aureus* is the most commonly reported cause of hospital-acquired infection. Patients with nosocomial *S. aureus* infection have approximately twice the length of hospital stay and are at an increased risk for dying during the hospitalization. The widespread transmission of strains resistant to beta-lactam antibiotics is of particular concern. Virtually all of the isolates recovered from both hospital and community-acquired infections are resistant to penicillin and as many as 50% of isolates from hospitals and long-term care facilities are resistant to methicillin. Methicillin-resistant *S. aureus* is becoming increasingly common in the community setting as well.

ETIOLOGY AND PATHOGENESIS

S. aureus is a is very robust organism, able to persist on surfaces at wide ranges of temperature, pH, and salt concentrations. Several bacterial products are associated with the ability of the organism to persist in the environment and cause disease. These are grouped into substances that allow the organism to persist on surfaces in vivo and toxins and enzymes that appear to be important in tissue invasion and destruction

A hallmark of *S. aureus* infection is its ability to colonize and persist on both implanted and indwelling foreign bodies such as intravenous catheters or prosthetic joints. The organism is also commonly found on disrupted native endovascular epithelium such as abnormal cardiac valves or thrombosed blood vessels. Attachment of the organism is mediated by a number of bacterial products including teichoic acid. Once the organism adheres to a surface, its persistence at that site is supported by several factors that interfere with immune clearance. These include factors that inhibit neutrophil access to the organisms (coagulase), limit phagocytosis (capsule/slime layer), inhibit opsonization (clumping factor and protein A), and interfere with intracellular killing (catalase).

Following adherence, a group of enzymes and toxins allow the organism to destroy involved tissue. These include several extracellular enzymes that are directly involved in tissue destruction through a disruptive effect on cellular membranes.

Secreted toxins that act at a distance and are responsible for many of the clinical manifestations of *S. aureus* infection are particularly important. These toxins are grouped into those that produce tissue destruction directly (α–, β–, γ–, and δ–toxins) or act by producing immune dysregulation (toxic shock syndrome toxins, enterotoxins, and exfoliative toxins). Many of the staphylococcal toxins act as superantigens. These bacterial proteins interact with major histocompatibility class II receptors outside of the antigen-binding groove. This high-affinity binding activates a large number of T lymphocytes, which in turn produce large amounts of cytokines. Elaboration of these cytokines plays a critical role in the pathogenesis of many of the clinical manifestations of *S. aureus* infection including the toxic shock syndrome, scalded skin syndrome, and staphylococcal food poisoning syndromes.

CLINICAL PRESENTATION

The clinical manifestations of *S. aureus* infection are protean and reflect the interaction between host and bacterial factors. Host factors predispose a patient to infection as well as influence the course of the disease and its presentation. Quantitative and qualitative defects in phagocytic function and conditions that disrupt the integrity of the skin increase the risk of infection. Among patients with phagocytic defects, those with deficiencies in neutrophil chemotaxis (e.g., Job's syndrome and Chediak-Higashi syndrome) and intracellular killing (e.g., chronic granulomatous disease) are at greatest risk. Patients with poorly controlled diabetes mellitus are also at increased risk for serious infection.

Skin and Soft Tissue Infections

Staphylococcal infection of the skin and soft tissues presents with a range of syndromes. Most characteristic is the tendency of the organism to form abscesses. Infections may progress from superficial, relatively benign infections of the hair follicle (folliculitis) to invasion of the tissue surrounding the follicle (furuncles). These small abscesses may coalesce and form larger collections of pus (carbuncles). Uncommonly, the underlying muscle and fascia become involved (pyomyositis and necrotizing fasciitis). Patients experiencing these deep-seated syndromes are generally febrile, complain of pain in the involved area, and appear ill. They require surgical intervention as well as appropriate antibiotic therapy. Staphylococcal wound infections associated with the presence of a foreign body such as a suture or surgical drain are of particular concern. The milder manifestations may be treated conservatively with oral antibiotics. Myositis and necrotizing fasciitis require aggressive surgical intervention for drainage and removal of infected tissue.

Staphylococcal Scalded Skin Syndrome

A bullous disease seen almost exclusively in children, staphylococcal scalded skin syndrome is associated with infection with an exfoliative toxin-producing *S. aureus*. Pathologically, the disease is associated with splitting of the granular layer of the epidermis. Generally, infected children are younger than 5 and present with fever and irritability. Sloughing of apparently uninvolved skin (Nikolsky's sign) is characteristic. Upon rupture of the fluid-filled bullae, large areas of epidermis may be disrupted, producing potentially serious volume and electrolyte losses, particularly in very young children. Therapy includes antibiotics and supportive care for electrolyte and volume loss.

Staphylococcal Toxic Shock Syndrome

This toxin-mediated syndrome was initially described in menstruating women using tampons (Figure 83-1). Staphylococcal toxic shock syndrome (TSS) has since been recognized in men and in women who are not menstruating. TSS initially presents as rash, fever, myalgias, diarrhea, and a depressed level of consciousness. Renal failure, hepatitis, and shock may rapidly follow these initial signs and symptoms within 24 to 48 hours. The shock may be severe and produce digital necrosis. TSS is often accompanied by the appearance of a desquamative rash, commonly on the hands and feet.

Unlike menses-associated TSS seen most commonly in young women, non-menstrual TSS is often associated with surgical procedures and may occur in the absence of frank evidence of active infection. A high level of suspicion for TSS must be maintained for patients with a "sunburn" appearing rash and a rapidly evolving shock picture following a surgical intervention. Patients with TSS should receive antibiotics active against *S. aureus* as well as supportive care for shock and organ failure. Any potential site of ongoing bacterial replication and toxin production (i.e., infected surgical suture, tampon) should be removed.

Figure 83-1

Toxic Shock Syndrome
Etiology and Pathogenesis

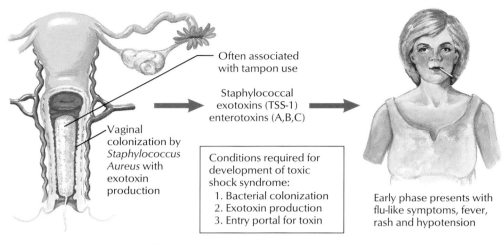

Often associated with tampon use

Staphylococcal exotoxins (TSS-1) enterotoxins (A,B,C)

Vaginal colonization by *Staphylococcus Aureus* with exotoxin production

Conditions required for development of toxic shock syndrome:
1. Bacterial colonization
2. Exotoxin production
3. Entry portal for toxin

Early phase presents with flu-like symptoms, fever, rash and hypotension

Clinical Features of Toxic Shock Syndrome

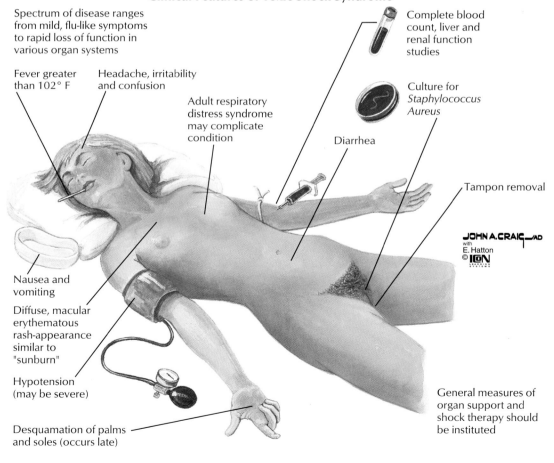

Spectrum of disease ranges from mild, flu-like symptoms to rapid loss of function in various organ systems

Complete blood count, liver and renal function studies

Fever greater than 102° F

Headache, irritability and confusion

Adult respiratory distress syndrome may complicate condition

Culture for *Staphylococcus Aureus*

Diarrhea

Tampon removal

Nausea and vomiting

Diffuse, macular erythematous rash-appearance similar to "sunburn"

Hypotension (may be severe)

Desquamation of palms and soles (occurs late)

General measures of organ support and shock therapy should be instituted

JOHN A. CRAIG AD
with
E. Hatton
© ICON

Staphylococcal Food Poisoning

S. aureus is associated with approximately 10% to 20% of the reported outbreaks of food-borne disease in the United States. The syndrome results from ingestion of any of the several heat-stable bacterial exotoxins. Because the preformed toxin is present in the food and does not require ongoing bacterial replication, rapid onset and resolution of symptoms mark the illness. Nausea and vomiting usually occur within 6 hours of ingesting the contaminated food and symptoms generally resolve within 12 hours. Patients are not febrile, but may appear quite ill from the hypovolemia associated with often explosive diarrhea and vomiting. Outbreaks are usually associated with the ingestion of partially cooked food (e.g., potato salad). Therapy is supportive; antibiotics are not required.

Pneumonia

S. aureus is an important cause of purulent pneumonia (Figure 83-2). The organism gains access to the lungs either through aspiration of nasopharyngeal contents colonized with staphylococci or via hematogenous spread (e.g., metastatic spread from bacteremia or septic emboli from right-sided endocarditis). Staphylococcal pneumonia tends to be fulminant and is often associated with infiltrative lesions that progress to cavitation as well as pleural empyemas. *S. aureus* is also a common cause of secondary bacterial pneumonia following infection with influenza virus. Antistaphylococcal antibiotics are usually effective in producing a cure; however, surgical drainage may be required in cases of pleural empyema.

Endocarditis

S. aureus, the second most common etiologic agent in infective endocarditis, is responsible for between 20% and 30% of the cases (Figure 83-3). Although the aortic and mitral valves are most likely to be involved, there is an increased prevalence of tricuspid valve involvement among intravenous drug users. As is the case for other organisms, *S. aureus* is more likely to infect heart valves with underlying abnormalities (e.g., degenerative valvular disease, rheumatic heart disease, or congenital abnormalities). However, the valves may be normal in as many as one third of all cases.

Staphylococcal endocarditis is also associated with the use of indwelling vascular catheters.

In comparison with endocarditis due to the viridans streptococci, staphylococcal endocarditis tends to be more aggressive and has an acute presentation. Myocardial abscesses are more frequent in the setting of *S. aureus* endocarditis as are valve ring abscesses, which often require surgical repair. Emboli to large organs occur in nearly half of all cases.

Treatment includes antibiotics active against the organism. Surgical replacement of the valve may be required because of serious conduction disturbances, myocardial abscesses, evidence of valvular instability, multiple large organ emboli, ongoing bacteremia on appropriate antibiotic therapy, and refractory congestive heart failure.

DIFFERENTIAL DIAGNOSIS/ DIAGNOSTIC APPROACH

Infection with *S. aureus* may be indistinguishable from other bacterial infections. Culture of the organism from infected tissue or blood is the basis of diagnosis. Given the aggressive nature of many staphylococcal infections, however, a high level of suspicion should be maintained in the presence of predisposing conditions such as defects in phagocytic function and in patients with diabetes mellitus.

MANAGEMENT AND THERAPY

Drainage of infected material and antibiotics are the mainstays of therapy. Organisms resistant to many of the available antimicrobial agents are routinely recovered in the hospital as well as the community setting.

Resistance may be due to either elaboration of beta-lactamase or alterations in one of the penicillin-binding proteins (PBPs). Beta-lactamase production is usually mediated by genes encoded on plasmids that are transferred between organisms. The enzyme is secreted extracellularly and acts by cleaving the beta-lactam ring, thereby inactivating the compound. Organisms using this mode of resistance may be treated with beta-lactamase–stable antibiotics such as nafcillin or oxacillin.

Penicillins and cephalosporins are ineffective against staphylococci with altered PBPs, the target enzyme for the beta-lactam antibiotics. These methicillin-resistant *S. aureus* are virulent and are

Figure 83-2

Staphylococcal Pneumonia

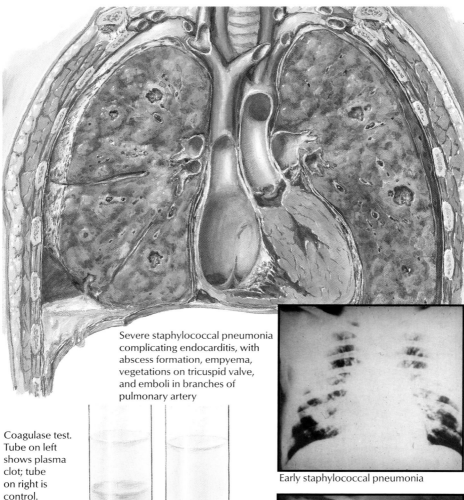

Severe staphylococcal pneumonia complicating endocarditis, with abscess formation, empyema, vegetations on tricuspid valve, and emboli in branches of pulmonary artery

Coagulase test. Tube on left shows plasma clot; tube on right is control.

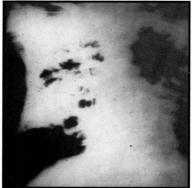

Early staphylococcal pneumonia

Staphylococcal and polymorphonuclear leukocytes in sputum (Gram's stain)

Late staphylococcal pneumonia with abscesses and pneumothorax

Figure 83-3

Bacterial Endocarditis
Early Lesions

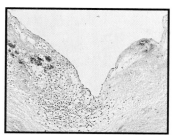

Deposit of platelets and organisms (stained dark), edema, and leukocytic infiltration in very early bacterial endocarditis of aortic valve

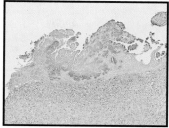

Development of vegetations containing clumps of bacteria on tricuspid valve

Early vegetations of bacterial endocarditis on bicuspid aortic valve

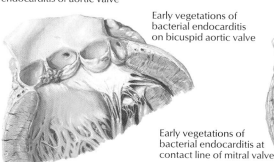

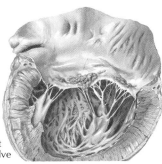

Early vegetations of bacterial endocarditis at contact line of mitral valve

Advanced Lesions

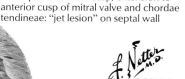

Advanced bacterial endocarditis of aortic valve: perforation of cusp; extension to anterior cusp of mitral valve and chordae tendineae: "jet lesion" on septal wall

Vegetations of bacterial endocarditis on under-aspect as well as on atrial surface of mitral valve

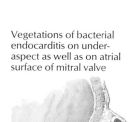

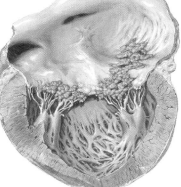

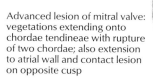

Advanced lesion of mitral valve: vegetations extending onto chordae tendineae with rupture of two chordae; also extension to atrial wall and contact lesion on opposite cusp

a major cause of nosocomial infection.

The appearance of strains of *S. aureus* that have reduced susceptibility to the glycopeptide antibiotics (e.g., vancomycin) is a particular concern. Several isolates have been reported from Japan and the United States. Thus far, these organisms show only intermediate levels of resistance to vancomycin and retain susceptibility to the newest classes of antistaphylococcal antibiotics, the oxazolidinones and quinupristin/dalfopristin.

FUTURE DIRECTIONS

Studies are likely to yield a more thorough understanding of the pathogenetic mechanisms. Of special interest are insights that should arise from studies of whole bacterial genomes. The introduction of two classes of agents with activity against gram-positive organisms, the oxazolidinones and quinupristin/dalfopristin, has enhanced the ability to treat resistant strains of *S. aureus*. Both agents act at the 50s bacterial ribosome, have good anti-staphylococcal activity, and appear to be effective against vancomycin-resistant enterococci. Resistance to these agents appears to be very uncommon; however, it is anticipated that resistant organisms will become prevalent as the use of these antibiotics becomes widespread.

REFERENCES

Chambers HF. Methicillin resistance in staphylococci: molecular and biochemical basis and clinical implications. *Clin Microbiol Rev.* 1997;10:781–791.

Crossley KB, Archer GL. *The Staphylococci in Human Disease.* New York, NY: Churchill Livingstone; 1997.

Dresser LD, Rybak MJ. The pharmacologic and bacteriologic properties of oxazolidinones, a new class of synthetic antimicrobials. *Phamacotherapy.* 1998;18:456–462.

Mandell GL, Bennett JE, Dolin R, eds. *Mandell, Douglas, and Bennett's Principles and Practice of Infectious Diseases.* 5th ed. Philadelphia, Pa: Churchill Livingstone; 2000.

Rubinstein E, Bompart F. Activity of quinupristin/dalfopristin against gram-positive bacteria: clinical applications and therapeutic potential. *J Antimicrob Chemother.* 1997;39(suppl A):139–143.

Chapter 84

Varicella-Zoster Infections

Adaora A. Adimora

Varicella zoster virus (VZV), a large DNA virus, belongs to the family Herpesviridae and, like all herpesviruses, induces lifelong latent infection. VZV causes two clinical syndromes: varicella (chickenpox), a highly contagious childhood rash illness due to primary infection with VZV; and herpes zoster (shingles), a dermatomal vesicular rash caused by reactivation of latent VZV infection. Varicella is usually benign in immunocompetent children but causes substantially greater morbidity and mortality in adults and immunocompromised hosts. Herpes zoster can cause severe and prolonged pain and, like varicella, is sometimes much more severe in compromised hosts.

ETIOLOGY AND PATHOGENESIS

Primary infection occurs through airborne transmission of infectious droplets from vesicular skin lesions or respiratory secretions resulting in infection of the upper respiratory tract, followed by viral replication in regional lymph nodes, viremia, and subsequent infection of endothelial cells of the skin and the epidermis. The rash of varicella-zoster infection is characterized initially by clear vesicles that contain infectious virus results. Vesicles become pustular with migration of polymorphonuclear cells (PMNs) and subsequently either rupture or resorb.

After primary VZV infection, the virus becomes latent in dorsal root ganglia. The factors that promote reactivation and subsequent development of clinical herpes zoster are poorly understood.

CLINICAL PRESENTATION

Varicella is extremely contagious; the reported attack rate among persons without previous infection exceeds 90%. Children aged 5 through 9 are affected most commonly. Approximately 90% of the U.S. population over the age of 15 has had VZV infection. Illness, characterized by rash, malaise, and fever, appears 10 to 21 days after infection. The rash, varicella's hallmark, begins as a vesicular eruption that occurs in crops of lesions over several days and spreads from the head to the trunk and finally to the extremities (Figure 84-1). The skin lesions undergo a characteristic series of changes as vesicles umbilicate, and then evolve into pustules and finally crusted papules. Varicella is contagious 1 or 2 days before the onset of rash and until all lesions have formed crusts.

Varicella is usually a benign illness in immunocompetent children; however, it is generally more severe in older adolescents and adults. In the neonate, it is associated with high mortality risk when maternal disease develops within 5 days before or 2 days after delivery. Disease may be severe in immunocompromised hosts of all ages.

Complications include secondary skin infections, usually due to *Staphylococcus aureus* or *Streptococcus pyogenes*, which occur as a result of scratching the pruritic lesions. Pneumonia is uncommon in children, but occurs in approximately 16% to 20% of adults usually about 3 to 5 days after the onset of illness (Figure 84-1). Pneumonia is often associated with dyspnea, cough, and fever, but radiographic evidence of pneumonitis may also occur in the absence of respiratory symptoms. Common radiographic findings include interstitial and nodular infiltrates. Morbidity is especially severe in pregnant women with varicella and pneumonia. CNS complications, such as cerebellar ataxia, aseptic meningitis, encephalitis, Guillain-Barré syndrome, Reye's syndrome, and transverse myelitis can occur. Myocarditis, hepatitis, nephritis, and arthritis may also complicate varicella.

Herpes zoster occurs at all ages, but incidence rises with old age and the waning of cell-mediated immunity. The first symptom is pain, followed within 48 to 72 hours by eruption of a unilateral maculopapular rash in a dermatomal distribution that subsequently becomes vesicular. The thoracic and lumbar dermatomes are most frequently involved. Lesions usually persist for 10 to 15 days, but skin

Figure 84-1

Varicella Pneumonia

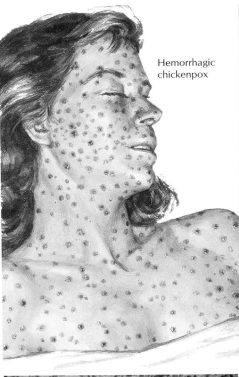

Hemorrhagic chickenpox

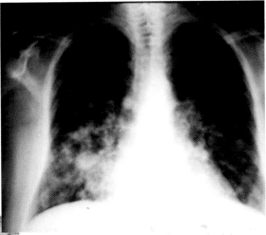

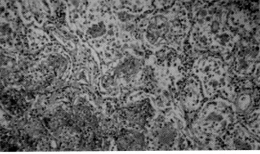

Varicella pneumonia. Nodular infiltrates in both lower lobes, more marked and coalescing on right side.

Pulmonary histology, low power. Alveoli filled with fibrin, fluid, and cellular exudate.

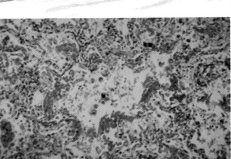

High power: Mononuclear infiltrate in interstitium and fibrin lining alveoli.

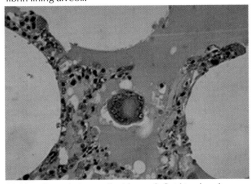

Multinucleated giant cell with much fluid in alveolus.

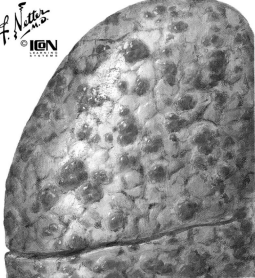

Pleural hemorrhagic pocks

Figure 84-2

Varicella Zoster with Probable Keratitis

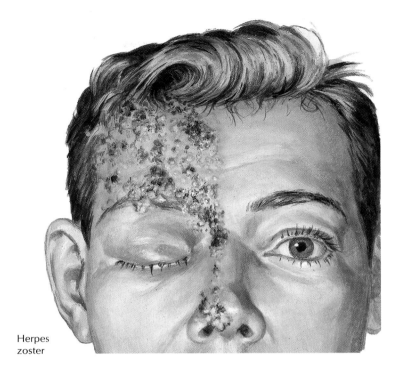

Herpes
zoster

may not become completely normal for several weeks. Involvement of the trigeminal nerve may cause eye involvement (herpes zoster ophthalmicus) and is a potentially sight-threatening condition (Figure 84-2). Zoster-associated pain and post-herpetic neuralgia are the most troublesome symptoms, and may be incapacitating, especially in persons older than 50. Pain is especially severe in the areas overlying the site of previous blisters. Risk factors for post-herpetic neuralgia include increased age, sensory loss, and severity of pain. Prompt treatment with antiviral agents appears to decrease the risk of post-herpetic neuralgia. Central nervous system involvement may occur as manifested by meningoencephalitis or encephalitis. Herpes zoster is more severe in immunocompromised hosts than in normal hosts. Patients with lymphoma, for example, are at increased risk for cutaneous dissemination and visceral involvement.

DIFFERENTIAL DIAGNOSIS

Diagnostic considerations include disseminated herpes simplex virus, coxsackievirus, echovirus, atypical measles, but these infections more often cause a morbilliform rash than vesicular lesions. Appearance of impetigo can be similar to varicella, but unroofing of impetigo lesions should reveal Gram-positive cocci due to *S. aureus* or *S. pyogenes*.

DIAGNOSTIC APPROACH

History and physical examination are usually sufficient for diagnosis. A characteristic skin rash in multiple stages of development should raise suspicion of varicella, especially in a person with a history of exposure. Similarly, diagnosis of herpes zoster should be considered for a dermatomally distributed vesicular rash. Laboratory testing can be useful in equivocal cases.

Vesicular skin lesions are scraped to obtain material for viral culture or performance of direct fluorescent antibody staining. Antibody testing with immune adherence hemagglutination assay, fluorescent antibody to membrane antigen assay, or enzyme-linked immunosorbent assay (ELISA) are occasionally helpful in demonstrating seroconversion or diagnostic rises in titer. Tzanck smears of lesions may reveal characteristic multinucleated giant cells, but sensitivity is only 60%. Such smears do not distinguish herpes simplex virus from VZV. PCR assays to detect VZV DNA in CSF may be helpful in the diagnosis of central nervous system involvement.

MANAGEMENT AND THERAPY

Maintenance of good hygiene with bathing is important to decrease the risk of complications in patients with varicella. Fingernails should be cut closely to reduce risk of secondary infection. Dressings and antipruritic drugs can decrease itching. Oral acyclovir (800 mg 4 times daily by mouth for 5 days) decreases the duration and number of lesions and reduces fever when given within 24 hours of onset and should be given to adults and adolescents. Children at high risk for complications should also be treated.

In patients with varicella zoster, antiviral therapy with famciclovir (500 mg thrice daily for 7 days), valacyclovir (1 g thrice daily for 7 days), or acyclovir (800 mg 5 times daily for 7 to 10 days) speeds resolution of lesions and pain, but is most efficacious when given within 3 days of onset of rash. The addition of prednisone to acyclovir improved pain and other quality-of-life measurements in one study; however, it should be used with caution in patients with diabetes mellitus and others at risk for complications of corticosteroid use. Amitriptyline, desipramine, and gabapentin may be useful in decreasing post-herpetic neuralgia.

PREVENTION

Varicella vaccine, a live attenuated virus vaccine, has at least a 95% to 99% efficacy and is approved for use in healthy children at least 12 months old and for susceptible adolescents and adults. All children should be routinely vaccinated between 12 and 18 months, and susceptible children should be vaccinated before their 13th birthday. Varicella zoster immune globulin (VZIG) should be given following exposure to persons at high risk for complications (eg, immunocompromised persons, pregnant women, premature infants [born at less than 28 weeks' gestation or birth weight of less than 1,000 g]). VZIG must be given within 96 hours of exposure.

FUTURE DIRECTIONS

Introduction and widespread use of the varicella vaccine is likely to change the epidemiology of varicella infection. Long-term follow-up will be required to determine whether re-vaccination is necessary and if there are new or different clinical manifestations in people whose waning vaccine immunity allows illness. Herpes zoster may present different clinical manifestations as a result of the vaccine and new types of immunosuppressive therapy.

REFERENCES

Grose C, Zaia J. Varicella-zoster virus. In: Gorbach SL, Bartlett JG, Blacklow NR, eds. *Infectious Diseases.* 2nd ed. Philadelphia, Pa: WB Saunders Co; 1998:2120–2125.

Whitley R. Varicella-zoster virus. In: Mandell GL, Bennett JE, Dolin R, eds. *Mandell, Douglas, and Bennett's Principles and Practice of Infectious Diseases.* 5th ed. Philadelphia, Pa: Churchill Livingstone; 2000:1580–1586.

Whitley R. Varicella-zoster virus infections. In: Braunwald E, Fauci AS, Kasper DL, Hauser SL, Longo DL, Jameson JL, eds. *Harrison's Principles of Internal Medicine.* 15th ed. New York, NY: McGraw-Hill; 2001.

Section X

SEXUALLY TRANSMITTED DISEASES

Chapter 85

Acquired Immune Deficiency Syndrome (AIDS)

Charles van der Horst and Yoshihiko Murata

Infection with the human immunodeficiency virus (HIV) causes a continuum of diseases, from the acute (primary) HIV infection to prolonged periods of asymptomatic infection to AIDS. The diagnosis of AIDS implies that there has been significant damage to the immune system and is a surveillance case definition established by the Centers for Disease Control and Prevention (CDC) as part of the classification of the clinical status of HIV-infected patients.

To date, two human immunodeficiency viruses, HIV-1 and HIV-2, have been identified as the causative agents of AIDS. There are several subtypes (clades) of HIV-1 with varying distributions throughout the world, while HIV-2 is more prevalent in Western Africa. The pandemic of HIV continues to be a serious international problem. As of the year 2000, there were approximately 34.4 million people worldwide living with HIV/AIDS.

ETIOLOGY AND PATHOGENESIS

HIV predominantly infects T cells bearing the CD4 surface protein and other cells associated with the immune system. HIV exhibits a cytopathic effect on the vast majority of infected cells, but it can also establish a latent state in cells that can be reactivated years after the initial infection.

Most patients with HIV experience a slow, progressive decline in the CD4+ T cell count and become increasingly at risk for opportunistic infections and certain types of malignancies.

HIV is transmitted by blood and other blood-derived products, through sexual contact, and from infected mothers to infants during the intrapartum or perinatal periods or via breastfeeding. There is no evidence to suggest that HIV is transmitted by casual social contact.

CLINICAL PRESENTATION

From 40% to 90% of patients with primary HIV infection present with symptomatic illness, including fever, fatigue, a rash (typically maculopapular), headaches, lymphadenopathy, pharyngitis, nausea, vomiting, and diarrhea. These symptoms usually last for less than 2 weeks. (Figure 85-1)

Thereafter, patients infected with HIV can remain asymptomatic for up to several years while their immune system becomes slowly depleted of CD4+ lymphocytes. Once the CD4+ cell count reaches between 200 and 500 cells/μL, certain infections may develop, including varicella zoster, hairy leukoplakia, oral thrush, and esophageal or vaginal candidiasis (Figures 85-2, 85-3, and 85-4). These patients are also at higher risk for malignancies, including Kaposi sarcoma and lymphoma, and may experience unexplained weight loss, sinusitis, diarrhea, and fatigue. Once the CD4+ T cell count becomes less than 200 cells/μL, patients are at greater risk of opportunistic infections and certain malignancies, and can present with a number of symptoms, including fever, headaches, weakness, cough, shortness of breath, nausea, vomiting, and diarrhea. A careful history and physical examination should be performed, and a high index of suspicion for HIV should be maintained because of the varied clinical presentation in HIV disease.

DIFFERENTIAL DIAGNOSIS

The presentation of primary HIV infection can mimic other viral diseases, including infectious mononucleosis, rubella, herpes simplex infection, and secondary syphilis.

Patients with rare congenital immune deficiencies may present with opportunistic infections. However, the serologic tests for HIV should be sufficient to identify those patients infected with HIV.

Figure 85-1

Sexually Transmitted Infections: Human Immunodeficiency Virus

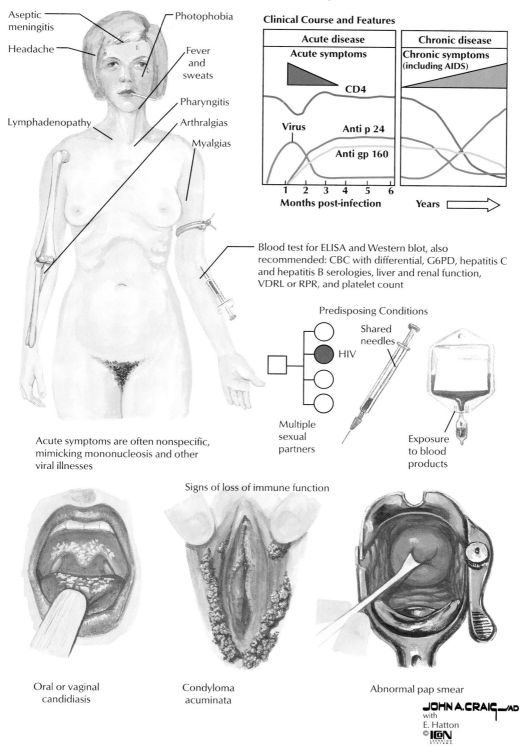

Aseptic meningitis

Photophobia

Headache

Fever and sweats

Lymphadenopathy

Pharyngitis

Arthralgias

Myalgias

Clinical Course and Features

Acute disease

Acute symptoms

CD4

Virus

Anti p 24

Anti gp 160

1 2 3 4 5 6
Months post-infection

Chronic disease

Chronic symptoms (including AIDS)

Years

Blood test for ELISA and Western blot, also recommended: CBC with differential, G6PD, hepatitis C and hepatitis B serologies, liver and renal function, VDRL or RPR, and platelet count

Predisposing Conditions

HIV

Shared needles

Multiple sexual partners

Exposure to blood products

Acute symptoms are often nonspecific, mimicking mononucleosis and other viral illnesses

Signs of loss of immune function

Oral or vaginal candidiasis

Condyloma acuminata

Abnormal pap smear

JOHN A. CRAIG—AD
with
E. Hatton
© ICON
LEARNING SYSTEMS

Figure 85-2   Hairy Leukoplakia of the Tongue

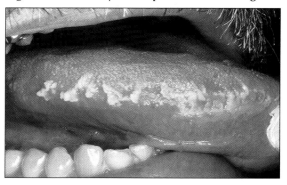

With permission from Mandel G., ed. *Essential Atlas of Infectious Diseases, 2nd ed.,* 2002; 21.

Figure 85-3   Disseminated Herpes Zoster

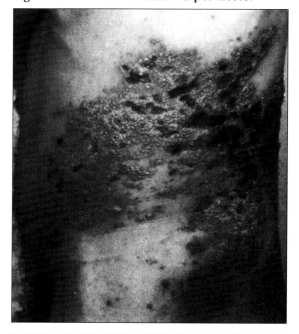

With permission from Cohen PR, Beitrani VP, Grossman ME. Disseminated herpes zoster in patients with human immunodeficiency virus infection. *Am J Med* 1988; 84: 1076-1080.

DIAGNOSTIC APPROACH

Diagnosis of HIV infection requires a careful history to identify potential high-risk behavior and physical examination to seek clinical evidence of opportunistic infections and malignancies.

Laboratory confirmation of HIV infection requires detection of antibodies against HIV-derived proteins by ELISA (enzyme-linked immunosorbent assay) fol-

Figure 85-4   Pseudomembranous Candidiasis of the Palate

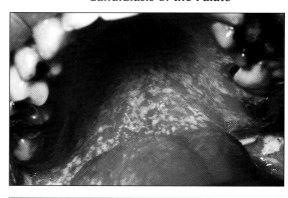

With permission from Mandel G., ed. *Essential Atlas of Infectious Diseases, 2nd ed.,* 2002; 27.

lowed by a confirmatory Western blot, or detection of the HIV-derived p24 antigen.

To assess prognosis and monitor the effectiveness of antiretroviral therapy, quantification of HIV RNA levels ("viral load") and the CD4+ T cell counts are used. At this time, the use of the HIV RNA level quantification test is not approved by the US Food and Drug Administration (FDA) for diagnosis of primary HIV infection.

The diagnosis of AIDS is confirmed by presumptive diagnosis of opportunistic infections by clinical and/or radiographic means in the presence of HIV infection, or definitive diagnosis of opportunistic infection or certain malignancies by microscopy, histologic studies, or culture. The 1993 revised CDC classification for AIDS in HIV-infected adults is shown in on page 565.

MANAGEMENT AND THERAPY
Therapy for HIV Infection

There is no known cure for HIV infection. The current principle of therapy is the use of 3 or more antiretroviral agents to maintain reduced viral load and thus allow some regeneration of the immune system. This approach prevents progression of HIV disease and significantly improves survival. Moreover, the concurrent use of multiple antiretroviral agents reduces the risk of early emergence of HIV that may be resistant to one or more agents.

Currently, there are three FDA-approved classes of antiretroviral agents: the nucleoside reverse transcriptase inhibitors (NRTIs), the non-nucleoside reverse transcriptase inhibitors (NNR-

TIs), and the protease inhibitors (PIs) (Table 85-1). Almost all of these agents can cause nausea, vomiting, and/or diarrhea to varying degrees.

Side effects associated with specific antiretroviral agents are listed in Table 85-1. More importantly, class-specific side effects have recently been noted. NRTIs have been implicated in mitochondrial dysfunction and rare but potentially life-threatening lactic acidosis and liver failure. Use of PIs and a subset of NRTIs has been associated with lipodystrophy with peripheral fat wasting and central fat accumulation with hyperlipidemia in up to 50% of patients after 1 year of therapy. In a subset of these affected patients, type 2 diabetes mellitus has also been noted.

There is some debate as to when antiretroviral therapy should be initiated. The most recent guidelines issued by the US Department of Health and Human Services suggest that the antiretroviral therapy be initiated when the CD4+ T cell count decreases below 350/µL. Because the initiation of antiretroviral therapy is a major therapeutic decision, it is essential that there is a strong mutual commitment between the patient and the physician to long-term, full adherence to therapy.

The decision to use specific antiretroviral agents for combination therapy should consider multiple factors, including previous exposure to antiretroviral drugs (and thus a chance to harbor resistant strains of HIV), the status of the patient's immune system, the patient's ability to adhere to drug treatment, and the potential side effects and drug-drug interactions.

Currently, patients are usually started on a combination of at least two NRTIs, in combination with another NRTI, a PI or one of the NNRTIs (e.g., nelfinavir, zidovudine, lamivudine or nevirapine, zidovudine, lamivudine). Some drug combinations, such as zidovudine and stavudine are to be avoided. In certain instances, low-dose ritonavir (100 to 200 mg orally twice daily) may be used to enhance the pharmacokinetic profile of other PIs. Ideally, HIV-viral load assays and CD4+ T cell counts are obtained before therapy and at 4 and 8 weeks after initiation of treatment, and thereafter followed at 3 to 4 month intervals. If the treatment is effective, the viral load should decrease to below 400 copies/mL, or on the more sensitive assay, less than 50 copies/mL within 4 to 6 months. Patients should be closely mon-

---

Conditions Included in the 1993 AIDS* Surveillance Case Definition

- Candidiasis of bronchi, trachea, lungs, or esophagus
- Cervical cancer, invasive
- Coccidioidomycosis, disseminated or extrapulmonary
- Cryptococcosis, extrapulmonary
- Cryptosporidiosis, chronic intestinal (greater than 1 month duration)
- Cytomegalovirus disease (other than liver, spleen or nodes; including cytomegalovirus retinitis with loss of vision)
- Encephalopathy, HIV-related
- Herpes simplex: chronic ulcer(s)(greater than 1 month duration) or bronchitis, pneumonitis, or esophagitis
- Histoplasmosis, disseminated or extrapulmonary
- Isosporiasis, chronic intestinal (greater than 1 month duration)
- Kaposi sarcoma
- Leukoencephalopathy, progressive multifocal
- Lymphoma, Burkitt (or equivalent form), immunoblastic (or equivalent form), or primary of brain
- *Mycobacterium avium* complex or *M. kansasii*, disseminated or extrapulmonary
- *Mycobacterium tuberculosis*, pulmonary or extrapulmonary
- Mycobacterium, other species or unidentified species, disseminated or extrapulmonary
- *Pneumocystis carinii*
- Pneumonia, recurrent
- Salmonella septicemia, recurrent
- Toxoplasmosis of brain
- Wasting syndrome due to HIV

* Patients infected with HIV and whose CD4+ T cell count is less than 200 are classified as having AIDS.

Adapted from 1993 AIDS Surveillance Case Definition. *CDC Mobidity and Mortality Weekly Report,* Vol 41 (RR-17) 12/18/1992.

---

itored for potential side effects of therapy. Consider performing the following laboratory studies at each clinic visit: serum chemistries, liver function tests, amylase, lipase, complete blood cell count with differential, viral load, and CD4+ T cell count.

Management of HIV-Associated Infections

The following baseline labs should be obtained prior to therapy: hepatitis A, B and C serologies;

Table 85-1
Summary of Antiretroviral Agents

	Usual Dosage	Major Side Effects (besides nausea, vomiting, and diarrhea)
NRTIs		
Zidovudine (AZT)	300 mg po bid	Anemia, granulocytopenia, headaches, myopathy
Lamivudine (3TC)	150 mg po bid	Pancreatitis (in pediatric trials), headaches
Abacavir (ABC)	300 mg po bid	Hypersensitivity reaction (including fever, respiratory symptoms, GI upset, rash) — DO NOT RECHALLENGE — anemia, neutropenia, headache
Didanosine (ddI)	>60 kg: 200 mg po bid or 400 mg po qd; <60 kg: 125 mg po bid or 250 mg po qd	Pancreatitis, peripheral neuropathy
Stavudine (d4T)	>60 kg: 40 mg po bid; <60 kg: 30 mg po bid	Pancreatitis, peripheral neuropathy
Tenofovir Disoproxil Fumarate	300 mg po qd	Asthenia, headaches
Zalcitabine (ddC)	0.75 mg po tid	Peripheral neuropathy, oral ulcers, rash
NNRTIs		
Nevirapine	200 mg po qd x 2 wk, then 200 mg po bid	Hepatotoxicity, rash
Delavirdine	400 mg po tid	Skin rash, headaches
Efavirenz	600 mg po qhs	Dizziness, insomnia, somnolence, abnormal dreams, rash, teratogen in animal models— AVOID PREGNANCY, monitor LFTs in patients with underlying hepatitis B or C
PIs		
Amprenavir	>50 kg: 1,200 mg po bid; <50 kg: 20 mg/kg bid	Rash
Indinavir	800 mg po q8h	Nephrolithiasis
Nelfinavir	1,250 mg po bid or 750 mg po tid	
Ritonavir	Hard capsules: 600 mg po tid (see text for reduced dosing); Soft capsules: 1200 mg po tid	Bitter aftertaste, perioral paresthesias
Saquinavir	1,200 mg po tid	
Lopinavir/Ritonavir	400 mg/100 mg po bid	

Adapted from Gilbert DN, Moellering RC Jr, Sande MA, eds. *The Sanford Guide to Antimicrobial Therapy.* 31st ed. Hyde Park, VT: Antimicrobial Therapy, Inc.; 2001: 108-111.

cytomegalovirus (CMV) IgG; toxoplasma IgG; and RPR. If a baseline Pap smear is abnormal, repeat smears every 6 months; if normal, then every 12 months.

Based on the CD4 count, the following algorithm may be used in initiating prophylaxis for serious opportunistic infections in HIV-infected patients:

· CD4 count 100 to 200 cells/μL: obtain baseline ophthalmologic examination, start *Pneumocystis carinii* pneumonia (PCP) prophylaxis with trimethoprim-sulfamethoxazole (TMP-SMX) 1 double-strength tablet daily or dapsone 100 mg orally once daily (check baseline glucose-6-phosphatase dehydrogenase) or atovaquone 1,500 mg orally once daily or aerosolized pentamidine monthly.

· CD4 count less than 100cells/μL: If toxoplasma IgG+, start either TMP/SMX single- or double-strength daily or dapsone 100 mg daily and pyrimethamine 50 mg daily with folinic acid 10 mg twice weekly.

· CD4 count less than 50 cells/μL: Ophthalmologist examination every 3 months, prophylaxis against *Mycobacterium avium* complex (MAC) with azithromycin 1,200 mg weekly or clarithromycin 500 mg orally twice daily.

In evaluating HIV-positive patients, particularly those with CD4 count <200 cells/μL who have the following clinical complaints, consider:

· Respiratory symptoms: PCP, tuberculosis, and histoplasmosis. Obtain chest X-ray, ABG, sputum culture, early referral for bronchoscopy if clinically warranted.

· Headache: CT scan, lumbar puncture. The differential diagnosis includes toxoplasmosis if toxoplasma IgG+ and CD4 cell count <100 cells/μL, CNS lymphoma, meningitis (bacterial, cryptococcus, syphilis, tuberculosis).

· Diarrhea: salmonella, giardia, shigella, campylobacter, and yersinia. Obtain stool culture and ova/parasite screen; consider cryptosporidia, isospora, MAC, microsporidia, CMV, *Clostridium difficile*.

· Rash: always consider drug-induced rash, most commonly from antiretroviral agents and TMP-SMX.

For specific treatments for these and other HIV-associated opportunistic infections, early referral to specialists is essential.

PREVENTION OF INFECTION AND TRANSMISSION

Physicians should emphasize preventive education to all patients, especially those who are sexually active or engage in high-risk behavior such as intravenous drug abuse. Offer HIV testing (which requires patient consent) with pre- and post-test counseling to patients who request such tests and also to those at increased risk for HIV and other sexually transmitted diseases.

HIV-infected patients should be carefully counseled to avoid transmission of HIV by practicing safer sexual behaviors and informing past and future partners of their HIV status, never sharing needles, and informing those involved in their care of the HIV status.

FUTURE DIRECTIONS

Management of HIV infection continues to change rapidly, as new potential therapeutic agents are being studied in clinical trials. Analysis of viral genotype for mutations that confer resistance against specific antiretroviral agents is available and should facilitate the selection of optimum therapeutic combinations in treatment-naïve and treatment-experienced patients. Numerous strategies to generate a vaccine against HIV are being tested.

REFERENCES

Guidelines for the use of antiviral agents in HIV-infected adults and adolescents. The Panel on Clinical Practices for Treatment of HIV Infection. 2002.

AIDSinfo Web site. Available at: http://www.aidsinfo.nih.gov. Accessed January 13, 2003.

Carr A, Cooper DA. Adverse effects of antiretroviral therapy. *Lancet.* 2000;356:1423-1430.

Hirsch MS, Brun-Vezinet F, D'Aquila RT, et al. Antiretroviral drug resistance testing in adult HIV-1 infection: recommendations of an International AIDS Society-USA Panel. *JAMA.* 2000;283:2417-2426.

Johns Hopkins AIDS Service Web site. Available at: http://www.hopkins-aids.edu. Accessed January 13, 2003.

Medscape Infectious Diseases Web site. Available at: http://www.medscape.com/infectiousdiseaseshome. Accessed January 13, 2003.

Chapter 86
Genital Warts

Peter Leone

Genital infection with human papilloma virus (HPV) is extremely common. Most infections are benign and result in no disease. The spectrum of genital HPV infection ranges from asymptomatic infection to warts and cervical cancer. Over 80 types of HPV have been identified with the more than 30 causing genital infection divided into low and high risk for the development of malignant cellular changes such as cervical and anal cancer. The clinical expression of low-risk types is genital warts, a problem that is increasing in incidence worldwide. The genital subgroups of HPV have a predilection for the anogenital squamous epithelium. Their primary mode of transmission is sexual, and genital warts are only one manifestation of a broad spectrum of clinical diseases associated with HPV, including a strong association with genital neoplasia.

Accurate incidence figures for genital warts in the United States are not available. It is estimated that approximately 50% of sexually active women are infected with HPV. More than 70% of the adult population have been or are currently infected with HPV. A 1996 report by the Centers for Disease Control and Prevention (CDC) estimated that 24 million Americans are infected with HPV, and that 500,000 to 1 million new cases of condylomata acuminata occur annually. This means that approximately 1% of sexually active persons in the United States have visible genital warts at any one time. The majority, approximately 80%, are caused by HPV 6. HPV 11 and HPV 6 account for >90% of genital warts. Epidemiological studies indicate that those at risk for HPV infection include adolescents, young adults, and persons with multiple sex partners.

ETIOLOGY AND PATHOGENESIS

HPV is a protein encapsulated, non-enveloped icosahedral virus. It contains 8 to 10 genes that are circular, double-stranded DNA. The early region's products control viral replication, transcription, and cellular transformation, and encode for the oncoproteins E6 and E7. The late region encodes for structural proteins, while the long-control region contains transcription enhancer genes and promoter elements.

HPV infects stratified squamous epithelial cells. HPV-containing cells do not undergo cell lysis and are shed from the surface of the skin. Upon infection with HPV, epithelial cells are transformed to proliferate into benign tumors known as warts. In nonkeratinized squamous epithelium, the exophytic growths are known as condylomata acuminata.

CLINICAL PRESENTATION

In addition to the classic cauliflower-like proliferations, HPV infection may also manifest as smooth flat lesions (pigmented or nonpigmented), papular warts (flesh-colored, dome-shaped papules), keratotic warts (thick, crust-like layer), or as subclinical infections. The lesions most commonly are multiple, but may be single, scattered, or confluent. They are seen most often in young adults. The incubation period is 2 to 3 months, although the latency period from exposure to disease development varies greatly. The entire genital tract, including the vulva, vagina, cervix, penis, perianal area, rectum, and urethra, are susceptible to HPV infection.

Clinical Features in Males

The classic condylomata acuminata (Figure 86-1) predominate in moist areas, the inner surfaces of the prepuce, coronal sulcus, frenum, and may spread to the perianal area. More rounded papular warts are seen in drier areas of the penile shaft or perineal skin. Other clinically apparent lesions include sessile lesions and flat keratotic plaques with a roughened variably pigmented surface. Condylomata may also involve the urethra and urethral meatus, resulting in hematuria and dysuria or discharge.

Figure 86-1

Condyloma Acuminata of Penis

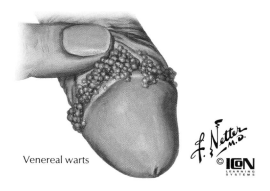

Venereal warts

Clinical Features in Females

Condylomata usually first appear at the posterior part of the introitus and adjacent labia and may involve other parts of the vulva, perineum, and anus, but rarely the adjacent thighs. The vagina (upper and lower third) may be involved and, infrequently, the cervix (Figure 86-2). More commonly, HPV infection of the cervix is subclinical, visible only after application of 5% acetic acid as flat acetowhite epithelium at colposcopy, or evident on PAP smears (2% to 3% of which are currently positive for warty changes). Subclinical HPV infection can occur elsewhere in the genital tract. Vaginal warts are usually asymptomatic, but occasionally present as vaginal discharge, pruritus, or postcoital bleeding.

In pregnancy and in immunosuppressed women, lesions may become exuberant. Occasionally, vaginal delivery may be threatened by obstruction or hemorrhage; however, lesions usually regress or disappear during the puerperium. The natural history of subclinical HPV infection of the vulva and vagina is poorly understood; in the cervix, a proportion will regress but a group will progress to dysplasia, intraepithelial neoplasia, or frank cancer.

Clinical Features in Children

Genital warts are rare in children. When present, there may be a history of maternal genital warts during pregnancy. In older children, molestation should be considered. Maternal genital warts during pregnancy may, in rare cases, cause laryngeal papillomatosis in infants. This may not become clinically apparent until the second decade of life.

DIFFERENTIAL DIAGNOSIS

Other papillomatous lesions that must be differentiated from anogenital warts include: (1) anatomical variants (e.g., papillae coronae glandis or the pearly penile papules); (2) infective conditions (e.g., condylomata lata of secondary syphilis [broader and flatter lesions; positive serological test for syphilis and dark field microscopy of lesions] and, in the tropics, donovanosis); and (3) benign and malignant neoplasias (e.g., intraepithelial carcinoma or invasive carcinoma).

DIAGNOSTIC APPROACH

HPV-associated lesions demonstrate specific changes recognized at colposcopy, cytology (Pap stain of ectocervical and endocervical smears), and histology of biopsy materials. Although HPV cannot be cultivated in vitro, recent advances in molecular biological techniques utilizing DNA probes can identify HPV DNA. Such techniques show that over 100 different types of HPV exist, and a subgroup of these (HPV types 6, 11, 16, 18 and less often 31, 33, 35) specifically infects the genital area. HPV types 6 and 11 have a predilection for the external anogenital skin, usually producing the exophytic condyloma of the vulva and perianal area, although occasionally causing subclinical infections or condylomata on the cervix.

HPV types 16 and 18 are associated most often with subclinical lesions of mucosal surfaces, especially the cervix. They have been implicated in oncogenic progression of tissue changes (benign warty to dysplasia, to intraepithelial neoplasia, to invasive carcinoma) in the penis, vulva, vagina, and, especially, the cervix. Other cofactors apart from HPV are no doubt involved in oncogenicity.

MANAGEMENT AND THERAPY

· Other associated sexually transmitted diseases should be excluded, especially condyloma lata of secondary syphilis.
· Warts should be treated as described on pages 570 and 571. All warts show unpredictable behavior and may regress spontaneously, enlarge and spread, or recur.
· Review weekly or biweekly for treatment and

Figure 86-2

Condylomata Acuminata in Females

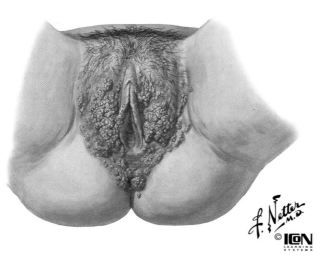

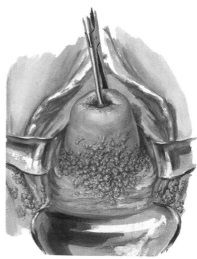

follow-up until lesions have resolved.

- It is important to evaluate for coexisting cervical dysplasia (Pap smear). Repeat Pap smears every 6 to 12 months thereafter.
- Refer for colposcopy if there is evidence of cervical dysplasia or if there is persistent cervical HPV infection.
- Ensure examination of sexual partner(s) and treat those with warts.
- Advise use of condoms until no lesions apparent.
- Obtain a biopsy specimen of any atypical wart.

Pharmacologic Agents

There is no specific antiviral therapy available for HPV and no one method of treatment that is superior to all others. Therapy often involves methods that attempt to nonspecifically destroy infected tissue. Most of these cytodestructive therapies are painful and require multiple visits to a provider or require adherence to daily application of a medication. The efficacy of cytodestructive therapies has not been verified in placebo-controlled trials and has highly variable reported rates of success and high recurrence rates. Newer therapies involving pharmacologic approaches that stimulate immunologic or antiviral responses offer promise of higher response rates and lower rates of recurrence. Pharmacologic agents available for treat-

ment include cytotoxic agents (podophyllin), destructive agents (trichloroacetic acid), and immunological agents (interferon, imiquimod). Therapies can be divided into two categories: patient-applied and provider-administered.

Provider-Administered Therapies

Podophyllin resin is used for penile and vulvar warts. It should not be used in well-vascularized areas such as the vagina or anus. The major disadvantages of podophyllin are: skin irritation if not properly applied, and systemic toxicity and potential oncogenicity with use of large amounts and/or repeated application. Its use is contraindicated in pregnancy and if dysplasia/neoplasia is present. Given current treatment options and the toxicities associated with podophyllin therapy, there is little clinical indication for its use.

5-Fluorouracil (5-FU) is used topically as a 5% cream for treatment of vaginal lesions and urethral condylomata, and for prophylaxis in immunocompromised patients. Its disadvantages are that an extensive erosive dermatitis may occur with incorrect application, and that its use requires a reliable patient to follow instructions. Pregnancy is a contraindication to 5-FU treatment. The 2002 Sexually Transmitted Diseases Treatment Guidelines does not recommend the use of 5-FU for the treatment of genital warts.

Trichloroacetic acid (TCA) and dichloracetic acid (DCA) are applied undiluted (25% to 85% solution) and washed off after 12 hours. They are weak destructive agents and are sometimes effective against small condylomata. They may be applied weekly for up to 6 weeks. Petroleum jelly or lanolin should be applied around the lesions to prevent spill onto surrounding normal tissue.

Interferon has antiviral, antiproliferative, and immunomodulating properties, and has been used for persistent or resistant disease. It is administered by intralesional or intramuscular injection 3 times weekly. However, it is expensive, nonspecific, and may cause multiple side effects (e.g., flu-like symptoms).

Patient-Applied Therapies

Imiquimod cream 5% is an immune-response modifier capable of inducing a variety of cytokines, including interferon alfa and tumor necrosis factor alpha. It is applied 3 times weekly to affected areas and washed off after 8 hours. Clinical response may take 2 to 8 weeks, and therapy may be continued for up to 16 weeks. Side effects include local inflammatory reactions with no systemic reactions.

Podofilox 0.5% solution or gel, an antimitotic agent purified from podophyllin resin, is less likely to cause systemic toxicity. It is approved for self-treatment in both men and women. It is applied twice daily for 3 days; this course can be repeated after 4 days and continued for up to 4 weeks if necessary. Safety for use in pregnant patients has not been established.

Other Treatment Methods

These include electrocautery and curettage under local or general anesthesia, depending on the site and extent of the lesions. Cryotherapy is effective for both genital and anal warts, provided they are not too large. Apply probe of the cryocautery to each wart for 30 to 60 seconds (no anesthetic necessary). Alternatively, freeze warts with liquid nitrogen. Cautery or cryosurgery are the methods of choice for keratinized warts or for warts refractory to other forms of treatment, or they can be used as primary treatment of mucosal warts. Surgical excision or carbon dioxide laser destruction under general anesthesia may be used for extensive lesions.

Optimum Treatment
Exophytic Condylomata of External Genitals

If lesions are nonextensive, options should be discussed with the patient; the patient's ability to adhere to treatment regimen as well as the location and number of warts should be considered. For provider-applied therapy, cryotherapy (weekly until lesions gone) or trichloroacetic/dichloracetic acid (applied twice weekly) should be used. For patient-applied therapy, imiquimod 5% cream or podofilox 0.5% solution or gel are options as well. If lesions are extensive, laser therapy, cautery, or surgical excision are alternatives. In females, cervical HPV infection (cytology), and in men who have sex with men, rectal HPV infection (anoscopy and rectal cytology) should be excluded.

Cervical HPV Infection

Patients with cervical HPV infection should be referred for colposcopic evaluation with directed biopsy of abnormal areas.

Pregnant Patients

Trichloroacetic acid or cryotherapy should be used for isolated lesions, or laser therapy for extensive lesions. Careful cytological and colposcopic follow-up is essential. Vaginal delivery, unless obstructed by lesions, is necessary because caesarean section does not prevent infant infection.

Specialist Referral

Referral is advisable for urethral or cervical warts; associated cervical HPV changes on cytology, dysplasia, or neoplasia; immunodeficient patients (who do not respond to conventional treatment); refractory warts; and condylomata in children.

FUTURE DIRECTIONS

Progress continues to be made on the development of prophylactic and therapeutic vaccines. One novel approach involves the use of a papillomavirus virus-like particle vaccine composed of a major structural viral protein, L1, to confer protection against infection. Initial vaccine development is focusing on types of HPV associated with the development of cervical cancer. It is unknown if vaccinating females alone will be sufficient to stop the HPV epidemic. To permit an HPV vaccine to be marketable as protective against an STD, and marketable to males and females, the vaccine will also have to be protective against types that cause warts. Progress is also being made in the development of therapeutic vaccines that may prove effective against persistent HPV infection, warts, and/or premalignant lesions.

REFERENCES

Auborn KJ, Carter TH. Treatment of human papillomavirus gynecologic infections. *Clin Lab Med.* 2000;20:407-422.

Beutner KR, Reitano MV, Richwald GA, Wiley DJ. External genital warts: report of the American Medical Association Consensus Conference. AMA Expert Panel on External Genital Warts. *Clin Infect Dis.* 1998;27:796-806.

Beutner KR, Spruance SL, Hougham AJ, Fox TL, Owens ML, Douglas JM Jr. Treatment of genital warts with an immune-response modifier (imiquimod). *J Am Acad Dermatol.* 1998;38:230-239.

Centers for Disease Control and Prevention. Sexually transmitted diseases treatment guidelines 2002. *MMWR Recomm Rep.* 2002;51:1-78.

Koutsky L. Epidemiology of genital human papillomavirus infection. *Am J Med.* 1997;102:3-8.

Langley PC, Richwald GA, Smith MH. Modeling the impact of treatment options in genital warts: patient-applied versus physician-administered therapies. *Clin Ther.* 1999;21:2143-2155.

Chapter 87

Gonorrhea

P. Frederick Sparling

Gonorrhea is a sexually transmitted disease known since biblical times, characterized by superficial or deep infection of mucosal surfaces, especially the genital mucosa, by the organism *Neisseria gonorrhoeae* (the gonococcus, [GC]). Untreated infection often results in deeper complications, including salpingitis or epididymitis, and occasionally bacteremia and arthritis, meningitis, or endocarditis. Although antibiotic resistance is more common than in earlier decades, treatment is still highly efficacious. The primary problem is in case detection. Because some infections may have few symptoms, infected persons can be missed without attention to risk factors in a patient's history and knowledge of the epidemiology pertinent to gonorrhea. Excellent new noninvasive diagnostic tests are readily available in the United States.

Most cases of gonorrhea are sexually transmitted. Infection in neonates may be from the mother's birth canal. Infection of prepubescent children should be assumed to be the result of sexual abuse. Infection is most common in adolescents and young adults, with peak prevalence in women aged 15 to 19 and men aged 21 to 25. Prevalence is much higher in the United States among African Americans, which probably reflects a complex mixture of socioeconomic, behavioral, health-care seeking, and health-care access factors. Rates of infection are particularly high in many rural southeastern states and in certain large cities. In general, risk is increased among the young and unmarried, and those having a new sex partner or multiple sex partners or a sex partner with multiple partners. The prevalence of infection has declined in the past decade, but is increasing in certain groups, including young men who have sex with men, among whom rectal GC is increasing in some locales. Condoms probably are quite effective in prevention of transmission by genital sex. The risk of infection after unprotected genital sex with an infected partner is approximately 30% for men and 70% to 80% for women. Antibiotic-resistant strains are becoming more common, but distribution is uneven; multiple resistances including resistance to ciprofloxacin are found, particularly in isolates from persons from southeast Asia or parts of Africa.

ETIOLOGY AND PATHOGENESIS

The gonococcus is a gram-negative diplococcus that grows only in humans and does not survive long outside of the body. It attaches to epithelial surfaces by several adherence ligands that interact with specific receptors. Attachment is followed by local invasion and sometimes by penetration of deeper tissues and bacteremia. Although much is known about molecular pathogenesis, there is no current vaccine candidate; earlier attempts to develop a vaccine based on the pilus adherence ligand failed. Strains may be serotyped on the basis of reactions with a panel of monoclonal antibodies against the porin (major outer membrane) protein. They also may be typed on the basis of differences in nutritional requirements on defined media or by a variety of other methods including genotyping, but these are only available in research laboratories.

CLINICAL PRESENTATION

In men, purulent urethritis with dysuria and small amounts of yellow or greenish mucoid discharge develops, especially in the early morning before urination, within 2 to 7 days of exposure (Figure 87-1). In 5% to 10% of men, a persistent low-grade or asymptomatic infection of the urethra may develop. These men do not present for health care and may transmit infection to their sexual partners. Epididymitis in men younger than

Figure 87-1 **Urethritis in Men**

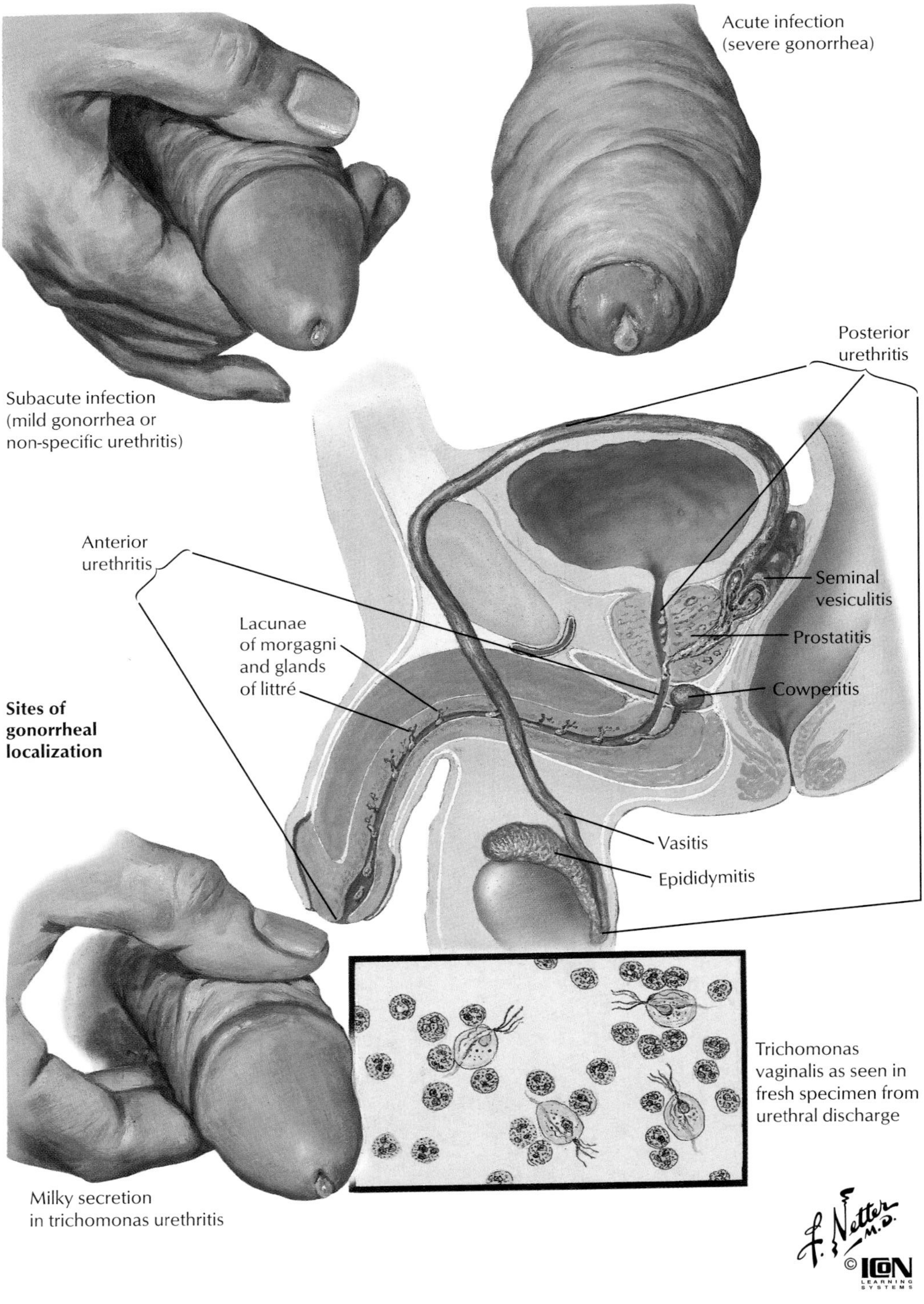
Acute infection
(severe gonorrhea)
Subacute infection
(mild gonorrhea or
non-specific urethritis)
Posterior
urethritis
Anterior
urethritis
Seminal
vesiculitis
Lacunae
of morgagni
and glands
of littré
Prostatitis
Cowperitis
Sites of
gonorrheal
localization
Vasitis
Epididymitis
Trichomonas
vaginalis as seen in
fresh specimen from
urethral discharge
Milky secretion
in trichomonas urethritis
F. Netter M.D.
© ICON LEARNING SYSTEMS

Figure 87-2

Gonorrhea in Women

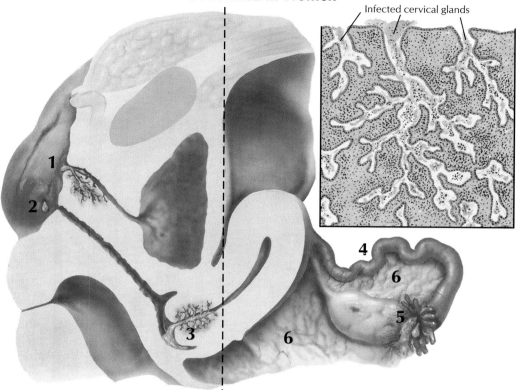

Infected cervical glands

Primary sites of infection
1. Urethra and Skene's glands
2. Bartholin's glands
3. Cervix and cervical glands

Subsequent sites of infection
4. Fallopian tubes (salpingitis)
5. Emergence from tubal ostium (tubo-ovarian abscess and peritonitis)
6. Lymphatic spread to broad ligaments and surrounding tissues (frozen pelvis)

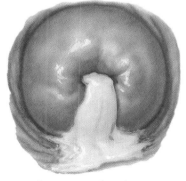

Appearance of cervix
in acute infection

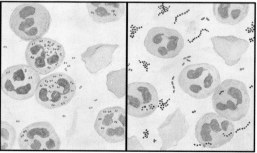

Gonorrheal infection
(Gram stain)

Non-specific infection
(Gram stain)

35 is usually due to either gonococcal or genital chlamydia infection.

Asymptomatic or oligosymptomatic cervical infection may develop in 50% of women; others have increased vaginal discharge or dysuria (Figure 87-2). Physical examination often reveals mucopurulent cervical discharge. Low-grade infection of the endometrium is relatively common. Approximately 10% to 15% of untreated genital infections in women are followed by salpingitis, with adnexal pain, and sometimes with fever and leukocytosis. Risk of salpingitis is increased in very young women (15 to 16 years) and in those who have had it previously. The severity of illness is variable, ranging from mild to acute; some patients may be treated as outpatients, while others require hospitalization. Physical examination may reveal cervical motion tenderness and adnexal tenderness or fullness. Salpingitis may be followed by tubal scarring and infertility, or increased risk for ectopic pregnancy. (Figure 87-2)

Infection of the pharynx is found in up to 20% of patients with genital gonorrhea, but there usually are no symptoms. Rectal gonorrhea is found in up to 40% of women with cervical gonorrhea, also without symptoms and, presumably, reflecting spread of infection from the contiguous genital site. In contrast, rectal gonorrhea in men who have sex with men is often quite symptomatic with pain, discharge, and tenesmus.

Bacteremia develops in approximately 1% of patients, particularly in those infected by strains that are highly resistant to human serum complement. Persons with homozygous deficiency of late complement components are susceptible to recurrent gonococcal or meningococcal bacteremias; approximately 5% of patients with the disseminated gonococcal infection (DGI) syndrome are lacking one of the late complement components C5 through C9. A CH50 test will detect such individuals, although it is best done after the acute infection has subsided. DGI presents in several forms, but patients usually are not acutely or severely ill, in contrast to meningococcal bacteremia. Approximately half of patients with DGI do not have fever. Many have a typical rash distributed over the periphery, especially the hands, with a small number (fewer than 30) of pustular or hemorrhagic tender lesions. This may be accompanied by polyarticular arthralgias or monoarticular arthritis, typically involving major joints; rash may be absent in patients with arthritis. DGI frequently follows asymptomatic genital or pharyngeal infection.

Typically, infection in neonates presents as purulent conjunctivitis, which was a major cause of blindness, but is now rare. Infection in young females most often presents as vulvovaginitis.

DIFFERENTIAL DIAGNOSIS

Gonococcal urethritis must be differentiated from *Chlamydia trachomatis* urethritis and from other causes of urethritis including *Mycoplasma genitalis* and, occasionally, *Herpes simplex virus* or *Trichomonas vaginalis* (Figure 87-1). Gonococcal urethritis tends to have a more profuse and purulent discharge, but this is not helpful in individual patients. The differential diagnosis for epididymitis includes chlamydia epididymitis and testicular torsion. Gonococcal cervicitis with mucopurulent discharge must be differentiated from chlamydia cervicitis, which may produce an indistinguishable clinical picture. Many diseases, including ectopic pregnancy and appendicitis, may mimic salpingitis. The DGI syndrome may mimic Reiter's syndrome, bacterial endocarditis, and other types of acute arthritis.

DIAGNOSTIC APPROACH

The diagnosis of gonorrhea depends on awareness of patient risk factors, including a sexual history. Urethral discharge or mucopurulent cervicitis suggests gonococcal or chlamydia infection. In women, it is important to differentiate vaginal discharge and vaginitis from cervicitis; gonococci do not cause vaginitis except in prepubescent girls.

In men with purulent urethral discharge, a Gram stain showing intracellular gram-negative diplococci (Figure 87-2) is both sensitive and specific, and cultures or other tests are not usually necessary. In infected men without frank discharge, Gram stain is no more than 60% sensitive, and diagnosis is best achieved either by culture of a urethral swab or fresh urine sediment, or by use of a molecular amplification (hybridization, LCR or PCR) test. PCR testing on urine is more than 98% sensitive and 98% specific, but cost may be a limiting factor for some patients or practices. Culture specimens should be plated on selective chocolate agar media containing antibiotics to inhibit the normal flora or placed in transport media for prompt transfer to the laboratory. There are no serologic tests for gonorrhea.

Women ordinarily require either cervical culture or a PCR test of urine or vaginal introitus. Gram stains of cervical discharge are only 50% sensitive and not sufficiently specific for accurate diagnosis in most clinics. The PCR test is highly sensitive and specific. The PCR test does not allow for antibiotic sensitivity testing or serotyping; the latter may be important legally in cases of rape or sexual abuse. In patients with possible salpingitis, it may be helpful to seek consultation and to perform vaginal ultrasound to examine the anatomy of the fallopian tubes. A CT of the pelvis and laparoscopy may be needed. Pregnancy tests should be obtained, and if culture materials are available from the tubes, they should be sent for testing for anaerobic and aerobic bacteria.

If DGI is suspected, culture specimens should be obtained from blood, genital, pharyngeal, and rectal sites, and PCR performed on urine. Culture specimen results from infected joints are positive in only about one third of patients, and skin lesion culture results are rarely positive. Obtain a total serum hemolytic complement, especially in patients with recurrent DGI.

Sexual partners of patients with any type of gonorrhea should be seen or referred for proper diagnostic evaluation. Asymptomatic carriers are important vectors for transmission. Urine-based PCR is the best test for detecting asymptomatic genital infection. Any patient with gonorrhea should be presumed to have other STDs, and appropriate tests should be undertaken including a serologic test for syphilis and a screening test for HIV.

MANAGEMENT AND THERAPY

For uncomplicated genital gonorrhea in adults, several regimens are highly effective, including a single IM injection of 125 mg ceftriaxone, or a single oral dose of ciprofloxacin 500 mg, cefixime 400 mg, levofloxacin 250 mg, or ofloxacin 400 mg. These regimens provide adequate therapy for rectal or pharyngeal infection as well. Penicillins and tetracycline should not be used because resistance has increased substantially, both due to plasmid-mediated genes and a variety of chromosomal mutations. Resistance to ciprofloxacin is becoming a clinical problem in areas of Asia and Africa, and there are reports of small pockets of resistance in the United States. Resistance is growing rapidly in Hawaii and California. Ciprofloxacin should be avoided if there are epidemiologic reasons to suspect that the infection might have been acquired in areas of significant resistance. In most cases, therapy against chlamydia should be added because of the frequency of coinfection by genital chlamydia; this can be in the form of either a single oral dose of azithromycin 1 g or doxycycline 100 mg orally twice daily for 7 days. For patients with complicated infections, including either salpingitis or DGI, consult standard texts for approaches to therapy.

Sex partners of patients should be screened and treated for probable gonorrhea. Patients and their contacts can be referred to local health departments for assistance. If possible, diagnostic tests for gonorrhea should be performed on contacts before treatment, but there may be circumstances where it is most practical to provide medication for treatment of the partners. Failure to treat infected sexual contacts results in repeated "ping-pong" infections. Report infections to the public health authorities.

Every STD, including gonorrhea, is an opportunity to counsel patients about the risks of unprotected sex, particularly with multiple or high-risk partners. Proper counseling of such patients may prevent other more serious STDs, including HIV.

FUTURE DIRECTIONS

Despite decades of research into the molecular basis of pathogenicity of gonorrhea, there is still no vaccine candidate in site. Previous attempts to create a vaccine against pilin protein failed, and more recent attempts to use porin protein as a vaccine have stalled in early stages of clinical development. A vaccine would be useful not only because gonorrhea is an important disease in its own right, especially regarding women's health, but also because it is a cofactor for transmission and acquisition of HIV.

Prevention depends on better sexual behaviors (abstinence, fewer partners, less risky partners, use of condoms in all but stable monogamous sexual relationships) and screening to detect infected persons who have yet to seek treatment. Implementation of screening in women was associated with better control of infection in the US, but prevalence has stabilized and is increasing in certain communities and groups. Use of the urine-based PCR test provides a noninvasive, patient-friendly means to screen groups at high risk, including adolescents, persons with a new sexual partner, and emergency room and jail populations.

Dramatic declines in the prevalence of gonorrhea in much of the industrialized world outside the United States shows that vaccines are not necessary for disease control. The success of gonorrhea control in these other countries undoubtedly is multifactorial, but includes better healthcare access and less inhibited use of media to promote healthy sexual behaviors, including use of condoms.

REFERENCES

Centers for Disease Control and Prevention. Sexually transmitted diseases treatment guidelines 2002. *MMWR Recomm Rep.* 2002;51:1-78.

Fleming DT, Wasserheit JN. From epidemiological synergy to public health policy and practice: the contribution of other sexually transmitted diseases to sexual transmission of HIV infection. *Sex Transm Infect.* 1999;75:3-17.

Sparling PF. Biology of *Neisseria gonorrhoeae*. In: Holmes KK, Sparling PF, Mårdh P-A, et al, eds. *Sexually Transmitted Diseases.* 3rd ed. New York, NY: McGraw-Hill; 1999:433-450.

Sparling PF. Gonococcal infections. In: Goldman L, Bennett JC, eds. *Cecil Textbook of Medicine.* 21st ed. Philadelphia, Pa: WB Saunders Co; 2000.

Sparling PF, Handsfield HH. *Neisseria gonorrhoeae.* In: Mandell GL, Bennett JE, Dolin R, eds. *Mandell, Douglas, and Bennett's Principles and Practice of Infectious Diseases.* 5th ed. Philadelphia, Pa: Churchill Livingstone; 2000:2242-2258.

Chapter 88
Nongonococcal Urethritis

Peter Leone

Urethritis, inflammation of the urethra, is a syndrome characterized by a urethral discharge and dysuria, but it may be asymptomatic. Urethritis is defined as the presence of an increased number of polymorphonuclear leukocytes (PMNs) from the anterior urethra. It is sexually acquired primarily and has many infectious etiologies. In general, the infectious etiologies are classified as either gonococcal or nongonococcal urethritis (NGU). Mucopurulent cervicitis is the female equivalent. Noninfectious etiologies include chemical and physical irritants. As with most sexually transmitted infections, NGU is most prevalent in the 19- to 24-year age group, a time when changing sexual relationships are common. A minor disorder in most cases, NGU is clinically important for three reasons: 1) the potential for complications, particularly pelvic inflammatory disease (PID) associated with decreased fertility in female partners when *Chlamydia trachomatis* is the underlying pathogen; 2) its damaging influence on interpersonal relationships, especially when the condition is not adequately understood; and 3) prolonged anxiety when symptoms, although mild, are slow to resolve or when there are recurrences.

ETIOLOGY AND PATHOGENESIS

Chlamydia trachomatis is the most common known causative organism and can be isolated from the urethra in 30% to 50% of men with NGU. Unlike most bacteria, this organism is dependent on the energy-producing metabolic activities of the host cells and thus is an obligate intracellular parasite.

Often, the causes of NGU are not elucidated, but recently defined pathogens include *Ureaplasma urealyticum*, *Mycoplasma genitalium*, *Trichomonas vaginalis*, Candida species, and *N. meningitides* (Figure 88-1). Genital herpes simplex virus (HSV) can cause urethritis in approximately 30% of men with primary genital infection, but it is seen in a much lower percentage of men with recurrent genital HSV infection. Often, *Ureaplasma urealyticum* is isolated from the urethra of men with NGU, and differential antibiotic studies support the view that it sometimes has a pathogenic role. However, this organism is often isolated from the urethra in healthy men, and there is no simple way of identifying those cases in which it is pathogenic. Between 20% and 30% of men with NGU have no detectable organisms. Recent observations have found an association of NGU with bacterial vaginosis and oral sex. Asymptomatic urethritis, without a visible discharge but with evidence of increased PMNs on smear, may have a different etiology from symptomatic disease. *C. trachomatis* is detected less frequently in this situation.

Noninfectious etiologies include chemical irritants, (e.g. spermicides, bath products), physical irritants, urethral stricture, foreign bodies, bacterial urinary tract infections, repeated vigorous urethral stripping, and heavy crystalluria or calculous gravel in the urine.

CLINICAL PRESENTATION

In the typical patient, symptoms include dysuria, urethral discharge (mucoid or purulent), and penile irritation. Urethral discharge, which may be present on examination or on a urethral smear in a significant number of asymptomatic individuals, is a sign of NGU (Figure 88–1).

The patient first notices symptoms from several days to several weeks after infection; 2 or 3 weeks is a common incubation period. Urethral inflammation will often give rise to a discharge and dysuria, and the patient may experience urinary frequency. When the posterior urethra is involved, symptoms are usually mild and may be intermittent or transient, lasting only 1 to 2 days. The absence of symptoms does not exclude the diagnosis of NGU. There is a high incidence of asymptomatic infection of the urethra with *C. trachomatis*.

Figure 88-1

Urethritis

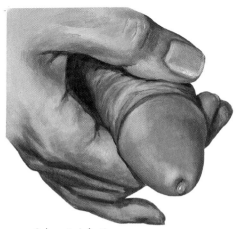

Subacute infection
(mild gonorrhea or
non-specific urethritis)

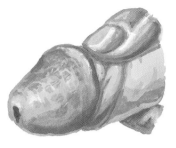

Candidal inflammation
of glans and prepuce

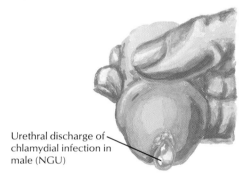

Urethral discharge of
chlamydial infection in
male (NGU)

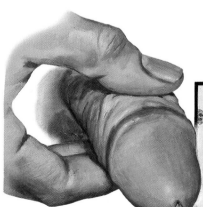

Milky secretion in
trichomonas urethritis

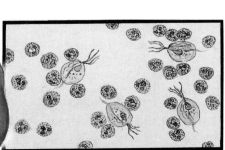

Trichomonas vaginalis as seen in fresh specimen
from urethral discharge

Spotty balanitis caused by candidal overgrowth in uncircumcised men is the most common complication of NGU. Men presenting with balanitis should always be checked for NGU, even when there are no symptoms. Hyperglycemia should be excluded because diabetes mellitus sometimes presents with candidal balanitis. Other complications include epididymitis, orchitis, acquired reactive arthritis, and Reiter's syndrome.

Epididymitis occurs less commonly. Swelling and tenderness begins in the lower pole. The groove between the epididymis and the testis is accentuated at first but then becomes obscured as the condition progresses. Occasionally, patients will complain of blood-stained semen due to seminal vesiculitis. Reiter's disease is a rare complication, which presents 10 to 30 days after the sexual contact. Patients may have an acute arthritis affecting one or more large peripheral joints. Conjunctivitis may also be present.

DIAGNOSTIC APPROACH

The diagnosis is confirmed by the demonstration of PMNs in the anterior urethra and by the absence of gram-negative diplococci on Gram's stain with a negative culture/test result for N. gonorrhea. Excessive PMNs can be confirmed by a Gram-stained urethral smear with >2 PMNs per high-powered microscopic field (×1000), or a Gram-stained preparation from a first-pass urine specimen containing >9 PMNs per high-powered microscopic field (×1000). Leukocyte esterase activity on first-pass urine correlates with the presence of urethritis but lacks sufficient sensitivity to be considered a reliable diagnostic test for NGU. The quality of the smear is dependent on how the specimen is collected.

Five or more PMNs per high-powered field (magnification, ×1000) is the generally accepted criterion. The absence of PMNs in a single urethral smear does not exclude the diagnosis, particularly if the patient urinated before the examination. There is no information on the optimal time between micturition and specimen collection, but 2 to 4 hours is preferred with a minimum of 30 minutes. Obtain specimens using a 5mm plastic loop or cotton-tipped swab. There is no information suggesting the superiority of either method, although the loop appears to be less physically and psychologically traumatic to the male patient.

Symptomatic patients without evidence of inflammation should be tested for an etiologic diagnosis. In most clinical settings, this includes testing for N. gonorrheae and C. trachomatis. Reexamination the following morning, having the patient not urinate overnight, may increase the diagnostic yield of the Gram stain. Empiric treatment is in order for those individuals with an observable purulent discharge, those at high risk for infection (e.g., patients in a sexually transmitted disease clinic, adolescent males in a juvenile detention center) or individuals unlikely to return for reevaluation. The minimum time between exposure and the development of a detectable inflammatory response, by urethral smear or microscopic study of a urine sample, is not known, but it is reasonable to allow 1 week after a risk contact before accepting a negative result as conclusive. The 2-glass test, because of its low sensitivity and specificity, is not recommended to diagnose NGU or to differentiate it from urinary tract infection.

MANAGEMENT AND THERAPY

The diagnosis should be established by demonstrating that urethral inflammation is present and by excluding gonorrhea; all patients should have testing for N. gonorrhea. C trachomatis testing, although preferable, may be deferred in men with inflammation on urethral smear when resources are limited. Urethral smears without evidence of significant PMNs should be tested for C. trachomatis in symptomatic men. The provider should take a detailed sexual history to identify all sexual partners requiring assessment and treatment, and should treat sexual partners considered to be at risk even if there are no signs of infection. Chlamydia cerviatis or PID can develop suddenly and without warning in a female partner. It is better to treat unnecessarily if exposure to infection has occurred, rather than risk this complication. A full course of antibiotics should be completed even when the symptoms resolve within a few days. Alcohol in moderation will not affect the outcome. Sexual activity should be avoided until the inflammation has resolved.

Treatment should be administered at the time of diagnosis with medications that are highly effective against Chlamydia (cure rate for C. trachomatis of >95%), easy to use (preferably single-dose therapy, but not more then twice-daily therapy), have a low incidence of side effects, and minimally interfere with lifestyle. The preferred medication regimens are: azithromycin 1 g orally in a single dose or doxycycline 100 mg orally twice daily for 7 days. Alternative regimens include erythromycin 500 mg orally 4 times daily for 7 days, erythromycin 500 mg orally twice daily for 14 days, ofloxacin 300 mg twice daily or 400 mg orally once daily for 7 days, levofloxacin 500 mg once daily for 7 days, or tetracycline 500 mg orally 4 times a day for 7 days.

Sulfamethoxazole/trimethoprim (co-trimoxazole) is active against Chlamydia but is not effective in the treatment of nongonococcal urethritis.

Recurrent or Persistent Nongonococcal Urethritis

In recurrent/persistent NGU, the urethral inflammation is usually mild and will resolve over several days with appropriate antibiotic therapy. Persistence occurs in 20% to 60% of men treated for acute NGU; however, resolution may take several weeks. Occasionally relapse occurs, even in the absence of reinfection. Relapse is most common in the first 3 months after the initial episode. The pathologic basis of these relapses is not understood and is probably multifactorial.

When relapse occurs in the context of a stable relationship, it is important to exclude the possibility of reinfection by confirming that the sexual partner has completed an appropriate course of antibiotics. Careful explanation is also necessary because relapse sometimes leads to the erroneous conclusion that there has been a sexual contact outside of the relationship.

Female partners of men with persistent/recurrent NGU do not appear to be at increased risk for the development of PID, provided they received appropriate therapy as a contact.

Minor sensations of urethral irritation may persist for some time after resolution of NGU, and the patient will often feel that the infection is still present. It is important to document definite urethral inflammation before prescribing another course of antibiotics.

After confirming persistent inflammation on urethral smear, alternative antibiotic therapy should be considered. If the patient has not adhered to initial therapy, consider switching to single-dose therapy. Azithromycin or doxycycline failure may be due to resistant *U. urealyticum* or to *Trichomonas vaginalis*. If the patient is symptomatic, was compliant with the initial regimen, and has not had sexual contact with an untreated partner, consider therapy with erythromycin 500 mg orally 4 times daily for 7 days plus a single oral dose of metronidazole 2 g. Some isolates of *U. urealyticum* are resistant to erythromycin but may respond to ofloxacin 300 mg every 12 hours orally for 7 days. Persistent NGU following 2 courses of therapy requires other diagnostic considerations (i.e., cystitis and prostatitis) and urological evaluation to rule out foreign bodies, strictures, and periurethral abscess. *Mycoplasma genitalium* may cause persistent NGU and require a 6-week course of erythromycin. If no cause for persistent NGU can be found, a 6-week course of empiric doxycycline or erythromycin is rational.

Sexual contacts and partners, including all partners/contacts of symptomatic men 2 weeks before the onset of symptoms and those of asymptomatic men 6 months before diagnosis, should be evaluated and offered empiric therapy. The treatment regimen should be consistent with that used for the partner and, at a minimum, be effective for uncomplicated chlamydia infection. Female contacts of men with chlamydia urethritis should be treated regardless of the results of chlamydia testing. Concurrent treatment is preferred and may result in improved clinical response in men with chlamydia-negative NGU.

Referral to a specialist clinic is advisable if there is reluctance to give a detailed sexual history. Treatment of all partners who may be at risk, if symptoms persist after two courses of antibiotics or if complications develop, should be arranged.

FUTURE DIRECTIONS

The use of urine-based nucleic acid amplification tests (NAAT) for the diagnosis of gonococcal and chlamydial urethral infections may warrant reclassification of urethritis into three categories: gonococcal, chlamydial, and nongonococcal-nonchlamydial urethritis. Diagnostic testing for *C. trachomatis* will be strongly recommended as the cost of NAAT continues to decrease because chlamydia infection has significant public health implications. Other developments include clarification of the role of *M. genitalium* in NGU and the development of screening algorithms for men at increased risk for recurrent NGU.

REFERENCES

Arya OP, Mallinson H, Andrews BE, Sillis M. Diagnosis of urethritis: role of polymorphonuclear leukocyte counts in gram-stained urethral smears. *Sex Transm Dis.* 1984;11:10-17.

Centers for Disease Control and Prevention. Sexually transmitted diseases treatment guidelines 2002. *MMWR Recomm Rep.* 2002;51:1-78.

Janier M, Lassau F, Casin I, et al. Male urethritis with and without discharge: a clinical and microbiological study. *Sex Transm Dis.* 1995;22:244-252.

Podgore JK, Holmes KK, Alexander ER. Asymptomatic urethral infections due to Chlamydia trachomatis in male US military personnel. *J Infect Dis.* 1982;146:828.

Root TE, Edwards LD, Spengler PJ. Nongonococcal urethritis: a survey of clinical and laboratory features. *Sex Transm Dis.* 1980;7:59-65.

Stamm WE, Hicks CB, Martin DH, et al. Azithromycin for empirical treatment of the nongonococcal urethritis syndrome in men. A randomized double-blind study. *JAMA.* 1995;274:545-549.

Stamm WE, Koutsky LA, Benedetti JK, Jourden JL, Brunham RC, Holmes KK. Chlamydia trachomatis urethral infections in men. Prevalence, risk factors, and clinical manifestations. *Ann Internal Med.* 1984;100:47-51.

Taylor-Robinson D, Horner PJ. The role of Mycoplasma genitalium in non-gonococcal urethritis. *Sex Transm Infect.* 2001;77:229-231.

Chapter 89
Syphilis

P. Frederick Sparling

Syphilis, an infectious disease caused by *Treponema pallidum,* usually is sexually transmitted, but may be transmitted transplacentally from an infected mother to her infant. Once very common, affecting as much as 10% or more of the general population, it became much less prevalent after the discovery of penicillin. Rates of infection declined steadily in the United States except for a rise among men having sex with men (MSM) at the onset of the HIV era, and a brief period in the late 1980s and early 1990s due to an epidemic of trading heterosexual sex for crack cocaine. The infection continues to be a plague and is a recognized cofactor for HIV transmission, warranting the serious attention of clinicians and investigators. In the United States, the infection is more common in some population groups, particularly African Americans who may have disease rates 30 times those of Whites. This probably reflects differences in several behaviors including sexual and health-seeking behaviors, availability of appropriate health-care access, and a complex mix of socioeconomic factors that help to determine behaviors. There has been recent progress in reducing the prevalence of syphilis in African Americans, and the disease is now at an all-time low. A recent upsurge in MSM is worrisome.

ETIOLOGY AND PATHOGENESIS

T. pallidum is a spirochetal bacterium whose genome has now been sequenced, but is less well understood than many bacterial pathogens because it has been impossible to grow it successfully in vitro other than in animals. It is a slender, spiral-shaped organism that cannot be seen by ordinary Gram stain, but can be visualized by dark field microscopy and has a characteristic motility that facilitates diagnosis from early infectious lesions. Relatively rare outer sheath proteins include proteins that are under intense current investigation because they appear to undergo rapid variation, possibly helping to account for the ability of the organism to persist in vivo despite an immune response. The organism does not survive drying, and its only natural host is humans, accounting for the usual necessity of contact with lesions in an infected sexual partner for disease transmission.

The median infective dose (ID50, the dose required to infect 50% of subjects) is approximately 10 organisms. Rate of growth in humans and animals is slow, with a doubling time of about 24 hours, which accounts for the slow progression of disease and helps explain the need for prolonged treatment to effect cure.

The intermittent, relapsing, slowly evolving nature of untreated syphilis suggests a delicate balance between the pathogen and the host immune system. There is partial immunity in late-acquired or congenital syphilis, as demonstrated in human prison volunteers 50 years ago. Immunity can be developed, albeit with difficulty, in experimental rabbit syphilis. Some of the lesions of late syphilis appear to be the result of a hypersensitivity response to infection, perhaps explaining the granulomatous reaction of some lesions (particularly gummas) of late syphilis. Typically, there is a vasculitis of the vasa vasorum, which may account for some late manifestations, including aortitis and some of the central nervous system lesions.

Women may transmit infection transplacentally for up to 6 or 7 years after untreated infection, but during approximately the last 3 months of gestation only, due to breakdown of placental barriers later in pregnancy. Routine testing and treatment of pregnant women during the first two trimesters should prevent congenital syphilis.

CLINICAL PRESENTATION

Syphilis is generally divided into primary, secondary, latent, and late stages. The disease is the result of contact with infected lesions. *T. pallidum* enters the skin or mucosa and then disseminates early to many organs, including the skin, central

Figure 89-1

Genital Lesions of Primary Syphilis

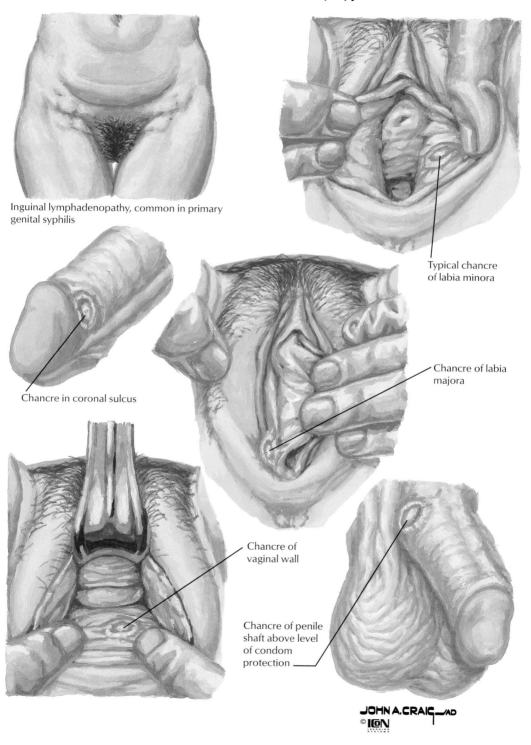

Inguinal lymphadenopathy, common in primary genital syphilis

Typical chancre of labia minora

Chancre in coronal sulcus

Chancre of labia majora

Chancre of vaginal wall

Chancre of penile shaft above level of condom protection

JOHN A. CRAIG AD
© ICON

Figure 89-2

Extragenital Lesions of Primary Syphilis

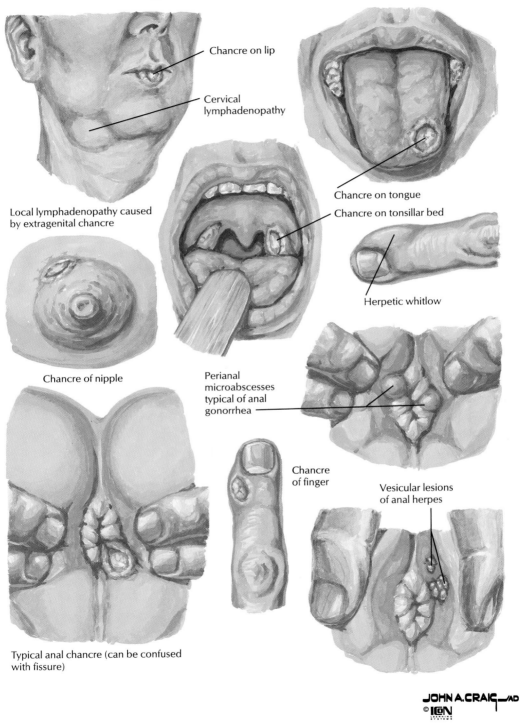

Chancre on lip

Cervical lymphadenopathy

Local lymphadenopathy caused by extragenital chancre

Chancre on tongue

Chancre on tonsillar bed

Herpetic whitlow

Chancre of nipple

Perianal microabscesses typical of anal gonorrhea

Chancre of finger

Vesicular lesions of anal herpes

Typical anal chancre (can be confused with fissure)

JOHN A. CRAIG—AD
© ICN

nervous system, and others. The illness progresses from a lesion at the site of inoculation to a more generalized disease, punctuated by periods of clinical well-being. Primary and secondary syphilis are termed early syphilis. This is followed by a latent period with no abnormalities other than immunologic evidence of infection. Late or tertiary types of clinical disease develop in approximately one third of untreated persons. The interval between initial infection and recognized onset of late syphilis may be remarkably long, up to 20 years or more, depending on the type of syndrome.

Primary Syphilis

After an incubation period of approximately 10 to 21 days, there typically is a papule that evolves into a painless ulcer termed chancre. Approximately 10% of chancres are extragenital, especially around or in the mouth and anal areas (Figure 89-1). A classical chancre has rolled margins and a clean non-tender base, often with satellite adenopathy. Perirectal or oral chancres may have atypical presentations and may be missed without strong suspicion (Figure 89-2. Untreated infection heals spontaneously in approximately 3 weeks.

Secondary Syphilis

Lesions of secondary syphilis occasionally coincide with the primary lesion, but more often occur weeks or months later, up to 6 months from onset of infection (Figure 89-3). A primary lesion may not have been recognized. The secondary rash heals spontaneously in approximately 3 weeks, but may relapse one or more times over the next 2 years if untreated. The cardinal sign of secondary syphilis is a rash on the mucosa or skin. Often, it starts on the trunk, but spreads to involve much of the body, including the palms and soles. Early rash may be subtle and can be missed in persons with dark pigmentation. It varies from copper to brown macules to papulosquamous lesions to nodules, but in adults almost never is vesicular or bullous or pruritic. Rash on moist mucosal surfaces may be hyperplastic (condyloma acuminata, or syphilitic warts) or may be flat plaques as in the gray mucous patches of the mouth or elsewhere. Mucosal lesions are quite infectious, but the cutaneous rash is minimally infectious. At this point, the disease is systemic, and there often is fever, sore throat, and generalized adenopathy. Meningitis with headache and a CSF mononuclear pleocytosis occurs in approximately 30% of patients. Occasional patients have clinical hepatitis or immune-deposit glomerulopathy.

Latent Syphilis

By definition, this is a stage where the patient is infected and has positive serologic tests for syphilis, but is clinically normal, including normal CSF findings. It is divided into early (first year) and late (more than 1 year) latency, for epidemiologic reasons because the risk of transmission to sexual partners is essentially zero after 1 year of untreated infection. Untreated, approximately two thirds of patients do not progress beyond latency, but late syphilis develops in one third.

Late Syphilis

Late syphilis may involve many organs, but can be divided into three general types: gumma, neurosyphilis, and cardiovascular syphilis. *Gumma* usually presents as granulomatous or destructive ulcerative or mass lesions of the skin or viscera. Once common, it is now rare, probably because it responds readily to antibiotics. In the past decade, multiple cases have been documented in patients with HIV infection.

In *cardiovascular syphilis,* inflammation of the ascending aorta results in aortic wall weakness and aneurysm formation, which may lead to aortic valve insufficiency and, on occasion, occlusion of the coronary arteries. Clinical onset usually is a decade or more after infection, with presentation as aortic insufficiency.

Involvement of the nervous system takes many forms in neurosyphilis, with variable onset after initial infection. Meningitis (headache, stiff neck) may occur coincident with secondary syphilis or in the next 5 or 6 years. The CSF formula is indistinguishable from other causes of aseptic meningitis, but the CSF VDRL test is positive. *Meningovascular syphilis* occurs within the first 12 years of infection, with occlusion of small to medium vessels and stroke syndrome. It should be considered in young persons with no obvious cause for stroke. The form of stroke varies from isolated cranial nerve palsies, including the eighth cranial nerve, to hemispheric lesions. The CSF test results are abnormal, and CSF serologic tests for syphilis

Figure 89-3

Secondary Syphilis

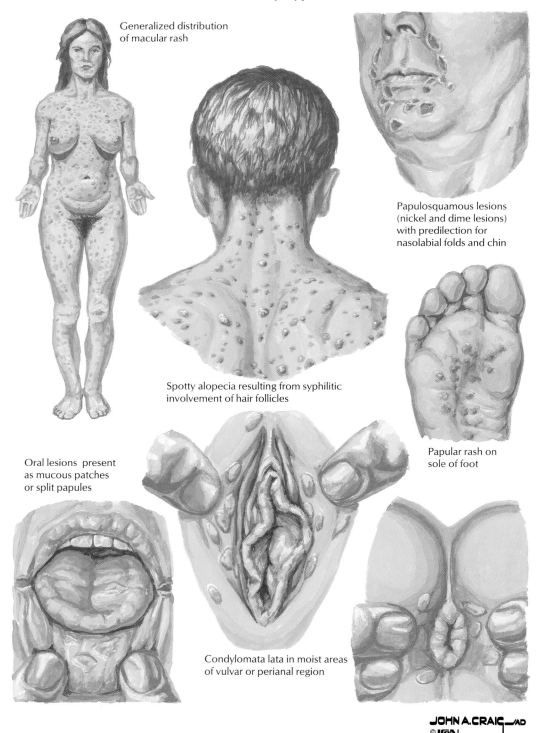

Generalized distribution of macular rash

Papulosquamous lesions (nickel and dime lesions) with predilection for nasolabial folds and chin

Spotty alopecia resulting from syphilitic involvement of hair follicles

Papular rash on sole of foot

Oral lesions present as mucous patches or split papules

Condylomata lata in moist areas of vulvar or perianal region

JOHN A. CRAIG—AD
© ICON

usually are positive. *General paresis* occurs from 10 to 20 years after infection, with involvement of the cerebral hemispheres and various signs and symptoms including dementia, paranoia, and delusions of grandeur. Often, the CSF test results are abnormal, but there may not be a pleocytosis, and the serologic test results for syphilis are not always positive. *Tabes dorsalis* affects the posterior columns of the spinal cord, with loss of proprioception, often with associated severe sharp intermittent radicular pains of the extremities or abdomen. There may be associated optic atrophy, and Argyll-Robertson pupils (small pupils that accommodate but do not react to light). The CSF test results often are abnormal (high protein, increased mononuclear cells, positive VDRL), but one or more of these findings may be absent. Tabes typically has late onset. Some of the classical clinical forms may be indistinct or overlap.

Syphilis in Patients with Human Immunodeficiency Virus Infection

Anecdotal evidence suggests that syphilis presents differently in the presence of HIV, but there have been no confirmatory studies to substantiate this observation. Serologic tests and response to therapy approximate those in non-HIV-infected patients. Neurosyphilis may present a particular dilemma, however, because patients with advanced HIV infection have myriad causes of abnormal CSF test results and neurologic illness.

DIFFERENTIAL DIAGNOSIS

In primary syphilis, the principal differential involves other causes of genital ulcer syndrome, particularly herpes simplex virus (HSV); HSV more often has multiple ulcers, and they are usually painful and tender, whereas the syphilitic chancre is painless unless secondarily infected (Figure 89-2). In other parts of the world, chancroid (*Hemophilus ducreyi*) is a common cause of single or multiple, usually tender, genital ulcers. Secondary syphilis has a very broad differential diagnosis, including mononucleosis, drug reactions, and many more, depending on the particular presentation. Late syphilis also has a broad differential diagnosis, but in current practice, the usual problems are limited to neurologic diseases. CNS syphilis is a common question in elderly persons with abnormal syphilis serology and abnor-

mal CNS function, and the most extensive workup may not provide definitive answers because of the lack of sensitivity of many of the CSF tests for neurosyphilis.

DIAGNOSTIC APPROACH

There are two principal diagnostic tests: the darkfield examination, by which motile spirochetes may be seen in lesions from primary syphilis; and serology, by which various antibodies are detected. In many centers, it also is possible to obtain polymerase chain reaction (PCR) molecular amplification tests for *T. pallidum*. Darkfield examination requires a special microscope and is used less frequently than in earlier times. A mail-in variation that uses fluorescent antibodies to detect *T. pallidum* on slides has not been widely deployed.

Serologic tests are of two general types: those that detect "nonspecific" antibodies against diphosphatidyl glycerol, a normal tissue component, and those that detect specific antibodies against *T. pallidum*. Nonspecific tests include the VDRL and rapid plasma reagin (RPR) test. These tests are inexpensive and easy to use; the levels of antibodies detected rise in acute disease and fall after successful treatment. Presumably, antibodies rise in syphilis because the spirochete binds host diphosphatidyl glycerol, increasing its immunogenicity. Reasons for false-positive test results include other infections and autoimmune diseases; in the latter, the test results are positive chronically (more than 6 months). Old age is another cause of a chronic false-positive VDRL test result, and a positive test result in a patient older than 80 should ordinarily be ignored.

Specific tests include the fluorescent treponemal antibody absorbed (FTA-ABS) and microhemagglutination against *T. pallidum* (MHA-TP) test, and other variants. There are few false-positive results, but because some studies showed that 1% of persons without any risks for STDs had a positive FTA-ABS test result, these tests are not used as screening tests. The titers do not fall after therapy; therefore, these tests are not useful for following response to therapy.

In primary syphilis, the VDRL-type test results are positive in approximately 80% of patients, and the specific treponemal test results are positive in slightly more (approximately 85%). All test results are positive in blood in patients with secondary syphilis, and the treponemal test results remain positive in almost all patients with late syphilis. The nonspecific test results may be negative in some patients with late syphilis; therefore, a negative blood RPR or VDRL does not rule out late syphilis.

A diagnostic dilemma may occur in patients with possible neurosyphilis. A positive CSF VDRL test result in the absence of a traumatic tap is specific for neurosyphilis, but a negative test result does not rule out the diagnosis because as few as 30% to 40% of patients have a positive CSF VDRL test result. The CSF FTA-ABS appears to be more sensitive than the VDRL, but there are worries that this may reflect passive transfer from blood. Cells or protein may be normal in CSF of patients with neurosyphilis.

MANAGEMENT AND THERAPY

The first principle of management is to make a diagnosis, which requires consideration of syphilis in young or old persons with an ulcerative lesion, rash and adenopathy, unexplained stroke or unexplained neurologic disease, among other syndromes. Assessment of risk is enhanced by a knowledgeable sexual history. In practice, a very common problem is how to diagnose and treat patients with nonspecific neurological findings and a positive VDRL or MHA-TP test result, and patients with positive serologic studies but no evidence of clinical syphilis. Careful examination and history, and examination of CSF, are helpful in management of problem cases.

T. pallidum is sensitive to many antibiotics, and there is no evidence for antimicrobial resistance. Standard therapy of early syphilis is one IM injection of benzathine penicillin 2.4 MU; some experts give two injections a week apart. Alternatively, ceftriaxone 1 g IM or IV daily for 8 to 10 days may be given, although this is not completely safe in patients with penicillin allergy. Doxycycline 100 mg orally twice daily for 14 days is an acceptable substitute in patients who cannot tolerate penicillin or ceftriaxone. Latent or late syphilis is treated with 3 IM injections of 2.4 MU benzathine penicillin at weekly intervals.

If there is evidence of symptomatic neurosyphilis, most experts advocate intravenous aqueous crystalline penicillin G 4 MU every 4 hours for at least 10 days because benzathine penicillin provides low serum levels, and undetectable CSF levels of penicillin. Similar considerations apply to patients with HIV who also have any type of neurosyphilis, including asymptomatic neurosyphilis, based on anecdotal evidence of poor response and persistent *T. pallidum* in CSF after benzathine penicillin therapy. This is a controversial issue because there is good evidence that patients with early syphilis are cured after benzathine therapy even though one third have abnormal CSF. In patients allergic to penicillin, referral to experts for desensitization to penicillin is recommended because no other therapy has been proven efficacious.

Patients treated for syphilis should be observed at 3-month intervals for 6 months and then at 6-month intervals to complete a second year. VDRL titers decrease at least 4-fold if therapy was successful and the patient did not reacquire infection. If titers persist unchanged or fall and then rise at least 4-fold, retreatment should be given and CSF should be examined if not done previously. Some patients, especially those with latent or late disease, may continue to have persistently positive VDRL test results in low titer for years. All infections should be reported to the public health authorities so that partners can be evaluated and treated.

FUTURE DIRECTIONS

Prevention requires adoption of better sexual behaviors by the at-risk public, including condom use, and better coordination between private and public medicine. Prevention campaigns focused on the highest risk groups, including men who have sex with men and socioeconomically deprived African Americans, hope to essentially eliminate syphilis in this country, but eradication will require a vaccine to be effective. A vaccine may be possible in the distant future.

REFERENCES

Centers for Disease Control and Prevention. Sexually transmitted diseases treatment guidelines 2002. *MMWR Recomm Rep.* 2002;51:1-78.

Scheck DN, Hook EW III. Neurosyphilis. *Infect Dis Clin North Am.* 1994;8:769-795.

Sparling PF. *Natural history of syphilis.* In: Holmes KK, Sparling PF, Mårdh P-A, et al, eds. *Sexually Transmitted Diseases.* 3rd ed. New York, NY: McGraw-Hill; 1999:473-478.

Section XI

DISORDERS OF THE REPRODUCTIVE SYSTEM

Chapter 90

Cervical Neoplasia

John F. Boggess

Since its adoption in the United States in the 1940s, universal screening using the Pap smear has decreased death from cervical cancer by more than 70%. Cervical cancer screening is the most successful cancer screening program in history.

Although the Pap smear has reduced cervical cancer deaths in the United States, many challenges remain. The most significant barrier is lack of compliance with screening recommendations, particularly in older women, the uninsured, ethnic minorities, and women in rural areas. In the United States, 50% to 70% of cervical cancer cases occur among women who have never been screened or who have not been screened within the past 5 years. Significant racial disparity exists in both incidence and death from cervical cancer, with the highest-risk ethnic group being Vietnamese women. While cervical cancer accounts for only 2% of all cancer deaths in women, it ranks second among women aged 20 to 39 years.

Prevention of cervical cancer and cervical cancer mortality is feasible because (1) progression from early cellular abnormalities, termed low-grade dysplasia (LGSIL), through more severe dysplasia (high-grade dysplasia [HGSIL]), to carcinoma in situ (CIS) and invasive cancer is generally slow, allowing time for detection; (2) associated cellular abnormalities can be identified; and (3) effective treatment is available for premalignant lesions. While screening has been successful in reducing squamous cancer incidence and mortality, the incidence of glandular or adenocarcinoma is increasing.

ETIOLOGY AND PATHOGENESIS

Most cervical cancer develops within the cervical transformation zone, the region where the epithelial cells of the cervix and vagina undergo metaplastic transformation to the columnar epithelium that lines the endocervical glands. Figure 90-1 demonstrates the findings in this area, visualized during colposcopy. The susceptibility of women to squamous cancer is due to the fragility of this tissue in combination with its direct exposure to environmental carcinogens, the most important being the human papilloma virus.

Human papilloma virus (HPV) plays a central role in the development of cervical cancer. Ninety-five percent to 99% of squamous cell cervical cancers and 75% to 95% of high-grade CIN lesions have detectable HPV DNA. HPV is transmitted primarily by sexual intercourse, and can persist in vulvar, vaginal, and cervical tissue throughout a woman's lifetime. As a group of over 100 viral types, HPV viruses cause a diverse spectrum of diseases. HPV types 6 and 11 cause warts, and types 16 and 18 cause cancer. Among women without cervical cytology abnormalities at baseline, those with high-risk HPV types have a relative risk of developing high-grade cervical lesions that is 58- to 71-fold higher than those without detectable HPV.

HPV DNA must integrate into the host genomic DNA to promote the changes that lead to cervical cancer. This event appears to be rare, but it is essential for cancer progression. In the absence of viral integration, the normal viral life cycle produces morphological changes in the cervical epithelium characteristic of LGSIL. With viral integration, cellular changes characteristic of HGSIL and ultimately cancer are observed (Figure 90-2). Interrelated host factors such as age, nutritional status, immune function, smoking, and possibly silent genetic polymorphisms modulate incorporation of viral DNA. It is estimated that nearly 100% of carcinoma in-situ and cancer lesions have integrated HPV DNA compared to a small minority of low-grade dysplastic lesions. The transition time from simple viral infection to integration of DNA and oncogenesis is unknown and may be influenced by the patient's risk profile.

Figure 90-1

Colposcopy

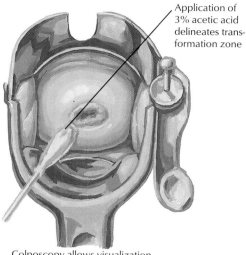

Application of 3% acetic acid delineates transformation zone

Colposcopy allows visualization of cervical transformation zone

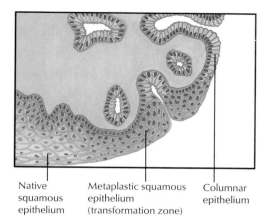

Native squamous epithelium   Metaplastic squamous epithelium (transformation zone)   Columnar epithelium

Section of transformation zone at cervical os

Variations in location of transformation zone

Prepubertal   Reproductive   Postmenopausal

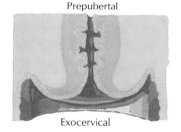 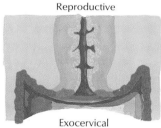 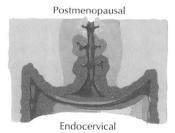

Exocervical   Exocervical   Endocervical

Features of normal transformation zone

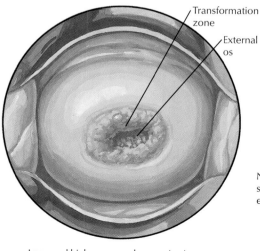

Transformation zone

External os

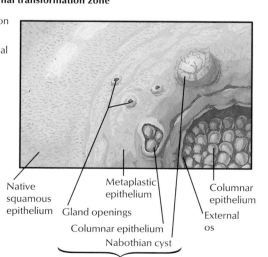

Native squamous epithelium   Gland openings   Metaplastic epithelium   Columnar epithelium   External os

Columnar epithelium

Nabothian cyst

Transformation zone

Low- and high-power colposcopic views of normal transformation zone

JOHN A. CRAIG—AD
© ICON

Natural history studies confirm that, in the majority of cases, the course of infection and cervical abnormalities progress in an orderly fashion from less to more severe lesions. Thus, the sequence of changes associated with HPV infection and the development of cervical cancer parallel the cytological changes observed and are amenable to surveillance with Pap smears.

In the United States, peak incidence and prevalence of HPV infection occurs among women under age 25; however, more than 30% of postmenopausal women have detectable HPV DNA using PCR detection methods. Because most cervical cancers are associated with HPV infection, independent of age of cancer incidence, screening for epithelial changes caused by the virus is indicated in all age groups.

CLINICAL PRESENTATION

Cervical cancer develops a clinically visible lesion when invasive, and, when deeply invasive, it spreads by local extension, via lymphatics or the bloodstream (Figure 90-3). Preinvasive cervical neoplasias are rarely associated with symptoms. With progression to invasive cervical cancer, women are more likely to complain of abnormal vaginal discharge and intermenstrual bleeding, specifically after douching or coitus. Pain, loss of appetite, and weight loss are all late manifestations. Back pain may indicate ureteral obstruction related to pelvic sidewall involvement by tumor. Involvement of the bladder or rectum may present with bleeding as well as fistula formation.

DIFFERENTIAL DIAGNOSIS

Many cervical conditions, including genital tract infection, can influence Pap smear interpretation, and may result in false-positive findings. Certain benign conditions such as leiomyomata, primary herpes infection, endometriosis, and cervical polyps, can cause a palpable or visible cervical mass. Uterine cancer can extend to the cervix and vagina and needs to be considered in the differential diagnosis.

MANAGEMENT AND THERAPY
Screening

Pap smear screening is recommended in women who are sexually active or age 18 or older. After 3 or more consecutive annual exami-

nations with normal findings, the Pap test may be performed less frequently at the discretion of the physician. In asymptomatic women who have undergone hysterectomy, and who do not have a history of genital dysplasia or cancer, Pap smears are not necessary.

Conventional Triage of Abnormal Pap Smears

Treatment and management of screening cytologic abnormalities begins with referral to a specialist trained in colposcopy and therapy of preinvasive cervical dysplasia. Documented cases of invasive cervical cancer should be referred to a gynecologic oncologist. Understanding the triage of abnormal Pap smears requires an understanding of the current Bethesda classification of Pap smear abnormalities (Table 90-1). Women with 2 ASCUS or LGSIL Pap smears should undergo colposcopy and directed biopsy. A single HGSIL or cancer Pap smear should prompt immediate referral for colposcopic evaluation. Whenever a clinically suspicious lesion or ulceration of the cervix is observed, referral for examination with colposcopy and biopsy should occur, irrespective of the Pap smear result. Colposcopy includes magnified examination of the cervix after the application of dilute acetic acid, which accentuates dysplastic epithelium by turning it white. Directed punch biopsies of the cervix of all "acetowhite" lesions and any ulcerative areas showing atypical vascular patterns are performed to determine which patients require treatment and which require routine or close follow-up (Figure 90-4).

Curettage of the endocervix is performed when the entire transformation zone cannot be visualized or when a visible lesion extends within the cervical canal. In most cases, histologically proven LGSIL is benign and Pap smear screening at frequent intervals is acceptable for compliant patients. HGSIL lesions are much more likely to develop into invasive cancer, and therefore are treated. If the whole lesion is visible on colposcopy, removal of all abnormal epithelium together with the whole transformation zone is performed by cryotherapy, laser ablation, or loop electrical excision (LEEP). If the lesion is not totally visible or if it is large, cold knife conization is preferred.

Follow-up of patients with LGSIL lesions or who have undergone definitive treatment includes Pap

Figure 90-2

Cervical Cell Pathology in Squamous Tissue
•
Grades and Cell Types

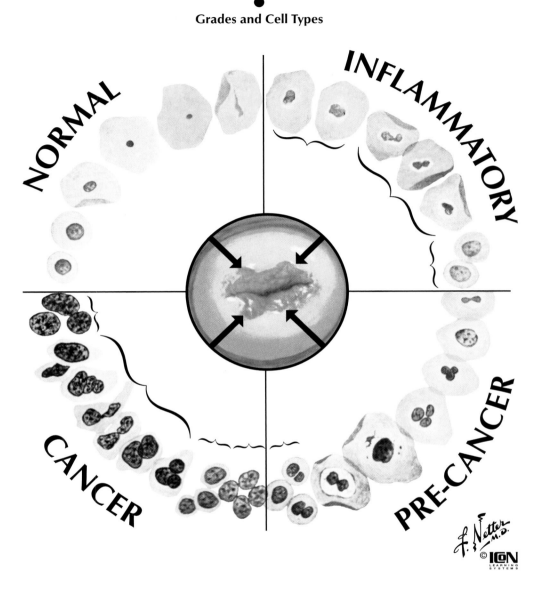

NORMAL

INFLAMMATORY

CANCER

PRE-CANCER

smear assessment every 3 to 6 months until 3 normal Pap smears are obtained. Yearly screening should be continued thereafter. Cytologic abnormalities detected on follow-up screening should be re-evaluated with colposcopy.

Hysterectomy may be appropriate for certain women who have completed childbearing and desire definitive treatment. Care must be taken to exclude invasive disease.

Treatment of Invasive Lesions

The current staging system of the International Federation of Gynecology and Obstetrics (FIGO) is presented in Table 90-2. Early stage disease is amenable to both surgical and radiation therapy. The choice of method is based upon many social and clinical factors. For tumors stage II and greater, radiation is the mainstay of therapy with chemotherapy added to potentiate the efficacy of the radiation.

Figure 90-3

Cancer of Cervix
Various Stages and Types

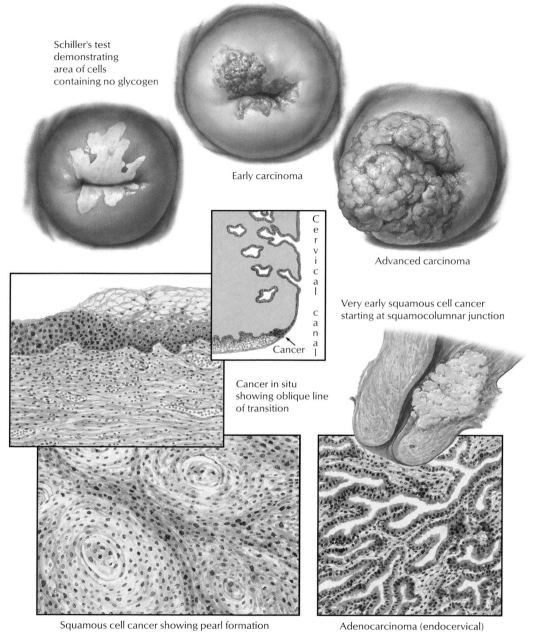

Schiller's test demonstrating area of cells containing no glycogen

Early carcinoma

Advanced carcinoma

Cervical canal

Cancer

Cancer in situ showing oblique line of transition

Very early squamous cell cancer starting at squamocolumnar junction

Squamous cell cancer showing pearl formation

Adenocarcinoma (endocervical)

Table 90-1
The 2001 Bethesda System (Abridged)

Specimen Adequacy
Satisfactory for evaluation (note presence/absence of endocervical/transformation zone component)
Unsatisfactory for evaluation . . . *(specify reason)*
Specimen rejected/not precessed *(specify reason)*
Specimen processed and examined, but unsatisfactory for evaluation of epithelial abnormality because of
(specify reason)

General Categorization *(Optional)*
Negative for intraepithelial lesion or malignancy
Epithelial cell abnormality
Other

Interpretation/Result
Negative for intraepithelial lesion or malignancy
Organisms
Tichomonas vaginalis
Fungal organisms morphologically consistent with *Candida* species
Shift in flora suggestive of bacterial vaginosis
Bacteria morphologically consistent with *Actinomyces* species
Cellular changes consistent with herpes simplex virus
Other non-neoplastic findings *(Optional to report; list not comprehensive)*
Reactive cellular changes associated with
inflammation (includes typical repair)
radiation
intrauterine contraceptive device
Glandular cells status posthysterectomy
Atrophy
Epithelial cell abnormaities
Squamous cell
Atypical squamous cells (ASC)
of undetermined significance (ASC-US)
cannot exclude HSIL (ASC-H)
Low-grade squamous intraepithelial lesion (LSIL)
encompassing: human papillomavirus/mild dysplasia/cervical intraepithelial neoplasia (CIN) 1
High-grade squamous intraepithelial lesion (HSIL)
encompassing: moderate and severe dysplasia, carcinoma in situ; CIN 2 and CIN 3
Squamous cell carcinoma
Glandular cell
Atypical glandular cells (AGC) *(specify endocervical, endometrial, or not otherwise specified)*
Atypical glandular cells, favor neoplastic *(specify endocervical, or not otherwise specified)*
Endocervical adenocarcinoma in situ (AIS)
Adenocarcinoma
Other *(List not comprehensive)*
Endometrial cells in a woman ≥40 years of age

Automated Review and Ancillary Testing *(Include as appropriate)*

Educational Notes and Suggestions *(Optional)*

Adapted from Solomon D, Davey D, Kurman R, et al. The 2001 Bethesda System: Terminology for reporting results of Cervical Cytology. *JAMA*. 2002; 287(16): 2116, Copyright © 2002, American Medical Association.

DISORDERS OF THE REPRODUCTIVE SYSTEM

Figure 90-4   ## Colposcopic Views of Abnormal Cervical Changes

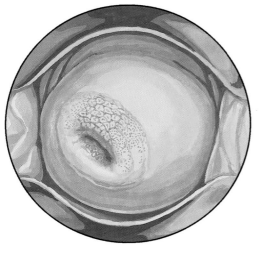

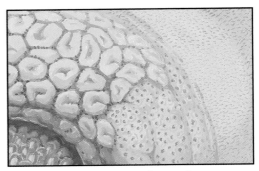

Coarse mosaicism and punctation
in transformation zone

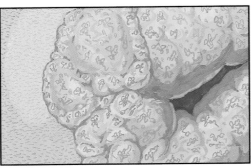

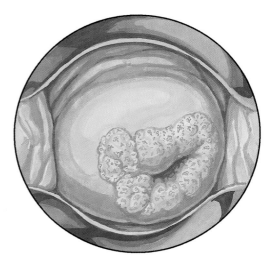

Papilloma of cervix. Some papillomas
may predispose to cervical malignancy

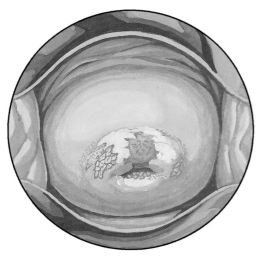

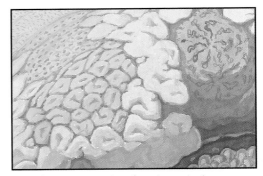

Changes suggestive of carcinoma in situ.
Abnormal vasculature with leukoplakia,
mosaicism, and punctation

JOHN A. CRAIG—AD
© ICON

Table 90-2
Staging of Cervical Cancer

Stage I
The carcinoma is strictly confined to the cervix (extension to the corpus should be disregarded).

Stage IA: Invasive cancer identified only microscopically. All gross lesions even with superficial invasion are Stage IB cancers. Invasion is limited to measured stromal invasion with maximum depth of 5.0 mm and no wider than 7.0 mm.

Stage IA1: Measured invasion of stroma no greater than 3.0 mm in depth and no wider than 7.0 mm.

Stage IA2: Measured invasion of stroma greater than 3.0 mm and no greater than 5.0 mm and no wider than 7.0 mm. The depth of invasion should not be more than 5.0 mm taken from the base of the epithelium, either surface or glandular, from which it originates. Preformed space involvement (vascular or lymphatic) should not alter the staging but should be specifically recorded so as to determine whether it should affect treatment decisions in the future.

Stage IB: Clinical lesions confined to the cervix or preclinical lesions greater than IA.

Stage IB1: Clinical lesions no greater than 4.0 cm in size.

Stage IB2: Clinical lesions greater than 4.0 cm in size.

Stage II
The carcinoma extends beyond the cervix but has not extended to the pelvic wall. The carcinoma involves the vagina but not as far as the lower third.

Stage IIA: No obvious parametrial involvement.

Stage IIB: Obvious parametrial involvement.

Stage III
The carcinoma has extended to the pelvic wall. On rectal examination, there is no cancer-free space between the tumor and the pelvic wall. The tumor involves the lower third of the vagina. All cases with a hydronephrosis or nonfunctioning kidney are included unless they are known to be due to other causes.

Stage IIIA: No extension to the pelvic wall.

Stage IIIB: Extension to the pelvic wall and/or hydronephrosis or nonfunctioning kidney.

Stage IV
The carcinoma has extended beyond the true pelvis or has clinically involved the mucosa of the bladder or rectum. A bullous edema as such does not permit a case to be allotted to Stage IV.

Stage IVA: Spread of the growth to adjacent organs.

Stage IVB: Spread to distant organs.

Adapted from Modifications in the staging for stage I vulvar and stage I cervical cancer. Report of the FIGO Committee on Gynecologic Oncology. *Int J Gynaecol Obslet.* Aug 1995;50(2):215–216.

Radiation therapy can be used in all stages of disease, but surgery alone is limited to patients with stage I and IIa disease. The 5-year survival rate for stage I cancer of the cervix is approximately 85% with either radiation therapy or radical hysterectomy. The advantage of surgical management is evident in younger women where conservation of ovarian function is important.

The governing principle behind treating invasive cervical lesions surgically is based upon the observation that cervical cancer typically spreads locally and to regional lymph nodes in a stepwise and predictable manner. En-bloc resection of the primary tumor with margins requires radical dissection of both parametrial tissues and excision of a 2- to 3-cm vaginal margin. The degree of resection is tailored to the primary lesion size. If significant extracervical disease is demonstrated in the parametrial tissues or lymph nodes, hysterectomy is abandoned in favor of radiation therapy. Postoperative assessment of the hysterectomy specimen and lymph nodes for occult lymph node metastasis, parametrial involvement, or extensive lymphatic space invasion is critical in selecting which patients would benefit from adjuvant radiation therapy.

Radiation therapy can be administered by both external beam to a total pelvic dose of 5,000 rads, and as brachytherapy applied transvaginally to the cervix, and vaginal and parametrial tissues to boost the total dose to the tumor to 7,500 rads. In selected patients with large tumors or known pelvic lymph node involvement, the radiation fields are extended to include the paraaortic lymph nodes.

Recent reports of increasing the efficacy of radiation therapy with the infusion of low-dose platinum chemotherapy have led to this regimen becoming the standard of care for extracervical disease.

Local/regional cervical cancer recurrences can often be salvaged with some long-term survivors. Following primary surgical management, pelvic recurrences can be treated with radiation therapy with curative intent if no distant metastatic disease is present. Isolated lung metastasis can be treated with surgical excision with good results in patients without other sites of recurrence. Chemotherapy for advanced or recurrent disease yields short-lived responses of 30%.

FUTURE DIRECTIONS

Given the pathogenetic role of human papilloma virus in cervical cancer and the virus prevalence among sexually active women, research is underway to develop a vaccine. While newer screening technologies offer promise, the major failure in preventing cervical cancer death in the United States remains lack of compliance with screening. Studies show that the strongest influence on compliance is whether physicians emphasize the importance of screening. Racial disparity still exists in outcomes of treatment. Finally, the National Cancer Institute (NCI) has recognized that the identification of biomarkers, which might better identify those cytologic abnormalities that are clinically significant, would dramatically improve the cost effectiveness of current screening algorithms. A consequence of the improved sensitivity of current screening methods is a loss of specificity. The number of women with an "abnormal" Pap smear has increased significantly since the Bethesda system was adopted in 1988. Screening techniques, like liquid-based cytology and computer-assisted analysis, have greater sensitivity, but their cost is prohibitive for many patients.

Based on a recent study of minimally abnormal Pap smears, the NCI has concluded that women with ASCUS smears who do not have high-risk HPV may be screened yearly. The results of this study are significant given that ASCUS is the most common Pap smear abnormality, but correlates with biopsy-proven dysplasia in fewer than half of women with the finding.

Cervical cancer prevention will require a "look forward" to new technology while continuing to "look back" and fully implement what has been to date the most successful cancer prevention strategy adopted.

REFERENCES

Berek JS, Hacker NF, eds. *Practical Gynecologic Oncology.* 3rd ed. Philadelphia, Pa: Lippincott Williams & Wilkins; 2000.

National Cancer Institute Web site. Available at: http://www.cancer.gov. Accessed January 15, 2003.

Rock JA, Thompson JD, eds. *Te Linde's Operative Gynecology.* 8th ed. Philadelphia, Pa: Lippincott-Raven Publishers; 1997.

US Preventive Services Task Force. *Guide to Clinical Preventive Services.* 2nd ed. Washington, DC: US Dept of Health and Human Services; 1996.

Chapter 91

Common Problems in Pregnancy

M. Cristina Muñoz

Pregnancy is a time of extraordinary maternal adaptation. Some symptoms of pregnancy, such as nausea, breast tenderness, low back pain, and fatigue, occur almost universally. These so-called "minor discomforts of pregnancy" cause significant morbidity. Benign conditions such as constipation, hemorrhoids, nasal congestion, and carpal tunnel syndrome are very common in pregnancy, but are treated in the same way as in nonpregnant individuals. Other common problems encountered in pregnancy are presented in Table 91-1.

MANAGEMENT AND THERAPY—THE RATIONAL USE OF MEDICATIONS IN PREGNANCY

Prescribing medications for pregnant women is difficult because the provider must tread a narrow path between excessively restrictive practices that deny women needed therapies and an excessively casual approach that assumes most pregnancies will turn out fine. The following are general guidelines for treatment of women with routine pregnancies. Women with significant medical illness or pregnancy complications should be referred to a perinatologist. It is never a mistake to call a specialist for management advice because informal consultations give the consultant an opportunity to intervene early and to identify those cases where complex management and transfer of care are necessary.

Plan for Pregnancy

Ideally, planning for use of medications in pregnancy begins before conception, especially in women with chronic illness. In conditions such as phenylketonuria, diabetes mellitus, hypertension, smoking, and obesity, the desire for a healthy baby may spur marked improvements in lifestyle and disease management. In these conditions, pre-conceptional improvements in maternal health status correlate with improved pregnancy outcomes, such as lower rates of miscarriage, fetal malformations, gestational hypertension, or delivery complications. For diseases such as hypertension or diabetes mellitus where there are several effective therapies but some are believed to be safer in pregnancy, it is best to switch therapies before attempted conception.

Expect the Unexpected Pregnancy

In all women of reproductive age, it is worthwhile to explore plans and desires for future pregnancy. Because over half of pregnancies in the United States are unplanned, a realistic assessment of the risk of pregnancy, including contraceptive choice, correct use of the method chosen, and sexual activity, is helpful for those who do not plan pregnancy. A multivitamin containing 400 µg of folic acid is recommended for all women of reproductive age. Women who do not expect to become pregnant may have delayed entry into prenatal care and prolonged exposure to medications that may be harmful in pregnancy. Alternatively, women may discontinue medications in early pregnancy in hopes of protecting their child, although in some cases, this can be harmful to both the woman and the developing embryo.

Current Prescriptions, Over-the-Counter Drugs, Herbs, and Drugs of Abuse

Pregnant women often assume that drugs they used before pregnancy, especially those sold over-the-counter, are safe in pregnancy; however, these often contain aspirin, NSAIDs, or other medications that are not recommended in pregnancy. Compound medications, such as antihistamine-decongestant combinations, are also problematic. Because these drugs are sold by brand name, many prescribers are unaware of the exact doses of each agent contained in the drug. Popular cold remedies may contain many different drugs, when a patient's symptoms could be treated with just 1 or 2. Herbal preparations are a concern because

Figure 91-1

Ectopic Pregnancy I
Tubal Pregnancy

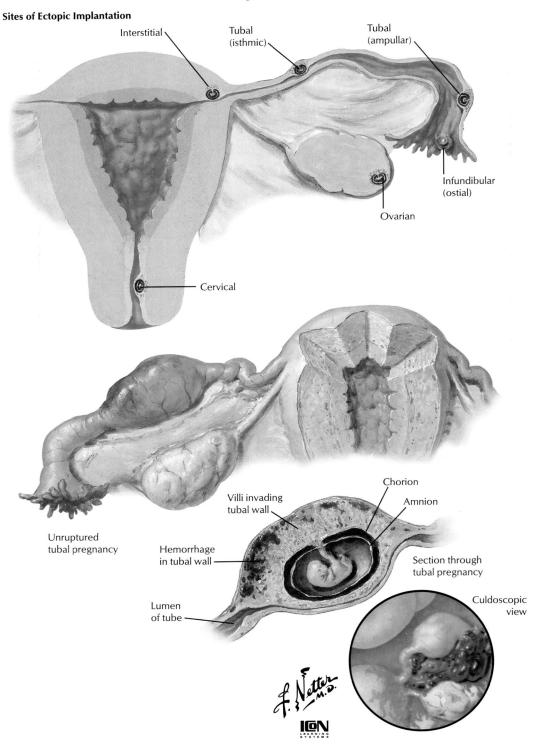

Sites of Ectopic Implantation

Interstitial

Tubal (isthmic)

Tubal (ampullar)

Infundibular (ostial)

Ovarian

Cervical

Unruptured tubal pregnancy

Villi invading tubal wall

Hemorrhage in tubal wall

Lumen of tube

Chorion

Amnion

Section through tubal pregnancy

Culdoscopic view

Table 91-1
Common Problems in Pregnancy

Common Pregnancy Problems	Etiology, Pathogenesis	Clinical Presentation, Differential Diagnosis, Diagnostic Approach	Serious Conditions to Consider	Management and Therapy
First trimester vaginal bleeding	Cervical bleeding: inflammation or polyp. Uterine bleeding: implantation of zygote, threatened pregnancy loss.	Ultrasound shows location of gestational sac/embryo, and findings should correlate with quantitative b-hCG and gestational age. In early gestation, β-hCG doubles every 48 to 72 hours; decreasing or plateauing level indicates abnormal pregnancy.	Threatened, incomplete, or completed spontaneous abortion, ectopic pregnancy, ruptured hemorrhagic ovarian cyst. (Figure 91-1)	*Threatened abortion:* observation; many continue with no sequelae. *Incomplete abortion:* suction curettage. *Inevitable abortion:* suction curettage. *Missed abortion or blighted ovum:* expectant management, misoprostol, or curettage. *Ectopic:* methotrexate or surgery.
Third trimester vaginal bleeding	"Bloody show" may occur as result of cervical changes in labor.	Avoid digital examination of cervix if location of placenta is unknown. Doppler ultrasound may show vessels.	Placenta previa, vasa previa, abruptio placentae.	For hemorrhage from placenta previa or abruption, emergency cesarean section and transfusion.
Contractions	Uterine muscular activity.	Braxton-Hicks contractions are painless and irregular; may increase with dehydration.	Regular, painful contractions, especially when accompanied by bloody show or rupture of membranes, usually signal labor.	Fluid boluses are helpful if the patient is dehydrated. Tocolytics may prolong pregnancy temporarily while steroids are given to improve neonatal outcome.
Rapid heartbeat	Increased cardiac output.	Sustained tachycardia is usually of supraventricular origin.	High-risk conditions include Marfan syndrome, aortic stenosis, pulmonary hypertension, and New York Heart Association class III or IV, regardless of etiology. Thyrotoxicosis may present with tachycardia, palpitations, and anxiety.	Reassurance, caffeine restriction, and change in activities if transient/mild. Cardiology evaluation (EKG, Holter monitor) if severe/persistent.

there is a dearth of research on their risks in pregnancy, and physicians are often unaware of the available data. Other drugs to consider include alcohol and illicit drugs. For many illnesses and discomforts of pregnancy, there are non-pharmacologic treatments that are effective. These include foods, reassurance, social support, rest periods or alteration in working conditions, postural changes, local heat or ice, and use of braces or supports.

Use Minimum Effective Dose

Pharmacokinetic changes in pregnancy may require upward or downward adjustments in dosing. These changes include increased plasma vol-

Table 91-1 Common Problems in Pregnancy (continued)

Common Pregnancy Problems	Etiology, Pathogenesis	Clinical Presentation, Differential Diagnosis, Diagnostic Approach	Serious Conditions to Consider	Management and Therapy
Nausea and vomiting of pregnancy	Central effect of β-hCG, estrogen.	Begins by 10 weeks, not accompanied by fever, headache, abdominal pain or jaundice.	Hyperemesis gravidarum: weight loss >5% of prepregnancy weight, large ketonuria. May occur in multiple gestation or molar pregnancy.	Frequent small, bland, or salty meals, high in carbohydrate, low in fat. Ginger or peppermint. Avoid rapid position changes, odors, and iron pills. Acupuncture/ acupressure wrist bands. Vitamin B₆, doxylamine, phenothiazines. Severe vomiting: metoclopramide, ondansetron, droperidol, or corticosteroids. IV fluids, hyperalimentation as needed.
Indigestion (heartburn, reflux)	Progesterone relaxes lower esophageal sphincter.	Worse after meals, improved by keeping head elevated.	HELLP (hypertension, elevated liver enzymes, low platelets) syndrome: right upper quadrant pain, nausea, vomiting from liver involvement, or fatty liver.	Small meals, elevate head of bed. Antacids, H₂-receptor antagonists, metoclopramide.
Dyspnea of pregnancy	Progesterone increases respiratory rate, uterus restricts diaphragmatic excursion.	Worse in late pregnancy, better with sitting.	Cough or fever may indicate asthma or infection. Severe symptoms, blood-tinged sputum, or acute change may indicate pulmonary embolus.	Reassurance. Asthma treatment is similar to nonpregnant; adequate treatment prevents intrauterine growth retardation, death.
Fatigue, syncope	Decreased blood pressure, hormonal effects.	Worst in first and third trimesters. Screen for anemia if persistent.	Hypovolemic shock (ectopic pregnancy, ruptured hemorrhagic cyst).	Arise slowly, remain well hydrated.
Anemia	Volume expansion, iron use by fetus.	Detected on routine screening.	Screen for thalassemia or sickle cell disease in high-risk populations.	Iron-containing foods, oral iron supplements.
Headache	Hormonal (vasodilation), postural.	Headache frequency (including migraine) may increase or decrease in pregnancy.	Preeclampsia: headache accompanied by hypertension, proteinuria.	Rest, massage, postural change, acetaminophen, narcotics. (Avoid NSAIDs due to risk of bleeding and closure of fetal patent ductus arteriosus.)
Back pain	Mechanical strain.	Worse in late pregnancy.	CVA tenderness may indicate pyelonephritis. Preterm contractions may be felt in low back.	Erect posture, avoid high heels, use elastic support for uterus, acetaminophen.

Table 91-1 Common Problems in Pregnancy (continued)

Common Pregnancy Problems	Etiology, Pathogenesis	Clinical Presentation, Differential Diagnosis, Diagnostic Approach	Serious Conditions to Consider	Management and Therapy
Abdominal/ pelvic pain	Mechanical (stretching of round ligament and other structures).	Common with walking or arising.	Wavelike contractions may indicate labor. Pain of appendicitis may be in abnormal location in pregnancy.	Reassurance.
Varicose veins, dependent edema	Expanded blood volume, uterus impedes venous return.	Worse in late pregnancy.	Deep venous thrombosis: unilateral pain, redness, swelling. Nerve compression may cause weakness or numbness in lower extremities.	Elastic stockings, or pad to compress vulvar varices, rest in horizontal position.
Leg cramps	Cause unknown.	Worse in late pregnancy.		Calcium supplements, magnesium oxide.
Respiratory infections	Viral or bacterial infection, may be more symptomatic in pregnancy.	Incidence similar to nonpregnant state.	Suspect pulmonary embolus if patient has been sedentary or symptoms are severe.	May use acetaminophen, antihistamines, guaifenesin, saline nasal spray. Pneumonia in pregnancy requires hospitalization.
Urinary tract infections	Stasis caused by increased GFR, compression of ureters, relaxed smooth muscle tone, glycosuria.	Frequent urination is normal in first and third trimester. Asymptomatic bacteriuria common in pregnancy, diagnosed by routine urinalysis.	Pyelonephritis with costovertebral angle tenderness and fever.	Penicillins, cephalosporins are safe. Trimethoprim-sulfamethoxazole and nitrofurantoin are effective, but may cause neonatal jaundice. Pyelonephritis in pregnancy requires hospitalization.
Vaginal discharge	Estrogen increases physiologic discharge. Bacterial vaginosis is an alteration of vaginal flora	Patient complaint.	Amniotic fluid leakage may cause watery discharge.	Topical azole antifungals are preferred to oral forms for Candida. Metronidazole treats bacterial vaginosis or trichomonas; some providers defer treatment until second trimester. Bacterial vaginosis increases risk of preterm rupture of membranes, preterm labor and delivery, and amnionitis.

ume and cardiac output, increased glomerular filtration rate, decreased protein binding, delayed gastric transit, altered hepatic metabolism, and other changes.

Stop Ineffective Drugs Rapidly

Prenatal visits in the first trimester are usually scheduled at 4- to 6-week intervals. When a drug is prescribed, the effectiveness of the therapy is

Table 91-1 Common Problems in Pregnancy (continued)

Common Pregnancy Problems	Etiology, Pathogenesis	Clinical Presentation, Differential Diagnosis, Diagnostic Approach	Serious Conditions to Consider	Management and Therapy
Dental problems	Edema and hyperemia of gums lead to gingivitis.	Dental examination and radiography (with abdomen shielded) should be done as early as possible, so preventive care can begin.	Periodontal infection may cause preterm labor.	Dental cleaning, extractions, and other needed treatments may be done in pregnancy
Dermatologic problems	Hormonal changes cause hyperpigmentation, skin tags. Abdominal distension causes striae.	Common dermatoses of pregnancy include pruritic urticarial papules and plaques of pregnancy, which cause an abdominal rash with intense itching, prurigo of pregnancy (itchy papules on extremities.) Check liver function tests with itching to rule out cholestasis.	Herpes gestationis (large blisters) may increase risk of premature delivery.	Most changes improve after delivery. Antihistamines or topical fluorinated steroids are used for pruritus.
Anxiety, depression	Multifactorial, including adjustment to new roles and body changes, hormonal influences, and social factors.	Substance abuse is common in pregnancy; diagnosis often missed in non-minority patients. Domestic violence crescendos in pregnancy, in all social classes.	Previous mood disorder or mental illness can recur in pregnancy or postpartum, with risk of suicide or infanticide.	Reassurance and social support are needed in each pregnancy. Antidepressant, antipsychotic, or anxiolytic medications are used for mental illness that cannot be controlled without drugs. Victims of abuse may initially decline help, but later accept help from battered women's shelter, hospital, or police.

often known in just a few days, but patients may obediently use an ineffective medication until the next scheduled visit. Rapid follow-up after starting a new medication is preferred, whether it is accomplished by a telephone call or an office visit.

Know a Few Drugs Well

Doctors who regularly care for pregnant women should have a personal formulary of treatments that they are comfortable prescribing, rather than relying only on the FDA's risk categories. It is reasonable to start with a few drugs

(e.g., acetaminophen, doxylamine, vitamin B_6, penicillins, cephalosporins, folic acid, and levothyroxine) and add only those drugs for which the literature shows effectiveness and not harm. The best approach favors drugs for which evidence has accumulated over years, rather than new drugs that have not previously been used in pregnancy.

Look Up What You Don't Know

Drug information changes rapidly, and recent policy changes will allow both better research on therapeutics in pregnancy and improved descriptive labeling of drugs. Textbooks and review articles may assist with the choice of a drug, and there are excellent reference texts of drug risks in pregnancy and lactation. The Organization of Teratology Information Services and its member organizations in several states offer free information to providers and patients, as well as informative fact sheets that can be printed directly from the Internet. Well-known teratogens include alcohol; radioactive iodine; lithium; mercury; thalidomide; isotretinoin; ACE inhibitors; coumarins; misoprostol; methimazole; penicillamine; tetracyclines; sex steroids, such as diethylstilbestrol and androgens; anti-epileptic drugs, such as phenytoin, trimethadione, carbamazepine, and valproic acid; and many antineoplastic agents.

This process is particularly important and complex in pregnancy. Although the developing fetus is at risk of teratogenesis, and the available information is woefully inadequate, a policy of complete abstinence from drugs is dangerous. For certain diseases, the benefit of treatment may significantly outweigh the risk. The benefit may accrue to the fetus (treatment of severe maternal fever with antipyretics) or to the mother (treatments for nausea and vomiting of pregnancy) or both (treatment of asthma, varicella, hyperthyroidism, hypothyroidism, and HIV disease). When assessing the risks of a drug, they should not be considered in isolation; the available alternatives should also be considered. A drug that is "bad" for a pregnant woman or her developing child may be far less bad than untreated disease, preterm delivery for maternal indications, or untested treatments. In such cases, it may be best to stay with the drug that has been effective previously.

FUTURE DIRECTIONS

Research on pregnant women had long been hampered by the perception that women's symptoms were "minor discomforts" and by hesitancy to include pregnant women and their fetuses in research trials. The generally good outcomes of pregnancies also contributed to acceptance of traditional methods of care without critical review. The current trend toward evidence-based medicine should help us determine what is effective care and what should be abandoned.

REFERENCES

Nausea and Vomiting of Pregnancy [CME module]. Washington, DC: Association of Professors of Gynecology and Obstetrics; 2001. APGO Educational Series on Women's Health Issues.

Briggs GG, Freeman RK, Yaffee SJ. *Drugs in Pregnancy and Lactation: A Reference Guide to Fetal and Neonatal Risk.* 6th ed. Philadelphia, Pa: Lippincott Williams & Wilkins; 2001.

Cunningham FG, Gant NF, Leveno KJ, Gilstrap LC III, Hauth JC, Wenstrom KD, eds. *Williams Obstetrics.* 21st ed. New York, NY: McGraw-Hill; 2001.

Enkin M, Keirse MJNC, Renfrew M, et al, eds. *A Guide to Effective Care in Pregnancy and Childbirth.* 3rd ed. Oxford, England: Oxford University Press; 2000.

Gleicher N, Buttino L, Elkayam U, et al, eds. *Principles & Practice of Medical Therapy in Pregnancy.* 3rd ed. Stamford, Conn: Appleton & Lange; 1998.

Youngkin EQ, Davis MS, eds. *Women's Health: A Primary Care Clinical Guide.* 2nd ed. Stamford, Conn: Appleton & Lange; 1998.

Chapter 92

Diabetes in Pregnancy

Kenneth J. Moise, Jr.

Diabetes mellitus (DM) complicating pregnancy can precede the onset of pregnancy (*pre-gestational diabetes,* PGDM) or present during gestation with resolution by 6 weeks after delivery (*gestational diabetes mellitus,* GDM). DM complicates 2% to 3% of all pregnancies with 90% of cases represented by GDM. Intensive management with home glucose monitoring and insulin therapy has virtually eliminated perinatal mortality. However, an increased rate of congenital anomalies and fetal macrosomia with resultant birth injury continue to challenge modern-day obstetrics.

ETIOLOGY AND PATHOGENESIS

Significant increases in placental hormones including progesterone, estradiol, prolactin, and human somatomammotropin alter pregnancy to become a diabetogenic state (Figure 92-1). Estrogen increases insulin binding at the cellular level; however, decreased binding secondary to progesterone and cortisol offsets this effect. A postbinding defect in insulin action is also caused by progesterone, cortisol, prolactin, and human somatomammotropin. In an effort to offset these changes, there is a marked increase in insulin secretion that peaks in the third trimester.

GDM shares many of the same features as type 2 diabetes mellitus. Hyperglycemia is related to 2 defects. First, there is a reduction in insulin secretion as compared to that in normal pregnancy. This is evidenced by a diminished first-phase insulin response and a delay and reduced incremental response to a peak in serum glucose after oral loading. Second, insulin sensitivity is reduced to almost one third of the non-pregnant state.

DIAGNOSTIC APPROACH

Significant controversy remains regarding universal screening for GDM (Table 92-1). Low-risk women (<25 years old; not a member of an ethnic/racial group with a high prevalence of DM such as Hispanic, American Indian, South or East Asian, Pacific Islander, African American; BMI <25; no history of abnormal glucose tolerance; no history of adverse obstetric outcomes related to GDM; and no first-degree relative with DM) probably do not need to be screened. Patients with high-risk factors, including morbid obesity, previ-ous unexplained fetal death, a previous infant weighing more than 4 kg, and a history of GDM or glycosuria warrant screening early in pregnancy after 12 weeks' gestation. All other patients are usually screened between 24 and 28 weeks' gestation.

Typically a 50-g oral glucose load is given with a plasma glucose measurement performed 1 hour later. The patient need not be in the fasting state. A value >140 mg% warrants evaluation with a 3-hour glucose tolerance test after a 100-g glucose load. Some centers choose to use a threshold of 130 mg% because the higher threshold is 10% less sensitive for the diagnosis of GDM. Several diagnostic thresholds have been proposed.

MANAGEMENT AND THERAPY
Pre-conceptual Counseling

Patients with PGDM contemplating pregnancy should be under tight glucose control before conception. Because more than 50% of pregnancies are unplanned, the primary care physician caring for the woman of reproductive age must inquire about contraceptive practices and plans for conception at each visit. Hemoglobin A1C levels should be measured and be well within the normal range. A multivitamin containing a minimum of 0.4 mg of folate taken daily for at least 3 months before conception has been shown to reduce the risk of neural tube defects, cleft lip, and certain congenital heart diseases. If the patient is taking an angiotensin-converting enzyme (ACE)-inhibitor for co-existing hypertension, consider changing to a calcium channel blocker because ACE-inhibitors are associated

Figure 92-1

Diabetes in Pregnancy

Relevant Pathophysiology

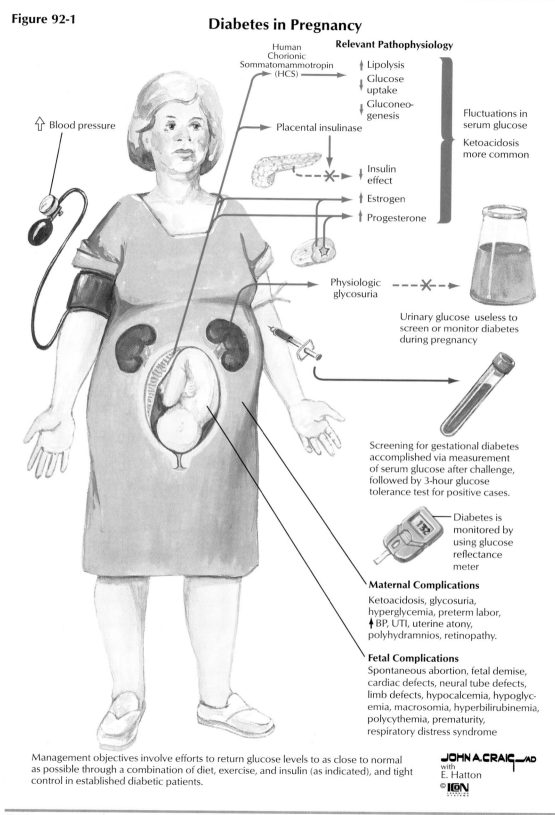

Human Chorionic Sommatomammotropin (HCS)

↑ Lipolysis
↓ Glucose uptake
↓ Gluconeo-genesis

Placental insulinase

↓ Insulin effect

↑ Estrogen

↑ Progesterone

Fluctuations in serum glucose

Ketoacidosis more common

⇧ Blood pressure

Physiologic glycosuria

Urinary glucose useless to screen or monitor diabetes during pregnancy

Screening for gestational diabetes accomplished via measurement of serum glucose after challenge, followed by 3-hour glucose tolerance test for positive cases.

Diabetes is monitored by using glucose reflectance meter

Maternal Complications
Ketoacidosis, glycosuria, hyperglycemia, preterm labor, ↑BP, UTI, uterine atony, polyhydramnios, retinopathy.

Fetal Complications
Spontaneous abortion, fetal demise, cardiac defects, neural tube defects, limb defects, hypocalcemia, hypoglycemia, macrosomia, hyperbilirubinemia, polycythemia, prematurity, respiratory distress syndrome

Management objectives involve efforts to return glucose levels to as close to normal as possible through a combination of diet, exercise, and insulin (as indicated), and tight control in established diabetic patients.

JOHN A. CRAIG—AD
with
E. Hatton
© ICON
LEARNING SYSTEMS

Table 92-1
Diagnostic Criteria for Gestational Diabetes

Parameter	National Diabetes Data Group[*][†]	Carpenter and Coustan[*]
WHO Oral glucose dose (g)	100	100
Fasting	105	95
1 hr	190	180
2 hr	165	155
3 hr	145	140
Criteria for diagnosis	2 or more values exceeded	2 or more values exceeded

[*] Endorsed by the American College of Obstetricians and Gynecologists.
[†] Most commonly used in the United States.

with fetal renal damage especially if taken in the second trimester of pregnancy.

Glucose Control
Diet

The patient with PGDM or newly diagnosed GDM should undergo dietary counseling. Table 92-2 can be used to calculate the total caloric needs.

Although traditional recommendations call for 50% to 60% of calories to be in the form of carbohydrate, recent studies indicate that limiting carbohydrates to 40% of calories results in less fetal macrosomia. Protein should comprise approximately 20% of calories with fats comprising the remaining 40%. More frequent intake makes for smoother glycemic control with one suggestion to distribute calories as follows: breakfast, 10% to 15%; morning snack, 0% to 10%; lunch, 20% to 30%; afternoon snack, 0% to 10%; supper, 30% to 40%; and bedtime snack, 0% to 10%.

Insulin

Pregestational Diabetes Mellitus: Patients taking oral hypoglycemics are usually switched to twice-daily insulin therapy using a combination of regular and NPH formulations. Typical needs involve a total daily dose of 0.5 U/kg from conception until 12 weeks, 0.8 U/kg from 12 to 28 weeks, and 1

Table 92-2
Calculation of Caloric Needs for the Gestational Diabetic

Weight Category	Body Weight Index[*]	Caloric Needs[†]
Underweight	<19.8	40 kcal/kg
Normal weight	19.8–26.0	30 kcal/kg
Obese	26.0–29.0	24 kcal/kg
Morbidly obese	>29.0	12 kcal/kg

[*] Actual weight at start of pregnancy.
[†] Based on weight in pregnancy when diet is prescribed.

U/kg thereafter. Caution should be exercised in patients on insulin pump therapy. Decreased appetite in the first trimester and changing sleep patterns related to pregnancy place the patient at increased risk for hypoglycemia. Instruct patients on a protocol for oral glucose supplementation with early signs of hypoglycemia. Family members should be educated on the proper use of a glucagon pen. Home glucose monitoring is undertaken daily with 4 to 7 measurements. The motivated patient can use e-mail messages or fax to report her values weekly for insulin adjustment.

Gestational Diabetes Mellitus: Many practitioners use once-weekly fasting and 2-hour postprandial plasma venous glucose determinations performed in the office, despite studies indicating a higher incidence of fetal macrosomia as compared to the use of home glucose monitoring. The decision to begin insulin therapy should be based on home capillary glucose monitoring using reflectance meters. Use of memory chips and computerized software to calculate mean glucose values allow for ease and accuracy of reporting. A minimum of 4 daily values should be obtained fasting and 2 hours after each meal. The use of postprandial values to target the dose of maternal insulin has proven more efficacious in preventing neonatal macrosomia than using preprandial values. A more intensive surveillance program includes preprandial values (7 determinations daily) with calculation of a daily mean glucose value. When measurements conducted on a daily basis confirm good control, the patient can decrease to 3 times a week determinations. Repetitive fasting values > 95 mg% or 2-hour postprandial values >120 mg% warrants insulin therapy. A total insulin dose of 0.7 U/kg actual body weight is calculated and divided into 2 daily injections given before breakfast and before supper. The morning dose usually consists of a 2:1 ratio of regular and NPH insulin; the evening dose consists of a 1:1 mix of these preparations. On some occasions, a persistently elevated fasting value may require that the PM NPH dose be moved to bedtime and only regular insulin given before supper. Target capillary glucose values should include fasting <95 mg%, preprandial <95 mg%, 2-hour postprandial <115 mg%, and mean glucose values of 90 to 100 mg%.

Oral Hypoglycemics

Until recently, oral hypoglycemics were not used in pregnancy due to concerns regarding fetal anomalies and neonatal hypoglycemia. The finding that GDM and type 2 diabetes have a similar pathophysiology has led to renewed interest in oral hypoglycemics for the treatment of GDM. Newer agents such as glyburide are tightly bound to protein and have a short elimination half-life, thereby minimizing fetal exposure. Recent studies in GDM have noted equivalent rates of macrosomia and neonatal hypoglycemia when compared to insulin

therapy. Metformin, on the other hand, has been associated with a 9-fold increase in perinatal mortality and a 4.5-fold increase in the rate of preeclampsia as compared to rates with insulin.

Other Prenatal Care

All PGDMs should undergo baseline ophthalmic examination to determine the presence of retinopathy. If proliferative changes are noted, photocoagulation can be undertaken during pregnancy. Benign retinopathy requires follow-up each trimester, as institution of tight glycemic control has been associated with rapid deterioration. A baseline urine culture as well as determination of 24-hour protein excretion and creatinine clearance should be assessed early in gestation.

Fetal Surveillance

Because PGDM is associated with a higher incidence of congenital anomalies, a first trimester hemoglobin A1C level should be obtained. All patients with PGDM should be offered maternal serum screening at 16 to 18 weeks' gestation for neural tube defects and chromosomal abnormalities. In addition, a comprehensive ultrasound should be done between 18 and 20 weeks' gestation. If the hemoglobin A1C is elevated in the first trimester, a fetal echocardiogram at 22 weeks should be undertaken to assess for congenital heart disease. Antenatal testing may be warranted as early as 28 weeks' gestation in the patient with poorly controlled diabetes or other complicating conditions such as hypertension. In most cases, testing is initiated by 32 weeks' gestation. Many centers use a modified biophysical profile consisting of a non-stress test performed in conjunction with an ultrasound determination of amniotic fluid volume; others prefer to use the non-stress test alone. Testing is undertaken at least weekly, although for the type 1 diabetic or the gestational diabetic requiring insulin, twice-weekly testing may be preferable.

Delivery

Optimal time for delivery in the patient with diabetes is debated. In the case of poor metabolic control and documentation of fetal lung maturity by amniocentesis, induction of labor should be undertaken by 38 weeks' gestation. Some studies have confirmed a reduced incidence of fetal macrosomia with routine induction at 38 weeks' gestation. However, most centers will not allow the diabetic (PGDM or GDM) to proceed past 40 weeks' gestation even in light of good metabolic control and reassuring antenatal fetal testing.

Fetal macrosomia is probably the most feared complication of diabetes secondary to its association with shoulder dystocia and subsequent Erb's palsy in the neonate. Only 10% to 50% of fetuses that weigh more than 4,500 g experience a shoulder dystocia at the time of vaginal delivery. Erb's palsy will develop in 4% to 8% of macrosomic infants delivered vaginally, but only 10% to 20% of cases persist after age 1. Current clinical and ultrasonographic techniques are poor predictors of fetal macrosomia. However, because of medical-legal concerns, the prevailing practice is to offer the diabetic patient delivery by cesarean section if the estimated fetal weight is 4,500 g or greater.

Neonatal hypoglycemia can be reduced when maternal glucose levels are tightly controlled in labor. A dextrose-containing intravenous fluid prevents ketosis. Continuous low-dose insulin infusion, in conjunction with hourly capillary glucose measurements, is then used to maintain the maternal glucose at less than 100 mg%.

Postpartum Care
Glucose Control

Because of the acute loss of placental hormones during delivery, the type 1 diabetic is extremely sensitive to insulin in the first 24 hours postpartum. Permissive hyperglycemia is allowed with maintenance of glucose levels <200 mg%. Typically the patient will only require half of her pre-pregnancy dose in the first 24 hours; a sliding scale can be used for additional control. By the second postpartum day, she can be placed back on her full pre-pregnancy dose if oral intake is adequate. If the patient is nursing, caloric intake should be increased by 500 kcal over her pre-gestation caloric needs. Patients who were taking oral hypoglycemic agents before pregnancy are maintained on low-dose insulin while breastfeeding because these agents are readily excreted into the breast milk and can cause profound neonatal hypoglycemia.

The patient with GDM requires no glucose monitoring in the postpartum period unless type 1 diabetes is suspected. In the typical GDM patient, a 75-g oral glucose tolerance test is taken at the 6-week postpartum visit. A fasting value $\geq$126 mg% or a 2-hour glucose measurement $\geq$200 mg% are provisional diagnostic criteria for diabetes . An impaired fasting glucose is defined as a value between 110 and 125 mg% while impaired glucose tolerance is defined as a 2-hour post-glucose value of 140 to 199 mg%. These patients require careful follow-up because they are at high risk for the development of overt diabetes .

Contraception

Today's oral contraceptives contain reduced amounts of estrogen and progestin and therefore have minimal effect on glucose control; their use in the diabetic patient is acceptable with monitoring of glucose and lipid levels. New intrauterine devices are not contraindicated in the diabetic patient. Injectable or implantable progestins can also be used. One study has indicated a higher rate of progression to type 2 DM in Hispanic patients with GDM who were taking progestin-only birth control pills due to breastfeeding.

Long-Term Outcome
Maternal

Women in whom GDM develops are at substantial risk for the subsequent development of type 2 DM. The rate of development is dependent on several factors, most notably race/ethnic background. Approximately 10% of white women will have type 2 DM within the first decade postpartum; the rate increases to 30% to 40% by the third decade. In contrast, 50% of Latina women with GDM will have type 2 DM within 5 years of delivery. Although parity does not seem to influence the risk, women with GDM in successive pregnancies are at increased risk for the development of type 2 DM. In contrast, women who have GDM in one pregnancy but do not manifest GDM in a subsequent gestation are at decreased risk. Obesity also is a major risk factor. The risk of DM increases almost 2-fold with each 10-pound weight gain over the patient's postpartum weight.

Neonatal

Macrosomia, hypoglycemia, hyperbilirubinemia, and polycythemia are the short-term detrimental effects of poorly controlled maternal DM.

More concerning are the results of long-term studies that indicate that detrimental in utero modeling occurs when there is poor maternal metabolic control. A higher incidence of obesity, persisting into adolescence; glucose intolerance; and even poorer intellectual and psychomotor development have been noted.

FUTURE DIRECTIONS

Randomized trials are desperately needed regarding therapeutic interventions in GDM and the relationship to short- and long-term neonatal outcome. In addition, newer treatment modalities such as intranasal insulin and new types of oral hypoglycemics should be studied in pregnancy.

REFERENCES

Dornhorst A, Rossi M. Risk and prevention of type 2 diabetes in women with gestational diabetes. *Diabetes Care.* 1998;21 (suppl 2):B43-B49.

The Expert Committee on the Diagnosis and Classification of Diabetes Mellitus. Report of the Expert Committee on the Diagnosis and Classification of Diabetes Mellitus. *Diabetes Care.* 2003;26(suppl 1):S5-S20.

Kuhl C. Etiology and pathogenesis of gestational diabetes. *Diabetes Care.* 1998;21(suppl 2):B19-B26.

Langer O. Maternal glycemic criteria for insulin therapy in gestational diabetes mellitus. *Diabetes Care.* 1998;21(suppl 2):B91-B98.

Silverman BL, Rizzo TA, Cho NH, Metzger BE. Long-term effects of the intrauterine environment. The Northwestern University Diabetes in Pregnancy Center. *Diabetes Care.* 1998;21(suppl 2):B142-B149.

Chapter 93
Endometriosis

AnnaMarie Connolly

A benign gynecologic condition with occasional invasive properties reminiscent of malignancies, endometriosis has long frustrated both physicians and patients. Defined as the presence and growth of both endometrial glands and stroma outside the endometrial cavity, endometriosis can lead to symptom manifestations of cyclical pelvic pain, dyspareunia, dysmenorrhea, and less frequently, abnormal uterine bleeding and gastrointestinal and urinary tract symptoms. There is speculation about the relationship between endometriosis and fertility.

The true incidence and prevalence of endometriosis are unknown because it is identified often incidentally at surgery for other indications. Estimates commonly cited include a 5% to 15% incidence in reproductive-aged women with active endometriosis found in approximately one third of women with chronic pelvic pain.

ETIOLOGY AND PATHOGENESIS

No single theory has emerged as dominant for the pathogenesis of endometriosis. It is unclear why endometriosis develops in some, but not all, women. Proposed explanations include anatomic (retrograde menstruation, vascular and lymphatic dissemination), histologic (coelomic metaplasia), immunologic, and other theories, as well as genetic predisposition.

Retrograde menstruation, found in up to 90% of women in any particular cycle, is clearly a common occurrence. Implantation of endometriotic cells shed during menstruation may lead to the development of endometriosis. Viable endometrial cells have been demonstrated in both menstrual effluent and in peritoneal fluid of reproductive-aged women. Supporting evidence for this theory includes work demonstrating endometriosis in women with genital tract outflow obstruction (up to 10% of teenagers with congenital outflow obstruction) and the fact that endometriotic implants most frequently appear in areas immediately adjacent to the tubal ostia and in the dependent regions of the pelvis (Figures 93-1 and 93-2).

Endometriosis may arise from metaplasia of the multipotential coelomic epithelium. This epithelial metaplasia may occur in response to "an inducing event" such as exposure to menstrual effluent, estrogen, and progesterone. Supporting evidence includes ovarian surface epithelium differentiation into a variety of histologic cell types; peritoneal decidual reaction during pregnancy; and the rare occurrence of endometriosis in prepubertal girls and women with congenital absence of the uterus.

Research is continuing on the relationship between endometriosis and the immune response. The failure of the immune response may involve decreased cellular immunity with impaired natural killer cell cytotoxicity and decreased humoral response with impaired secretory product elaboration from B-cell lymphocytes. Combined, these defects in both cellular-mediated and humoral-mediated immunity likely contribute to faulty clearance of ectopic endometriotic implants and subsequent development of the disease. The exaggerated response may involve overactive peritoneal macrophages that secrete multiple growth factors and cytokines and exhibit impaired phagocytic properties in patients with endometriosis.

Lymphatic and vascular dissemination have been proposed to explain the development of endometriosis in sites distant from the pelvis including the lung, brain, and spinal column. Endometriotic involvement of pelvic lymph nodes has been reported in 30% of women with the disease. Iatrogenic spread has been implicated to explain the appearance of endometriosis in the anterior abdominal wall after abdominal surgery and, more rarely, in episiotomy scar sites.

Genetic predisposition has also been described.

Figure 93-1

Endometriosis
Laparoscopic views

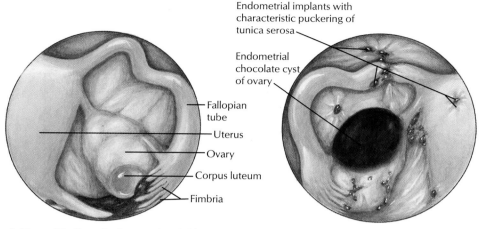

Endometrial implants with characteristic puckering of tunica serosa

Endometrial chocolate cyst of ovary

Fallopian tube

Uterus

Ovary

Corpus luteum

Fimbria

A. Normal findings. (Indigo carmine visible at end of tube)

B. Endometriosis. (Involving ovary and distorting fallopian tube)

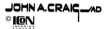

A study has shown a 7-fold increase in the incidence of endometriosis in relatives of women with the disease and that 1 in 10 women with severe disease have a mother or sister with symptomatic disease.

CLINICAL PRESENTATION

The heterogeneity of endometriosis symptom expression should not be overlooked with as many as one third of patients lacking symptoms. The classical presentation is that of cyclical pelvic pain 2 to 4 days before the onset of menses. A more traditional clinical picture of endometriosis includes secondary dysmenorrhea, dyspareunia, infertility, a fixed retroverted uterus, and tender nodularity of the cul-de-sac. However, in a Brisbane study, only 5% of 717 patients with endometriosis had this complete clinical picture. Moreover, clinicians have often observed an inverse relationship between extent of observable endometriotic disease and extent of pain.

Symptoms include cyclical pelvic pain, secondary dysmenorrhea, dyspareunia, abnormal uterine bleeding, constitutional symptoms, and infertility. Cyclical pelvic pain may result from cyclical swelling of endometriosis implants with blood extravasation into surrounding tissues. Secondary dysmenorrhea, described as a constant pain, may occur in 30% of patients and is a dominant symptom in adolescents. Dyspareunia, a deep pelvic pain during intercourse, occurs in approximately 30% of patients, and may be secondary to immobility of pelvic organs or stretching of scarred tissues and uterine support tissues. Abnormal bleeding occurs in up to 15% of patients and may be secondary to ovulatory dysfunction, coincidental fibroids, or adenomyosis. Constitutional symptoms such as cyclical gastrointestinal complaints (cyclical diarrhea or constipation, abdominal pain) or urinary complaints (urinary frequency, hematuria, or dysuria) are experienced in as many as 15% of patients. Infertility may accompany endometriosis; however, in the work of O'Connor, this was observed in a minority of patients (13%).

Findings on examination include fixed uterine retroversion (up to 15% of patients); tenderness and nodularity in the cul-de-sac and rectovaginal septum (up to 30% of patients), best confirmed by rectovaginal examination; and uterine tenderness or enlargement with adnexal swelling (up to 20% to 30% of patients).

Figure 93-2

Endometriosis
Pelvis — Sites of Implantation

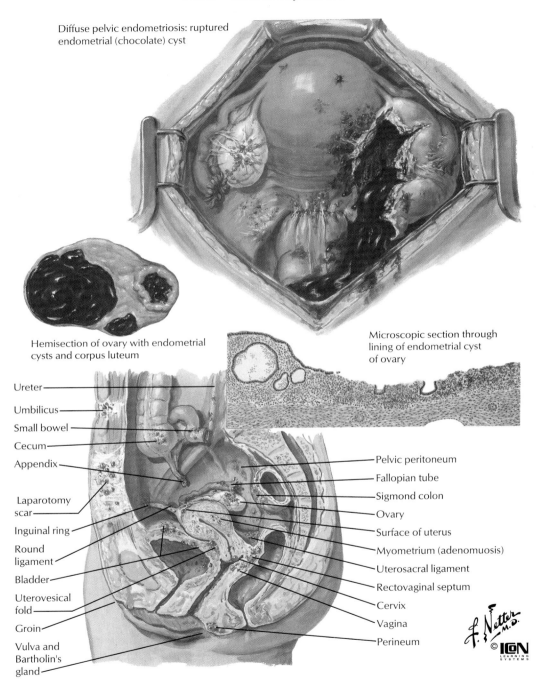

Diffuse pelvic endometriosis: ruptured endometrial (chocolate) cyst

Hemisection of ovary with endometrial cysts and corpus luteum

Microscopic section through lining of endometrial cyst of ovary

Ureter

Umbilicus

Small bowel

Cecum

Appendix

Laparotomy scar

Inguinal ring

Round ligament

Bladder

Uterovesical fold

Groin

Vulva and Bartholin's gland

Pelvic peritoneum

Fallopian tube

Sigmond colon

Ovary

Surface of uterus

Myometrium (adenomuosis)

Uterosacral ligament

Rectovaginal septum

Cervix

Vagina

Perineum

DIFFERENTIAL DIAGNOSIS

The differential diagnosis includes pelvic inflammatory disease, ovarian neoplasms, intermittent ovarian torsion, hemorrhagic ovarian cysts, uterine myomas with degeneration, adenomyosis, primary dysmenorrhea, and functional bowel disease such as irritable bowel syndrome.

DIAGNOSTIC APPROACH

Although symptoms are strongly suggestive of the disease process, definitive diagnosis requires biopsies taken at the time of laparoscopy or laparotomy to confirm the presence of extrauterine endometrial glands and stroma. Staging is based on the updated scoring system from the American Society for Reproductive Medicine.

MANAGEMENT AND THERAPY

The goal of therapy is relief of pain and preservation of fertility. Both medical and surgical options have been effective in relief of pain when compared to expectant management. Medical options include gonadotrophin-releasing hormone agonists, oral contraceptives and other hormonal treatments, and danazol. Surgical options include ablation or excision of implants, excision of endometriomas, lysis of adhesions, and even appendectomy. The appendix is involved in up to 13% of cases. Other procedures include presacral neurectomy and uterosacral nerve ablation. The surgical approach can involve laparoscopy or laparotomy. Lastly, definitive surgical management, when other options have proven unsuccessful in symptom relief, requires total abdominal hysterectomy with or without bilateral salpingo-oophorectomy.

Medical Therapy

While the ultimate goal of endometriosis therapy is pain relief and protection of fertility, the goal of medical therapy is amenorrhea. Available medical therapies appear equally effective for treatment of symptoms, improvement in American Fertility staging of disease scores, and in recurrence rates when compared to placebo. Recurrence rates after discontinuation of therapy have been reported as 5% to 15% in the first year and as high as 40% to 50% in 5 years. Recurrence appears directly related to the extent of the original disease — 35% in women with minimal disease and 75% in women with severe disease. Side effect profile appears to be the primary factor in selection of the medical option utilized.

Gonadotropin-releasing hormone (GRH) agonists bind to receptors leading to decreased gonadotropin secretion and subsequent decreased ovarian steroidogenesis. Therapy is usually recommended for 6 months. Agents available (leuprolide acetate, nafarelin acetate, and goserelin acetate) can be administered via intramuscular, intranasal, and subcutaneous routes. Medical oophorectomy leads to endometriosis pain relief in 75% to 90% of women with disease. Bothersome side effects include hot flashes, vaginal dryness, insomnia, headaches, diminished libido, mood swings, and breast changes. Bone density may decrease by 2% to 7% during the 6-month course of treatment but completely recovers by 12 to 24 months after completion of therapy. "Add-back" therapy with low doses of estrogen and progesterone has been used to ease side effects associated primarily with estrogen deficiency and appears to attenuate loss of bone mineral density while not interfering with the effectiveness on GRH agonist therapy.

Oral contraceptives taken continuously to induce amenorrhea are effective therapy for endometriosis. While 80% of women experience symptom improvement, side effects most common with this therapy include weight gain and breast tenderness. Other hormonal therapies include daily medroxyprogesterone (30 mg orally each day) and depo-medroxyprogesterone (150 to 200 mg intramuscularly every 3 months). The antiprogesterone mifepristone (RU486) has also demonstrated success in inducing amenorrhea.

Danazol, an attenuated androgen, is a derivative of 17-alpha ethinyltestosterone. While its mechanism of action is not entirely clear, danazol binds to androgen and progesterone receptors as well as to sex hormone-binding globulin, inhibiting ovarian steroidogenesis as well as mid-cycle luteinizing hormone release. Amenorrhea is usually induced within 6 to 8 weeks of initiating therapy. Side effects include acne, hot flashes, depression, headaches, weight gain, and altered libido. Other androgen-related effects such as increased facial hair, clitoral hypertrophy, and voice changes are experienced by 80% of patients. As a result, 20% of women discontinue treatment.

Surgical Therapy

Surgical therapy is often used for diagnostic purposes and after the failure of medical therapy. Conservative therapy includes diagnostic laparoscopy accompanied by laser or electrocautery ablation of implants. Laser ablation has been effective in 95% of women at 18 months after surgery. Midline pelvic pain has been relieved by laparoscopic uterosacral nerve ablation and presacral neurectomy; however, there are no evidence-based studies comparing these procedures to placebo or sham procedures. More definitive surgical therapy includes hysterectomy with preservation of one or both ovaries for women in their 20s and 30s. In women for whom future fertility is not a consideration, definitive surgical therapy via total abdominal hysterectomy with bilateral salpingo-oophorectomy may be warranted.

FUTURE DIRECTIONS

The remarkable heterogeneity of endometriosis provides both a diagnostic and management challenge. While therapy at this time is focused on steroidogenesis suppression or surgical ablation or excision, future therapies may be directed toward some of the multiple immunologic mediators potentially involved in endometriosis development. Evidence-based medicine should guide therapy based on trials designed to study the effectiveness of current therapies, including the comparison of medical and surgical approaches. With this information, both the patient and her clinician can make better-informed treatment decisions in dealing with this common and at times disabling condition.

REFERENCES

Revised American Society for Reproductive Medicine classification of endometriosis: 1996. *Fertil Steril.* 1997;67:817-821.

Farquhar C, Sutton C. The evidence for the management of endometriosis. *Curr Opin Obstet Gynecol.* 1998;10:321-332.

Fedele L, Parazzini F, Bianchi S, Arcaini L, Candiani GB. Stage and localization of pelvic endometriosis and pain. *Fertil Steril.* 1990;53:155-158.

Halme J, Hammond MG, Hulka JF, Raj SG, Talbert LM. Retrograde menstruation in healthy women and in patients with endometriosis. *Obstet Gynecol.* 1984;64:151-154.

Kruitwagen RF, Poels LG, Willemsen WN, de Ronde IJ, Jap PH, Rolland R. Endometrial epithelial cells in peritoneal fluid during early follicular phase. *Fertil Steril.* 1991;55:297-303.

O'Connor, DT. *Endometriosis (Current Reviews in Obstetrics and Gynaecology).* Edinburgh, Scotland: Churchill Livingstone; 1987.

Simpson JL, Elias S, Malinak LR, Buttram VC Jr. Heritable aspects of endometriosis. I. Genetic studies. *Am J Obstet Gynecol.* 1980;137:327-331.

Stenchever MA, Droegemueller W, Herbst AL, Mishell DR Jr. *Comprehensive Gynecology.* 4th ed. St Louis, Mo: Mosby; 2001.

Chapter 94
Erectile Dysfunction

Culley C. Carson III

Erectile dysfunction (ED) is the inability to achieve, and/or maintain an erection adequate for sexual intercourse. Based on extrapolated data from the Massachusetts Male Aging Study, ED affects some 20 to 30 million American men, most of who are older than 50. This epidemiologic study of a homogeneous suburban Boston community surveyed 1,709 men and reports 52% of men aged 40 to 70 had erectile dysfunction: 10% had complete ED, 25% moderate, and 17% minimal. The prevalence of ED increases with age, with moderate and complete ED increasing most markedly. The percentages of ED were increased substantially in men with risk factors including cardiac disease, antihypertensive and vasoactive drug use, and tobacco use.

PHYSIOLOGY OF ERECTIONS

Sexual stimulation causes release of the neurotransmitter nitric oxide (NO) from nerve endings in the corpus cavernosum, in turn increasing blood flow to the corpora cavernosa (Figure 94-1). NO production results in relaxation of the corpus cavernosum smooth muscle tissue. The venous structures beneath the tunica albuginea are compressed, inhibiting venous outflow and producing a rigid erection. In the penis, NO is available from nitrergic nerve and endothelial cells. By stimulating the guanylate cyclase system and increasing cyclic guanicine monophosphate (cGMP), nitric oxide causes an efflux of calcium from the smooth muscle cell, producing relaxation. cGMP is broken down by the enzyme phosphodiesterase (PDE5). The PDE inhibitors such as sildenafil, papaverine, and newer PDE inhibitors, prolong the presence of cGMP and facilitate the relaxation of corpus cavernosum smooth muscle. The predominate PDE type in corpus cavernosum is type 5 (PDE5).

ETIOLOGY AND PATHOGENESIS

ED has both organic and psychogenic etiologies with 60% of patients having organic ED caused by vasculogenic, neurogenic, hormonal, or smooth muscle abnormalities (Figure 94-2). Fewer than 40% of patients have pure psychogenic ED. It is unclear why men with psychogenic ED demonstrate erectile dysfunction. We do know that stress disorders and depression produce an over-activity of alpha agonists in the corpus cavernosum smooth muscle tissue, and this imbalance of alpha stimulation may inhibit smooth muscle relaxation.

CLINICAL PRESENTATION
Risk Factors

Risk factors for ED include systemic diseases that produce vascular abnormalities, including hyperlipidemia, diabetes mellitus, the results of hypertension and antihypertensive therapy, and atherosclerosis.

Neurogenic erectile dysfunction is seen with multiple sclerosis, diabetes mellitus, paraplegia, and following radical pelvic surgery or radiation for pelvic malignancy such as prostate, colon, or bladder cancer.

Hormonal abnormalities and hypogonadism are also risk factors for ED, producing not only central nervous system abnormalities and low libido, but also local changes in corpus cavernosum smooth muscle relaxation.

Psychologic causes are significant, and ED is frequently associated with depression, even of mild degree. Treatment for depression using SSRI medication further enhances ED by decreasing and delaying ejaculatory function.

Evaluation

A careful general and sexual history is the cornerstone in the evaluation and treatment of patients with erectile dysfunction. History should include information regarding age of onset, associated lifestyle changes at onset, speed of onset,

Figure 94-1

Cellular Mechanisms of Penile Smooth Muscle Relaxation

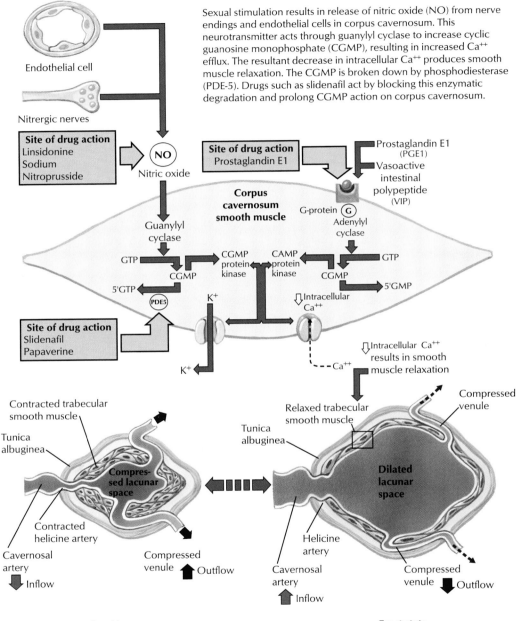

Sexual stimulation results in release of nitric oxide (NO) from nerve endings and endothelial cells in corpus cavernosum. This neurotransmitter acts through guanylyl cyclase to increase cyclic guanosine monophosphate (CGMP), resulting in increased Ca^{++} efflux. The resultant decrease in intracellular Ca^{++} produces smooth muscle relaxation. The CGMP is broken down by phosphodiesterase (PDE-5). Drugs such as slidenafil act by blocking this enzymatic degradation and prolong CGMP action on corpus cavernosum.

Flaccid state
Contracted trabecular smooth muscle limits inflow of blood into lacunar spaces while venous outflow is high enough to prevent lancular dilation

Erect state
Relaxed trabecuilar smooth muscle allows increased inflow of blood, dilated lacunar spaces compress venules against tunica albuginea, decreasing outflow

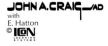

JOHN A. CRAIG—AD
with
E. Hatton
© ICON

and the presence or absence of erections with other partners, during masturbation, and at night and in the early am. Patients should be asked about ejaculatory function, post-ejaculatory pain, and ejaculatory volume. Careful questioning regarding decreased libido may suggest a hormonal cause, but more often is associated with clinical depression.

Patients who present with organic ED most often have a gradual onset beginning with intermittent loss of erections, decreased duration, and difficulty with maintaining erections until ejaculation. History is the most proficient method of identifying patients complaining of premature ejaculation who may also present for evaluation of ED.

Psychogenic ED most often begins with abrupt onset precipitated by psychologic abnormalities such as depression, anxiety disorder, changes in lifestyle, or relationship problems. These men usually have preserved nocturnal and morning erections, and may be functional with masturbation. Patients with organic ED also have secondary psychologic ED. Patients with pure loss of libido or with other symptoms of androgen deficiency of the aging male can be identified by a hormone profile.

Physical Examination

The physical examination is focused on secondary sex characteristics, hair distribution, and genitalia. Evaluation of peripheral pulses, neurologic reflexes such as the bulbocavernosus reflex and anal sphincter tone may help to identify some patients with peripheral neuropathy from nerve injury or diabetes. Changes in testicular size and consistency may be associated with primary hypogonadism. General physical examination of blood pressure, lower extremity reflexes and pulses, and visual fields (to evaluate pituitary tumors) may suggest underlying systemic causes for erectile dysfunction.

DIAGNOSTIC APPROACH
Laboratory Investigation

Because ED may be the first symptom of diabetes, hypercholesterolemia, hypertension, or other systemic disease, it is important to evaluate patients thoroughly for each of these disorders. A hormone profile should include a morning total testosterone. If the total testosterone is abnormal, a follow-up repeat total testosterone, free testosterone, LH, and prolactin may identify patients with androgen deficiency, pituitary tumors, or other causes of hypogonadism. Testosterone is typically low and prolactin high in patients who have pituitary tumors or chronic renal failure on hemodialysis. A lipid profile, hemoglobin A1C, and other general medical studies may be helpful.

For patients requiring additional investigation prior to surgical reconstruction or vascular bypass, specialized investigation such as Doppler penile blood flow studies following injection of vasoactive agents, nocturnal penile tumescence monitoring studies, and pelvic angiography may be helpful. Candidates for vascular bypass are usually young men with solitary pelvic artery lesions and a strong history of perineal or pelvic trauma. Vascular bypass surgery in older patients is rarely successful, especially if ED is associated with hypercholesterolemia, diabetes, hypertension, or smoking.

Nocturnal penile tumescence monitoring studies may be helpful in differentiating organic and psychogenic ED in some patients.

MANAGEMENT AND THERAPY

Initial treatment should focus on modifying medication and lifestyle abnormalities. Smoking cessation, managing diabetes, hypercholesterolemia, and hypertension may improve erectile function and facilitate medical treatment.

Modifying antihypertensive medications to include "erection-hospitable agents" such as alpha-blockers, ace inhibitors, and calcium channel blockers may maintain antihypertensive therapy with restoration of erectile function. Patients with low testosterone should receive injectable or topical testosterone supplements.

If depression or relationship issues are a significant problem, sexual counseling may be helpful in addition to pharmacologic treatment. Office counseling with patient and partner may facilitate understanding of the probable causes of erectile dysfunction, treatment alternatives, and expectations.

First-Line Therapy

The introduction of oral agents such as sildenafil in 1998 has revolutionized first-line treatment of erectile dysfunction. Sildenafil, as well as some newer agents in development, are selective phosphodiesterase type 5 (PDE5) inhibitors that facilitate cGMP and subsequent corpus cavernosal smooth muscle relaxation. There is improvement in erectile function 30 to 60 minutes following ingestion of sildenafil. The most popular starting dose is 50 mg although most patients respond best to 100 mg. As many as 8 trials may be required for full success and effectiveness. Side effects include headache, dyspepsia, facial flushing, and blue vision. Sildenafil has been reported to be significantly better in producing erections than placebo in patients with diabetes mellitus, spinal cord injury, hypercholesterolemia, depression, cardiac disease, following radical prostatectomy, and in psychogenic erectile dysfunction. While sildenafil is effective in virtually all etiologies and severities of ED, it is least effective in patients with severe vascular disease. Sildenafil is generally an extremely safe drug; however, it does have additive affects with nitrate agents used for coronary artery disease, producing severe transient hypotension. *The use of sildenafil with nitrate drugs is absolutely contraindicated.* In patients taking sildenafil following radical prostatectomy, results are best in those receiving a bilateral nerve-sparing radical prostatectomy. Sildenafil treatment following non-nerve-sparing prostatectomy or pelvic radiation therapy is often unsuccessful.

Second-Line Therapy

Additional therapeutic alternatives are available if oral agents fail to improve erectile function. Intracavernosal pharmacotherapy is most effective in producing physiologic erections. This therapy can be carried out with prostaglandin E1 (PGE1) or a combination of papaverine and phentolamine. PGE1 can be administered by intracavernosal injection or transurethral pellet.

Transurethral PGE1 is available in 250, 500, or 1,000 mcg. Its effectiveness is approximately 30% in large clinical studies. A small applicator with a pellet of prostaglandin E1 is placed in the urethra. After the pellet is deposited and the applicator removed, the patient stimulates the urethra to allow PGE1 to enter the corpus cavernosum. Erection usually occurs in 10 to 15 minutes and is maintained for as long as 40 minutes. Rarely, side effects include prolonged erection or priapism,

and significant penile pain, aching and urethral burning can occur. While this agent is an excellent addition to patients with penile prostheses for further engorgement, its success in patients with erectile dysfunction of significant organic etiology has been disappointing.

Intracavernosal injection of PGE1 has been widely used for over a decade. It appears to be safe, although penile aching and occasional prolonged erections do occur. Initial dose of PGE1 varies from 2.5 to 5 mcg. Patients with significant vasculogenic erectile dysfunction require higher starting and maintenance doses. After an initial in-office titration to a dose that produces a firm erection satisfactory for sexual intercourse that lasts no longer than 60 minutes, many men may require at-home dose adjustment. If erections last more than 4 hours, patients should be advised to go to the emergency room for treatment using an alpha agonist such as intracavernosal phenylephrine or aspiration therapy. While this complication is rare, early treatment will preserve future erectile function. If intracavernosal PGE1 is ineffective or produces excessive pain, a combination of papaverine with or without phentolamine and PGE1 may produce satisfactory erectile function with less penile discomfort. Side effects from this combination include prolonged erections and priapism, corpus cavernosum fibrosis, and occasional transient hypotension.

In addition to prolonged erections and priapism, side effects from PGE1, as well as papaverine and phentolamine, include penile pain. This complication is most marked with PGE1 and occurs in approximately 20% of injections. Patients may also observe hematoma, edema, and occasional corpus cavernosum fibrosis (<5%). Despite initial success rates in excess of 70%, few patients continue injection therapy for more than 3 to 4 years. The reasons for discontinuation include mental anxiety, inadequate erections, penile pain, and poor patient and partner satisfaction. Several series have reported a less than 50% continuation rate at 60 months.

DEVICES FOR TREATMENT OF ERECTILE DYSFUNCTION

For many years, vacuum erection devices have been used to stimulate, facilitate, and prolong duration of erections. These external devices cre-

Figure 94-2

Etiology and Pathogenesis
of Erectile Dysfunction

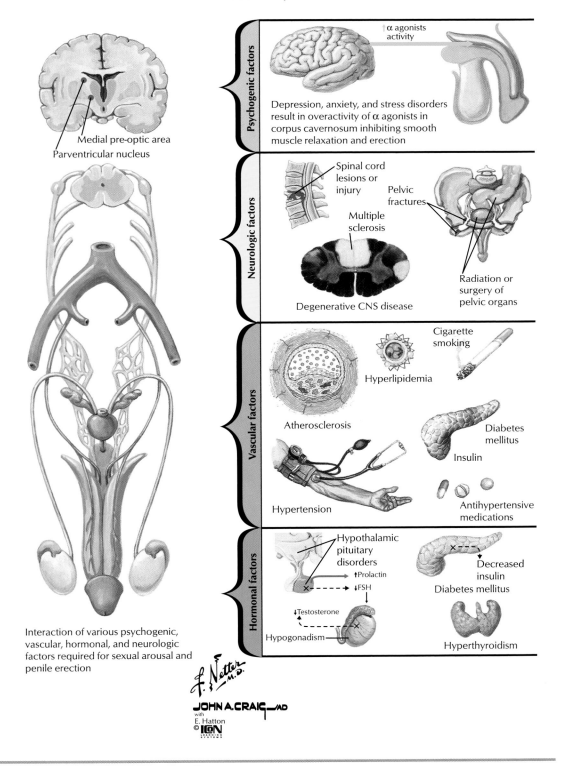

Medial pre-optic area
Parventricular nucleus

Interaction of various psychogenic, vascular, hormonal, and neurologic factors required for sexual arousal and penile erection

Psychogenic factors

↑α agonists activity

Depression, anxiety, and stress disorders result in overactivity of α agonists in corpus cavernosum inhibiting smooth muscle relaxation and erection

Neurologic factors

Spinal cord lesions or injury

Pelvic fractures

Multiple sclerosis

Degenerative CNS disease

Radiation or surgery of pelvic organs

Vascular factors

Cigarette smoking

Hyperlipidemia

Atherosclerosis

Diabetes mellitus

Insulin

Hypertension

Antihypertensive medications

Hormonal factors

Hypothalamic pituitary disorders

↑Prolactin

↓FSH

Decreased insulin

Diabetes mellitus

↓Testosterone

Hypogonadism

Hyperthyroidism

JOHN A. CRAIG—AD
with
E. Hatton
©ICON

ate a vacuum around the penis to produce engorgement and tumescence, maintained by a constrictive ring placed at the base of the penis. While the erections that ensue are less natural for stimulating erectile function, they are satisfactory for vaginal penetration and sexual intercourse. The constriction devices may produce penile pain, bruising, scarring, and Peyronie's disease. They may also inhibit ejaculations. While the cost is low, patient satisfaction is limited. Counseling and careful instruction prior to initiating use can increase patient satisfaction.

Implantation of penile prostheses is a successful, important method for restoring erectile function in severe ED, and for reconstructing the penis of patients with significant Peyronie's disease or priapism. These surgically implanted devices are most often of the inflatable variety and consist of two hollow cylinders placed in the corpora cavernosa of the penis and connected to a small pump device placed in the scrotum. Fluid (normal saline or water) is supplied by a reservoir placed beneath the rectus muscles of the abdomen. Patients can feel and compress the pump device in the scrotum, fill the cylinders of the corpora cavernosa, and maintain an erection of normal sensation and rigidity throughout sexual intercourse. The device can then be deflated for concealment with excellent cosmetic results. The longevity of these devices is quite satisfactory with 93% of devices functional at 3 years, 86% at 5 years, and 76% at 10 years after implantation. Mechanical malfunction is treated with device replacement. Patient satisfaction has been reported in excess of 90%.

Androgen Replacement Therapy

In patients with androgen deficiency of the aging male or hypogonadism, testosterone replacement is necessary to enhance libido and facilitate other medical treatment. Testosterone replacement therapy is carried out using long-acting injectable agents, such as testosterone enanthate or cypionate 200 mg every 2 to 3 weeks, and topical testosterone patches or gel. Topical treatment is more physiologic with high testosterone levels in the morning and low in the evening, similar to the testosterone levels of young sexually active males. Similarly, testosterone metabolites estradiol and dihydrotestosterone are maintained best with the topical prepa-

rations. The goal of testosterone replacement therapy is to restore testosterone levels to the normal physiologic range. The use of testosterone in eugonadal men with psychogenic erectile dysfunction, while raising testosterone beyond normal levels, is both ineffective and associated with significant potential complications. Testosterone supplementation can be associated with activation of carcinoma of the prostate, increased hematocrit and lipid levels, as well as increased benign prostatic hyperplasia. Patients treated with testosterone supplementation should be carefully evaluated twice yearly with digital rectal examination, PSA, lipid profile and hematocrit. For patients with chronic renal failure or macroprolactinomas, normalization of prolactin prior to testosterone treatment is critical. Use of agents such as bromocriptine or cabergoline, in addition to testosterone replacement, will produce the best subsequent results.

FUTURE DIRECTIONS

The treatment of ED was revolutionized by the introduction of sildenafil in 1998. Newer agents are currently being investigated and will provide additional methods of treatment for patients with ED. Newer PDE5 inhibitors such as vardenafil and tadolafil are in late stages of clinical investigation and will be marketed soon. Central nervous system acting agents will also be available for stimulating erections. The first of these agents, apomorphine SL, is currently approved and in use in Europe. This agent, which stimulates dopamine receptors in the erectile center of the mid-brain, has been demonstrated in phase 3 clinical trials to be effective in producing erectile function with minimal side effects. Side effects include nausea, vomiting, and syncope in small numbers of patients with predominate first dose effect. Additional central nervous system acting agents are currently in clinical trials and should be available as first-line therapy in addition to PDE5 agents in patients with inadequate response. Newer injectable agents are also being investigated including the novel potassium channel opener, which requires no refrigeration and has little penile discomfort associated with treatment. Topical preparations of PGE1 have completed clinical trials and will soon be available for general use.

Active research is underway to evaluate the feasibility and effectiveness of gene therapy for erectile dysfunction. Gene therapy to restore nitric oxide synthase concentrations, endothelial cell function, and potassium channel function in the corpus cavernosum smooth muscle appears, in animal models, to be an excellent method for restoring erectile function lost through diabetes, hypercholesterolemia, and other causes of vascular disease. This mode of therapy may provide a long-term solution for many patients with erectile dysfunction.

Despite the strides made in pharmacologic treatment, many patients will still require surgical reconstruction using penile prostheses. The currently available penile implant and prostheses have been modified and improved over the past 25 years to provide safe, reliable reconstruction for penile abnormalities and erectile dysfunction with low expected complications and morbidity, and high patient satisfaction.

REFERENCES

Carson CC III. Erectile dysfunction: diagnosis and management with newer oral agents. *BUMC Proceedings.* 2000;13:356-360.

Carson CC III, Kirby RS, Goldstein I, eds. *Textbook of Erectile Dysfunction.* Oxford, England: Isis Medical Media; 1999.

Feldman HA, Goldstein I, Hatzichristou DG, Krane RJ, McKinlay JB. Impotence and its medical and psychosocial correlates: results of the Massachusetts Male Aging Study. *J Urol.* 1994;151:54-61.

Goldstein I, Lue TF, Padma-Nathan H, Rosen RC, Steers WD, Wicker PA. Oral sildenafil in the treatment of erectile dysfunction. Sildenafil Study Group. *N Engl J Med.* 1998;338: 1397-1404.

Morales A, Heaton JP, Carson CC III. Andropause: a misnomer for a true clinical entity. *J Urol.* 2000;163:705-712.

Chapter 95

Infertility

William R. Meyer and Ringland S. Murray, Jr

Primary infertility is the absence of conception after 1 year of unprotected intercourse. Secondary infertility is a similar malady in a couple that has previously borne at least one child. The risk of infertility in those age 35 to 45 is twice that of those who are 30 to 34 years old. Infertility affects 10% to 15% of couples and, although the cause may be attributed to abnormalities solely in the female or in the male, in many cases, it represents an abnormality in the reproductive potential of both partners. Hence, infertility is a disorder of "the couple" and should be approached from this perspective.

Deferment of marriage and postponement of pregnancy within the marriage are the most obvious reasons for an increase in infertility seen worldwide. The decline in fertility among married couples with advancing age is well documented. All couples need to be aware of the normal time necessary to achieve a pregnancy (Table 95-1).

ETIOLOGY AND PATHOGENESIS/ DIAGNOSTIC APPROACH

The evaluation of infertility focuses on three primary areas that reflect etiology and pathogenesis: oocyte production, sperm production, and the presence of tubal or other pelvic factors. Many couples have more than 1 factor at work, and the assessment is designed to reveal problems in these 3 areas. Only 10% of affected couples have unexplained infertility.

Diagnosis of Ovulation

Women who have regular monthly menstrual cycles are almost always ovulatory (Figure 95-1). Indirect confirmation of ovulation can be obtained by 1) basal body temperature (BBT) graphing, 2) serum progesterone levels, 3) urinary luteinizing hormone (LH) monitoring, or 4) endometrial biopsy. BBT is obtained by the patient using a special thermometer that magnifies the physiological range of normal body temperatures taken before rising from bed before any physical activity. A rise in temperature of one half of a degree coincides with progesterone levels greater than or equal to 4 ng/mL, and occurs 2 to 3 days after the serum LH peak.

Home urinary LH testing is used to assist in timing coitus after ovulation has been confirmed. Optimal timing for coitus starts 2 days before ovulation. An endometrial biopsy taken approximately 10 days after presumed ovulation is a reliable, yet expensive and invasive assessment of ovulation. The biopsy is used more often after ovulation has been confirmed to diagnose a luteal phase deficiency, as evidenced by delayed endometrial maturation in excess of 2 days.

Serum progesterone levels less than 3 ng/mL do not confirm ovulation; a luteal phase progesterone value greater than 6.5 ng/mL is required. If ovulation cannot be confirmed by these tests, the patient is experiencing some form of anovulation.

Anovulation

Ovulation relies on the cyclic interplay between the hypothalamus, the pituitary gland,

Table 95-1
Average Time to Conception in Couple Attaining Pregnancy

Months of Exposure	Pregnant
3	57%
6	72%
12	85%
24	93%

Adapted from Speroff, Leon. *Clinical Gynecologic Endocrinology and Infertility.* 6th ed. LWW, 1999: 1021 and Guttmacher AF, Factors affecting normal expectancy of conception. *JAMA.* 1956;161:855

Figure 95-1

Assessment of Ovulation

Ovulatory phase
Hormonal and physical findings indicate ovulation occurred

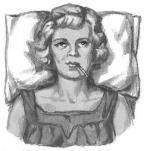

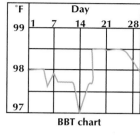

°F | Day
BBT chart

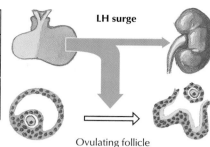

LH surge

Ovulating follicle

Basal body temperature (BBT). Detects signs of ovulation

Preovulatory follicle

Ruptured follicle

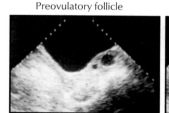

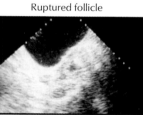

Positive reading

Ovulation detection kit detects urinary metabolites of luteinizing hormone (LH)

Serial follicular ultrasonography. Monitors follicular rupture

Luteal phase

↑ Serum progesterone

Corpus luteum

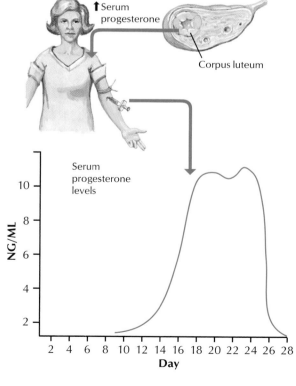

Serum progesterone levels

NG/ML

10
8
6
4
2

2 4 6 8 10 12 14 16 18 20 22 24 26 28
Day

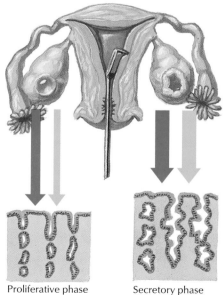

Proliferative phase

Secretory phase

Endometrial biopsy and dating. Provides evidence of functioning corpus luteum and end organ response

JOHN A. CRAIG—AD
© ICN

Figure 95-2

Causes of Ovulatory Dysfunction

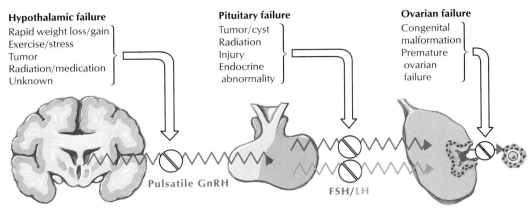

Hypothalamic failure
Rapid weight loss/gain
Exercise/stress
Tumor
Radiation/medication
Unknown

Pituitary failure
Tumor/cyst
Radiation
Injury
Endocrine
abnormality

Ovarian failure
Congenital
malformation
Premature
ovarian
failure

Pulsatile GnRH

FSH/LH

Hypothalamic dysfunction is most common cause of ovulatory dysfunction

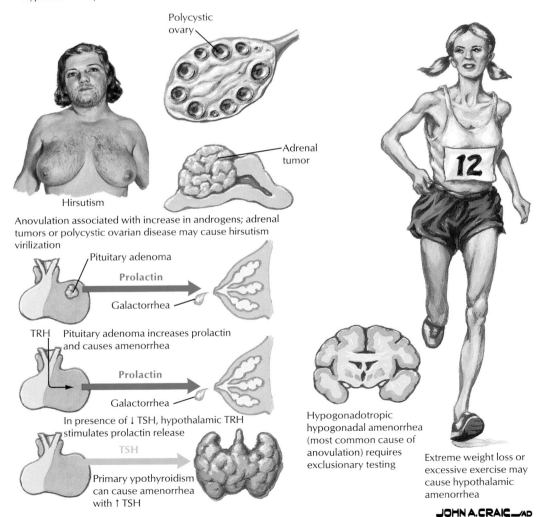

Polycystic
ovary

Adrenal
tumor

Hirsutism

Anovulation associated with increase in androgens; adrenal
tumors or polycystic ovarian disease may cause hirsutism
virilization

Pituitary adenoma

Prolactin

Galactorrhea

Pituitary adenoma increases prolactin
and causes amenorrhea

TRH

Prolactin

Galactorrhea

In presence of ↓ TSH, hypothalamic TRH
stimulates prolactin release

TSH

Primary ypothyroidism
can cause amenorrhea
with ↑ TSH

Hypogonadotropic
hypogonadal amenorrhea
(most common cause of
anovulation) requires
exclusionary testing

Extreme weight loss or
excessive exercise may
cause hypothalamic
amenorrhea

JOHN A. CRAIG—AD
© ICON

and the ovary. A malfunction at any point in this axis may lead to anovulation (Figure 95-2). Anovulation is a type of ovulatory dysfunction that is distinct from ovarian failure; the ovary is capable of producing eggs, but the hormonal milieu makes ovulation difficult. Often, the specific underlying cause is not known. The most common cause of anovulation occurs in chronic hyperandrogenic anovulation syndrome, known as polycystic ovarian syndrome (PCOS) that affects up to 10% of reproductive-aged women.

Once anovulation has been confirmed, the anovulation workup can be simplified into an algorithmic approach to pinpoint the disruption. The investigation begins with a serum pregnancy test followed by serum levels of thyroid-stimulating hormone and prolactin and finally 17-hydroxyprogesterone. A 24-hour urine cortisol to rule out Cushing's syndrome should be considered in the hirsute patient. An elevation in any of these levels may pinpoint the source of infertility.

A progesterone withdrawal test helps determine if the patient is anovulatory or if the ovary is unresponsive. If a woman has an induced bleed after taking progesterone for 10 days, her ovaries are producing adequate estrogen to build her uterine endometrial lining, and she should be able to ovulate with appropriate treatment. If she does not have menses, either the ovary has failed (ovarian failure, premature menopause), or she has a hypothalamic-pituitary disorder and the ovary is not receiving satisfactory gonadotropin stimulation to produce estrogen. Infrequently, patients who fail to bleed have Asherman's syndrome, scarring of the uterine lining due to previous uterine surgery.

Ovarian failure is confirmed by measuring a serum follicle-stimulating hormone (FSH) level. A level >40 mIU/mL is consistent with menopause. PCOS is a diagnosis of exclusion and is made by the presence of oligoovulation and hirsutism. Testing for insulin resistance, which may affect 80% of obese and 25% of thin PCOS patients, is becoming standard as the association between hyperinsulinemia and hyperandrogenism is clarified. A fasting glucose: insulin (mIU/mL) ratio less than 4.5 suggests insulin resistance.

Treatment of Anovulation

Clomiphene citrate (Clomid) is a drug so commonly prescribed by primary care physicians that its proper use deserves discussion. Clomiphene citrate is a partial agonist/antagonist at the estrogen receptor that competitively opposes the actions of the more potent estradiol. It induces ovulation by decreasing the effects of estrogen at the pituitary gland, thereby reducing feedback inhibition and allowing for greater FSH production.

Clomiphene citrate, standard therapy for PCOS patients desiring fertility through ovulation induction, is successful in 70% of patients; although a significant number of patients are resistant or cannot tolerate the anti-estrogen side effects of clomiphene. Other side effects result from the anti-estrogen effect on the hypothalamus–pituitary axis (hot flushes, emotional lability) and uterus (poor endometrial development and decreased cervical mucus). Informed use should include discussions of multiple gestations and the risk of ovarian cancer.

Of patients who take clomiphene citrate, 80% will ovulate and 50% will conceive. The risk of multiple gestations is approximately double the baseline of 2%; most multiples are twins. There have been concerns over a theoretical increased risk of ovarian cancer with prolonged use (greater than 12 months). Once ovulation is documented, clomiphene citrate should not be used for more than a 6-month trial.

Clomiphene citrate requires proof of ovulation (LH kit or serum progesterone) and an intact hypothalamic-pituitary-ovarian axis to be effective. The empirically derived starting dose is 50 mg daily on cycle days 5 to 9, cycle day 1 being the first day of bleeding. If the patient does not ovulate, increase the dose by 50 mg each month to a maximum of 250 mg daily; 70% of women who ovulate respond before the 150-mg dose. To confirm ovulation, an LH surge should be documented and a serum progesterone level should be greater than 6.5 ng/mL after the surge. A false-positive LH surge may be detected if monitoring occurs within 3 days of completion of clomiphene citrate.

If the patient does not respond at the 150-mg dose, adjunctive therapies dictate referral to a reproductive endocrinologist. Amelioration of hyperinsulinemia (insulin resistance) in patients with PCOS results in lower ovarian androgen production and a subsequent increased rate of spontaneous (or clomiphene induced) ovulation.

The combination use of clomiphene and metformin, an oral biguanide associated with improvements in insulin sensitivity and lower plasma insulin levels, to induce ovulation in insulin-resistant women is becoming popular. Nestler studied the effects of metformin in obese PCOS patients and reported that 19 of 21 women ovulated using both metformin and clomiphene citrate compared with only 2 of 25 (8%) women who used clomiphene citrate only.

Premature Ovarian Failure

Failure to experience a withdrawal uterine bleed after progesterone administration suggests ovarian failure. An elevated serum FSH level confirms the diagnosis. Premature ovarian failure is usually idiopathic, but chromosomal evaluation in patients with primary or secondary ovarian failure before age 35 is suggested. Estrogen/progestin hormone replacement is the treatment of choice. Childbearing can result only from oocyte donation. Evaluation of adrenal and thyroid function has proven futile because polyglandular failure is rare.

Hypothalamic Pituitary Disorders

Hypothalamic pituitary disorders are of idiopathic origin most commonly. The lack of progestin withdrawal bleeding accompanied by normal, low, or immeasurable serum gonadotropin levels suggests the diagnosis. MRI of the pituitary gland is recommended in idiopathic cases. Estrogen/progestin hormone therapy is the treatment of choice. For the infertile woman, the use of exogenous gonadotropins is necessary to induce ovulation. Additional exogenous LH is often required to induce ovulation in women with hypogonadotropic hypogonadism (Figure 95-2).

Hyperprolactinemia

Hyperprolactinemia may cause dysfunctional ovarian function (oligoovulation). A fasting serum prolactin level, if elevated, should be repeated to confirm the diagnosis. Excess prolactin may occur with primary hypothyroidism due to a compensatory increase in thyrotropin-releasing hormone that stimulates prolactin release. Transitory elevations of prolactin may result in oligoovulation and galactorrhea. Breast manipulation, sexual relations, exercise, stress, and heavy protein meal ingestion may result in transitory hyperprolactine-

mia. Many psychotropic drugs also result in an elevated prolactin level. Head MRI that includes the pituitary fossa may be required to exclude an adenoma in patients with moderately elevated prolactin levels. Dopamine agonists remain the mainstay of treatment. Bromocriptine should be initiated at bedtime (1.25 mg) due to potential initial episodes of orthostatic hypotension. Increasing dosages are used weekly to normalize prolactin levels. Cabergoline, a dopamine agonist, is as effective as bromocriptine in lowering prolactin values with fewer side effects. Oral dopamine agonists are usually discontinued once the patient has conceived. Continuation of therapy during pregnancy may be recommended when a known pituitary macroadenoma (greater than 10 mm) is present (Figure 95-2).

Diminished Ovarian Reserve

When the evaluation of the infertile couple yields no clear etiology, diminished ovarian reserve should be excluded. The clomiphene challenge test involves checking baseline (day 3) serum estradiol and FSH, administration of clomiphene citrate 100 mg per day, days 5 to 9, then repeat measurement of FSH on day 10. Elevated baseline or day 10 values (i.e., FSH >10 mIU/mL, estradiol >75 pg/mL, dependent on assay used) suggest compromised ovarian function and decreased fecundity.

Tubal Damage

Tubal damage may be responsible for up to 50% of cases of infertility in women. The hysterosalpingogram is the most practical means of diagnosing tubal disease. The care provider should treat unilateral or bilateral partial distal obstruction with a short course of antibiotics after a hysterosalpingogram (Figure 95-3). Tubal disease most commonly results from previous pelvic infection, pelvic surgery, or endometriosis and is usually classified as proximal or distal. Distal tubal occlusions may lead to dilated, fluid-filled tubes (hydrosalpinges). Reparation of hydrosalpinges, done through the laparoscope most commonly, results in a maximum pregnancy rate of 30%. Ectopic pregnancy is not an infrequent sequela of reparative tubal surgery. Proximal tubal disease may be treated by microsurgical tubal reimplantation into the uterus or by hysteroscopic tubal

Figure 95-3   **Tests for Tubal Patency**

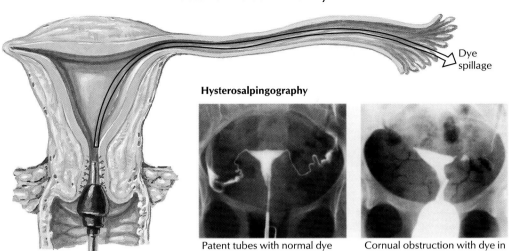

Dye
spillage

Hysterosalpingography

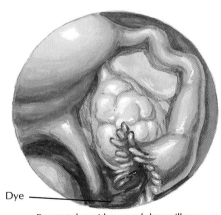

Radiopaque dye injected into uterus;
tubal filling and spillage monitored
with fluoroscopy

Patent tubes with normal dye
spillage

Cornual obstruction with dye in
uterus only

Laparoscopy

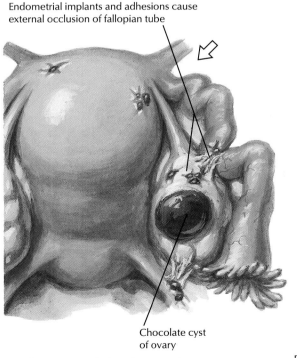

Endometrial implants and adhesions cause
external occlusion of fallopian tube

Chocolate cyst
of ovary

Endometriosis with chocolate cyst of ovary

Dye

Patent tube with normal dye spillage

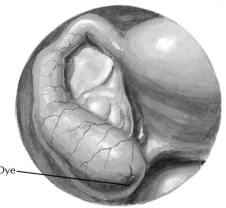

Dye

Obstructed tube with dye retention

JOHN A.CRAIG—AD
©ICN

cannulization. In-vitro fertilization, a means to bypass the fallopian tube, is the treatment of choice when tubal disease is bipolar, resulting in both proximal and distal obstruction.

Recent evidence suggests that fluid collected in a hydrosalpinx via transudation may adversely affect embryo implantation during in-vitro fertilization (Figure 95-4). In patients contemplating in-vitro fertilization (IVF), extirpative tubal surgery to prevent retrograde uterine spill is often recommended.

Endometriosis

The mechanism of how endometriosis affects fertility is unknown. The disease may impact fertility by promoting intraperitoneal inflammatory processes and modifying cytokine action. Treatment of endometriosis for infertility by a medicinal approach is recommended only in those cases accompanied by pelvic pain. During surgery for endometriosis, ablation and removal of implants may augment pregnancy rates. Uterine abnormalities are associated with pregnancy wastage more frequently than infertility and occur in the second trimester most commonly.

Developmental Abnormalities of the Uterus

Developmental abnormalities of the uterus are diagnosed by pelvic examination, hysteroscopy, or hysterosalpingography. Fibroids and uterine septae are abnormalities of the uterus that cause infertility. Hysteroscopic reparation of both conditions may increase fecundity.

Male Infertility

Significant advancement in the diagnosis and treatment of infertile couples allows men who had little chance of having a biological child previously to succeed in having one. Take a thorough history; post-pubertal mumps, testicular torsion, diabetes mellitus, prostate surgery, or history of hernia repair warrant investigation. Medications, including calcium channel blockers, or exposure to toxic agents such as heavy metals, polycarbons, and other organic solvents may impede fertilization. The physical examination is most pertinent for the genital area; evaluate for the presence of enlarged symptomatic veins around the testes (varicoceles).

Semen analysis is the central component of the evaluation. Traditionally, a normal semen analysis included an ejaculate volume between 1.5 and 5 cc, a sperm density greater than 20 million per milliliter, motility greater than 60%, and normal morphology greater than 70%. More recently, sperm morphology has been recognized as most predictive of male factor infertility. This "Kruger" morphology requires just 4% normal sperm based on strict standards.

A reduction in sperm production can be severe and result in azoospermia, or it can be milder and induce only oligospermia. When no sperm are seen in the ejaculate, the care provider should evaluate the patient for cystic fibrosis. Semen white blood cells have been associated with genitourinary infections and/or inflammation. Blood cells may be implicated in the release of reactive oxygen species, thus evidence of elevated levels of white blood cells in the semen should lead to a semen culture. Antisperm antibodies commonly seen after reversal of a vasectomy have been associated with genitourinary infections, testicular trauma, thermal injury, and genital tract obstruction. Greater than 20% of the sperm having antibodies especially to the head region is clinically significant and possibly associated with deficits in the sperm function. Couples who have suboptimal semen analysis may be candidates for artificial insemination, a procedure in which the semen is processed, concentrated, and inserted through the cervix. In psychogenic ejaculatory failure, intravaginal ejaculation is impossible but ejaculation via masturbation is usually possible. In some cases, vibratory stimulation is necessary when psychogenic ejaculatory failure is present. Donor sperm is the alternative treatment when adequate sperm cannot be obtained. In men with a normal hormonal profile who are azospermic due to ductal obstruction, a testicular biopsy or an epididymal tap may be performed to obtain spermatozoa for intracytoplasmic sperm injection (ICSI) procedure.

ICSI is a modification of the routine in-vitro fertilization procedure. ICSI is similar to IVF except instead of incubating the sperm and egg together, the egg is stabilized under a special microscope using a microsuction instrument while a very fine pipette injects a selected sperm into the egg. ICSI has made it possible for couples with impairments in sperm counts, motility, morphology, and a degree of sperm maturity to conceive.

Figure 95-4

In Vitro Fertilization

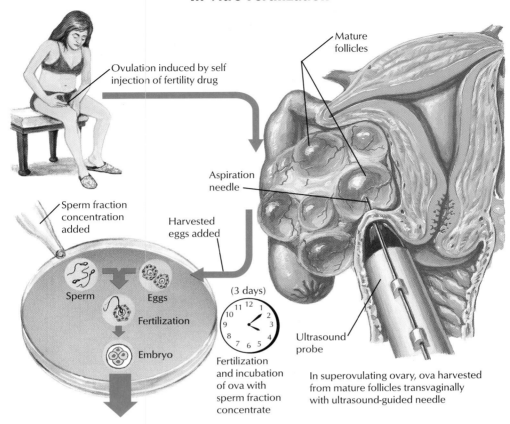

Ovulation induced by self injection of fertility drug

Mature follicles

Aspiration needle

Ultrasound probe

Sperm fraction concentration added

Harvested eggs added

Sperm

Eggs

Fertilization

Embryo

(3 days)

Fertilization and incubation of ova with sperm fraction concentrate

In superovulating ovary, ova harvested from mature follicles transvaginally with ultrasound-guided needle

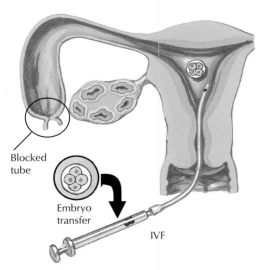

Blocked tube

Embryo transfer

IVF

Ova fertilized in vitro (IVF) with sperm fraction concentrate. Embryo transferred directly into uterus, bypassing tubal occlusion

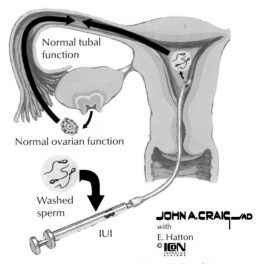

Normal tubal function

Normal ovarian function

Washed sperm

IUI

JOHN A. CRAIG__AD
with
E. Hatton
©ICON

For IUI, sperm are first washed and placed in sterile medium and concentrated to a small volume, then injected direct into ovary

Figure 95-5 Evaluation of the Infertile Couple

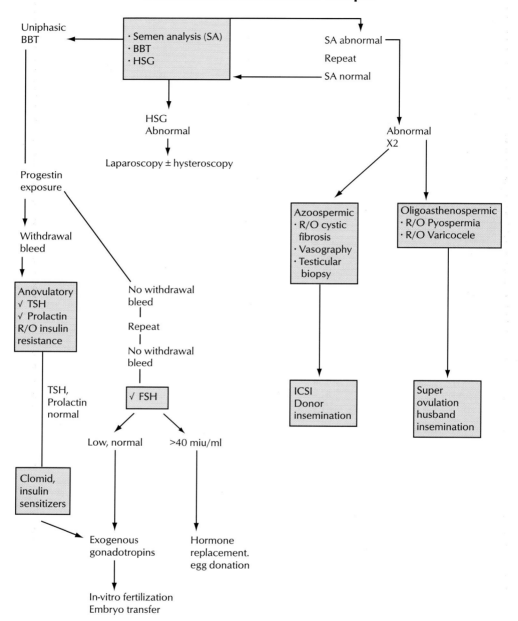

SUMMARY

The basic infertility workup consists of the systematic evaluation of 3 key areas: ovulation, sperm production, and pelvic factors. This can be accomplished in the primary care setting with ancillary testing done by radiology and the clinic laboratory (semen analysis). If the workup does not reveal an obvious cause for the infertility, laparoscopy or referral to a reproductive endocrinologist may be warranted. Figure 95-5 outlines a reasonable, stepwise approach.

One should emphasize to the couple that infertility is not a problem of just one partner. Many couples have more than one obstacle to overcome. Even in cases where there is a known cause for infertility, there may be other forces at work. Not uncommonly, couples have infertility for unknown reasons. A man whose wife has PCOS may have a subtle yet crucial disorder that testing fails to identify.

Pay attention to the emotional needs of patients. Infertility can be a dispiriting, withering process that may lead to profound depression. Some patients may feel isolated and defective, and even avoid social functions where they could encounter children. Some investigators have theorized that a patient's poor coping mechanisms and/or depression compound the problem and make conception even more difficult. Professional counseling or even pharmacologic remedies may be appropriate.

FUTURE DIRECTIONS

Reproductive science is advancing on several fronts that hold potential for infertility patients. Preimplantation genetics may one day prevent aneuploid embryos from being implanted and significantly increase IVF success rates. Investigators are also working on ovarian and uterine transplants, correction of embryo implantation defects, and microsurgical techniques. The use of thiazolidinediones, a new class of insulin sensitizing agents, in ovulation induction in PCOS is in its initial investigative stages. These compounds enhance peripheral insulin action without directly stimulating insulin secretion. Advances such as these may not only improve diagnostic skills but offer hope to women with refractory or unexplained infertility.

REFERENCES

Boer-Meisel ME, te Velde ER, Habbema JD, Kardaun JW. Predicting the pregnancy outcome in patients treated for hydrosalpinx: a prospective study. *Fertil Steril.* 1986;45:23-29.

Carr BR, Blackwell RE, eds. *Textbook of Reproductive Medicine.* 2nd ed. Stamford, Conn: Appleton & Lange; 1998.

Demyttenaere K, Bonte L, Gheldof M, et al. Coping style and depression level influence outcome in in vitro fertilization. *Fertil Steril.* 1998;69:1026-1033.

Dunaif A. Insulin resistance and the polycystic ovary syndrome: mechanism and implications for pathogenesis. *Endocr Rev.* 1997;18:774-800.

Gorlitsky GA, Kase NG, Speroff L. Ovulation and pregnancy rates with clomiphene citrate. *Obstet Gynecol.* 1978; 51:265-269.

Kee BS, Jung BJ, Lee SH. A study on psychological strain in IVF patients. *J Assist Reprod Genet.* 2000;17:445-448.

Nestler JE, Jakubowicz DJ, Evans WS, Pasquali R. Effects of metformin on spontaneous and clomiphene-induced ovulation in the polycystic ovary syndrome. *N Engl J Med.* 1998; 338:1876-1880.

Speroff L, Glass RH, Kase NG, eds. *Clinical Gynecologic Endocrinology and Infertility.* 6th ed. Philadelphia, Pa: Lippincott Williams & Wilkins; 1999.

Shoham Z, Howles CM, Jacobs HS, eds. *Female Infertility Therapy: Current Practice.* London, England: Martin Dunitz Ltd; 1999.

Chapter 96

Menopause

AnnaMarie Connolly

Menopause is technically defined as the permanent cessation of menses, although the term is commonly used in association with the clinical manifestations and consequences of ovarian failure. Menopause is a physiological event in the lives of all women. The clinical manifestations and consequences vary in type and intensity. The age of onset is genetically predetermined and independent of factors such as race, education, socioeconomic status, as well as weight, height, and age at time of last pregnancy. Cigarette smoking has been shown consistently to hasten menopause by approximately 1 year. The average age of menopause in the United States is 51 years and, while this is normally distributed with 95% confidence limits between 45 and 55 years of age, approximately 1% of women experience menopause before age 40. The climacteric, the time during which women transition from reproductive years to postmenopausal years, usually lasts 4 years. The average life expectancy in the United States is 78 years; most women will live one third of their lives in the postmenopausal state. It is estimated that there are 60 million women in the United States older than 50 years.

ETIOLOGY AND PATHOGENESIS

Ovarian failure leads to menopause (Figure 96-1). Diminished ovarian function is present several years before the permanent cessation of menstruation. The number of ovarian follicles and follicular cell production of the glycoprotein inhibin, which functions to inhibit pituitary production of follicle stimulating hormone (FSH), decrease with age, causing FSH levels to rise. Because FSH release is primarily controlled by inhibin, FSH levels should not be observed to determine "therapeutic doses" of postmenopausal estrogen replacement because FSH levels will remain elevated even with the administration of large doses of exogenous estrogen. Granulosa and thecal cells degenerate with ovarian estradiol secretion waning significantly up to 1 year before menopause, while stromal cells continue to produce the androgens androstenedione and testosterone.

Premature ovarian failure, or ovarian failure before the age of 40 years, occurs in up to 1% of women with X chromosome abnormalities, accounting for most cases. Women with a family history of early menopause may have as much as 6 times the likelihood of menopause before age 46, with the strongest association seen in women who had mothers or sisters undergoing menopause before age 40. Surgical removal of the ovaries can induce menopause and associated postmenopausal symptoms.

CLINICAL PRESENTATION

Although hot flushes and vaginal dryness are commonly associated with the postmenopausal state, change in menstrual cycle length is one of the first signs of menopause. A consequence of waning ovarian function, this change in cycle length reflects increasing anovulatory cycles and can occur up to 4 years before menopause.

Hot flushes, which occur in up to 50% of women, likely result from a central nervous system-mediated change in hypothalamic thermoregulation. Frequency of severity of this symptom corresponds to the magnitude of estrogen level fluctuation; the greater the estrogen level fluctuation, the more frequent and severe the hot flushes. The incidence of flushes declines with time with only 20% of women reporting such symptoms 4 years after menopause. Obesity leads to fewer complaints of hot flushes given increased peripheral aromatization of androstenedione to estrone in adipose tissues.

Vaginal dryness and genitourinary atrophy are frequent complaints of women in the climacteric. Estrogen deficiency may lead to atrophy of vaginal epithelium, causing the symptoms of itching, light vaginal discharge, dyspareunia, and even

Figure 96-1

Pituitary and Ovarian Hormone Changes in Menopause

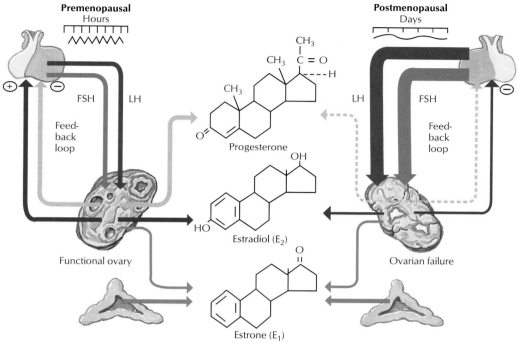

Premenopausal
Hours

Postmenopausal
Days

FSH   LH

Feed-back loop

Progesterone

Estradiol (E$_2$)

Estrone (E$_1$)

Functional ovary

LH   FSH

Feed-back loop

Ovarian failure

Hormone levels increase and decrease cyclically during menstrual cycle. Modulation occurs by pulsatile release of gonadotropins and positive and negative feedback loops.

In postmenopausal period, gonadotropin levels increase and ovarian hormone levels decrease secondary to ovarian failure. Endogenous estrogen is primarily of adrenal origin, and E$_1$ to E$_2$ ratio is reversed.

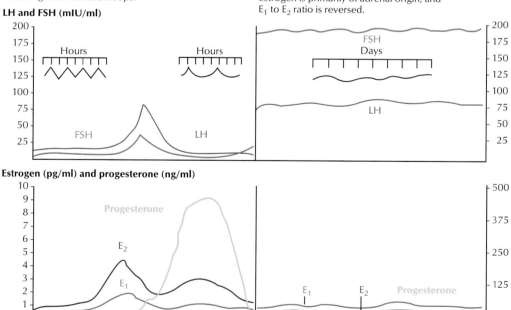

LH and FSH (mIU/ml)

Hours   Hours

FSH
Days

FSH   LH

LH

Estrogen (pg/ml) and progesterone (ng/ml)

Progesterone

E$_2$

E$_1$

E$_1$ E$_2$ Progesterone

Days   7   14   21

JOHN A. CRAIG—AD

© ICON

Figure 96-2   **Target Organ Changes in Menopause**

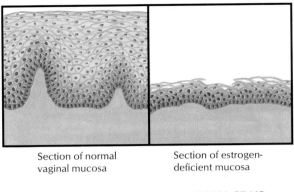

Section of normal
vaginal mucosa

Section of estrogen-
deficient mucosa

JOHN A.CRAIG—AD
© ICN

vaginal bleeding (Figure 96-2). Decreased libido has also been associated with menopause. Decreased collagen content associated with estrogen deficiency may lead to loss of support of the vaginal walls and uterus. Other estrogen-deficiency related symptoms include urinary urgency, frequency, nocturia, and dysuria as estrogen-dependent lower urinary tract epithelial tissues atrophy.

Menopause is also associated with change in body weight and total body fat. The randomized Postmenopausal Estrogen/Progestin Interventions (PEPI) study reported less weight gain in women on hormone replacement as compared to placebo. A reduced shift in body fat to the abdominal area was also noted, a factor associated with higher cardiovascular morbidity and mortality.

Other symptoms include increased insomnia, anxiety, mood lability, and depression. What is unclear is whether estrogen administration, which has been shown to improve such symptoms, works directly on the symptom of concern or alleviates hot flushes, allowing women to sleep better, thus leading to resolution of symptoms. Migraine headaches may improve with menopause while tension headaches remain unchanged. Cognitive function may also be affected. In one study, reported mental status examination scores of postmenopausal women taking estrogen were significantly higher than those of women not on estrogen.

DIFFERENTIAL DIAGNOSIS

The differential diagnosis for menopausal symptoms is narrow. The most common additional diagnosis to consider is anxiety.

DIAGNOSTIC APPROACH

The diagnosis of menopause relies primarily on the history. Menstrual cycle irregularity secondary to oligo-ovulation or anovulation is commonly reported. Intermittent hot flushes secondary to fluctuating estrogen levels may lead to interrupted sleep, fatigue, irritability, anxiety, and/or depression. Personal and family history regarding cardiovascular and osteoporosis risk factors is important.

Physical examination should include weight, height, and blood pressure. Pelvic examination may reveal atrophic changes of the external genitalia, including thinning of the labial tissues and/or fusion of labial minora folds with the labia majora. Thinning of vaginal mucosa with loss of rugation commonly occurs, as does decreased vaginal pH. Serum FSH and LH concentrations are elevated.

Yearly Pap smears and mammograms should be obtained in all postmenopausal women over the age of 50 presenting for annual care. The frequency of Pap smears can be decreased after 3 consecutive negative smears.

MANAGEMENT AND THERAPY

Why attempt to manage and/or treat a physiological condition? This is a question posed to clinicians by many patients. The answer lies in the appreciation of the health problems of postmenopausal women and the preventative measures available. Two major health problems for which preventative measures are available include cardiovascular disease and osteoporosis.

Cardiovascular Disease

Responsible for more postmenopausal deaths than all other causes of death combined, cardiovascular disease is 3 times as common in men than women before menopause. This ratio of myocardial infarction in women to men older than 50 changes to 2:1. So, it is important that postmenopausal women address cardiovascular risk factors aggressively, including control of hypertension, hypercholesterolemia, diabetes mellitus, and cessation of cigarette smoking.

Controversy in the literature over the use of estrogens to reduce cardiac risk has existed for many years. On the basis of observational and epidemiological studies and strong experimental data, estrogen therapy was recommended by many for cardiac risk reduction in women. The recent Women's Health Initiative Randomized Controlled Trial demonstrated a small but significantly increased cardiac risk for postmenopausal women taking combination (estrogen/progestin) hormone replacement therapy. Thus, it is not currently recommended to initiate combination hormone replacement therapy solely for prophylaxis against myocardial infarction. The results of ongoing research will guide future recommendations regarding estrogen-only therapy for MI prevention.

Osteoporosis

Characterized by decreased bone mass, osteoporosis is usually asymptomatic and often not detected until fracture occurs. In the United States, approximately 800,000 fractures occur per year; 300,000 of these are hip fractures, with 15% of hip fractures in women older than 80 being fatal within 6 months. Fractures may occur many years after onset of the disease. The underlying pathophysiology in postmenopausal women is increased osteoclastic activity associated with a normal rate of bone formation. Dual-energy X-ray absorptiometry is currently the most accurate test for measurement of bone density, although 25%

of bone needs to be lost before osteoporosis can be detected by routine examination. Markers of bone resorption, such as urinary excretion of collagen degradation products, are of limited use in the diagnosis of osteoporosis.

The most rapid phase of bone mass accrual occurs during puberty into the mid-20s. Bone mineral density may continue to improve until women reach their mid-30s, when peak bone mass is reached. After menopause, bone density decreases by 1% to 2% per year, more rapidly in trabecular than in cortical bone, with 25% of White and Asian women experiencing vertebral compression fractures by age 60 if not taking hormone replacement. Risk factors include family history, race (White, Asian), body type, sedentary lifestyle, dietary calcium deficiencies, and tobacco use. Notably, these risk factors, only identify 30% of women with osteoporosis.

While weight-bearing exercise is important for overall health, exercise alone does not prevent postmenopausal bone loss. Recommendations from the National Institutes of Health (NIH) consensus panel of 1994 include that postmenopausal women take 1,000 to 1,500 mg of calcium per day along with vitamin D, 400 to 800 IU. Current data suggest that this level is too high and that calcium supplementation is necessary only for those women ingesting less than 500 mg per day if they are taking estrogen replacement therapy. NIH recommendations remain in place at this time.

Estrogen replacement appears to retard bone resorption though estrogen and progesterone receptors have been identified in osteoblasts. Decreased postmenopausal bone loss and a decreased incidence of hip and spine fracture have been reported. The minimum estrogen dose observed to prevent bone loss was 0.625 mg of conjugated equine estrogens, 0.5 mg of esterified estrogens, or 0.3 mg of conjugated equine estrogen in the presence of 1,500 mg of calcium each day, or 0.05 mg of transdermal estrogen. The addition of progestins to hormone replacement regimens does not appear to attenuate this bone-protective effect.

When hormone replacement is not an option, bisphosphonates such as alendronate and risedronate are available to decrease bone resorption and reduce fracture incidence. Calcitonin via nasal spray is also available for osteoporosis treatment and has been shown to increase vertebral bone mass. Lastly, the selective estrogen receptor modulator (SERM) raloxifene has been shown to increase vertebral bone mass although data available at this time do not demonstrate protective effects against hip fracture.

Hormone Replacement Therapy

Preventative measures such as balanced diet, multivitamin and calcium supplementation, and regular exercise are important factors in postmenopausal health. Hormone replacement therapy with either estrogen alone in those women who have undergone hysterectomy or with estrogen/progestin combination in women with an intact uterus has been the mainstay of postmenopausal medical management. Relief from symptoms of urogenital atrophy such as vaginal dryness, dyspareunia, and urinary frequency is a clear benefit. Regimens are numerous. In the United States, continuous and cyclical regimens are most commonly used. The continuous regimen utilizes conjugated equine estrogen, 0.625 mg, and medroxyprogesterone acetate, 2.5 mg, given daily. The cyclical regimen uses 0.625 mg conjugated equine estrogen given on days 1 to 25 and cyclic 5 mg of medroxyprogesterone acetate given on days 14 to 25. On the continuous regimen, women may frequently have some degree of irregular spotting for up to 3 months after initiating therapy. On the cyclical regimen, most women will demonstrate withdrawal bleeding. Contraindications to estrogen replacement therapy include unexplained vaginal bleeding, the presence of breast or endometrial cancer, active liver disease, and active thrombophlebitis. The full impact of the recently-released Women's Health Initiative Randomized Controlled Trial on the prescription of postmenopausal estrogen remains uncertain at this time.

FUTURE DIRECTIONS

Postmenopausal health is impacting an ever-increasing number of women in the United States, and preventative health care is, at long last, becoming a focus for women and health-care providers alike. The health benefits of hormone replacement have been outlined; however, concerns remain regarding breast cancer risks, particularly in long-term users. The Women's Health Initiative Randomized Controlled Trial will hopefully provide helpful insight into this problem regarding estrogen-only and combination hormone replacement therapy. The development and longer-term use of agents such as the SERMs may also provide preventative health advantages without the potential adverse effects on endometrium and breast. Evidence-based medicine will continue to provide guidance in efforts to optimize the health care of postmenopausal women.

REFERENCES

Precis V: An Update in Obstetrics and Gynecology. Washington, DC: American College of Obstetricians and Gynecologists; 1994.

Cramer DW, Xu H, Harlow BL. Family history as a predictor of early menopause. *Fertil Steril.* 1995;64:740-745.

McKinlay SM, Brambilla DJ, Posner JG. The normal menopause transition. *Maturitas.* 1992;14:103-115.

Stanford JL, Hartge P, Brinton LA, Hoover RN, Brookmeyer R. Factors influencing the age at natural menopause. *J Chronic Dis.* 1987;40:995-1002.

Steffens DC, Norton MC, Plassman BL, et al. Enhanced cognitive performance with estrogen in nondemented community-dwelling older women. *J Am Geriatr Soc.* 1999;47:1171-1175.

Stenchever MA, Droegemueller W, Herbst AL, Mishell DR Jr. *Comprehensive Gynecology.* 4th ed. St Louis, Mo: Mosby; 2001.

The Writing Group for the PEPI Trail. Effects of estrogen or estrogen/progestin regimens on heart disease risk factors in postmenopausal women. The Postmenopausal Estrogen/Progestin Interventions (PEPI) Trial. *JAMA.* 1995;273:199-208.

Chapter 97

Menstrual Disorders

M. Cristina Muñoz

Menstruation is a normal event that signals sexual maturity, fertility, and good health for many women, but it may be accompanied by significant morbidity. The most important menstrual complaints are excessive bleeding, bleeding that occurs too frequently or too infrequently, painful menstruation, and premenstrual syndrome.

The menstrual cycle (Figure 97-1) is described in terms of ovarian hormonal events or in terms of endometrial responses to hormonal changes. The first day of bleeding is defined as day 1 of the cycle. The ovarian cycle begins with the *follicular phase*, in which several follicles (an oocyte surrounded by estrogen-producing granulosa cells) begin maturing in response to follicle-stimulating hormone (FSH) and luteinizing hormone (LH) secreted by the anterior pituitary gland. Through positive feedback, the follicle that secretes the most estradiol (the dominant follicle) becomes more sensitive to FSH stimulation and enlarges to about 2 cm in diameter, while others atrophy. The hypothalamus and pituitary gland respond to ovarian hormones with a surge in LH and FSH secretion. Ovulation occurs within 24 to 48 hours of the LH surge. After ovulation, the granulosa and theca cells of the ovulatory follicle become the corpus luteum and produce estrogen and progesterone during the *luteal phase*. Rising ovarian hormone levels exert negative feedback on FSH and LH production. As FSH and LH fall (in the absence of pregnancy), the corpus luteum degenerates.

The uterus responds to ovarian or pharmacologic hormonal stimulation in a stereotypical fashion. During menstruation, there is shedding of the hormonally responsive upper zone of the endometrium due to declining hormonal support. While the lining sheds down to its basal layer, estrogen stimulation from ovarian follicles causes new proliferation, or thickening, of endometrial glands and stroma, the *proliferative phase*. After ovulation, progesterone and estrogen cause increased tortuosity of endometrial glands and secretion from the gland lumen, the *secretory phase*.

The length of the average menstrual cycle is 28 days, with ovulation occurring on day 14. While this is a useful approximation of normal cycle length, there is considerable variation in cycle length among women, and a significant chance that a woman will experience long or short cycles each year. Women age 20 to 40 usually have regular cycles. The chance of irregular cycles is increased for 2 to 5 years after menarche and before menopause.

The duration of bleeding in ovulatory menses averages 3 to 6 days, with the heaviest bleeding usually on day 2. Average blood loss is 30 to 40 mL per cycle.

DISORDERS OF TIMING AND AMOUNT OF BLEEDING

Menstruation may be excessive in flow, frequency, or duration, or a combination of these. *Menorrhagia* (hypermenorrhea) is prolonged (over 7 days) or heavy (greater than 80 mL/menses) bleeding, occurring at regular intervals. *Polymenorrhea* is regular menses occurring more often than every 21 days. *Metrorrhagia* or *menometrorrhagia* refer to irregularly timed, frequent bleeding. *Amenorrhea* is the absence of bleeding. *Oligomenorrhea* refers to irregularly timed, infrequent periods. *Dysfunctional uterine bleeding* (DUB) refers to abnormal bleeding for which an organic cause cannot be found.

Etiology and Pathogenesis

Ovulatory DUB, heavy but regular bleeding, is often due to an anatomical distortion of the uterus (Figure 97-2). Submucous leiomyomata uteri (uterine fibroids), adenomyosis, and endometrial polyps can lead to heavy bleeding by increasing endometrial surface area or another (unknown) mechanism. Nonhormonal intrauterine devices cause local foreign-body reactions and heavier, longer periods. Coagulation disorders (e.g., von Willebrand's dis-

Figure 97-1

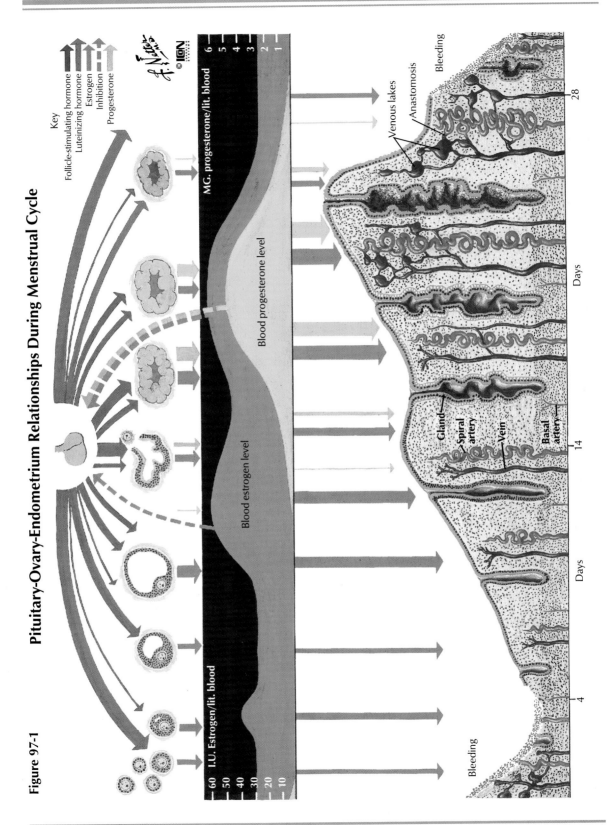

Pituitary-Ovary-Endometrium Relationships During Menstrual Cycle

ease) and alterations in clotting from use of anticoagulants or aspirin also increase menstrual blood loss. *Anovulatory DUB,* irregularly timed excessive bleeding, may be due to threatened or incomplete abortion, ectopic pregnancy, or molar pregnancy. Endometritis causes irregular uterine bleeding and uterine tenderness from inflammation. Anatomical distortions such as fibroids, polyps, and carcinoma can cause irregular bleeding.

Bleeding from the cervix or vagina (e.g., cervicitis, ectropion, invasive cancer, severe atrophic vaginitis, or trichomoniasis) may be confused with uterine bleeding. Rectal or anal bleeding, or gross hematuria is occasionally misinterpreted as genital in origin.

Causes of *amenorrhea* include hyperprolactinemia, hypothyroidism or adrenocorticotropic hormone deficiency, hypogonadotropic hypogonadism, menopause or premature ovarian failure, anorexia nervosa, sudden weight loss, severe stress, strenuous exercise, and numerous medications.

Anovulation, such as that seen with *polycystic ovary syndrome* (PCOS) is a common cause of amenorrhea followed by menorrhagia. Patients with PCOS have obesity, acne, hirsutism, amenorrhea, and multiple cysts of the ovaries. Women with less severe symptoms whose ovaries are not polycystic are said to have *hyperandrogenic chronic anovulation.* In PCOS, elevated pituitary LH secretion and excessive ovarian androgens prevent follicle maturation in the ovary. Ovarian androstenedione is converted peripherally to estrone, which stimulates further LH release, and a vicious cycle ensues. Estrogens cause prolonged proliferation of the endometrium, but without ovulation, normal menstruation does not occur. Eventually the thick endometrium breaks down, causing heavy bleeding. PCOS may be associated with elevated serum lipids, centripetal obesity, insulin resistance, and an increased risk of future development of diabetes mellitus and heart disease.

Clinical Presentation

Patients complain when their menstrual pattern changes, when they pass large clots, or when bleeding overflows sanitary protection. Chronic menorrhagia frequently causes iron deficiency anemia. Occasionally, women with severe anemia from menstrual bleeding do not recognize that their periods are abnormal. Absence of anemia does not exclude menorrhagia because women may compensate for significant losses by increasing iron consumption.

Diagnostic Approach

A menstrual history should include an estimate of the timing, duration, and amount of bleeding (size of clots, the type of protection needed, and the time needed to soak a maxi pad or tampon.) Age at menarche and the presence of perimenopausal symptoms such as hot flashes and night sweats help to diagnose age-appropriate anovulatory cycles. The history should address diseases or medications that can affect the hypothalamic-pituitary-ovarian axis. Galactorrhea, hirsutism, acne, and weight gain or loss are important associated symptoms. Rapidly progressive virilization (deepening voice, clitoral enlargement, temporal balding, and increased muscle mass or libido) raises concern about ovarian or adrenal neoplasms. A family history of menstrual disorders, hysterectomy, and bleeding disorders is notable. Physical examination should assess height, weight, blood pressure, hair distribution, and acne. Speculum examination may demonstrate vaginal inflammation, cervical erosion, tumor, or cervical polyps. Bimanual examination reveals firm lump texture with leiomyomas. Tenderness to uterine palpation may occur with infection or adenomyosis, and enlarged ovaries or cysts may develop in patients with anovulation. In obese patients, the ovaries are often not felt. In menopausal women, it is abnormal to palpate the ovaries; any palpable ovary must be evaluated by ultrasound.

Useful laboratory tests include a sensitive pregnancy test, complete blood cell count, ferritin and serum iron levels for women with menorrhagia, and PT and PTT in women suspected of bleeding disorders. In amenorrheic patients, measurement of prolactin, thyroid-stimulating hormone, FSH, and estradiol are helpful. Suspected PCOS warrant evaluation for elevated serum testosterone, dehydroepiandrosterone sulfate (DHEA-S), and LH/FSH ratio. Endometrial biopsy may show polyps, infection, endometrial hyperplasia, or carcinoma. "Dating" the endometrium by its histologic appearance may document ovulation or determine hormonal causes of irregular menses. Ultrasound shows the total uterine size and the thickness of the endometrial stripe, as well as

Figure 97-2

Causes of Abnormal Uterine Bleeding

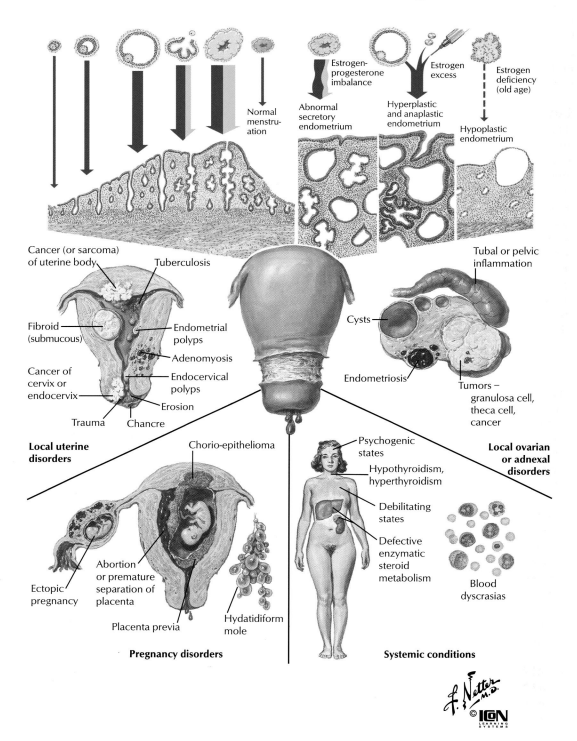

Normal menstru-ation

Estrogen-progesterone imbalance

Estrogen excess

Estrogen deficiency (old age)

Abnormal secretory endometrium

Hyperplastic and anaplastic endometrium

Hypoplastic endometrium

Cancer (or sarcoma) of uterine body

Tuberculosis

Tubal or pelvic inflammation

Fibroid (submucous)

Endometrial polyps

Cysts

Adenomyosis

Cancer of cervix or endocervix

Endocervical polyps

Endometriosis

Erosion

Trauma

Chancre

Tumors – granulosa cell, theca cell, cancer

Local uterine disorders

Chorio-epithelioma

Psychogenic states

Hypothyroidism, hyperthyroidism

Local ovarian or adnexal disorders

Debilitating states

Abortion or premature separation of placenta

Defective enzymatic steroid metabolism

Ectopic pregnancy

Placenta previa

Hydatidiform mole

Blood dyscrasias

Pregnancy disorders

Systemic conditions

leiomyomas and ovarian cysts or polycystic ovaries. Hydrosonography and hysterosalpingography outline lesions in the endometrial cavity. Hysteroscopy allows visualization of the uterine cavity, and many lesions, such as submucous or pedunculated leiomyomata, or endometrial polyps, can be treated during the same procedure.

Management and Therapy

Hormonal treatment is useful in treating excessive bleeding, even that due to non-hormonal causes. Estrogen stops bleeding by stimulating growth of new tissue to cover the denuded endometrium. Progestins mature the uterine lining, making it compact and ready to slough off after the drug is withdrawn, mimicking the normal changes that occur in the secretory phase of the menstrual cycle. In anovulation, cyclic use of progestins prevents the buildup of a thick endometrium by allowing regular withdrawal bleeding. High doses of combined (estrogen/progestin) oral contraceptive pills will arrest heavy bleeding, and normal doses will establish predictable withdrawal bleeding every 28 days. The programmed "period" in pill users, and breakthrough bleeding, are both effects of the drug, and they represent neither normal menstruation nor a menstrual abnormality. Oral contraceptives can be taken continuously (without placebos) to prevent withdrawal bleeding and blood loss. A levonorgestrel-containing intrauterine device, and implanted or injected progestins also decrease menstrual blood loss, although irregular bleeding in the first months of use is expected. NSAIDs decrease the total amount of uterine bleeding and pain associated with menses. They may be used in conjunction with oral contraceptives or cyclic progestins. Antifibrinolytic agents effectively reduce menstrual blood loss, but are not used in the United States.

Surgical treatments include curettage, numerous procedures to ablate or resect the endometrial lining, myomectomy and destructive procedures for fibroids, and hysterectomy.

DYSMENORRHEA AND PREMENSTRUAL SYNDROME

Menstrual discomfort affects 30% to 60% of women. Approximately 5% have symptoms severe enough to interfere with daily activities. Premenstrual syndrome (PMS), a group of physical and emotional symptoms that occur in the luteal phase of the cycle, affects more than half of menstruating women intermittently, although severe symptoms occur in only 2% to 3% of women.

Etiology and Pathogenesis

Primary dysmenorrhea is caused by prostaglandin F2α, which causes uterine contractions. Secondary dysmenorrhea is caused by inflammation in acute or chronic pelvic infection, excessive prostaglandin production in endometriosis and adenomyosis, or by cervical stenosis. The physical symptoms of premenstrual syndrome, such as bloating and breast tenderness, are hormonal in origin. Emotional symptoms, such as anger, irritability, and depression, are serotonin-mediated.

Clinical Presentation

Presentation is straightforward because the patient notes a symptom pattern and requests treatment.

Differential Diagnosis

PMS and premenstrual dysphoric disorder (PMDD) must be distinguished from mood disorders. Because mental illness is stigmatized, women with depression or anxiety often seek treatment for PMS. However, the emotional symptoms of PMS and PMDD occur only in the luteal phase, clearing during the menstrual and follicular phases.

Diagnostic Approach

Menstrual history is important to elucidate the age at onset, symptom changes with age, contraceptive use, pregnancy and lactation, associated symptoms such as backache or dyspareunia, and response to previous treatments. Ideally, a menstrual calendar is used to document symptoms over several cycles. Family history of menstrual disorders may affect a woman's response to menstruation, while a history of endometriosis or adenomyosis increases suspicion of these conditions. Pelvic examination may demonstrate cervical motion tenderness or adnexal tenderness in infection, uterosacral nodularity in endometriosis, or a boggy, tender uterus in adenomyosis.

Management and Therapy

Menstrual pain can be treated with NSAIDs, which decrease prostaglandin production, hypertonic uterine contractions, and menstrual blood loss. Oral contraceptives also decrease menstrual pain in 90% of users and can be used together with NSAIDs. Heat, transcutaneous electrical nerve stimulation, acupuncture, and acupressure are also effective. Severe pain refractory to treatment should be evaluated with laparoscopy, and endometriotic lesions can be fulgurated simultaneously. Presumed endometriosis can be empirically treated with gonadotropin-releasing hormone agonists. Improvement with this treatment does not confirm a diagnosis of endometriosis because ablation of menstruation treats several menstrual disorders. Pregnancy and vaginal delivery are associated with lower rates of dysmenorrhea, but the stress of parenting may increase PMS. Hysterectomy is effective in relieving pure dysmenorrhea. Chronic pelvic pain often recurs after hysterectomy even if the pain is localized to the uterus on examination.

The physical symptoms of PMS can be effectively treated with mild diuretics and analgesics. Emotional symptoms may improve with selective serotonin reuptake inhibitors (SSRIs), (dosed continuously or in the luteal phase only), anxiolytics, tricyclic antidepressants, or suppression of menses with danazol, gonadotropin-releasing hormone (GnRH) agonists, or oral contraceptives.

FUTURE DIRECTIONS

We have poor understanding of the epidemiology of menstruation, the considerable variability in cycles among women in different cultures and circumstances, and the effects of life events on the cycle. The role of overweight and insulin resistance in anovulation, and the response to dietary changes and exercise are all being studied. Because hysterectomy is expensive and has significant operative morbidity, many less invasive surgical alternatives have been proposed. Research is needed to distinguish which women will benefit most from medical therapies, versus destruction or removal of the endometrium, versus hysterectomy.

REFERENCES

Harlow SD, Ephross SA. Epidemiology of menstruation and its relevance to women's health. *Epidemiol Rev.* 1995;17:265-286.

Lethaby A, Augood C, Duckitt K. Nonsteroidal anti-inflammatory drugs for heavy menstrual bleeding. *Cochrane Database Syst Rev.* 2000;CD000400.

Mishell DR Jr. Abnormal uterine bleeding: ovulatory and anovulatory dysfunctional uterine bleeding, management of acute and chronic excessive bleeding. In: Stenchever MA, Droegemueller W, Herbst AL, Mishell DR Jr. *Comprehensive Gynecology.* 4th ed. St Louis, Mo: Mosby; 2001.

Speroff L, Glass RH, Kase NG, eds. *Clinical Gynecologic Endocrinology and Infertility.* 6th ed. Philadelphia, Pa: Lippincott Williams & Wilkins; 1999.

Section XII
NEUROLOGIC DISORDERS

Chapter 98

Bell's Palsy

Benjamin J. Copeland and Harold C. Pillsbury III

The muscles of facial expression are intimately involved in our ability to communicate emotions with those around us. Acute unilateral facial palsy, also known as Bell's palsy after Sir Charles Bell who described the disorder in 1821, is the most common cause of facial weakness and the most common cranial neuropathy. Traditionally, a diagnosis of exclusion attributed to idiopathic origins, recent investigations have implicated herpetic viral infection with associated inflammation as the source of the paresis or paralysis. Bell's palsy shows no gender or seasonal predilection and occurs with an incidence of approximately 20 per 100,000 population. The majority of afflicted patients recover fully with supportive care; however, 15% suffer sequelae such as contracture and synkinesis (unintentional movements). There is evidence of decreased complete recovery and increased sequelae with advancing patient age.

ETIOLOGY AND PATHOGENESIS

An understanding of the anatomy of the facial nerve is critical to the understanding of Bell's palsy. The facial nerve primarily carries fibers for motor control to the muscles of facial expression, the stapedius muscle, and the posterior belly of the digastric muscle. In addition to these motor fibers, sensory branches and parasympathetic fibers course within the facial nerve. Taste sensation fibers from the anterior two thirds of the tongue joins the facial nerve via the chorda tympani branch. Parasympathetic fibers reach the lacrimal and submandibular glands via the greater superficial petrosal nerve and the chorda tympani, respectively. Loss of nerve conduction in the facial nerve may potentially disrupt all of these fibers (Figure 98-1).

The facial nerve travels through the temporal bone housed in a bony canal (fallopian canal), entering the temporal bone at the internal auditory canal and exiting from the stylomastoid foramen. The narrowest segment of the bony canal is located at the lateral end of the internal auditory canal. Acute unilateral facial palsy is thought to arise from perineural inflammation and edema within the rigid bony canal surrounding the facial nerve.

A large body of evidence implicates herpes simplex virus (HSV) infection as the primary cause of acute unilateral facial palsy. Nucleic acids from HSV have been demonstrated in the geniculate ganglion of the facial nerve, and HSV DNA has been detected in the endoneural fluid of the

nerve in patients with acute paralysis who are undergoing surgical decompression. Another herpes virus, varicella zoster virus, is associated with acute facial nerve palsy in the Ramsey Hunt syndrome. A double-blind placebo-controlled prospective trial has shown improvement in outcome when antiviral therapy is added to treatment regimens.

CLINICAL PRESENTATION

Typically, the onset of Bell's palsy is acute with the progression of weakness in several hours to overnight (Figure 98-2). Complete hemifacial paralysis may occur at onset or, more commonly, progress from hemifacial weakness initially to complete paralysis over several days. Many patients describe pain behind the affected ear as a prodrome and a sensation of "numbness" on the affected side of the face, although this sensation appears to be secondary to the lack of motion. Dysgeusia (disturbed taste), hyperacusis (sounds are too loud in the affected ear), and difficulty drinking are also common complaints.

Physical examination reveals unilateral paresis or paralysis of the muscles of facial expression involving both the upper and lower face on the affected side (lower motor neuron lesion pattern). When severe, the affected hemiface shows no voluntary movements and obvious asymmetry at rest. The House-Brackmann scale, which incorporates gross facial appearance, symmetry at rest, and symmetry of the forehead, eye and mouth in

Figure 98-1

Facial (VII) Nerve

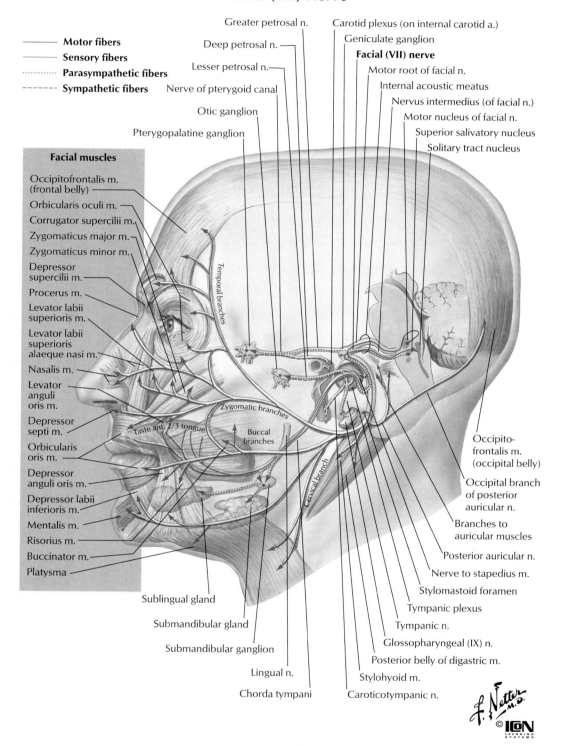

——— **Motor fibers**
——— **Sensory fibers**
·········· **Parasympathetic fibers**
------ **Sympathetic fibers**

Greater petrosal n.
Deep petrosal n.
Lesser petrosal n.
Nerve of pterygoid canal
Otic ganglion
Pterygopalatine ganglion

Carotid plexus (on internal carotid a.)
Geniculate ganglion
Facial (VII) nerve
Motor root of facial n.
Internal acoustic meatus
Nervus intermedius (of facial n.)
Motor nucleus of facial n.
Superior salivatory nucleus
Solitary tract nucleus

Facial muscles
Occipitofrontalis m. (frontal belly)
Orbicularis oculi m.
Corrugator supercilii m.
Zygomaticus major m.
Zygomaticus minor m.
Depressor supercilii m.
Procerus m.
Levator labii superioris m.
Levator labii superioris alaeque nasi m.
Nasalis m.
Levator anguli oris m.
Depressor septi m.
Orbicularis oris m.
Depressor anguli oris m.
Depressor labii inferioris m.
Mentalis m.
Risorius m.
Buccinator m.
Platysma

Temporal branches
Zygomatic branches
Taste ant. 2/3 tongue
Buccal branches
Cervical branch

Occipitofrontalis m. (occipital belly)
Occipital branch of posterior auricular n.
Branches to auricular muscles
Posterior auricular n.
Nerve to stapedius m.
Stylomastoid foramen
Tympanic plexus
Tympanic n.
Glossopharyngeal (IX) n.
Posterior belly of digastric m.
Stylohyoid m.
Caroticotympanic n.

Sublingual gland
Submandibular gland
Submandibular ganglion
Lingual n.
Chorda tympani

Figure 98-2

Bell's Palsy

Course and distribution of facial (VII) nerve

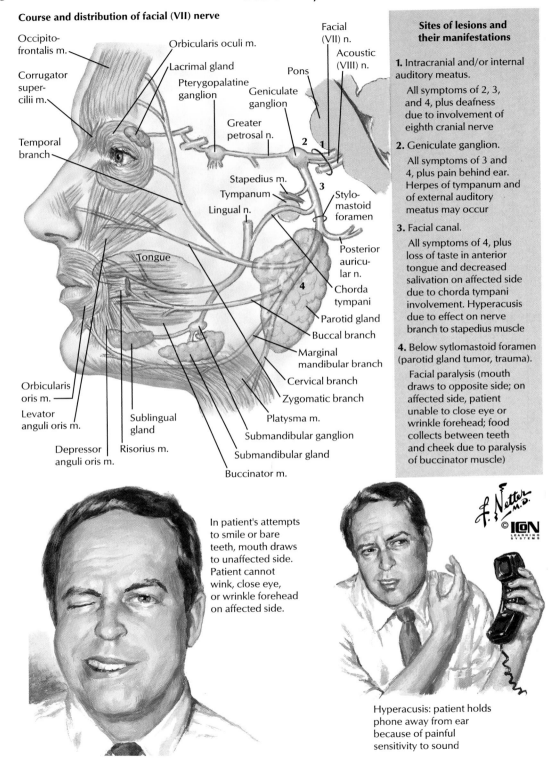

Occipito-frontalis m.

Orbicularis oculi m.

Lacrimal gland

Corrugator super-cilii m.

Pterygopalatine ganglion

Temporal branch

Greater petrosal n.

Facial (VII) n.

Acoustic (VIII) n.

Pons

Geniculate ganglion

Stapedius m.

Tympanum

Lingual n.

Stylo-mastoid foramen

Tongue

Posterior auricu-lar n.

Chorda tympani

Parotid gland

Buccal branch

Marginal mandibular branch

Cervical branch

Zygomatic branch

Platysma m.

Submandibular ganglion

Submandibular gland

Buccinator m.

Orbicularis oris m.

Levator anguli oris m.

Sublingual gland

Depressor anguli oris m.

Risorius m.

Sites of lesions and their manifestations

1. Intracranial and/or internal auditory meatus.

All symptoms of 2, 3, and 4, plus deafness due to involvement of eighth cranial nerve

2. Geniculate ganglion.

All symptoms of 3 and 4, plus pain behind ear. Herpes of tympanum and of external auditory meatus may occur

3. Facial canal.

All symptoms of 4, plus loss of taste in anterior tongue and decreased salivation on affected side due to chorda tympani involvement. Hyperacusis due to effect on nerve branch to stapedius muscle

4. Below sytlomastoid foramen (parotid gland tumor, trauma).

Facial paralysis (mouth draws to opposite side; on affected side, patient unable to close eye or wrinkle forehead; food collects between teeth and cheek due to paralysis of buccinator muscle)

In patient's attempts to smile or bare teeth, mouth draws to unaffected side. Patient cannot wink, close eye, or wrinkle forehead on affected side.

Hyperacusis: patient holds phone away from ear because of painful sensitivity to sound

Table 98-1
House-Brackmann Facial Nerve Grading System

Grade	Description	Findings
I	Normal	Normal facial function in all areas
II	Mild dysfunction	Gross: slight weakness on close inspection, very slight synkinesis
		At rest: normal symmetry and tone
		In motion: forehead — moderate to good function; eye — complete closure with minimal effort; mouth — slight asymmetry
III	Moderate dysfunction	Gross: obvious but not disfiguring difference between sides; noticeable but not severe synkinesis
		At rest: normal symmetry and tone
		In motion: forehead — slight to moderate movement; eye — complete closure with effort; mouth — slightly weak with maximal effort
IV	Moderately severe dysfunction	Gross: obvious weakness or disfiguring asymmetry
		At rest: normal symmetry and tone
		In motion: forehead — no movement; eye — incomplete closure; mouth — asymmetric with maximal effort
V	Severe dysfunction	Gross: barely perceptible motion
		At rest: asymmetry
		In motion: forehead — no movement; eye — incomplete closure; mouth — slight movement
VI	Total paralysis	No movement

Adapted from House JW and Brackmann DE. Facial Nerve Grading System. *Otolaryngol Head Neck Surg.* 1985;83:146–7.

motion, is used to quantify the degree of facial paralysis (Table 98-1). The skin surrounding the affected side of the mouth is displaced to the opposite side with smiling. Often, the affected eye cannot be completely closed with maximal effort, and the globe rolls upward into the orbit, revealing sclera (Bell's phenomenon).

Complete physical examination is critical to establishing the diagnosis. The parotid glands are palpated for masses, and the otoscopic examination must establish clear tympanic membranes with no evidence of infection or lesions. Often, examination of the tongue reveals inflammation of the fungiform papillae on the affected side. Lacrimation in the affected eye may be decreased. Audiometric assessment will often reveal stapedial muscle dysfunction and hyperacusis on the affected side.

DIFFERENTIAL DIAGNOSIS

The differential diagnosis for unilateral facial palsy includes infectious, inflammatory, traumatic, neoplastic, and metabolic disorders.

Infectious etiologies, including varicella zoster virus facial paralysis (Ramsey Hunt syndrome), the second most common cause of hemifacial palsy, must be excluded. The severity and prognosis for recovery of facial function is much graver in varicella-zoster infection. Acute otitis media may present as unilateral facial palsy. Suppurative or coalescent mastoiditis may alter neural conduction through the facial nerve in its vertical segment in the temporal bone. Facial paralysis is the most common head and neck manifestation of Lyme disease. Traumatic injury to the facial nerve includes recent surgeries involving the parotid gland, middle ear, or internal auditory canal as well as closed head injuries involving temporal bone fractures. Parotid gland neoplasms and paragangliomas of the middle ear cavity may cause hemifacial paresis or paralysis. Temporal bone malignancy, primary or metastatic, may also present in a similar fashion. Central nervous system insults, such as cerebrovascular accident, multiple sclerosis, and brain tumor, may present with facial paralysis. Bilateral facial palsy suggests systemic disorders such as Guillain-Barré syndrome, meningitis, leprosy, sarcoidosis, or polyneuropathy.

DIAGNOSTIC APPROACH

When suspicion for another etiology of facial paralysis is high after careful physical examination, radiographic study of the brain and the course of the facial nerve is indicated. CT is the study of choice; when this is not possible, an MRI may yield sufficient information. Further testing for infectious and inflammatory etiologies includes complete blood cell counts, Lyme disease titers, erythrocyte sedimentation rate, and examination of the cerebrospinal fluid. Severe pain or sensorineural hearing loss should raise suspicion of varicella zoster virus infection.

MANAGEMENT AND THERAPY

The management of Bell's palsy should focus on decreasing presumed inflammation of the facial nerve, preventing potential complications, and establishing the prognosis for recovery. Corticosteroid therapy increases the liklihood of complete recovery of facial function. A typical regimen involves initial doses equivalent to 1 mg/kg prednisone daily for 1 week, tapering to zero over a second week of therapy. Antiviral therapy improves outcome when given in conjunction with corticosteroids, in a dose equivalent to 1,000 mg of acyclovir daily for 7 to 10 days.

For patients unable to fully close the affected eye (House-Brackmann grade IV or higher), protection and care includes the liberal use of artificial tears and lubricating ointment multiple times daily until the protective function of eye closing returns. Taping or patching the affected eye closed before bed prevents inadvertent damage or desiccation to the exposed cornea during sleep. Rarely, a tarsorrhaphy may be required to prevent eye damage.

An audiogram should be obtained to ascertain the nature of any hearing loss and assess the presence or absence of the stapedial reflex. The presence of sensorineural hearing loss raises the possibility of varicella zoster virus infection as the likely etiology.

Electrical testing, by stimulating the trunk of the facial nerve as it exits the stylomastoid foramen with measurement of compound muscle action potential amplitude of the muscles of facial expression, may be helpful in establishing prognosis. This test, electroneurography (ENOG), is only beneficial between days 3 and 21 after complete loss of voluntary movements. Patients with >90% degeneration on ENOG compared to the contralateral side and no evidence of motor unit potentials on electromyography by day 14 of paralysis, have a poorer prognosis for return of facial function. Surgical decompression should be considered.

The role for surgical decompression of the facial nerve in acute paralysis has generated much debate. The surgical approach involves a middle cranial fossa craniotomy with selected decompression of the perigeniculate region of the facial nerve by an experienced otolaryngologist or neurosurgeon. In carefully selected patients with clearly defined electrical findings, this directed decompression has improved the final House-Brackmann grade of facial nerve function.

Generally, recovery from paresis or paralysis is satisfactory. Surgical procedures may help restore function in patients with poor recovery at 3 to 6 months after onset. A variety of re-animation and re-innervation operations are available to restore the muscles of facial expression.

FUTURE DIRECTIONS

The current evidence linking HSV infection to Bell's palsy is strong, although our understanding of when and why the latent infection causes symptoms is poorly understood. Further investigations may identify those patients at risk for Bell's palsy and increase our understanding of the stressors that may precipitate an episode of facial paralysis.

REFERENCES

Adour KK, Ruboyianes JM, Von Doersten PG, et al. Bell's palsy treatment with acyclovir and prednisone compared with prednisone alone: a double-blind, randomized, controlled trial. *Ann Otol Rhinol Laryngol.* 1996;105:371–378.

Friedman RA. The surgical management of Bell's palsy: a review. *Am J Otol.* 2000.21:139–144.

Gantz BJ, Rubinstein JT, Gidley P, Woodworth GG. Surgical management of Bell's palsy. *Laryngoscope.* 1999;109:117–1188.

Ramsey MJ, DerSimonian R, Holtel MR, Burgess LP. Corticosteroid treatment for idiopathic facial nerve paralysis: a meta-analysis. *Laryngoscope.* 2000;110:335–341.

Steiner I, Mattan Y. Bell's palsy and herpes viruses: to (acyclo)vir or not to (acyclo)vir? *J Neurol Sci.* 1999;170:19–23.

Chapter 99
Epilepsy

Bradley V. Vaughn and Robert S. Greenwood

Epilepsy has been described for more than 2,500 years. Hippocrates, in "On the Sacred Disease," described detailed seizure types and localized seizures as a disorder of the brain. The term *epilepsy* is a derivative of the Greek word for "to take hold of" (epilepsia). Throughout time individuals with epilepsy have been regarded as having special powers or being possessed. Yet, historical figures such as Julius Caesar, VanGogh, Napoleon, and Dostoyevsky, who lived with epilepsy, demonstrate that individuals with epilepsy can make tremendous contributions to society.

ETIOLOGY AND PATHOGENESIS

The broad definition of seizure includes any sudden onset of morbid symptoms. This includes syncope, cataplexy, or even psychogenic events. Epileptic seizures, a more narrowly defined paroxysmal form of seizures, are events resulting from excessive pathological synchronous neuronal activity in a large population of neurons. They are one of the most common symptoms of disturbed brain function. Approximately 10% of the population will have a seizure by age 80 years. Some seizures are self-limited as part of an acute medical condition, illness, or exposure to epileptogenic substances; other epileptic seizures are a sign of abnormal neuronal physiology and networks.

Epilepsy is a chronic disorder that is hallmarked by recurrent, unprovoked seizures. The diagnosis is based on historical features and can be made after the second unprovoked epileptic seizure. The patient may have multiple seizure types. A patient with juvenile myoclonic epilepsy, for example, may display absence, generalized tonic-clonic, and myoclonic seizures. Yet, all of these seizure types occur in one type of epilepsy.

Classification of Seizures

Seizures are classified by behavioral symptoms (semiology) and electroencephalographic data (Table 99-1). There are fundamentally 2 types: focal onset (partial) or diffuse onset (primary generalized). Approximately two thirds of epilepsy patients have partial seizures, which are further divided into simple partial and complex partial. Simple partial seizures are defined by the retention of consciousness or memory. Complex partial seizures are defined by the impairment of consciousness or the loss of memory during the seizure. Focal onset seizures may evolve into generalized seizures, and these secondarily generalized seizures are the most common generalized seizures in adults.

Table 99-1
Seizure Classification

Generalized Seizures of Non-focal Origin
    Tonic-Clonic
    Tonic
    Clonic
    Absence
    Atonic/akinetic
    Myoclonic

Partial Seizures
    Simple partial (without loss of consciousness)
      · With motor symptoms
      · With sensory symptoms
      · With autonomic symptoms
      · With psychic symptoms
      · Compound forms
    Complex partial (impaired consciousness)
      · Simple partial onset followed by impairment of consciousness
      · With impairment of consciousness at onset
      · With or without automatisms
    Partial seizures evolving to complex partial seizures or secondary generalization

Unclassified Seizures

Adapted from Commission on the Classification and Terminology of the International League Against Epilepsy. Proposal for Classification of Epilepsies and Epileptic Syndromes. *Epilepsia*. 1985;26:268–278.

Primary generalized seizures begin simultaneously across the whole brain and may comprise various types of behavior. Behavioral pauses associated with a 3-per-second generalized spike and wave discharge characterize absence seizures. These seizures occur in children typically, last less than 20 seconds and are associated with no postictal confusion. A sudden loss of muscle tone characterizes atonic seizures, which often cause patients to fall and sustain injuries. Tonic seizures produce generalized stiffening and often result in falls. Repetitive quick jerks with a slow relaxation phase are observed during clonic seizures. Tonic seizures may develop into clonic seizures, and clonic seizures may progress into tonic and then clonic seizures. Single quick jerks of the whole body or a portion of the body characterizes myoclonic seizures. The minority of myoclonus is of epileptic origin so that myoclonus often does not have an EEG correlate. Only myoclonus with an EEG correlate is considered epileptic.

Classification of Epilepsy

The classification of the epilepsies is based on age, family history, seizure types, associated clinical findings, and laboratory abnormalities, especially the EEG characteristics and neuroimaging abnormalities. Etiology, anatomic correlates, age of onset, associated neurological signs, precipitating factors, prognosis, circadian cycles, and seizure type are important features used in classification. The epilepsies are divided into 2 principal groups: localization-related and generalized events (Table 99-2). Plans to revise this classification are underway.

Causes of Seizures and Epilepsy

Focal seizures begin as an autonomous electrochemical discharge of a group of neurons that recruit surrounding neurons into a rhythmical firing pattern. Although many theories have been postulated about how focal seizures begin, most likely multiple factors are responsible. At the cellular level, the characteristic interictal abnormality of an epileptic focus is the paroxysmal depolarization shift (PDS). The PDS is an abnormal cellular event characterized intracellularly by a large membrane depolarization, which produces a burst of action potentials followed by hyperpolar-

Table 99-2
Epilepsy Classification

Localization-related (focal)
- Idiopathic, age-related onset: genetic, often associated with normal intelligence
- Symptomatic: seizures arise from a known lesion or site
- Cryptogenic: no identified symptomatic cause

Generalized
- Idiopathic, with age-related onset
- Cryptogenic or symptomatic
- Symptomatic

Undetermined whether focal or generalized

Special syndromes

Adapted from Commission on the Classification and Terminology of the International League Against Epilepsy. Proposal for Classification of Epilepsies and Epileptic Syndromes. *Epilepsia.* 1981;22:489–501.

ization of the neuron. On the surface of the brain or scalp, the PDS is seen as a spike followed by a slow wave. With the occurrence of a seizure, the intracellular depolarization and bursting persist, and no hyperpolarization occurs. A clinical seizure occurs only when a large number of neurons synchronously display this activity. The spread of seizures from the focus is usually prevented by a surround inhibition manifested intracellularly by hyperpolarization of the neurons. This inhibition is mediated predominately by gamma-aminobutyric acid (GABA). The mechanisms of the generalized epilepsies involve many neurons in a large portion of the brain.

Potential causes that lead to these epileptic changes can be age-dependent (Figure 99-1). The age of onset may give clues to the underlying cause of the seizures and epilepsy. Yet, any significant injury to cortical structures can evoke seizures. More than two thirds of patients have no clear cause for their seizures. The most common identifiable causes by age include:

Newborn: perinatal hypoxia and ischemia, drug withdrawal, hypocalcemia, hypomagnesemia, hyperbilirubinemia, hypoglycemia, water intoxication, intracranial hemorrhage, intracranial birth injury, newborn errors in metabolism, pyridoxine dependency, congenital malformations of the brain, intracranial infections, and sepsis.

Figure 99-1

Causes of Seizures

Primary

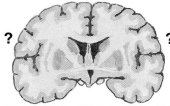

?   ?   Unknown (genetic or biochemical predisposition)

Intracranial

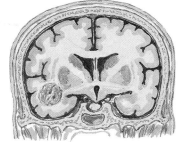

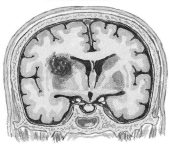

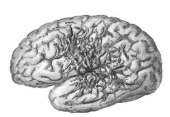

Tumor   Vascular (infarct or hemorrhage)   Arteriovenous malformation

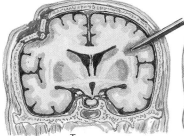

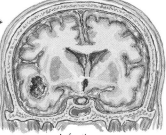

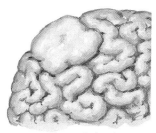

Trauma
(depressed fracture,
penetrating wound)   Infection
(abscess,
encephalitis)   Congenital and
hereditary diseases
(tuberous sclerosis)

Extracranial

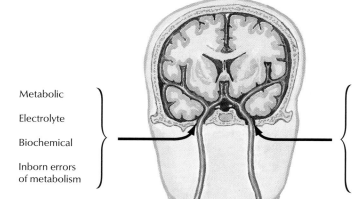

Metabolic

Electrolyte

Biochemical

Inborn errors
of metabolism

Anoxia

Hypoglycemia

Drugs

Drug withdrawal

Alcohol withdrawal

Table 99-3
Gene Defects in Genetic Epilepsy

Epilepsy	Inheritance	Gene Abnormality	Protein
Benign familial neonatal convulsions	AD	20q- BFNC1 8q- BFNC2	voltage-sensitive K+ channel
Juvenile myoclonic epilepsy	AD (variable penetrance)	6p21.2 15q14 2q22-q23 5q34-q35	Nicotinic ACh receptor α_4 subunit (nACh R) voltage-dependent Ca++ channel GABA receptor
Progressive myoclonus epilepsy	AR	21q22.3	cystatin
Nocturnal frontal lobe epilepsy	AD	20q13	nicotinic ACh receptor 4 subunit
Pyridoxine-dependent seizures	AR	2q31	Deficiency of pyridoxine as a co-factor for glutamic dehydrogenase
Gen. Epilepsy with febrile seizures +	AD (variable penetrance)	19q13 2q24 5q31-q33	Voltage-gated Na+ channel subunits $6\alpha\beta\alpha(\alpha)$ receptor extracellular loop
Familial Frontal Lobe Epilepsy	Type 1 AD Type 2 AD Type 3 AD	chromosome 20q13.2. chromosome 15q24 chromosome 1	neuronal nicotinic acetylcholine receptor subunit mutations neuronal nicotinic acetylcholine receptor β2 subunit mutation
Familial adult myoclonic epilepsy	AD	chromosome 8q24	Unknown
Lafora's disease	AD	chromosome 6q24, EPM2A	Laforin

nACh R, Acetylcholinesterase receptor; AD, autosomal dominant; AR, autosomal recessive.

Infancy: congenital defects, inborn errors in metabolism, acute infection, trauma, febrile convulsions, idiopathic.

Childhood: trauma, congenital defects, intracranial hemorrhage/arterial venous malformation, CNS infection, idiopathic.

Adolescence/Young Adult: trauma, drug and alcohol withdrawal, intracranial hemorrhage/arterial venous malformation, brain tumor, idiopathic.

Older Adult: alcoholism, brain tumor, cerebrovascular disease, trauma, metabolic disorders, uremia, hepatic failure, electrolyte abnormalities, hypoglycemia, CNS infection, idiopathic.

Most epilepsies with defined gene abnormalities are abnormalities of membrane channels. Only a few of the known genetic causes of epilepsy have been shown to be abnormalities of neurotransmitters (Table 99-3).

CLINICAL PRESENTATION

Individuals with epilepsy present with a wide variety of symptoms (Figures 99-2, 99-3, and 99-4). The key clinical feature of a seizure is the paroxysmal nature of discrete stereotypic events.

Figure 99-2 **Partial Motor and Somatosensory Seizures**

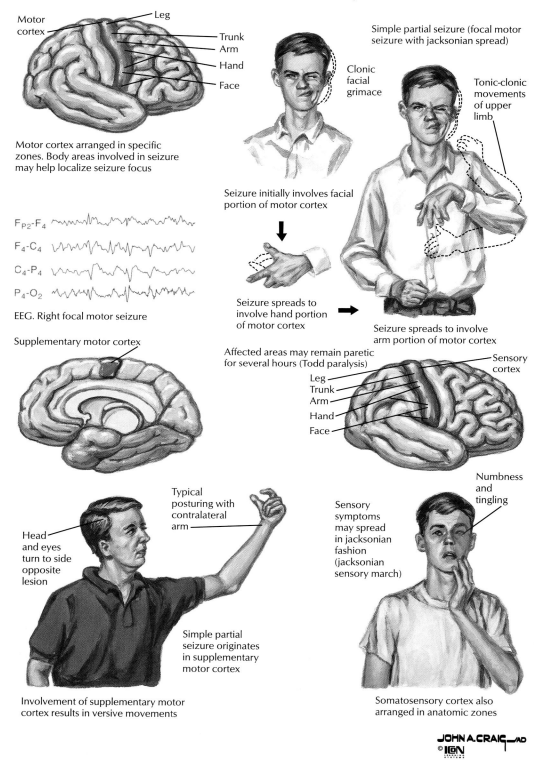

Motor cortex
Leg
Trunk
Arm
Hand
Face

Motor cortex arranged in specific zones. Body areas involved in seizure may help localize seizure focus

F_{P2}-F_4

F_4-C_4

C_4-P_4

P_4-O_2

EEG. Right focal motor seizure

Supplementary motor cortex

Simple partial seizure (focal motor seizure with jacksonian spread)

Clonic facial grimace

Tonic-clonic movements of upper limb

Seizure initially involves facial portion of motor cortex

Seizure spreads to involve hand portion of motor cortex

Seizure spreads to involve arm portion of motor cortex

Affected areas may remain paretic for several hours (Todd paralysis)

Leg
Trunk
Arm
Hand
Face

Sensory cortex

Head and eyes turn to side opposite lesion

Typical posturing with contralateral arm

Simple partial seizure originates in supplementary motor cortex

Involvement of supplementary motor cortex results in versive movements

Sensory symptoms may spread in jacksonian fashion (jacksonian sensory march)

Numbness and tingling

Somatosensory cortex also arranged in anatomic zones

JOHN A. CRAIG—MD
© ICON

Figure 99-3

Generalized Tonic-Clonic Seizures

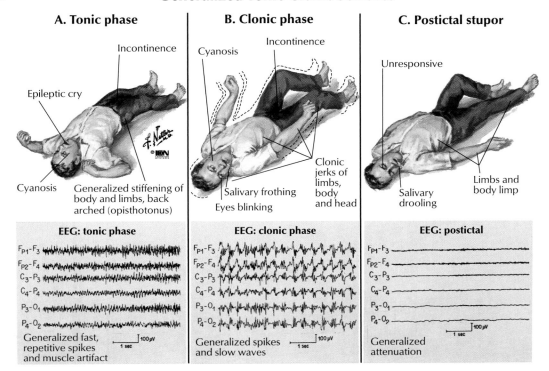

A. Tonic phase

Incontinence

Epileptic cry

Cyanosis

Generalized stiffening of body and limbs, back arched (opisthotonus)

B. Clonic phase

Cyanosis

Incontinence

Clonic jerks of limbs, body and head

Salivary frothing

Eyes blinking

C. Postictal stupor

Unresponsive

Limbs and body limp

Salivary drooling

EEG: tonic phase

F_{P1}-F_3
F_{P2}-F_4
C_3-P_3
C_4-P_4
P_3-O_1
P_4-O_2

Generalized fast, repetitive spikes and muscle artifact

$\boxed{}$ 100 µV 1 sec

EEG: clonic phase

F_{P1}-F_3
F_{P2}-F_4
C_3-P_3
C_4-P_4
P_3-O_1
P_4-O_2

Generalized spikes and slow waves

$\boxed{}$ 100 µV 1 sec

EEG: postictal

F_{P1}-F_3
F_{P2}-F_4
C_3-P_3
C_4-P_4
P_3-O_1
P_4-O_2

Generalized attenuation

$\boxed{}$ 100 µV 1 sec

An accurate description of a seizure may require reports from many sources and, at times, even a videotape of the events because the patient may be unaware of the events. Most seizures last less than 5 minutes.

In partial onset seizures, the behavior exhibited during a seizure is determined by the affected region of brain (Figure 99-2). Nearly any function performed by the brain may occur as part of a seizure. These symptoms range from motor involvement or sensory involvement to complex automatisms, repetitive motor activities that are purposeless, undirected, and inappropriate, which can be done without awareness (e.g., lip smacking, sucking, swallowing, chewing, repetitive hand movement, picking at clothes, or fidgeting), or hallucinations. Thus, a patient with occipital lobe seizures may have visual symptoms, or a patient with temporal lobe seizures may smell something burning or have a rising sensation in the chest. Patients with frontal lobe seizures may have unusual motor manifestations such as turning or bicycling movements. In the postictal period that

follows the seizure, patients are frequently confused and disoriented. These symptoms and behaviors are important in helping to define the seizure type and subsequent therapy.

Primary generalized seizures involve both cerebral hemispheres from the onset and require the interaction of cerebral hemispheres, thalamus, and possibly the brain stem. They are subcategorized into specific types. The most common is generalized tonic-clonic convulsion (previously called grand mal) (Figure 99-3). These seizures begin as tonic stiffening of the limbs in the extended position followed by synchronous clonic jerking of the muscles. Occasionally patients have pure tonic or pure clonic seizures. Following the seizure, the patient is very lethargic, confused, and disoriented.

Absence seizures (previously called petite mal) are characterized by staring spells lasting less than 20 seconds and often associated with eye blinking (Figure 99-4). Patients have no warning of oncoming seizures and also have no postictal period. Frequently they will have no memory for the event but may note a brief loss of time.

Figure 99-4

Absence (Petit Mal) Seizures

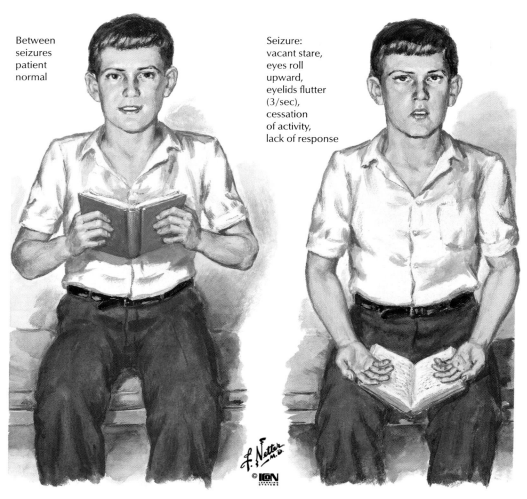

Between seizures patient normal

Seizure: vacant stare, eyes roll upward, eyelids flutter (3/sec), cessation of activity, lack of response

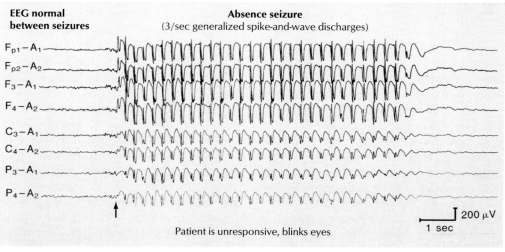

EEG normal between seizures

Absence seizure
(3/sec generalized spike-and-wave discharges)

$F_{p1} - A_1$
$F_{p2} - A_2$
$F_3 - A_1$
$F_4 - A_2$
$C_3 - A_1$
$C_4 - A_2$
$P_3 - A_1$
$P_4 - A_2$

200 µV
1 sec

Patient is unresponsive, blinks eyes

Patients usually have hundreds of these per day. These seizures usually occur in children and many times are first noticed in school. Frequently, hyperventilation can be used to provoke absence seizures. The characteristic generalized 3-per-second spike and wave pattern on EEG is the hallmark for this seizure type.

Atonic seizures are drop attacks or brief periods of loss of postural body tone. Patients may have clusters of seizures causing injury from the falls. These patients frequently wear helmets to avoid serious head injury.

Myoclonic seizures are rapid, brief, usually bisynchronous contractions of the musculature. Patients may have frequent jerks occurring in bursts and have minimal impairment of consciousness.

DIFFERENTIAL DIAGNOSIS

The differential diagnosis for paroxysmal events can be divided into several categories: vascular, endocrine, metabolic, neurologic, and psychiatric events (Table 99-4). The clinician should use a relatively wide differential before presuming the diagnosis. Frequently, non-epileptic paroxysmal events can be misinterpreted for epileptic seizures.

DIAGNOSTIC APPROACH

The goals of evaluation of the patient with seizures are to 1) identify the type of seizure that occurred, 2) look for potential causes, 3) elucidate risk factors that may promote recurrence, 4) review previous therapies, 5) define psychological and psycho-social impact of seizures on the patient, and 6) recognize the patient's goals. The history is the most important feature of the evaluation. A clear description of the events as witnessed by an observer increase the likelihood of obtaining a correct diagnosis. Particular attention is given to events leading up to the seizures, during the seizures, and following the seizures. The patients may have certain risk factors such as significant head trauma, stroke, febrile seizures, developmental delay, or family history of seizures. The physical examination should focus on the cardiac and vascular systems. A complete neurological examination should be performed. Most patients with epilepsy have a normal neurological examination, so the absence of neurological deficits does not exclude the diagnosis.

All patients with epilepsy should have had an

Table 99-4
Differential Diagnosis of Paroxysmal Disorders

Category	Cause
Vascular	Cardiac arrhythmia, transient ischemic attack, syncope, migraine, hyperventilation
Endocrine	Hypoglycemia, thyroid storm
Movement disorders	Paroxysmal vertigo, tics, alternating hemiplegia
Sleep disorders	Cataplexy, sleep paralysis, hypersomnia
Metabolic	Hypoxia, periodic paralysis
Toxic	Drugs
Psychiatric	Panic attacks, psychosis, conversion disorders, fugue states

EEG. This study records the electrical fields generated over the scalp. Although approximately 40% of patients with epilepsy will have a normal routine EEG, a second EEG performed with the subject asleep will increase the yield of abnormalities to 80%. The classic epileptiform abnormalities are spikes, sharp waves, or spike and slow wave complexes. These waveforms are the electrical signature of epilepsy; however, the incidence of these abnormalities in the people without seizures may be as high as 2%.

Patients with possible focal-onset epilepsy should undergo MRI of the brain, which demonstrates the cortex in great detail and allows for the detection of small structural abnormalities.

MANAGEMENT AND THERAPY

The goals for managing a patient with epilepsy are to have the patient completely seizure-free, with no side effects of therapy and to reverse any untoward effects of the epilepsy. These goals are not obtainable in all patients; an estimated 25% to 44% of patients are not completely controlled by medication. The general principles of medication therapy are to start a single medication at a low dose, slowly titrate the medication until the

Table 99-5
Medications

Focal Onset Seizures
- Phenytoin
- Carbamazepine
- Phenobarbital
- Primidone
- Methsuximide
- Valproate
- Gabapentin
- Lamotrigine
- Felbamate
- Topiramate
- Tiagabine
- Zonisamide
- Oxcarbazepine
- Levetiracetam
- Clorazepate
- Clonazepam
- Lorazepam

Primary Generalized Seizures
- Valproate
- Lamotrigine
- Ethosuximide (for absence seizures)
- Felbamate

patient is seizure-free or has untoward side effects that do not abate with drug manipulation. If the first medication does not succeed, a second medication is added and titrated to an efficacious dose before the tapering off of the first medication. Medications should be given ample trial time especially to allow side effects to improve with time (Table 99-5).

If medications are not helpful, consider reevaluating the patient. Confirmation of the diagnosis with video-EEG monitoring may prove helpful.

Additionally, this monitoring may demonstrate if the patient would be a candidate for evaluation for epilepsy surgery. Resection of the epileptic focus in some cases can cure the epilepsy. Success rates as high as 85% have been reported in resection of the seizure foci from the temporal lobes. Unfortunately, resections from other areas of the brain have not been as fruitful. Alternatively, neuronal stimulation therapy is available. The vagus nerve stimulator is also a proven therapy for patients with intractable epilepsy.

FUTURE DIRECTIONS

Epilepsy research is striving toward curing epilepsy and the epileptic process. . Although seizures are the defining component of the epilepsies, further research is needed to completely characterize the effect the epileptic process has upon the brain and the body. Development of new therapies such as cortical or deep brain stimulation provides exciting avenues to seizure control. Whatever the method of treatment, we know we must strive to selectively treat the neurons participating in the seizure focus while not altering normal brain function. This will ultimately provide a path for us to unlock the mysteries of neuronal networking and plasticity.

REFERENCES

Engel J Jr, Pedley TA, Aicardi J, et al, eds. *Epilepsy: A Comprehensive Texbook*. Philadelphia, Pa: Lippincott-Raven; 1997.

Levy RH, Mattson RH, Meldrum BS, Perucca E, eds. *Antiepileptic Drugs*. 5th ed. Philadelphia, Pa: Lippincott Williams & Wilkins; 2002.

Pellock JM, Dodson EW, Bourgois BFD, eds. *Pediatric Epilepsy: Diagnosis and Therapy*. 2nd ed. New York, NY: Demos Medical Publishing; 2001.

Wyllie E, ed. *The Treatment of Epilepsy: Principles and Practice*. 3rd ed. Philadelphia, Pa: Lippincott Williams & Wilkins; 2001.

Chapter 100
Migraine Headache

Kevin A. Kahn and Alan G. Finkel

Migraine is a prevalent disorder that has been documented throughout the record of human history. Neolithic humans (7000 B.C.) bore holes (trephination) into the skulls of presumed headache sufferers, and the Egyptians (1200 B.C.) wrapped a clay crocodile to the heads of headache patients with cloth bearing the names of the gods. It was Arateus of Cappodocia (second century A.D.) who is given credit for first identifying many of the features of migraine described in later history. Galen (A.D. 200) named the illness using the Greek *hemicrania* from which the term *migraine* derives its name.

Today, we know migraine to be a disabling disorder with a lifetime prevalence of 18% in females and 6% in males in the United States. In 1988, the International Headache Society published guidelines for classification of all recognized headaches types. Shortly thereafter, Stewart and Lipton published the American Migraine Study, recognized for its generalized approach and reproducibility in other countries throughout the world.

Migraine disability has been estimated to cost the United States between $5 billion and $17 billion annually. Fifty percent of migraineurs miss work 2 days per month and have reduced work efficiency for 6 days per month. Two thirds of migraineurs recognize that the disease has adversely affected their family life. Classifiable migraine is diagnosed by physicians in only 52% of sufferers. These facts underscore the importance of the physician in recognizing, diagnosing, and treating migraine in the workplace and at home.

ETIOLOGY AND PATHOGENESIS

Migraine was considered a purely vascular disorder until the mid-1980s when Moskowitz proposed the *Trigeminovascular Theory* of migraine. With use of animal models, Moskowitz demonstrated that electrical stimulation of the trigeminal nucleus caudalis in the pons causes plasma protein extravasation from dural blood vessels. He concluded that the generation of migraine depended on serotonin-mediated increases in neuronal excitation, not primary vascular reactivity. Thus, the pain results in inflammation of

blood vessels, although its source is a *neurogenic* cause localized to trigeminal nuclear centers. In humans, trigeminal stimulation during neurosurgery has resulted in the expression of recognized inflammatory and pronociceptive substances (calcitonin gene-related peptide, NKA, substance P) within the extracranial circulation similar to those produced in the animal studies (Figure 100-1).

Migraine aura occurs consistently in 15% to 25% of migraineurs. Aura is a localizable and fully reversible neurologic deficit preceding head pain, which results from progressive neuronal dysfunction spreading across the cerebral cortex. A similar 'spreading cortical depression' occurs in experimental animals after chemical or electrical irritation of the brain surface. Studies including single-photon emission computed tomography (SPECT), PET, fMRI, magnetic resonance spectroscopy (MRS), and magnetoencephalography have bolstered this hypothesis. Decreased blood flow does not reach levels severe enough to qualify as ischemia. Other systems including serotonergic, noradrenergic, and dopaminergic pathways, hormonal (e.g., estrogen), hypothalamic, and deep brainstem structures are involved in the ultimate expression of migraine. Thus, migraine can be described as neuronal sensitization and neurogenic inflammation in a milieu of multiple neurochemical influences. The goal of migraine treatment is to attenuate neuronal irritability and neurogenic inflammation while keeping in mind the importance of the contributions of these other central mechanisms.

Figure 100-1

Mechanisms in Migraine

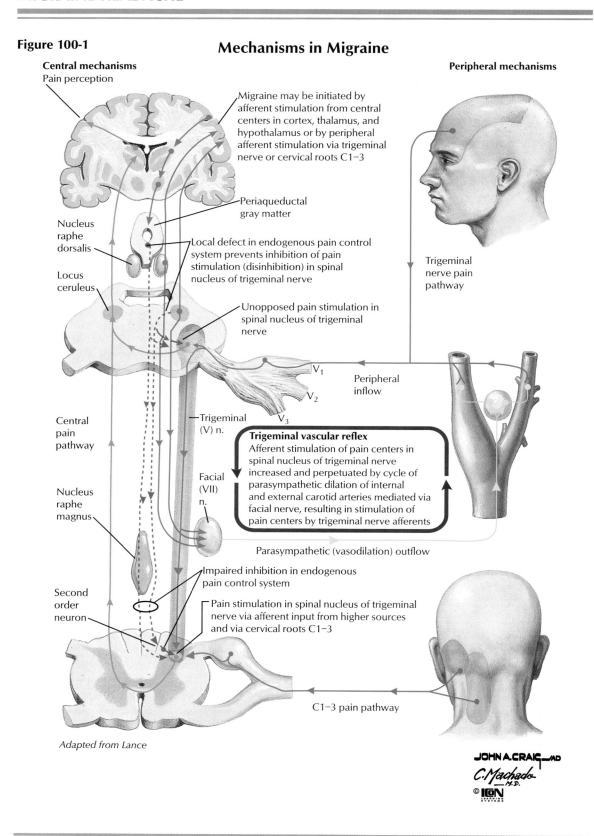

Central mechanisms
Pain perception

Migraine may be initiated by afferent stimulation from central centers in cortex, thalamus, and hypothalamus or by peripheral afferent stimulation via trigeminal nerve or cervical roots C1–3

Peripheral mechanisms

Periaqueductal gray matter

Nucleus raphe dorsalis

Local defect in endogenous pain control system prevents inhibition of pain stimulation (disinhibition) in spinal nucleus of trigeminal nerve

Locus ceruleus

Trigeminal nerve pain pathway

Unopposed pain stimulation in spinal nucleus of trigeminal nerve

V_1

Peripheral inflow

V_2

Central pain pathway

Trigeminal (V) n.

V_3

Trigeminal vascular reflex
Afferent stimulation of pain centers in spinal nucleus of trigeminal nerve increased and perpetuated by cycle of parasympathetic dilation of internal and external carotid arteries mediated via facial nerve, resulting in stimulation of pain centers by trigeminal nerve afferents

Facial (VII) n.

Nucleus raphe magnus

Parasympathetic (vasodilation) outflow

Impaired inhibition in endogenous pain control system

Second order neuron

Pain stimulation in spinal nucleus of trigeminal nerve via afferent input from higher sources and via cervical roots C1–3

C1–3 pain pathway

Adapted from Lance

JOHN A. CRAIG—MD
C. Machado—M.D.
© ICON LEARNING SYSTEMS

Figure 100-2

Migraine
Aura

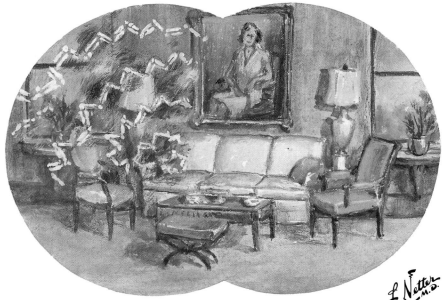

Visual disturbances, most common element of migraine aura:
blurred cloudy vision, scotomas, scintillating zigzag lines
(fortification spectrum), flashes of light, etc.

CLINICAL PRESENTATION

Migraine presents in a variable fashion, but it can be divided into two groups: with aura (classic migraine) and without aura (common migraine). A prodrome may occur up to 24 hours preceding headache. Prodromal features may include hunger, thirst, euphoria, mania, depression, drowsiness, psychomotor slowing, or irritability. Aura is present in only 15% to 25% of migraineurs. Aura symptoms may include visual scotomata (dark spots), photopsias (bright spots), fortification spectra (jagged bright lines), numbness, tingling, weakness, confusion, or aphasia (Figures 100-2, 100-3, 100-4). Triggers include environmental stimuli such as intense light, sound, or odors; certain foods (nitrates, sulfites, monosodium glutamate, alcohol); irregular sleep or nutrition; exercise; stress; and hormonal fluctuations (Figure 100-5). The International Headache Society proposed the following guidelines in 1988 to diagnose migraine:

Diagnostic Criteria for Migraine Without Aura (Common Migraine)—No single feature is required

or sufficient for diagnosis. At least 5 attacks, each lasting 4–72 hours should have occurred. Headache has at least 2 of the following characteristics: 1) unilateral location, 2) pulsating quality, 3) moderate or severe intensity (inhibits or prohibits daily activities), 4) aggravation by routine physical activity. At least 1 of the following during headache: 1) nausea or vomiting, 2) photophobia (light sensitivity), 3) phonophobia (sound sensitivity). History and examination do not support evidence of organic disease that could cause headaches, or if disease is present, then headaches should not have originated in close temporal relation to the disease.

Diagnostic Criteria for Migraine with Aura (Classic Migraine) — At least 2 attacks. Aura must exhibit at least 3 of the following characteristics: 1) fully reversible and indicative of focal cerebral cortical or brainstem dysfunction, 2) gradual onset, 3) lasts less than 60 minutes, 4) followed by headache with a free interval of less than 60 minutes, 5) headache may begin before or simultaneously with the aura. (If history and examination do

Figure 100-3

Migraine Prodromes

Scintillating scotoma and fortification phenomena

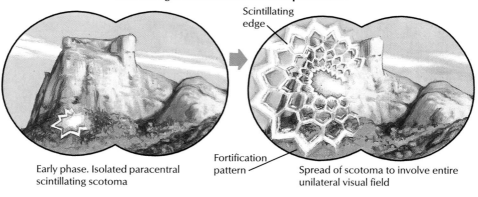

Scintillating edge

Early phase. Isolated paracentral scintillating scotoma

Fortification pattern

Spread of scotoma to involve entire unilateral visual field

Wavy lines (heat shimmers)

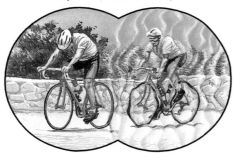

Wavy line distortions in part of visual field similar to shimmers above hot pavement

Metamorphopsia

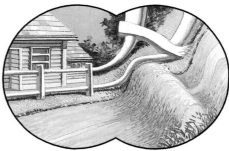

Distortions of form, size, or position of objects or environment in part of visual field

Figure 100-4

Focal Neurologic Phenomena

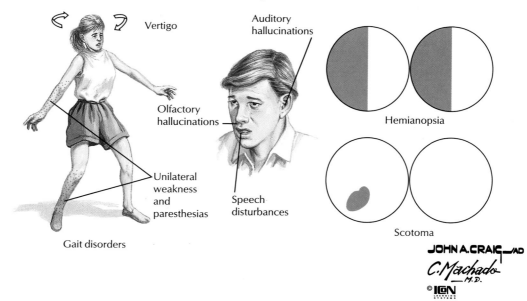

Vertigo

Auditory hallucinations

Olfactory hallucinations

Unilateral weakness and paresthesias

Speech disturbances

Gait disorders

Hemianopsia

Scotoma

JOHN A. CRAIG—MD

C. Machado —M.D.

©ICN

not support evidence of organic disease that could cause headaches or if disease is present, then headaches should not have originated in close temporal relation to the disease).

DIFFERENTIAL DIAGNOSIS

Migraine must be differentiated from secondary causes of headache to rule out more lethal causes of severe head pain. Other primary headache disorders, tension-type headache, cluster headache, and cluster variants, are often confused with migraine. Tension-type headache typically does not cause nausea and does not present with *both* photophobia and phonophobia. There is considerable debate on whether tension-type headache is an independent disorder or if it represents a part of a migraine continuum. Nevertheless, tension-type headache may co-exist with migraine, and the presence of a tension headache does not preclude the possibility of migraine. *Cluster headache* derives its name from the pattern of recurrent groups of headaches within a finite period of days to months. It is characterized as an excruciating, typically retro-orbital or temporal pain with duration of 15 to 180 minutes and typically affects males more than females (Figure 100-5). The headache attack may recur at specific times of the day with remarkable consistency. It is differentiated from migraine by its short duration and difference in behavior of the patient during the attack; the patient cannot be still during the event, whereas the migraine patient prefers immobility and hibernation. In addition, it must present with at least 1 of the following features: lacrimation, rhinorrhea, ptosis, miosis, nasal congestion, conjunctival injection, eyelid edema, or forehead/facial sweating abnormalities. Cluster variants include those headaches with similar features to cluster but with shorter duration. *Chronic paroxysmal hemicrania*, a cluster variant, affects women more than men and has an absolute response to indomethacin.

Secondary causes of headache disorders include head trauma, vascular disorders (e.g., hemorrhage, stroke, vasculitis), intracranial disorders (e.g., neoplasm, increased or decreased intracranial pressure), substance withdrawal, infection, metabolic disorders (e.g., hypoxia, hypercapnia, hypoglycemia, dialysis), and disorders of other structures of the head and neck (e.g., cervical spine, eyes, ears, nose and sinuses, temporomandibular joints). Most of these disorders can be elucidated by a careful history and examination; however, sometimes it is necessary to perform diagnostic procedures if suspicion for these disorders is raised.

DIAGNOSTIC APPROACH

There is no specific diagnostic test for migraine, but investigations are mandated if secondary causes of headache are of concern. Secondary headaches should be suspected when the patient reports a "worst headache," has an abnormal neurologic examination, has a new-onset headache, or when there has been a dramatic change in headache pattern. To rule out an acute hemorrhage, non-contrast CT scan is preferred due to speed of the procedure and sensitivity. Lumbar puncture (LP) may be necessary to detect xanthochromia in patients with normal CT scan results and high index of suspicion for bleeding (worst headache of life). LP may also be helpful in assessing causes of headache related to pressure (position affects headache) or infection (nuchal rigidity plus photophobia or altered mental status). However, if intracranial masses are suspected, then contrast-enhanced MRI is preferred. Abnormalities in the posterior fossae are associated with headaches with coughing, straining, bending, etc. Contrast-enhanced magnetic resonance angiography (MRA) may be helpful in assessing vasculitis or the presence of an aneurysm, but traditional angiography should be considered if suspicion is high and MRA results are normal. Carotid Doppler assessment may be helpful in acute-onset headache with Horner's syndrome to rule out carotid dissection. EEG assessment should be performed in those patients with paroxysmal headache with cognitive or behavioral changes to rule out epilepsy.

MANAGEMENT AND THERAPY

Treatment of migraine begins with clear diagnosis and knowledge of its pathophysiology. Acute treatment of headache should be stratified to level of disability in the patient. Non-specific therapies include NSAIDs, sympathomimetics (e.g., caffeine), or analgesics (e.g., acetaminophen, opiates). Frequent use of many of these agents has been associated with substance withdrawal

Figure 100-5

Migraine Headache
Attack

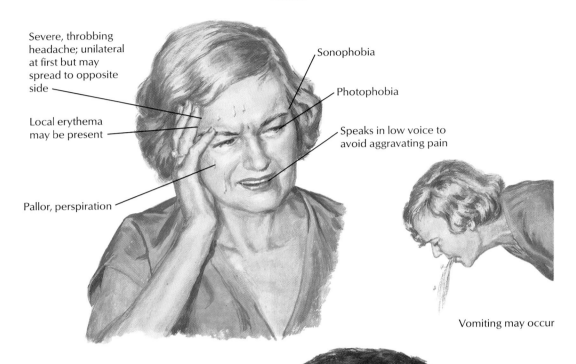

Severe, throbbing headache; unilateral at first but may spread to opposite side

Local erythema may be present

Pallor, perspiration

Sonophobia

Photophobia

Speaks in low voice to avoid aggravating pain

Vomiting may occur

Cluster Headache

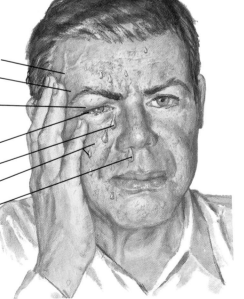

Temporal artery bulging and pulsating

Severe headache, pain behind eye

Unilateral ptosis, swelling and redness of eyelid

Myosis, conjunctival injection

Tearing

Flushing of side of face, sweating

Nasal congestion, rhinorrhea

Figure 100-6

Triggers of Migraine

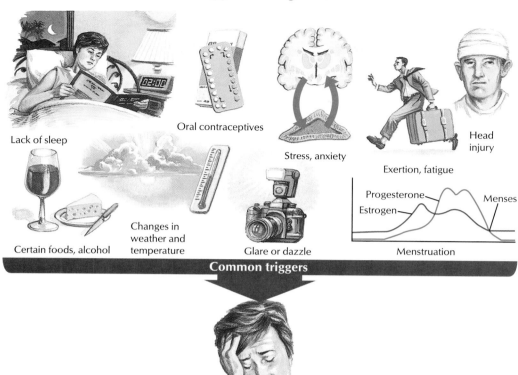

Lack of sleep

Oral contraceptives

Stress, anxiety

Head injury

Exertion, fatigue

Certain foods, alcohol

Changes in weather and temperature

Glare or dazzle

Progesterone

Estrogen

Menses

Menstruation

Common triggers

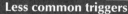

Less common triggers

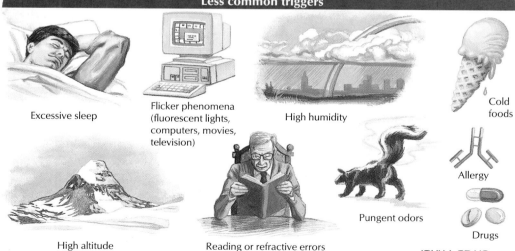

Excessive sleep

Flicker phenomena (fluorescent lights, computers, movies, television)

High humidity

Cold foods

Allergy

High altitude

Reading or refractive errors

Pungent odors

Drugs

JOHN A. CRAIG—MD

C. Machado—M.D.

© ICN

headache and analgesic rebound. For moderate to severely disabling headache, specific medication should be used. The most specific of these are triptans. They bind specifically to serotonin receptors on trigeminal nerve endings to halt neurogenic inflammation in addition to binding to dural blood vessels to reduce painful swelling. There is no 'class effect' of triptans, and if one is not effective, then another may be tried. They are contraindicated in patients with uncontrolled hypertension and history of coronary artery disease but are generally extremely safe and effective. Triptans are more costly than nonspecific therapy but economic analyses point to cost savings and decreased disability when triptans are used in patients with moderate-to-severe headache.

Patients should be offered preventive treatment if untreatable headaches occur more than twice per month or if the patient is willing to use a daily medication to prevent headache. Preventive medication usually provides benefit after 2 to 3 months of administration. FDA approved preventive treatment for migraine includes valproic acid, propranolol, and methysergide. There is evidence to support the use of other agents including other anticonvulsants (decrease neuronal irritability), other ß-blockers (modulate noradrenergic system and vascular system), tricyclic antidepressants (modulate serotonin and norepinephrine), calcium channel blockers (vascular and central factors), and hormonal manipulation. Oral chelated magnesium and high-dose (400 mg/day) oral riboflavin have been reported to be effective in double-blinded studies.

Non-pharmacologic approaches include the avoidance of migraine triggers (e.g. foods, missed meals), biofeedback and self-hypnosis, psychological counseling to improve stress management skills, regular exercise, good sleep hygiene, and balanced diet. All these measures serve to decrease neuronal irritability and thereby reduce the frequency of migraine.

FUTURE DIRECTIONS

The future of migraine management lies in the development of pharmacologic and non-pharmacologic strategies that follow advances in migraine pathophysiology. Genetic studies have linked hemiplegic migraine (aura of reversible hemiplegia) to a defect on chromosome 19p 13, which encodes voltage-gated P/Q type calcium channels. Genetic polymorphism studies have implicated alterations in the gene for serotonin receptors in migraine without aura and in dopamine receptors with migraine with aura. Such studies may provide clues about why migraineurs are predisposed to central sensitization and neurogenic inflammation. Neuroimaging studies may continue to provide links between the animal and human models. Non-pharmacologic therapies are just beginning to be subjected to evidence-based medicine trials. Pending such studies there will likely be a place in migraine therapy for neurohypnosis, acupuncture, music therapy, and other complementary medical approaches. Education of health-care professionals is an important part of management of migraine because nearly half of all cases of migraine remain undiagnosed. Proactive and educated health-care providers will serve to improve the quality of life in migraineurs and will lessen the impact of this prevalent and disabling disease.

REFERENCES

Classification and diagnostic criteria for headache disorders, cranial neuralgias and facial pain. Headache Classification Committee of the International Headache Society. *Cephalalgia.* 1988;8(suppl 7):1-96.

Lipton RB, Silberstein SD. The role of headache-related disability in migraine management: implications for headache treatment guidelines. *Neurology.* 2001;56(suppl 1):S35–S42.

Olesen J, Tfelt-Hansen P, Welch KMA, eds. *The Headaches.* 2nd ed. Philadelphia, Pa: Lippincott Williams & Wilkins; 2000.

Silberstein SD, Lipton RB, Goadsby PJ. *Headache in Clinical Practice.* 2nd ed. London, England: Martin Dunitz Ltd; 2002.

Chapter 101
Multiple Sclerosis

J. Douglas Mann and Susan A. Gaylord

Multiple sclerosis (MS) is a disease of central nervous system (CNS) white matter that afflicts young adults with a peak incidence between ages 20 and 50. Prevalence of the disease in the United States is close to 300,000. The impact of MS is considerable given the age at onset, lost work and family time, and the overall reduction in quality of life.

Diagnosis is based on a careful history and neurological examination combined with confirmatory lumbar puncture and MRI. Although treatment is largely symptomatic, there have been major advances in our understanding of the immunology of MS with some translation into effective immune-modifying therapies. There is no known cure.

ETIOLOGY AND PATHOGENESIS

Risk of developing MS is based in part on geographical location during the first 15 years of life. The condition is progressively more common with distance from the equator in both hemispheres. Those of northern European ancestry are at relatively high risk, while African Americans exhibit half the risk of whites. Asians and Hispanics in the United States carry a low overall risk.

Genetic influences are reflected in twin studies where the monozygotic concordance rate is 30%, while the dizygotic rate is 5%. First-degree relatives carry at least a 20% increased risk of the disease compared to an age-matched population. Those with major histocompatibility subtypes HLA-DR2, B7, and A3 are at greater risk. MS is not contagious

Although seasonal variations in disease activity have been reported, the pace of the illness is largely independent of environmental factors. Physical trauma, emotional stress, and upper respiratory infections have been implicated and may precipitate attacks. Elevated body temperature temporarily brings out latent and reversible neurological deficits secondary to impaired neural transmission through affected white matter.

Recent advances in the treatment of MS have come through a better understanding of immune-mediated damage to the nervous system. Multiple lines of evidence point to a cascade of events that result in perivascular demyelination of CNS white matter through an autoimmune inflammatory process. Mechanisms of remyelination are incompletely effective, accounting for partial recovery and accumulation of deficits with repeated attacks over time. Specific mechanisms of initiation, maintenance, and cessation of attacks are under intensive investigation.

CLINICAL PRESENTATION

Typically, multiple attacks occur over a period of years, involving multiple areas of CNS white matter in a process of plaque formation (Figure 101-1). Several patterns of attack are encountered. Relapsing-remitting (R-R) MS occurs in approximately 85% of cases, is more common in younger females, and often starts with prominent sensory/visual symptoms (Figure 101-2). The average attack frequency is less than 1 per year in that group. Chronic progressive (CP) MS without remitting features is seen in up to 10% of patients, typically later in onset and frequently in males. A progressive component of the illness develops in half of those with R-R MS after 10 years, termed secondary progressive (SP) MS. A fulminant course without remission is encountered rarely. Cases of single attacks without further progression occur. The risk of developing MS following a single episode of optic neuritis or transverse myelitis is 30% to 60%.

Symptoms in the R-R form develop over hours to days and are followed by variable recovery over days to weeks. Vertigo, monocular blindness (Figure 101-2) double vision, paresthesias, numbness, incoordination, intention tremor, focal weakness, and bladder dysfunction lead the symptom list. Multiple symptoms, reflecting

Figure 101-1   Multiple Sclerosis: Central Nervous System Plaques

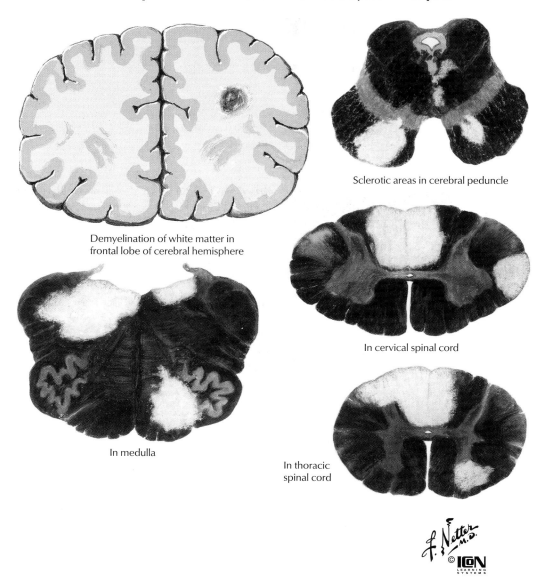

Demyelination of white matter in
frontal lobe of cerebral hemisphere

Sclerotic areas in cerebral peduncle

In cervical spinal cord

In medulla

In thoracic
spinal cord

involvement of multiple areas of white matter, can appear during a single attack. First attacks, especially if vision is not involved, tend to be unnoticed except in retrospect, being attributed to viral causes, stress, or minor trauma. Some patients will experience recurrent episodes involving the same brain region. The timing of attacks and degree of recovery are highly variable and may change abruptly during the course of the illness. Pregnancy tends to be protective.

Chronic fatigue is very common and difficult to treat. An elevation in core temperature will worsen fatigue that, in turn, restricts exercise in many patients.

Pain at presentation is uncommon, although two thirds of patients with MS will have significant pain at some time during their illness. Pain syndromes include central neuropathic pain with burning dysesthesias and radicular pain similar to trigeminal neuralgia. Lhermitte's sign is a painful shock-like sensation, usually experienced in the neck, upper

Figure 101-2

Multiple Sclerosis

Ocular Manifestations of Multiple Sclerosis

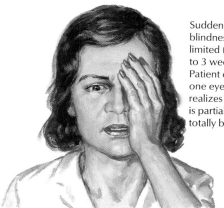

Sudden unilateral blindness, self-limited (usually 2 to 3 weeks). Patient covering one eye, suddenly realizes other eye is partially or totally blind.

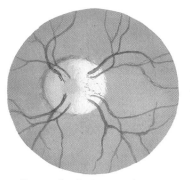

Temporal pallor in optic disc, caused by delayed recovery of temporal side of optic (II) nerve

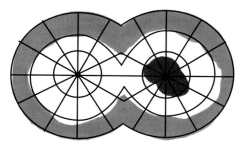

Visual fields reveal central scotoma due to acute retrobulbar neuritis

Internuclear Ophthalmoplegia

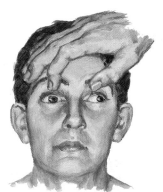

Eyes turned to left, right eye lags

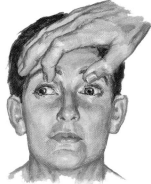

Eyes turned to right, left eye lags (to lesser degree)

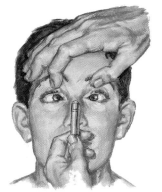

Convergence unimpaired

back or limbs, occurring spontaneously or with neck movement. Spasticity can lead to painful muscle contractions, and autonomic nervous system impairment leads to painful distention of bladder and bowel. Headache is more common (27%) than in an age-matched population (12%). Optic neuritis can be painful before and during the episode. Seizures attributable to MS are twice the number seen in a matched population but are uncommon overall. Constipation and bladder dysfunction require careful management. Emotional lability and cognitive deficits associated with accelerated cortical atrophy are noted in all forms of MS.

Prognosis

The average duration of MS is 30 years from diagnosis. Overall life expectancy is reduced by 7 years. Death from complications of MS is more common in males with progressive forms of the illness. Pneumonia and loss of respiratory drive are associated causes in those patients. Depression is common. The suicide rate is increased 7-fold, especially in younger patients early in the clinical course.

MS is benign in 40% with few limiting deficits after 15 years. Favorable prognostic factors include younger age at onset, dominance of sensory and visual symptoms, female gender, a R-R pattern of attacks, and sparing of spine and bladder. Poor prognosis is associated with age at onset above 35, early motor impairment, male gender, a chronic progressive pattern, and cerebellar and spinal involvement.

Brain atrophy is present in mild-to-moderate MS and is likely to progress when enhancing MRI lesions are present at onset.

DIFFERENTIAL DIAGNOSIS

Recurrent exacerbations of CNS vasculitis mimic MS. Atypical features such as psychosis, seizures, and gray matter lesions on MRI assist in making the correct diagnosis. Behçet's disease and Sjögren's syndrome can manifest as multifocal CNS disease. Behçet's disease is suspected when there are multiple cranial nerve deficits in combination with oral or genital ulcers, uveitis, and meningoencephalitis. A diagnosis of Sjögren's syndrome can be made with a lip or parotid gland biopsy. Vitamin B_{12} deficiency can present with progressive spinal cord symptoms that correlate with white matter lesions in the posterior columns seen on MRI. Adrenoleukodystrophy and tropical spastic paraparesis can also resemble MS, but are rare. Transverse myelitis in combination with optic neuritis suggests Devic's disease, especially when the spinal fluid is relatively benign and there are no lesions noted on MRI of the head. Vascular disease with multiple transient ischemic attacks or infarctions generally occurs in an older population or with significant risk factors and is not often mistaken for MS. Sarcoid, lues, and tumors round out the differential and are diagnosed with MRI and CSF studies when suspected. The diagnosis can be difficult with a first attack of MS that has atypical features (e.g. face pain, confusion, seizures, fever, or headache). An antecedent systemic infection that triggers an attack can cause further confusion.

DIAGNOSTIC APPROACH

The diagnosis rests on a history of multiple episodes of CNS dysfunction, occurring over a period of months to years with variable recovery, combined with a neurologic examination revealing abnormal signs referable to multiple CNS locations. Lumbar puncture, MRI, and evoked potential studies are useful in confirming the clinical impression and ruling out other conditions.

Definite MS is characterized by 2 distinct attacks with 2 or more lesions confirmed by examination or laboratory studies. Anything less must be considered probable or possible MS.

MRI of brain and spinal cord, with and without contrast material, is used to define active lesions (contrast positive) and older lesions, seen especially well on T2-weighted images in 90% of those with definite MS.

CSF will test positive for oligoclonal bands or elevated IgG/albumin CSF/serum ratios in 90% with a disease duration greater than 1 year. The CSF may be normal with the first attack (Figure 101-3).

In definite MS, visual-evoked potentials are abnormal in 90% of cases, while auditory and somatosensory studies are abnormal in 60% to 80%. Evoked potentials are useful in uncovering clinically silent white matter lesions that may confirm the diagnosis by establishing multiple sites of CNS involvement (Figures 101-3 and 101-4).

MANAGEMENT AND THERAPY

It is helpful to inform patients of the high degree of variability of attack and recovery patterns in MS as well as the considerable amount of research devoted to this condition, which is leading to effective treatment strategies.

Acute Exacerbations

Although steroids may shorten an attack, they have no effect on long-term outcome. Side effects limit their use, and chronic steroids must be avoided.

Methylprednisolone: One gram IV daily for 3 consecutive days followed by a 2-week tapering course of oral prednisone starting at 60 mg daily for 5 days, 40 mg for 4 days, 30 mg for 3 days, 20 mg for 2 days, and 10 mg for the last day. Preventive treatment for gastric bleeding is started and continued during each course of therapy.

Prednisone: A slightly longer course of oral steroids starting with 60 mg daily for the first week, followed by 40 mg daily for a week, 20 mg for a week, then 10 mg and 5 mg per day for the last 2 weeks, respectively.

ACTH: This older therapy is used for those not responding to the above medications for exacerbations. Forty mg is given twice per day IV for the first week followed by a weekly taper to 40 mg, 20 mg, and then 10 mg per day given IM.

Suppression of Exacerbations

Interferon-beta 1a and interferon-beta 1b reduce the number of attacks in R-R forms of MS by an average of 35%. Reduction in numbers of active lesions noted on MRI is also reported with their use. Their mechanism of action is complex and includes inhibition of suppressor cell function and T cell migration across the blood-brain barrier and enhanced production of anti-inflammatory cytokines. Dosing is either by weekly IM injection (interferon-beta 1a) or every-other-day subcutaneous (SC) injection (interferon-beta 1b). Side effects include flu-like symptoms; depression; injection site reactions; and rarely thyroiditis, lupus, or rheumatoid symptoms. Neutralizing antibodies occur 30% of the time and are associated with reduction in treatment efficacy.

Glatiramer acetate (copolymer 1) is a 4-amino acid molecule that acts by reducing reactivity to CNS antigens. Given daily by SC injection, it reduces exacerbations by one third in R-R MS.

Side effects include injection site pain, fatigue, nausea, chest pain, anxiety, and flushing.

Azathioprine, methotrexate, cladribine, and *cyclosporin A* have limited benefit in patients with rapidly progressive MS. Significant side effects limit their use.

Hyperbaric oxygen, lymphoid cell irradiation, plasmapheresis, and *oral myelin* have not been found to be effective.

Complications

Use of medications for complications arising from MS is limited by frequent major side effects. Quality of life, autonomy, and the frequency of depression and cognitive deficits must be considered when recommending specific therapies. Treatments that enlist patient enthusiasm and participation carry highest priority.

Fatigue: Regular exercise, the addition of complex carbohydrates to the diet, and multivitamin supplements reduce chronic fatigue. Amantadine 100 mg up to 3 times a day is the only proven medication-based therapy for this problem.

Spasticity: Physical therapy, massage, osteopathy, yoga, acupuncture, mindfulness meditation, and biofeedback are helpful singly or in combination. Electromyographic-guided motor point injections can reduce spasticity significantly but with some reduction in power. Baclofen starting at 5 mg 3 times daily and 10 mg at bedtime can be helpful for painful muscle spasms. Drowsiness and fatigue are notable side effects.

Bladder dysfunction: Therapy for significant urinary incontinence or retention is guided by urodynamic studies when possible. Urgency, frequency, or a "no-warning" bladder are treated with anticholinergic agents such as propantheline bromide up to 60 mg per day in 3 or 4 divided doses, or penthienate bromide up to 50 mg daily. When urodynamics reveal problems with bladder emptying, cholinergic agents are used, including bethanechol chloride 10 mg to 15 mg 3 to 4 times per day. Baclofen can reduce urethral sphincter spasm when the spasm limits voiding. Biofeedback training is useful for both types of problems and avoids drug side effects.

Pain: Burning dysesthesias and lancinating, tic-like pain may respond to gabapentin up to 600 mg 4 times a day, carbamazepine up to 400 mg three times a day, or alpha-lipoic acid 200 mg

Figure 101-3

Multiple Sclerosis: Diagnostic Tests I

Somatosensory evoked responses (SER)

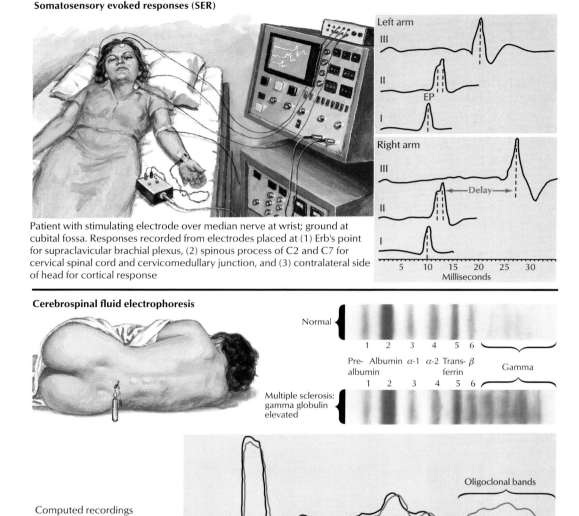

Patient with stimulating electrode over median nerve at wrist; ground at cubital fossa. Responses recorded from electrodes placed at (1) Erb's point for supraclavicular brachial plexus, (2) spinous process of C2 and C7 for cervical spinal cord and cervicomedullary junction, and (3) contralateral side of head for cortical response

Left arm

Right arm

Delay

Milliseconds

Cerebrospinal fluid electrophoresis

Normal

Pre-albumin   Albumin   α-1   α-2   Trans-ferrin   β   Gamma

Multiple sclerosis: gamma globulin elevated

Oligoclonal bands

Computed recordings

Normal

Multiple sclerosis

Prealbumin   Albumin   Alpha−1   Alpha−2   Trans-ferrin   Beta   Gamma globulin

twice daily. Muscular pain responds to slow stretch exercise, massage, and cooling. Transcutaneous nerve stimulation and trigger point injections are also useful for muscle pain. Muscle relaxants may worsen depression and chronic fatigue and cause drowsiness. Use of tricyclic antidepres-

sants for pain is limited by aggravation of bladder and bowel symptoms.

Depression/Anxiety: Depression is encountered in more than 50% of patients at some time in their disease, particularly in younger patients early in the illness. Counseling combined with a selective

Figure 101-4

Multiple Sclerosis: Diagnostic Tests II

Visual evoked response (VER)

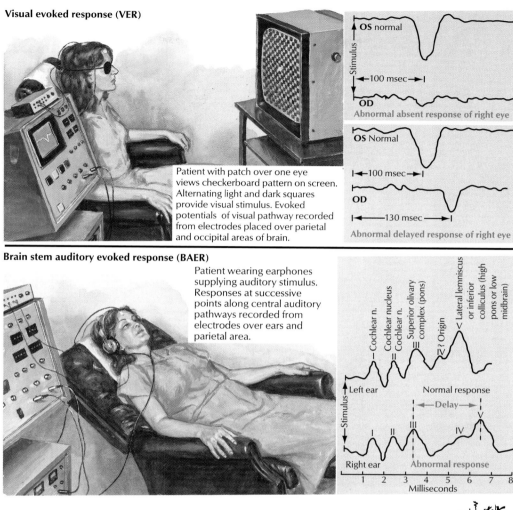

Patient with patch over one eye views checkerboard pattern on screen. Alternating light and dark squares provide visual stimulus. Evoked potentials of visual pathway recorded from electrodes placed over parietal and occipital areas of brain.

OS normal

←100 msec→

OD

Abnormal absent response of right eye

OS Normal

←100 msec→

OD

←130 msec→

Abnormal delayed response of right eye

Brain stem auditory evoked response (BAER)

Patient wearing earphones supplying auditory stimulus. Responses at successive points along central auditory pathways recorded from electrodes over ears and parietal area.

Cochlear n.
Cochlear nucleus
Cochlear n.
Superior olivary complex (pons)
? Origin
Lateral lemniscus or inferior colliculus (high pons or low midbrain)

Left ear   Normal response
←Delay→

Right ear   Abnormal response

1 2 3 4 5 6 7 8
Milliseconds

serotonin reuptake inhibitor drug St, John's Wort can ameliorate symptoms that are often chronic and difficult to treat. Guided imagery, self-hypnosis, and mindfulness meditation practices are very helpful in treating anxiety and are clearly superior to anxiolytics, which usually worsen depression.

FUTURE DIRECTIONS

Major areas of investigation include further definition of key steps in the immune process leading to plaque formation, reversing activation of T cells and limiting their penetration into the CNS; enhancement of ameliorating cytokine production; stem cell therapy for damaged oligodendroglia; orally effective interferons; definition of predisposing and precipitating factors; genetic precursors; the role of diet and stress in disease maintenance and healing; and establishing the role of complementary therapies including supplements, herbals, dietary fats, homeopathic remedies, and mind-body approaches in the control of symptoms.

REFERENCES

Andrews KL, Husmann DA. Bladder dysfunction and management in multiple sclerosis. *Mayo Clin Proc*. 1997;72: 1176–1183.

Bowling AC. *Alternative Medicine and Multiple Sclerosis*. New York, NY: Demos Medical Publishing; 2001.

Filippi M, Tortorella C, Bozzali M. Normal-appearing white matter changes in multiple sclerosis: the contribution of magnetic resonance techniques. *Mult Scler*. 1999;5: 273–282.

Hogancamp WE, Rodriguez M, Weinshenker BG. The epidemiology of multiple sclerosis. *Mayo Clin Proc*. 1997;72:871–878.

Offenbacher H, Fazekas F, Schmidt R, et al. Assessment of MRI criteria for a diagnosis of MS. *Neurology*. 1993;43:905–909.

Schapiro RT. *Symptom Management in Multiple Sclerosis*. 3rd ed. New York, NY: Demos Medical Publishing; 1998.

Schwid SR, Thornton CA Pandya S, et al. Quantitative assessment of motor fatigue and strength in MS. *Neurology*. 1999;53:743–750.

Weintraub MI, ed. *Alternative and Complementary Treatment in Neurologic Illness*. New York, NY: Churchill Livingstone; 2001.

Wingerchuk DM, Lucchinetti CF, Noseworthy JH. Multiple sclerosis: current pathophysiological concepts. *Lab Invest*. 2001;81:263–281.

Chapter 102
Myasthenia Gravis

James F. Howard, Jr.

Myasthenia gravis (MG) is the most common primary disorder of neuromuscular transmission. The usual cause is an acquired immunological abnormality, but some cases result from genetic abnormalities at the neuromuscular junction. The estimated incidence of MG is 9 per million per year with a prevalence of 14 per million population; however, MG is probably underdiagnosed. Previous studies showed that women are more often affected than men. The most common age at onset is the second and third decades in women and the seventh and eighth decades in men. As the population ages, the average age at onset has increased correspondingly, and now males are more often affected than females, and the onset of symptoms is usually after age 50.

ETIOLOGY AND PATHOGENESIS

The normal neuromuscular junction releases acetylcholine (ACh) from the motor nerve terminal in discrete packages (quanta). These ACh quanta diffuse across the synaptic cleft and bind to specific receptors on the folded muscle end-plate membrane. Stimulation of the motor nerve releases many ACh quanta that depolarize the muscle end-plate region and the muscle membrane, causing muscle contraction. In acquired MG, the post-synaptic muscle membrane is distorted and simplified, having lost its normal folded shape. The concentration of ACh receptors (AChRs) is reduced on the muscle end-plate membrane, and antibodies attach to the membrane. ACh is released normally, but its effect on the post-synaptic membrane is reduced, lessening the probability that any nerve impulse will cause a muscle action potential.

Thymic abnormalities are associated with MG, but the nature of the association is uncertain. Ten percent to 15% of patients with MG have a thymic tumor, and 70% have hyperplastic changes (germinal centers) that indicate an active immune response. These are areas within lymphoid tissue where B cells interact with helper T cells to produce antibodies. Because the thymus is the central organ for immunologic self-tolerance, it is reasonable to suspect that thymic abnormalities cause the breakdown in tolerance that produces an immune-mediated attack on AChR in MG. The thymus contains all the necessary elements for the pathogenesis of MG: myoid cells that express the AChR antigen, antigen-presenting cells, and immunocompetent T cells. Thymus tissue from patients with MG produces AChR antibodies when implanted into immunodeficient mice. It is still uncertain whether the role of the thymus in the pathogenesis of MG is primary or secondary.

Most thymic tumors in patients with MG are benign, well differentiated, and encapsulated, and can be removed completely at surgery. It is unlikely that thymomas result from chronic thymic hyperactivity because MG can develop years after thymoma removal, and the HLA haplotypes that predominate in patients with thymic hyperplasia are different from those with thymomas. Patients with thymoma usually have more severe disease, higher levels of AChR antibodies, and more severe electromyographic (EMG) abnormalities than patients without thymoma. Almost 20% of patients with MG whose symptoms began between the ages of 30 and 60 years have thymoma; the frequency is much lower when symptom onset is after age 60.

CLINICAL PRESENTATION

Patients with MG complain of specific muscle weakness rather than generalized fatigue. Ocular motor disturbances, ptosis or diplopia, are the initial symptom of MG in two thirds of patients; almost all have both symptoms within 2 years (Figure 102-1). Oropharyngeal muscle weakness (difficulty chewing, swallowing, or talking), is the initial symptom in one sixth of patients, and limb

Figure 102-1

Myasthenia Gravis

Pathophysiologic concepts

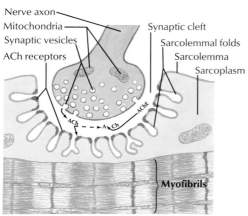

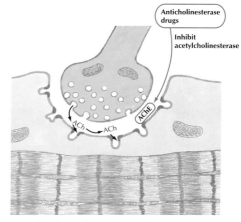

Normal neuromuscular junction: Synaptic vesicles containing acetylcholine (ACh) form in nerve terminal. In response to nerve impulse, vesicles discharge ACh into synaptic cleft. ACh binds to receptor sites on muscle sarcolemma to initiate muscle contraction. Acetylcholinesterase (AChE) hydrolyzes ACh, thus limiting effect and duration of its action.

Myasthenia gravis: Marked reduction in number and length of subneural sarcolemmal folds indicates that underlying defect lies in neuromuscular junction. Anticholinesterase drugs increase effectiveness and duration of ACh action by slowing its destruction by AChE.

Clinical manifestations

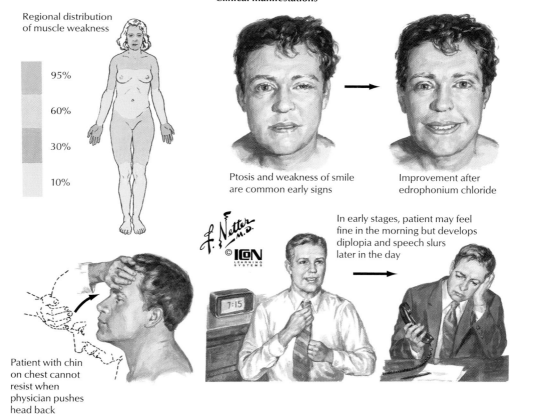

Regional distribution of muscle weakness

95%
60%
30%
10%

Ptosis and weakness of smile are common early signs

Improvement after edrophonium chloride

In early stages, patient may feel fine in the morning but develops diplopia and speech slurs later in the day

Patient with chin on chest cannot resist when physician pushes head back

Figure 102-2

Complimentary Exams

Thymus gland abnormality in myasthenia gravis

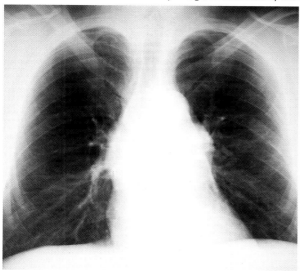

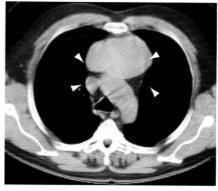

CT scan clearly demonstrates same large tumor anterior to aortic arch (arrowheads)

X-ray film shows large mediastinal tumor, which localized to anterior compartment (view not shown)

Repetitive nerve stimulation

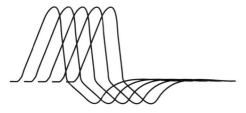

No decremental response is seen to slow rates of stimulation (1,2,3,5,Hz) in normal individuals

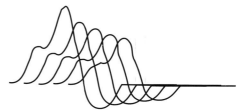

Decremental responses are seen to slow rates of stimulation in patients with abnormal synaptic transmission

Single fiber electromyography

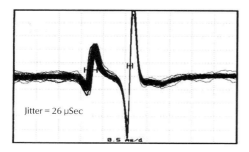

Jitter = 26 μSec

0.5 ms/d

Normal neuromuscular jitter (variation in single action potential intervals) in normal individuals

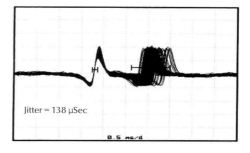

Jitter = 138 μSec

0.5 ms/d

Increased neuromuscular jitter in patients with abnormal synaptic transmission

weakness occurs in only 10%. Initial weakness is rarely limited to single muscle groups such as neck or finger extensors or hip flexors. The severity of weakness fluctuates during the day, usually being least severe in the morning and worse as the day progresses, especially after prolonged use of affected muscles.

The course of disease is variable but usually progressive. Weakness is restricted to the ocular muscles in approximately 10% of cases. The rest have progressive weakness during the first 2 years involving oropharyngeal and limb muscles. Maximum weakness occurs during the first year in two thirds of patients. Before corticosteroids were used for treatment, approximately one third of patients improved spontaneously, one third became worse, and one third died of the disease. Spontaneous improvement occurred early in the course. Symptoms fluctuated over a relatively short time and then became progressively severe for several years. Myasthenic symptoms are made worse by emotional upset, systemic illness (especially viral respiratory infections), hypothyroidism or hyperthyroidism, pregnancy, the menstrual cycle, drugs affecting neuromuscular transmission, and increases in body temperature.

DIFFERENTIAL DIAGNOSIS

The differential diagnosis of muscle weakness is broad; however, in typical cases, the diagnosis is apparent to the clinician. Variable eyelid ptosis and fluctuating ophthalmoparesis are unique to MG. In less typical cases, one must consider diseases of the motor neuron and the muscle membrane (mitochondrial myopathies). Rarely, neurotoxins as well as central nervous system disorders involving the brain stem, and cavernous sinus thrombosis must be considered. Careful neurologic examination and appropriate diagnostic testing should clarify each diagnosis.

DIAGNOSTIC APPROACH

Weakness caused by abnormal neuromuscular transmission characteristically improves after intravenous administration of edrophonium chloride. Often, it is diagnostic in patients with ptosis or ophthalmoparesis, but it is less useful when other muscles are weak. Some patients, particularly infants and children, who do not respond to intravenous edrophonium chloride may respond to intramus-

cular neostigmine because of the longer duration of action. In some patients, a therapeutic trial of daily oral pyridostigmine produces improvement that cannot be appreciated after a single dose of edrophonium chloride or neostigmine.

Serum antibodies that bind human AChR are found in 74% of patients with acquired generalized myasthenia and 54% with ocular myasthenia. The serum concentration of AChR antibody varies widely among patients with similar degrees of weakness and cannot predict the severity of disease. Approximately 10% of patients who do not have binding antibodies, have other antibodies that modulate the turnover of AChR in tissue culture. The concentration of binding antibodies may be low at symptom onset and become elevated later. They are rarely increased in patients with systemic lupus erythematosus, inflammatory neuropathy, amyotrophic lateral sclerosis, rheumatoid arthritis patients taking D-penicillamine, thymoma without MG, and in normal relatives of patients with MG. False-positive test results are reported when blood is drawn within 48 hours of a surgical procedure using general anesthesia and muscle relaxants. An elevated concentration of AChR binding antibodies in a patient with compatible clinical features confirms the diagnosis of MG, but normal antibody concentrations do not exclude the diagnosis.

The amplitude of the compound muscle action potential elicited by repetitive nerve stimulation (RNS) is normal or only slightly reduced in patients without MG. The amplitude of the fourth or fifth response to a train of low frequency nerve stimuli falls at least 10% from the initial value in myasthenic patients (Figure 102-2). This decremental response to RNS is seen more often in proximal muscles, such as the facial muscles, biceps, deltoid, and trapezius, than in hand muscles and more severe generalized weakness. A significant decrement to RNS is found in approximately 60% of patients with MG.

Single fiber EMG (Figure 102-2), the most sensitive clinical test of neuromuscular transmission, shows increased jitter in some muscles in almost all patients with MG. Jitter is greatest in weak muscles but may be abnormal even in muscles with normal strength. In mild or purely ocular muscle weakness, increased jitter may be in facial muscles only. Increased jitter is a nonspecific sign of abnormal neuromuscular transmission and is seen in other motor unit diseases. Normal jitter in a weak muscle excludes abnormal neuromuscular transmission as the cause of weakness.

MANAGEMENT AND THERAPY

There are numerous treatment options for MG. All recommended regimens are empirical, and experts disagree on treatments of choice. Treatment decisions should be based on knowledge of the natural history of disease in each patient and the predicted response to a specific form of therapy. Treatment goals must be individualized according to the severity of disease, the patient's age and gender, and the degree of functional impairment. The response to any treatment is difficult to assess because the severity of symptoms fluctuates. Spontaneous improvements, even remissions, occur without specific therapy, especially during the early stages of the disease.

Cholinesterase (ChE) inhibitors retard the enzymatic hydrolysis of ACh at cholinergic synapses so that ACh accumulates at the neuromuscular junction and its effect is prolonged. ChE inhibitors cause considerable improvement in some patients and little to none in others. Strength rarely returns to normal. Pyridostigmine bromide and neostigmine bromide are the most commonly used ChE inhibitors. No fixed dosage schedule suits all patients. The need for ACh inhibitors varies from day to day and during the same day in response to infection, menstruation, emotional stress, and hot weather. Different muscles respond differently; with any dose, certain muscles get stronger, others do not change, and still others become weaker. Adverse effects of ChE inhibitors may result from ACh accumulation at muscarinic receptors on smooth muscle and autonomic glands and at nicotinic receptors of skeletal muscle. CNS side effects are rarely seen with the doses used to treat MG. Gastrointestinal complaints (queasiness, loose stools, nausea, vomiting, abdominal cramps, and diarrhea) are common. Increased bronchial and oral secretions are a serious problem in patients with impaired swallowing or respiratory insufficiency. Symptoms of muscarinic overdosage may indicate that nicotinic overdosage (weakness) is also occurring. Excessive nicotinic receptor over-

dosage results in myasthenic crisis characterized by severe generalized weakness and respiratory failure.

Thymectomy is recommended for most patients with MG. Most reports do not correlate the severity of weakness before surgery and the timing or degree of improvement after thymectomy. The maximal favorable response generally occurs 2 to 5 years after surgery; however, it is relatively unpredictable, and significant impairment may continue for months or years after surgery. The best responses to thymectomy are in young people early in the course of their disease, but improvement can occur even after 30 years of symptoms. Patients with disease onset after the age of 60 rarely show substantial improvement from thymectomy. Patients with thymomas do not respond as well to thymectomy as do patients without thymoma.

Marked improvement or complete relief of symptoms occurs in more than 75% of patients treated with prednisone, and some improvement occurs in most of the rest. Much of the improvement occurs in the first 6 to 8 weeks, but strength may increase to total remission in the months that follow. The best responses occur in patients with recent onset of symptoms, but patients with chronic disease may also respond. The severity of disease does not predict the ultimate improvement. Patients with thymoma have an excellent response to prednisone before or after removal of the tumor. The most predictable response to prednisone occurs when treatment begins with a daily dose of 1.5 to 2 mg/kg/day. Approximately one third of patients become weaker temporarily after starting prednisone, usually within the first 7 to 10 days, and lasting for up to 6 days. Treatment can be started at low dose to minimize exacerbations; the dose is then slowly increased until improvement occurs. Exacerbations may also occur with this approach, and the response is less predictable. The major disadvantages of chronic corticosteroids are the side effects.

Several immunosuppressive medications are used in treatment of MG. Mycophenolate mofetil and azathioprine reverse symptoms in most patients. The effect is delayed by 6 to 8 months with azathioprine. Once improvement begins, it is maintained for as long as the drug is given, but symptoms recur 2 to 3 months after the drug is discontinued or the dose is reduced below therapeutic levels. Patients who fail corticosteroids may respond to other immunosuppressive drugs, and the reverse is also true. Some respond better to treatment to corticosteroids with another immunosuppressive drug than to either alone. Because the response to azathioprine is delayed, both drugs may be started simultaneously with the intent of rapidly tapering prednisone when azathioprine becomes effective. Approximately one third of patients have mild dose-dependent side effects that may require dose reductions but do not require stopping treatment.

Cyclosporine inhibits predominantly T-lymphocyte–dependent immune responses and is sometimes beneficial in treating MG. Most patients improve 1 to 2 months after starting cyclosporine, and improvement is maintained as long as therapeutic doses are given. Maximum improvement is achieved 6 months or longer after starting treatment. After achieving the maximal response, the dose is gradually reduced to the minimum that maintains improvement. Renal toxicity and hypertension are the most concerning adverse reactions. Many drugs interfere with cyclosporine metabolism and should be avoided or used with caution.

Cyclophosphamide is used intravenously and orally for the treatment of MG. More than half of patients become asymptomatic after 1 year. Side effects are common. Life-threatening infections are an important risk in immunosuppressed patients and patients with invasive thymoma. The long-term risk of malignancy is not established.

Plasma exchange is used as a short-term intervention for patients with sudden worsening of myasthenic symptoms for any reason, to rapidly improve strength before surgery, and as a chronic intermittent treatment for patients who are refractory to all other treatments. The need for plasma exchange and its frequency of use is determined by the clinical response. Almost all patients with acquired MG improve temporarily following plasma exchange. Maximum improvement may be reached as early as after the first exchange or as late as the 14th. Improvement lasts for weeks or months, and then the effect is lost unless the exchange is followed by thymectomy or immunosuppressive therapy. Most patients who respond to the first plasma exchange will respond again to subsequent courses. Repeated exchanges do not have a cumulative benefit.

Favorable response to high-dose (2 g/kg infused over 2 to 5 days) infusions of intravenous immunoglobulin (IVIG) has been reported. Improvement occurs in 50% to 100% of patients, usually within 1 week and lasting for several weeks or months. The common adverse effects of IVIG are related to the rate of infusion. The mechanism of action is not known, but is probably nonspecific downregulation of antibody production.

FUTURE DIRECTIONS

The future of MG lies in the elucidation of the molecular immunology of the anti-acetylcholine receptor response with the goal of developing a rational treatment for the illness that will cure the abnormality in the immune system that results in the AChR immune response. To this end, six broad categories of theoretical treatment strategies need to be explored. First, those treatments that target the antigen specific B-cells; second, those treatments that target the antigen specific CD4+ T-cells; third, those treatments that interfere with co-stimulatory response for antigen presentation; fourth, treatments aimed at inducing tolerance or anergy of the CD4+ T-cell to the autoantigen or the CD4+ epitopes; fifth, those treatments designed to stimulate those immunological circuits that activate CD8+ cells specific for the activation antigens expressed by CD4+ cells; and sixth, those treatments that intervene with cytokine function and discourage autoimmune-mediated inflammatory responses.

REFERENCES

Conti-Fine BM, Protti MO, Bellone M, Howard JF. *Myasthenia Gravis: The Immunology of an Autoimmune Disease.* Austin, Tex: RG Landes Co; 1997.

Howard JF Jr. Adverse drug effects on neuromuscular transmission. *Semin Neurol.* 1990;10:89–102.

Howard JF Jr, Sanders DB, Massey JM. The electrodiagnosis of myasthenia gravis and the Lambert-Eaton myasthenic syndrome. *Neurol Clin.* 1994;12:305–330.

Sanders DB, Howard JF Jr. Disorders of neuromuscular transmission. In: Bradley WG, Daroff RB, Fenichel GM, Marsden CD, eds. *Neurology in Clinical Practice: Principles of Diagnosis and Management.* 3rd ed. Boston, Mass: Butterworth-Heinemann; 2000:2167–2185.

Vincent A, Palace J, Hilton-Jones D. Myasthenia gravis. *Lancet.* 2001;357:2122–2128.

Chapter 103

Parasomnias

Bradley V. Vaughn

Parasomnias have attracted the interest of scholars and writers for centuries. Lady Macbeth, in Shakespeare's *Macbeth*, is perhaps the most famous literary example of sleepwalking and sleep talking. Differentiation of a sleep-related phenomenon, nocturnal seizures, and psychogenic events can be difficult because of the frequent overlap of clinical descriptions and lack of diurnal findings.

ETIOLOGY AND PATHOGENESIS

Wakefulness, non-rapid eye movement (NREM) sleep, and rapid eye movement (REM) sleep are recognized as normal states of being. They are defined by the physiologic measures of the EEG, eye movement, and muscle tone. The change between these states is not necessarily a "flick of a switch" phenomenon, but involves activation of several neuronal networks that can be disrupted to produce a mixture of states with behaviors that usually accompany one state intruding into another. Other pathological nocturnal phenomena, such as seizures or nocturnal psychogenic events, may occur during the sleep period.

Most NREM sleep parasomnias are disturbances of arousal (confusional arousals, sleepwalking, and sleep terrors), and have features of both wakefulness and NREM sleep. Others, including sleep starts, are normal phenomena associated with the transition from sleep to wakefulness and wakefulness to sleep.

Stress and sleep deprivation commonly precipitate parasomnias in susceptible individuals, and prescription and nonprescription drug use may contribute in some instances. Psychopathology is sometimes a factor in nightmares, but many common parasomnias, such as sleep terrors and REM sleep behavior disorder, are not associated with major psychiatric disturbances. In adult patients, sleep disorders such as obstructive sleep apnea or periodic limb movements may trigger parasomnia events.

Neuropathological abnormalities have not been identified in most of the common parasomnias; however, approximately one half of patients with REM sleep behavior disorder have CNS disorders, such as Parkinson's disease, spinocerebel-

lar atrophy, multiple system atrophy, or Lewy body disease. Some patients, who are neurologically normal at the time of diagnosis of REM sleep behavior disorder, later develop Parkinsonism. REM sleep behavior disorder (RBD) can be induced by medication, and cases of tricyclic antidepressants, monoamine oxidase inhibitors, and serotonin reuptake inhibitors causing RBD-like behavior have been reported. Acute forms of RBD can occur during alcohol withdrawal and, potentially, with benzodiazepine withdrawal.

Nocturnal paroxysmal dystonia, a distinct parasomnia, is now considered a form of frontal lobe epilepsy. Australian and Italian familial forms are categorized as Autosomal Dominant Nocturnal Frontal Lobe Epilepsy. The Australian form has been linked to chromosome 20q 13.2 and causes an abnormality of the neuronal nicotinic acetylcholine receptor 4 subunit.

CLINICAL PRESENTATION
NREM Sleep Events

Disorders of arousal, such as sleepwalking, sleep talking, confusional arousals, and night terrors, are defined by the incomplete arousal from NREM stage 2 or NREM stages 3 and 4 (slow wave) sleep. Patients demonstrate behaviors associated with wakefulness while still asleep. These events are more common in children (6% to 65%) than in adults (2% to 5 %). Frequently, there is a positive family history. NREM events are more common in the first half of the night, although spells can occur at any time. Most patients have no memory of the event; however, some report memory of vague visual imagery and auditory perceptions.

Sleep walking events can be very elaborate and involve dressing, unlocking locks, cleaning, cooking,

Table 103-1
Distinguishing Features of Nocturnal Events

	NREM Parasomnia	REM Behavior Disorder	Nocturnal Seizures	Psychogenic Events
Time of Occurrence	First third of the night	During REM	Anytime	Anytime
Memory of Event	Usually None	Dream recall	Usually none May have memory	Usually none
Stereotypical Movements	No	No	Yes	No
PSG findings	Arousals from deep NREM sleep	Excessive EMG tone during REM	Potentially epileptiform activity	Occur from awake state

and driving. Typically, they are arousals from slow wave sleep that occur during the first third of the sleep period. Patients usually have little or no memory of the event. A potential variant of this behavior is *nocturnal eating disorder* in which patients arise in the night and eat high calorie food. Generally, the quantity and type of food eaten differs from usual daytime habits, and the patient has no memory of the event.

Sleep terrors are a more intense form of sleepwalking; most patients with sleep terror also have sleepwalking events. The predominance of autonomic expression during sleep terrors distinguishes them from other partial arousals of NREM sleep. This arousal starts with a piercing scream or cry accompanied by autonomic and behavioral manifestation of intense fear. Onset, usually in the first third of the sleep period, is abrupt; tachycardia, tachypnea, flushing, diaphoresis, and mydriasis are common. The patients are confused and disoriented, and can become violent, resulting in injury to patients and bed partners. Patients have no or minimal memory of the events.

Confusional arousals can occur with any arousal from NREM sleep and are characterized by disorientation, slow speech and mentation, or inappropriate behavior. Patients have impaired memory of the event, which can be induced with forced arousal. The course of these events usually improves with age, but can persist in adulthood.

REM Sleep Behavior Disorder

REM sleep behavior disorder (RBD) was origi-

nally postulated by Jouvet as a result of lesional experiments in cats in 1965. The human clinical correlate was described in 1986 by Schenck and Mahowald. RBD is characterized by intermittent loss of REM sleep muscle atonia and by the appearance of elaborate motor activity (punching, kicking, leaping, running, talking, and yelling) associated with dream mentation (Table 103-1). Bed partners are injured frequently, and patients may go to great lengths to prevent injury to themselves or bed partners. Usually, there is vivid recall of the actual dreams that correlate to the behavior; however, dream recall is not uniformly noted, and patients may not be willing to talk about the dream that led them to seek medical attention. Events are more commonly in the later half of the night, but can occur any time that the patient enters REM sleep. Most cases begin in late adulthood.

Rhythmic Movement Disorder

Patients present with complaints of rocking movements, which occur before sleep onset. The movements are stereotyped, involving large muscles, usually of the head and neck, and are sustained into light sleep. Movements may include head banging, body rocking, leg rolling, humming, and chanting. Some patients are relatively unaware of the movement, and others describe the movement as having a calming effect or as a compulsion. Frequently, this behavior diminishes with age and is more common in individuals with mental handicaps or autism.

Psychogenic States

Psychogenic phenomena can present as nocturnal events. This broad class of behavioral processes denotes a lack of pathological findings and can be subdivided into by underlying psychological classifications: dissociative disorders, conversion disorders, panic disorders, depression, or anxiety. These events can occur at any time during the night, and memory retainment is variable. Wakefulness before onset, as seen on polysomnography, is the hallmark for these events. Patients labeled as having psychogenic events can still have unrecognized parasomnias or epilepsy, and the diagnosis should always be considered with skepticism.

Nocturnal Seizures

Sleep related seizures could be confused with other parasomnias or psychiatric conditions, especially if the patient has no diurnal findings. Witnesses may describe the cardinal epileptic features: stereotyped behavior and repetitive nature of the events. Usually, patients do not have memory of the seizures, which can occur at any time in the sleep period (day or night). Patients can exhibit a variety of nocturnal behaviors (ambulation, confused wondering, or screaming), which appear similar to events of sleepwalking or sleep terrors. Most nocturnal seizures occur in NREM sleep, whether they are of temporal or frontal onset. Rare REM-related seizures involving recurrent dreams and dream enactment similar to REM sleep behavior disorder have been described. Nocturnal paroxysmal dystonia (NPD) and Autosomal Dominant Nocturnal Frontal Lobe Epilepsy are sleep related epilepsies. NPD, previously known as hypnogenic paroxysmal dystonia, is characterized by multiple dystonic or dyskinetic episodes occurring at night with few EEG changes. Occasionally, patients may vocalize and appear confused, yet they recall the event. NPD is a form of frontal lobe epilepsy. Autosomal dominant nocturnal frontal lobe epilepsy, a rare, inherited form of epilepsy, is characterized by recurrent brief tonic movements, vocalizations, nocturnal wandering, or brief epileptic arousals. Often, the EEG demonstrates no epileptic changes during the spells, and daytime EEGs are normal.

DIFFERENTIAL DIAGNOSIS

The differential diagnosis depends on the symptoms and signs associated with the particular disorder. Consider nocturnal seizures in patients with rhythmic, repetitive, or stereotyped behaviors or movements. Psychiatric events such as panic attacks, conversion disorders, or fugue states can occur during the sleep period. Consider other conditions associated with nocturnal pain, gastroesophageal reflux, asthma, or cardiac impairment, particularly in infants or developmentally disabled individuals, who cannot describe nocturnal symptoms.

DIAGNOSTIC APPROACH

Determining the cause of these events can be difficult and requires a high index of suspicion. Keep an open mind about the validity of the diagnosis, limitations of technology, and lack of understanding about these unusual phenomena. The diagnostic workup is highly dependent on the type and frequency of symptoms. Many parasomnias can be diagnosed on the basis of the history and physical examination, but the clinician needs to delineate between a "benign" parasomnia and a nocturnal event that is a symptom of another problem. Indications for polysomnography include: 1) atypical presentation for a parasomnia (time of night, behavioral description); 2) events are injurious or have significant potential for injury; 3) significant disturbance to patient's home life; 4) begin at an unusual age; 5) events are stereotyped or repetitive; 6) unusual frequency of the events; 7) excessive daytime sleepiness or complaints of insomnia; 8) complaints suggestive of sleep apnea or periodic limb movements. Evaluations include 1 or 2 nights of recording in a sleep laboratory by personnel experienced in studying parasomnias. Simultaneous polysomnographic-audio-video monitoring is essential, often with additional physiologic measures beyond the minimum required for standard polysomnography. Consider video-EEG monitoring if the events are stereotypic or repetitive, occur frequently, and have not responded to medication trials.

MANAGEMENT AND THERAPY

Management for children with typical, noninjurious disorders of arousal consists of reassurance that a particular nocturnal symptom is normal. Patient education, non-pharmacologic treatment, and medications are important parts of therapy for most NREM parasomnias. Stress management, counseling, and avoidance of cognitively impairing medications may lessen the frequency of the events. Patients with the potential for injury and their families need to be counseled in methods to reduce risk for injury (e.g., protective material across windows, lack of access to potential weapons). Underlying sleep disorders such as obstructive sleep apnea or periodic limb movements should be treated to decrease the potential for sleep disruption. Some patients may require medication therapy for their nocturnal events. Patients with NREM related events might respond to diazepam, temazepam, or clonazepam, and benefit from treatment with imipramine.

Individuals with REM sleep behavior disorder frequently respond well to clonazepam. Some may improve with L-dopa/carbidopa or dopamine agonists, whereas others may respond to selective serotonin reuptake inhibitors, although this therapy may provoke attacks in some patients. Treatment regimens for paroxysmal nocturnal dystonia and episotic wandering include anticonvulsants typically used for the focal onset epilepsies. Carbamazepine, lamotrigine, topiramate, and valproate have all been tried to ameliorate the nocturnal seizures.

FUTURE DIRECTIONS

As we elucidate the underlying processes involved with many of these unusual nocturnal events, we will gain a better understanding of the mechanisms of differentiation of state and consciousness. Future research directed at identifying the genetic components and methods to modify these neurochemical processes will aid in treatment of nocturnal events and other sleep-related disorders.

REFERENCES

Aldrich MS. *Sleep Medicine*. New York, NY: Oxford University Press; 1999.

Chokroverty S, ed. *Sleep Disorders Medicine: Basic Science, Technical Considerations, and Clinical Aspects*. 2nd ed. Boston Mass: Butterworth-Heinemann; 1999.

Kryger MH, Roth T, Dement WC, eds. *Principles and Practice of Sleep Medicine*. 3rd ed. Philadelphia, Pa: WB Saunders Co; 2000.

Chapter 104

Parkinson's Disease

Peter Lars Jacobson and J. Douglas Mann

Parkinson's disease (PD) is a chronic, progressive neurodegenerative disorder of unknown etiology that can cause significant disability and early mortality. The incidence of PD is believed to be 20 new cases per 100,000 persons each year with a prevalence of 100 to 150 per 100,000 persons. Increasing age is a risk factor for PD with the first symptoms and signs of the disease usually appearing in middle age with a marked acceleration in prevalence among persons over the age 65 (2,000 cases per 100,000 persons over 65 years).

The impact of PD is reflected in a marked reduction in life expectancy with a mortality rate that is 2 to 5 times that of age-matched controls. Slowly progressive disability occurs despite symptomatic relief with new medications and possible surgical interventions.

ETIOLOGY AND PATHOGENESIS

The neurodegeneration of the substantia nigra is the most distinctive neuropathological finding. Progressive neuronal loss occurs in the dopaminergic neurons of the pars compacta of the substantia nigra. Regional loss of striatal dopamine is believed to contribute to the clinical symptoms and signs of PD, and many of the medications are aimed at the dopaminergic systems for motor control. In most cases, residual neurons have eosinophilic intracytoplasmic inclusions called Lewy bodies that are found predominately in the basal ganglia, brain stem, spinal cord, and sympathetic ganglia. No specific cause for PD has been identified. Speculation on etiology includes:

Viral infections: Theories are based primarily on the epidemic of encephalitis lethargica or von Economo disease between 1919 through 1926; a parkinsonian syndrome could appear in patients immediately or up to 10 years after the illness.

Neurotoxins: Theories are based on the parkinsonian syndrome that is found in persons exposed to N-methyl-phenyl-1,2,3,6-tetrahydropyridine (MPTP), which targets dopaminergic neurons. MPTP raises concern about the role of free radicals in neuronal death found in PD.

Genetic predisposition: A familial form of PD has been identified in 5% of patients. The lifetime risk of first-degree relatives of patients with PD is twice the risk of age-matched controls. Several loci have been related to PD, but no specific "Parkinson's disease gene" has been identified.

CLINICAL PRESENTATION

The classic clinical triad of PD is tremor, bradykinesia, and rigidity (Figure 104-1). Tremor is the most obvious symptom and sign identified by both patient and family. The tremor occurs at rest and usually has a frequency of 4 to 7 Hz. The tremor may start in one extremity but can spread to include the arms, legs, head, and even the voice. Physical and emotional stress are exacerbating factors.

Bradykinesia is a progressive slowing of motor function. Handwriting is affected with difficulty in initiating hand movement and a gradual reduction in the size of the writing (micrographia). Ambulation is slowed with decreased arm swing. Poor turning ability, decreased reaction time, and shuffling gait increase the risks of falls and subsequent trauma. Facial immobility occurs (mask-like facies); the frequency of spontaneous eye blinks is reduced. Speech also slows and the volume softens and fades.

Rigidity is reflected in increased muscle tone. A progressive stiffening of the body with resistance to passive movement of the extremities is often found on examination. Rigidity contributes to generalized immobilization and is also a component of the stooped posture and gait (Figure 104-1, Stage 3). The passive movement of an extremity by the examiner produces cogwheel rigidity, which appears to combine rigidity with tremor.

Additional findings in PD include drooling, facial seborrhea, and mild dementia, which may progress. Comorbid depression may be present similar to other chronic illnesses.

The neurological examination can demonstrate the mask-like facies, decreased eye blinks, resting tremor, cogwheel rigidity, micrographia, bradykinesia in movements, decreased arm swing, and stooped posture with shuffling gait. The examination also has a significant absence of abnormal findings with normal tendon reflexes, no lateralized weakness, no sensory changes, and the absence of cerebellar signs. Frontal lobe reflexes may be present with mild memory disturbance.

DIFFERENTIAL DIAGNOSIS

Drug effects: Extrapyramidal side effects of medications (e.g., phenothiazines) may produce findings suggestive of PD.

Depression: Flat affect, psychomotor retardation, and pseudodementia may be present, but the primary findings of PD are not evident.

Head trauma: Lateralized tendon reflexes, motor weakness, and sensory findings help to distinguish traumatic injury from PD (e.g., subdural hematomas).

Stroke: Vascular injury to the brain can produce parkinsonian signs and symptoms.

Wilson's disease: Family history, Kayser-Fleischer rings on eye examination, liver dysfunction, abnormal serum ceruloplasmin, and elevated levels of copper in serum and urine facilitate the diagnosis.

Progressive supranuclear palsy: Bradykinesia and rigidity may be present, but the loss of voluntary eye movement, particularly upward gaze, is characteristic.

Intracranial tumors: The neurological examination should help in identifying signs that are not consistent with PD.

Viral: Neurological examination suggests a more diffuse brain involvement with other physical symptoms and signs.

Normal pressure hydrocephalus: Gait may be more suggestive of apraxia ("stuck foot"), and urinary incontinence is a major component in the history.

Huntington's disease: Family history, choreiform movements, and dementia are predominant.

Multisystem atrophy including Shy-Drager syndrome: Parkinsonian features may be present, but autonomic insufficiency and postural hypotension are major components of illness.

DIAGNOSTIC APPROACH

The diagnosis of PD is based on clinical criteria including the classic triad (resting tremor, rigidity, and bradykinesia), asymmetry of symptoms and signs at initial presentation, and usually a good clinical response to levodopa (greater than 90% of patients with PD will improve). Currently, no biologic marker is definitive in establishing the diagnosis. MRI can confirm changes in the substantia nigra and eliminate other causes in the differential diagnosis (e.g., mass lesions, stroke, etc.). Laboratory tests should include thyroid and parathyroid functions, and, if younger than 50 at onset with positive family history, serum ceruloplasmin.

MANAGEMENT AND THERAPY
Medications

Symptomatic treatment is not indicated unless or until the symptoms or signs of PD are affecting the patient's quality of life or limiting activities of daily living.

Levodopa, a precursor of dopamine, remains the most effective medication to control the symptoms of PD. Levodopa is thought to help replenish dopamine in the dopamine-depleted regions of the brain. Approximately 90% of patients with PD will demonstrate a positive response to it. Both short-term and long-term side effects are noted with levodopa. Initial side effects include nausea, postural hypotension, and rarely cardiac arrhythmias. Long-term side effects include dyskinesias, akathisia, and confusion. Dose adjustments need to be regularly monitored. The long-term side effects appear to be related to fluctuations in blood levels and possible neuronal receptor sensitivity. "Wearing off" is an expected loss of effectiveness of levodopa before the next dose is needed. "On-off phenomena" are unpredictable sudden losses of levodopa response in long-term users. Prolonged use of levodopa can cause various abnormal involuntary movements. Motor fluctuations occur in approximately 50% of patients after 5 years on levodopa with an increase to 70% after 15 years. Blood tests are not required.

Carbidopa (dopa-decarboxylase inhibitor) is combined with levodopa to reduce the peripheral breakdown of levodopa before transport into the brain through the blood-brain barrier. It

Figure 104-1

Parkinson's Disease

Clinical signs of Parkinson's Disease

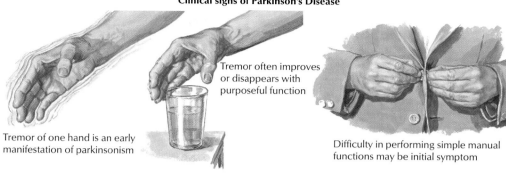

Tremor often improves or disappears with purposeful function

Tremor of one hand is an early manifestation of parkinsonism

Difficulty in performing simple manual functions may be initial symptom

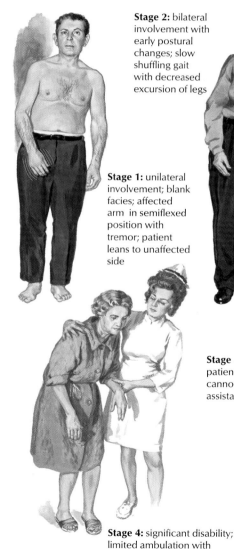

Stage 2: bilateral involvement with early postural changes; slow shuffling gait with decreased excursion of legs

Stage 1: unilateral involvement; blank facies; affected arm in semiflexed position with tremor; patient leans to unaffected side

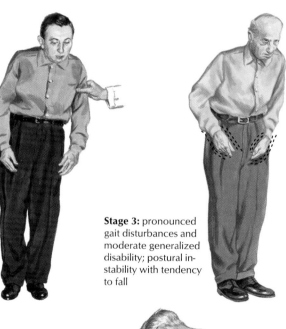

Stage 3: pronounced gait disturbances and moderate generalized disability; postural instability with tendency to fall

Stage 5: complete invalidism; patient confined to bed or chair; cannot stand or walk even with assistance

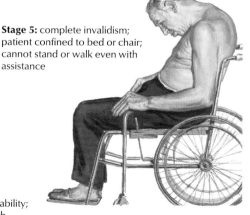

Stage 4: significant disability; limited ambulation with assistance

JOHN A. CRAIG—MD
C. Machado—M.D.
©ICON

increases levodopa availability to the brain and reduces the peripheral side effects of levodopa, which can include severe nausea.

Dopamine agonists are effective medications through direct action on the dopamine receptors in the brain. As additive therapy to levodopa, the benefits include reducing the fluctuating responses to levodopa. Older dopamine agonists (bromocriptine and pergolide) are ergot derivatives with major side effects including delusions, hallucinations, and hypotension, and pulmonary and retroperitoneal fibrosis. Newer dopamine agonists, ropinirole and pramipexole, are non-ergot derivatives with decreased risk of vascular problems and pleural/pulmonary fibrosis. Ropinirole and pramipexole can cause postural hypotension, peripheral edema, nausea, dyskinesias, and confusion. Excessive somnolence may require discontinuation of the medication. The new dopamine agonists may be helpful as an initial therapy in patients with early PD, but the major role remains adjunctive.

Selective catechol-o-methyl transferase inhibitors (COMT inhibitors) improve levodopa availability to the brain by reducing the conversion of levodopa to 3-o-methyldopa; 3-o-methyldopa competes with levodopa for transport across the blood-brain barrier. COMT inhibitors reduce fluctuations in response to levodopa with more "on" time. The use of COMT inhibitors requires a 20% to 30% reduction in the daily dosage of levodopa to avoid side effects. Tolcapone and entacapone are COMT inhibitors. Tolcapone has been associated with acute hepatic failure in a small number of patients, and a transient effect on liver function tests (LFTs) has occurred; monitoring of LFTs is required. Entacapone is preferred because its hepatic side effects are less than those with tolcapone. LFTs are still monitored before and up to 3 months after the start of therapy. Side effects include diarrhea, abdominal pain, sleep disturbance, and postural hypotension.

Anticholinergic agents, benztropine and trihexyphenidyl, may relieve tremor and may also reduce drooling. Small dosages are used due to the significant side effects of these medications in patients with PD. The benefit/side effect ratio limits the use of these agents because they are prone to cause blurred vision, urinary retention, memory disturbance, hallucinations, and confusion.

Amantadine is effective in PD, but the response may not last. The mode of action of amantadine is not known, but a clinical response has been well documented. Side effects may include peripheral edema, urinary retention, livedo reticularis, restlessness, confusion, dizziness, and insomnia.

Monoamine oxidase B inhibitor, selegiline, may slow disease progression and have a "neuroprotective" effect. Because selegiline has a small effect on the symptoms of PD, this concept has been questioned. Selegiline may reduce both fluctuations in the levodopa response and the daily dosage of levodopa. Selegiline does not have the dietary restrictions of monoamine oxidase A inhibitors, but does interact with meperidine, tricyclic antidepressants, and selective serotonin reuptake inhibitors.

Diet

Restricting dietary protein improves the gastrointestinal uptake of levodopa and also improves transport of levodopa across the blood-brain barrier. High protein diets increase amino acids that compete with levodopa for transport and may produce fluctuations in levodopa levels. Vitamin E (tocopherol) acts on free radicals, but a large study did not confirm benefit in PD.

Physical Therapy

Physical therapy helps patients maintain flexibility and strength through an exercise program. Speech therapy may help patients with their speech volume and clarity.

Neurosurgical Treatment

Ablative procedures for tremor have included the placement of a lesion in the contralateral ventral intermediate nucleus of the thalamus. Ablative procedures are being replaced by high frequency thalamic stimulation. Early reports suggest better results with less morbidity and mortality. When compared to ablative procedures, medications still have priority over surgical intervention.

FUTURE DIRECTIONS

Several new dopamine agonists are under evaluation and development. In addition, new medication transport mechanisms are needed to supplement the oral route. Transdermal patches and other forms for administration of PD medications are being studied. For example, apomorphine is water- soluble and may be administered through intravenous, subcutaneous, intranasal, or sublingual routes.

Cell therapy for PD has been evaluated, and further research is progressing. Recently, transplantation of embryonic dopamine neurons for severe PD showed some clinical benefit for patients who are 60 or younger. Transplantation of stem cells in animal models is in progress. More details on the role of genetics in PD will be available with the advancement of our understanding of the human genome.

REFERENCES

Aminoff MJ. Parkinson's disease. *Neurol Clin.* 2001;19:119–128.

Fischbach GD, McKhann GM. Cell therapy for Parkinson's disease. *N Engl J Med.* 2001;344:763–765.

Freed CR, Greene PE, Breeze RE, et al. Transplantation of embryonic dopamine neurons for severe Parkinson's disease. *N Engl J Med.* 2001;344:710–719.

Jankovic J. New and emerging therapies for Parkinson disease. *Arch Neurol.* 1999;56:785–790.

Lang AE, Lozano AM. Parkinson's disease. First of two parts. *N Engl J Med.* 1998;339:1044–1053.

Lang AE, Lozano AM. Parkinson's disease. Second of two parts. *N Engl J Med.* 1998;339:1130–1143.

National Institute of Neurological Disorders and Stroke Web site. Available at: http://www.ninds.nih.gov. Accessed Feb. 28, 2003.

Chapter 105
Peripheral Neuropathy

James F. Howard, Jr.

Peripheral neuropathies are common conditions that result from abnormalities of structure and function of motor, sensory and/or autonomic neurons. Neuropathies are broadly classified into disorders that primarily affect myelin, or those that affect the axon. They may be either acquired or hereditary. Within each subgroup are numerous causes. Alternatively, neuropathies may be classified etiologically and encompass those secondary to hereditary, toxic-metabolic, traumatic, entrapment, and systemic disease causes.

ETIOLOGY AND PATHOGENESIS

The causes of neuropathy are very diverse, and numerous pathogenic mechanisms exist. Broadly, one may consider acquired neuropathies and those that are hereditary. The acquired neuropathies are those due to the following: 1) metabolic disorders (e.g., critical care neuropathy, diabetes mellitus, renal disease, vitamin B_{12} deficiency (Figure 105-1); 2) toxins (e.g., heavy metals, industrial toxins) (Figure 105-2); 3) infectious causes (e.g., leprosy, herpes zoster, HIV disease); 4) pharmaceutical agents (e.g., vinca alkaloids, ddC, ddI, pyridoxine, amiodarone, cisplatin); 5) vasculitic processes and connective tissue disorders (e.g., lupus) (Table 105-3); immune system aberrations (e.g., Landry-Guillain-Barré Syndrome (GBS), acute (AIDP) and chronic (CIDP) inflammatory demyelinating neuropathy; 7) underlying malignancy (e.g., paraproteinemias, lymphoma, a variety of solid cell tumors); 8) compressive-entrapment situations (e.g., carpal tunnel, cubital tunnel syndromes, peroneal nerve compression at the fibular head).

Hereditary neuropathies are less common and may be of autosomal dominant or recessive or X-linked inheritance. In some instances, they are the major feature of the illness (e.g., Charcot-Marie-Tooth disease) or may be a manifestation of a more widespread disorder (e.g., metachromatic leukodystrophy, adrenoleukodystrophy, Fabry's disease, Refsum's disease).

CLINICAL PRESENTATION

The prototypical neuropathy is a distal symmetrical motor-sensory process that produces a stocking more than glove distribution of sensory disturbance and muscle weakness. The clinical presentations of neuropathy are varied, but often stereotypical, and fall under the broad categories of motor weakness, sensory disturbance, and autonomic dysfunction.

The predominant motor symptom is muscle weakness. The pattern of distribution and severity depends on the cause of the neuropathy. Symptoms of weakness begin distally and may cause the patient to trip, particularly when walking on uneven terrain, across door thresholds, or when walking on rugs. There may be difficulties with fine motor movements of the fingers such as opening jars and manipulating small objects.

Sensory symptoms may be quite varied. Positive symptoms include tingling, paresthesias (pins and needles), neuropathic pain and dysesthesias (unpleasant painful or uncomfortable symptoms). Negative symptoms include numbness or loss of sensation.

Autonomic dysfunction ranges from specific enzymatic deficiencies to selective efferent pathway abnormalities to more global dysfunction affecting the entire autonomic pathway.

A distal symmetrical abnormality of motor and sensory function with associated diminution of muscle stretch reflexes is the most common pattern of involvement. Weakness and muscle wasting predominate in the distal muscles of the hands and feet. Sensory loss follows the classic "glove-stocking" distribution, and reflex loss follows a similar pattern. Other disorders have a proximal pattern of muscle weakness. GBS is the most well known, and it can be seen in porphyric neuropathy. Sensory loss is less common in this pattern of abnormality.

Figure 105-1

Peripheral Neuropathies:
Metabolic, Toxic and Nutritional

Etiology

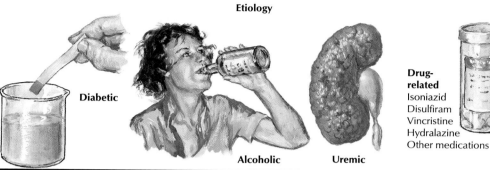

Diabetic

Alcoholic

Uremic

Drug-related
Isoniazid
Disulfiram
Vincristine
Hydralazine
Other medications

Clinical manifestations

Graduated glove-and-stocking hypesthesia

Loss of ankle jerk

Impaired vibration sense

Foot drop

Patient walks gingerly due to loss of position sense and/or painful dysesthesia

Patient sleeps with covers off feet because of burning sensation

Diabetic third cranial nerve palsy

Figure 105-2   ### Peripheral Neuropathy Caused by Heavy Metal Poisoning

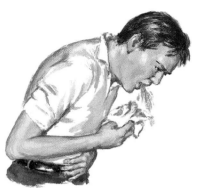

History of nausea and vomiting may suggest arsenic poisoning in patient with peripheral neuropathy

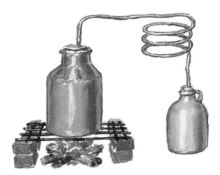

Antique copper utensils (eg, still for bootleg liquor) and runoff waste from copper smelting plant may be sources of arsenic poisoning

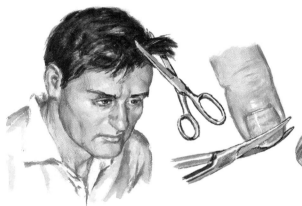

Although 24-hour urinalysis is best diagnostic test for arsenic, hair and nail analysis may also be helpful

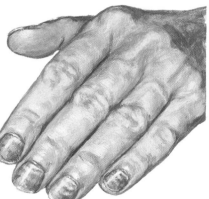

Mees' lines on fingernails are characteristic of arsenic poisoning

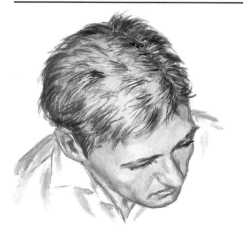

Spotty alopecia associated with peripheral neuropathy characterizes thallium poisoning

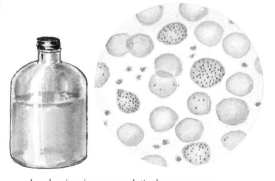

Lead poisoning, now relatively rare, causes basophilic stippling of red blood cells. 24-hour urinalysis is diagnostic test

A selective or predominant pattern of sensory loss suggests a paraneoplastic syndrome but may also be seen in diabetes, vitamin B_6 deficiency, leprosy, and hereditary sensory neuropathy. Those neuropathies that have motor involvement predominantly include GBS, selective hereditary motor neuropathies, diphtheria, and lead intoxication. Autonomic dysfunction is a feature of hereditary sensory-autonomic neuropathies and diabetic polyneuropathy.

Neuropathies with very rapid evolution are GBS, those of vasculitic or ischemic origin or heavy metal intoxication (arsenic) typically. They may also follow acute compression resulting from hemorrhage (e.g., within the carpal tunnel or anterior compartment syndrome), direct trauma, or exposure to extreme cold. Subacute neuropathies, evolving over many days to a few weeks are characteristic of toxin exposure, critical illness, Lyme disease, HIV, and nutritional disorders. A chronic time course is typical of hereditary disorders, nutritional deficiencies, paraproteinemias, and some forms of inflammatory and HIV neuropathies.

DIFFERENTIAL DIAGNOSIS

The differential diagnosis is made more easily once the localization and characterization within the peripheral nervous system are defined. This requires a carefully elicited history and a thorough examination. The presence of sensory loss and diminished or absent muscle stretch reflexes is the *sine qua non* of neuropathy. The neuropathy of childhood onset and insidious progression is likely to be of genetic origin. Similar progression in late adult life suggests a paraneoplastic or paraproteinemic disorder. Acute or subacute demyelinating neuropathies suggest an inflammatory process. The patient with marked disturbances of sensation suggests diabetes, heavy metal intoxication, pyridoxine abnormalities, or alcohol as the probable cause. Pure sensory neuropathies in an age-appropriate individual suggest a paraneoplastic disorder.

There are situations in which differentiation from motor neuropathy may be difficult. Motor neuron disease (e.g., spinal muscular atrophy, polio/postpolio syndrome, amyotrophic lateral sclerosis) may be difficult to distinguish from axonal motor neuropathies. Careful history and electrodiagnostic and laboratory examination differentiate these dis-

orders. The initial presentation of a spinal cord syndrome may be confused for a sensory neuropathy because of the distal paresthesiae. The presence of a definable upper sensory limit and the presence of corticospinal tract involvement should differentiate them. On rare occasions, isolated motor cranial neuropathies may be confused with myasthenia gravis. However, diurnal fluctuation of these signs and the tendency of the symptoms to worsen toward the end of the day in myasthenia gravis should aid in the proper diagnosis. Rarely, myopathies may present with a distal pattern of weakness. The preservation of muscle stretch reflexes, the absence of sensory abnormalities and the typical laboratory (increased CK) and electrodiagnostic findings should clarify the problem.

DIAGNOSTIC APPROACH

Nearly 75% of patients with neuropathic symptoms have a specific diagnosis if evaluated by neuromuscular centers. Establishing a correct diagnosis is based on the optimal utilization of clinical, electrodiagnostic, and laboratory information. In some situations, pathological examination of a peripheral nerve is necessary.

The role of routine screening blood laboratory studies has not been established. The most useful studies include measurement of the vitamin B_{12} level, serum protein and immune protein electrophoresis, and glycosylated hemoglobin. Other "routine" studies may be of benefit in carefully screened patients to confirm a diagnosis, for example thyroid function studies, vitamin B_6 levels, Lyme titer, urine heavy metals, collagen vascular studies.

Specific serum antibodies directed towards gangliosides and glycoproteins have been implicated in several motor and sensory neuropathies. These include anti-MAG, anti-GM_1, anti-GM_2, anti-GD1a and b, anti-GQ1b, anti-sulfatide and anti-Hu antibodies; however, the diagnostic and prognostic value of these antibodies remains unclear. Although their presence enhances the likelihood of an immune-mediated or paraneoplastic neuropathy, many patients with identical clinical syndromes are seronegative, and some individuals express low levels of these antibodies. The role of antibody testing in neuropathy patients is limited. Anti-GM1 antibody is useful in situations of suspected treatable motor neuropathy that cannot be distinguished from amyotrophic lateral sclero-

Figure 105-3

Signs and Symptoms Consistent with Neuropathy

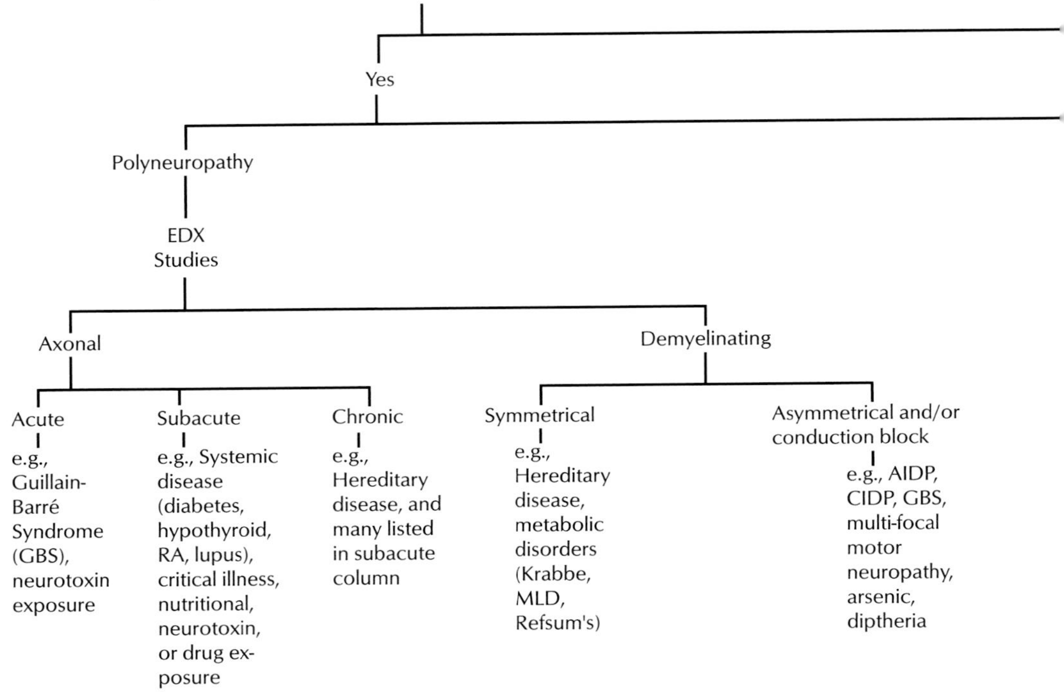

Yes

Polyneuropathy

EDX Studies

Axonal

Acute
e.g., Guillain-Barré Syndrome (GBS), neurotoxin exposure

Subacute
e.g., Systemic disease (diabetes, hypothyroid, RA, lupus), critical illness, nutritional, neurotoxin, or drug exposure

Chronic
e.g., Hereditary disease, and many listed in subacute column

Demyelinating

Symmetrical
e.g., Hereditary disease, metabolic disorders (Krabbe, MLD, Refsum's)

Asymmetrical and/or conduction block
e.g., AIDP, CIDP, GBS, multi-focal motor neuropathy, arsenic, diptheria

sis, or in those patients in whom pure motor neuropathies are associated with a paucity of upper motor neuron findings. Anti-GQ1b antibodies may be helpful in confirming the suspected Miller-Fisher variant of GBS. Anti-Hu antibody is useful in patients with asymmetrical proximal sensory findings or in those patients with a predominantly sensory neuropathy and strong smoking history because this may be the earliest manifestation of an underlying malignancy. Modest to marked elevations of anti-GM1 antibody suggest an immune-mediated motor neuropathy.

The electrophysiological examination involves nerve conduction studies (NCS), needle electromyography (EMG) and, in selected situations, autonomic function testing. Electrodiagnostic (EDX) studies provide information about the distribution of neuropathy, the elements involved (e.g,. motor, sensory, autonomic or combinations thereof), and determine whether the neuropathy pri-

marily involves disease of myelin or disease of axon. EDX studies may help distinguish between acquired and hereditary diseases. Disorders characterized by disease of myelin typically have modest to marked slowing of conduction velocity, whereas those of predominant axonal origin preserve conduction velocity; or it is only minimally slowed but the amplitude of the response elicited by nerve stimulation is reduced. Needle EMG examination typically is normal in demyelinating disorders and demonstrates the findings of denervation and reinnervation in axonal disorders.

Nerve biopsy is rarely useful in making a diagnosis of neuropathy. It is most helpful in acquired disorders such as vasculitis and amyloidosis, in instances of tumor infiltration of the nerve sheath, and in small fiber neuropathy in which electrodiagnostic studies are usually normal, as well as in the hereditary disorders of polyglucosan body neuropathy and Charcot-Marie-Tooth disease.

Signs and Symptoms Consistent with Neuropathy (continued)

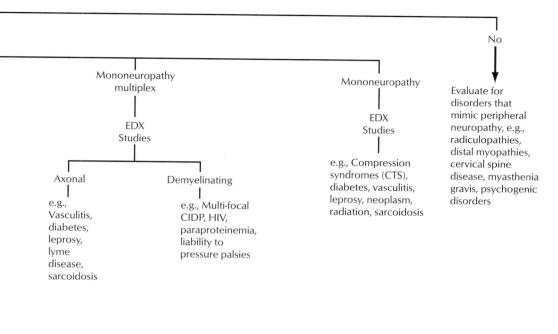

Abbreviations: AIDP – acute inflammatory demyelinating polyneuropathy; CIDP – chronic inflammatory demyelinating polyneuropathy; CTS – carpal tunnel syndrome; EDX – electrodiagnostic; GBS – Guillain-Barré syndrome; HIV – human immunodeficiency virus; MLD – metachromatic leukodystrophy; RA – rheumatoid arthritis

The role of nerve biopsy in hereditary disorders will become less useful as the molecular genetics of these disorders are elucidated. Typically the sural nerve is the most common nerve biopsied. Because this is a sensory nerve, it is not useful in disorders that only affect motor or autonomic function.

MANAGEMENT AND THERAPY

The treatment of neuropathy depends on its cause and can either be directed toward the underlying disease process or a specific symptom. For example, therapy may be directed toward the improvement of a particular symptom, usually pain or a skilled function that is disabling. The symptomatic treatment of pain control is evolving. Many of the newer anticonvulsant agents have been shown to be beneficial in treating neuropathic pain.

Entrapment neuropathies are best treated through discontinuation of those activities that worsen or precipitate symptoms. In some situations surgical intervention is necessary. Many of the metabolic and toxic neuropathies require correction of the underlying problem (e.g, B_{12} replacement, control of diabetes mellitus or the thyroid state, collagen vascular associated neuropathies), or removal or avoidance of the toxic agent. Inflammatory (e.g., CIDP, AIDP) or paraproteinemic neuropathies can be successfully treated with corticosteroids, intravenous immunoglobulin (IVIg), immunosuppressive therapy, or therapeutic apheresis (PLEX). GBS improves with IVIg and PLEX. Physical therapy and the use of adaptive equipment is of benefit in more severe forms of neuropathies. Similarly, these modalities are all that are available in the management of hereditary neuropathies.

Patients with significant sensory loss (e.g., diabetic neuropathy) as the result of their neuropathy are at risk for orthopedic and dermatologic injury of their limbs. The foot is most likely to be affected because patients are not able to perceive painful stimuli and their feet are subjected to repetitive trauma. The resulting painless, often overlooked, ulcers that develop may become secondarily infected resulting in cellulitis and osteomyelitis. Charcot joints may develop in the most severe cases.

FUTURE DIRECTIONS

Advances in the treatment of neuropathy will come on three broad fronts: the identification of the gene and gene product of hereditary neuropathies, the elucidation of the immunopathology in several autoimmune mediated acquired neuropathies, and the control of pain.

As understanding of the immune-mediated basis for several of the neuropathic disorders evolves, newer immunosuppressive regimens will be developed. The goal is to develop specific or tar-geted therapies that are non-toxic and that quickly and permanently remove the abnormal immune response. The role of interferons, and cytokines, and the ability to interfere with antigen presentation or co-stimulatory processes will be studied. Because pain is a prominent feature of many neuropathies, extensive work is being carried out on the role of neural growth factors to modulate pain perception and to promote neuronal survival.

REFERENCES

Bromberg MB. Peripheral neurotoxic disorders. *Neurol Clin.* 2000;18:681-694.

England JD. Entrapment neuropathies. *Curr Opin Neurol.* 1999;12:597-602.

Keller MP, Chance PF. Inherited peripheral neuropathy. *Semin Neurol.* 1999;19:353-362.

Leger JM, Salachas F. Diagnosis of motor neuropathy. *Eur J Neurol.* 2001;8:201-208.

Vedeler CA. Inflammatory neuropathies: update. *Curr Opin Neurol.* 2000;13:305-309.

Chapter 106
Sleep Disorders

Bradley V. Vaughn and Brian A. Boehlecke

Sleep is a universal process found in all animals. Sleep promotes the ability to attain high levels of cognition, although the underlying physiological purpose remains a mystery. Disordered sleep has a significant impact on individuals and societies. Individuals with inadequate or disrupted sleep are more likely to have accidents, higher health insurance claims, lower workplace productivity, and poorer quality of life.

One in 3 individuals will present a sleep-related complaint to his or her physician. The International Classification of Sleep Disorders divides sleep disorders into *dyssomnias, parasomnias, sleep disorders associated with medical and psychiatric disorders, and proposed sleep disorders.* Dyssomnias, disorders that result in either excessive daytime sleepiness or insomnia, include intrinsic sleep disorders (e.g., obstructive sleep apnea [see Chapter 122], restless legs syndrome, periodic limb movement disorder, and narcolepsy); extrinsic sleep disorders (e.g., insufficient sleep, inadequate sleep hygiene, or alcohol-dependent sleep disorder); and circadian rhythm sleep disorders (e.g., shift-work sleep disorder or jet lag syndrome). Parasomnias are events that occur in association with sleep such as sleepwalking, night terrors, or rapid eye movement (REM) sleep behavior disorder (See Chapter 103). Other medical and psychiatric disorders such as gastroesophageal reflux disease, heart failure, arthritis, or affective disorders can also disrupt sleep.

ETIOLOGY AND PATHOPHYSIOLOGY

A symphony of neuronal processes determines the sleep-wake state. Sleep is typically divided into stages based on EEG features, eye movements (electro-oculography [EOG]) and muscle tone (electromyography [EMG]). Stages 1 through 4 are called collectively non-rapid eye movement (NREM) sleep. Stage 1 sleep is frequently associated with the perception of drowsiness, and is characterized by EEG features of mild slowing and Vertex sharp waves. Stage 2, light sleep, is characterized by the presence of K complexes or sleep spindles. In stages 3 and 4, high-amplitude slow-wave EEG activity is the prominent feature. During these "deeper" stages, stronger stimuli are needed to produce arousal. Rapid eye movement (REM) sleep is characterized by a low amplitude mixed frequency pattern on the EEG, absence of muscle tone in voluntary muscles, and intermittent rapid eye movements. Dreams can occur in all stages of sleep but are more vivid and recalled more frequently from REM sleep. All of these stages have other physiological correlates, NREM sleep has relatively constant respiration, cardiac rhythm, and autonomic function, while REM sleep demonstrates variation in respiration, cardiac function, and an absence of thermal regulation.

Healthy adults display a reproducible pattern of sleep organization. They enter sleep through stage 1, progress to stage 2, and after 20 to 30 minutes to stages 3 and 4; the first REM sleep period occurs after 90 minutes. This pattern repeats approximately every 90 minutes throughout the sleep period with progressively less deep sleep and longer REM sleep periods in each cycle.

Both extrinsic and intrinsic factors may contribute to disordered sleep. Extrinsic sleep disorders include environmental disturbances such as noise or bright light, which acutely disrupt the continuity of sleep. Intrinsic disorders are prompted by the physiological state change of sleep. Obstructive sleep apnea and periodic limb movements of sleep are excellent examples of disorders that become evident once the CNS has changed to the sleep state (Figure 106-1). Other sleep disorders such as narcolepsy are abnormalities in the mechanism of sleep-wake differentiation. Narcolepsy has a strong linkage to HLA DQB1*0602, DR2 (DR15) major histocompatability complex and a weaker link to DQW1. Recently, it has been linked to a depletion of

Figure 106-1

Sleep Disorders

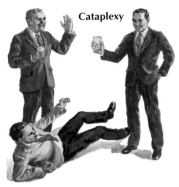

Cataplexy

Sudden loss of muscular-postural
tone with laughter or fright

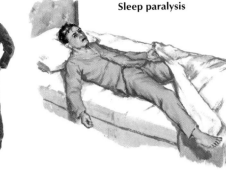

Sleep paralysis

Momentary paralysis on awakening
lasts seconds to minutes

Orexin-producing neurons in the hypothalamus. Alteration of the circadian rhythm can also disrupt sleep-wake determination. This internal clock allows the body to anticipate periods that are likely to be active or inactive. Thus, certain times are associated with a greater "circadian pressure" to sleep (for example, 4:00 A.M. in persons normally active during daylight hours). A complex interaction of proteins and genes produce this chemical rhythm, which can be affected by many stimuli including bright light, activity level, and social interactions. Some individuals have a circadian preference for morning (morning larks) and others for evening (night owls).

CLINICAL PRESENTATION

Typically, patients present with one of three major complaints: excessive daytime sleepiness, difficulty initiating or maintaining sleep, or unusual events occurring during the night. Patients may focus on one symptom, yet have features that suggest several processes are contributing to dysfunctional sleep. Below are commonly recognized sleep disorders.

Sleep Deprivation

Chronic reduction in total sleep time interferes with normal daytime function. Most often sleep deprivation is voluntary; societal pressures push adults to perform with less time for sleep. This shortened sleep time increases the "homeostatic pressure" for sleep and increases the likelihood for an individual to fall asleep at inappropriate

times. Attempts to "make up" sleep fail because of the accumulation of a large sleep debt and the lack of synchronization of the sleep period with the body clock. Sleep debt accumulates over decades and may result in decreased productivity and increased risk for accidents.

Narcolepsy

Narcolepsy, a disorder of the control of sleep, particularly REM sleep, is an inherited nonprogressive disorder that appears in early adolescence typically, and persists throughout life. Patients have difficulty controlling the onset of sleep and have the intrusion of fragments of sleep. The traditional tetrad of symptoms is excessive daytime sleepiness, cataplexy, sleep paralysis, and hypnagogic hallucinations (Figure 106-2). Excessive daytime sleepiness occurs despite a relatively normal total sleep time and may be described as irresistible bouts of sleep ("sleep attacks"). Cataplexy is an abrupt decrease in muscle tone without loss of consciousness provoked by strong emotional stimuli or exercise; individuals may fall or experience varied degree of weakness. Sleep paralysis occurs in the transition from sleep to wakefulness with the retention of the atonia of REM sleep and can be accompanied by the feeling of impending doom and occasionally hallucinations. Hypnagogic hallucinations are visual imagery just before the onset of sleep that may be difficult to distinguish from reality. Cataplexy and sleep paralysis are the atonia of REM sleep, and hypnagogic hallucinations are the visual imagery

Figure 106-2

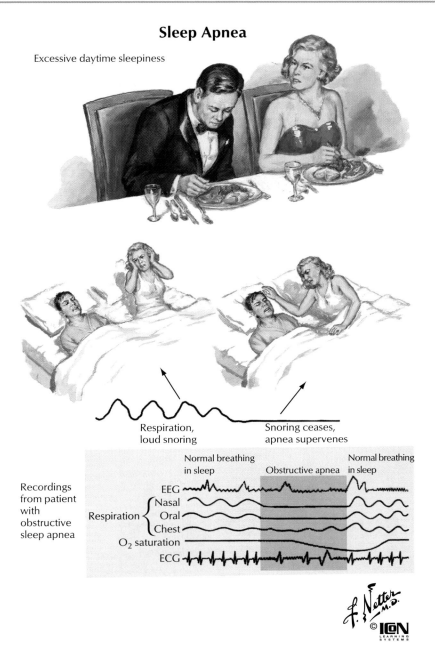

Sleep Apnea

Excessive daytime sleepiness

Respiration, loud snoring

Snoring ceases, apnea supervenes

Recordings from patient with obstructive sleep apnea

Respiration { Nasal, Oral, Chest

Normal breathing in sleep

Obstructive apnea

Normal breathing in sleep

EEG

O_2 saturation

ECG

occurring with REM sleep. Many patients also complain of insomnia and disrupted nighttime sleep.

Periodic Limb Movements of Sleep

Periodic limb movements of sleep are repetitive stereotyped movements of the upper or lower extremities lasting 0.5 to 4.0 seconds, occurring at 20- to 120-second intervals, and sometimes asso-

ciated with arousals. Patients may be unaware of the movements and few have sleep complaints. Bed partners usually note the movements. Iron deficiency, anemia, uremia, peripheral vascular disease, arthritis, peripheral neuropathy, and spinal cord lesions have been associated with the disorder. The use of tricyclic antidepressants, selective serotonin reuptake inhibitors, dopamine antagonists, and caffeine may exacerbate movements. More recently, a connection has been drawn between low stores of central nervous system iron and periodic limb movements. *Restless legs syndrome*, characterized by unpleasant crawling, deep aching sensations in the extremities that improve with movement, is frequently related to periodic limb movements. Patients complain of the need to continuously move their legs while sitting or resting and, often, they have periodic limb movements during sleep. The same factors that provoke periodic limb movements increase the symptoms of restless legs syndrome.

Circadian Rhythm Disorders

The desynchronization of behavioral and neural sleep cycles, which commonly occurs when traveling across time zones or changing work schedules, may result in excessive daytime sleepiness or disrupted nocturnal sleep. Some individuals have chronic desynchronization of the body clock with their surrounding environment. Delayed sleep phase syndrome, characterized by an inability to fall asleep until past midnight and trouble waking in the morning, is seen commonly in adolescents. Advanced sleep phase syndrome is more common among elderly individuals who fall asleep early in the evening and awake in the early morning hours. Individuals with a free-running schedule, common in patients who are blind, have a lack of entrainment of the endogenous 24.3-hour circadian clock. Patients with hypothalamic dysfunction may have an irregular sleep-wake schedule due to a loss of the rhythm generators.

Primary Disorders of Initiation or Maintenance of Sleep

Insomnia is the difficulty initiating or maintaining sleep, combined with daytime sleepiness or impairment of daytime performance. Most adults have an occasional night of poor sleep often linked to events of the day or sudden changes in medical condition. For a smaller group of patients, insomnia persists for weeks, months, or years and leads to significant psychological and medical symptoms. Primary insomnias account for more than one third of cases. *Psychophysiological insomnia* is characterized by somatized tension and learned sleep-preventing associations; individuals typically sleep well in a new environment

Table 106-1
Dyssomnias

Intrinsic Sleep Disorders
- Obstructive sleep apnea
- Central sleep apnea
- Narcolepsy
- Periodic limb movement disorder
- Restless legs syndrome
- Psychophysiologic insomnia
- Sleep state misperception
- Idiopathic insomnia
- Idiopathic hypersomnia
- Recurrent hypersomnia
- Posttraumatic hypersomnia
- Central alveolar hypoventilation
- Intrinsic sleep disorder

Extrinsic Sleep Disorders
- Inadequate sleep hygiene
- Environmental sleep disorder
- Altitude insomnia
- Adjustment sleep disorder
- Insufficient sleep syndrome
- Limit-setting sleep disorder
- Sleep onset association disorder
- Food allergy insomnia
- Hypnotic dependent sleep disorder
- Stimulant dependent sleep disorder
- Alcohol dependent sleep disorder
- Toxin-induced sleep disorder

Circadian Rhythm Disorders
- Delayed sleep phase syndrome
- Advanced sleep phase syndrome
- Non-24-hr sleep-wake syndrome
- Irregular sleep-wake pattern
- Jet lag syndrome
- Shift work sleep disorder

away from associations that remind them of the difficulty of sleeping. *Sleep state misperception* is the inability to recognize the occurrence of sleep. Patients have normal sleep as measured by polysomnography, but report being unaware that they have slept. *Idiopathic insomnia*, an abnormality in the physiological ability to attain adequate sleep, typically starts in childhood and persists as fragmented and unrefreshing sleep through adulthood.

DIFFERENTIAL DIAGNOSIS

The differential diagnosis is divided into intrinsic sleep disorders, extrinsic sleep disorders, medical disorders, and psychiatric disorders (Tables 106-1 and 106-2). Patients with sleep apnea, peri-

Table 106-2
Sleep Disorders with Medical/Psychiatric Disorders

Associated with Medical Disorders
    Chronic pulmonary disease
    Sleep-related asthma
    Nocturnal cardiac ischemia
    Sleep-related gastroesophageal reflux
    Peptic ulcer disease
    Sleeping sickness

Associated with Neurologic Disorders
    Cerebral degenerative disorders
    Dementia
    Parkinsonism
    Sleep-related headaches
    Fatal familial insomnia

Associated with Psychiatric Disorders
    Psychoses
    Mood disorders
    Anxiety disorders
    Panic disorder
    Alcoholism
    Fibrositis syndrome

odic leg movements of sleep, and circadian rhythm disorders may or may not complain of sleepiness despite severe sleep disruption. Patients with medical disorders such as congestive heart failure, renal failure, arthritis, and pain syndromes may complain of poor sleep or fatigue. Psychiatric disorders are often preceded by insomnia; frequently, sleep disturbance outlasts the mood disturbance of affective disorders.

DIAGNOSTIC APPROACH

The diagnostic evaluation should focus on several key points. Complaints should be separated into categories of excessive daytime sleepiness, insomnia, or unusual events at night. A detailed history, including information regarding the clinical course, the degree of impact on daytime function, the sleep-wake pattern, perception of sleep quality, report from bed partner, dietary habits (especially caffeine and alcohol intake), activity changes, drug use (including over-the-counter agents, herbs, and home remedies), and medical conditions, is crucial. It is important to distinguish between fatigue and true sleepiness. The clinician should look for potential causes of sleep disturbance from four groups: intrinsic sleep disorder, extrinsic sleep disturbance,

circadian rhythm disorder, and other medical, neurological or psychiatric disorders.

The potential for multiple etiologies should be considered. To sleep well, one needs a conducive environment, psychological preparedness for sleep, an adequate sleep period, and the neurophysiological mechanisms for sleep. Most patients with chronic insomnia have a set of factors that predispose, initiate, and perpetuate insomnia. Gender, age, and coping mechanisms may predispose one to insomnia, while poor sleep hygiene, substance abuse, and performance anxiety may perpetuate it. Question patients for cardinal symptoms of intrinsic sleep disorders, such as snoring, leg kicking, or sleep-related activities.

Many disorders can be elucidated with objective evaluation of the patient's sleep. Consider referring a patient for polysomnography at a qualified and experienced sleep laboratory when he or she has symptoms of a sleep-related breathing disorder, movement disorder, narcolepsy, paroxysmal arousals, or behaviors that are potentially injurious or typical for parasomnia. Patients being evaluated for excessive daytime sleepiness may require a multiple sleep latency test to measure the degree of daytime sleepiness and the potential to enter REM sleep inappropriately during the wake period. This test is especially useful for evaluating the possibility of narcolepsy and the complaint of hypersomnolence that has no clear etiology.

MANAGEMENT AND THERAPY

The treatment of patients with sleep disorders requires close follow-up and clearly established therapeutic goals. Causes of extrinsic sleep disruption should be identified before expensive polysomnographic investigation is performed. Successful management depends on identifying underlying causes of sleep disruption and initiating specific therapeutic interventions. CNS active medications should be used to affect specific neurochemical processes. Stimulants, such as modafinil, methylphenidate, dextroamphetamine, and pemoline, can be used to treat the excessive sleepiness in narcolepsy or idiopathic hypersomnolence.

Benzodiazepines and antidepressants have been used for the treatment of insomnia; however, zolpidem and zaleplon, newer hypnotic agents, induce sleep with fewer psychomotor side effects and lower the chance of rebound insomnia. For insomnia, behavioral modification and cognitive therapies, in addition to the medication therapies, are helpful in improving sleep. . Most patients need clinical monitoring and education to reinforce therapies and behaviors conducive for good sleep.

FUTURE DIRECTIONS

Our understanding of the mechanisms involved in determining the sleep-wake state is rapidly expanding. Application of molecular biological techniques to determine novel neuroactive substances and receptors has opened new understanding of state determination. Understanding these mechanisms provides opportunities for molecularly targeted therapies to manipulate sleep and wake states.

REFERENCES

Aldrich MS. *Sleep Medicine*. New York, NY: Oxford University Press; 1999.

Chesson AL Jr, Ferber RA, Fry JM, et al. The indications for polysomnography and related procedures. *Sleep*. 1997;20:423–487.

Chokroverty S, ed. *Sleep Disorders Medicine: Basic Science, Technical Considerations, and Clinical Aspects*. 2nd ed. Boston Mass: Butterworth-Heinemann; 1999.

Kryger MH, Roth T, Dement WC, eds. *Principles and Practice of Sleep Medicine*. 3rd ed. Philadelphia, Pa: WB Saunders Co; 2000.

Chapter 107

Stroke and Transient Ischemic Attacks

Albert R. Hinn

Stroke is a general term for focal brain injury of vascular origin that lasts more than 24 hours. Strokes can be further characterized as ischemic or hemorrhagic (Figure 107-1). This chapter concentrates on ischemic strokes. Transient ischemic attacks (TIAs) are defined as focal ischemic cerebrovascular events lasting less than 24 hours.

ETIOLOGY AND PATHOGENESIS

Most ischemic strokes are thrombotic or embolic in origin, and the result of underlying atherosclerotic disease involving the extracranial and/or intracranial cerebrovascular vessels, or underlying cardiac disease. The major modifiable stroke risk factors are hypertension, atrial fibrillation, cardiac disease, smoking, alcohol abuse, and diabetes mellitus. Hypercholesterolemia does not have as clear of an association with cerebrovascular disease s it does with cardiovascular disease. A number of medical conditions (e.g., polycythemia vera, meningovascular syphilis, bacterial endocarditis) can result in cerebrovascular events as well, but these conditions are found less commonly (Figure 107-2). Lacunar strokes are usually the result of lipohyalinosis involving the small subcortical penetrating arteries of the brain.

CLINICAL PRESENTATION

The presenting symptoms are a reflection of the underlying cerebrovascular distribution of the event.

Carotid Artery Territory

Common symptoms and findings are monocular visual loss, contralateral weakness or sensory disturbance, dysarthria, language impairment with dominant hemisphere involvement, denial or neglect with nondominant hemisphere involvement, other higher cortical deficits, and visual field loss. (Figure 107-3)

Subcortical Lacunar Strokes

This type of stroke results in various syndromes including pure motor hemiplegia, pure sensory stroke, dysarthria, clumsy hand syndrome, and ataxic hemiparesis.

Vertebrobasilar Artery Distribution

Common symptoms and findings are unilateral or bilateral weakness or sensory disturbance, crossed motor or sensory findings (i.e., symptoms on one side of the face and the contralateral side of the body), dysarthria, pupil abnormalities, ophthalmoplegia, other cranial nerve deficits, Horner's syndrome, ataxia, various visual field deficits, and altered level of consciousness (Figure 107-4). Named brainstem syndromes describe the findings seen with involvement of specific vascular distributions, and are best understood in terms of the specific nuclei and anatomical pathways involved by the event.

DIFFERENTIAL DIAGNOSIS

Many medical conditions may be confused for cerebrovascular events including partial seizures and migrainous auras; syncope/near-syncope; peripheral vestibulopathies; hypoglycemia; brain tumors, subdural hematomas, and other intracranial mass lesions. Consider systemic infection, metabolic disorders, and medication intoxication/overdose, particularly in the patient without focal neurologic symptoms.

DIAGNOSTIC APPROACH

Rapid diagnosis and early treatment are essential. Initial evaluation involves a careful history and neurologic examination. Attention should be given to the ABCs, and supplemental oxygenation given if indicated. Vascular access should be

Figure 107-1

Diagnosis of Stroke

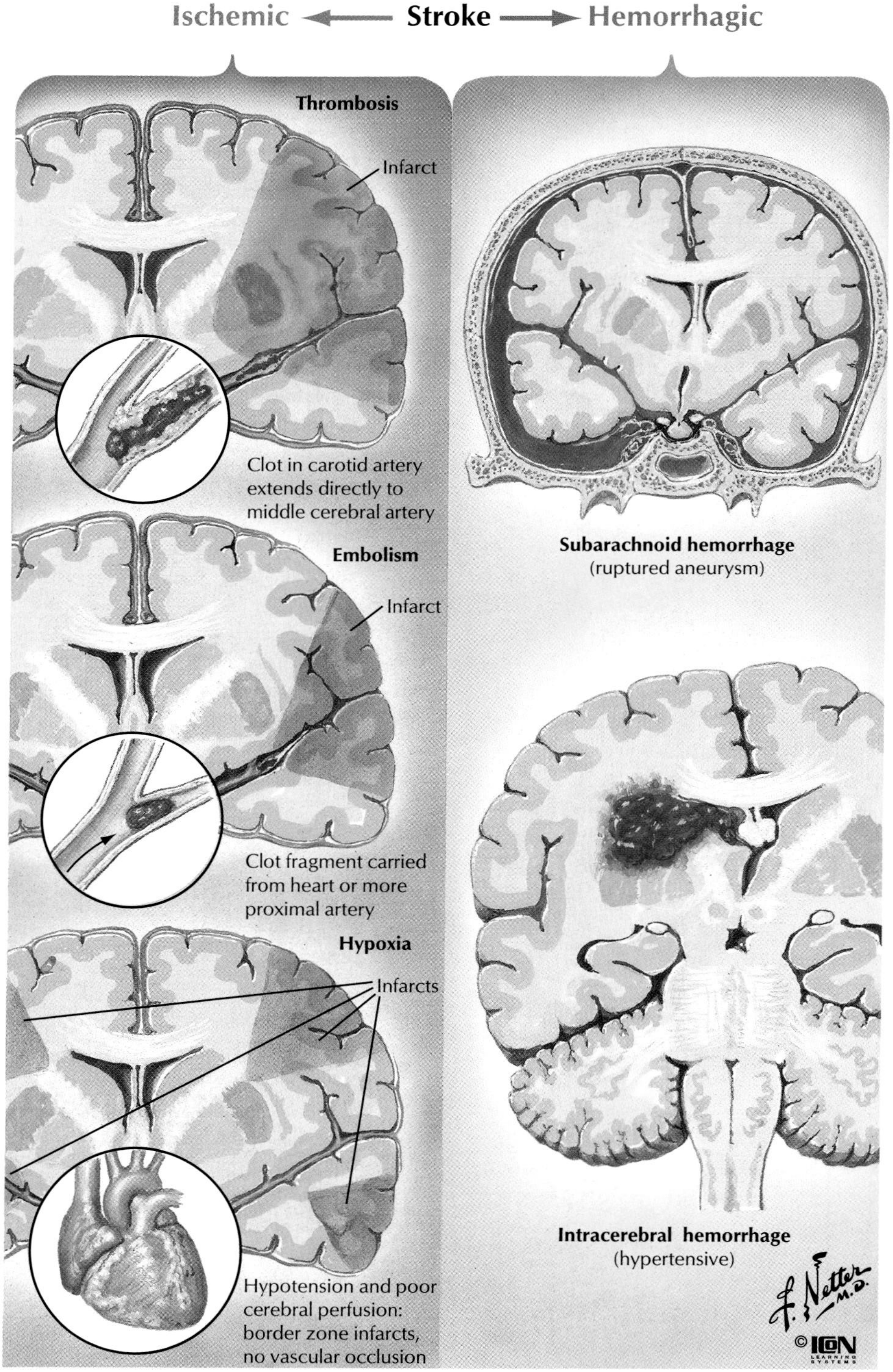

Ischemic ⟵ Stroke ⟶ Hemorrhagic

Thrombosis

Infarct

Clot in carotid artery extends directly to middle cerebral artery

Embolism

Infarct

Clot fragment carried from heart or more proximal artery

Hypoxia

Infarcts

Hypotension and poor cerebral perfusion: border zone infarcts, no vascular occlusion

Subarachnoid hemorrhage
(ruptured aneurysm)

Intracerebral hemorrhage
(hypertensive)

obtained. A CT scan of the head is indicated emergently, particularly if the patient presents within the 3-hour time window considered acceptable or administration of recombinant tissue plasminogen activator (rt-PA). Generally, the CT can be performed without the use of contrast material. If concerned or an underlying mass lesion exists, then plain and contrast-enhanced studies should be ordered. Blood specimens should be drawn for routine metabolic studies, glucose, CBC, sedimentation rate, VDRL/RPR, and coagulation studies. Additional laboratory studies may be indicated to rule out systemic infection and medication intoxication/overdose. In the young stroke patient, further laboratory evaluation may be indicated, including antithrombin III activity, protein C and S activity, sickle cell screen, lupus inhibitor, anticardiolipin antibody, antinuclear antibody, homocysteine level, and a urine toxicology screen. The evaluation should also include a 12-lead electrocardiogram (ECG), transthoracic echocardiography, and carotid Doppler study. ECG telemetry monitoring can be useful, particularly if concern exists about undetected cardiac arrhythmias. Additional studies such as an MRI of the brain, MR angiography (MRA) of the intracranial and/or extracranial vasculature, cerebral angiography, and transesophageal echocardiography may be helpful, depending on the clinical situation. MRI with diffusion-weighted images is very useful in demonstrating acute ischemic infarcts.

MANAGEMENT AND THERAPY

Currently, acute ischemic stroke therapy is largely limited to the use of intravenous thrombolytic therapy. Alteplase (rt-PA) is the only approved therapy for the treatment of acute ischemic stroke. The National Institute of Neurological Disorders and Stroke (NINDS) study documented an approximately 30% relative and 12% absolute increase in patients having a good outcome with minimal to no disability at 3 months when compared with the placebo group. This was despite an absolute increase of 6% in the occurrence of symptomatic intracerebral hemorrhage in the rt-PA treated patients. Treatment must be initiated within 3 hours after the onset of stroke symptoms,and only after exclusion of intracranial hemorrhage by a CT scan or other diagnostic imaging method. Onset of symptoms is defined as the time

since the patient was last known to be symptom-free. For patients awakening with deficits, one must use the time they were last awake, and without symptoms. The recommended dose of rt-PA is 0.9 mg/kg (maximum of 90 mg) infused over 60 minutes with 10% of the total dose administered

---

Contraindications to IV rt-PA Therapy

- Etiology for deficits is other than acute ischemic stroke
- Minor neurologic deficit or rapidly improving symptoms before the start of therapy
- Initiation of rt-PA would be more than 3 hours after onset of stroke symptoms
- Intracranial hemorrhage evident on pretreatment CT scan
- Subarachnoid hemorrhage is suspected.
- Intracranial surgery, serious head trauma, or a prior stroke within the previous 3 months
- History of intracranial hemorrhage
- Intracranial neoplasm, arteriovenous malformation, or aneurysm
- Recent surgery (e.g., coronary artery bypass graft, obstetrical delivery, organ biopsy, or puncture of noncompressible vessels within the preceding 14 days)
- Gastrointestinal or genitourinary bleeding within the preceding 21 days
- Recent lumbar puncture
- Active internal bleeding
- Uncontrolled hypertension at time of treatment (i.e., systolic BP >185 mmHg or diastolic BP >110 mmHg)
- Seizure at the onset of the event
- A blood glucose <50 mg/dL or >400 mg/dL
- Hematocrit <25
- Current use of oral anticoagulants with an International Normalized Ratio (INR) >1. 7
- Administration of heparin within 48 hours preceding the onset of the stroke, and an elevated activated PTT at presentation
- Platelet count <100,000/mm3
- Patients with major early infarct signs on the CT scan (e.g., substantial edema, mass effect, or midline shift) are at increased risk of intracerebral hemorrhage with use of rt-PA, and generally should not receive thrombolytic therapy.

Figure 107-2

Uncommon Etiologic Mechanisms in Stroke

Cardiac emboli

 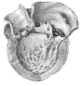 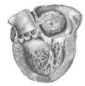 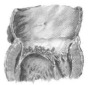

Myocardiopathy with thrombi

Mitral valve prolapse with clots

Atrial myxomatous tumor emboli

Marantic emboli

Probe-patent foramen ovale transmitting venous clots

Carotid or intracerebral arterial disorders

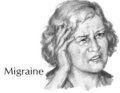 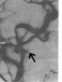

Migraine

Angiogram showing dissection of carotid artery, with high-grade stenosis and pseudo-aneurysm

Intracerebral aneurysm. Spasm in distal vessel

Giant-cell arteritis

Drug-induced mechanisms

Birth control pills

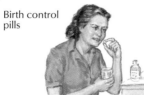

Drug addiction ("mainliner")

Monoamine oxidase (MAO) inhibitors (potentiated by wine and cheese)

Hematologic disorders

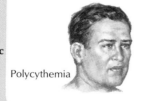 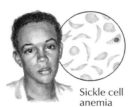 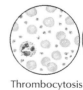 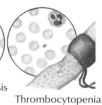

Polycythemia

Sickle cell anemia

Thrombocytosis

Thrombocytopenia

Infectious diseases

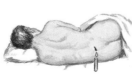 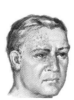

Herpes zoster (ophthalmic)

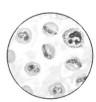

CNS syphilis

Meningitis

Malaria

Figure 107-3

Ischemia in Internal Carotid Artery Territory:
Clinical Manifestations

A. Ocular

Transient blindness in one eye from temporary occlusion by platelet-fibrin or cholesterol emboli (on side of involved artery)

Internal carotid a.

Ophthalmic a.

Central retinal a.

Partial blindness may be detected by covering one eye at a time to determine if defect is monocular or binocular

B. Cerebral hemisphere

Occasional headache (usually supraorbital or temporal)

Homonymous (partial) visual field defects

Language defect (partial or complete) only when dominant hemisphere is involved

Hemiparesis or hemiplegia (only arm or leg may be affected); may be fleeting, transient, or permanent and may appear with or without sensory deficits

On side opposite involved artery

Patient may awaken from sleep unable to move affected side

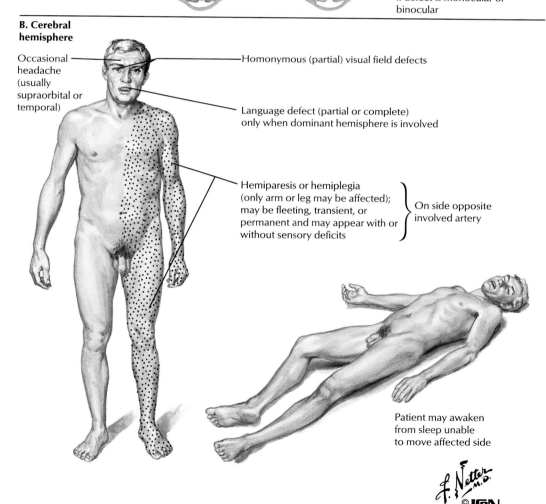

Figure 107-4

Ischemia in Vertebrobasilar Territory:
Clinical Manifestations

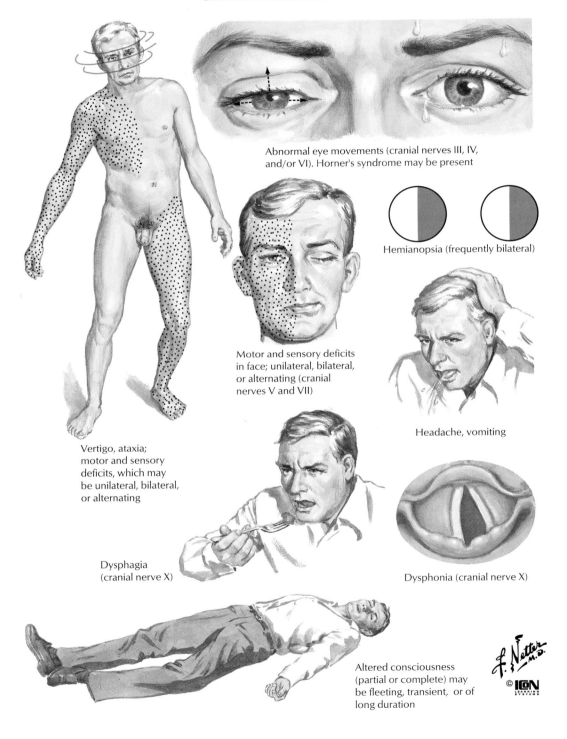

Abnormal eye movements (cranial nerves III, IV, and/or VI). Horner's syndrome may be present

Hemianopsia (frequently bilateral)

Motor and sensory deficits in face; unilateral, bilateral, or alternating (cranial nerves V and VII)

Headache, vomiting

Vertigo, ataxia; motor and sensory deficits, which may be unilateral, bilateral, or alternating

Dysphagia (cranial nerve X)

Dysphonia (cranial nerve X)

Altered consciousness (partial or complete) may be fleeting, transient, or of long duration

as an initial intravenous bolus over 1 minute.

Patients treated with rt-PA should be admitted to a monitored bed and closely observed with frequent vital sign and neurologic checks. Blood pressure should be monitored frequently for the first 24 hours, and actively controlled (<180/105 mm Hg) with appropriate medication if indicated.

If serious bleeding occurs, rt-PA should be discontinued immediately. Blood should be drawn for CBC, PT, PTT, fibrinogen level, and type and cross. The administration of 5 to 10 units of cryoprecipitate should be considered for serious bleeding, and packed RBCs and platelets should be transfused if required. If an intracranial hemorrhage is suspected, rt-PA should be discontinued and an emergency head CT scan obtained. Neurosurgery should be consulted for any intracranial hemorrhage that occurs in patients treated with rt-PA for acute ischemic stroke.

Patients receiving rt-PA should not receive aspirin, dipyridamole, ticlopidine, clopidogrel, heparin, or warfarin during the first 24 hours. Patients who have been taking aspirin or other antiplatelet agents are eligible for treatment with rt-PA if they meet all other criteria for therapy.

Although anticoagulation with heparin has commonly been done for patients presenting with an acute ischemic stroke, there is no convincing evidence for a clinical benefit from such an approach. It is possible that subsets of patients might benefit, but this is unproven. Intravenous heparin administration is commonly done for patients with progressing stroke symptoms (stroke-in-evolution), but this is also of unproved benefit.

Noncardioembolic Infarcts

Therapy aimed at prevention of recurrent strokes should begin with risk-factor reduction.

Most patients with noncardioembolic infarcts should be placed on antiplatelet therapy. Aspirin 50 to 325 mg once daily the combination agent of aspirin 25 mg and extended-release dipyridamole 200 mg administered twice daily, and clopidogrel 75 mg once daily are all acceptable initial options. Ticlopidine is used less commonly because of adverse events associated with its use. These include a 1% risk of severe neutropenia and the occurrence of thrombotic thrombocytopenic purpura. Headache is the most common side effect associated with the use of the combination agent of aspirin 25 mg and extended-release dipyridamole 200 mg. The combination of clopidogrel and aspirin is frequently used, but the benefits and safety of this treatment regimen in the long-term treatment of patients with cerebrovascular disease are unknown.

Cardioembolic Infarcts

Anticoagulation with warfarin is effective, with a goal of an INR in the range of 2.0 to 3.0. For high-risk patients with atrial fibrillation, long-term anticoagulation with warfarin is generally recommended. High risk factors include previous stroke/TIA or systemic embolus, hypertension, poor left ventricular systolic function, age >75 years, rheumatic mitral valve disease, and prosthetic heart valve. Moderate risk factors include age between 65 and 75 years, diabetes mellitus, and coronary artery disease with preserved left ventricular systolic function. For patients with atrial fibrillation and age <65 years, and with no other evidence of cardiovascular disease, aspirin therapy is recommended.

Carotid Atherosclerotic Disease

Surgical management is generally indicated for patients with symptomatic carotid artery stenosis of 70% to 99%. A more moderate reduction in the risk of stroke is seen for patients with symptomatic carotid artery stenosis of 50% to 69% and in those patients with asymptomatic carotid artery stenosis of >60% who undergo a caroid endarterectomy.

Prevention of Complications

An elevated blood pressure is commonly found in patients with acute ischemic stroke. Optimal management has not been established. In general, antihypertensive drugs should be withheld acutely, unless the calculated mean arterial blood pressure is greater than 130 mm Hg or the systolic blood pressure is greater than 220 mm Hg. Deep venous thrombosis (DVT) and pulmonary embolism (PE) can occur as a complication of immobility associated with strokes. For this reason, DVT/PE prophylaxis is recommended for all stroke patients with immobility. Early mobilization of the patient is another important measure in preventing medical complications. The involvement of speech therapy, physical therapy, occupational therapy, and rehabilitative medicine is important in preventing complications and maximizing recovery of the stroke patient.

FUTURE DIRECTIONS

Diagnostically, newer brain imaging modalities will be used to define the areas of cerebral perfusion abnormality and the degree of ischemic injury. This will allow physicians to better define which patients might benefit from specific acute stroke therapies. Research continues in the areas of both intravenous and intra-arterial thrombolytic therapy. In addition, mechanical methods of clot disruption are being developed. To date, attempts at limiting the extent of neuronal injury with neuroprotective agents have been disappointing. Research in this area of acute stroke treatment continues.

REFERENCES

Adams HP Jr, Brott TG, Furlan AJ, et al. Guidelines for thrombolytic therapy for acute stroke: a supplement to the guidelines for the management of patients with acute ischemic stroke. A statement for healthcare professionals from a Special Writing Group of the Stroke Council, American Health Association. *Circulation*. 1996;94:1167–1174.

Albers GW, Amarenco P, Easton JD, Sacco RL, Teal P. Antithrombotic and thrombolytic therapy for ischemic stroke. *Chest*. 2001;119(suppl):300S–320S.

Albers GW, Hart RG, Lutsep HL, Newell DW, Sacco RL. AHA Scientific Statement. Supplement to the guidelines for the management of transient ischemic attacks: a statement from the Ad Hoc Committee on Guidelines for the Management of Transient Ischemic Attacks, Stroke Council, American Heart Association. *Stroke*. 1999;30:2502–2511.

Brott T, Bogousslavsky J. Treatment of acute ischemic stroke. *N Engl J Med*. 2000;343:710–722.

Goldstein LB, Adams R, Becker K, et al. Primary prevention of ischemic stroke: a statement for healthcare professionals from the Stroke Council of the American Heart Association. *Circulation*. 2001;103:163–182.

Chapter 108

Tremor

Xuemei Huang and Colin D. Hall

Tremor is defined as involuntary, rhythmic oscillations of a body part. The involved body part can be proximal (e.g., head tremor) or distal (e.g., hand tremors). The tremor may be fine or coarse, fast or slow, exist at rest, when maintaining a posture, or with movement. The 1998 Movement Disorder Society consensus paper on clinical classification serves as a guide for this chapter.

ETIOLOGY AND PATHOGENESIS

Tremor is a nonspecific finding that can result from a variety of nervous system lesions and a number of underlying disease processes. Lesions in the basal ganglia, the cerebellum, or certain areas of the brainstem are particularly likely to result in tremor. Some fairly common tremors have no clear localization (*vide infra*), and a number have metabolic or toxic causes.

CLINICAL PRESENTATION

Observation is a key to identify the etiology and should include a description of the body parts involved, type of tremor, tremor frequency (e.g., low [<4 Hz], medium [4 to 7 Hz], or high [>7 Hz]), and the factors that exacerbate or suppress the tremor. (Figure 108-1).

Phenomenology of Tremor
Physiologic Tremor

An 8- to 12-Hz tremor is inherent in the normal nervous system. It is the result of physiologic subtetanic recruitment of motor units and is not generally clinically obvious. Enhanced physiologic tremor (PT) involves more prominent responses in stressful situations (e.g., fatigue, anxiety, fever, and some hypermetabolic states) or after certain medications. Enhanced PT is easily visible when arms are held outstretched, or during writing or drinking from a cup. There should be no evidence of underlying neurologic disease, and the tremor should be reversible as soon as the offending factor is removed.

Rest Tremor

Rest tremor is usually 4 to 5 Hz, often called parkinsonian tremor, and occurs in a limb that is not voluntarily activated. It is suppressed with voluntary movement, and may appear as "pill rolling" (thumb rubbing across the palm or fingers). In early Parkinson's disease (PD), rest tremor can be intermittent and obvious only under emotional or physical stress. As with almost all movement disorders, it disappears with sleep.

Action Tremor

Action tremor is accentuated by voluntary contraction of muscle. This group includes postural, kinetic, and isometric tremor. *Postural tremor* is seen when maintaining a position, such as with the arms outstretched. *Kinetic tremor* occurs during voluntary movement and is subdivided into *simple kinetic tremor* (during non-target-directed movement), *intention tremor* (exacerbated as the hand or foot approaches the target of a voluntary movement, such as finger-to-nose), and *task-specific tremor*. *Isometric tremor* occurs with muscle contraction against a stationary object (e.g., queezing the examiner's fingers).

Localization and Etiology of Different Clinical Tremor Syndromes

The tremor elements (*vide supra*) can be combined into the following clinical syndromes with specific causes that are useful for clinical diagnosis and treatment.

Rest tremor (Parkinsonian tremor) occurs most commonly with diseases of the extrapyramidal system, most commonly with idiopathic PD. The diagnosis of PD is usually established by concomitant findings, such as bradykinesia (e.g., slow movement, facial masking), rigidity (including cogwheel phenomenon from tremor superimposed on rigidity), and gait disorder (e.g., shuffling, lack of arm swing on

Figure 108-1

Tremor

Rest tremor

Usually called parkinsonian tremor, occurs in a limb that is not voluntarily activated. It is suppressed with voluntary movement. It may appear as "pill rolling."

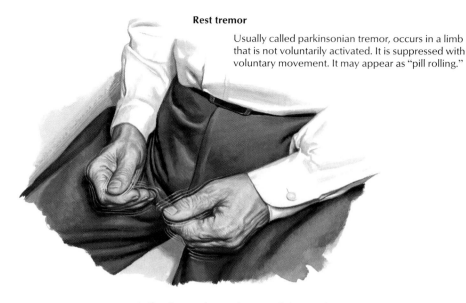

Action tremor (example: essential tremor)

Typically bilateral, this movement disorder is the most common. It may be accentuated with goal-directed movement of the limbs. Essential tremor affects the hands and facial musculature (in this order of prevalence). Most common presentation is the association of hand tremor and tremor in cranial musculature.

However considered benign, it can become incapacitating. In the severe forms the patient may not be able to perform essential daily activities, such as drinking from a cup or dressing.

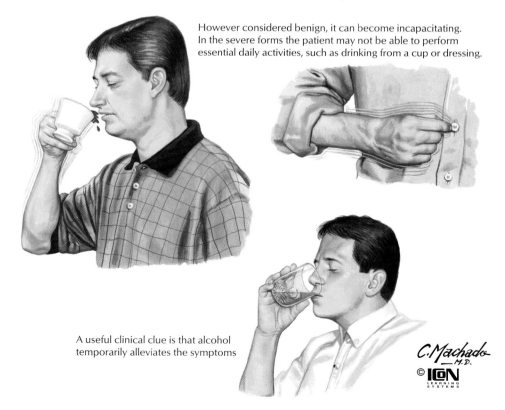

A useful clinical clue is that alcohol temporarily alleviates the symptoms

walking). Other causes for rest tremor include both primary (e.g., progressive supranuclear palsy, multiple system atrophy) and secondary parkinsonism (e.g., stroke lesions of the basal ganglia, carbon monoxide intoxication, mitochondrial diseases).

In *action tremor* (cerebellar tremor), postural and kinetic tremor are common features of disease involving the deep cerebellar nuclei and the cerebellar tracts in the brainstem. There may be a striking intention component that is particularly incapacitating. Other findings such as nystagmus, scanning dysarthria, dysrhythmia, and truncal ataxia help in cerebellar localization. Accompanying cranial nerve and pyramidal tract involvement also suggest brainstem disease. Many disease processes involving these structures may result in tremor, including neoplastic and paraneoplastic, hereditary and sporadic degenerative, demyelinating, traumatic, infectious, and cardiovascular. Alcohol is among the best-known toxicants causing this tremor.

Although of unknown etiology, essential tremor (ET) is the most common movement disorder (prevalence of 0.4% to .09%), presenting typically as bilateral, largely symmetric postural tremor that may be accentuated with goal-directed movement of the limbs. Severe ET also can manifest as rest tremor. ET most frequently affects the hands, and next the cranial musculature. Although tongue, head, or voice may be affected in isolation, it is most common for the tremor in cranial musculature to occur in association with hand tremor. The legs and trunk are least affected, and usually only in the later stages of the illness.

ET may be sporadic or familial. It may appear at any age, but is more frequent in early adulthood. The onset of ET may be earlier in the familial than the sporadic form. The course is unpredictable, but may be static for many years, or progress with a slow decline. While usually considered benign, it can become incapacitating, particularly in occupations that require precise hand movements. In the severe form, patients may not be able to perform essential daily activities such as dressing or drinking from a cup. A family history will assist the diagnosis of ET, although the expression may be extremely varied in different members. A useful clinical clue is if alcohol temporarily alleviates the

symptoms. As with most other tremor, ET remits during sleep.

Dystonic tremor is described as postural, localized, and irregular, decreased during muscle relaxation and accentuated by positioning the dystonic body part opposite to the direction of dystonia. The tremor caused by cervical dystonia is usually present as "no-no" kind of head shaking. The hand-and-head dystonic tremor can be difficult to differentiate from ET, but failure to respond to treatment for ET, or any dystonic feature in other body parts, may suggest the diagnosis.

Primary orthostatic tremor (OT) is an uncommon condition, also called "shaky leg syndrome," and starts in late adulthood. The patient has a feeling of tremulousness in the legs when standing. This may lead to falls, but generally disappears on movement and is not present when sitting or lying. The diagnosis is helped by specific surface electromyographic evaluation showing a 14- to 18-Hz oscillating tremor in the musculature of the legs when standing, disappearing with rest or movement. The etiology is unknown. While suggested to be a variant of ET, it is probably a distinct entity because of the difference in age of onset, involvement of different parts (ET rarely affects legs), lack of family history, and lack of response to alcohol.

Holmes' tremor syndrome combines features of rest, intention, and postural tremor. The amplitude while resting may be small, but may become uncontrollable while attempting to hold a posture, even worse when attempting a movement. In 1904, Holmes first described this as "rubral" tremor, but later it was called midbrain or thalamic tremor. Holme's tremor is now preferred because the syndrome can occur with lesions affecting not only the red nucleus and rubral spinal tract in the brainstem, but also the cerebellum and thalamus. The tremor may appear weeks to months after a known lesion (e.g., stroke), and some patients have associated dystonia. Identifying this tremor always warrants evaluation for an underlying focal lesion.

A tremor is considered drug- or toxicant-induced if it occurs in a reasonable timeframe following ingestion or exposure. The tremor can take any form, but the most common clinical manifestation is enhanced PT, which can be caused by sympathomimetic agents, such as bronchodilators, xanthines (e.g., caffeine), and epinephrine; centrally acting agents (e.g., valproate, lithium, tricyclic and other antidepressants, cocaine); antiarrhythmics (e.g., mexiletine, procainamide, and amiodarone); steroids (e.g., adrenocorticosteroids, tamoxifen, and progesterone); and cyclosporin and antimetabolites, such as vincristine. Withdrawal from medications such as benzodiazepines or alcohol may also precipitate enhanced PT. Parkinsonian tremor can be caused by neuroleptic and dopamine-blocking drugs (e.g., haloperidol or metoclopramide), or dopamine-depleting agents (e.g., reserpine). Cerebellar tremor may occur after intoxication by lithium or alcohol. Environmental toxicants such as organophosphates and or other insecticides, toxic metals, and some industrial chemicals can also cause or exacerbate tremor.

Tremor in lower motor neuron diseases and peripheral neuropathy may accompany diseases of the anterior horn cell (e.g., amytrophic lateral sclerosis) and peripheral neuropathies. Demyelinating and particularly dysglobulinemic neuropathies are particularly likely to be associated with tremor, usually postural and/or kinetic. It is unclear if tremor associated with peripheral neuropathy is due to enhanced PT secondary to weakness, or to an abnormality in the central nervous system, or both.

Psychogenic tremor can take almost any form, and at times is difficult to diagnosis. Psychogenic origin should be suspected when features of other recognized forms of tremor are not found. Clues to psychogenic etiology include sudden onset, bizarre fluctuations in the frequency and direction, increase when attention is drawn to the movement, history of secondary gain, and response to placebo. As always, it must be remembered that psychogenic disease may coexist in patients with organic disease.

DIFFERENTIAL DIAGNOSIS

Tremor must be differentiated from other movement disorders.
- Clonus, unlike tremor, is increased by passive stretch of the muscle.
- Myoclonus, while difficult to distinguish and may have an EEG correlate, is generally more dysrhythmic with visible pauses between the jerks.

- Epilepsy partialis continua may continue through sleep and generally has EEG correlates.
- Asterixis (also called negative myoclonus) is characterized by a sudden loss of a maintained posture, followed by recovery, rather than an active movement.

DIAGNOSTIC APPROACH

History should focus on the onset of tremor, family history, alcohol sensitivity, spreading sequence, associated disease, medication or chemical exposure, and possible drug abuse. The neurologic examination should assess akinesia/bradykinesia, muscle tone, postural abnormalities, dystonia, cerebellar signs, pyramidal signs, neuropathic signs, gait, and stance. Consideration should not be limited to the nervous system because tremor may result from endocrine disease, hepatic failure, or neoplasm.

A history of relapsing and remitting neurologic symptoms or the findings of other neurologic abnormalities associated with action tremor may suggest evaluation for multiple sclerosis, mass lesions, or stroke. Effective treatments for some tremor-inducing conditions (thyroid dysfunction or Wilson's disease) make it reasonable to check thyroid function in all patients with movement disorder, and ceruloplasmin levels in young patients. Holme tremor requires an extensive workup to identify local lesions in the brainstem, cerebellum, or thalamus pathway. If the tremor is bilateral and symmetric but not associated with other clinical abnormalities, imaging of the head is unlikely to be revealing.

MANAGEMENT AND THERAPY

Effective treatment of the underlying disease is generally the most appropriate initial approach. Early in the course of PD, tremor may respond to anticholinergic medications (amantadine, trihexyphenidyl), or later to levodopa and dopamine agonists. The most often utilized drug treatment for essential tremor is propranolol, primidone, or a combination of these agents. Isolated reports also suggest relief from gabapentin, clonidine, clozapine, topiramate, acetazolamide, or methazolamide.

Primary OT is sometimes treated by clonazepam, phenobarbital, primidone, or valproate, although careful studies are not available. Neither alcohol nor propranolol is helpful. Treatment of dystonia with botulinum toxin often results in significant improvement of tremor (e.g., in cervical dystonia), but dystonic tremor may also respond to benzodiazepines (e.g., clonazepam 0.25 to 2 mg/day). The overall treatment for cerebellar tremor remains unsatisfactory. While appending weights to the wrist may damp the amplitude of cerebellum, dystonic, and ET, this rarely results in sustained functional improvement.

Stereotactic surgical ablation and deep-brain stimulation (DBS) of the thalamus or basal ganglia are reserved for patients with severely disabling and medically intractable rest, essential, or intention tremor. Trained and experienced multidisciplinary teams, appropriate patients, and clearly identified neuroanatomic targets are the critical factors for successful outcome.

FUTURE DIRECTIONS

It is likely that surgical ablation and DBS will become more useful as targets and methods are refined. Similarly, a wealth of new knowledge becoming available about the chemical neurocircuitry of the brain should also lead to better mechanistic understanding, as well as new pharmacotherapeutic agents.

REFERENCES

Britton TC, Thompson PD. Primary orthostatic tremor. *BMJ.* 1995;310:143–144.

Deuschl G, Bain P, Brin M. Consensus statement of the Movement Disorder Society on Tremor. Ad Hoc Scientific Committee. *Mov Disord.* 1998;13(suppl 3):2–23.

Koller WC, Hristova A, Brin M. Pharmacologic treatment of essential tremor. *Neurology.* 2000;54(suppl 4):S30–S38.

Marsden CD. Origins of normal and pathological tremor. In: Findley LJ, Capildeo R, eds. *Movement Disorders: Tremor.* New York, NY: Oxford Unversity Press; 1984:37–84.

Chapter 109

Trigeminal Neuralgia

Wesley Caswell Fowler and Elizabeth Bullitt

Trigeminal neuralgia (TGN) or tic douloureux is a clinical entity consisting of episodes of brief lancinating facial pain in the sensory distribution of the trigeminal nerve. Episodes are often triggered by specific sensory stimuli such as chewing, light touch, or shaving. No other symptoms accompany the pain episodes, and their presence should alert the examiner to entertain other diagnoses such as tumor. Most cases occur in patients in their fifth decade or beyond, with an incidence ranging from 1 to 4 per 100,000 persons per year, females predominating over males.

ETIOLOGY AND PATHOGENESIS

The exact cause of TGN is unclear. In 1934, Walter Dandy published a series of 215 cases of TGN. Although Dandy did not discuss presenting symptoms, he found that in the majority of cases there was vascular compression of the sensory component of the nerve, most commonly by the superior cerebellar artery, or no obvious abnormality. Mass lesions such as tumors and intrinsic white matter disease such as multiple sclerosis may produce facial pain as well. However, the pain is often of a different character than that of TGN and is usually accompanied by other neurologic deficits. Currently, the leading etiologic theory holds that the sensory root entry zone of the trigeminal nerve is particularly susceptible to mechanical compression, most commonly by the superior cerebellar artery. Microscopically, the root entry zone adjacent to the brainstem is an area of transition from central myelin to peripheral myelin. Pathophysiologically, this mechanical disturbance may result in ephaptic transmission and the conduction of painful stimuli.

CLINICAL PRESENTATION

Patients presenting with idiopathic TGN complain of brief, recurrent episodes of lancinating, burning pain in a specific facial dermatome (Figure 109-1). Most commonly, the V2 (maxillary) and V3 (mandibular) dermatomes are involved unilaterally. Fewer than 6% of cases involve V1 (ophthalmic). The pain is often induced by certain triggers and may spontaneously remit. Episodes tend to become more frequent and more severe with time, which may lead to malnutrition and poor hygiene of the affected region. Bilateral symptoms occur in approximately 5% of patients and should alert the examiner to the possibility of multiple sclerosis. The presence of pain awakening the patient at night, numbness, weakness, or other neurologic abnormalities should call the diagnosis into question.

DIFFERENTIAL DIAGNOSIS

Presence of any neurologic deficit should alert the physician to consider diagnoses other than idiopathic TGN. Secondary TGN, accompanied by neurologic deficits, may be caused by a variety of mass lesions including tumors, infection, aneurysms, other vascular malformations, multiple sclerosis, and possibly skull base abnormalities. A minority of patients with underlying mass lesions may present without neurologic deficit, complaining only of lancinating, paroxysmal pain episodes inseparable from those of TGN. In their series of 2,000 patients with facial pain, Bullitt and Tew found that 16 of these patients' symptoms were secondary to tumors. These patients exhibited either subtle or no neurologic findings. The investigators concluded that some tumors, particularly those located in the posterior fossa, could present with pain identical to TGN without neurologic deficit. Other cranial neuralgias including geniculate, glossopharyngeal, occipital, and sphenopalatine neuralgia may mimic some aspects of TGN but can usually be distinguished based on history and physical examination. Specifically, geniculate neuralgia, consisting of pain in the external ear canal and tympanic membrane, often occurs secondary to the herpes virus, and evidence of vesicles is present (Ramsay Hunt syndrome). Primary geniculate neuralgia can be diagnosed by the otologic location of the pain, although the character of the pain may be identical to that of TGN. Similarly, the pain of glossopharyngeal neuralgia mimics TGN; however, the location of the pain in the pharynx, ear, and throat, as well as its trigger mechanisms of swallowing and tactile stimulation of the tonsillar pillars, allow its distinction from TGN. Sphenopalatine (Sluder's) neuralgia is accompanied by sinus congestion, salivation, and lacrimation in addition to an aching maxillary and retroorbital pain. The location of occipital neuralgia in the posterior region of the scalp differentiates the 2 diagnoses. Cluster headaches are characterized by sharp retro-orbital pain, typically occur in men, and follow a remitting, relapsing pattern. Episodes occur at night and are often accompanied by other neurologic findings including Horner's syndrome, lacrimation, and nasal congestion. Postherpetic trigeminal neuralgia frequently follows the V1 dermatome, is continuous and burning, is worse at night, and is accompanied by evidence of vesicles.

Dental disease and temporomandibular joint (TMJ) disease may also simulate TGN. Like postherpetic neuralgia, the character of the pain tends to be steady and aching rather than lancinating. As with TGN, pain can be induced by chewing and occasionally by pressure over the TMJ or diseased tooth, but other signs of TMJ disease or dental disease are present. Atypical facial pain is associated with a normal neurologic examination. Distinguishing characteristics include an aching pain that is long-standing, is poorly localized, is often bilateral, is more severe at night, is without trigger points, and is often associated with depression.

DIAGNOSTIC APPROACH

Strict attention to the clinical history and the physical examination is the key to successful diagnosis of both primary and secondary TGN. Attention to the defining characteristics of the pain is critical. Specifically, the exact location, the precise quality, the duration and timing, as well as triggering and alleviating factors of pain should be

noted. Finally, any neurologic deficit found on physical examination should point to diagnoses other that idiopathic TGN.

MANAGEMENT AND THERAPY

Having completed the history and physical examination, the physician must begin the search for treatment. If the history and physical examination findings indicate diagnoses other than primary TGN, steps must be taken for their further definition. If the diagnosis of primary TGN is entertained, an MRI of the brain with attention to the trigeminal nerve should be undertaken, remembering that a small percentage of patients may harbor tumor. A negative MRI result helps solidify the diagnosis and will be needed in the event of surgical therapy. The goal of treatment is to alleviate the patient's pain with a minimum of side effects.

Treatment begins with medicinal therapy. First-line therapy is carbamazepine, which provides relief in 70% to 75% of patients initially. Dosing should be titrated to effect from 200 mg a day, in increments of 100 to 200 mg, to a maximum of 1,200 mg per day. Side effects occur in 30% of patients and include dizziness, sedation, nystagmus, hepatic and bone marrow toxicity, syndrome of inappropriate antidiuretic hormone secretion, CHF, and rashes. Periodic monitoring of CBC and blood chemistries is required. If carbamazepine fails, gabapentin may be added or substituted. It should begin at 300 mg, then, on the second day, 300 mg twice a day, followed by 300 mg 3 times a day on the third day. The dosage may be titrated to effect to 1.8 to 2.4 g per day. Because of its low side effect profile and effectiveness in relief of pain, gabapentin may be used as a first-line agent. Phenytoin can be used if other therapies fail. If there is no response to anticonvulsants or if breakthrough pain occurs, then baclofen may be added or substituted with a long-term response rate of less than 50%. Dosing should begin at 5 mg 3 times a day, increasing 5 mg per dose every 3 days to a maximum of 80 mg per day.

Failure to respond to medical therapy mandates surgery. Surgical approaches fall into 3 categories: percutaneous ablative procedures, microvascular decompressive procedures, and stereotactic radiosurgical procedures.

Various ablative procedures have been used for

Figure 109-1

Trigeminal Neuralgia

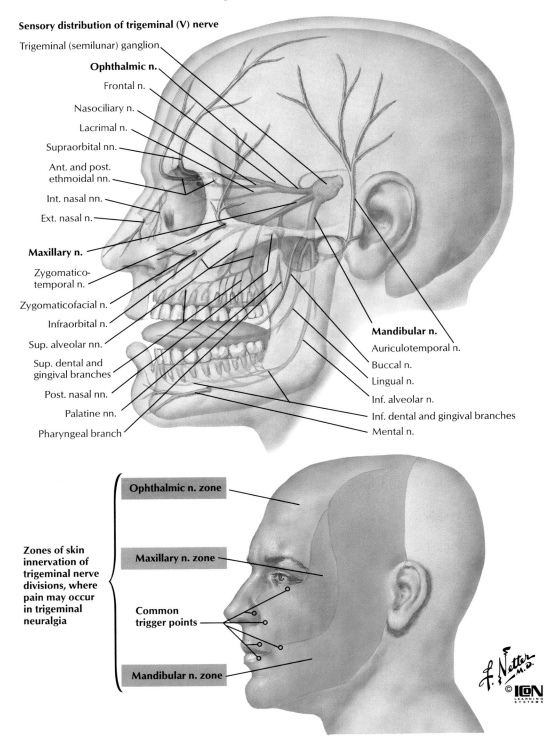

Sensory distribution of trigeminal (V) nerve

Trigeminal (semilunar) ganglion

Ophthalmic n.

Frontal n.

Nasociliary n.

Lacrimal n.

Supraorbital nn.

Ant. and post. ethmoidal nn.

Int. nasal nn.

Ext. nasal n.

Maxillary n.

Zygomatico-temporal n.

Zygomaticofacial n.

Infraorbital n.

Sup. alveolar nn.

Sup. dental and gingival branches

Post. nasal nn.

Palatine nn.

Pharyngeal branch

Mandibular n.

Auriculotemporal n.

Buccal n.

Lingual n.

Inf. alveolar n.

Inf. dental and gingival branches

Mental n.

Ophthalmic n. zone

Maxillary n. zone

Zones of skin innervation of trigeminal nerve divisions, where pain may occur in trigeminal neuralgia

Common trigger points

Mandibular n. zone

the treatment of TGN. All result in some degree of facial numbness. The most common procedures include percutaneous retrogasserian glycerol injection, percutaneous balloon compression of the trigeminal ganglion, and percutaneous radiofrequency trigeminal rhizotomy (PTR). In each procedure, the foramen ovale is cannulated percutaneously via a needle introduced through the cheek ipsilateral to the patient's symptoms Patient selection includes those failing medical management, patients older than 70, patients in poor health, patients feeling they can tolerate facial numbness, and patients with symptoms excluding the V1 distribution. Taha and Tew, in their prospective 15-year follow-up study of 154 patients undergoing PTR for TGN, found that 99% of patients had initial pain relief after 1 procedure. A 25% recurrence rate was estimated at 14 years. Forty-six percent of patients experienced postoperative facial analgesia, 42% dense hypalgesia, and 17% mild hypalgesia. Dysesthesia developed in 36% of patients with postoperative analgesia, in 15% of patients with dense hypalgesia, and in 7% of patients with mild hypalgesia. Pain recurrence occurred in 18% of patients with postoperative analgesia, 21% of patients with dense hypalgesia, and 47% of patients with mild hypalgesia. No mortality occurred. Taha and Tew concluded that PTR is safe and effective and that a lesion producing dense postoperative hypalgesia is optimum.

Microvascular decompression (MVD) of the trigeminal nerve is more invasive than the percutaneous procedures, but offers the advantage of preserving facial sensation. It should be entertained in younger patients, in patients with symptoms in the V1 distribution primarily, and for patients unable to tolerate facial numbness. Barker and Jannetta evaluated their long-term results of MVD in 1,185 patients with TGN. They found that in 75% of cases, the superior cerebellar artery compressed the trigeminal root, while a vein accounted for compression in 12% of cases. Immediate pain relief occurred in 82% of patients. Ten years following surgery, 70% continued to have excellent pain relief. The rate of facial numbness was 1% and, of dysesthesia requiring treatment, 0.3%. As reported by Barker et al., major complications included 2 deaths (0.2%), one brainstem infarction (0.1%), and 16 ipsilateral hearing losses (1%). Factors predictive of long-

term operative success included male gender, a duration of preoperative symptoms less than 8 years, absence of venous compression, and immediate postoperative relief.

Tew compared the different surgical procedures for the treatment of TGN and found that immediate relief of pain for all procedures ranged from 91% for glycerol rhizotomy to 97% to 98% for MVD and PTR. The recurrence rate was highest for glycerol injection (54%) and lowest for MVD (15%), with PTR having a 20% to 23% recurrence rate. Major dysesthesia occurred in 2% to 10% of PTR procedures, 55% of glycerol injections, and 0.3% of MVD procedures. Perioperative mortality occurred in 0.6% of the MVD procedures and 0% of percutaneous procedures.

In summary, the diagnosis of TGN should be made based on the history and physical examination and with the aid of MRI. Medical therapy should then be initiated with carbamazepine or gabapentin. Failure to respond requires additional therapy with other anticonvulsants such as phenytoin or with baclofen. When all medical therapies have been exhausted, surgical therapy can be entertained. The choice of surgical therapy depends on the distribution of the pain, patient characteristics, and patient preference.

FUTURE DIRECTIONS

Recently, stereotactic radiosurgery (SRS) has been used in the treatment of TGN. SRS, least invasive of the surgical approaches, consists of the application of a stereotactic head frame under local anesthetic followed by MRI and focused-beam radiation therapy. Its true effectiveness is not yet known because most cases have involved patients refractory to other medical and surgical therapies, because new techniques including 2 isocenters and higher radiation doses are being used, and because of lack of sufficient time for follow-up. Results of SRS for the treatment of TGN to date are encouraging. SRS may represent a minimally invasive, effective choice of surgical therapy for the treatment of TGN associated with very low complication rates.

REFERENCES

Barker FG II, Jannetta PJ, Bissonette DJ, Larkins MV, Jho HD. The long-term outcome of microvascular decompression for trigeminal neuralgia. *N Engl J Med.* 1996;334: 1077–1083.

Bullitt E, Tew JM, Boyd J. Intracranial tumors in patients with facial pain. *J Neurosurg.* 1986;64:865–871.

Dandy WE. Concerning the cause of trigeminal neuralgia. *Am J Surg.* 1934;24:447–455.

Maesawa S, Salame C, Flickinger JC, Pirris S, Kondziolka D, Lunsford LD. Clinical outcomes after stereotactic radiosurgery for idiopathic trigeminal neuralgia. *J Neurosurg.* 2001;94:14–20.

McQuay H, Carroll D, Jadad AR, Wiffen P, Moore A. Antipconvulsant drugs for management of pain: a systematic review. *BMJ.* 1995;31:1047–1052.

Taha JM, Tew JM Jr, Buncher CR. A prospective 15-year follow up of 154 patients with trigeminal neuralgia treated by percutaneous stereotactic radiofrequency thermal rhizotomy. *J Neurosurg.* 1995;83:989–993.

Tew JM, Taha JM. Treatment of trigeminal and other facial neuralgias by percutaneous techniques. In: Youmans, JR, ed. *Neurological Surgery: A Comprehensive Reference Guide to the Diagnosis and Management of Neurosurgical Problems.* 4th ed. Philadelphia, Pa: WB Saunders Co; 1996: 3376–3403.

Chapter 110

Vertigo

Benjamin J. Copeland and Harold C. Pillsbury III

Vertigo is not a disease, but a symptom describing disturbance of the peripheral vestibular system or its central nervous system connections. Vertigo is the chief complaint in approximately 10% of all patients in a primary care setting and 20% of patients seen by otolaryngology and neurology practices. True vertigo is the illusion or perception of motion. In typical practice, terms as varied as 'lightheadedness,' 'off-balance,' and 'dizziness' are often lumped together under the umbrella of vertigo.

ETIOLOGY AND PATHOGENESIS

Acute vestibulopathy is the sudden failure of the balance system. A viral etiology is suspected. Termed labyrinthitis when associated with hearing loss, and vestibular neuritis when hearing is preserved, the CNS receives conflicting or absent signals from the impaired side, resulting in central incompatibility of signals and subsequent vertigo. (Figures 110-1, 110-2, and 110–3)

Endolymphatic hydrops (Meniere's disease) is believed to be caused by excessive accumulation of endolymph in the endolymphatic sac secondary to impaired resorption. The exact pathophysiologic mechanism remains unknown.

Episodic vertigo associated with *perilymph fistula* may be caused by a leak of perilymph from the otic capsule from a damaged oval or round window. The episodic nature of the vertigo and associated sensorineural hearing loss reflects the intermittent leak from the defect and the subsequent exposure of the inner ear to ambient pressure changes. Superior semicircular canal dehiscence is also consistent with the findings of a perilymph fistula. Trauma to the ear (direct, surgical, or barometric) is the most common etiology for perilymph fistula.

Benign paroxysmal positional vertigo results from canalolithiasis, an accumulation of otoconial debris displaced into the (typically posterior) semicircular canal system, resulting in limited-duration gravity-dependent stimulation with changes in head position.

Vestibular schwannomas (acoustic neuromas) are benign tumors arising from the vestibular nerve which eventually encroach other structures in the internal auditory canal and cerebellopon-

Table 110-1
Common Causes of Vertigo

Peripheral

Acute vestibulopathy (vestibular neuritis or labyrinthitis)

Endolymphatic hydrops (Meniere's disease) Perilymph fistula

Benign paroxysmal positional vertigo

Vestibular schwannoma (acoustic neuroma)

Chronic middle ear disease (cholesteatoma)

Central

Multiple sclerosis

Migraine

Vascular disease

Brainstem neoplasms

tine angle. Increasing tumor size and resulting local compression cause increased vestibular deficit, tinnitus, and sensorineural hearing loss.

Chronic middle ear disease, either infection or cholesteatoma, causes vertigo by local destruction and erosion into the otic capsule, creating a fistula into the perilymph-filled system. The pathophysiology is similar to that of perilymph fistula. Serous labyrinthitis associated with the chronic suppurative process may exacerbate vertigo.

Vertigo is often associated with flares of *multiple sclerosis.* The etiology may be plaque formation in the pontine region of the brainstem or proximal eighth nerve. Central vertigo may result from interruption of the medial longitudinal fasciculus and resulting disconjugate eye movements (internuclear ophthalmoplegia).

Figure 110-1

Vestibulocochlear (VIII) Nerve

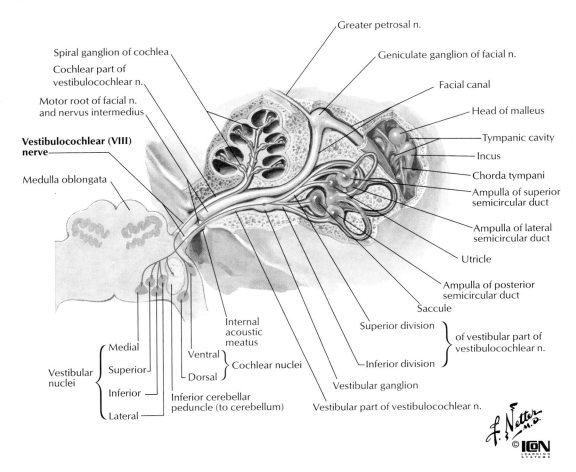

Migraine may produce vertigo through poorly understood mechanisms. Vertigo may precede the headache (aura equivalent) or replace it (migraine equivalent). Recent genetic discoveries have implicated ion channel mutations as a potential link with the vestibular system; however, definitive pathophysiology remains elusive.

Vascular disease in the vertebrobasilar system may induce vertigo by compromising posterior circulation via occlusive or embolic processes. The anterior inferior cerebellar artery, posterior inferior cerebellar artery, and superior cerebellar artery are most commonly affected. Severe arthritic changes to the cervical spine are thought to be related to vascular insufficiency in the vertebrobasilar system. There is evidence that aberrant vessel anatomy compresses the eighth nerve com-

plex, resulting in vertigo and pulsatile tinnitus.

Brainstem neoplasms involving the cerebellopontine angle (meningiomas, epidermoids, lipomas, gliomas, astrocytomas) may cause vertigo. The etiology of the vertigo is usually compression of adjacent structures, either via direct extension of the neoplasm upon the eighth nerve complex/brainstem or resulting hydrocephalus.

CLINICAL PRESENTATION

A careful and thorough patient history is critical to reaching a reasonable differential diagnosis in the vertiginous patient. The clinical features of common causes of vertigo are summarized in Table 110-2.

Acute vestibulopathy typically presents as an attack of prolonged incapacitating vertigo with nausea and vomiting that can persist for greater

Figure 110-2

Bony and Membranous Labyrinths

Bony and membranous labyrinths: schema

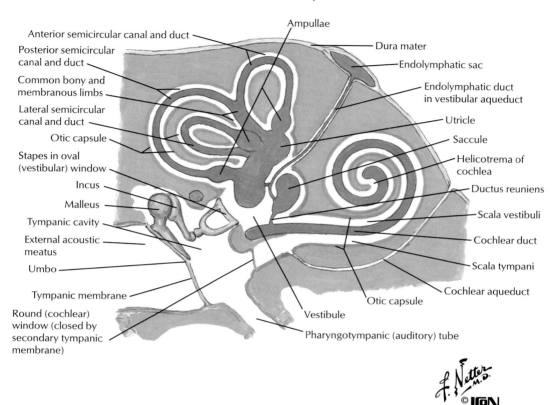

Anterior semicircular canal and duct

Posterior semicircular canal and duct

Common bony and membranous limbs

Lateral semicircular canal and duct

Otic capsule

Stapes in oval (vestibular) window

Incus

Malleus

Tympanic cavity

External acoustic meatus

Umbo

Tympanic membrane

Round (cochlear) window (closed by secondary tympanic membrane)

Ampullae

Dura mater

Endolymphatic sac

Endolymphatic duct in vestibular aqueduct

Utricle

Saccule

Helicotrema of cochlea

Ductus reuniens

Scala vestibuli

Cochlear duct

Scala tympani

Cochlear aqueduct

Otic capsule

Vestibule

Pharyngotympanic (auditory) tube

than 24 hours, gradually subsiding over the following days to weeks. Patients often describe a history of antecedent upper respiratory infection, and hearing is variably affected. Approximately 20% of patients will experience recurrent episodes that are often less severe than the initial presentation.

Endolymphatic hydrops episodes are characterized by fluctuating sensorineural hearing loss, vertigo, and tinnitus and usually last several hours. A sensation of aural fullness is often present during or before an attack. Episodes occur at irregular intervals for many years and may become bilateral as the disease progresses. Late Meniere's disease is characterized by permanent severe sensorineural hearing loss and less severe vertiginous attacks.

Perilymph fistulas present as episodic vertigo with episodic sensorineural hearing loss of vari-

able degree. Vertigo is least noticeable early in the morning or after lying down, then progresses with upright posture and activities through the day. Symptoms are exacerbated by Valsalva maneuvers (nose blowing, heavy lifting, straining, vomiting) and can often be reproduced with pneumatic otoscopy. An inciting traumatic event can often be elicited with a careful history (e.g., diving, head injury, direct ear trauma, childbirth, extreme straining, or lifting).

Benign paroxysmal positional vertigo presents as short vertiginous episodes associated with changes in head position. Predictable changes in head position routinely precipitate the symptom (e.g., rolling over in bed, looking up to the top shelf) and latency in the onset of vertigo of up to 1 minute is common. No hearing loss is reported,

Figure 110-3   **Causes of Vertigo**

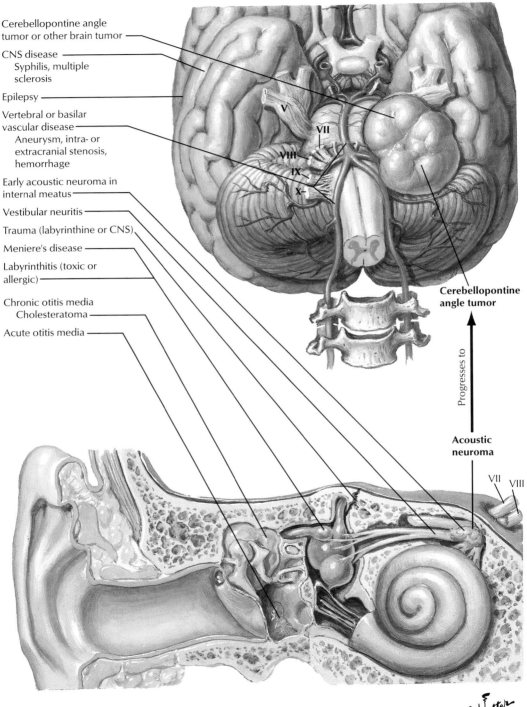

Cerebellopontine angle tumor or other brain tumor

CNS disease
    Syphilis, multiple sclerosis

Epilepsy

Vertebral or basilar vascular disease
    Aneurysm, intra- or extracranial stenosis, hemorrhage

Early acoustic neuroma in internal meatus

Vestibular neuritis

Trauma (labyrinthine or CNS)

Meniere's disease

Labyrinthitis (toxic or allergic)

Chronic otitis media
    Cholesteratoma

Acute otitis media

V

VII

VIII

IX

X

Cerebellopontine angle tumor

Progresses to

Acoustic neuroma

VII   VIII

Table 110-2
Clinical Features of Common Causes of Vertigo

Clinical Features	Vestibular Neuritis	Labyrinthitis	Meniere's Disease	Perilymph Fistula	BPPV	Vestibular Schwannoma	Chronic Otitis Media
Vertigo intensity duration	Days	Days	Hours	Variable, worsens through day	Seconds	Imbalance	Variable
Nausea vomiting	Yes	Yes	Yes	No	Yes	No	No
Hearing loss	No	SNHL	SNHL, fluctuates	Mild SNHL	No	SNHL, unilateral, progressive	CHL
Symptom-free interval	No	No	Yes	Lessens with rest	Yes	No	No
Tinnitus present	No	No	Yes	Variable	No	Yes	Variable
Associated findings			Aural fullness	Barotrauma, ear surgery	Positional		Otorrhea
Study of choice	ENG	ENG	ECOG	Pneumatic otoscopy	Dix-Hallpike	MRI/CT	CT

BPPV, benign paroxysmal positional vertigo; CHL, chronic hearing loss; CT, computed tomography; ECOG, electrocochleography; ENG, electronystagmogram; MRI, magnetic resonance imaging; SNHL, sensorineural hearing loss.

and fatigable torsional nystagmus with latency onset may be reproduced by Dix-Hallpike positioning maneuvers.

Vestibular schwannoma most often presents as progressive unilateral sensorineural hearing loss with symptoms of imbalance and tinnitus. The vestibular system often is able to compensate over time for the tumor growth, so vertigo is often absent. The hearing loss may be sudden in up to 20% of patients. With large tumors, ipsilateral facial nerve function may be compromised.

Chronic middle ear disease classically presents as a persistently draining and painful ear, often with visible tympanic membrane perforation. The otorrhea is often malodorous in the chronic state. Often, the tympanic membrane is heavily scarred with visible perforation. Pearly white cholesteatoma matrix may be seen deep to the tympanic membrane remnant. As with perilymph fistula, pneumatic otoscopy may reproduce associated vertigo.

Multiple sclerosis (MS) is characterized by neurologic deficits separated by space and time. Vertigo and hearing fluctuate as plaques are formed. Nearly half of patients with MS present with vertigo at some point, and examination often reveals internuclear ophthalmoplegia. An MS flare involving vertigo typically persists for days to weeks before adequate central compensation is achieved.

Vertigo associated with *migraine* is difficult to categorize. It may replace the aura of the migraine headache, the headache itself, or happen in the interval between headaches. The duration of migraine-associated vertigo is highly variable.

Occlusive or embolic vascular disease affecting the posterior circulation results in severe postural instability, direction-shifting nystagmus without suppression by visual fixation, and multiple neurologic findings, particularly if the brainstem is involved. Vascular insufficiency is typically associated with a lightheaded or pre-syncopal sensation exacerbated by neck extension with no related hearing loss. By contrast, vascular compression or impingement of the eighth nerve complex presents typically as pulsatile tinnitus with hypacusis, often exacerbated by head position. Vertigo in this case is typically a result of progressive functional loss and less severe due to central compensation.

Brainstem neoplasms presenting with vertigo are large and produce symptoms of cerebellar compression and hydrocephalus. There is often hearing loss, and patients may complain of otalgia, diplopia, and headaches.

DIFFERENTIAL DIAGNOSIS

Vertigo can have a myriad of presentations. A careful history and physical examination are essential to narrow the diagnostic possibilities.

The effect of medications deserves special consideration. Aminoglycoside antibiotics, in particular, are highly ototoxic. Susceptibility to aminoglycoside ototoxicity is variable and develops despite normal peak and trough levels of the drug. Individual susceptibility appears to be an inherited mitochondrial DNA mutation.

Less common causes of vertigo include labyrinthine concussion (head trauma), autoimmune inner ear disease (systemic lupus erythematosus), congenital malformations of the membranous labyrinth (TORCH viruses), inflammatory lesions (petrous apex cholesterol granuloma), infections (syphilis), metabolic disorders (otosclerosis, Wernicke's encephalopathy, hypoglycemia), neurologic conditions (epilepsy and palatal myoclonus), and structural abnormalities (Arnold-Chiari malformation and normal pressure hydrocephalus).

Consider "light-headedness" and pre-syncopal dizziness in any patient with the complaint of vertigo. Hyperventilation, decreased cardiac output states, orthostatic hypotension, and vasovagal episodes may all be interpreted as true vertigo by patients and need to be distinguished early by careful history, physical examination, and adjunctive testing.

DIAGNOSTIC APPROACH

A thorough patient history is essential. The description of the balance disturbance should include duration and chronicity of symptoms, exacerbating and relieving factors, description of the initial episode, related or concurrent symptoms (such as changes in vision, muscle tone,

hearing, somatic sensation), and what was experienced during the episode.

Physical examination includes complete otoscopic evaluation with pneumatic otoscopy, cranial nerve testing, ophthalmoscopic examination, assessment of eye movement and presence of nystagmus, cerebellar examination, Romberg and gait testing, and auscultation of the neck and heart. Additional examinations may include orthostatic vital signs, muscle strength, proprioception, visual acuity, and positional testing with Dix-Hallpike maneuvers. (Figure 110-4)

Adjunctive testing is often helpful in distinguishing causes of vertigo. A pure tone audiogram can assess related hearing loss. An auditory brainstem response helps define retrocochlear pathology. Caloric testing and an electronystagmogram (ENG) frequently identify unilateral vestibular weakness and help distinguish nystagmus of peripheral and central origin. Electrocochleography (ECOG) aids in the diagnosis of Meniere's disease. Dynamic posturography is used to localize balance disorders when multiple systems are involved. Laboratory evaluation usually has a limited role and may include complete blood cell count, erythrocyte sedimentation rate, antinuclear antibody titers, rapid plasma reagin or VDRL screening, and evaluation of thyroid function. Cerebrospinal fluid analysis may aid in the diagnosis of multiple sclerosis.

Radiographic imaging may be helpful. For middle ear disease and temporal bone pathology or trauma, CT is beneficial in highlighting bony anatomy. For soft tissue examination (e.g., cerebellopontine angle masses, vestibular schwannoma, multiple sclerosis plaques), MRI is the study of choice. For suspected vascular disease, transcranial Doppler, MRA, or selected arterial angiography may be diagnostic.

MANAGEMENT AND THERAPY

Treatment is aimed at controlling acute symptoms and maximizing remaining vestibular function. Acute episodes often require labyrinthine sedatives (e.g., diazepam or meclizine) alone or in combination with antiemetics (e.g., promethane, prochlorperazine). Chronic use of these compounds should be avoided as central compensation may be slowed or inhibited. Vestibular rehabilitation exercises should be initiated as soon as

Figure 110-4

Test for Positional Vertigo

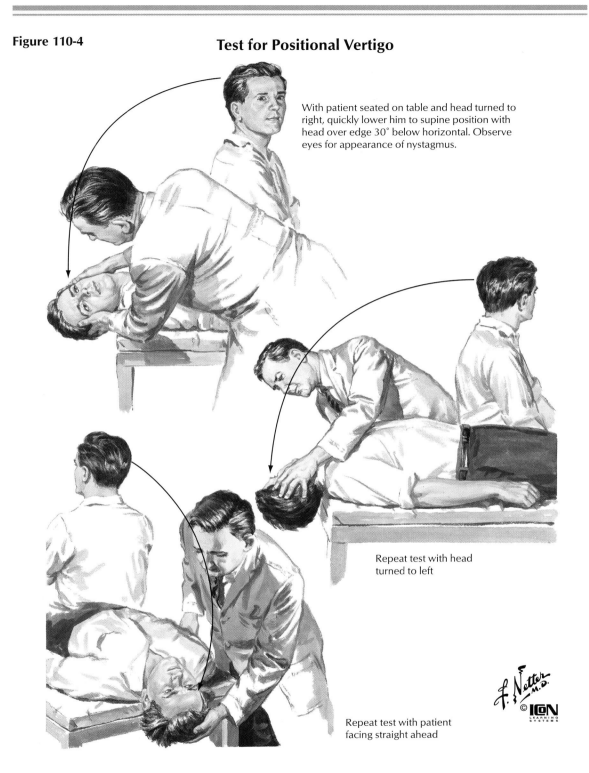

With patient seated on table and head turned to right, quickly lower him to supine position with head over edge 30° below horizontal. Observe eyes for appearance of nystagmus.

Repeat test with head turned to left

Repeat test with patient facing straight ahead

possible after acute symptoms subside to facilitate central compensation. Once a definitive diagnosis is made, specific therapies should be pursued.

Acute vestibulopathy is treated acutely with labyrinthine sedatives and antiemetics. Medications should be withdrawn as soon as possible to allow effective central adaptation. Vestibular rehabilitation exercises and early mobilization improve final outcomes.

Endolymphatic hydrops is treated with a salt-restricted (1 to 2 mg/day) diet and diuretic therapy with labyrinthine sedatives for acute exacerbations. In early disease with serviceable hearing, transmastoid endolymphatic sac decompression is efficacious. Vestibular nerve section may improve control of vertigo while preserving hearing. In late disease with poor hearing, transtympanic gentamicin instillation or labyrinthectomy improves control of vertigo.

Suspected *perilymph fistula* may be initially managed with strict bedrest and lack of exertion or straining. If symptoms persist or if hearing loss ensues, middle ear exploration with identification of the fistula and subsequent tissue grafting over the oval or round window is indicated.

Benign paroxysmal positional vertigo is successfully treated with a series of positional maneuvers to relocate the otoconial debris from the semicircular canal (Epley or Semont maneuvers). Patients remain upright while sleeping for several days to avoid reaccumulation of displaced particles. If repeated positioning maneuvers fail, posterior canal occlusion or singular neurectomy may control symptoms.

Vestibular schwannoma is treated with surgical resection. Stereotactic radiation therapy is an alternative treatment if surgery is not desired or the patient is at risk for a general anesthetic.

Chronic middle ear disease treatment typically involves surgery to remove erosive cholesteatoma or infected tissue, repairing hearing loss, and preventing further intratemporal or intracranial complications.

MS often responds to high-dose pulse corticosteroids with shortened duration of symptoms. Additionally, gabapentin may reduce resultant nystagmus and vertigo.

Migraine therapy involves behavioral as well as pharmacologic interventions. Serotonin receptor antagonists have proven effective as aborting agents, and prophylaxis has been demonstrated for beta-blockers, tricyclic antidepressants, valproic acid, and calcium-channel blockers.

Vascular disease requires addressing risk factors as well as instituting antiplatelet therapy. For significant stenosis, consider anticoagulation with warfarin.

Brainstem neoplasms usually require resection and adjunctive therapy as dictated by histopathology.

FUTURE DIRECTIONS

An understanding of the vestibular system and its pathophysiology is essential for the treatment of vertigo. The diagnosis still heavily depends on the history of symptoms, but several areas show promise for future research. Reliable objective testing for perilymph fistula could streamline its diagnosis and treatment. Improved imaging modalities could pinpoint vascular lesions without the present risks of invasive angiography. Research into the underlying pathophysiology of Meniere's disease continues and may one day explain its constellation of findings. Even as more discoveries are made, patients with vertigo will continue to challenge the clinician's knowledge and skills.

REFERENCES

Fetter M. Assessing vestibular function: which tests, when? *J Neurol.* 2000;247:335–342.

Luxon LM. The medical management of vertigo. *J Laryngol Otol.* 1997;111:1114–1121.

Strupp M, Arbusow V. Acute vestibulopathy. *Curr Opin Neurol.* 2001;14:11–20.

Weber PC, Adkins WY Jr. The differential diagnosis of Meniere's disease. *Otolaryngol Clin North Am.* 1997; 30:977–986.

Section XIII

DISORDERS OF THE KIDNEY AND URINARY TRACT

Chapter 111

Acute Renal Failure

Michelle C. Whittier and William F. Finn

Acute renal failure (ARF) occurs when the function of the kidneys declines by a variable degree over a period of hours to days. As a result, there are progressive increases in plasma concentrations of urea and creatinine, disruption of fluid and electrolyte balance, acid-base derangement, and impairment of metabolic functions of the kidney such as erythropoietin production and vitamin D metabolism. Often, ARF is accompanied by oliguria, with a reduction in urine volume to less than 600 mL per day.

The actual incidence of ARF is difficult to determine because of its many diverse etiologies, the complexity of the conditions that existed before its development, and ambiguity in the definition of ARF itself. In most instances, ARF occurs in the hospital and may affect 5% of all inpatients, with a higher percentage of those in intensive care units affected. ARF also may be community-acquired and represents a great diagnostic challenge.

In contrast to those with chronic renal failure (CRF) where compensatory and adaptive changes in glomerular and tubular function obscure the severity of the condition, individuals with ARF exhibit a high level of morbidity and mortality. The mortality rate for those requiring renal replacement therapy with dialysis may exceed 50%. There are few parameters by which to predict the severity or the prognosis of ARF; however, a prompt diagnosis and an aggressive treatment strategy are mandatory to preserve renal function and to avoid serious complications.

ETIOLOGY AND PATHOGENESIS

ARF is often classified as prerenal, postrenal, and intrinsic, which is further categorized on the basis of the proximate cause of the renal injury. Each of these conditions has different mechanisms of injury.

Prerenal Acute Renal Failure

Prerenal ARF is marked by an elevation in the blood urea nitrogen (BUN) out of proportion to the rise in the serum creatinine (S_{Cr}). As a result, the BUN:S_{Cr} ratio exceeds the usual 10:1 to 15:1. The increase in BUN may be a result of accelerat-ed urea generation in response to increased protein intake, absorption of blood from the gastrointestinal tract, increased tubular reabsorption, or the reduction in the GFR due to a disturbance in systemic or renal hemodynamics. Absolute volume depletion such as in severe dehydration, blood loss, and septic shock are frequent causes of prerenal ARF. In other circumstances, such as decompensated liver disease or congestive heart failure, there is a functional rather than an absolute decrease in the effective blood volume leading to acute changes in renal function.

In advanced liver disease, the fall in GFR is often masked because poor nutrition and the decline in the hepatic production of urea limit the rise in BUN. A loss of muscle mass may restrict the rise in S_{Cr}. In some circumstances, the renal function deteriorates to the point that renal replacement therapy with dialysis is necessary. This often signifies the development of the hepatorenal syndrome (HRS) (Figure 111-1). Distinguishing the HRS from other causes of prerenal ARF, such as gastrointestinal bleeding, diuretic overuse and other causes of fluid loss, is imperative because of the substantial difference in prognosis. These individuals are at high risk for the development of intrinsic ARF. In HRS, the use of a transvenous internal portosystemic shunt (TIPS) may result in an improvement in renal function. Overall prognosis is poor unless the liver failure resolves or liver transplantation occurs.

Prerenal ARF may also be present in individuals with congestive heart failure as a result of an increase in renal vascular resistance (RVR) and a decrease in renal blood flow (RBF). At times, renal perfusion is so severely compromised that an ischemic component of ARF develops. Edema formation is a common component of this condition.

Prerenal ARF may also occur with certain medications, especially diuretics, angiotensin-converting enzyme inhibitors, and NSAIDs.

Postrenal Acute Renal Failure

Typically, urinary tract obstruction is an infrequent cause of ARF, although the incidence is higher in selected populations. Postrenal ARF may result from obstruction at any point along the urinary tract system (Figure 111-2).

Excluding individuals with solitary kidneys and those with significantly impaired renal function due to underlying renal parenchymal disease, ureteral obstruction must be bilateral to produce clinically apparent abnormalities. If the obstruction is partial, urine flow may remain normal as a result of elevated pressures proximal to the site of the obstruction. Ureteral obstruction may be from a calculus, mass lesion, or sloughed papilla in papillary necrosis. The latter may occur in individuals with sickle cell disease or diabetes mellitus, and in those with excessive analgesic use. Urethral obstruction occurs more commonly in men with prostatic hypertrophy.

Intrinsic Acute Renal Failure

The pathogenesis of ARF associated with ischemic and nephrotoxic injury is complex, and a spectrum of abnormalities accounts for the fall of the glomerular filtration rate (GFR) (Figure 111-3). In most circumstances, an increase in RVR results in both a decrease in RBF and in the hydrostatic pressure within glomerular capillaries. If severe, primary glomerular filtration failure occurs. Independent of RBF and glomerular hydrostatic pressure, the permeability of the glomerular capillary membranes may be altered, contributing to glomerular filtration failure. In both ischemic and nephrotoxic ARF, renal tubular epithelial cells are injured, and some may undergo necrosis or apoptosis. With severe tubular injury, debris accumulates within tubules causing obstruction of fluid flow; tubules then dilate and compress nearby peritubular capillaries causing greater ischemic damage. Necrosis may even permit passage of the filtrate into the renal interstitium causing a disruption in the solute concentrating function of the kidney.

CLINICAL PRESENTATION

The clinical course of ARF is highly variable, ranging from a transient, self-limited disturbance of kidney function to prolonged and often life-threatening renal failure. The classical pattern involves three phases: initial, maintenance, and recovery. The *initial phase* begins with a specific renal insult and continues until functional abnormalities of the kidney develop. These abnormalities may include azotemia, metabolic acidosis, hyperkalemia, and fluid overload. Time from injury to renal impairment during the initial stage depends on the severity of the injury. Oliguria or anuria (oliguric ARF) may accompany the *maintenance phase*. In some instances, however, the urine volume remains normal (non-oliguric ARF), although the quality of the urine is poor, the GFR is severely reduced, and the BUN and S_{Cr} rise. Characteristically, the maintenance phase lasts for 10 to 14 days depending on the nature of the injury to the kidney, although longer courses have been described. The final phase of ARF is the *recovery phase*. In oliguria, there may be a dramatic increase in urine volume at a relatively constant rate, ranging anywhere from hours to days. The degree of the diuresis is dependent on the volume status of the individual and inversely related to the duration of the maintenance phase. In non-oliguric individuals, improvement in the quality of the urine heralds recovery. Late in recovery, glomerular and tubular function is restored, and the renal function returns to or toward the pre-existing level. The likelihood of complete renal recovery is influenced by many factors. Poor prognostic indicators include the presence of pre-existing renal disease, advanced age during the onset of renal injury, and persistent oliguria. As many as 10% to 15% of individuals will not recover adequate renal function, and CRF develops in up to one third of patients.

DIFFERENTIAL DIAGNOSIS

Among the conditions that may precipitously disrupt renal function resulting in ARF, ischemic injury and exposure to nephrotoxic agents account for a significant proportion. Injury resulting in ARF may involve any or all of the 4 histologic components of the kidney, the glomeruli, the tubules, the interstitium, and the

Figure 111-1

Renal Failure in Liver Disease

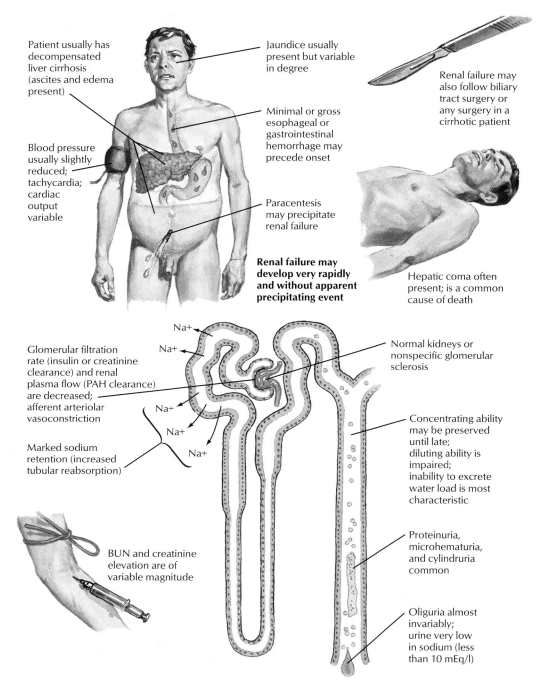

Patient usually has decompensated liver cirrhosis (ascites and edema present)

Jaundice usually present but variable in degree

Renal failure may also follow biliary tract surgery or any surgery in a cirrhotic patient

Minimal or gross esophageal or gastrointestinal hemorrhage may precede onset

Blood pressure usually slightly reduced; tachycardia; cardiac output variable

Paracentesis may precipitate renal failure

Renal failure may develop very rapidly and without apparent precipitating event

Hepatic coma often present; is a common cause of death

Glomerular filtration rate (insulin or creatinine clearance) and renal plasma flow (PAH clearance) are decreased; afferent arteriolar vasoconstriction

Na+
Na+

Na+
Na+
Na+

Normal kidneys or nonspecific glomerular sclerosis

Marked sodium retention (increased tubular reabsorption)

Concentrating ability may be preserved until late; diluting ability is impaired; inability to excrete water load is most characteristic

BUN and creatinine elevation are of variable magnitude

Proteinuria, microhematuria, and cylindruria common

Oliguria almost invariably; urine very low in sodium (less than 10 mEq/l)

Figure 111-2

Obstructive Uropathy: Etiology

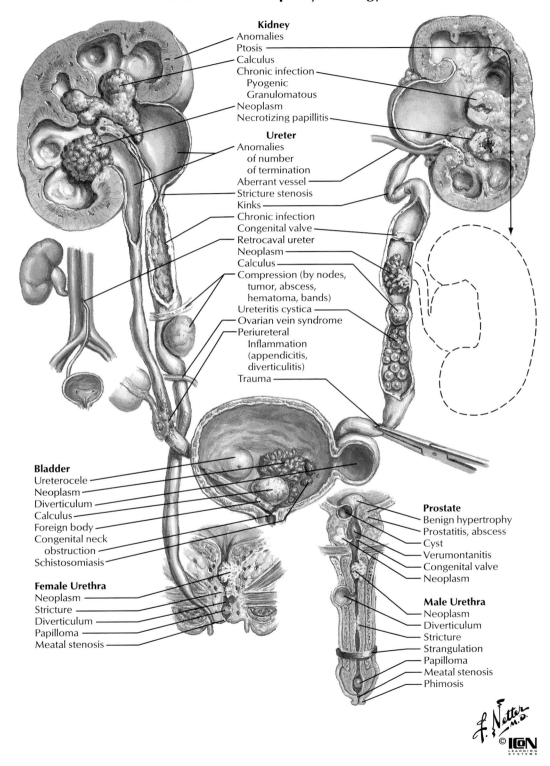

Kidney
Anomalies
Ptosis
Calculus
Chronic infection
  Pyogenic
  Granulomatous
Neoplasm
Necrotizing papillitis

Ureter
Anomalies
  of number
  of termination
Aberrant vessel
Stricture stenosis
Kinks
Chronic infection
Congenital valve
Retrocaval ureter
Neoplasm
Calculus
Compression (by nodes,
  tumor, abscess,
  hematoma, bands)
Ureteritis cystica
Ovarian vein syndrome
Periureteral
  Inflammation
  (appendicitis,
  diverticulitis)
Trauma

Bladder
Ureterocele
Neoplasm
Diverticulum
Calculus
Foreign body
Congenital neck
  obstruction
Schistosomiasis

Female Urethra
Neoplasm
Stricture
Diverticulum
Papilloma
Meatal stenosis

Prostate
Benign hypertrophy
Prostatitis, abscess
Cyst
Verumontanitis
Congenital valve
Neoplasm

Male Urethra
Neoplasm
Diverticulum
Stricture
Strangulation
Papilloma
Meatal stenosis
Phimosis

Figure 111-3

Hemolytic-Uremic Syndrome

Intravascular coagulation, hemolytic-uremic syndrome, and thrombotic microangiopathy

Common electron microscopic findings: Deposits (D) and mesangial cell cytoplasmic processes (M) in the subendothelial space; endothelium (E) swollen; both mesangial (MC) and endothelial cells (EN) contain many vacuoles and dilated rough endoplasmic reticulum; lumen (L) narrowed (may be "slitlike"); red blood cells (RC) may or may not be present; basement membrane (B) often wrinkled; epithelial foot processes (F) partly fused.

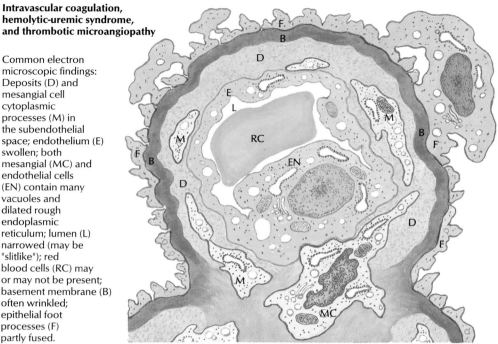

vasculature (Table 111-1).

Sustained episodes of prerenal ARF due to protracted decreases in arterial blood pressure (ABP) and RBF may evolve into post-ischemic ARF where tubular injury predominates. With profound ischemia, glomerular damage and cortical necrosis may develop. Cortical necrosis may also result from intraglomerular microthrombi as occurs with the hemolytic-uremic syndrome or other types of thrombotic microangiopathies. (Figure 111-3)

Other instances of post-ischemic ARF happen in severe crushing injuries from trauma, resulting in rhabdomyolysis and myoglobinuria. This is a significant cause of ARF following earthquakes and military conflicts. ARF may also occur with hemolysis and hemoglobinuria.

A number of substances (xenobiotics) have been identified as capable of producing significant renal injury. The most common agents caus-

ing nephrotoxic ARF are medications, including antibiotics, especially the aminoglycosides, antifungal and chemotherapeutic agents; diagnostic agents such as iodinated radiocontrast dye; and environmental substances including organic solvents and heavy metals.

Analgesics, certain antibiotics, and several diuretics may be associated with a diffuse acute interstitial nephritis (AIN) that differs from post-ischemic and nephrotoxic ARF because of evidence of an allergic reaction.

Less frequently intrinsic ARF occurs with multiple myeloma where light chains and uric acid may deposit in the renal tubules, resulting in "cast nephropathy."

DIAGNOSTIC APPROACH

The diagnosis of ARF requires a careful and systematic approach to identify and manage potentially reversible conditions. After a history and

Table 111-1
Causes of Acute Renal Failure

Diseases of the Renal Vasculature
Renal artery occlusion
  Thromboemboli
  Atheroemboli
  Thrombosis
  Dissecting aortic aneurysm
  Renal artery stenosis
  Vasculitis
Renal vein thrombosis
  Dehydration (infants)
  Hypercoagulable state
  Neoplasms

Diseases of the Renal Cortex
Bilateral cortical necrosis
  Obstetrical accidents
  Abruptio placentas
  Placentas previa
Gram-negative septicemia
Ischemia
Hyperacute renal allograft rejection
Gastroenteritis (children)

Acute Tubulointerstitial Diseases
Acute pyelonephritis
Acute allergic interstitial nephritis
Hypokalemic nephropathy
Hypercalcemia
Acute uric acid nephropathy
Multiple myeloma

Acute Glomerular Diseases
Acute glomerulonephritis
  Postinfectious glomerulonephritis
  Bacterial endocarditis
  Henoch-Schönlein Purpura
  Hypersensitivity angiitis
Rapidly progressive glomerulonephritis
  Systemic lupus erythematosus
  Wegener's granulomatosis
  Goodpasture's syndrome

Thrombotic Microangiopathy
Hemolytic-uremic syndrome
Thrombotic thrombocytopenic purpura
  Scleroderma
Malignant hypertension

Diseases of the Renal Medulla
Bilateral papillary necrosis
Analgesic abuse
  Sickle cell disease
Diabetes mellitus

Urinary Obstruction
Intrarenal abnormalities
Ureteral obstruction
Diseases of bladder or urethra

Post-ischemic Acute Renal Failure

Nephrotoxic Acute Renal Failure

physical examination, urine and plasma measurements are useful for further investigation of the etiology. The urine examination includes a microscopic examination of the urinary sediment and electrolyte measurements. The urine sediment is typically normal in prerenal and postrenal ARF except for the presence of hyaline casts. In intrinsic ARF, the urine sediment may be quite active with muddy brown granular casts, free renal tubular epithelial cells (RTE) and casts, white blood cells (WBCs), and red blood cells (RBCs).

The urinary sodium concentration and osmolality help to differentiate prerenal failure from ARF due to intrinsic renal disease. In prerenal ARF, the fractional excretion of sodium (FE_{Na}) is low and the urinary osmolality and specific gravity are high. In post-ischemic and nephrotoxic ARF, the urinary sodium is high and the urinary osmolality

and specific gravity are closer to that of plasma. Intrinsic ARF is associated with a high FE_{Na}, usually greater than 1% and often more than 3%, thus helping to distinguish it from the prerenal causes of ARF. Plasma measurements of electrolytes, BUN, and S_{Cr} indicate the severity of the ARF.

Renal ultrasonography is highly recommended in the evaluation of ARF because of the importance of diagnosing postrenal ARF quickly. Less commonly, plain radiographs of the abdomen are performed to evaluate for urinary calculi. Renal biopsy is indicated if the diagnosis of the ARF is in question, if a systemic illness is suspected, and to help guide therapy.

MANAGEMENT AND THERAPY
The management and therapy of ARF are largely supportive. All potential reversible causes

should be identified and corrected. In prerenal ARF, volume repletion to correct circulatory abnormalities will restore renal function. In all patients, the cessation of nephrotoxic agents is recommended. For mild cases of ARF that fail to resolve quickly, conservative medical management may be all that is required. This includes careful monitoring of fluid and electrolyte intake, in addition to potassium-binding resins and sodium bicarbonate for non–life-threatening hyperkalemia and metabolic acidosis, respectively. For persistent oliguria, a trial of diuretics after volume repletion has been suggested, although the benefit is controversial. Treatment with so-called renal dose dopamine has not been shown to be useful and carries with it some risk. For more relentless episodes, renal replacement therapy with dialysis is often essential until the renal function is restored. Hemodialysis using "biocompatible" filters has been suggested to avoid secondary injury. In addition, daily hemodialysis may shorten the course of ARF and increase the survival rate.

FUTURE DIRECTIONS

The continued high mortality rate in individuals with ARF and the failure of many who survive to recover normal renal function has placed considerable importance on understanding the mechanisms by which the kidney responds to injury.

Despite attempts to identify one or more biomarkers to judge the events occurring within the kidney, none have demonstrated widespread clinical usefulness. Additional insight into the details of the cell cycle and the application of the tools of molecular biology may eventually lead to the development of pharmacologic agents that protect the kidney from injury or promote its full recovery. A better understanding of the causes and effects of ARF may require further investigation by way of anatomical studies with the application of new technologic methods.

REFERENCES

Bellomo R, Chapman M, Finfer S, Hickling K, Myburgh J. Low-dose dopamine in patients with early renal dysfunction: a placebo-controlled randomised trial. Australian and New Zealand Intensive Care Society (ANZICS) Clinical Trials Group. *Lancet.* 2000;356:2139-2143.

Guevara M, Gines P, Bandi JC, et al. Transjugular intrahepatic portosystemic shunt in hepatorenal syndrome: effects on renal function and vasoactive systems. *Hepatology.* 1998;28:416-422.

Molitoris BA, Finn WF, eds. *Acute Renal Failure: A Companion to Brenner & Rector's The Kidney.* Philadelphia, Pa: WB Saunders Co; 2001.

Schiffl H, Lang SM, Fischer R. Daily hemodialysis and the outcome of acute renal failure. *N Engl J Med.* 2002;346:305-310.

Thadhani R, Pascual M, Bonventre JV. Acute renal failure. *N Engl J Med.* 1996;334:1448-1460.

Chapter 112

Bladder Function Disorders

Kathryn A. Copeland and Ellen C. Wells

Bladder symptoms are a common presenting complaint in the primary care setting. Many of these symptoms are the result of infectious or inflammatory processes of the lower urinary tract. Others represent abnormalities in bladder storage and emptying. Urinary incontinence is a common and distressing symptom within this group, affecting between 25% and 38% of the female population. Many women do not seek treatment due to embarrassment and lack of knowledge of treatment options.

Adequate bladder storage and emptying depends on the anatomical relationships of the lower genitourinary system and the neurologic control of micturition. It is also influenced by other systemic medical conditions and medications.

ETIOLOGY AND PATHOGENESIS

Continence requires that the urethral closure pressure exceeds the intravesical pressure. (Figure 112-1) Urethral closure pressure is maintained by smooth and striated muscle, urethral vasculature, and the elasticity of the urethral tissue. It is also influenced by abdominal pressure due to the intraabdominal location of the proximal urethra. Intravesical pressure increases with increases in intraabdominal pressure and with detrusor contractions. With normal pelvic anatomy, intraabdominal pressure is transmitted equally to the bladder and proximal urethra.

Neurologic control of urethral closure depends on stimulation of alpha receptors within the smooth muscle of the urethral sphincter by the sympathetic nervous system. In addition, the sympathetic system aids in storage of urine by relaxing the detrusor through stimulation of beta receptors by norepinephrine. The parasympathetic system aids in voiding by contracting the detrusor muscle through stimulation of receptors by acetylcholine.

The act of micturition is controlled by a system of complex neurologic loops that involve the cerebral cortex, brain stem, sacral micturition center, detrusor muscle, and urethral sphincter. The integrity of these loops is necessary for proper storage and emptying of the bladder. Consequently, varied neu-

rologic disorders, systemic diseases, and medications can affect these functions.

DIFFERENTIAL DIAGNOSIS OF STORAGE AND EMPTYING DISORDERS

Urinary incontinence can be a symptom about which patients complain, a sign that can be demonstrated, or a diagnosis confirmed by studies. As a symptom, urinary incontinence is defined as the involuntary loss of urine, which is objectively demonstrable and is a social or hygienic problem. (Figure 112-2)

Genuine stress urinary incontinence (GSI) is defined as urinary incontinence associated with physical exertion, plus the observation of involuntary urine loss per urethra with an increase in abdominal pressure in the absence of a detrusor contraction. Patients complain of loss of urine with maneuvers such as coughing, sneezing, or running. This is caused by inadequate support of the proximal urethra usually as a result of childbirth, repeated Valsalva maneuvers, or atrophy due to advancing age. In women who have lost this support, the proximal urethra is displaced inferiorly out of its normal intraabdominal location. Consequently, an increase in intraabdominal pressure causes a greater increase in the intravesical pressure than the intraurethral pressure, thus favoring incontinence. Physical examination often reveals a cystourethrocele. The cotton swab test (described below) reveals hypermobility of the urethrovesical angle.

Intrinsic sphincter deficiency (ISD) is urinary incontinence associated with a urethra that does

Figure 112-1

Bladder Function

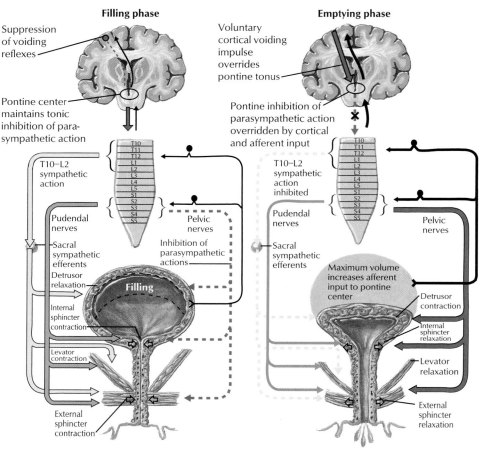

Filling phase

Suppression of voiding reflexes

Pontine center maintains tonic inhibition of para-sympathetic action

T10–L2 sympathetic action

Pudendal nerves

Sacral sympathetic efferents

Detrusor relaxation

Internal sphincter contraction

Levator contraction

External sphincter contraction

Pelvic nerves

Inhibition of parasympathetic actions

Filling

Emptying phase

Voluntary cortical voiding impulse overrides pontine tonus

Pontine inhibition of parasympathetic action overridden by cortical and afferent input

T10–L2 sympathetic action inhibited

Pudendal nerves

Sacral sympathetic efferents

Maximum volume increases afferent input to pontine center

Pelvic nerves

Detrusor contraction

Internal sphincter relaxation

Levator relaxation

External sphincter relaxation

Tonic relaxation of detrusor muscle and contraction of sphincters and levator muscles allow bladder filling. Accomplished via parasympathetic inhibition and stimulation of sympathetic and pudendal nerves

Voiding initiated by afferent input to cortical centers from stretch receptors in bladder wall. Parasympathetic inhibition released by pontine center. Sphincter and levator relaxation with detrusor contraction culminate in voiding.

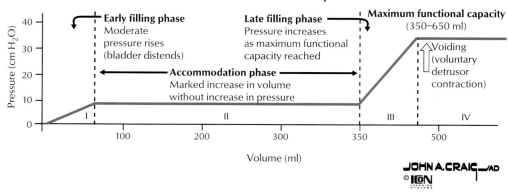

Pressure and volume relationships

Early filling phase
Moderate pressure rises (bladder distends)

Late filling phase
Pressure increases as maximum functional capacity reached

Maximum functional capacity
(350–650 ml)

Voiding (voluntary detrusor contraction)

Accommodation phase
Marked increase in volume without increase in pressure

I   II   III   IV

Pressure (cm H$_2$O): 0, 10, 20, 30, 40

Volume (ml): 100, 200, 300, 350, 500

JOHN A. CRAIG—AD
© ICON

Figure 112-2   ## Causes of Incontinence

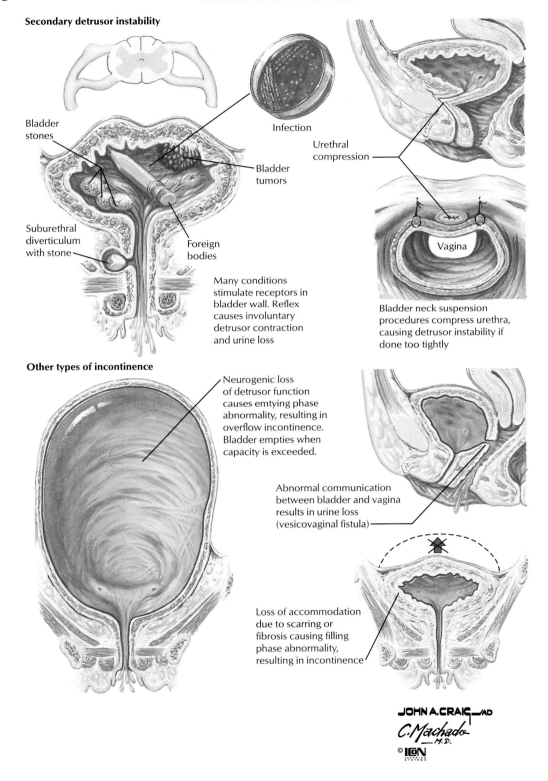

Secondary detrusor instability

Bladder stones

Infection

Urethral compression

Bladder tumors

Suburethral diverticulum with stone

Foreign bodies

Vagina

Many conditions stimulate receptors in bladder wall. Reflex causes involuntary detrusor contraction and urine loss

Bladder neck suspension procedures compress urethra, causing detrusor instability if done too tightly

Other types of incontinence

Neurogenic loss of detrusor function causes emtying phase abnormality, resulting in overflow incontinence. Bladder empties when capacity is exceeded.

Abnormal communication between bladder and vagina results in urine loss (vesicovaginal fistula)

Loss of accommodation due to scarring or fibrosis causing filling phase abnormality, resulting in incontinence

JOHN A. CRAIG—MD

C. Machado
—M.D.

©ICON

Figure 112-3

Rectocele and Enterocele

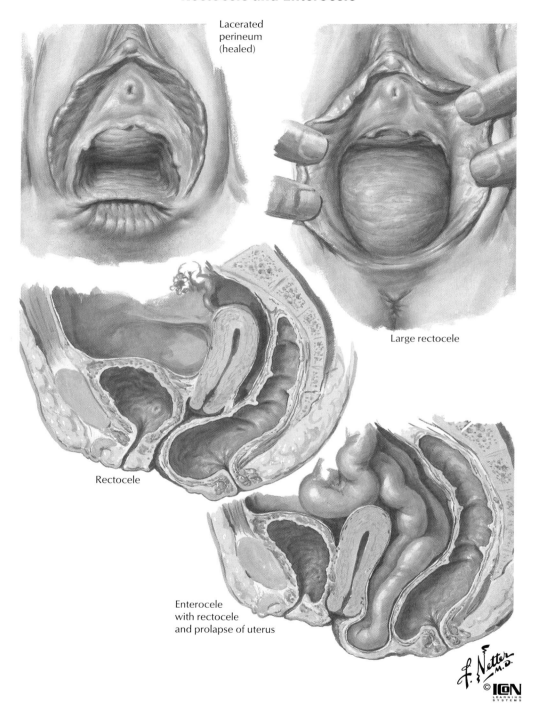

Lacerated
perineum
(healed)

Large rectocele

Rectocele

Enterocele
with rectocele
and prolapse of uterus

Table 112-1
Systemic Illnesses That
Can Affect Bladder Function

Diabetes mellitus
Myasthenia gravis
Parkinson's disease
Multiple sclerosis
Cerebrovascular disease
Central nervous system mass
Spinal cord injury or mass
Dementia

Table 112-2
Medications That Can
Affect Bladder Function

Diuretics	Caffeine
Alcohol	Anticholinergic agents
Narcotic analgesics	Antidepressants
Antipsychotics	Sedatives/hypnotics
Alpha or beta blockers or agonists	Calcium-channel blockers

not coapt properly to prevent leakage of urine. Urethral closure pressure is diminished. Patients complain of frequent loss of urine even with small increases in intraabdominal pressure. ISD can be caused by denervation injury, radiation, neurologic disorders, or scarring. Cotton swab tests can show a normal or hypermobile urethrovesical junction with strain. Diagnosis requires more sophisticated testing than office cystometrics. It is thought that many surgical procedure failures for GSI may be due to undiagnosed ISD.

Urge incontinence (UI) is the involuntary loss of urine associated with a strong need to void. UI is due to involuntary detrusor contractions. Patients often complain of large volumes of urine loss, nocturia, urinary frequency (more than 7 times a day with normal fluid intake), enuresis, and a sense of urgency with fear of urinary leakage. Urge incontinence is suggested by office cystometrics (described below) if, during filling of the bladder, the fluid level in the syringe rises. Possible etiologies include decreased central inhibition due to disease or tumor, spinal lesions, dietary irritative substances, or infection. Often UI is considered idiopathic and the term *detrusor instability* is used. If UI is due to a neurologic disorder or central nervous system pathology, the term *detrusor hyperreflexia* is used. *Detrusor hyperreflexia with impaired contractility* is a condition found in the elderly where detrusor instability coexists with urinary retention due to detrusor weakness.

Overflow incontinence (OI) occurs when incomplete emptying and/or decreased sensation of fullness are present and result in the bladder being filled to maximum capacity from which the patient constantly leaks. A high post-void residual (usually greater than 300 cc) supports this diagnosis. Patients may complain of a sense of incomplete emptying, a slow urine stream, or the need to use abdominal strain to void. OI can be due to obstruction such as with an enlarged prostate gland or due to an inadequate detrusor contraction. The latter can be due to neurologic diseases, diabetes mellitus, medications, or aging.

Functional incontinence occurs in individuals who have normal emptying capabilities but are incontinent due to decreased mobility or decreased cognitive function. Congenital ectopic ureters may present in children who are not able to toilet train. Urinary tract fistulas can result from pelvic surgery and inflammatory conditions such as inflammatory bowel disease and can present as incontinence. Patients complain of constant loss of urine from the vagina. Orange coloring on a tampon in the vagina after a patient has taken oral Pyridium can document the vaginal fluid as urine. Urethral diverticulae are outpocketings of the urethral mucosa that can fill with urine during micturition and then drain when the patient stands up, thus presenting with post-void dribbling. On physical examination, urethral diverticulae can occasionally be palpated or purulence can be milked from the urethra. Often a double-balloon radiologic study is necessary to confirm the diagnosis.

Systemic illnesses or medications can disrupt the neurologic loops that control micturition and storage (Tables 112-1 and 112-2).

DIAGNOSTIC APPROACH

When evaluating a patient who complains of urinary incontinence, a thorough guided history and physical examination are essential. Important information includes duration, frequency, estimated volume, nocturia, enuresis, sensation of incomplete emptying, post-void dribbling, impact on quality of life, history of urinary tract infections or urolithiasis, dysuria, hematuria, and associations with the loss of urine, (e.g., coughing, laughing, running water). Pertinent parts of the history include medications; general medical history; previous surgeries, particularly gynecologic or urologic procedures; and an obstetric history including methods of delivery, birth weights, and delivery complications. A functional status evaluation is important to determine if a patient is able to get to the toilet and to comply with treatment options. Smoking, caffeine, and alcohol intake are important variables to consider. A review of systems should include the gastrointestinal system with particular emphasis on history of constipation. A review of systems should also probe for underlying neurologic or medical diseases that can affect proper bladder function. A diary that tracks the amount and kind of fluid intake as well as the timing and volume of urinary voids and leaking episodes should be kept for 3 to 7 days.

A complete pelvic examination that includes testing pelvic floor muscle strength, reflexes, and sensation should be performed. The presence and degree of pelvic organ prolapse should be assessed. A bimanual examination is done to evaluate for gynecologic pathology and should include palpating the urethra for masses or tenderness. A cotton swab test is performed by placing the cotton end of a cotton swab through the urethra to the level of the vesical neck. The angle between the cotton swab and the horizontal when the patient is lying flat is measured at rest and with Valsalva maneuvers; 30 degrees or greater with strain indicates hypermobility of the urethrovesical angle. A rectal examination is performed to ensure that fecal impaction is not present. A lower extremity neurologic examination should be performed.

A urinalysis and urine culture should be sent. A pad test can be performed to quantify the amount of leaking by placing a pad on the patient's perineum for 1 hour while maneuvers are performed. An increase in the weight of the pad by 2 g indicates incontinence. Pyridium can be used to confirm that the fluid is urine. Office cystometrics are performed as follows: The patient voids and a post-void residual is obtained by transurethral catheterization. The bladder is filled by gravity through this catheter with water via a 50-mL syringe without the plunger. During filling, sensation and capacity are documented. In the absence of an increase in abdominal pressure, a rise in the column of water during filling indicates a detrusor contraction. The catheter is removed and the patient coughs while standing, and any leaking is noted.

Multichannel urodynamic studies are performed largely at academic institutions. Patients who warrant referral for these studies include those who describe mixed symptoms or have a history of failed anti-incontinence surgery. Other indications include the desire to rule out detrusor instability when history is suggestive of its presence but simple cystometry is negative, to identify risk factors for surgical failure (e.g., ISD), and to determine the voiding mechanism to attempt to predict those who will have postoperative urinary retention.

MANAGEMENT AND THERAPY

Conservative measures for GSI include pelvic floor muscle exercises (Kegel exercises), biofeedback with or without electrical stimulation, weighted vaginal cones, and/or placement of a vaginal pessary. Surgical procedures to correct GSI stabilize the urethrovesical angle. The anterior colporrhaphy, once a common surgical procedure for GSI, is no longer preferred due to high rate of failure. Urethropexy and pubovaginal slings are the preferred surgical procedures for GSI.

Intrinsic sphincter deficiency with hypermobility of the urethrovesical junction can be managed surgically with a pubovaginal sling to help support and coapt the urethra. ISD without urethrovesical hypermobility can be managed with injection of periurethral bulking agents such as collagen. Conservative measures as listed under GSI can also be attempted, but often are not as successful.

Detrusor instability/urge incontinence can be managed through pelvic floor muscle exercises, bladder retraining programs, and behavioral techniques based on patterns identified from the voiding diary. Bladder infections are treated with antibiotics. Bladder irritants such as alcohol and caffeine should be avoided. Nocturia, often associated with DI, can also be due to mobilization of lower extremity edema upon becoming supine. Elevation of the legs during the day or compression stockings can decrease this problem.

Overflow incontinence due to obstruction requires correction of the obstruction. OI due to an incontractile bladder usually requires self-catheterization, Crede, or an abdominal strain technique. Functional incontinence requires assistance in the form of a bedside commode, assistance with mobility, or verbal prompts to void. Fistulas and diverticulum require surgical excision/repair. Underlying neurologic and medical diseases should be optimally treated. Medications can be changed or the dosage or timing can be altered. For all forms of urinary incontinence, conservative methods should be tried before surgical procedures.

FUTURE DIRECTIONS

Areas of active investigation into bladder function disorders include new surgical techniques and medications. Surgical management currently centers on the belief that restoring anatomy will help restore function, but other procedures are under development that focus on nerve modulation or local enhancement of urethral closure. Sacral nerve stimulators help to modulate reflexes and may improve emptying or storage of urine in patients who have incomplete emptying or detrusor hyperreflexia. Other periurethral bulking agents are being tested that may last longer than the currently used collagen for ISD. Various mechanical devices are being designed with the goals of being inexpensive, effective, easy to use, and without major side effects.

Women are becoming educated and aware that treatment options are available for urinary incontinence. They are presenting to their primary care physicians in increasing numbers, complaining of urinary incontinence, no longer as inhibited by embarrassment. This has resulted in increased and improved research involving not only management options but also the pathophysiology, etiology, and prevention of urinary incontinence. The next decade will undoubtedly bring many new and exciting options for individuals suffering from urinary incontinence.

REFERENCE

American College of Obstetrians and Gynecologists. *Urinary Incontinence.* Washington, DC: American College of Obstetricians and Gynecologists; 1995. Technical bulletin 213.

Chapter 113
Chronic Renal Failure

Kevin O'Reilly and Gerald A. Hladik

The number of patients with end-stage renal disease (ESRD) receiving dialysis is growing rapidly. In 1973, approximately 10,000 patients were in the Medicare ESRD program. By 1997, this increased to 304,083, and by 2,010 the number is projected to be 651,330, a 114.2% increase. The incidence of ESRD has doubled in the past decade and is projected to be 129,200 in 2010, a 63.3% increase from 1997.

The ESRD population consumes a large proportion of health-care resources. In 2010, Medicare costs for ESRD are projected to be $28.29 billion, a 162% increase from 1997. Despite this large utilization of resources, morbidity (substantially higher hospitalization rates) and mortality (the life expectancy of dialysis patients is only 16% to 37% of the age-, gender-, and race-matched population) remain high. It is hoped these outcomes can be improved with better detection and treatment of renal insufficiency.

There are various recommendations on when to refer a patient to a nephrologist. A 1994 National Institutes of Health (NIH) consensus statement on morbidity and mortality in dialysis patients recommended that patients be referred when the serum creatinine (Scr) reaches 1.5 mg/dL in women and 2.0 mg/dL in men. The Clinical Practice Guidelines of the Canadian Society of Nephrology recommend referral when the Scr is greater than 2.3 mg/dL. Given the increasing number of patients with kidney disease, primary care providers should remain current in the care of patients with chronic renal insufficiency and in interventions that can slow the progression of renal disease.

ETIOLOGY AND PATHOGENESIS

Per U.S. Renal Data System (USRDS) data available from 1998 (319,515 patients), causes of ESRD included:

Diabetes mellitus	31.8%
Hypertension	20.2%
Glomerulonephritis	17.8%
Polycystic kidney	5.3%
Urologic	3.7%
Unknown or unidentified	21.2%

In most patients with renal disease, renal function declines progressively after sufficient parenchymal damage has occurred to increase the Scr to 1.5 to 2 mg/dL (Figure 113-1). In the Modification of Diet in Renal Disease study, 85% of patients with non-diabetic renal disease had a persistent decline in glomerular filtration rate (GFR) averaging 4 mL/minute/year. In patients with untreated diabetic nephropathy, the decline in GFR may approach 12 mL/minute/year. It is postulated that the progressive decline in GFR, regardless of the original disease, enters a "final common pathway" of glomerular sclerosis and intraglomerular hypertension, which further reduces functional renal mass. Studies have demonstrated that angiotensin-converting enzyme (ACE) inhibitors not only reduce blood pressure, but also glomerular hypertension and fibrosis. These drugs have been shown to slow, and in some cases halt, progression of renal failure and to reduce mortality.

CLINICAL PRESENTATION

Chronic renal failure is a slowly progressive disease that is frequently asymptomatic until the GFR decreases to 5 to 10 mL/minute, at which point the uremic syndrome (Table 113-1) becomes apparent and dialysis is necessary to maintain life.

Often, chronic renal insufficiency is diagnosed unexpectedly with routine serum chemistries demonstrating azotemia (increased Scr or blood urea nitrogen [BUN]), hyponatremia, hyperkalemia, metabolic acidosis, hypocalcemia, or hyperphosphatemia. Chronic renal failure may also be diagnosed for the first time during the clin-

Figure 113-1

Chronic Renal Failure

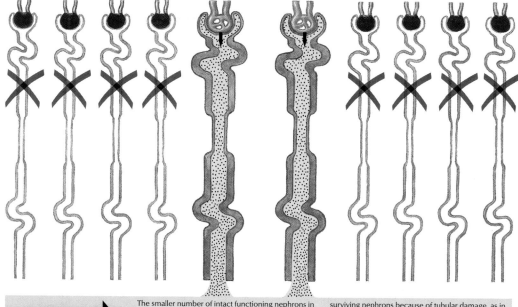

Water excretion in renal insufficiency: Intact nephron theory

The smaller number of intact functioning nephrons in the diseased kidneys excrete practically the same amount of solute as did all the nephrons of the normal kidney. Thus the solute excreted per surviving nephron is increased, resulting in osmotic diuresis, i.e., rise in urine flow and reduction in concentration. (Diminished water reabsorption capacity of the surviving nephrons because of tubular damage, as in pyelonephritis, may also play a part.) Ability to dilute the urine is lost later, but the few surviving nephrons may not be able to excrete the same total amount of water as did all the nephrons of the normal kidney, resulting in impaired ability to excrete a water load.

---

ical evaluation of hypertension, anemia, edema, malnutrition, fatigue, or depression.

DIFFERENTIAL DIAGNOSIS/ DIAGNOSTIC APPROACH

The etiology of renal insufficiency may be readily apparent, such as in patients with long-standing diabetes mellitus and hypertension complicated by end-organ damage in other vascular beds. The differential diagnosis is broader in patients presenting with hematuria, proteinuria, and renal insufficiency, and includes those entities that present as the nephritic or nephrotic syndromes. In these situations, diagnosis, and specific treatment, may require a renal biopsy; early referral to a nephrologist is essential.

MANAGEMENT AND THERAPY
Renoprotective Therapy

Control blood pressure. Sitting systolic blood pressure should ideally be less than 125 mm Hg. This goal is particularly important if there is proteinuria in excess of 3.0 g/day.

ACE inhibitor or angiotensin receptor blocker therapy. In patients with proteinuria, these agents should be considered even in the setting of normotension. Renoprotection has been demonstrated with low- to moderate-dose ACE inhibitor therapy, although the optimum dose is unknown. If proteinuric, the goal is to reduce proteinuria to <1.0 g/day. The caregiver should:

Assure optimal control blood glucose in diabetics.

Table 113-1
Uremic Syndrome: Clinical Alterations

Nervous System

Stupor, coma	Polyneuritis
Fatigue	Seizures
Dementia	Motor weakness
Malaise	Asterixis
Sleep disturbances	Headache
Cramps	Restless legs

Gastrointestinal System

Stomatitis	Nausea, vomiting
Gastritis	Ulcers
Anorexia	

Hematologic System

Anemia	Bleeding

Cardiovascular System

Pericarditis	Hypertension
Atherosclerosis	Cardiomyopathy
Edema	Diastolic dysfunction

Pulmonary System

Pleuritis	Pulmonary edema
Uremic lung	

Skin

Pruritus	Melanosis
Retarded wound healing	Nail atrophy

Bone Disease

Osteodystrophy	Amyloidosis
Hyperparathyroidism	Adynamic bone disease

Miscellaneous

Thirst	Uremic fetor
Weight loss	Hypothermia
Erectile dysfunction	

Adapted from *The Primer on Kidney Disease, 3rd edition.* Greenberg, Cheung, Coffman, Falk, and Jennette. Uremic Syndrome: Clinical Alterations, 2001:392, with permission from Elsevier.

Control blood lipids. The goal is an LDL cholesterol <120 mg/dL (<100 mL/dL if atherosclerosis is present or suspected).

Discontinue use of tobacco products.

Avoid NSAIDs and the newer cyclooxygenase (COX- 2) inhibitors.

Control plasma homocysteine. Folic acid (5 to 10 mg daily may be required). Vitamin B_6 and B_{12} supplementation may be necessary.

Correct anemia.

Control hyperphosphatemia.

Prevention of Uremic Complications

Malnutrition. Hypoalbuminemia at the time dialysis is initiated is a strong predictor of early death and increased morbidity. It can result from multiple causes, including derangements in protein metabolism and spontaneous dietary protein restriction secondary to anorexia. Modifiable practice patterns that could reduce the prevalence of hypoalbuminemia include early referral to a nephrologist for initiation of dialysis, referral to a nutritionist, and a protein intake of 0.8 to 1.0 g/kg/day. If malnutrition is present, the protein intake should be increased to 1 to 1.2 g/kg/day.

Anemia. Patients with a creatinine clearance of less than 30 mL/minute should have their hemoglobin levels checked at least every 3 to 6 months. Based on the Dialysis Outcomes Quality Initiative (DOQI) guidelines, the desired hemoglobin level is 11 to 12.5 g/dL. A hemoglobin level less than 10 g/dL justifies treatment with erythropoietin (EPO). Iron stores also require close monitoring; current recommendations are for the transferrin saturation to be greater than 20% and for the ferritin level to be greater than 100 ng/mL. Oral supplementation of iron should be started when EPO therapy is initiated. Some patients may require therapy with IV iron.

Renal Osteodystrophy

Chronic renal insufficiency (CRI) is associated with many bone disorders including osteitis fibrosa cystica, the classic lesion of secondary hyperparathyroidism, osteomalacia due to vitamin D deficiency or aluminum toxicity, and adynamic bone disease due to over suppression of parathyroid hormone (PTH) with calcitriol or excess aluminum. Metabolic changes that result in renal osteodystrophy occur early in renal insufficiency; increased PTH levels have been found when the GFR falls below 60 to 80 mL/minute. Metabolic acidosis can also contribute to bone disease. The skeletal changes and parathyroid hyperplasia are not easily reversed; therefore, careful monitoring and early intervention are critical to prevent secondary hyperparathyroidism and to control metabolic acidosis. (Figures 113-2 and 113-3)

Hyperphosphatemia and Hypocalcemia

Dietary phosphate restriction to 60 mmol/day should be instituted at the earliest manifestation

Figure 113-2

Vascular and Soft Tissue Calcification in Secondary Hyperparathyroidism of Chronic Renal Disease

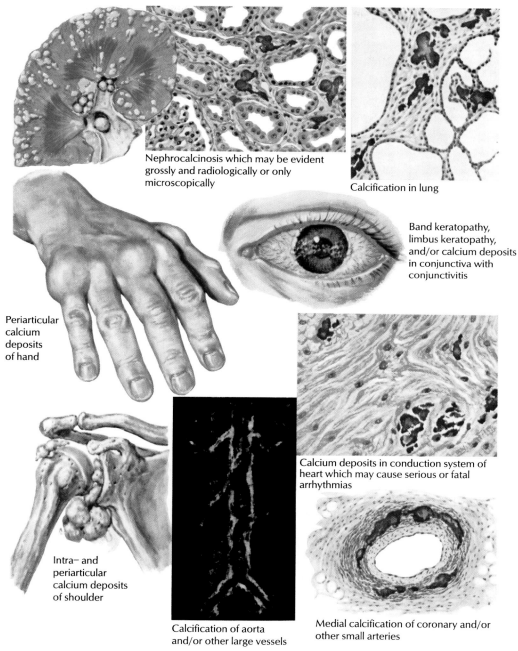

Nephrocalcinosis which may be evident grossly and radiologically or only microscopically

Calcification in lung

Band keratopathy, limbus keratopathy, and/or calcium deposits in conjunctiva with conjunctivitis

Periarticular calcium deposits of hand

Intra– and periarticular calcium deposits of shoulder

Calcium deposits in conduction system of heart which may cause serious or fatal arrhythmias

Calcification of aorta and/or other large vessels

Medial calcification of coronary and/or other small arteries

Bone Manifestations of Secondary Hyperparathyroidism in Chronic Renal Disease

Figure 113-3

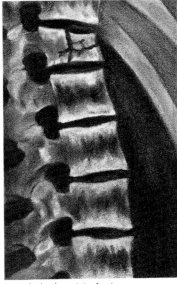

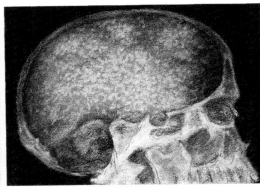

Spotty demineral-ization of skull

"Banded sclerosis" of spine, sclerosis of upper and lower margins of vertebrae with rarefaction between. Note compression fracture

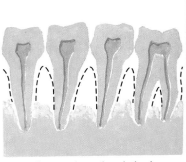

Loss of lamina dura of teeth (broken lines indicate normal contours)

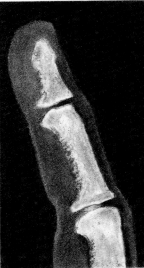

Subperiosteal resorption of phalanges (chiefly on palmar aspect of middle phalanx)

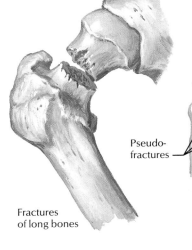

Pseudo-fractures

Fractures of long bones

Resorption of lateral end of clavicle; rib fractures

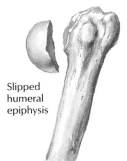

Slipped humeral epiphysis

of azotemia. When dietary changes are insufficient, therapy with calcium-containing phosphate binders should be initiated. Calcium carbonate 1.25 g with meals is indicated when the creatinine clearance falls to less than 30 mL/minute. Aluminum-containing binders should be reserved for extreme hyperphosphatemia (e.g., if the calcium-phosphate product is greater than 60). These should not be used any longer than necessary to avoid the complications of aluminum accumulation (osteomalacia and adynamic bone disease). The use of the newer calcium-free phosphate binders, sevelamer for example, is likely to increase as concern for adverse vascular effects from excess vascular calcification grows (Figure 113-2). Calcitriol supplementation, usually at doses of 0.25 to 0.5 µg/day, should be used to prevent and treat hyperparathyroidism, with a goal PTH level of 200 to 300 pg/mL. Careful monitoring, initially every 4 to 8 weeks, then quarterly, is important to prevent development of an increased calcium-phosphate product, hypercalcemia, or over suppression of PTH, that could cause adynamic bone disease.

Preparation for Renal Replacement Therapy

Discussions regarding the need for renal replacement therapy (RRT) and choice of modality should begin at least 6 months before the anticipated start of dialysis. The appropriate mode of dialysis should be determined as well as suitability for transplant. Patients electing peritoneal dialysis (PD) should have a PD catheter inserted 2 to 4 weeks prior to the anticipated need for dialysis. Patients going on hemodialysis (HD) should have a functioning, permanent vascular access at the time RRT is initiated. A native arteriovenous fistula (AVF) is preferred as there are fewer infectious and thrombotic complications and, possibly, better patient survival rates compared to arteriovenous grafts (AVG). Vascular access should ideally be placed once the Scr is greater than 4 mg/dL or the estimated GFR falls to less than 25 mL/minute. A maturation time of at least 3 months is recommended. Patients with indwelling central venous catheters have the highest rates of complications and mortality and often receive a lower dose of hemodialysis compared to those with AVFs or AVGs. Patients should be instructed to "save" an arm (usually the nondominant) for future access placement. Instruct the patient and medical staff to avoid phlebotomies and IV lines in that arm, as well as central lines in the subclavian vein.

Timing of Initiation of Dialysis

The current recommendation of the DOQI PD Adequacy Work Group is to begin dialysis when the weekly Kt/V_{urea} (calculated by dividing the weekly urea clearance [in liters] by the estimated volume of total body water [in liters]) for residual renal function drops below 2.0. Patients may start later if they have stable or increasing edema-free body weight, their normalized protein-equivalent of total nitrogen appearance is greater than 0.8 g/kg/day, and if there are no signs or symptoms of uremia. Current Medicare guidelines are for patients with diabetes mellitus to begin renal replacement therapy at a GFR of 15 mL/minute (as determined by the average of creatinine and urea clearance from a 24-hour urine) and at a GFR of 10 mL/minute for other patients.

Discussions are ongoing as to whether outcomes would improve with an earlier start of dialysis compared with currently recommended levels of renal function. There are no randomized trials that address this issue; however, several observations support this approach. Earlier dialysis protects against malnutrition and its related morbidity and mortality. Poor volume control and solute clearance can lead to increased complication rates. Some studies suggest that the severity of certain uremic complications, and morbidity and mortality correlate inversely with residual renal function at the time of initiation of dialysis.

FUTURE DIRECTIONS

Patients with CRI constitute a large population, and more in-depth research is needed to further define optimal therapy. There are few studies of prognostic variables in CRI and little information regarding the impact of therapy during CRI on morbidity and mortality as these patients reach ESRD.

Interventions to increase the rate of earlier referral that are directed at both patients and physicians should be studied in randomized trials. The detrimental effects of late referral include increased morbidity and mortality, increased costs, decreased utilization of PD and home HD, and fewer patients with permanent vascular accesses. Early referral is associated with earlier initiation of dialysis, greater probability of a permanent vascular access, less anemia, and less malnutrition.

Identifying and managing complications and comorbidity should be a priority. The prevention or correction of anemia in patients with CRI should receive special attention, especially given the effect of anemia on left ventricular hypertrophy (LVH) and the high risk of cardiovascular death in patients on HD. The optimal level of hemoglobin to prevent and/or reverse LVH without adverse effects on blood pressure control or progression of renal disease should be studied in a randomized clinical trial. Regarding hyperparathyroidism, alternatives to calcium-containing phosphate binders such as sevelamer and calcimimetic agents to suppress PTH should be studied in CRI patients.

Clinical practice guidelines in Canada and the United States recommend earlier initiation of dialysis than is usually the case. These recommendations are based only on observational studies, and a randomized clinical trial should be done.

REFERENCES

NKF-DOQI clinical practice guidelines for vascular access. National Kidney Foundation-Dialysis Outcomes Quality Initiative. *Am J Kidney Dis.* 1997;30(suppl 3):S150-S191.

Bonomini V, Feletti C, Scolari MP, Stefoni S. Benefits of early initiation of dialysis. *Kidney Int Suppl.* 1985;17:S57-S59.

Goodman WG, Goldin J, Kuizon BD, et al. Coronary-artery calcification in young adults with end-stage renal disease who are undergoing dialysis. *N Engl J Med.* 2000;342:1478-1483.

Lindberg J, Churchill DN, Fishbane S. Research directions: new clinical frontiers. *Am J Kidney Dis.* 2000;36(suppl 3):S52-S61.

Sesso R, Belasco AG. Late diagnosis of chronic renal failure and mortality on maintenance dialysis. *Nephrol Dial Transplant.* 1996;11:2417-2420.

Taal MW, Brenner BM. Renoprotective benefits of RAS inhibition: from ACEI to angiotensin II antagonists. *Kidney Int.* 2000;57:1803-1817.

US Renal Data System. USRDS 2002 Annual Data Report: *Atlas of End-Stage Renal Disease in the United States.* Bethesda, Md: National Institutes of Health, National Institute of Diabetes and Digestive and Kidney Diseases; 2002.

Chapter 114

Glomerulonephritis

Patrick H. Nachman and Ronald J. Falk

Glomerulonephritis refers to injury of glomeruli typically due to inflammation. Glomerular damage results in hematuria, proteinuria, edema, hypertension, and azotemia. There are dozens of glomerular diseases, each with its own characteristic pathologic features, natural history, and response to treatment; however, many different types of glomerular disease can result in the same clinical syndrome. For instance, asymptomatic microscopic hematuria is a consequence of several different pathologic entities, most commonly thin basement membrane nephropathy and IgA nephropathy. Thus, when evaluating patients with glomerulonephritis, it is best to group them according to general categories, and then dissect the different diseases within each group described in Table 114-1.

ETIOLOGY AND PATHOGENESIS

There are several pathogenetic mechanisms of glomerulonephritis. The most common cause is an inflammatory injury of the glomeruli as a result of immune complex formation or deposition within the glomerular basement membrane or the mesangium (Figure 114-1). These immune complexes initiate many phlogistic pathways, in particular, complement activation, and cytokine and chemokine generation and release. As a consequence, circulating inflammatory cells, including neutrophils, monocytes, and lymphocytes infiltrate the glomeruli and the surrounding tubulointerstitial compartments. Immune deposits may result from the deposition of circulating immune complexes (e.g., lupus nephritis), from antigens deposited in the glomeruli with subsequent in situ immune complex formation (e.g., peri-infectious disorders), or from antibodies that react to intrinsic components of the glomerulus (e.g., anti-glomerular basement membrane [anti-GBM] diseases). The mesangial cell response to injury is marked by proliferation, production and deposition of extracellular matrix, and, eventually, glomerular scarring. Glomerular endothelial cells are the target of injury is some diseases, such as hemolytic-uremic syndrome and the vasculitides.

Hereditary nephritides include Alport's syndrome and thin basement membrane disease. *Alport's syndrome*, which results from mutations in the α5 chain of type IV collagen, is a genetically heterogenous disease that can be transmitted in an X-linked, autosomal recessive or dominant pattern. *Thin basement membrane disease,* a relatively common autosomal dominant disorder, is also due to a mutation in type IV collagen. Although both syndromes present with asymptomatic glomerular hematuria, they diverge in their natural history. Thin basement membrane disease (also referred to as "benign familial hematuria") is associated with an excellent long-term outcome, whereas Alport's syndrome causes a progressive loss of renal function.

CLINICAL PRESENTATION

The clinical expression of disease correlates with the pathologic features; the more aggressive the pathologic injury, the more severe the illness. Some patients present with asymptomatic hematuria and recurrent gross hematuria. Hematuria, defined as more than 3 red blood cells per high-power field observed in centrifuged urine sediment, can be of either glomerular or non-glomerular origin. Chemical stress of red blood cells as they pass along the nephron results in morphologic changes and dysmorphic red blood cells. The most diagnostic of these, acanthocytes ("Mickey Mouse" cells), are virtually pathognomonic of glomerular bleeding. In combination with red blood cell casts and other cylindruria and proteinuria, these abnormalities suggest glomerular bleeding as opposed to urinary tract hematuria. (Figure 114-2)

The most common causes of asymptomatic hematuria are listed in Table 114-1. Patients with *IgA nephropathy* present with 1 of 3 syndromes.

Table 114-1
Clinical Presentation of Various Glomerulonephritides

Asymptomatic Microscopic Hematuria
Thin basement membrane nephropathy
IgA nephropathy
Mesangioproliferative GN
Alport's syndrome

Recurrent Gross Hematuria
Thin basement membrane nephropathy
IgA nephropathy
Alport's syndrome

Acute Nephritis
Acute diffuse proliferative GN
Poststreptococcal GN
Poststaphylococcal GN
Focal or diffuse proliferative GN
IgA nephropathy
Lupus nephritis
Membranoproliferative GN

Rapidly Progressive Nephritis
Crescentic GN
Anti-GBM GN
Immune complex GN
ANCA-GN

Pulmonary-Renal Vasculitic Syndrome
Goodpasture's (anti-GBM) syndrome
Immune complex vasculitis
Lupus nephritis
ANCA vasculitis
   Microscopic polyangiitis
   Wegener's granulomatosis
   Churg-Strauss syndrome

Renal-Dermal Vasculitic Syndromes
Immune Complex Vasculitis
ANCA vasculitis
Cryoglobulinemia
Henoch-Schönlein purpura

Chronic Renal Failure
Chronic Sclerosing GN

Approximately one half have a history of episodic macroscopic hematuria associated with an infection of the upper respiratory tract that may recur with subsequent episodes of pharyngitis, febrile illness, or heavy exertion. Patients are typically asymptomatic; hypertension and peripheral edema are uncommon. *Asymptomatic microscopic hematuria with proteinuria*, the second most common presentation, is associated with the worst long-term prognosis. A third presentation is part of the vasculitic syndrome *Henoch-Schönlein purpura*, which develops most commonly in children. The periinfectious nephritic syndrome of IgA nephropathy is differentiated from poststreptococcal glomerulonephritis in that it occurs only 1 to 2 days after the onset of the infection, as opposed to the 10- to 14-day delay in poststreptococcal glomerulonephritis.

Acute glomerulonephritis usually presents with the sudden onset of proteinuria, hematuria, and urine sediment containing dysmorphic red blood cells, casts, and cellular debris. Patients typically have edema, hypertension, oliguria, and renal insufficiency (Figure 114-3). In the most severe form, *rapidly progressive glomerulonephritis* (RPGN), the serum creatinine concentration rises in a matter of days to weeks, resulting in profound renal insufficiency. Structurally, RPGNs are usually associated with the formation of glomerular crescents that result from the proliferation of both glomerular epithelial cells and mononuclear phagocytes in Bowman's space. Crescents are not indicative of a specific cause of glomerular injury, but may result from many different pathogenetic mechanisms.

All forms of acute nephritis, including RPGN, may be a consequence of streptococcal or staphylococcal infections or immunologic diseases. The illness is characterized by the sudden onset of edema, and oliguria with heavy proteinuria and hematuria. Hypertension, cardiac enlargement, and pulmonary edema may be present. In the Western world, the types of infections resulting in postinfectious glomerulonephritis have changed so that glomerulopathies associated with a variety of gram-negative organisms develop in patients with underlying immunocompromised states, including cirrhosis, malignancy, and transplantation.

Recently, the role of the *hepatitis C virus* was recognized in the pathogenesis of membranoproliferative glomerulonephritis type I and cryoglobulinemia. Hepatitis C viral antigens were found in the cryoglobulins of some affected patients. A clinical syndrome of mixed cryoglobulins is char-

Figure 114-1

Hypothesis of Pathogenesis of Acute Glomerular Injury by Circulating Immune Complexes (Schematic)

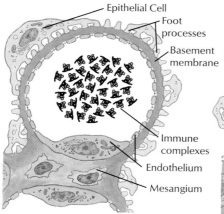

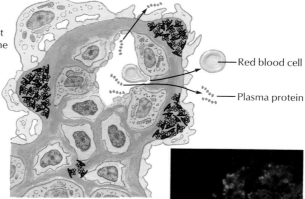

Epithelial Cell
Foot processes
Basement membrane
Immune complexes
Endothelium
Mesangium

Red blood cell
Plasma protein

A: Circulating immune complexes, formed anywhere in the body, consisting of antigen, antibody, and complement components, arrive at glomerular capillaries in large amounts over a short period of time

B: Complexes penetrate endothelium and basement membrane of glomerular capillaries and form large isolated deposits (humps); foot processes fuse; mesangial and endothelial cells swell and proliferate, invading capillary lumen; fibrillar basement membranelike material (mesangial matrix) is deposited between cells; increased porosity of capillary walls permits escape of plasma proteins and blood cells, causing proteinuria and hematuria

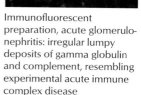

Immunofluorescent preparation, acute glomerulonephritis: irregular lumpy deposits of gamma globulin and complement, resembling experimental acute immune complex disease

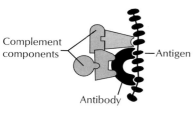

Complement components
Antigen
Antibody
Composition of complexes

acterized by purpura, weakness, arthralgias, and in some cases, glomerular disease.

Systemic lupus erythematosus (SLE) is the prototypic cause of acute nephritis associated with immunologic injury. The characteristic renal lesion of SLE is a consequence of the accumulation of immune complexes in the mesangium and along the glomerular capillary wall. SLE ranges from almost no lesion to a severe diffusely proliferative and crescentic lesion. The clinical spectrum of disease ranges from normal renal function with minimal proteinuria (<1 g/24 hours) to a rapidly progressive glomerulonephritis and severe proteinuria. Almost all patients have hematuria. Other causes of diffuse proliferative glomerulonephritis

include IgA nephropathy, membranoproliferative glomerulonephritides, and fibrillary glomerulonephritis.

The most common causes of RPGN associated with crescent formation include the immune complex-mediated diseases and diseases associated with *anti-neutrophil cytoplasmic autoantibodies* (ANCA). An uncommon, but explosive, disease is caused by *antibodies to the glomerular basement membrane* (anti-GBM). Pulmonary hemorrhage in addition to anti-GBM-mediated nephritis defines *Goodpasture's syndrome*. There is a bimodal age distribution of patients with peaks in the third and sixth decades. One third of patients have isolated glomerular disease.

Figure 114-2

Urinary Sediment: Organized Elements

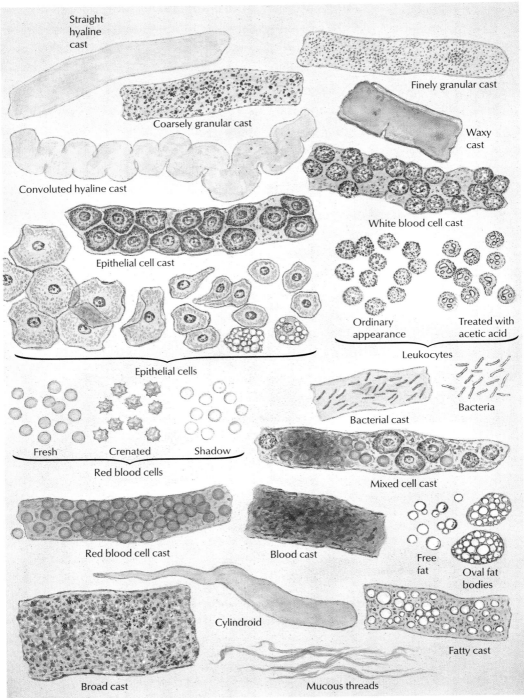

Straight hyaline cast

Finely granular cast

Coarsely granular cast

Waxy cast

Convoluted hyaline cast

White blood cell cast

Epithelial cell cast

Ordinary appearance

Treated with acetic acid

Leukocytes

Epithelial cells

Bacteria

Fresh   Crenated   Shadow

Bacterial cast

Red blood cells

Mixed cell cast

Red blood cell cast

Blood cast

Free fat

Oval fat bodies

Cylindroid

Fatty cast

Broad cast

Mucous threads

Malaise, fatigue, and weight loss are common.

In a patient with a glomerulonephritis, it is most important to determine whether it is part of a systemic disorder resulting from an infection or due to an immunologic disorder. One approach is to determine whether a patient has a pulmonary-renal or dermal-renal syndrome. Pulmonary-renal vasculitic syndromes are due to Goodpasture's syndrome, the ANCA vasculitides (including microscopic polyangiitis, Wegener's granulomatosis, and Churg-Strauss syndrome), or immune complex vasculitis, especially SLE and cryoglobulinemia. In renal-dermal vasculitic syndromes, the glomerulonephritis is associated with a number of skin manifestations, including petechiae, purpura, hives, livedo reticularis, and ecchymoses. These diseases are usually attributable to SLE, ANCA-vasculitis, Henoch-Schönlein purpura, or cryoglobulinemia.

DIFFERENTIAL DIAGNOSIS

The differential diagnosis is broad and includes other causes of hematuria or azotemia. Glomerulonephritides account for only about 5% of hematuria in the adult population where urinary tract stones, infections, and malignancies predominate. Azotemia may be due to tubulointerstitial disease (e.g., acute tubular necrosis or acute interstitial nephritis), thrombotic microangiopathies, or urinary tract obstruction. The presence of dysmorphic erythrocyturia, red blood cell casts, and proteinuria >500 mg/day are strong clues for a glomerular cause of hematuria. Extra-renal manifestations of disease identified on a thorough review of systems and physical examination provide clues for the presence of systemic infections or autoimmune diseases associated with glomerulonephritis.

DIAGNOSTIC APPROACH

The initial diagnostic approach in anyone with kidney disease is to examine the urine for the presence of glomerular hematuria, proteinuria, or other formed elements. This simple study allows the inclusion or exclusion of many renal processes. Multisystem disease is usually associated with constitutional signs and symptoms of inflammation including arthralgias, myalgias, fever, and weight loss. A history and physical examination provide clues for a differential diagnosis of organ distribution of injury, and the presence of pulmonary-renal or renal-dermal syndromes. Serologic tests help in the diagnosis of glomerular diseases. It is possible to separate glomerular diseases on the basis of whether the patient has circulating immune complexes such as cryoglobulins; antibodies to nuclear antigens including anti-double–stranded DNA, ANCA, hypocomplementemia; or evidence for infectious diseases including assays for hepatitis C, hepatitis B, and streptococcal disease (DNase B and antistreptolysin O testing). (Figure 114-4)

The evaluation of pathologic features on a renal biopsy specimen is usually required for diagnosis. Light, immunofluorescence, and electron microscopy are used to establish the precise pattern of injury. The definitive diagnosis frequently depends on an integrated synthesis of the clinical features of disease, serologic tests, and pathologic findings. For example, glomerulonephritides associated with proliferative lesions are attributable to infections, lupus nephritis, or IgA nephropathy and require serologic tests to differentiate among them. In addition to its diagnostic value, the renal biopsy specimen also allows an estimation of prognosis and treatment options. Generally, a renal biopsy is indicated in any patient with renal disease when the cause cannot be adequately determined by the clinical pattern of disease or laboratory findings, the differential diagnosis results in differing prognoses/treatment, or signs and symptoms suggest intrinsic renal disease that can be diagnosed by the biopsy.

Contraindications to renal biopsy include the presence of a solitary kidney, an uncooperative patient, bleeding disorders of any kind, severe hypertension, multiple cysts within the kidney, obstructive uropathy, renal neoplasm, and a very thin cortex (usually indicative of end-stage renal disease) in which case a biopsy is no longer useful.

MANAGEMENT AND THERAPY

All forms of glomerular disease require supportive care. The treatment of hypertension is a cornerstone of therapy. Angiotensinconverting enzyme inhibitors or angiotensin receptor blockers are the agents of choice because they control blood pressure, reduce proteinuria, and slow the rate of decline of creatinine clearance. Other supportive measures include management of edema

Figure 114-3

Clinical Course of Acute Glomerulonephritis

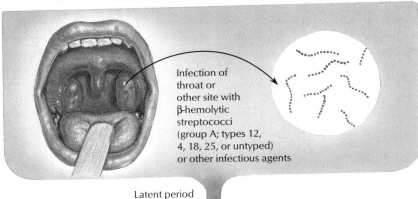

Infection of throat or other site with β-hemolytic streptococci (group A; types 12, 4, 18, 25, or untyped) or other infectious agents

Latent period 1 to 3 weeks

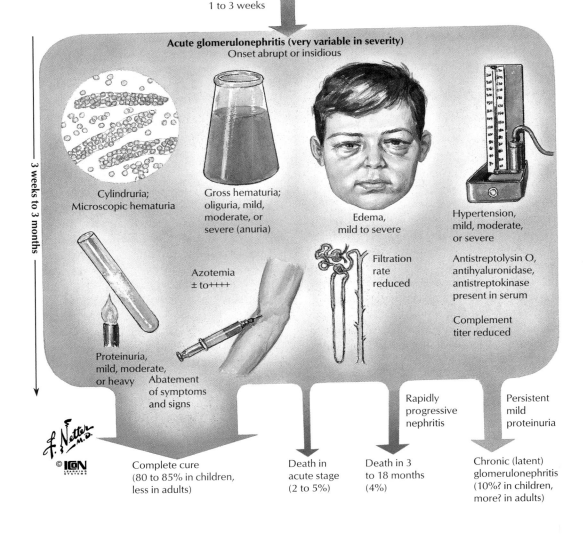

Acute glomerulonephritis (very variable in severity)
Onset abrupt or insidious

3 weeks to 3 months

Cylindruria; Microscopic hematuria

Gross hematuria; oliguria, mild, moderate, or severe (anuria)

Edema, mild to severe

Hypertension, mild, moderate, or severe

Azotemia ± to++++

Filtration rate reduced

Antistreptolysin O, antihyaluronidase, antistreptokinase present in serum

Complement titer reduced

Proteinuria, mild, moderate, or heavy

Abatement of symptoms and signs

Rapidly progressive nephritis

Persistent mild proteinuria

Complete cure (80 to 85% in children, less in adults)

Death in acute stage (2 to 5%)

Death in 3 to 18 months (4%)

Chronic (latent) glomerulonephritis (10%? in children, more? in adults)

Figure 114-4

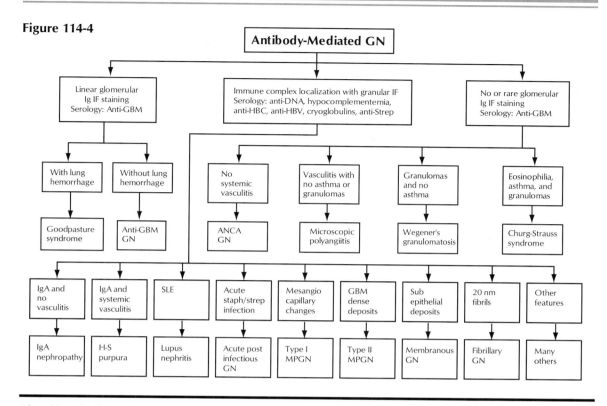

Adapted from The *Kidney*, 6th ed., Brenner & Rector, 2000: 1314; with permission from Elsevier.

with diuretics, diminution of hyperlipidemia, prevention of osteoporosis from glucocorticoids, and a moderate restriction of protein intake (avoiding protein malnutrition in patients with severe proteinuria).

Some diseases require observation alone, including thin basement membrane disease, Alport's syndrome, and mild glomerular injury. Post-streptococcal glomerulonephritis typically resolves spontaneously, but other peri-infectious diseases may require specific treatment of the underlying infection, including antiviral therapy in hepatitis C-associated conditions. Glucocorticoid therapy, usually given orally, is useful in patients with many types of acute nephritis, especially those in whom renal impairment may ensue. Glucocorticoids are usually started at 1 mg/kg/day of prednisone for the first 2 to 4 weeks, and then rapidly titrated to an alternate-day regime, and discontinued by the end of 3 to 4 months. This approach is used in treating lupus nephritis, ANCA glomerulonephritis, and milder forms of other types of glomerulonephritis. The use of cyclophosphamide is indicated for patients with severe lupus nephritis, anti-GBM disease, Goodpasture's syndrome, and ANCA-glomerulonephritis or vasculitis. The method in which cyclophosphamide is administered has varied, although monthly intravenous doses for at least 6 months has been recommended for the treatment of lupus nephritis. A "consolidation treatment" is extended for an additional 18 months to preserve renal remission in severe lupus nephritis. Similarly, both intravenous cyclophosphamide and oral cyclophosphamide have been used in the treatment of ANCA glomerulonephritis. The duration and intensity of therapy must match the intensity and severity of the underlying glomerular/systemic inflammation. Data do not allow for specific recommendations, but generally 6 to 12 months is usually sufficient for almost all forms of glomerulonephritis.

Some conditions are life-threatening as a consequence of pulmonary hemorrhage or rapidly progressive glomerulonephritis. In these most aggressive forms of disease, induction therapy

Figure 114-5 **Clinical Course of Chronic Glomerulonephritis**

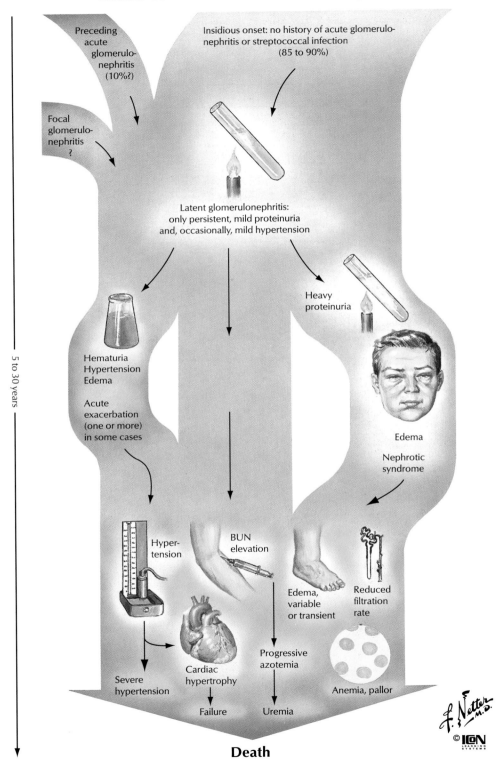

with intravenous methylprednisolone at a dose of 7 mg/kg on 3 consecutive days is useful adjunctive therapy. Pulmonary hemorrhage is treated with plasmapheresis in addition to glucocorticoids and cyclophosphamide.

The outcome of patients with aggressive forms of glomerulonephritis depends on a prompt diagnosis and the early institution of therapy. The milder the inflammation and the lower the serum creatinine at the time of initiation of therapy, the smaller is the risk of progression to end-stage renal disease. Delay in diagnosis and therapy adversely affects long-term outcome in all forms of glomerular inflammation. (Figure 114-5)

FUTURE DIRECTIONS

Very little is known about the precise pathogenesis of any form of glomerulonephritis, so it is difficult to target therapy on the basis of the actual cause of these disorders. New pharmaceutic agents are on the horizon that interfere with specific portions of the immune system's effector arm. Specific drugs that block the effect of cytokines, including tumor necrosis factor, IL-1, and IL-8, and transforming growth factor-β as well as complement component inhibitors are at various stages of development. Agents that inhibit T and B cells are available and have been experimentally used in glomerular diseases, including cyclosporine, tacrolimus, and mycophenolate mofetil. The precise role of these agents in the treatment of glomerular disease remains under investigation.

Precisely targeted therapy will have to await the understanding of proximal causes of glomerular inflammation, while the ultimate goal will be their prevention altogether. Assessment of populations at risk will require a careful understanding of the genes and environmental conditions that spawn glomerular injury.

REFERENCES

Falk RJ, Jennette JC, Nachman PH. Primary glomerular disease. In: Brenner BM, ed. *Brenner and Rector's The Kidney.* 6th ed. Philadelphia, Pa: WB Saunders Co; 2000.

Jennette JC, Falk RJ. Glomerular clinicopathologic syndromes. In: Greenberg A, Cheung AK, Coffman TM, Falk RJ, Jennette JC, eds. *Primer on Kidney Diseases.* 3rd ed. San Diego, Calif: Academic Press; 2001:129-142.

Mandal AK, Jennette JC. The syndrome of glomerulonephritis. In: Mandal AK, Jennette JC, eds. *Diagnosis and Management of Renal Disease and Hypertension.* 2nd ed. Durham, NC: Carolina Academic Press; 1994.

Chapter 115

Urinary Stone Disease (Nephrolithiasis)

Cynthia J. Denu-Ciocca and Romulo E. Colindres

Nephrolithiasis is a common disorder with an annual incidence of 0.1% to 0.4%. The peak age of onset is from ages 20 to 30, and 3 to 4 males are affected for each female affected. Rates of stone formation may be affected by genetic, nutritional, and environmental factors. The relative risk of nephrolithiasis for patients with a positive family history may be as great as 2.5. In the United States, the prevalence of stones is greatest among those who live in the southern latitudes. This may be due to differences in diet and water composition, as well as ambient and sunlight exposure. An estimated 28% to 50% of patients will experience a recurrence at 5 years.

ETIOLOGY AND PATHOGENESIS
Calcium Stones

Approximately 75% to 80% of all kidney stones contain calcium. The majority are composed of calcium oxalate alone or in combination with calcium phosphate. Calcium oxalate stones are brown or gray, small, and well circumscribed on radiographs. Calcium oxalate crystals may appear as dumbbells or pyramids (Figure 115-1). Calcium phosphate stones are beige or white and form brushite crystals. Calcium stones may form in urine that is supersaturated from excess excretion of calcium, oxalate, or uric acid. Diminished citrate in the urine may also lead to calcium stone formation. Hypercalciuria, the most common metabolic disorder in people in whom stones form, affects 50% of patients. Hypercalciuria is classified as absorptive, renal leak, or hormonal.

Absorptive Hypercalciuria

Absorptive hypercalciuria is the most common cause of abnormal calcium excretion. These patients tend to absorb and excrete a higher proportion of dietary calcium than normal people. The disorder is familial and affects both sexes equally.

Renal Leak

Renal leak or renal hypercalciuria is a syndrome of inappropriate renal wasting of calcium. This wasting leads to the stimulation of parathyroid hormone (PTH) and subsequently 1,25 vitamin D in efforts to normalize the serum calcium.

Hormonal Hypercalciuria

Hormonal hypercalciuria may be caused by hyperparathyroidism of both primary and paraneoplastic origin. Granulomatous disorders such as sarcoidosis may also lead to hypercalciuria due to increased levels of 1,25 vitamin D.

Hypocitraturia

Citrate is an inhibitor of calcium stone formation that complexes with calcium, reducing its free urinary concentration, and subsequently decreases the saturation of calcium oxalate and calcium phosphate. *Hypocitraturia* may be idiopathic or secondary to metabolic acidosis, a metabolic state that reduces urinary citrate excretion by increasing its proximal reabsorption. Type I renal tubular acidosis is a defect in hydrogen ion secretion that leads to metabolic acidosis and inability to acidify the urine. More than half of these patients have nephrolithiasis, nephrocalcinosis, or both. Increased bone turnover due to the metabolic acidosis leads to increased filtration of calcium and phosphorus. The metabolic acidosis decreases calcium reabsorption and increases citrate reabsorption. Finally, the alkaline urine pH leads to supersaturation of calcium phosphate.

Hyperoxaluria

Primary hyperoxaluria types I and II are rare

genetic disorders caused by enzyme deficiencies that lead to massive oxaluria. Patients may excrete up to 300 mg per day and deposit calcium oxalate in multiple tissues including kidneys, heart, and blood vessels. *Enteric hyperoxaluria* occurs when small bowel absorption is altered, leading to increased intraluminal bile salts and fatty acids, which increase the permeability of the colonic mucosa to oxalate and bind to calcium. The end result is an increase in the free oxalate available for absorption. This is accompanied by a markedly reduced urinary citrate due to additional bicarbonate loss through the bowel and systemic acidosis.

Hyperuricosuria

There is an increased incidence of hyperuricosuria in calcium stone formers. Uric acid crystals may serve as a nidus for heterogeneous nucleation; 5% to 10% of calcium stones contain a uric acid core.

Uric Acid Stones

Uric acid stones account for 5% to 10% of stones, although in Mediterranean countries they may cause up to 30%. They are yellow or orange and transparent on plain radiography. Urate crystals take various shapes including rhomboids, rosettes, needles, or amorphous material (Figure 115-1). Hyperuricosuria, low urinary volume, and low urine pH predispose to uric acid nephrolithiasis. Excessive urinary excretion of uric acid may be secondary to increased dietary intake of purines, hyperuricemic disorders such as tumor lysis syndrome, or related to certain medications. Urine pH is the major determinant of uric acid supersaturation; an increase to 6.5 can increase the solubility markedly and possibly dissolve existing stones. Decreased urinary volume also increases uric acid supersaturation.

Struvite Stones (Magnesium Ammonium Phosphate)

"Infection stones" (10% to 15% of all stones), the most common cause of staghorn calculi, are more prevalent in women (Figure 115-2). They are light brown and appear laminated on radiograph. Struvite crystals have the classic coffin lid appearance (Figure 115-1). They are associated with infections of the urinary tract by urease-producing bacteria. Hydrolysis of urea sets up a cascade of events that leads to supersaturation of magnesium ammonium phosphate.

Cystine Stones

Less than 2% of all stones are composed of cystine. They are yellow-green and homogeneous on radiograph. Cystine crystals take a hexagonal form, and the stones are often bilateral and may cause staghorn calculi (Figure 115-2). Cystinuria is an autosomal recessive disease in which there is a tubular defect in dibasic amino acid transport. Affected patients excrete excessive amounts of cystine, ornithine, arginine, and lysine. Cystine has a low solubility (300 mg/L), and affected patients may excrete 480 to 3,600 mg/day.

CLINICAL PRESENTATION

The typical presentation of nephrolithiasis is renal colic caused by an acute obstruction of the urinary tract. Severe pain begins suddenly in the flank and radiates laterally around the abdomen to the groin, testicles, or labia (Figure 115-3). Urinary frequency and dysuria may occur when the stone reaches the ureterovesicular junction. Nausea and vomiting are common. Microscopic hematuria occurs in 75% of patients and gross hematuria in 20% or less.

DIAGNOSTIC APPROACH

The usual diagnostic approach is to obtain an imaging study. Radiography of the kidneys, ureters, and bladder (KUB) reveals most stones, with the exception of uric acid stones. Ultrasound of the urinary tract is noninvasive, identifies all stone types including uric acid stones, and can assess the presence of obstruction. Unfortunately, ureteral stones are not well visualized. Intravenous pyelography (IVP) provides information on the structure and function of the urinary tract, as well as determining the cause, site, and severity of obstruction. Recently, unenhanced helical CT has become the standard radiological test for evaluating patients with acute renal colic in many centers. CT requires less time to perform, has an excellent sensitivity and specificity (96% and 99%, respectively), it obviates the risks of intravenous contrast material, and detects extraurinary diseases that may present with symptoms similar to renal colic. Once a diagnosis of

Figure 115-1

Unorganized Elements Which May Be Found in Urinary Sediment

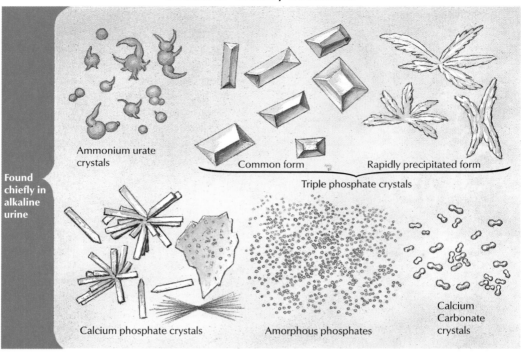

Found chiefly in alkaline urine

Ammonium urate crystals

Common form

Rapidly precipitated form

Triple phosphate crystals

Calcium phosphate crystals

Amorphous phosphates

Calcium Carbonate crystals

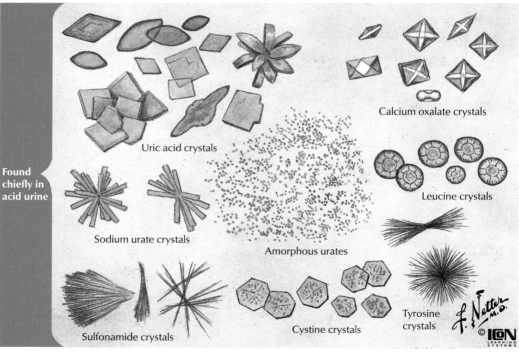

Found chiefly in acid urine

Uric acid crystals

Calcium oxalate crystals

Leucine crystals

Sodium urate crystals

Amorphous urates

Sulfonamide crystals

Cystine crystals

Tyrosine crystals

Figure 115-2

Renal Calculi

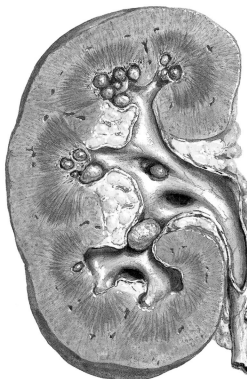

Multiple small calculi

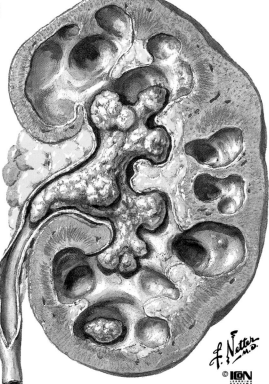

Plain film: multiple renal calculi

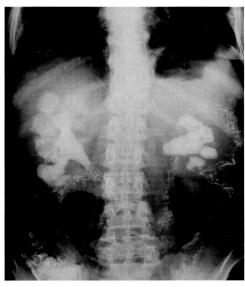

Bilateral staghorn calculi

Staghorn calculus plus smaller stone

Figure 115-3   ## Calculous Urinary Obstruction

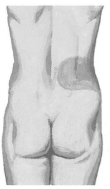
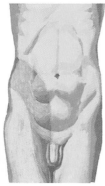

Distribution of pain in renal colic

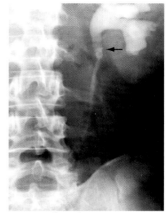

Ureteropelvic obstruction

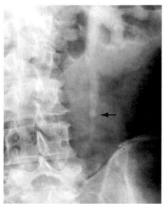

Midureteral obstruction

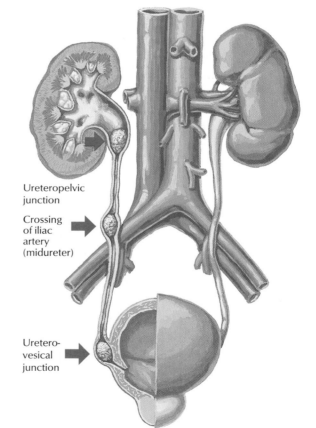

Ureteropelvic
junction

Crossing
of iliac
artery
(midureter)

Uretero-
vesical
junction

Distal ureteral obstruction

Common sites of obstruction

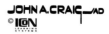

Table 115-1
Evaluation of Patients with Nephrolithiasis

History
  Stone history
  Medical diseases associated with stone disease:
    sarcoidosis, inflammatory bowel disease,
    malignancy
  Family history: age of onset, type of nephrolithiasis
  Medications: loop diuretics, indinovir
  Social history: occupation
  Diet: fluids, protein, purine, sodium, calcium,
    oxalate

Laboratory studies
  Stone analysis
  Urinalysis and culture
  Serum electrolytes, BUN*, creatinine, calcium,
    phosphorous, uric acid, PTH† if the calcium is
    elevated

Adapted from Bushinsky, DA. Nephrolithiasis. *Journal of the American Society of Nephrology.* 1998 9(5): 918, and *Seminars in Nephrology,* 16(5). Monk R., Clinical Approach to Adults. 375-388, 1996, with permission from Elsevier.
* BUN- blood urea nitrogen
† PTH-parathyroid hormone

Table 115-2
Normal 24-Hour Urinary Values

Volume	>2 – 2.5 L
Calcium	<300 mg in men, <250 mg in women
Uric acid	<800 mg in men, <750 mg in women
Oxalate	<40 mg
Citrate	>320 mg
Phosphorus	<1,000 mg
Sodium	<200 mEq
pH	5.0 to 7.0

Adapted from *Seminars in Nephrology,* 16(5). Monk R., Clinical Approach to Adults. 381, 1996, with permission from Elsevier.

nephrolithiasis has been made, an evaluation should be performed as outlined in Table 115-1.

Although some recommend further metabolic screening on all patients with nephrolithiasis, it is generally accepted that patients with recurrent stone disease, nephrocalcinosis, and all children should undergo a 24-hour urine collection to establish risk factors for nephrolithiasis. Obtaining at least two 24-hour urine samples on a normal diet is optimal. The normal values of all the constituents that should be tested are listed in Table 115-2.

MANAGEMENT AND THERAPY

In the acute phase of renal colic, the goal of management is to relieve pain, treat infection, and establish the size and location of the stone and presence of obstruction. Most ureteral stones less than 5 mm in diameter pass spontaneously. Stones 7 mm in diameter or greater rarely pass spontaneously, and urologic management including extracorporeal shock wave lithotripsy, ureteroscopic removal, or percutaneous nephrolithotomy (PCNL) may be needed.

To decrease the incidence of stone recurrence, all patients should be treated with nonspecific therapy. Urinary volume should exceed 2 L/day. Increased urinary volume alone has been shown to reduce the incidence of recurrent nephrolithiasis. Certain dietary restrictions have been shown to change urine constituents favorably. A low protein diet (0.8 g/kg/day) is recommended for stone formers because a high protein diet (2.0 g/kg/day) increases uric acid and calcium excretion and reduces citrate excretion. Multiple studies have shown that high dietary sodium intake increases sodium and calcium excretion, and low sodium diets have the opposite effect; therefore a modest sodium dietary restriction (2 to 3 g/day) is recommended. Dietary restriction of calcium is not recommended to prevent calcium stones. A recent study has shown a decreased risk of nephrolithiasis in patients with normal calcium intake. In addition to conservative measures, specific therapy should be tailored to patients with recurrent stone disease.

Calcium Stones

In *hypercalciuria*, thiazide diuretics decrease urinary calcium excretion by reducing intestinal calcium reabsorption and increasing renal tubular reabsorption. Thiazides are the first line of treatment for patients with renal leak syndrome and have been shown to be effective in reducing stone recurrence in patients with idiopathic hypercalciuria. Adding potassium citrate may be helpful to avoid associated hypokalemia, as well as offering the benefit of increasing citraturia. Parathyroid surgery is the treatment of choice for patients with primary hyperparathyroidism and nephrolithiasis. In *hypocitraturia*, potassium alkali salts significantly reduce the rates of stone recurrence. Potassium citrate or potassium magnesium citrate at doses of 15 to 30 mEq 2 to 3 times daily may be needed. The goal of treatment of calcium phosphate stones due to type I *renal tubular acidosis* is to reduce systemic metabolic acidosis, which in turn decreases bone resorption and urinary calcium excretion and increases citraturia. Potassium citrate or potassium bicarbonate may be used, but large doses are often required. A thiazide diuretic may be added if hypercalciuria persists. *Primary oxaluria* is treated with dietary oxalate restriction and increased urinary volume. Some patients may benefit from pyridoxine therapy. For *enteric hyperoxaluria,* calcium supplementation with meals will bind dietary oxalate. A low-fat diet and cholestyramine to bind bile acids may decrease oxalate absorption. For patients with metabolic acidosis due to diarrhea, potassium citrate may be a helpful adjuvant therapy. Dietary purine restriction and increasing urinary volume are first-line treatments for *hyperuricosuria*. If it persists, allopurinol should be added.

Uric Acid Stones

Conservative therapy including increased urinary volume and dietary restriction of protein and purine products may decrease uric acid supersaturation. Urinary alkalinization with potassium citrate or potassium bicarbonate to a pH of 6.0 to 7.0 may help dissolve existing stones and prevent recurrence. Add allopurinol if urinary pH remains low or if hyperuricosuria persists despite dietary modification.

Struvite Stones

Therapy is aimed at removing existing calculi,

which harbor the urease-producing bacteria, and eradicating infection. Acetohydroxamic acid, an inhibitor of urease production, has been shown to reduce the rate of stone growth but is poorly tolerated due to its multiple side effects.

Cystine Stones

The goal of therapy is to increase the solubility of cystine in the urine with hydration and alkalinization (pH 6.5 to 7.0) For patients with severe disease, more specific therapy with D-penicillamine may be necessary to reduce cystine excretion.

FUTURE DIRECTIONS

Two areas of interest in stone prevention include the use of potassium magnesium citrate and the study of urinary protein inhibitors. Potassium magnesium citrate may be a preferable agent given the fact that magnesium acts as an inhibitor of stone formation. Future research may investigate specific urinary proteins, such as fibronectin and osteopontin, and their role as inhibitors of calcium oxalate nephrolithiasis.

The trend in urologic treatment of nephrolithiasis is for fewer percutaneous procedures and more ureteroscopic approaches. Diagnostically, helical CT is widely used as the initial screening study for patients with renal colic. Magnetic resonance urography is being investigated as an alternative diagnostic test. While it offers the benefit of avoidance of intravenous contrast material, use may be limited by cost and availability.

REFERENCES

Bushinsky DA. Nephrolithiasis. *J Am Soc Nephrol.* 1998;9:917-924.

Chen MY, Zagoria RJ, Saunders HS, Dyer RB. Trends in the use of unenhanced helical CT for acute urinary colic. *AJR Am J Roentgenol.* 1999;173:1447-1450.

Coe FL, Parks JH, Asplin JR. The pathogenesis and treatment of kidney stones. *N Engl J Med.* 1992;327:1141-1152.

Monk RD. Clinical approach to adults. *Semin Nephrol.* 1996;16:375-388.

Pak CY. Kidney stones. *Lancet.* 1998;351:1797-1801.

Parks JH, Coe FL. Pathogenesis and treatment of calcium stones. *Semin Nephrol.* 1996;16:398-411.

Chapter 116

Nephrotic Syndrome

Patrick H. Nachman

The hallmark of the nephrotic syndrome is *proteinuria* of 3.5 g/day/1.73 m² body surface area or more, accompanied by *hypoalbuminemia, edema, hyperlipidemia,* and *lipiduria.*

ETIOLOGY AND PATHOGENESIS

The nephrotic syndrome presents as a diverse group of diseases, with various etiologies and pathogeneses. In general, it is due to a primary renal disease or secondary to an underlying systemic disease. Diabetes mellitus is the most common cause of secondary nephrotic syndrome. Other causes are infections, malignancies, connective tissue diseases, exposure to drugs or environmental agents, and hemodynamic or genetic abnormalities (Table 116-1 and Figure 116-1).

The exact mechanisms leading to the severe proteinuria are poorly understood in most cases of primary and secondary nephrotic syndrome. (Figure 116-2)

CLINICAL PRESENTATION

Edema is the most common presenting symptom. Reduced plasma oncotic pressure has long been considered the proximal cause of intravascular depletion resulting in salt and water retention by the kidney (Figure 116-3). This concept is challenged by the fact that some patients have an increased plasma volume and hypertension. Furthermore, in children with a relapse of minimal change glomerulopathy, sodium retention may precede the reduction in serum protein concentrations, and natriuresis can start before the hypoalbuminemia has resolved with treatment. Enhanced tubular sodium reabsorption is instead likely a function of multiple mediator systems including the activation of the renin-angiotensin-aldosterone pathway, the sympathetic nervous system, and the vasopressor system.

Hypercholesterolemia and hypertriglyceridemia (with increases in both LDL and VLDL) are thought to be the consequence of both increased synthesis and decreased catabolism, and may persist well after clinical remission has occurred. Hypercholes-terolemia is largely due to hepatic overproduction of lipoproteins and appears to be stimulated by the fall in oncotic pressure. An acquired defect in the LDL receptor results in a diminished clearance of LDL. *Lipiduria* is reflected by the presence of oval fat bodies in the urine. These are sloughed tubular epithelial cells engorged with excess lipids and lipoproteins. *Hypoalbuminemia* is a consequence of urinary losses and increased albumin catabolism, while hepatic albumin synthesis is increased.

As a consequence of the urinary losses of immunoglobulins and defects in the complement cascade, nephrotic patients have an increased susceptibility to infection, particularly peritonitis.

Several abnormalities of the coagulation system may result in venous and, less frequently, arterial thrombi. Thrombi may occur in virtually any venous bed, but have a predilection for the renal veins. The hypercoagulability is attributed to urinary losses of anti-coagulant factors such as proteins C and S and antithrombin III, as well as to intravascular consumption.

MAJOR FORMS OF PRIMARY NEPHROTIC SYNDROME
Minimal Change Glomerulopathy

Minimal change glomerulopathy (MCG) is most common in children. It accounts for 70% to 90% of cases of nephrotic syndrome in children under 10 years old, and 10% to 15% of cases of primary nephrotic syndrome in adults. MCG has no glomerular lesions by light microscopy and no staining with antisera specific for immunoglobulins or complement by immunofluorescence microscopy (Figure 116-4). Electron microscopy reveals effacement of visceral epithelial cell foot processes. Primary MCG is thought to be mediated by an as yet unidentified T cell lymphokine that increases glomerular permeability to protein. The

Table 116-1
Underlying Causes of the Nephrotic Syndrome and Associated Pathologic Findings

Underlying Cause	Disease
Infections	
HIV	Collapsing FSGS
Hepatitis C virus	MPGN > MGN
Hepatitis B virus	MGN > MPGN
Subacute bacterial infections (endocarditis, osteomyelitis)	MPGN, MGN
Malaria	proliferative GN > MGN
Syphilis	MGN > MPGN
Autoimmune	
Autoimmune thyroiditis	MGN
Systemic lupus erythematosus	MGN, MPGN
Allergic	
Food allergies	MCD
Malignancies	
Hodgkin's lymphoma	MCD
non-Hodgkin's lymphoma, leukemia	MGN
Solid tumors	MGN
Metabolic and hemodynamic	
Diabetes mellitus	Diabetic nephropathy
Obesity	FSGS
Sickle cell disease	FSGS
Cyanotic congenital heart disease	FSGS
Congenital pulmonary disease	FSGS
Nephron loss	FSGS
Exposures	
NSAIDs	MCG
Penicillamine, gold	MGN
Heroin, IV drug abuse	Collapsing FSGS
Genetic	Familial FSGS

FSGS, Focal segmental glomerulosclerosis; GN, glomerulonephritis; MCG, minimal change glomerulopathy; MGN, membranous glomerulopathy; MPGN, membranoproliferative glomerulonephritis; NSAIDs, nonsteroidal antiinflammatory drugs.

cardinal clinical feature of MCG is the abrupt onset of the nephrotic syndrome. Hypertension and renal insufficiency, while rare in children, may be seen in older adults.

Focal Segmental Glomerulosclerosis

Focal segmental glomerulosclerosis (FSGS) is a clinical-pathologic syndrome that likely encompasses diseases of multiple etiologies and pathogenic mechanisms. The incidence of FSGS has increased over the past 2 decades; it is the most common cause of nephrotic syndrome among African Americans. FSGS may be a primary renal disease, or it may be associated with a variety of other conditions (Table 116-1). On histologic studies, it is characterized by focal and segmental glomerular sclerosis. Although many specimens have nonspecific patterns of sclerosis, at least 3 major structural variants are recognized.

The perihilar variant is characterized by sclerotic lesions that have a predilection for the glomerular perihilar segments and are accompanied usually by hyalinosis and adhesions to Bowman's capsule. There is no staining for immunoglobulins or complement by immunofluorescence microscopy. Electron microscopy reveals focal foot process effacement.

The collapsing glomerulopathy variant may be seen in HIV nephropathy, with intravenous drug abuse, or as an idiopathic process. The characteristic feature is focal segmental or global collapse of glomerular capillaries with obliteration of capillary lumens. Visceral epithelial cells that overlie collapsed segments usually are enlarged and contain conspicuous resorption droplets.

The glomerular tip lesion variant is characterized by consolidation of the glomerular segment that is adjacent to the origin of, and may project into the lumen of the proximal tubule. Visceral epithelial cells adjacent to the consolidated segment are enlarged and contain clear vacuoles and hyaline droplets.

The pathogenesis of FSGS is poorly understood. Many theories suggest that podocyte injury is a component of the pathogenetic process. FSGS may result from the loss of nephrons, which causes compensatory intraglomerular hypertension and hypertrophy in the remaining glomeruli, although data from long-term studies of uninephrectomized individuals have demonstrated either none or only a small increase in mild proteinuria and systolic hypertension. An as yet poorly characterized permeability factor has been described in some patients with primary FSGS, especially in those with recurrent FSGS after transplantation. Microscopic hematuria occurs in over half of patients with FSGS, and approximately one third of patients present with

Figure 116-1

Multiple Etiologies of Nephrotic Syndrome

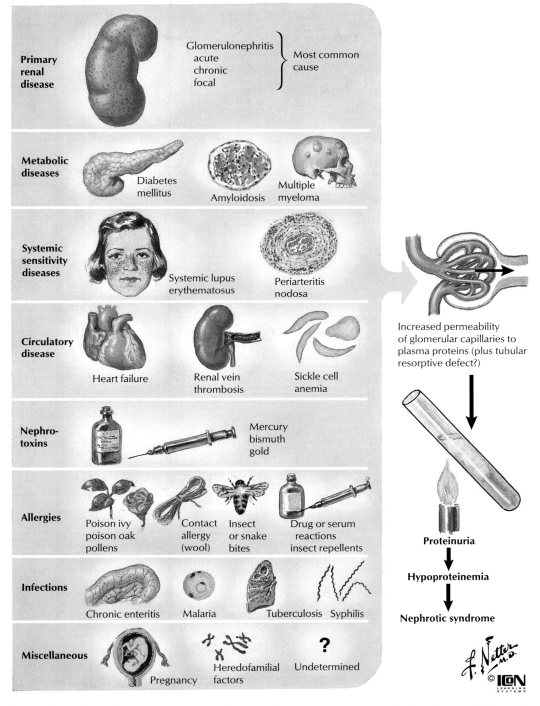

Primary renal disease
Glomerulonephritis
acute
chronic
focal
} Most common cause

Metabolic diseases
Diabetes mellitus
Amyloidosis
Multiple myeloma

Systemic sensitivity diseases
Systemic lupus erythematosus
Periarteritis nodosa

Circulatory disease
Heart failure
Renal vein thrombosis
Sickle cell anemia

Nephro-toxins
Mercury
bismuth
gold

Allergies
Poison ivy poison oak pollens
Contact allergy (wool)
Insect or snake bites
Drug or serum reactions insect repellents

Infections
Chronic enteritis
Malaria
Tuberculosis   Syphilis

Miscellaneous
Pregnancy
Heredofamilial factors
Undetermined

Increased permeability of glomerular capillaries to plasma proteins (plus tubular resorptive defect?)

Proteinuria

Hypoproteinemia

Nephrotic syndrome

some degree of renal insufficiency or hypertension. The collapsing variant often presents with more severe proteinuria and renal insufficiency, and carries a poorer prognosis than the perihilar variant. The glomerular tip lesion variant often presents with rapid onset of edema similar to that in MCG.

Figure 116-2 **Pathophysiologic Factors in Etiology of Nephrotic Edema**

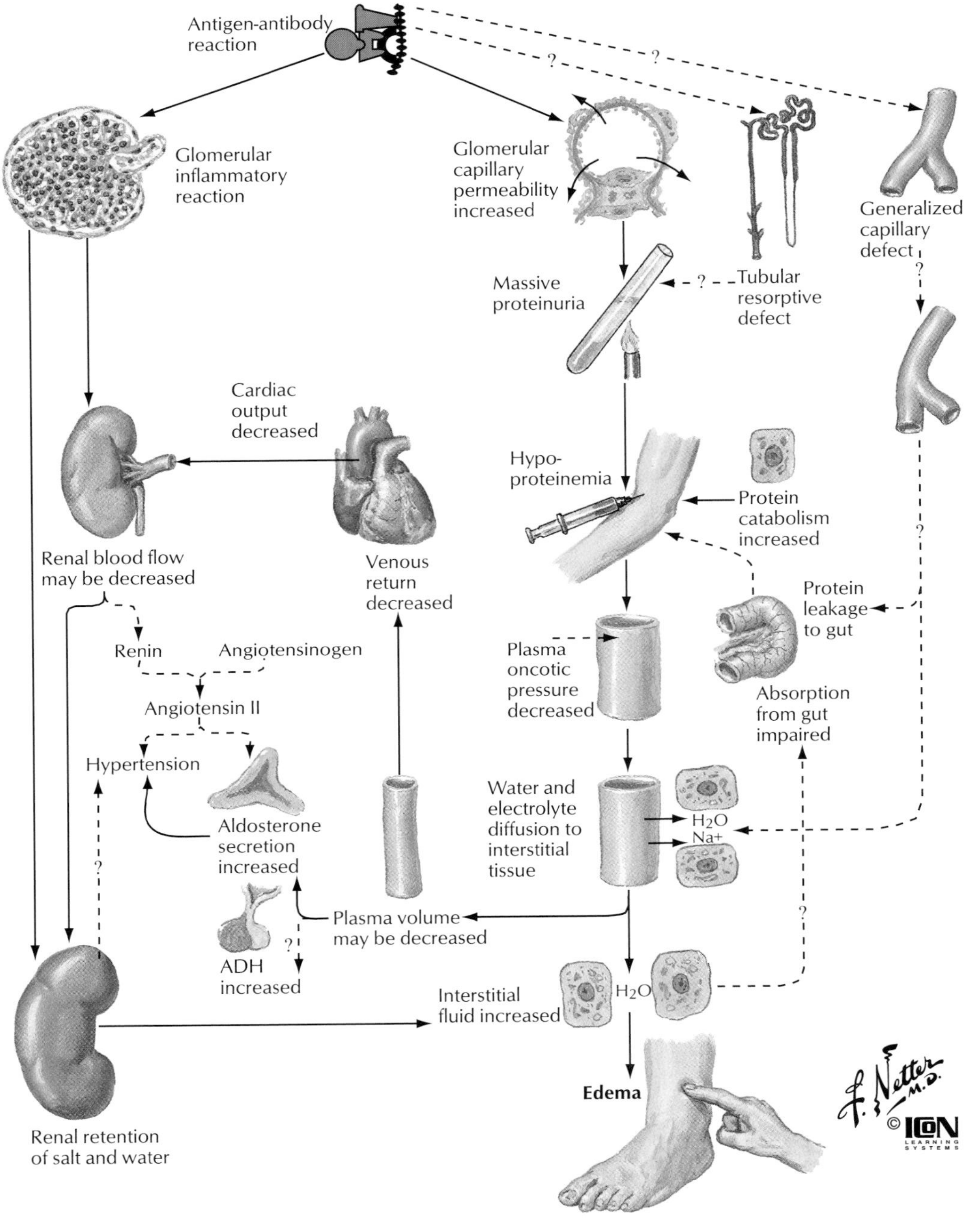
Antigen-antibody reaction
Glomerular inflammatory reaction
Glomerular capillary permeability increased
Generalized capillary defect
Massive proteinuria
Tubular resorptive defect
Cardiac output decreased
Hypo-proteinemia
Protein catabolism increased
Renal blood flow may be decreased
Venous return decreased
Protein leakage to gut
Renin
Angiotensinogen
Plasma oncotic pressure decreased
Angiotensin II
Absorption from gut impaired
Hypertension
Water and electrolyte diffusion to interstitial tissue
H_2O
Na+
Aldosterone secretion increased
Plasma volume may be decreased
ADH increased
Interstitial fluid increased
H_2O
Edema
Renal retention of salt and water
F. Netter M.D.
© ICON LEARNING SYSTEMS

Membranous Glomerulopathy

Membranous glomerulopathy, the most common cause for nephrotic syndrome in white adults, is uncommon in children. The peak incidence is in the fourth or fifth decade. It occurs as an idiopathic (primary) or secondary disease (Table 116-1). Infectious and autoimmune causes are more frequent in children, whereas underlying malignancies are

Figure 116-3

Clinical and Laboratory Findings Which
May Be Present in Nephrotic Syndrome

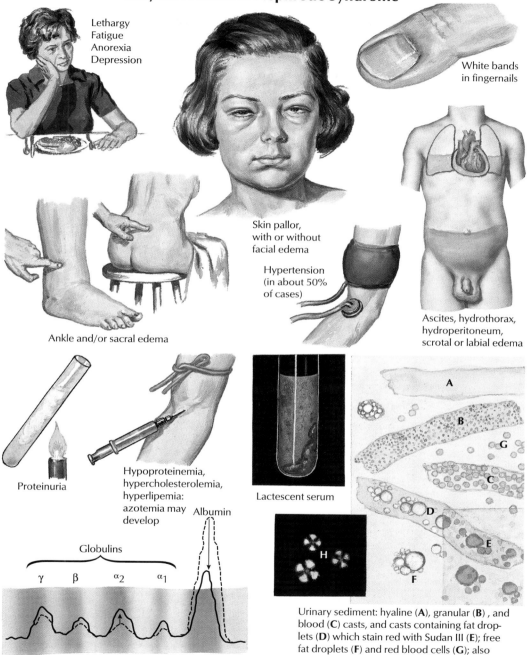

Lethargy
Fatigue
Anorexia
Depression

White bands
in fingernails

Skin pallor,
with or without
facial edema

Hypertension
(in about 50%
of cases)

Ankle and/or sacral edema

Ascites, hydrothorax,
hydroperitoneum,
scrotal or labial edema

Proteinuria

Hypoproteinemia,
hypercholesterolemia,
hyperlipemia:
azotemia may
develop

Lactescent serum

Albumin

Globulins

γ β α_2 α_1

Serum albumin decreased, α_2 – globulin increased
(broken line indicates normal)

Urinary sediment: hyaline (**A**), granular (**B**), and
blood (**C**) casts, and casts containing fat droplets (**D**) which stain red with Sudan III (**E**); free
fat droplets (**F**) and red blood cells (**G**); also
cholesterol ester crystals (maltese crosses)
(**H**) demonstrated by polarized light

Figure 116-4

Pathology of the Nephrotic Syndrome

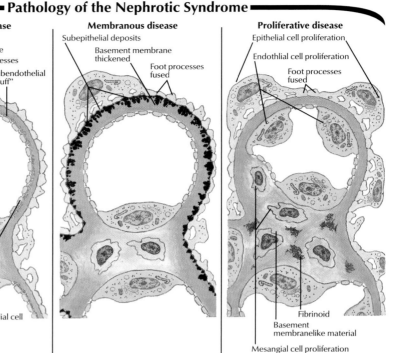

Minimal disease

Epithelial cell
Basement membrane
Foot procesesses fused
Subendothelial "fluff"
Glomerular capillary lumen
Endothelial cell
Mesangial cell

Membranous disease

Subepithelial deposits
Basement membrane thickened
Foot processes fused

Proliferative disease

Epithelial cell proliferation
Endothlial cell proliferation
Foot processes fused
Fibrinoid
Basement membranelike material
Mesangial cell proliferation

Electron microscopic findings: Only fusion of epithelial foot processes and some subendothelial "fluff"

Electron microscopic findings: Electron-dense deposits beneath epithelial cells, thickening of basement membrane, and fusion of foot processes

Electron microscopic findings: Epithelial, endothelial, and mesangial cell proliferation; little or no thickening of basement membrane, but variable amount of basement membranelike material (mesangial matrix) deposited in mesangium; foot processes fused

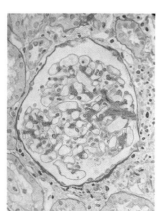

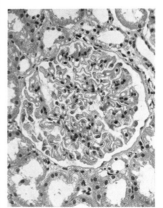

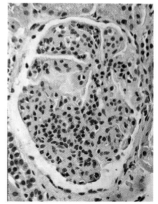

Light microscopic findings: Glomerulus appears normal; protein may be present in tubule lumina and lipoid droplets in tubule cells (pas, x 250)

Light microscopic findings: Basement membrane thickened and eosinophilic; prominence but no numerical increase of epithelial, endothelial, and mesangial cells (H. & E., x 250)

Light microscopic appearance: Cellular proliferation – epithelial, endothelial, and mesangial; very little, if any, basement membrane thickening (H. & E., x 250)

found in 20% to 30% of patients older than 60. The characteristic histologic abnormality is diffuse global capillary wall thickening associated with subepithelial immune complex deposits, in the absence of significant glomerular hypercellularity (Figure 116-4). By immunofluorescence microscopy, there is diffuse granular capillary wall staining for immunoglobulin and complement. In idiopathic membranous glomerulopathy, the nature of the antigen(s) involved in the subepithelial immune complexes is unknown. The immune complexes activate the complement pathway leading to the formation of the C5b to C9 membrane attack complex and injury to the epithelial cells. Patients usually present with normal or slightly decreased renal function. If progressive renal insufficiency develops, it is usually relatively indolent, resulting in end-stage renal disease in 25% of patients. Twenty-five percent of patients may have a complete spontaneous remission of proteinuria within 5 years.

Membranoproliferative Glomerulonephritis

Type I membranoproliferative glomerulonephritis (MPGN) is characterized by diffuse global capillary wall thickening and endocapillary hypercellularity with infiltrating mononuclear leukocytes and neutrophils (Figure 116-4). Immunofluorescence microscopy reveals a characteristic pattern of peripheral granular to band-like staining for complement, especially C3, and usually immunoglobulins. Electron microscopy reveals prominent subendothelial immune complexes with associated subendothelial mesangial interposition. The identity of the antigen(s) involved in the immune complexes is unknown in most cases.

Type II MPGN, also termed "dense deposit disease," is characterized by discontinuous electron dense bands within glomerular basement membranes. Immunofluorescence microscopy demonstrates intense capillary wall band-like staining for C3, with little or no staining for immunoglobulin. The pathologic findings suggest that the deposited immune complexes or complement result in the proliferation of mesangial and endothelial cells, and the recruitment of inflammatory cells, including neutrophils and monocytes.

Hypocomplementemia is a frequent feature of all types of MPGN. Complement activation occurs through the classical pathway initiated by immune complex formation in type I MPGN, and by the alternate pathway in type II MPGN. C3 nephritic factor (C3NeF), an autoantibody that binds to C3 convertase and prevents its inactivation, is found in more than 60% of patients with MPGN type II.

The clinical features of all forms of MPGN are usually that of the nephrotic syndrome but approximately 30% of patients (especially patients with type II) present with an acute nephritic syndrome with hematuria, hypertension, and renal insufficiency. In general, one third of patients with type I MPGN will have a spontaneous remission, one third will have progressive disease, and one third will have a disease process that will wax and wane but never completely disappear. The prognosis for type II disease is worse than that for type I, and clinical remissions are rare.

DIFFERENTIAL DIAGNOSIS

In the evaluation of patients with proteinuria, non-glomerular causes, such as *functional* or *transient* proteinuria, and *orthostatic* proteinuria should be excluded. These types of proteinuria rarely exceed 500 mg/day.

DIAGNOSTIC APPROACH

The diagnosis of the nephrotic syndrome begins with quantifying the proteinuria using a 24-hour urine collection measurement of protein and creatinine excretion. The latter allows verifying that the collection is adequate as the normal creatinine excretion is 20 to 25 mg/kg/day for males and 15 to 20 mg/kg/day for females.

Unless an underlying systemic disease is evident, a renal biopsy is usually required in adults to establish the specific diagnosis of the nephrotic syndrome and to assess the severity and acuity of the renal disease. This is accompanied by a serologic workup that includes testing for hepatitis B and C, HIV, syphilis, ANA, cryoglobulins, and hypocomplementemia. Based on the clinical presentation, testing for chronic infections such as subacute endocarditis is necessary. The search for occult malignancies is warranted, especially for older adults.

MANAGEMENT AND THERAPY

The management of edema requires dietary restriction of sodium intake and the judicious use of diuretics. Overzealous diuresis should be avoided as it may result in intravascular depletion, hypotension, and acute renal failure. Mild diuretics, including thiazides, may be sufficient with mild edema, while loop diuretics are typically used for moderate to severe edema.

The hyperlipidemia of the nephrotic syndrome predisposes to atherosclerotic cardiovascular disease and may contribute to the progression of renal disease. The treatment of hyperlipidemia is difficult, the most useful agents being the HMG-CoA reductase inhibitors and bile acids sequestrants. Because of their anti-proteinuric and nephroprotective effect, angiotensinconverting enzyme inhibitors and angiotensin receptor blockers are the agents of choice in treating nephrotic patients with hypertension.

The treatment of secondary forms of nephrotic syndrome depends on the underlying disease. When the syndrome is associated with the use of medicines such as NSAIDs, the proteinuria may resolve with cessation of the offending agent. Similarly, peri-infectious nephrotic syndrome typically responds to treatment of the underlying infection.

For the primary diseases causing the nephrotic syndrome, various therapies apply depending on the pathologic diagnosis.

Minimal change glomerulopathy is treated primarily with corticosteroids resulting in the disappearance of proteinuria in more than 90% of children within 4 to 6 weeks, but may take up to 15 weeks in adults. After the clinical response to initial treatment, as few as 25% of patients have a long-term remission, 25 to 30% have infrequent relapses (≤ one per year), and the remainder have frequent relapses, steroid-dependence or steroid-resistance. Frequently relapsing or steroid-dependent nephrotic patients may require the use of cyclophosphamide. Cyclosporine may lead to a partial or complete remission in up to 90% of patients with steroid-resistant MCG, but relapses are frequent once the drug is discontinued.

The treatment of patients with FSGS remains controversial. While some studies suggested that only 15% of patients responded to corticosteroids, more recent reports suggest that 40% to 55% of adult patients may attain some form of remission with the prolonged use of high dose corticosteroids. The data currently available do not take into account a careful assessment of the risk-benefit ratio of such treatments. Cyclosporine has been used with varying degrees of success and an elevated rate of relapse.

In patients with membranous glomerulopathy, a pooled analysis of randomized and prospective studies demonstrated a lack of benefit of corticosteroids in inducing a remission of the nephrotic syndrome or on renal survival. The current approach includes the use of an alkylating agent such as chlorambucil or cyclophosphamide, which improves the chance of a complete remission of proteinuria by fourfold to fivefold, but may not significantly alter the long-term renal survival. Cyclosporin A may also lead to a complete or partial clinical remission of proteinuria in as many as 75% of patients, but the rate of relapse after discontinuation of cyclosporin is high.

The treatment of patients with type I MPGN is based on the underlying cause of the disease process. In children, corticosteroid therapy improves renal survival. The addition of anticoagulant therapy with dipyridamole, aspirin, and warfarin is of questionable benefit. Unfortunately, there is no good therapy for type II MPGN.

FUTURE DIRECTIONS

Advances in the diagnosis and treatment of nephrotic syndrome will depend on a better understanding of the precipitating agents (e.g., infectious pathogens or toxins for secondary forms), and the pathogenetic mechanisms involved (e.g., characterization of the "permeability factor" in FSGS). This holds the promise of more specifically targeted therapies that will avoid the need for aggressive immunosuppression.

REFERENCES

Cattran DC. Idiopathic membranous glomerulonephritis. *Kidney Int.* 2001;59:1983-1994.

D'Amico G, Ferrario F. Mesangiocapillary glomerulonephritis. *J Am Soc Nephrol.* 1992;2(suppl):S159-166.

Donckerwolcke RA, Vande Walle JG. Pathogenesis of edema formation in the nephritic syndrome. *Kidney Int Suppl.* 1997;58:S72-S74.

Falk RJ, Jennette JC, Nachman PH. *Primary glomerular disease.* In: Brenner BM, ed. *Brenner and Rector's The Kidney.* 6th ed. Philadelphia, Pa: WB Saunders Co; 2000.

Glassock RJ. Secondary membranous glomeruloephritis. *Nephrol Dial Transplant.* 1992;7(suppl 1):64-71.

Kerjaschki D. Pathogenetic concepts of membranous glomerulopathy (MGN). *J Nephrol.* 2000;13(suppl 3):S96-S100.

Passerini P, Ponticelli C. Treatment of focal segmental glomerulosclerosis. *Curr Opin Nephrol Hypertens.* 2001;10:189-193.

Chapter 117
Urinary Tract Infection

William D. Mattern

Urinary tract infection (UTI) is a broad term describing microbial colonization of the urine and infection of any of the components of the urinary tract, including the urethra, bladder, ureters, renal pelvis, and kidneys. UTI is among the most common reasons for office visits in general medical practice; it is also among the most common predisposing causes for bacteremia and sepsis in hospitalized patients. UTI is divided into 4 categories: asymptomatic bacteriuria (AB), uncomplicated UTI, complicated UTI, and acute pyelonephritis. Uncomplicated UTIs are those that occur in otherwise healthy adult women who are not pregnant and who do not have underlying abnormalities of the urinary tract. Complicated infections are all others.

CLINICAL PRESENTATION, DIAGNOSTIC APPROACH, MANAGEMENT AND THERAPY
Asymptomatic Bacteriuria

In adult, non-pregnant healthy women of childbearing age, the prevalence of AB is approximately 6%, using a urine culture cutoff of >10^5/mL. The most common infecting organism is *Escherichia coli*. Epidemiologic studies have shown that AB may resolve spontaneously, but it is sometimes associated with an increased incidence of symptomatic UTI with the onset of sexual activity. Treatment is not indicated unless there is a history of highly recurrent UTI.

Screening and treatment for AB is an essential part of prenatal care because, untreated, it is associated with a 40% risk of UTI and a 20% to 60% risk of acute pyelonephritis in late pregnancy. AB is also associated with prematurity and low birth weight.

In diabetic women, the incidence of AB may be as high as 18%. Treatment is still not generally recommended because recurrence is extremely high, and no long-term benefit can be documented. Treatment is also not recommended in the elderly who live independently because no adverse effects have been documented. In those with long-term indwelling catheters who are colonized treatment tends to select out resistant strains and will not eradicate bacteriuria while the catheter remains in place.

Uncomplicated Urinary Tract Infection

Acute cystitis is extremely common. Approximately one half of adult women report having had at least one UTI. Young, sexually active women have approximately 0.5 episodes per person year. *E. coli* is responsible for infection in approximately 80% of episodes in healthy adult women, while *Staphylococcus saprophyticus* accounts for most of the rest. Cystitis develops when fecal flora from the rectum colonize the vaginal introitus and periurethral zone, colonize the urethra, ascend into and invade the bladder mucosa, proliferate in the urine, and incite an inflammatory response (Figure 117-1). The shorter urethra may help explain why women are more susceptible than men, but not why some women are more susceptible than others. Studies have indicated that uropathogens, such as *E. coli,* have special characteristics that facilitate this process of colonization and invasion, while other studies indicate that host factors also play a role. Of particular interest are the studies examining the role of behavioral or mechanical factors. In women otherwise predisposed to UTI, the frequency of sexual intercourse and the use of spermicide-containing contraceptives, particularly the diaphragm-spermicide combination, are clearly associated, as is a history of UTI. Perineal hygiene and the direction of wiping have not been shown to be associated.

The usual symptoms of cystitis are dysuria, along with frequency, urgency, suprapubic discomfort (and tenderness), and hematuria. The diagnosis is made by the history, physical examination (temperature, abdominal examination, and testing for costovertebral angle [CVA] tender-

Figure 117-1

Factors in Etiology of Cystitis

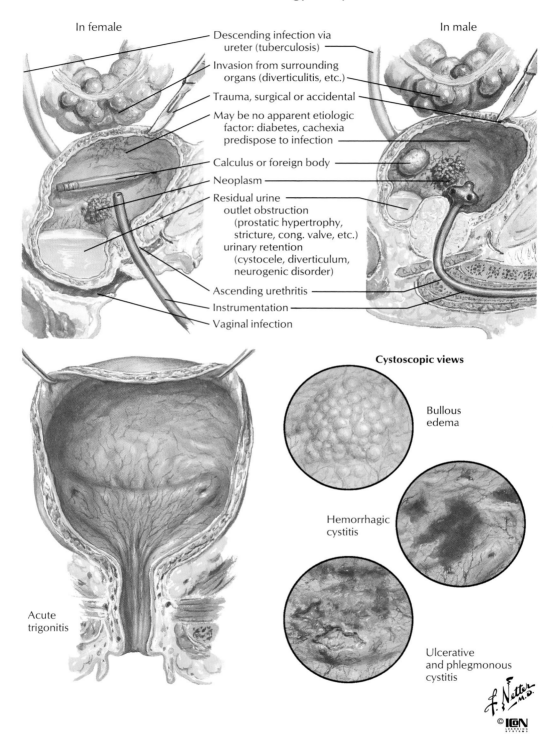

In female

In male

Descending infection via ureter (tuberculosis)

Invasion from surrounding organs (diverticulitis, etc.)

Trauma, surgical or accidental

May be no apparent etiologic factor: diabetes, cachexia predispose to infection

Calculus or foreign body

Neoplasm

Residual urine
  outlet obstruction
    (prostatic hypertrophy,
    stricture, cong. valve, etc.)
  urinary retention
    (cystocele, diverticulum,
    neurogenic disorder)

Ascending urethritis

Instrumentation

Vaginal infection

Cystoscopic views

Bullous edema

Hemorrhagic cystitis

Acute trigonitis

Ulcerative and phlegmonous cystitis

ness), and examination of the urine. Although the gold standard for pyuria is the finding of 10 to 20 leukocytes/mm^3 in an unspun, midstream urine using a counting chamber, examination of the urine sediment for white blood cells and bacteria is more routinely done. In practice, urine dipsticks that detect leukocyte esterase, indicating significant pyuria, and nitrite, indicating the presence of Enterobacteriaceae, which convert nitrate to nitrite, provide a reliable method for excluding and a rapid method for confirming the likelihood of infection. Urine cultures are not routinely done with uncomplicated UTI, unless it fails to resolve with treatment, relapses quickly after treatment, or frequently recurs. Imaging studies of the urinary tract are also unnecessary.

Patients presenting with dysuria as their predominant symptom have the broadest differential diagnosis. Hematuria makes cystitis more likely. Urethritis due to *Neisseria gonorrhea* or *Chlamydia trachomatis* is suggested by a history of sexually transmitted disease (STD), a new partner or one with urethral symptoms, a more gradual or uneven onset, and, when pyuria is present, with negative urine culture results. Pelvic examination is indicated to look for discharge from the urethral or cervical os. Although Gram stain and culture of discharge are still valuable in diagnosing gonococcal infection, DNA amplification tests on urine have now emerged as highly sensitive and specific tests for detection of both chlamydia and *N. gonorrhea*. In patients with dysuria, particularly when it is perceived as an external burning and is accompanied by symptoms of vaginitis (vaginal discharge or odor, pruritus, and dyspareunia), consider infection with *Candida albicans*, *Trichomonas vaginalis*, and *Gardnerella vaginalis*, especially in young, sexually active women. Urine culture results are negative, as above, but pyuria is less common. Pelvic examination to detect and characterize the vaginal discharge is indicated, as well as microscopic examination of the discharge to distinguish among the 3 common infecting organisms and to guide treatment. Three-day, short course antibiotic regimens for uncomplicated UTI, using trimethoprim-sulfamethoxazole, trimethoprim, or the fluoroquinolones (ofloxacin, ciprofloxacin, norfloxacin) are more effective than 1-day regimens, and equally as effective as 7-day regimens with lower cost and better compliance.

Nitrofurantoin, for 7 days, remains an established alternative. Many do not recommend the fluoroquinolones as initial drugs because of concerns about cost and the emergence of resistance. The increasing resistance of *E. coli* to trimethoprim-sulfamethoxazole needs to be kept in mind. No adverse effects on renal function or long-term morbidity have been documented as a consequence of uncomplicated UTI.

Recurrent Urinary Tract Infection

Most recurrent UTI in otherwise healthy women represent reinfection, not relapse or recurrence with the same strain. The epidemiology, organisms, clinical presentation, and treatment regimens are the same as those for initial episodes. Most recurrences occur within 3 months, and single recurrences are quite common. In those predisposed, the frequency of sexual intercourse and the use of the diaphragm-spermicide combination are strongly associated, as is recent antibiotic use and a history of UTI.

Highly recurrent infections, more than 2 within a year, indicate the need to consider preventive and prophylactic measures. Successful approaches, using trimethoprim-sulfamethoxazole, trimethoprim, or the fluoroquinolones (ofloxacin, ciprofloxacin, norfloxacin) have been reported using 3 regimens: continuous daily treatment for at least 6 months, and sometimes for an additional 2 years in the event of relapse; post-coital single-dose treatment if the episodes are temporally related to intercourse; and intermittent self-treatment at the first onset of symptoms in reliable, highly motivated patients. Decisions on which to use are based on physician and patient preference. Imaging studies are almost always unrevealing, and no long-term adverse consequences have been noted.

Complicated Urinary Tract Infection

These include UTI that occurs during pregnancy, in the presence of structural or functional abnormalities of the urinary tract (obstruction, stones, or indwelling urinary catheters), in those with underlying diseases such as diabetes who are immunosuppressed, in the institutionalized elderly, in men, and in children (Figure 117-1). The presence of underlying structural abnormalities determines the nature of invading organisms and choice of thera-

Figure 117-2

Pyelonephritis

Possible Routes of Kidney Infection

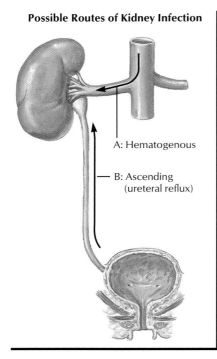

A: Hematogenous

B: Ascending
(ureteral reflux)

Predisposing Factors in Acute Pyelonephritis

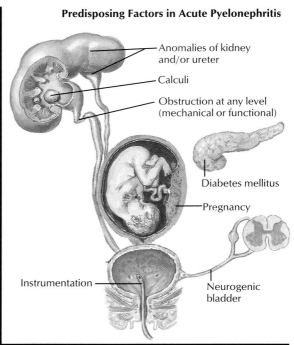

Anomalies of kidney
and/or ureter

Calculi

Obstruction at any level
(mechanical or functional)

Diabetes mellitus

Pregnancy

Instrumentation

Neurogenic
bladder

Common Clinical and Laboratory Features of Acute Pyelonephritis

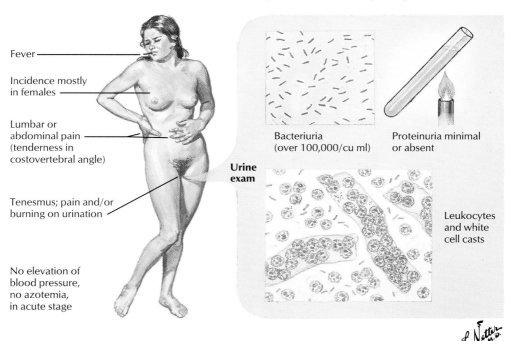

Fever

Incidence mostly
in females

Lumbar or
abdominal pain
(tenderness in
costovertebral angle)

Tenesmus; pain and/or
burning on urination

No elevation of
blood pressure,
no azotemia,
in acute stage

Urine
exam

Bacteriuria
(over 100,000/cu ml)

Proteinuria minimal
or absent

Leukocytes
and white
cell casts

Figure 117-3

Pyelonephritis
Acute Pyelonephritis: Pathology

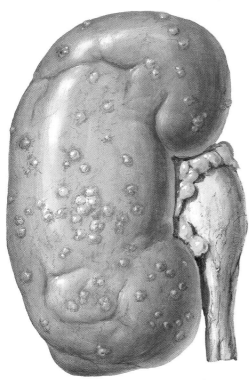

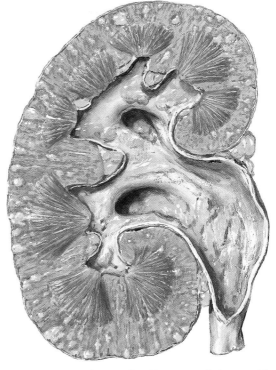

Surface aspect of kidney: Multiple minute abscesses (surface may appear relatively normal in some cases)

Cut section: Radiating yellowish gray streaks in pyramids and abscesses in cortex; moderate hydronephrosis with infection; blunting of calyces (ascending infection)

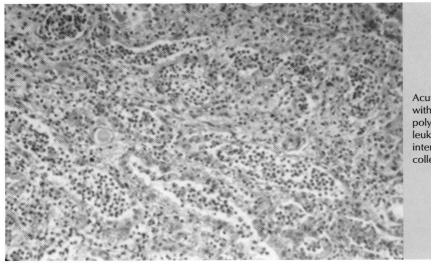

Acute pyelonephritis with exudate chiefly of polymorphonuclear leukocytes in interstitium and collecting tubules

py. Treatment of complicated infections remains difficult; it is most important to relieve obstruction, remove foreign bodies, such as stones and catheters, and restore complete emptying as opposed to eradicating organisms. The latter can include the more resistant strains of *E. coli*, enteric gram-negative organisms, Pseudomonas, *Staphylococcus aureus*, enterococci, yeast, and fungi.

In pregnancy, the focus is on detecting asymptomatic bacteriuria by urine culture and preventing the significant morbidity of UTI and acute pyelonephritis later in pregnancy. The same uropathogens are involved as in uncomplicated UTI. Predisposing factors include dilatation of the ureters and forward displacement of the bladder as the uterus enlarges, along with incomplete emptying. In regard to treatment, trimethoprim and the quinolones are not approved for use, and tetracycline is contraindicated because it concentrates in bone. The beta-lactam antibiotics and nitrofurantoin are highly effective. A single course of therapy is not always effective, and follow-up cultures are mandatory, including in the post-partum period where risk remains high. Abdominal and renal ultrasound studies are indicated in those in whom treatment repeatedly fails. Intravenous antibiotics, guided by urine culture, along with ultrasound studies are indicated for acute pyelonephritis.

In men, UTI may be asymptomatic or present with symptoms of cystitis, prostatitis, epididymitis, or pyelonephritis. Bacteriuria and symptomatic infections are uncommon in males under age 50 in the absence of urinary tract instrumentation or prostatitis. Organisms that persist in the prostate gland and intermittently colonize the bladder urine usually cause recurrent UTI in younger men. Prostatic infections are very difficult to eradicate, especially when prostatic stones are present. In older men, the organisms are those associated with complicated infection, usually in association with obstructive symptoms or use of indwelling catheters. Antibiotic selection should be guided by urine culture. Nitrofurantoin and beta lactams may not achieve predictable tissue concentrations. The fluoroquinolones provide the best initial coverage and adequate tissue levels. The site of infection, severity of symptoms, and frequency of recurrence determine the duration of therapy. Imaging studies are routine, except in younger males with uncomplicated presentations.

Patients with diabetes usually have uncomplicated UTI. However, some diabetics, mostly women with a history of recurrent UTI due to multiple resistant organisms, have an increased risk for severe acute cystitis and acute pyelonephritis, complicated by papillary necrosis, perinephric abscess, and bacteremia. Predisposing factors in these patients include impaired bladder emptying, impaired leukocyte function, and focal damage to the kidney as a consequence of diabetic microangiopathy. Initial therapy with a fluoroquinolone is recommended. Subsequent therapy is guided by cultures and imaging studies of the urinary tract and kidneys. Recurrences are difficult to prevent while impaired emptying persists.

In the elderly who live independently and void normally, UTI is usually uncomplicated and responds to treatment without increased morbidity or mortality. UTI in the more debilitated elderly is usually complicated, often by concomitant disease, by bladder malfunction, incontinence, or indwelling catheters. UTI accounts for more than 50% of episodes of bacteremia in the institutionalized elderly, often in those with long-term indwelling catheters. It is complicated by septic shock in one third of cases, and the fatality rate in patients with bacteremia approaches 20%. These infections may be resistant to multiple antibiotics and are difficult to treat if the underlying abnormalities are not corrected. Incontinence occurs in 5% to 10% of the elderly living independently and in 50% of those in long-term facilities. It should be managed without a catheter whenever possible, using "prompted voiding" in the more responsive or by diapers in women and condom catheters in men. The indwelling catheter is an independent risk factor for premature death.

Acute Pyelonephritis

Acute pyelonephritis presents with fever, flank pain, costovertebral angle tenderness, leukocytosis, pyuria with white cell casts in the urine sediment, positive urine culture results, and frequently, bacteremia (Figures 117-2 and 117-3). Most uncomplicated episodes occur in young women and respond to treatment with no residual damage. In all others, renal and bladder ultrasound studies are standard. These studies are rapid, noninvasive, and less expensive than other radiologic screening procedures, show the extent of renal involvement, eliminate obstruction and stones, and indicate the ability to empty the bladder. The differential diagnosis includes renal or ureteral stones, acute cholecystitis, appendicitis, diverticulitis, tubo-ovarian abscess, and acute pancreatitis. Hospitalization and intravenous drugs are indicated for patients with nausea and who cannot be treated at home; oral treatment is indicated otherwise. The usual duration of treatment is 10 to 14 days, and the fluoroquinolones are recommended for empiric therapy until cultures are available to guide treatment.

FUTURE DIRECTIONS

A better understanding of the factors that predispose to urethral colonization and bladder infection, particularly in otherwise healthy women is needed. Methods of restoring function of the urinary tract that do not predispose to complicated infection are also needed, particularly in the institutionalized elderly. Of course, there is always the need for new antibiotics as resistance emerges to today's standard regimens.

REFERENCES

Hooton TM, Scholes D, Hughes JP, et al. A prospective study of risk factors for symptomatic urinary tract infection in young women. *N Engl J Med*. 1996;335:468-474.

Hooton TM, Stamm WE. Diagnosis and treatment of uncomplicated urinary tract infection. *Infect Dis Clin North Am*. 1997;11:551-581.

Kunin CM. *Urinary Tract Infections: Detection, Prevention, and Management*. 5th ed. Baltimore, Md: Lippincott Williams & Wilkins; 1997.

Nicolle LE, Ronald AR. Recurrent urinary tract infection in adult women: diagnosis and treatment. *Infect Dis Clin North Am*. 1987;1:793-806.

Pappas PG. Laboratory in the diagnosis and management of urinary tract infections. *Med Clin North Am*. 1991;75:313-325.

Stamm WE, Hooton TM. Management of urinary tract infections in adults. *N Engl J Med*. 1993;329:1328-1334.

Warren JW, Abrutyn E, Hebel JR, Johnson JR, Schaeffer AJ, Stamm WE. Guidelines for antimicrobial treatment of uncomplicated acute bacterial cystitis and acute pyelonephritis in women. Infectious Diseases Society of America (IDSA). *Clin Infect Dis*. 1999;29:745-758.

Wong KC, Ho BS, Egglestone SI, Lewis WH. Duplex PCR system for simultaneous detection of Neisseria gonnorrhoeae and Chlamydia trachomatis in clinical specimens. *J Clin Pathol*. 1995;48:101-104.

Section XIV

DISORDERS OF THE RESPIRATORY SYSTEM

Chapter 118
Asthma

David C. Henke

Asthma is a syndrome with a chronic but variable clinical course and presentation. Its main features are: 1) reversible airflow obstruction, 2) nonspecific airways hyperreactivity, and 3) airways inflammation. The nonspecific nature of the hyperreactivity is perhaps a reflection of airway inflammation. It is airway hyperreactivity that predisposes patients to symptoms in a variety of environments.

Both children and adults develop asthma. The remission rate in adults is 10% to 15% but over 50% in children. Despite advances in the understanding of asthma and better medications, asthma morbidity and mortality have increased. Over the past 110 years, our understanding of asthma has changed greatly. It was long considered a disease of "twitchy" airways and a minor ailment that, according to Osler, allowed the patient to "pant into old age." Now, asthma is considered a disease of chronic fluctuating airways inflammation with a lethal potential of 5,000 deaths annually in the United States. It is a major public health problem that results in 1.8 million emergency room visits per year with approximately 10% requiring hospitalization.

ETIOLOGY AND PATHOGENESIS

Asthma manifests as inflammation in the central and peripheral airways. The inflammation results in structural changes in the airway called "remodeling" (e.g., muscle hypertrophy and thickening of the basement membrane) (Figure 118-1). These changes degrade airway function, causing respiratory symptoms and even death by suffocation.

There are clinical and epidemiologic links between asthma and IgE. Transcription factors, such as nuclear factor-KB and members of the signal transduction-activated transcription (STAT) factor family, act on genes encoding for inflammatory cytokines, such as interleukins (ILs), and appear to initiate and sustain airway (Figure 118-2) inflammation. Corticosteroids inhibit these transcription factors and airway inflammation.

A widely held mechanistic explanation holds that inhaled antigen activates mast cells and Th2 lymphocytes, causing mediator release that promotes a persistent eosinophilic airway inflammation. There is no clear understanding of which biologic influences lead to chronic eosinophilic airway inflammation and hyperresponsiveness in asthma. Genetic factors (e.g., polymorphism for the IgE receptor, beta receptor, matrix metalloproteinase, and CD14); environmental factors (e.g., "excessive hygiene" vaccinations); and triggers (e.g., viral infection, exposures to tobacco smoke, pollutants, allergens have all been implicated in the pathogenesis of asthma—see Figure 14-3 in Rhinitis chapter). Most asthmatics are atopic and have IgE-mediated disease, although there is evidence suggesting that "intrinsic" or "nonatopic" asthmatics may produce local, as opposed to circulating, IgE.

The estimates of the rate of decline in pulmonary function vary from those with no asthma from 22 to 35 mL/yr in forced expiratory volume in 1 second (FEV_1) to those with asthma from 38 to 160 ml/yr in FEV_1. Whether "remodeling" contributes to or causes the accelerated loss of pulmonary function is not known.

CLINICAL PRESENTATION

The clinical presentation for asthma is nonspecific (Figure 118-3). Prototypically, the chief complaint consists of the triad: wheezing, shortness of breath, and chest tightness. Symptoms vary in severity with time, sometimes changing in minutes or over many months, but commonly changing daily. Symptoms are typically worse at night. The hyperreactivity is associated with triggers such as respiratory infections and exposure to strong odors or cold air. Repeated allergen exposures lower the threshold for nonspecific hyperreactivity symptoms.

Occasionally, the sole presentation is dyspnea on exertion or cough. Cough-variant asthma is usually

Figure 118-1

Pathology of Asthma

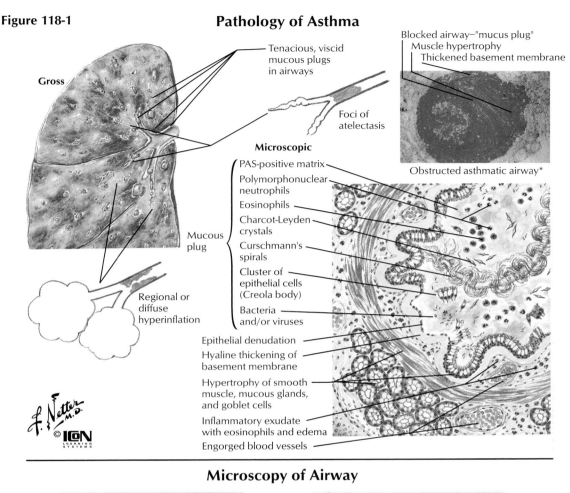

Gross

Tenacious, viscid mucous plugs in airways

Foci of atelectasis

Blocked airway–"mucus plug"
Muscle hypertrophy
Thickened basement membrane

Obstructed asthmatic airway*

Microscopic

PAS-positive matrix
Polymorphonuclear neutrophils
Eosinophils
Charcot-Leyden crystals
Curschmann's spirals
Cluster of epithelial cells (Creola body)
Bacteria and/or viruses

Mucous plug

Regional or diffuse hyperinflation

Epithelial denudation
Hyaline thickening of basement membrane
Hypertrophy of smooth muscle, mucous glands, and goblet cells
Inflammatory exudate with eosinophils and edema
Engorged blood vessels

Microscopy of Airway

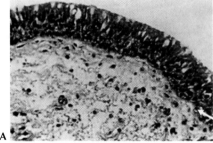

A

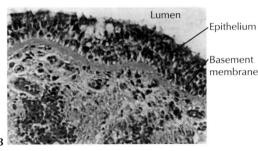

Lumen
Epithelium
Basement membrane

B

(**A**) Normal airway and airway appearance after control of hyperreactivity following high doses of inhaled steroids. (**B**) Asthmatic airway before therapy with high-dose inhaled steriods to control

Courtesy of Nizar N. Jarjour, MD, University of Wisconsin and with permission from Morgenroth, Newhouse, and Nolte. *Atlas of Pulmonary Pathology*. PVG Pharmazeutische Verlagsgesellschaft. 1982: 37.

unproductive. Occasionally, however, the patient produces copious sputum laden with eosinophils and eosinophilic debris, mucus casts of the small airways (Curschmann's spirals), airway epithelial cells (sometimes in clumps referred to as Creola bodies), and Charcot-Leyden crystals (protein from eosinophils) (Figure 118-4). Thirty percent or more of patients with chronic cough have asthma.

Acute exacerbations generally present, by patient history, as a sudden onset of respiratory

Figure 118-2

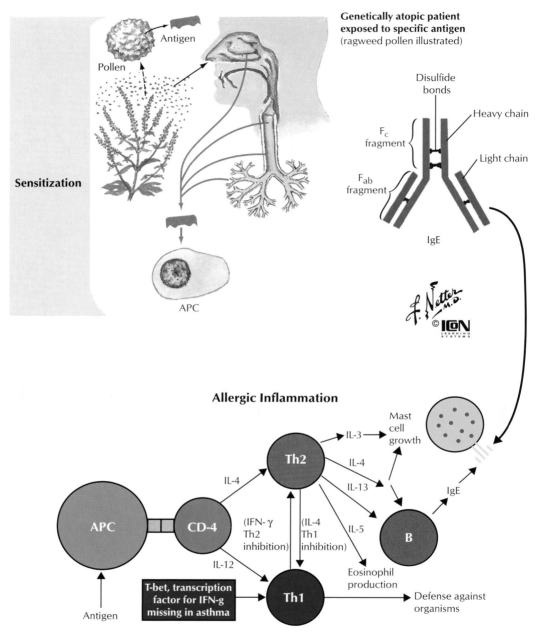

Extrinsic Asthma
Mechanism of Type 1 (Immediate) Hypersensitivity

APC, antigen presenting cell; CD-4 lymphocyte; Th2, Th2 lymphocyte; Th1, Th1 lymphocyte; B, B lymphocyte.
Adapted with permission from Busse WW, Lemanske RF. Advances in Immunology: Asthma. *N Engl J Med* 2001; 344(5): 353 and Schwartz RS. A new element in the mechanism of asthma. *N Engl J Med* 2002; 346 (11): 857. Copyright ©2001 and 2002 Massachusetts Medical Society. All rights reserved.

Figure 118-3

Clinical Features

Features common to both extrinsic allergic and intrinsic asthma:
Respiratory distress, dyspnea, wheezing, flushing, cyanosis, cough, flaring of alae, use of accessory respiratory muscles, apprehension, tachycardia, perspiration, hyperresonance, distant breath sounds and rhonchi, eosinophilia

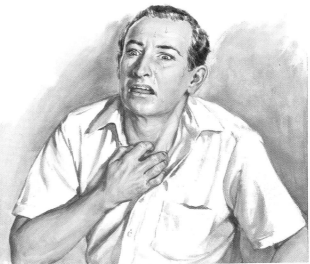

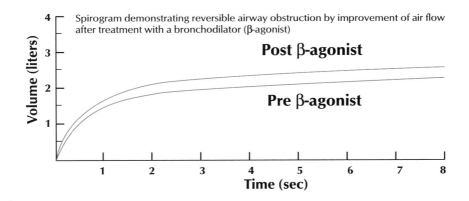

Spirogram demonstrating reversible airway obstruction by improvement of air flow after treatment with a bronchodilator (β-agonist)

Post β-agonist

Pre β-agonist

Volume (liters)

Time (sec)

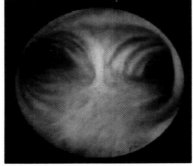

Normal airway seen through a broncho-scope looking at the main carina with the right main branches to the right

With permission from Stradling P. *Diagnostic Bronchoscopy*, 3rd ed. 1976: 42, with permission from Elsevier.

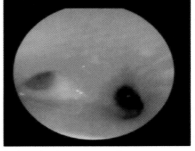

Asthmatic airway - same view as shown in the normal airway

With permission from Smalhout B, Hill-Vaughan AB. *The suffocating child; bronchoscopy: a guide to diagnosis and treatment.* Munich. Boehringer Ingelheim. 1979.

Figure 118-4

Sputum in Bronchial Asthma

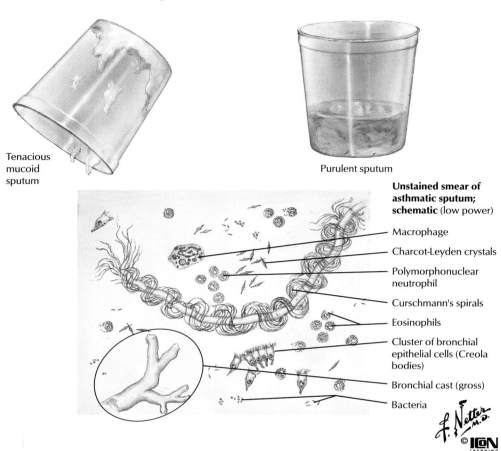

Tenacious
mucoid
sputum

Purulent sputum

**Unstained smear of
asthmatic sputum;
schematic** (low power)

— Macrophage

— Charcot-Leyden crystals

— Polymorphonuclear
neutrophil

— Curschmann's spirals

— Eosinophils

— Cluster of bronchial
epithelial cells (Creola
bodies)

— Bronchial cast (gross)

— Bacteria

distress. Following the resolution of the acute event, a history, either from the patient or from others who have observed the patient, often reveals that signs of disease activity have been present for many hours or days before the acute decompensation. However, actual sudden onset respiratory failure and death are reported with asthma. At autopsy these individuals demonstrate less "mucus" plugging and more neutrophilic, and less eosinophilic, airway infiltration. Death in this setting is associated with suffocation secondary to bronchospasm rather than "mucus" occlusion of the airways. Objective monitoring of signs of respiratory disease activity such as peak expiratory flows, nocturnal awakenings due to shortness of breath, chest tightness, and cough can be useful as a guide to early intervention (Figure 118-

5). Occasionally, lung infection or pneumothorax is associated with acute decompensation. These conditions require early detection and therapy in severely compromised individuals if they are to survive. Life-threatening signs include marked accessory muscle use, depressed mental status, diaphoresis, cyanosis, fatigue, pulsus paradoxus greater than 15 mm Hg, peak expiratory flows less than 100 L/min, and CO_2 retention.

Morbidity and mortality from asthma are increased in the elderly. Generally, there is less reversible airflow obstruction and eosinophilia. IgE concentrations are also less impressively elevated. The signs and symptoms are similar to those of younger patients, and response to therapy is good. Conditions that exacerbate asthma, such as congestive heart failure, hypothyroidism, and gas-

DISORDERS OF THE RESPIRATORY SYSTEM

Table 118-1
Stepwise Approach for Managing Asthma in Adults and Children Older than Five Years of Age: Treatment

Classify Severity: Clinical Features Before Treatment or Adequate Control			Medications Required to Maintain Long-Term Control
Classification	*Symptoms/Day* *Symptoms/Night*	*PEF or FEV1* *PEF Variability*	*Daily Medications*
STEP 1 Mild intermittent	≤ 2 days/week ≤ 2 nights/month	≥ 80% < 20%	· No daily medication needed. · Severe exacerbations may occur, separated by long periods of normal lung function and no symptoms. A course of systemic corticosteroids is recommended.
STEP 2 Mild persistent	> 2/week but < 1x/day > 2 nights/month	≥ 80% 20–30%	· Preferred treatment: − Low-dose inhaled corticosteroids · Alternative treatment: cromolyn, − leukotriene modifier, nedocromil, OR sustained release theophylline to serum concentration of 5–15 mcg/mL
STEP 3: Moderate persistent	Daily > 1 night/week	> 60% – < 80% > 30%	· Preferred treatment: − Low-to-medium dose inhaled corticosteroids and long-acting inhaled beta$_2$-agonists. · Alternative treatment: − Increase inhaled corticosteroids within medium-dose range OR − Low-to-medium dose inhaled corticosteroids and either leukotriene modifier or theophylline. If needed (particularly in patients with recurring severe exacerbations): · Preferred treatment: − Increase inhaled corticosteroids within medium-dose range and add long-acting inhaled beta$_2$-agonists · Alternative treatment: − Increase inhaled corticosteroids within medium-dose range and add either leukotriene modifier or theophylline
STEP 4: Severe persistent	Continual Frequent	≤ 60% > 30%	· Preferred treatment: − High-dose inhaled corticosteroids AND − Long-acting inhaled beta$_2$-agonists AND, if needed, − Corticosteroid tablets or syrup long term (2 mg/kg/day, generally do not exceed 60 mg per day). (Make repeat attempts to reduce systemic corticosteroids and maintain control with high-dose inhaled corticosteroids.)
QUICK RELIEF All patients			· Short-acting bronchodilator: 2–4 puffs short-acting inhaled beta$_2$-agonists as needed for symptoms. · Intensity of treatment will depend on severity of exacerbation; up to 3 treatments at 20-minute intervals or a single nebulizer treatment as needed. Course of systemic corticosteroids may be needed. · Use of short-acting beta$_2$-agonists >2 times a week in intermittent asthma (daily, or increasing use in persistent asthma) may indicate the need to initiate (increase) long-term control therapy.

Adapted from The National Heart, Lung, and Blood Institute's National Asthma Education and Prevention Program, *National Institutes of Health Expert Panel Report*, December 2002.

DISORDERS OF THE RESPIRATORY SYSTEM

Table 118-2
A Differential Diagnosis of Common Diseases That Produce Signs and Symptoms Associated with Asthma

Recurrent Episodic Dyspnea
· Chronic obstructive pulmonary disease
· Coronary artery disease
· Congestive heart failure
· Mitral stenosis
· Pulmonary Emboli
· Recurrent gastroesophageal reflux with aspiration
· Recurrent anaphylaxis
· Systemic mastocytosis
· Carcinoid syndrome
· Muscle weakness

Chronic Cough
· Rhinitis
· Sinusitis
· Otitis
· Bronchitis (chronic or postviral)
· Bronchiectasis
· GI reflux with or without aspiration
· Cystic Fibrosis
· Pneumonia
· Pulmonary fibrosis
· Eosinophilic pneumonia parasitic infections
· Drugs (e.g., ACE inhibitors)

Airflow Obstructive
· Chronic obstructive bronchiolitis and emphysema
· Bronchiolitis obliterans
· Cystic Fibrosis
· Organic or functioning laryngeal narrowing
· Extrinsic or intrinsic narrowing of trachea or main stem bronchus
· Airway tumors
· Churg-Strauss vasculitis
· Hypothyroidism aggravating asthma

Adapted from Murray JF, Nadel JA eds. *Textbook of Respiratory Medicine*. 3rd ed. Philadelphia, Pa: WB Saunders Co; 2000:1269.

troesophageal reflux, are more common in this population.

Asthma has many clinical forms. The syndrome has been classified by severity by the National Asthma Education and Prevention program (NAEPP) guidelines: intermittent asthma, requiring bronchodilator therapy less than twice weekly, and three degrees of persistent asthma: mild, moderate, and severe (Table 118-1).

Steroid-dependent asthma, steroid-resistant asthma, and difficult or brittle asthma are categories of severe asthma. Asthma is also classified into groups by presumed cause: intrinsic asthma with no apparent allergic sensitization, and extrinsic asthma demonstrating elevated IgE and skin test reactions to allergens and seasonal variability (Figure 118-2). Other categories separate asthma by the type of trigger for the exacerbation, such as exercise-associated asthma, nocturnal asthma, and drug-induced asthma (e.g., NSAIDs, angiotensin-converting enzyme inhibitors, and beta blockers). Asthmatic bronchitis is associated with chronic obstructive pulmonary disease (COPD) or an acute respiratory infection causing prolonged cough and sputum production. Allergic bronchopulmonary mycosis (ABPM) reflects a hypersensitivity to airway colonization with fungus such as Aspergillus (ABPA). Occupational asthma refers to new-onset asthma caused by work place exposures and asthma aggravated by exposure to factors in the work environment.

DIFFERENTIAL DIAGNOSIS
The causes of cough and dyspnea are legion and the adage that "all that wheezes is not asthma" is true (Table 118-2).

Establishing the diagnosis of asthma in the setting of COPD, which shares many signs and symptoms with asthma, can be challenging. Also, asthmatic smokers often can develop fixed airflow obstruction. However, even when no reversible airflow obstruction is demonstrated with spirometry, a clinical trial of corticosteroids and bronchodilators is appropriate. Another consideration is bacterial infections causing bronchial hyperreactivity in asthmatics, for example, *Mycoplasma pneumoniae* and *Chlamydia pneumoniae*. The functional disorder, "vocal cord dysfunction," is often initially confused with asthma. Underlying hypothyroidism aggravating asthma is also worth consideration in some clinical settings.

DIAGNOSTIC APPROACH
Patients with undiagnosed asthma often present with complaints of episodic attacks of wheezing, cough, and/or shortness of breath. The suspected diagnosis is supported when examination documents wheezing, and the history of asymptomatic intervals and precipitating "triggers" is elicited. Most often a chest X-ray is obtained to

Figure 118-5

Asthma Diary

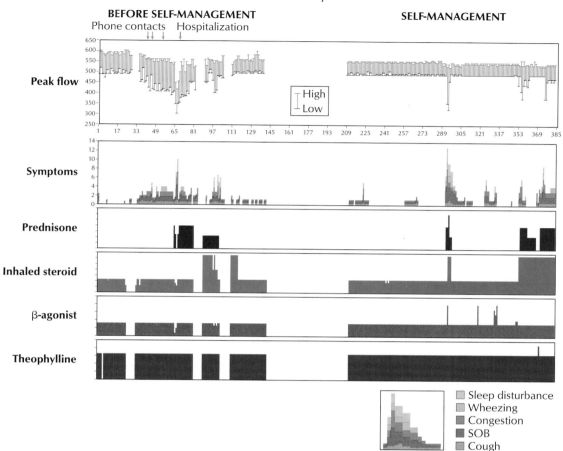

BEFORE SELF-MANAGEMENT — Phone contacts, Hospitalization

SELF-MANAGEMENT

Peak flow, Symptoms, Prednisone, Inhaled steroid, β-agonist, Theophylline

High / Low

Sleep disturbance, Wheezing, Congestion, SOB, Cough

exclude other pulmonary pathology. Generally, the chest X-ray in asthma is normal. Radiographs demonstrating hyperinflation during an acute attack are seen, but this finding is more often associated with COPD. Atelectasis with mucus plugging is associated with asthma (Figure 118-1). Pneumothorax is more common in asthmatics and can present as an asthma exacerbation.

Spirometry or peak expiratory flow rate (PEFR) measurements before and after administering a bronchodilator are usually obtained to demonstrate reversible airflow obstruction and to determine the severity of the acute disease (Figure 118-3). Chronic cough associated with normal spirometry and an elevated DLCO suggests the diagnosis of "cough asthma." Skin scratch testing may be useful diagnostically and is used when prescribing immunotherapy and designing avoid-

ance strategies. Other observations supporting the diagnosis of asthma include variability in home monitoring of PEFRs, improving PEFRs on asthma therapy, hyperreactivity to challenge testing with histamine or methacholine, peripheral blood eosinophilia, elevated IgE, and the characteristic sputum previously described. Generally, the diagnosis is made correctly using only spirometry and chest radiography to support the physical examination and history. Failure to respond to asthma therapy should prompt a search for other causes.

MANAGEMENT AND THERAPY

Asthma therapy focuses on the management of airway inflammation. The goal is to prevent exacerbations, minimize symptoms, and maintain near-normal lung function. Informed patient self-management, allergen and irritant avoidance strategies, and medications are keys to controlling asthma. Anti-inflammatory agents (e.g., inhaled corticosteroids) are the pharmacologic cornerstones for prevention. Bronchodilators such as beta agonists, however, remain the cornerstone of acute management of exacerbations. Severe exacerbations may require monitoring in an intensive care unit and mechanical ventilation. Grading chronic asthma severity, however, is difficult. It is clear that physical examination, symptoms and/or pulmonary function tests lack adequate predictive value. Even asthmatics with increasing PEFRs have died suddenly of their disease. Asthma deaths are equally distributed among asthmatics classified as mild, moderate, and severe.

Beta-2 Agonists

Beta agonists reverse smooth muscle bronchospasm regardless of the stimulus, inhibit histamine and other mediator release from inflammatory cells, inhibit cholinergic neurotransmission, inhibit airway vascular leakage, and increase mucociliary clearance. Although the anti-inflammatory effects of beta agonists in asthma have been difficult to demonstrate clinically, no other class of drug is as effective at relieving the acute symptoms of asthma. Racemic albuterol (R-albuterol) is a commonly used short-acting bronchodilator drug. Levalbuterol, the active component in R-albuterol, is available and may prove superior to albuterol. Short-acting beta agonists are used on an as-needed basis to relieve symptoms and not routinely in an effort to prevent them. The frequency of as-needed use, therefore, is a marker of disease control. A metered dose inhaler (MDI) with a spacer is as effective as wet nebulizer delivery of the drug when airflow is not extremely restricted. Parenteral beta agonist or wet nebulizers delivery should be considered if there is little air movement and if the MDI technique is inadequate. Intravenous epinephrine poses a cardiovascular risk in adults.

Long-acting beta agonists, such as salmeterol and formoterol are used in conjunction with inhaled steroids as preventive agents. This combination is more effective than doubling the dose of steroid. In vitro work demonstrates enhanced transport of the steroid receptor into the nucleus in the presence of a beta agonist. Whether this is an explanation for the clinical observation is not clear. Monotherapy with long- or short-acting

beta agonists does not control the clinical expression of persistant asthma and should not be used.

Steroids

Steroids are the most effective agents for preventing asthma symptoms through their role as inhibitors of inflammatory mediator production. They are the only class of medication demonstrated to decrease asthma mortality. Inhaled steroids are recommended to control chronic asthma when as-needed beta agonist rescue is required more than once or twice weekly. Potent inhaled steroids take days to weeks to produce significant clinical improvement. There is, however, reported effect in 2 hours with 4 puffs (1,000 µg) of flunisolide every 10 minutes for 3 hours by MDI with spacer, suggesting a role for inhaled steroid in acute exacerbations.

Inhaled steroids dosing by NAEPP guidelines is established by PF measurements and symptoms (Table 118-1). If, instead, dosing is based on control of hyperreactivity, as defined by challenge testing with histamine, for example. Much higher doses of inhaled steroid are employed, to achieve the clinical end point. Pulmonary function is enhanced and asthmatic lung remodeling improves (Figure 118-1).

Sixty milligrams of prednisone or 125 mg of methylprednisolone intravenously are commonly used to initiate therapy in severely ill asthmatics. Generally, there is good bioavailability of steroids orally; however, intravenous administration is used to ensure delivery in the acute situation. The onset of action is uncertain and variability reported as 1 to 24 hours. Oral prednisone as outpatient therapy following a severe exacerbation is generally used at a dose of 40 mg orally in the morning for 2 weeks. Tapering schedules are the norm. However, this dose is generally tolerated without a taper for 3 weeks. Intramuscular (IM) dosing is rarely required. It has not been studied as a long-term maintenance therapy. IM dosing may be useful for patients unable to comply with oral medications upon discharge from the emergency department.

Leukotriene Modifiers

Leukotrienes (LT) are elevated in asthmatics and are linked to relevant inflammatory changes in the lung. This class of agents inhibits both the early and to a lesser extent the late phase asthmatic response and blocks aspirin-induced asthma. LT modifiers improve lung function in chronic asthma and decrease beta agonist rescue, inhaled corticosteroid use, and exacerbations requiring oral steroids. They are no longer recommended as monotherapy in mild persistent asthma. They are used as added therapy when inhaled steroids alone fail. There is an unclear association between the use of LT modifiers to treat asthma and the risk of developing Churg-Strauss vasculitis. While inhaled steroids remain the preferred therapy for any degree of persistant asthma, leukotriene modifiers are an acceptable second choice. Long-acting bronchodilators (β-agonists) are the recommended therapy to be added when inhaled steroids do not control symptoms; leukotrienes are an acceptable second choice.

Ipratropium Bromide

Ipratropium bromide is a bronchodilator, but not as potent as beta agonists; its most accepted role in asthma therapy is as a rescue in asthmatics receiving beta blockers. It may prove useful in children and for severe adult exacerbations when routine agents fail.

Other Agents

Cromolyn and nedocromil are anti-inflammatory agents used primarily in children. Magnesium 2 g intravenously over 15 minutes is used in severely ill asthmatics to reverse bronchospasm. The phosphodiesterase inhibitor theophylline is a bronchodilator that also enhances respiratory muscle contraction and mucociliary clearance, decreases hypoventilation, and has anti-inflammatory properties. Its narrow therapeutic window and lack of dramatic efficacy limits its use. Mixtures of helium and oxygen, inhaled furosemide, inhaled anesthetics, and mucolytic agents have anecdotally been reported to be beneficial.

FUTURE DIRECTIONS

The focus for drug development in asthma is on interrupting its inflammatory cascade. Much effort is being made at the molecular level. Anti-IgE will be available soon. Anti-IL-5, while able to reduce blood eosinophilia, had no effect on clinical disease. Soluble IL-4 receptor, on the other hand, shows clinical promise. Other efforts target other cytokines, transcription factors, arachidonic acid metabolites, platelet-activating factor, cell-adhesion molecules, phosphodiesterase-4, and T-cell markers. Efforts using bacterial DNA repeats as adjuvants for vaccines, and immunotherapy may prove useful to direct inflammatory responses away from pathways that produce pathologic chronic atopic inflammation. Markers of asthmatic inflammation, for example, exhaled nitrous oxide (NO) may prove helpful in predicting exacerbations, grading disease severity, and judging therapeutic success. Finally, a mutation on chromosome 10, involving metalloproteinase matrix (MMPs) ADAM-33, has been linked to bronchial hyperactivity and presumptively to airway smooth muscle hypertrophy. MMPs were formally thought to be involved only with remodelling of the extracellular matrix. Recent speculations, however, suggest a role for MMPs in the clearing of cytokines and their receptors, and thus a role in immune modulation. This makes them a potential therapeutic target in asthma.

REFERENCES

Barnes PJ, Grunstein MM, Leff AR, Woolcock AJ, eds. *Asthma.* Vol 1. Philadelphia, Pa: Lippincott-Raven Publishers; 1997.

Busse WW, Lemnske RF Jr. Asthma. *N Engl J Med.* 2001;344: 350-362.

Horiuchi T, Castro M. The pathobiologic implications for treatment. Old and new strategies in the treatment of chronic asthma. *Clin Chest Med.* 2000;21:381-395.

Kay AB. Advances in immunology: allergic diseases-first of two parts. *N Engl J Med.* 2001; 344:30-37.

Shapiro SD, Owen CA. ADAM-323 surfaces on an asthma gene. *N Engl J Med.* 2002; 347: 936-938.

Chapter 119

Chronic Cough

Robert M. Aris

Chronic cough is the presence of cough that persists for longer than 1 month, often without a diagnosis being established. It is a common clinical problem, occurring in approximately 5% of individuals in the general population and 25% of smokers. Patients often present with a cough they have had for many years that has responded poorly to numerous therapies (mostly empirical) and interferes with normal activities. Smokers rarely report it as a symptom and may consider it a normal phenomenon.

Acute cough commonly results from upper respiratory viral infections and is usually considered a benign, self-limiting symptom. Chronic cough may not only be a clinical indicator of serious underlying illness, but may itself have clinical consequences—conjunctival bleeding, epistaxis, tussive or post-tussive syncope or vomiting, stress urinary incontinence, rib fractures, cervical disk herniation, abdominal hernias, esophageal rupture, cardiac arrhythmias and infarction, pulmonary barotrauma, and even cerebral air embolism. Therefore, chronic cough warrants a thorough evaluation to define a specific etiology and to avoid empiric therapy.

ETIOLOGY AND PATHOGENESIS

Approximately 75% of cases of chronic cough are due to a single cause with 20% due to 2 causes (e.g., allergic rhinitis and asthma). Fewer than 5% are due to more than 3 causes. Usually, smokers are excluded from chronic cough studies, a practice that leads to an underestimate of smoking-related diseases. More than 100 diseases are associated with chronic cough, but most are uncommon. Air pollution (ozone and particulates) is becoming an increasingly common cause of chronic cough, but the prevalence is not defined.

CLINICAL PRESENTATION

An adequate history is vital in establishing a diagnosis and initiating management. In smokers, the cough is considered due to cigarette-related disease until proven otherwise. Common causes of chronic cough in nonsmokers are bronchial asthma, post-infectious bronchial hyper-responsiveness, postnasal drip, chronic bronchitis, and gastroesophageal reflux disease

Table 119-1
Etiology of Chronic Cough with a Normal Chest Radiograph

Cause	Prevalence
Postnasal drip	28–41%
Asthma	24–33%
GERD*	10–21%
Chronic bronchitis Post-infectious (often, viral URI†) bronchial hyper-responsiveness	5–10% 10%
Bronchiectasis	4%
ACE†† inhibitors, tracheomalacia, eosinophilic bronchitis, psychogenic, etc.	5%

*GERD, gastroesophageal reflux disease; †URI, upper respiratory infection; ††ACE, angiotensin-converting enzyme

(GERD) (Table 119-1). Determining the precipitating factors for cough provides useful clues to the underlying etiology. The timing of cough is important [e.g., it might occur postprandially in GERD, or nocturnally in asthma or congestive heart failure (CHF)]. Patients with chronic bronchitis or bronchiectasis often cough most vigorously after awakening because secretions have pooled in the lung during sleep. Chronic productive coughs with purulent sputum are usually seen in chronic bronchitis and bronchiectasis and, less commonly, from lung abscesses. Productive coughs with

Figure 119-1

Causes of Chronic Cough

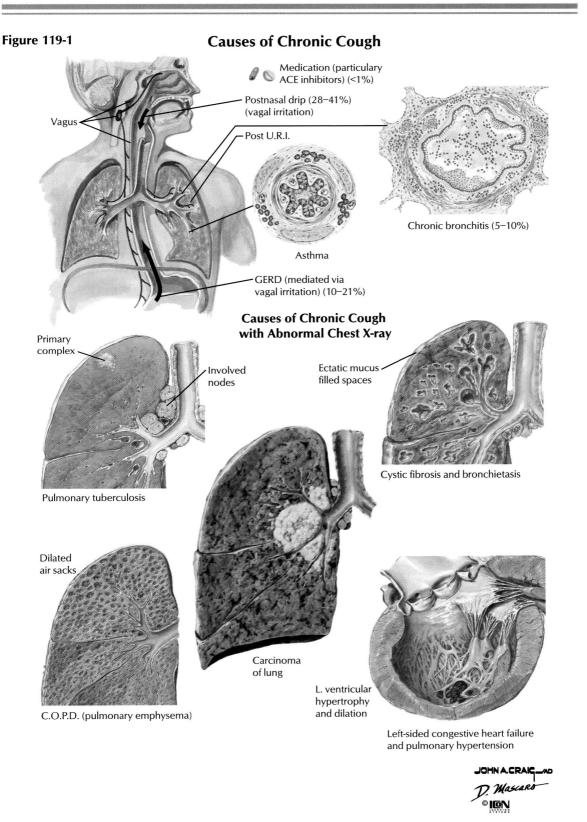

Medication (particulary ACE inhibitors) (<1%)

Postnasal drip (28–41%) (vagal irritation)

Post U.R.I.

Vagus

Chronic bronchitis (5–10%)

Asthma

GERD (mediated via vagal irritation) (10–21%)

Causes of Chronic Cough with Abnormal Chest X-ray

Primary complex

Involved nodes

Ectatic mucus filled spaces

Pulmonary tuberculosis

Cystic fibrosis and bronchietasis

Dilated air sacks

Carcinoma of lung

L. ventricular hypertrophy and dilation

C.O.P.D. (pulmonary emphysema)

Left-sided congestive heart failure and pulmonary hypertension

JOHN A. CRAIG—MD

D. Mascaro

©ICN

Table 119-2
Etiology of Chronic Cough with an Abnormal Chest Radiograph

· Bronchogenic carcinoma
· Interstitial lung disease (pulmonary fibrosis, sarcoidosis, etc.)
· Emphysema and chronic bronchitis
· Congestive heart failure
· Cystic fibrosis and/or bronchiectasis
· Tuberculosis
· Alveolar hemorrhage syndromes
· Pulmonary hypertension

white to off-white sputum may be seen in asthma or post-nasal drip. In the latter conditions, the secretions are usually from the upper respiratory tracts. Dry chronic coughs usually result from asthma (many sufferers never report wheezing), interstitial lung disease (ILD), CHF, and the use of ACE inhibitors.

Physical examination may detect some causes of chronic cough, including chronic airway obstruction (particularly in asthma) if expiratory rhonchi or wheezes are present. CHF and ILD present with "wet" or "dry" inspiratory crackles respectively. Inflamed nasal mucosa indicates the diagnosis of chronic sinusitis and post-nasal drip. Lower extremity edema and an abnormal heart exam point to the diagnosis of CHF, while extremity clubbing may lead to the diagnoses of lung malignancy, ILD, or bronchiectasis.

DIAGNOSTIC APPROACH

Diagnostic tests are unnecessary if the history and/or physical examination suggest benign or self-limiting causes. A cough caused by an ACE inhibitor is managed with a trial off the drug or, if mild, observation while therapy continues. Symptoms and signs suggestive of postnasal drip may also warrant a therapeutic trial before diagnostic testing. A chronic post-viral cough is managed with simple observation or a short anti-tussive therapy trial because it will probably spontaneously remit. Otherwise, diagnostic tests should be directed by the history and physical examination. A chest radiograph is essential early in the investigation because it may prevent unnecessary tests and has the potential to diagnose many seri-ous parenchymal lung diseases (e.g., bronchogenic malignancy, CHF, ILD, lung abscess, or emphysema with a bronchitic component) (Table 119-2 and Figure 119-1). Symptoms suggestive of asthma or chronic bronchitis are more effectively evaluated with pulmonary function tests (PFTs) than chest radiography. Patients with chronic cough from advanced lung disease related to the airways or parenchyma should undergo both an anatomical (chest radiograph) and physiologic (i.e., PFTs) workup.

A recommended diagnostic protocol is outlined below, but individualization based on the history and physical examination is important (Figure 119-2). A chest radiograph is usually the most sensitive test. If a cause is identified from the chest radiograph, the workup proceeds on the basis of the abnormality (Table 119-2). Sputum cultures are necessary if infection is suspected. Bronchoscopy or lung biopsy can confirm the presence of a malignant or an inflammatory entity. If the chest radiograph is normal or shows signs of a quiescent disease, spirometry before and after bronchodilator therapy should be obtained if airway diseases (e.g., asthma) are suspected. Many patients with asthma will show some evidence of airflow obstruction (forced expiratory volume in 1 second [FEV_1] <80% of predicted, FEV_1/forced vital capacity [FVC] ratio <80% of predicted, low forced expiratory flow [FEF] 25% to 75%, or a large [>10% increase in FEV_1] bronchodilator response). Additional PFTs, including diffusing capacity and lung volume measurements, may be useful in a subset of patients with normal spirometry or to better define the extent of disease in those with abnormal spirometry. If the chest radiograph is normal in a smoker or an individual exposed to occupational or seasonal antigens or environmental irritants, the patient should be encouraged to avoid the irritating factor before additional diagnostic testing. Unfortunately, many patients cannot or will not avoid potential irritants, and PFTs may prove useful in defining the disease and its severity (if only to reinforce the need for irritant avoidance).

If the history, physical examination, chest radiograph, and spirometry do not suggest a cause for the chronic cough, pulmonary consultation is indicated. If asthma remains a possibility with a normal examination and spirometry, home peak flow

Figure 119-2

Diagnostic Testing in Chronic Cough

Chest X-Ray

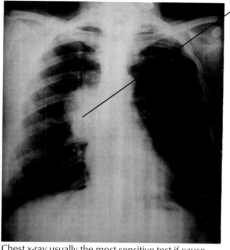

Hilar tumor demonstrated on chest x-ray

Chest x-ray usually the most sensitive test if cause identified by chest x-ray work-up proceeds on basis of abnormality.

Sputum Studies

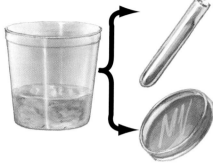

Sputum cultures should be obtained if infection is suspected

JOHN A. CRAIG—AD
C. Machado
—M.D.
© ICN

Bronchoscopy and lung biopsy

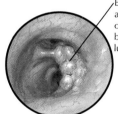

Endoscopic appearance of tumor in bronchial lumen

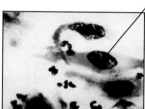

Malignant cells demonsrated on exam of scrapings

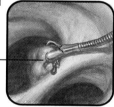

Endoscopic biopsy of bronchial lesion

Bronchoscopy or lung biopsy can confirm presence of malignant or inflammatory entity

Pulmonary function testing (Spirometry)

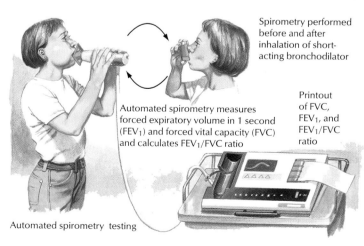

Spirometry performed before and after inhalation of short-acting bronchodilator

Automated spirometry measures forced expiratory volume in 1 second (FEV_1) and forced vital capacity (FVC) and calculates FEV_1/FVC ratio

Printout of FVC, FEV_1, and FEV_1/FVC ratio

Automated spirometry testing

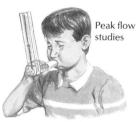

Peak flow studies

Test performed three times and results compared with best

If asthma remains a possibility after a normal exam and spirometry, home peak flow monitoring may demonstrate classic variability seen in asthma

If x-ray is normal or shows signs of quiescent disease, spirometry before and after bronchodilator use is updated if airway disease (asthma) suspected monitoring may prove valuable in demonstrating the classic variability seen in asthma. Methacholine challenge testing may be used to demonstrate bronchial hyperresponsiveness. High-resolution chest CT is the best diagnostic test if clinical suspicion for ILD exists or if the PFTs show a restrictive disorder (total lung capacity [TLC] <80% predicted or FVC <80% without concomitant obstruction). If GERD is suspected on the basis of indigestion or acid brash, 24-hour esophageal pH monitoring may prove diagnostic, but many clinicians opt for a trial of therapy to reduce gastric acidity with a proton pump inhibitor or H2 antagonist to determine if the cough improves. Cough associated with GERD is unlikely to result from aspiration and is more likely from stimulation of afferent limb of the cough reflex in the distal esophagus. Unsuspected sinus disease may be diagnosed with imaging studies. If patients give a history of an upper airway source of cough ("tickle" in the throat), fiberoptic laryngoscopy may exclude vocal cord nodules and lesions. Bronchoscopy or cardiac evaluation for poor left ventricular function is used as a last resort, but the diagnostic yield is low if other testing is negative.

MANAGEMENT AND THERAPY

The management of chronic cough depends on an understanding of the underlying cause. Because chronic cough has more than one cause in at least 20% of patients, add-on therapy should be considered if there is a poor response to initial, cause-directed therapy. The management principles for intractable cough of unknown etiology are not well defined. A reasonable approach has evolved from recent clinical trials. Some causes of cough are etiologically related to or trigger other causes of cough. For example, more than 80% of patients with asthma have been found to have significant GERD and, in turn, chronic cough from any cause has been found to precipitate GERD. Thus, the potential for a self-perpetuating cycle exists.

Specific Antitussive Therapy

Specific antitussive therapy has a high likelihood of success (>84%) because a specific cause for chronic cough is usually found (88%-100% based on previous studies). Postnasal drip usually results

from antigens or environmental irritants, and therapy is directed at the underlying cause(s). Allergic rhinitis can be treated successfully with intranasal corticosteroids, combination antihistamine/decongestants, and intranasal anticholinergic agents (e.g., ipratropium bromide). Infectious sinusitis should be treated with antibiotics directed against upper respiratory tract pathogens. Asthma therapy guidelines focus on obtaining disease control with inhaled corticosteroids, leukotriene modifiers (e.g., montelukast) or, less commonly, mast cell stabilizers (e.g., cromolyn sodium). Medications that provide acute relief (e.g., adrenergic bronchodilators) should be added for breakthrough symptoms; however, they do not treat the underlying nature of the disease. Some asthma patients cannot achieve good control without additional therapy for allergic rhinosinusitis or GERD.

Patients with chronic cough from GERD should use an anti-reflux regimen (weight loss; elevation of the head of the bed on blocks; avoidance of bedtime snacks, caffeine, and theophylline). A trial of anti-reflux medications is appropriate even if there are no other reflux symptoms. Ranitidine, a histamine H2-receptor antagonist, improves intractable cough in 85% of patients with proven GERD within 2 weeks. Most of the non-responders improve with omeprazole, a proton pump inhibitor. Controlled studies have not been carried out with other anti-reflux measures, although there are case reports of the prokinetic agent, metoclopromide, being effective. Other anti-reflux agents such as antacids and cytoprotective agents (e.g., sucralfate) have been disappointing in the management of cough.

Chronic bronchitis is successfully treated with smoking cessation alone in >90% of smokers. More than half the time, cough disappears within a month of cessation. For infectious exacerbations of chronic bronchitis and/or bronchiectasis, antibiotics and bronchodilators are the mainstay of therapy. Chest physiotherapy and drainage may help chronic cough in patients with chronic suppurative diseases (e.g., cystic fibrosis).

Nonspecific Antitussive Therapy

Medications in this category address cough as a symptom rather than the manifestation of an underlying disease. Ipratropium bromide by nebulizer or inhaler is effective in suppressing the cough reflex via the efferent limb and/or decreasing airway secretions. A trial of inhaled or oral corticosteroids is often used in patients with intractable cough. This therapy may be particularly valuable in undiagnosed asthmatics and in patients with eosinophilic bronchitis. Non-narcotic medications, such as dextromethorphan, nedocromil sodium, caramiphen, viminol, and levopropizine, are efficacious for acute cough, but may work in chronic cough as well. Narcotics in the phenanthrene group (codeine, morphine, etc.) are effective antitussive agents, but are reserved for intractable cough unresponsive to other measures.

FUTURE DIRECTIONS

Because cough is a common symptom of underlying respiratory and non-respiratory disease, much of the future research in this area will address the underlying pathologic processes rather than the symptoms. Studies measuring exhaled nitric oxide and inflammatory mediators in bronchoalveolar lavage samples may shed important light on the role of lung inflammation in the pathogenesis of chronic cough.

REFERENCES

Fujimura M. Eosinophilic bronchitis is an important cause of chronic cough. *Am J Respir Crit Care Med.* 2000;161:1764-1765.

Ing AJ, Ngu MC, Breslin AB. Chronic persistent cough and gastro-oesophageal reflux. *Thorax.* 1991;46:479-483.

Irwin RS, Boulet LP, Cloutier MM, et al. Managing cough as a defense mechanism and as a symptom. A consensus panel report of the American College of Chest Physicians. *Chest.* 1998;114(suppl 2):133S-181S.

Irwin RS, Curley FJ, French CL. Chronic cough. The spectrum and frequency of causes, key components of the diagnostic evaluation, and outcome of specific therapy. *Am Rev Respir Dis.* 1990;141:640-647.

Irwin RS, Widdicombe J. Cough. In: Murray JF, Nadel JA, eds. *Textbook of Respiratory Medicine.* 3rd ed. Philadelphia, Pa: WB Saunders Co; 2000.

Jatakanon A, Lalloo UG, Lim S, Chung KF, Barnes PJ. Increased neutrophils and cytokines, TNF-alpha and IL-8, in induced sputum of non-asthmatic patients with dry cough. *Thorax.* 1999;54:234-237.

Mello CJ, Irwin RS, Curley FJ. Predictive values of the character, timing, and complications of chronic cough in diagnosing its cause. *Arch Intern Med.* 1996;156:997-1003.

Pratter MR, Bartter T, Akers S, DuBois J. An algorithmic approach to chronic cough. *Ann Intern Med.* 1993;119:977-983.

Smyrnios NA, Irwin RS, Curley FJ, French CL. From a prospective study of chronic cough: diagnostic and therapeutic aspects in older adults. *Arch Intern Med.* 1998;158:1222-1228.

Chapter 120

Chronic Obstructive Pulmonary Disease

James F. Donohue

Chronic obstructive pulmonary disease (COPD) is a heterogeneous disorder that includes emphysema, chronic bronchitis, obliterative bronchiolitis, and asthmatic bronchitis. The definition of COPD includes the following: "a disease state characterized by airflow limitation that is not fully reversible. The airflow limitation is usually both progressive and is associated with an abnormal inflammatory response of the lungs to noxious particles or gases."

COPD may affect up to 31 million people in the United States, 17 million of whom have been diagnosed and 6 million of whom are on therapy. Cigarette smoking is the major risk factor for COPD, and the disease develops in up to 15% of chronic smokers. More than 80% of cases in the United States can be attributed to smoking. Other important risk factors include occupational and environmental insults such as bronchitis related to the workplace and air pollution.

A diagnosis of COPD should be considered in any patient who has symptoms of cough, sputum production, dyspnea, and/or a history of exposure to risk factors. The diagnosis is usually confirmed by spirometry, a test with standards that continue to evolve (Figure 120-1). The recent GOLD Guidelines used the presence of a postbronchodilator forced expiratory volume in 1 second (FEV_1) of <80% of the predicted value in combination with a ratio of 1-second forced expiratory volume to vital capacity (FEV_1/FVC ratio) <70% that confirms the presence of airflow limitation that is not fully reversible. Clinical symptoms and signs, including abnormal shortness of breath and increased forced expiratory time, are useful in diagnosis.

CLINICAL PRESENTATION

The clinical course of COPD is affected by multiple factors, including genetic susceptibility, low birth weight, maternal smoking, poor maternal nutrition, infections in the first years of life, asthma in childhood, and exposure to inhaled irritants in the workplace and environmental air pollution.

Lung function in most nonsmoking adults decreases gradually throughout life with a loss of about 20 cc per year from the FEV_1. Susceptible smokers may lose 50 to 60 cc of lung function each year, and those who have alpha-1 deficiency may lose up to 100 cc per year. Young smokers often have more frequent colds that settle in their chest. Usually, middle-aged smokers begin to lose the ability to exercise, and in their 50s begin to lose the ability to work. There is a great loss of quality of life and functional performance as the patient with COPD approaches 60. Many patients lose up to 15 years life expectancy due to this disease.

With far-advanced disease, structural changes result in chronic alveolar hypoxia, which in turn produces pulmonary hypertension and cor pulmonale. These patients are described as "blue bloaters"; they have cyanosis, edema, cardiomegaly, recurrent respiratory failure, hypoventilation, and carbon dioxide retention. Patients at this stage frequently require hospitalization and have a poor prognosis. Some have overlap with obstructive sleep apnea syndrome.

Patients in whom emphysema predominates have severe dyspnea and are called "pink puffers" because they maintain relatively normal arterial oxygen and carbon dioxide tension (Figure 120-2). These patients clearly have evidence of systemic disease. They are cachectic with marked weakness and fatigue and poor muscle function. They tend to be thin and barrel-chested without cyanosis or edema, until the terminal stage of the disease. Most patients fall into a "mixed" bronchitis-emphysema clinical category.

PATHOGENESIS

COPD is characterized by chronic inflammation throughout the airways, parenchyma, and pulmonary vasculature. Macrophages, CD8 lymphocytes, and neutrophils are increased. Activated inflammatory cells release a variety of mediators, including leukotriene B4 (LTB4), interleukin 8 (IL-8), and tumor necrosis factor-α (TNF-α), which damage lung structures. Also, important in the pathogenesis of COPD is an imbalance of proteinases and antiproteinases in the lung, and oxidative stress. This inflammation is attributable to exposure to inhaled noxious particles and gases including cigarette smoking and indoor air pollutants. These irritants directly inflame and damage the lungs.

PATHOLOGY

Pathologic changes are found in the central airways, pulmonary vasculature, peripheral airways, and lung parenchyma. In the central airways, there are enlarged mucus-secreting glands and an increase in the number of goblet cells, plus marked increase in inflammatory cells infiltrating the surface epithelium (Figure 120-3). In the peripheral airways, there is chronic inflammation with repeated cycles of injury and repair of the airway wall leading to remodeling. Structural remodeling of the airway wall with increased collagen content and scar tissue formation narrow the airways and produce fixed obstruction. In the parenchyma, there is often centrilobular emphysema plus dilatation and destruction of the respiratory bronchioles. In alpha-1 antitrypsin deficiency, these changes tend to be panlobular and involve the lower lobes. In cigarette smokers, centrilobular emphysema involves the upper lobes. The vessel walls are thickened with increased smooth muscle mass and infiltration of the vessel wall by inflammatory cells.

DIFFERENTIAL DIAGNOSIS

There is a considerable overlap between COPD and asthma. Both conditions are characterized by obstruction, airway inflammation, and bronchial hyperresponsiveness, and there is an overlap in the response to inhaled beta-adrenergic agonist bronchodilators. However, unlike obstruction in asthma, the obstruction in COPD in not completely reversible, and the inflammation is characterized predominantly by neutrophil, macrophage, and CD8 cellular infil-

trates. Hyperresponsiveness, while greater than that in the general population, is not nearly as marked in asthma. Other obstructive lung diseases that may mimic COPD include *bronchiectasis* with dilatation and inflammation of the small airways of the lungs with recurrent respiratory infections. *Cystic fibrosis*, an inherited disease primarily affecting children and younger adults, is different, with an abnormal sweat chloride test, susceptibility to repetitive infections, much thicker mucopurulent secretions, and a lack of a relationship to cigarette smoking. *Obliterative bronchiolitis* with obstruction of the airways is sometimes seen spontaneously but also as a feature of transplant rejection, and shares its features with COPD as does *panbronchiolitis* and *small airway obstructive disease* primarily seen in Asia.

DIAGNOSTIC APPROACH

The diagnosis of COPD should be considered in a patient with symptoms of cough, sputum production or dyspnea, and/or with a history of exposure to risk factors. Spirometry confirms the diagnosis and is useful for assessing severity. The recent GOLD guidelines classify patients in 4 stages. Management is largely symptom-driven and is in perfect correlation between the degree of airflow limitation and the presence of symptoms.

Stage 0: At risk — characterized by chronic cough and sputum production. The lung function is normal.

Stage I: Mild COPD — with mild airflow limitation with an FEV_1/FVC ratio of <70% but >80% of predicted. Some have cough and sputum production.

Stage II: Moderate COPD — characterized by worsening airflow limitation. 2A with an FEV_1 between 30% to 80% of predicted and 2B with 30% to 50% of predicted. Usually there is progression of symptoms with shortness of breath typically on exertion. Patients at this stage seek medical attention. There are more frequent exacerbations in patients who have an FEV_1 less than 50%. The frequent exacerbations have an impact on quality of life.

Stage III: Severe COPD — characterized by severe airflow limitations with an FEV_1 <30% of predicted or the presence of respiratory failure or clinical signs of right heart failure. Patients who

Figure 120-1

Pulmonary Function in Obstructive Disease

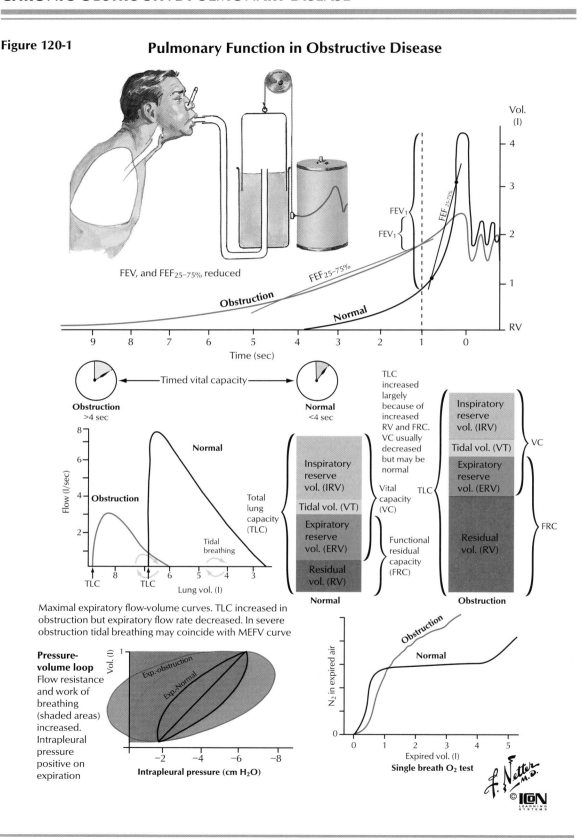

FEV, and FEF$_{25-75\%}$ reduced

Obstruction

Normal

FEV$_1$

FEV$_1$

FEF$_{25-75\%}$

Time (sec)

Timed vital capacity

Obstruction
>4 sec

Normal
<4 sec

TLC increased largely because of increased RV and FRC. VC usually decreased but may be normal

Maximal expiratory flow-volume curves. TLC increased in obstruction but expiratory flow rate decreased. In severe obstruction tidal breathing may coincide with MEFV curve

Pressure-volume loop
Flow resistance and work of breathing (shaded areas) increased. Intrapleural pressure positive on expiration

Exp-obstruction

Exp-Normal

Intrapleural pressure (cm H$_2$O)

Obstruction

Normal

N$_2$ in expired air

Expired vol. (l)

Single breath O$_2$ test

Normal

Inspiratory reserve vol. (IRV)

Tidal vol. (VT)

Expiratory reserve vol. (ERV)

Residual vol. (RV)

Vital capacity (VC)

Functional residual capacity (FRC)

Total lung capacity (TLC)

Obstruction

Inspiratory reserve vol. (IRV)

Tidal vol. (VT)

Expiratory reserve vol. (ERV)

Residual vol. (RV)

VC

TLC

FRC

Normal

Obstruction

Tidal breathing

Figure 120-2

Chronic Obstructive Pulmonary Disease
Interrelationship of Chronic Bronchitis and Emphysema

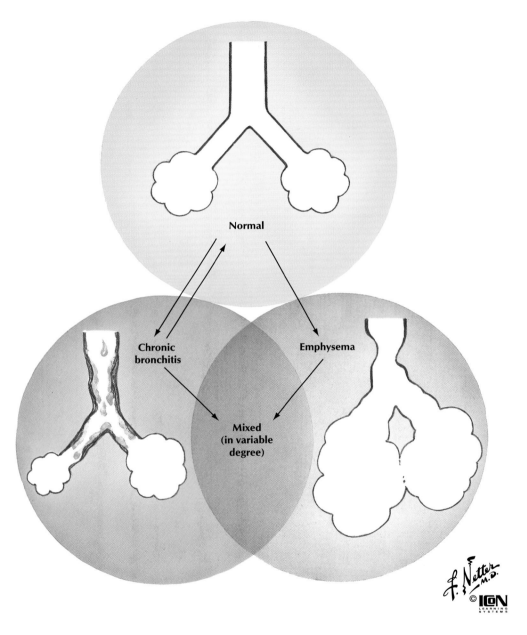

Normal

Chronic
bronchitis

Emphysema

Mixed
(in variable
degree)

have an FEV$_1$ less than 30% have a poor quality of life and more frequent exacerbations.

Laboratory evaluation by spirometry documents an FEV$_1$/FVC ratio <70% that does not completely reverse to normal following bronchodilator therapy.

The chest radiograph appears normal early in COPD and is not useful in the diagnosis. In chronic bronchitis, there are increased lung markings in the lower lobes (so-called dirty lungs). Findings in emphysema include hyperinflation with a low diaphragm, enlarged ret-

Figure 120-3

Chronic Obstructive Pulmonary Disease
Bronchitis

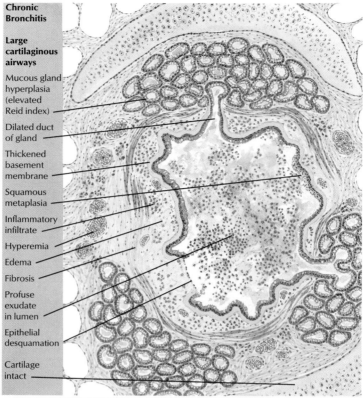

Chronic Bronchitis

Large cartilaginous airways

Mucous gland hyperplasia (elevated Reid index)

Dilated duct of gland

Thickened basement membrane

Squamous metaplasia

Inflammatory infiltrate

Hyperemia

Edema

Fibrosis

Profuse exudate in lumen

Epithelial desquamation

Cartilage intact

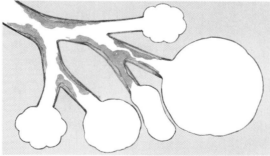

Airways partially or completely blocked or "one-way" valve effect by mucoid or mucopurulent secretions, with impaired or non-uniform distribution of ventilation

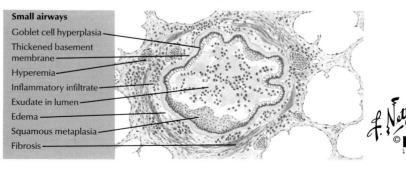

Small airways

Goblet cell hyperplasia

Thickened basement membrane

Hyperemia

Inflammatory infiltrate

Exudate in lumen

Edema

Squamous metaplasia

Fibrosis

rosternal space, hypovascularity, areas of hyper-lucency, and bullae formation.

Arterial blood gases are usually measured in patients with COPD with more severe disease, usually an FEV_1 <40%. However, baseline values are usually benchmarked for comparison during subsequent exacerbations. During the early stage, mild hypoxemia is usually seen. Later, due to ventilation-perfusion ratio abnormalities, severe arterial hypoxemia, respiratory acidosis, and hypoventilation are seen. Secondary poly-cythemia often results.

Electrocardiogram findings are nonspecific. With severe disease, changes of right ventricular hyper-trophy are seen along with atrial arrhythmias.

All patients with COPD, particularly those with early onset or those with a family history of either lung or liver disease should be screened for alpha-1 antitrypsin deficiency. This occurs in 1% to 2% of patients with emphysema. Deficient levels are seen in those who have <15% of the normal value.

MANAGEMENT AND THERAPY

Management of COPD involves 1) educating patients and their families; 2) retarding the progression of airflow limitation by early disease recognition and avoidance of risk factors; 3) minimizing airflow limitation by reducing the production and increasing the elimination of secretions; 4) utilizing bronchodilators effectively; 5) correcting the secondary physiological alterations including hypoxemia, hypercapnia, and pulmonary hypertension; and 6) optimizing functional lung capacity through exercise conditioning, muscle training, rest, nutrition, and psychosocial rehabilitation. The overall approach to managing stable COPD should be characterized by stepwise increase in treatment, dependent on the severity of the disease.

Bronchodilator medications are central to the symptomatic management of COPD. They are given on an as-needed basis or on a regular basis to prevent or reduce symptoms. The aerosol route particularly for longer-acting agents is preferred. Frequently, a long-acting beta-2 agonist, anticholinergics, and theophylline are combined. For mild COPD, only a short-acting as-needed bronchodilator is used. For those with stage 2A, 2B, or 3, regular treatment includes a long-acting bronchodilator often taken alone. Salmeterol, for-moterol, or anticholinergic agents, such as ipratropium bromide either alone or combined with a short-acting bronchodilator, are recommended. A short-acting beta-2 agonist, such as albuterol and terbutaline, can be used either on an as-needed basis or combined with other medications and used on a more regular schedule. These agents are frequently given by metered dose inhalers that elderly patients often find difficult to use. Patients with more severe disease often require nebulized albuterol. Increasing doses of these agents, are associated with cardiac arrhythmias. Usually albuterol, 90 μg per puff, is given 2 puffs 4 times a day.

Anticholinergic medications include ipratropium bromide oxitropium bromide (not available in the United States), and a new agent, tiotropium bromide. Anticholinergics are particularly useful in COPD, especially in patients who have smoked for many years and who have a low FEV_1. These agents are poorly absorbed systemically, do not cross the blood-brain barrier, and do not adversely affect cili-ary activity. The main side effect is cough. Because of their slow onset of action, they are not particularly useful for rescue mode. However, they are excellent and safe medications when used in chronic maintenance programs. Ipratropium can be administered either by metered dose inhaler or by a nebulized solution. Ipratropium is also effective in acute respiratory failure. Tiotropium is a new 24-hour agent with a selective anti-muscarinic and so far appears to be the most effective chronic bronchodilator for stable outpatients with COPD. It is now becoming more widely available.

Salmeterol and formoterol are 12-hour long-acting bronchodilators used as chronic maintenance therapy. Both of these agents are highly effective and are very safe in stable patients. The doses, in general, should not be increased. For-moterol has a more rapid onset of action. Salme-terol may be better tolerated. Both of these agents can easily be combined with theophylline or ipratropium bromide.

Theophylline, used previously in COPD as first-line therapy, is now secondary therapy. This agent has some anti-inflammatory effects and improves the strength of diaphragmatic contractility. It also improves mucociliary clearance and cardiac output. However, theophylline has substantial toxicity in patients with COPD. Elderly patients with preexisting abnormal cardiac function are at risk for cardiac arrhythmias, even if levels are in the high therapeutic range. Theophylline has important, potentially toxic, interactions with other drugs that are frequently used for COPD, including macrolide antibiotics, ciprofloxacin, and cimetidine. Most patients require somewhere between 100 and 400 mg per/day. The dose should be titrated to a serum level of 8 to 12.

Prolonged treatment with oral glucocorticosteroids is not recommended in COPD. The severe side effects of systemic glucocorticosteroids are well known and include steroid myopathy, osteopenia, and cataracts. Oral steroids administered as a short course, however, are very useful in acute exacerbations.

Prolonged treatment with inhaled corticosteroids does not modify the long-term decline in FEV_1. The GOLD Guidelines recommend regular treatment with inhaled steroids in those with an FEV_1 of <50% of predicted or those in stage III who have frequent exacerbations requiring treatment with antibiotics and oral corticosteroids. In this setting, there is preservation of quality of life and a reduced number of exacerbations. A therapeutic trial of up to 3 months with inhaled corticosteroids may identify patients who would benefit.

FUTURE DIRECTIONS

Research progress in COPD has been slow. Characterizations of human lung tissue by advanced molecular, biochemical, microbiologic, and histopathologic methods are ongoing. Identification of biomarkers and clinical end points is also essential because the studies of inflammation and the development of new anti-inflammatory agents might be highly effective. Knowledge of genetic determinants of COPD could lead to recognition of biochemical pathways that contribute to the disease and allow targeting of public health intervention to individuals at greatest risk. The causes and consequences of exacerbations need to be identified, and therapy directed at mucus gland metaplasia and excess mucus secretions is necessary. Finally, therapy that results in a stimulation of alveolar regeneration is an exciting possibility for disease-modifying therapy of emphysema. Clinical studies needing additional work include better tools for disease monitoring and more control studies to validate or revise current clinical practice.

REFERENCES

Standards for the diagnosis and care of patients with chronic obstructive pulmonary disease. American Thoracic Society. *Am J Respir Crit Care Med.* 1995;152:S77–S121.

Barnes PJ. Chronic obstructive pulmonary disease. *N Eng J Med.* 2000;343:269–280.

Pauwels RA, Buist AS, Calverley PM, Jenkins CR, Hurd SS, and the GOLD Scientific Committee. Global strategy for the diagnosis, management, and prevention of chronic obstructive pulmonary disease. NHLBI/WHO Global Initiative for Chronic Obstructive Lung Disease (GOLD) Workshop summary. *Am J Respir Crit Care Med.* 2001;163:1256–1276.

Snow V, Lascher S, Mottur-Pilson C, and the Joint Panel on Chronic Obstructive Pulmonary Disease of the American College of Chest Physicians and the American College of Physicians-American Society of Internal Medicine. Evidence base for management of acute exacerbations of chronic obstructive pulmonary disease. *Ann Intern Med.* 2001;134:595–599.

Chapter 121

Community-Acquired Pneumonia

David J. Weber and Meera K. Kelley

Community-acquired pneumonia (CAP) is an important source of morbidity and mortality in the United States. Each year, the 2 to 3 million cases of CAP result in approximately 10 million physician visits, 500,000 hospitalizations, and 45,000 deaths. The incidence of CAP requiring hospitalization is estimated to be 258 cases per 100,000 population and 962 cases per 100,000 persons aged ≥65 year. The mortality rate of persons hospitalized is approximately 14% (range, 2% to 30%).

Community-acquired pneumonia is an acute infection of the pulmonary parenchyma associated with symptoms of acute infection and accompanied by the presence of an acute infiltrate on a chest radiograph or auscultatory findings consistent with pneumonia (such as altered breath sounds and/or localized rales). It occurs in a patient who is not hospitalized or has not resided in an extended care facility for ≥14 days before the onset of symptoms. CAP in the normal host may be caused by a variety of pathogens with *Streptococcus pneumoniae* the most commonly identified (Table 121-1). The epidemiology, etiology, pathogenesis, and treatment of CAP differs from health-care–associated pneumonia, pneumonia in the immunocompromised host, and pneumonia associated with travel outside the United States. The following recommendations for the diagnosis and treatment of CAP are largely drawn from recent guidelines published by the Infectious Diseases Society of America, the Drug-Resistant *Streptococcus pneumoniae* Therapeutic Working Group, and the American Thoracic Society.

CLINICAL PRESENTATION

Pneumonia should be suspected in patients with newly acquired lower respiratory symptoms such as cough, sputum production, and/or shortness of breath. Fever and chills are frequent. Elderly and immunocompromised patients may not manifest the classic symptoms of CAP such as fever and cough; a high index of suspicion for CAP should be maintained if such patients exhibit a significant medical deterioration (e.g., decreased responsiveness, poor appetite, low-grade fever).

Cough is the hallmark of pneumonia. Initially, it may be nonproductive, only to become productive with disease progression. The sputum may be yellow to green as a result of the action of myeloperoxidase produced by polymorphonuclear white cells. Green sputum occurs most commonly as a result of bacterial infection, but it may result from invasive viral illness. Occasionally, pigment-producing *Pseudomonas spp.* may present with green-colored sputum. The neutropenic

Table 121-1
Common Etiologies of Community-Acquired Pneumonia Requiring Hospitalization

Pathogen	Frequency (%)
Streptococcus pneumoniae	20–60
Haemophilus influenzae	3–10
Aspiration pneumonia (mixed flora, especially anaerobes)	6–10
Staphylococcus aureus	3–5
Gram-negative bacilli	3–10
Viruses	2–15
Chlamydia pneumoniae	4–6
Mycoplasma pneumoniae	1–6
Legionella spp.	2–8

Figure 121-1

Pneumococcal Pneumonia

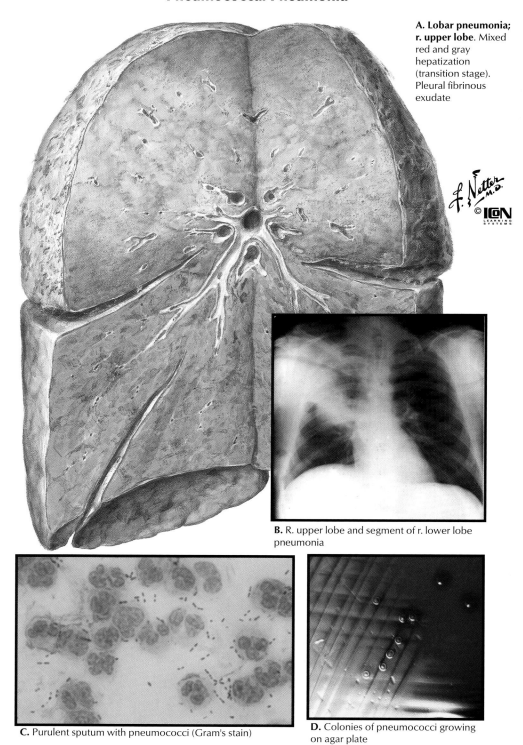

A. Lobar pneumonia; r. upper lobe. Mixed red and gray hepatization (transition stage). Pleural fibrinous exudate

B. R. upper lobe and segment of r. lower lobe pneumonia

C. Purulent sputum with pneumococci (Gram's stain)

D. Colonies of pneumococci growing on agar plate

patient will not produce purulent sputum even with a life-threatening pneumonia. Signs of pneumonia include elevated temperature, elevated respiratory and heart rates, use of accessory muscles, and generally ill appearance. Auscultatory signs of pneumonia result from alveolar infiltration and may include rales, decreased breath sounds, dullness to percussion, and egophony.

Pneumonia is traditionally divided into "typical" and "atypical" categories. Typical pneumonia is due to extracellular bacterial pathogens such as *Streptococcus pneumoniae, Haemophilus influenzae, Klebsiella pneumoniae,* and *Staphylococcus aureus* (Figures 121-1, 121-2, and 121-3). It is characterized by sudden onset, prominent pulmonary symptoms and signs, purulent sputum, and clinical and radiographic evidence of lobar consolidation. Atypical pathogens include viruses and intracellular bacteria such as *Legionella spp., Mycoplasma spp.,* and *Chlamydia pneumoniae* (Figures 121-4). Pneumonia due to "atypical" pathogens is characterized by a stepwise fever curve, prolonged prodrome, frequently extrapulmonary symptoms and signs, non-purulent sputum (i.e., dry cough), and diffuse infiltrate on chest radiography. Extrapulmonary symptoms include headache and/or bullous myringitis (blood blebs on the tympanic membrane) with *Mycoplasma spp.,* myalgias with viral influenza, and gastrointestinal symptoms (e.g., nausea, vomiting, diarrhea) with *Legionella spp.* Often the differentiation of "typical" from "atypical" pneumonia is not clear because patients present with overlapping symptoms.

DIFFERENTIAL DIAGNOSIS

The differential diagnosis of lower respiratory tract illness is extensive and includes both upper and lower respiratory tract infections as well as noninfectious disorders. Important noninfectious disorders that can mimic pneumonia include aspiration of blood or gastric contents, pulmonary emboli with or without pulmonary infarction, congestive heart failure, bronchiolitis obliterans with organizing pneumonia, primary pulmonary malignancy, metastatic cancer, respiratory distress syndrome, drug toxicity, sarcoidosis, and vasculitis (e.g., Wegener's granulomatosis). Many of these disorders may be associated with fever including aspiration of gastric contents, malignancy, pulmonary emboli with infarction, and vasculitis.

DIAGNOSTIC APPROACH

The diagnosis of CAP requires a combination of clinical and laboratory assessments (including microbiologic data). Differentiation of CAP from upper respiratory tract infection is important because most URIs and acute bronchitis are of viral origin and do not require antibiotic therapy; antimicrobial therapy is usually indicated for bacterial pneumonia. It is important to obtain a chest radiograph in persons with symptoms and signs suggestive of lower respiratory tract infection to substantiate the diagnosis of pneumonia because the likelihood of an abnormal chest radiograph ranges from 3% in a general outpatient setting to 28% in an emergency department. In addition, a chest radiograph may be useful for determining the etiologic diagnosis, the prognosis, and for raising suspicion for alternative diagnoses or associated conditions. Chest radiographs in patients with *Pneumocystis carinii* pneumonia (PCP) are normal (false-negative results) in up to 30% of infected patients. PCP should be considered in the differential diagnosis of pneumonia in the immunocompromised host, especially persons with HIV infection, steroid use, or hematologic malignancies.

MANAGEMENT AND THERAPY

The key decision concerning treatment is whether to treat patients as outpatients or in the hospital. Most patients, approximately 75%, can safely be treated with oral antibiotics on an outpatient basis. Investigators from the Pneumonia Patient Outcomes Research Team (PORT) have developed a prediction rule that stratifies patients into 5 classes by using a cumulative point system based on 19 variables. This rule has been validated and allows the identification of patients with CAP who are at increased risk for death and other adverse outcomes. These prediction rules are meant to contribute to rather than supersede the physicians' judgment. Outpatient treatment requires that the patient be able to both comply with therapy as well as to absorb oral antibiotics. Hospitalization may be required for persons with cognitive impairment, history of substance abuse, nausea and vomiting, or underlying disorders that

Figure 121-2

Klebsiella (Friedländer's) Pneumonia

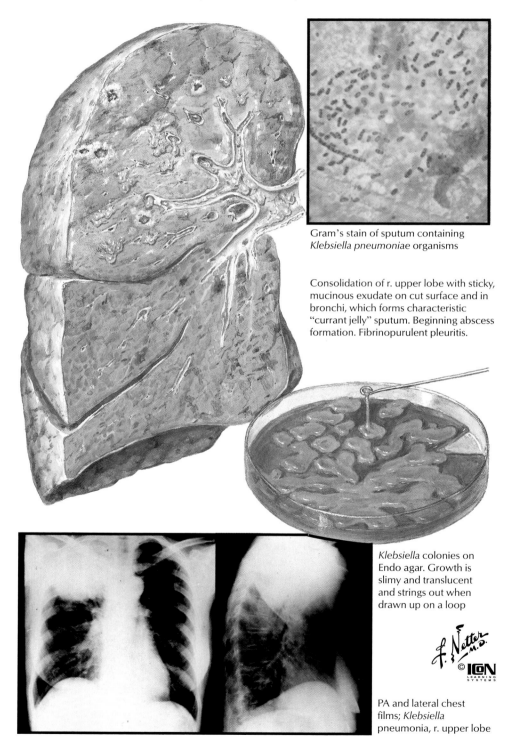

Gram's stain of sputum containing *Klebsiella pneumoniae* organisms

Consolidation of r. upper lobe with sticky, mucinous exudate on cut surface and in bronchi, which forms characteristic "currant jelly" sputum. Beginning abscess formation. Fibrinopurulent pleuritis.

Klebsiella colonies on Endo agar. Growth is slimy and translucent and strings out when drawn up on a loop

PA and lateral chest films; *Klebsiella* pneumonia, r. upper lobe

Figure 121-3

Staphylococcal Pneumonia

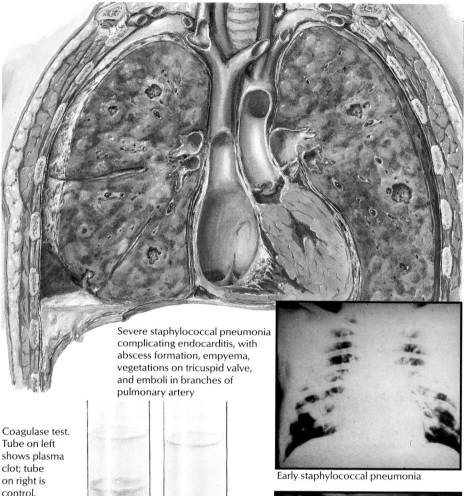

Severe staphylococcal pneumonia complicating endocarditis, with abscess formation, empyema, vegetations on tricuspid valve, and emboli in branches of pulmonary artery

Coagulase test. Tube on left shows plasma clot; tube on right is control.

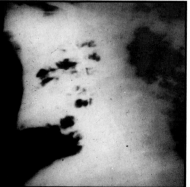

Early staphylococcal pneumonia

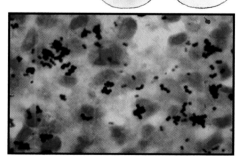

Staphylococcal and polymorphonuclear leukocytes in sputum (Gram's stain)

Late staphylococcal pneumonia with abscesses and pneumothorax

increase the risk of morbidity that are not included in the PORT rules.

Every effort should be made to establish an etiologic diagnosis. First, it permits optimal antibiotic selection specifically directed at the causative agent. Second, it allows for a rational basis for change from parenteral to oral therapy and for a change in therapy necessitated by an adverse drug reaction. Third, this specific diagnosis permits antibiotic selection that limits the consequences of injudicious antibiotic use in terms of cost, inducible resistance, and adverse drug reactions. Finally, this allows identification of pathogens of potential epidemiologic significance, such as *Legionella*, Hantavirus, and penicillin-resistant *S. pneumoniae*. A detailed history may be helpful in suggesting a diagnosis (Table 121-2).

Once a clinical diagnosis has been made, consider making a microbiologic diagnosis with bacteriologic studies of sputum and blood. Obtain sputum from a deep-cough specimen before antibiotic therapy for Gram stain (and culture) to aid in initial selection of antimicrobial therapy. Sputum is acceptable for culture if under low-power microscopy there are >25 polymorphonuclear cells and <10 to 25 squamous epithelial cells. The Gram-stain appearance of *S. pneumoniae* (lancet-shaped Gram-positive diplococci), *H. influenzae* (small Gram-negative coccobacilli), and *S. aureus* (clusters of Gram-positive cocci) are sufficiently distinctive to allow a tentative diagnosis. Blood culture results are positive in approximately 10% of patients hospitalized with pneumonia. Additional diagnostic tests including rapid tests for respiratory syncytial virus and/or influenza, special smears (acid fast smears) and culture for *M. tuberculosis*, urine antigen for *Legionella*, and serologic tests for *Mycoplasma pneumoniae*, *Legionella*, or *Chlamydia* may be indicated, depending on the presence of epidemiologic clues, chest radiographic pattern, severity of illness, and host defense abnormalities. Many additional tests are available to diagnose less common pathogens.

Bronchoscopy is rarely indicated in immunocompetent patients with CAP. It should be considered in patients with a fulminant course without a clear etiology who require admission to the intensive care unit, or have complex pneumonia unresponsive to antimicrobial therapy. Bronchoscopy is particularly useful for the detection of selected pathogens, such as *P. carinii*, *Mycobacterium spp.*, cytomegalovirus, and *Legionella spp.* Standard hematologic tests, chemistries, and oxygen saturation should be obtained to help assess the physiologic status of hospitalized patients and need for intensive care.

Therapy

Empiric antimicrobial therapy is guided by knowledge of likely pathogens (Tables 121-1 and 121-2) and local resistance patterns. Therapy guidelines have undergone recent changes due to the increase in antimicrobial resistance of common pathogens (e.g., *S. pneumoniae*). Therapy may need to be altered or modified by host factors including age, pregnancy, liver or renal dysfunction, use of other medications that interact with planned antimicrobial therapy, and allergies. Everything being equal, the least expensive therapy should be chosen. For oral therapy, also consider frequency of dosing (better compliance is achieved with once- or twice-daily administration), taste, and frequency of gastrointestinal irritation.

Antimicrobial therapy should be initiated promptly after the diagnosis is established with radiography, and Gram stain results are available to facilitate antimicrobial selection. For patients requiring hospitalization, initiate therapy within 4 hours (preferably after blood culture specimens have been obtained). Antibiotic therapy should not be withheld from acutely ill patients because of delays in obtaining appropriate specimens or the results of Gram stains and cultures. The empiric therapy recommended by the Infectious Diseases Society of America is summarized in Table 121-3. If an etiologic agent is isolated, therapy should be altered based on the known susceptibilities of the pathogen or in vitro testing. Drug resistance is a growing problem with *S. pneumoniae* (especially resistance to beta-lactam antibiotics, macrolides, and tetracyclines) and *S. aureus* (especially resistance to beta-lactam antibiotics, macrolides, quinolones, and tetracyclines). The duration of therapy is based on the pathogen, response to therapy, comorbid illness, and complications. In most cases, patients should receive therapy for 7 to 14 days (longer therapy required

Figure 121-4

Legionnaires' Disease
(Pneumonia Due to *Legionella* spp)

A. Small, blunt, pleomorphic intracellular and extracellular bacilli in lung of patient with Legionnaires' disease as shown by Dieterle silver impregnation stain, x 1500 (after Chandler, et al.)

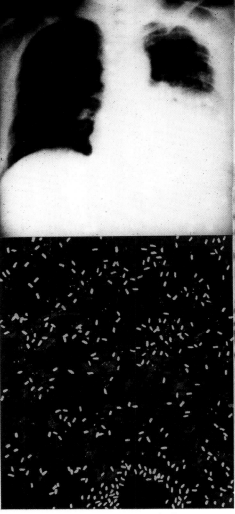

B. Chest x-ray film on fifth day of illness of 58-year-old man with serologically confirmed Legionnaires' disease. L. lower lobe consolidation the only involvement. Clinical improvement within 2 to 3 days of initiation of treatment with erythromycin. Radiologic changes did not completely disappear for 2 months.

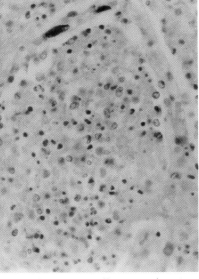

C. *Legionella* spp. dentified by specific fluorescent antibody stain

D. Histologic section of lung (H and E stain) from fatal case of Legionnaires' disease. Extensive intraalveolar exudate present, containing many large macrophages.

Table 121-2
Epidemiology Clues Related to Specific Pathogens with Selected Community-Acquired Pneumonia

Epidemiologic Clue	Pathogen (disease)
Associated with specific pathogen	
Poor dental hygiene; risk of aspiration (e.g., seizure disorder)	Anaerobes
Exposure to birds (especially psittacine birds)	*Chlamydia psittaci* (psitticosis)
Exposure in endemic area (southwest United States, northern Mexico)	*Coccidioides* spp. (coccidioidomycosis)
Exposure to infected farm animals or cats, especially parturient animals	*Coxiella burnetii* (Q fever)
Exposure to rabbits or infected ticks	*Francisella tularensis* (tularemia)
Exposure to bats or soil enriched with bird dropping in an endemic area	*Histoplasma capsulatum* (histoplasmosis)
Exposure to water sources (epidemic setting)	*Legionella* spp. (Legionnaires' disease)
Exposure to cats and less commonly to dogs	*Pasteurella multocida* (Pasteurellosis)
Exposure to infected fleas or host animals (e.g., ground squirrels) in an endemic area, or to persons with pneumonic plague	*Yersinia pestis* (plague)
Associated with multiple pathogens	
Alcoholism	*Streptococcus pneumoniae, Klebsiella pneumonaie,* anaerobes
Chronic obstructive pulmonary disease or smoking	*S. pneumoniae, Haemophilus influenzae, Moraxella catarhalis, Legionella* spp.
HIV* infection (early)	*S. pneumoniae, H. influenzae,* Mycobacterium tuberculosis
HIV* infection (late)	Above plus *P. carinii, Cryptococcus, Histoplasma* spp., *Coccidioides* spp.
Residence in an extended care facility	*S. pneumoniae,* Gram-negative bacilli, *H. influenzae, Staphylococcus aureus,* anaerobes, viral influenza, *Mycobacterium tuberculosis,* structural abnormalities of the lung (e.g., cystic fibrosis, bronchietasis) *S. aureus, Pseudomonas aeruginosa, Bulkholderia cepacia*

* HIV, human immunodeficiency virus.

Table 121-3
Empiric Therapy for Patients with Community-Acquired Pneumonia*

Outpatients

- General preferred (not in particular order)
  - Doxycycline
  - A macrolide: erythromycin, azithromycin, clarithromycin
  - A fluoroquinolone: levofloxacin, moxifloxacin, gatifloxacin
- Selection should be influenced by regional antibiotic susceptibility patterns for *S. pneumoniae* and the presence of other risk factors for drug-resistant *S. pneumoniae.*
- Penicillin-resistant pneumococci may be resistant to macrolides and/or doxycycline.
- For older patients or those with underlying disease, a fluoroquinolone may be a preferred choice; some authorities prefer to reserve fluoroquinolones for such patients.
- Hospitalized patients (general medical ward)
- Generally preferred are: an extended spectrum cephalosporin combined with a macrolide or a beta-lactam/beta-lactamase inhibitor combined with a macrolide, or a fluoroquinolone (alone)
- Extended spectrum cephalosporins: ceftriaxone, cefotaxime, cefepime
- Macrolides: Erythromycin, azithromycin
- Beta-lactam/beta-lactamase inhibitor combination: piperacillin/tazobactam, ampicllin/sulbactam
- Fluoroquinolone: levofloxacin, gatifloxacin, moxifloxacin

Hospitalized patients (intensive care unit)

- Generally preferred are: an extended-spectrum cephalosporin or beta-lactam/beat-lactamase inhibitor plus either fluoroquinolone or macrolide
- Alternatives or modifying factors
- Structural lung disease: antipseudomonal agents (pipercillin, piperacillin-tazobactam, imiperam or meraperam, or cefepime) plus a fluoroquinolone (including high-dose ciprofloxacin)
- Beta-lactam allergy: Fluoroquinolone $\pm$ clindamycin
- Suspected aspiration: Fluoroquinolone with or without clindamycin, metronidazole, or a beta-lactam/beta-lactamase inhibitor

---

* Dose may need to be adjusted for weight, or renal or hepatic failure

Adapted from Bartlett JG, Dowell SF, Mandell LA, File TM Jr, Musher DM, Fine MJ. Practice guidelines for the management of community-acquired pneumonia in adults. Infectious Diseases Society of America. *Clin Infect Dis.* 2000;31:347-382.

for *S. aureus* and enteric Gram-negative bacteria). In general, hospitalized patients can be switched from intravenous therapy to oral therapy when they experience clinical improvement, have been afebrile (<38.3°C) for 24 hours, and have a stable or improved chest radiograph.

Prevention

The annual impact of viral influenza is highly variable. During years in which influenza is epidemic, its impact on CAP is sizeable as a result both of primary influenza pneumonia and secondary bacterial superinfection. Influenza vaccine should be provided annually to persons at high risk for complications of illness and to all health-care workers as recommended by the Advisory Committee on Immunization Practices. The currently available 23-valent pneumococcal capsular polysaccharide vaccine is approximately 50% effective at preventing hospitalization and approximately 80% effective at preventing death from pneumococcal disease in immunocompetent adults. It should be offered to all adults who are >65 years of age and to younger persons who are at high risk of pneumococcal infection.

FUTURE DIRECTIONS

Recommendations for the therapy of CAP are likely to require frequent modifications based on emerging antimicrobial resistance of respiratory pathogens and introduction of new antimicrobial agents. Physicians providing primary care can help minimize the evolution of antimicrobial resistance by not prescribing antibiotics for non-bacterial respiratory tract infections.

REFERENCES

Bartlett JG, Dowell SF, Mandell LA, File TM Jr, Musher DM, Fine MJ. Practice guidelines for the management of community-acquired pneumonia in adults. Infectious Diseases Society of America. *Clin Infect Dis.* 2000;31:347–382.

Heffelfinger JD, Dowell SF, Jorgensen JH, et al. Management of community-acquired pneumonia in the era of pneumococcal resistance: a report from the Drug-Resistant *Streptococcus pneumoniae* Therapeutic Working Group. *Arch Intern Med.* 2000;160:1399–1408.

Niederman MS, Mandell LA, Anzueto A, et al, and the American Thoracic Society. Guidelines for the management of adults with community-acquired pneumonia. Diagnosis, assessment of severity, antimicrobial therapy, and prevention. *Am J Respir Crit Care Med.* 2001;163:1730–1754.

Chapter 122
Obstructive Sleep Apnea

Brian A. Boehlecke

The obstructive sleep apnea syndrome (OSAS) is characterized by recurrent episodes of complete or partial upper airway obstruction during sleep resulting in sleep disruption and excessive daytime sleepiness. OSAS is associated with significant morbidity including increased risk for auto accidents, mood disorders, and cognitive impairment. Even without excessive daytime somnolence, sleep-disordered breathing appears to cause an increased risk for hypertension and cardiovascular disorders. Appropriate management is important to improve quality of life and reduce morbidity.

ETIOLOGY AND PATHOGENESIS

Upper airway dilating muscle activity is reduced during sleep, causing increased pharyngeal wall compliance and reduced airway caliber. Gravitational forces in the supine position compress the upper airway, especially if there is excess fat in the neck. Large tonsils, uvula, or tongue or a retropositioned mandible can also narrow the upper airway. During sleep, partial or complete upper airway collapse causes recurring episodes of increased respiratory effort and brief arousals (microarousals) on EEG. Hypoxemia and hypercarbia from the reduction in ventilation during these episodes may also contribute to the arousals. Sleep disruption due to microarousals is likely the basis for the excessive daytime sleepiness. Arousals are associated with increased sympathetic nervous system activation with tachycardia and increased blood pressure, increasing the risk for sustained hypertension and cardiovascular disease.

Obesity is a risk factor, but its presence is neither necessary nor sufficient for the development of OSAS. Central fat deposition may be more important than peripheral obesity. Neck circumference is better correlated than overall weight. Men are at significantly greater risk for OSAS, and African Americans appear to have a greater risk for severe OSAS than Caucasians of similar weight. The prevalence of OSAS increases with age up to middle age, but shows no increase thereafter. It is not clear whether this is due to bias from selective survival in cross-sectional studies. Nasal obstruction, frequently found in patients with OSAS, may promote airway collapse by causing increased nega-

tive pressure in the upper airway during inspiration. Alcohol and sedating medications reduce upper airway muscle tone and predispose to airway collapse. Snoring may result in vibratory damage to upper airway soft tissues resulting in edema, worsening the obstruction. Excess upper airway tissue in conditions such as hypothyroidism and acromegaly may also increase risk. A combination of factors resulting in upper airway narrowing and increased collapsibility generally contributes to the development of OSAS.

CLINICAL PRESENTATION

Patients commonly present with loud snoring and excessive daytime sleepiness. The bed partner may also note snorting, gasping, or pauses in breathing and often repeatedly shakes the patient to be sure he or she will restart breathing (Figure 122-1). The patient may exhibit nocturnal jerking and frequent nocturia, or even enuresis. Excessive sleepiness may result in auto accidents, poor job performance, or social problems. Morning headaches, poor concentration and memory, depressed mood, and decreased libido or erectile dysfunction are common.

Patients with underlying coronary artery disease may have episodes of nocturnal angina possibly prompted by episodes of hypoxemia. High negative intrathoracic pressure during inspiratory efforts with a closed upper airway may exacerbate symptoms of gastroesophageal reflux.

Physical examination should include documentation of the body mass index and the neck circumference because both are correlated with the risk for OSAS. The nose should be examined

Figure 122-1

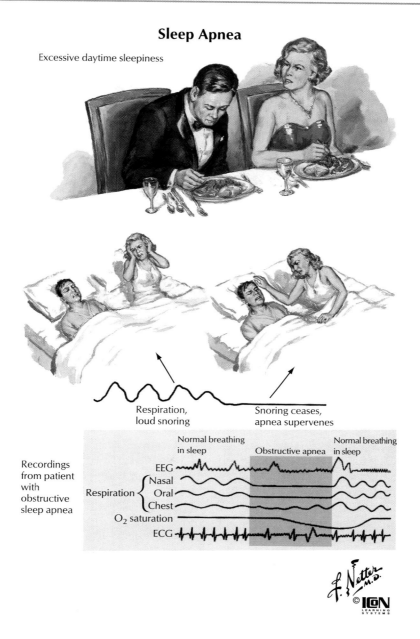

Sleep Apnea

Excessive daytime sleepiness

Respiration, loud snoring

Snoring ceases, apnea supervenes

Recordings from patient with obstructive sleep apnea

Respiration { Nasal / Oral / Chest

Normal breathing in sleep

Obstructive apnea

Normal breathing in sleep

EEG

O_2 saturation

ECG

for obstruction due to a deviated septum or swollen turbinates. Notable findings include the presence of retrognathia, dental overbite, an enlarged uvula, large tonsils, and macroglossia. However, the absence of anatomic upper airway obstruction does not rule out the diagnosis. Hypertension and otherwise unexplained lower extremity edema may be signs of repeated episodes of nocturnal hypoxemia and sympathetic nervous system stimulation.

DIFFERENTIAL DIAGNOSIS

It is important to distinguish true excessive daytime sleepiness (EDS) from fatigue, a common symptom in organic diseases such as congestive heart failure and in depression. However, periodic breathing with central apneas (Cheyne-Stokes respiration) associated with congestive heart failure and stroke can disrupt sleep and cause true EDS. Central sleep apnea (idiopathic or associated with Arnold-Chiari malformation) and CNS disorders such as narcolepsy and idiopathic hypersomnia cause excessive daytime sleepiness. Sleep disruption due to periodic limb movements of sleep, frequent urination, poorly controlled pain syndromes, gastroesophageal reflux, asthma attacks, medications, and external disturbances such as noise should also be considered. Shift in the time period during which the patient is most able to sleep (circadian rhythm disorders such as advanced sleep phase syndrome, common in the elderly, or delayed sleep phase syndrome, common in teenagers) may cause excessive sleepiness during certain periods of the day with normal alertness at other times. Insufficient sleep due to social activities or excessive school or work demands can cause EDS.

DIAGNOSTIC APPROACH

Confirmation of the diagnosis of OSAS is best accomplished by an overnight polysomnogram in a sleep laboratory. *Polysomnography* (PSG) includes recordings of the electroencephalogram, electro-oculogram, and chin electromyogram (EMG) to allow sleep stage scoring. Airflow measurement and some index of respiratory "effort" (e.g., chest and abdominal wall motion or esophageal manometry) detect and distinguish central and obstructive apneas (Figure 122-1). Arterial blood oxygen saturation measured with pulse oximetry, ECG, and pretibial EMG (to detect periodic limb movements of sleep) are monitored continuously.

Abnormal breathing events and arousals are scored and indexes of the number of events per hour of sleep calculated. Both apneas (complete cessation of airflow for 10 seconds or longer) and hypopneas (reductions in airflow associated with oxygen desaturations or arousals) are included in the respiratory disturbance index (RDI). Clinical grading of the severity of respiratory disturbance is somewhat controversial, but generally an RDI up to 5, or even 10, is considered normal. Values up to 20 indicate a relatively mild abnormality, over 20 to 40 moderate, and greater than 40 severe. Studies have demonstrated that severity of symptoms and risk for cardiovascular morbidity increase with a higher RDI.

Some patients with EDS have recurrent respiratory events with increasing effort terminated by arousal on EEG (respiratory-related arousals), but no overt apneas or hypopneas. This upper airway resistance syndrome may have the same consequences as OSAS.

Repetitive stereotypic limb movements may be associated with arousals (periodic limb movement disorder), but some patients have frequent spontaneous arousals indicating sleep disruption with no recognizable cause. Intrusion of alpha frequencies (8 to 13 cycles per second) into deeper stages of sleep (alpha-delta sleep) may indicate chronic pain or anxiety causing less than refreshing sleep.

If no cause of sleep disruption is found on PSG, a multiple sleep latency test (MSLT) is performed the following day to document objective sleepiness. The MSLT consists of four to five 20-minute naps 2 hours apart, starting 1 hour after the patient awakens from the PSG. Average sleep onset latency from lights off of 10 minutes or longer is considered normal. A sleep latency less than 5 minutes indicates definite excessive sleepiness. Patients with narcolepsy may have an average sleep latency of less than 2 minutes and may show rapid eye movement (REM) sleep in 2 or more of the naps. The latter finding can also occur as a rebound phenomenon after REM sleep deprivation due to alcohol, antidepressant drugs, or obstructive sleep apnea.

MANAGEMENT AND THERAPY

Although there is no consensus on the indications for treatment, patients with an RDI of 15 or higher are likely to experience significant symptoms and be at risk for increased morbidity. Patients with lower RDIs but with severe symptoms, or with objective findings consistent with consequences of sleep-disordered breathing, such as hypertension, should also be treated. The treatment of choice is the use of nasal continuous positive airway pressure (CPAP). Determination of the proper pressure requires titration during PSG. Although this may require a second PSG night, many laboratories try to establish the correct pressure during the latter portion of a single night study if the diagnosis of OSA is made during the first several hours. The CPAP is titrated to a pressure that abolishes apneas and hypopneas and prevents recurrent desaturations and arousals. Abolishment of snoring is also desirable. However, the optimal pressure for clinical management may not achieve complete resolution of all respiratory disturbances because higher pressures are less easily tolerated. Use of nasal CPAP for at least 4 hours per night usually produces a significant reduction in symptoms and improvement in quality of life. Patient education and early follow-up to deal with complications such as mask leaks or nasal drying is important to increase usage. Adequate humidification prevents ineffective CPAP due to nasal mucosal drying, irritation, and obstruction. Patients experiencing nasal congestion with room temperature humidifiers may benefit from a heated humidifier.

Factors contributing to upper airway collapse should also be addressed. Weight reduction is extremely important, but difficult to achieve. Patients should be encouraged to take advantage of the increased energy level and improved mood they experience by getting better sleep with CPAP to attempt to lose weight. Respiratory depressant medications such as sedating antihistamines and sleeping pills should be avoided. Alcohol should be avoided for several hours before bedtime. Using pillows or a foam wedge to maintain the lateral position or elevating the head of the bed slightly is also helpful. An adequate number of hours in bed is important because sleep deprivation worsens obstructive sleep apnea. Chronic rhinitis should be treated with a nasal steroid spray and possibly a nonsedating antihistamine. If anatomical nasal obstruction is present, consultation with an otolaryngologist for possible correction of septal deviation or submucous resection of enlarged nasal turbinates is indicated. A technique using high-frequency energy administered through a needle to shrink the turbinates shows some promise in reducing nasal obstruction. An oral-maxillofacial surgeon should evaluate patients with severe retrognathia to determine if jaw advancement would be beneficial.

Surgical removal of the tonsils, uvula, and "excess" tissue of the oropharynx, the uvulopalatopharyngoplasty procedure is used to treat OSAS. Although highly effective in reducing the loudness of snoring, the procedure is only approximately 50% effective in curing severe OSAS. This procedure may benefit patients with severe OSAS who cannot tolerate nasal CPAP. Tracheostomy can be curative for patients with serious consequences or who are at high risk for future morbid-

ity and have failed all other treatments.

Protriptyline in doses of 10 to 20 mg at bedtime may reduce symptoms, possibly by increasing upper airway tone. It may be used as an adjunct to nasal CPAP therapy to facilitate a reduction in pressure to improve tolerance if the patient is experiencing difficulty.

Common causes of persistent excessive daytime somnolence during CPAP treatment are ineffective pressure due to mask leaks or poor patient compliance. If symptoms persist after a good mask fit has been achieved and other causes such as inadequate hours of sleep have been considered, a repeat PSG is indicated to determine if the patient's current nasal CPAP setting is adequate. The PSG may detect other causes of sleep disruption such as periodic limb movements of sleep that were not noted on the first study because frequent respiratory events disrupted sleep.

Bilevel positive airway pressure with higher pressures during inspiration than during expiration may be better tolerated than nasal CPAP by some patients.

Intra-oral devices worn during the night to advance the mandible are available. These have been less adequately studied than CPAP but may be useful for patients who cannot tolerate CPAP. Patients who remain sleepy despite adequate therapy on CPAP and lack of other documented sleep disruptions may benefit from stimulant medication. Methylphenidate and dextroamphetamine, traditionally used in the treatment of narcolepsy, have bothersome side effects of nervousness and insomnia and potential for abuse. Modafinil increases alertness without the same propensity for these effects.

FUTURE DIRECTIONS

Screening studies with portable devices to facilitate earlier diagnosis are being reviewed and practice guidelines developed. The Sleep Heart Health Study, a long-term prospective study with in-home PSG, should provide significant insight into the thresholds for treatment and help identify the patients who are at greatest risk for cardiovascular complications. Computerized CPAP devices that automatically alter the pressure based on detection of flow limitation are available and may allow adequate diagnosis and titration to be done in non-laboratory settings in selected patients. Pharmacologic therapy to increase upper airway tone and to prevent upper airway collapse during sleep is under investigation. Results have been promising for serotonin agonists in animal models, but methods to deliver adequate concentrations to the appropriate CNS locations in ways clinically useful in humans are not yet available. Results of trials with available selective serotonin reuptake inhibitor antidepressant medications have been disappointing.

REFERENCES

Badr MS. Pathogenesis of obstructive sleep apnea. *Prog Cardiovasc Dis.* 1999;41:323-330.

Engleman HM, Kingshott RN, Wraith PK, Mackay TW, Deary IJ, Douglas NJ. Randomized placebo-controlled crossover trial of continuous positive airway pressure for mild sleep apnea/hypopnea syndrome. *Am J Respir Crit Care Med.* 1999;159:461-467.

Gottlieb DJ, Whitney CW, Bonekat WH, et al. Relation of sleepiness to respiratory disturbance index: the Sleep Heart Health Study. *Am J Respir Crit Care Med.* 1999;159:502-507.

Nieto FJ, Young TB, Lind BK, et al. Association of sleep-disordered breathing, sleep apnea, and hypertension in a large community-based study. Sleep Heart Health Study. *JAMA.* 2000;283:1829-1836.

Redine S, Strohl KP. Recognition and consequences of obstructive sleep apnea hypopnea syndrome. *Otalaryngol Clin North Am.* 1999;32:303-331.

Chapter 123

Pleural Effusion and Pneumothorax

M. Patricia Rivera

Typically, pleural effusions and pneumothoraces are secondary manifestations of other underlying disease states, such as empyema with pneumonia or spontaneous pneumothorax with emphysema. Less commonly, the pleura can be the primary site of disease, as with mesothelioma. Although much is known about the clinical patterns of pleural diseases, surprisingly little is understood about their pathogenesis.

PATHOPHYSIOLOGY

The pleural space, 10 to 20 μm in diameter, is filled with a thin layer of pleural fluid that acts as a lubricant. Both the visceral and parietal pleura are lined with a single layer of mesothelial cells overlying a layer of connective tissue and derive their blood supply from the systemic capillaries. Pleural fluid can originate in the interstitial spaces of the lung, the pleural capillaries, the intrathoracic lymphatics, or the peritoneal cavity. In normal individuals, the origin of most pleural fluid is the capillaries in the parietal pleura, and the amount of fluid produced each day is approximately 0.1 to 0.2 mL/kg of body weight. The pleural space is in communication with the lymphatic vessels in the parietal pleura by means of stomas in the parietal pleura. The capacity for lymphatic clearance of fluid is 20-fold to 30-fold greater than the rate of fluid influx. Normal fluid has a pH of 7.6, protein <1.5 g/dL, and a cell count of approximately 1,500 cells/mL with a predominance of monocytes.

Fluid accumulates when the rate of formation exceeds the rate of absorption; the most common cause is increased interstitial fluid in the lungs. Mechanisms for pleural fluid accumulation include increased hydrostatic pressure, decreased oncotic or pleural pressure, increased vascular permeability, transdiaphragmatic movement of ascitic fluid, and disruption of the thoracic duct. Obstruction of the lymphatics draining the parietal pleura and an elevation of systemic vascular pressures are the most common causes of decreased fluid absorption.

CLINICAL AND RADIOLOGIC PRESENTATION

Patients may present asymptomatically or with pleuritic chest pain, non-productive cough, and dyspnea. Examination of the chest reveals decreased tactile fremitus and diminished or absent breath sounds. When pleural effusions diminish in size spontaneously or as a result of treatment, a pleural rub may develop.

Obliteration of the posterior costophrenic angle by a meniscus-shaped homogenous shadow is a common finding on the upright chest radiograph. As more fluid accumulates, the diaphragm silhouette on the affected side is lost, and the fluid extends upward around the anterior, lateral, and posterior thoracic walls. The lateral decubitus radiograph helps to quantify the size of the effusion. Fluid that exceeds 10 mm in diameter from the inside margin of the rib to the outside margin of the lung is amenable to thoracentesis.

At times, substantial amounts of pleural fluid can be present in a subpulmonic location without spilling into the costophrenic sulci. The radiographic characteristics of a subpulmonic effusion include elevation of the diaphragm, lateral displacement of the dome of the diaphragm, diaphragmatic flattening, and if the effusion is on the left side, a gap greater than 2 cm between the left hemidiaphragm and the gastric bubble.

When the patient is in the supine position, pleural fluid gravitates to the posterior parts of the thoracic cavity. The supine radiograph reveals blunting of the costophrenic angle, loss of the hemidiaphragm silhouette, and increased homogenous density superimposed over the lung.

When the entire hemithorax is opacified due to a pleural effusion, the mediastinum shifts to the contralateral side. Shifting of the mediastinum toward the ipsilateral side implies either complete obstruction of the ipsilateral mainstem bronchus or a trapped lung as in mesothelioma. If no shift is

Table 123-1
Pleural Effusion and Pneumothorax

Transudates

Congestive heart failure, urinothorax, cirrhosis/ascites, myxedema, nephrotic syndrome, pulmonary embolism, peritoneal dialysis, malignancy, superior vena caval obstruction, atelectasis

Exudates

Infectious diseases: parapneumonic, empyema, tuberculosis, aspergillosis, blastomycosis, cryptococcosis, histoplasmosis, coccidioidomycosis, viral infections, nocardiosis, actinomycosis, paragonimiasis, amebiasis

Gastrointestinal diseases: pancreatitis, pancreatic pseudocyst, esophageal perforation, abdominal surgery, postsclerotherapy, abscess

Collagen vascular diseases: rheumatoid arthritis, systemic lupus, Sjögren's syndrome, Churg-Strauss vasculitis, familial mediterranean fever, immunoblastic lymphadenopathy

HIV disease: Kaposi's sarcoma, parapneumonic, tuberculosis, opportunistic infections, other malignancies

Malignancy: metastatic carcinoma, lymphoma, mesothelioma, leukemia, multiple myeloma

Lymphatic diseases: chylothorax, yellow nail syndrome, lymphangiomyomatosis

Drugs: nitrofurantoin, amiodarone, dantrolene, methysergide, procarbazine, drug-induced lupus, bromocriptine, minoxidil, bleomycin, methotrexate, mitomycin

Miscellaneous: pulmonary embolism, sarcoidosis, benign asbestos effusion, uremia, Meig's syndrome, radiation therapy, hemothorax, postthoracotomy

*HIV, Human immunodeficiency virus.

evident, the mediastinum is likely fixed due to fibrosis or malignant infiltration.

DIAGNOSTIC APPROACH
Pleural Fluid Analysis:
Transudate versus Exudate

A diagnostic thoracentesis is performed when the thickness of pleural fluid on the lateral decubitus radiograph is greater than 10 mm or when loculated fluid is demonstrated on ultrasound, unless the patient has typical congestive heart failure (CHF). Pleural effusions have classically been divided into transudates and exudates (Table 123-1).

A transudative effusion develops when systemic factors (hydrostatic or oncotic pressures) influencing the formation of fluid are altered. Vascular permeability is normal. Exudative effusions develop when the pleural surfaces or the capillaries in the location where the fluid accumulates are altered. Exudative pleural effusions meet at least one of the following criteria (Light's criteria): 1) fluid/serum protein ratio >0.5; 2) fluid/serum lactate dehydrogenase (LDH) ratio >0.6; 3) pleural fluid LDH >two thirds the upper limit of normal for serum LDH. Transudative effusions meet none of the criteria.

A confounding factor encountered with the diagnostic separation of transudates and exudates is seen in diuretic-treated CHF, where the fluid protein can be elevated in the range of 3 to 4 g/dL. In this instance, the pleural fluid to serum albumin gradient is useful; if it is greater than 1.2 g/dL, in all probability the pleural fluid is due to CHF.

Routine tests performed on all effusions include protein, LDH, glucose, pH, and cell count with differential. Additional studies include Gram stain and culture, potassium hydroxide preparation and fungal culture, acid-fast bacteria smear and culture, and cytology. In the appropriate clinical context, additional studies such as amylase, triglycerides, cholesterol, rheumatoid factor, and antinuclear antibody (ANA) may be helpful.

Turbid pleural fluid is usually associated with a chylothorax, elevated levels of cholesterol (pseudochylothorax), or empyema. Chocolate brown-colored fluid suggests amebiasis with a hepatobiliary fistula.

Clear or bloody viscous fluid (increases hyaluronic acid level) is suggestive of malignant mesothelioma. Yellow-green fluid is described with rheumatoid pleural effusions, and black fluid with *Aspergillus* infection. A feculent odor indicates an anaerobic infection; an ammonia scent is associated with urinothorax. A bloody effusion, red blood cell (RBC) count >100,000/mm³, suggests trauma, malignancy, or pulmonary embolism. When the hematocrit exceeds 50% of the blood value, a hemothorax is present and chest tube thoracostomy should be considered (Figure 123-1).

Differential white blood cell count is one of the most informative tests on pleural fluid. Neutrophils predominate in pleural fluid resulting from acute inflammatory processes such as bacterial infection, pancreatitis, and pulmonary embolism. Lymphocyte predominance implies malignancy or tuberculosis. The most common cause of pleural fluid eosinophilia (>10%) is the presence of air or blood in the pleural space; other causes include asbestos, drugs (dantrolene, nitrofurantoin, bromocriptine), parasitic infections (paragonimiasis, amebiasis), and Churg-Strauss syndrome. Basophilia (>10%) is most common with leukemic pleural involvement. The presence of mesothelial cells (>5%) excludes tuberculosis.

Specific tests may provide additional insight. A markedly elevated fluid protein (>7 g/dL) implies a paraproteinemia or multiple myeloma. A low pleural fluid glucose level (<60 mg/dL) indicates rheumatoid disease, empyema, parapneumonic effusions, malignancy, esophageal rupture, and occasionally tuberculosis. Pleural fluid amylase above the upper limits for serum indicates 1 of 4 problems: pancreatic disease, esophageal rupture, malignancy, or ruptured ectopic pregnancy. A pH below 7.30 is seen in esophageal rupture, empyema, rheumatoid effusion, malignant effusion, lupus pleuritis, tuberculosis, and systemic acidosis. In the evaluation of collagen vascular disease, measurement of a rheumatoid factor and ANA can be very helpful.

Transudative Effusions

The most common cause of pleural effusions is CHF; most patients (88%) have bilateral effusions. Unilateral right- and left-sided effusions are reported in 8% and 4%, respectively. Approximately 25% of patients with unilateral effusions attributable to CHF have concomitant pneumonia or pulmonary embolism. Patients with bilateral effusions and the accompanying physical findings of left ventricular dysfunction can safely be observed without thoracentesis. Failure of the effusion to respond to heart failure management, or the presence of pleuritic chest pain or fever mandates evaluation of the pleural fluid. Other causes of transudative effusions are listed in Table 123-1.

Exudative Effusions

The differential diagnosis of exudative pleural effusions is extensive (Table 123-1). The most common causes are infectious processes and malignancy (Figure 123-2).

Parapneumonic effusions, associated with bacterial pneumonia or lung abscess, are the most common cause of exudative effusions in the United States. Approximately 40% of cases of pneumonia have an associated pleural effusion. Typically, *uncomplicated parapneumonic effusions* have a pH of >7.30, glucose >60 mg/dL, and LDH <1000 IU/L and resolve spontaneously with antibiotic therapy. An *empyema* is pus in the pleural space, but it can also be defined by the presence of bacteria on a fluid Gram stain or bacterial growth from fluid culture. It warrants immediate drainage with tube thoracostomy. A *complicated parapneumonic* effusion lacks any of the criteria defining empyema, but has a pH of <7.0, glucose <40 mg/dL, and LDH >1,000 IU/ L. These effusions are not likely to respond to antibiotic therapy alone, and drainage with tube thoracostomy is necessary. The bacteriology of empyema focuses on Gram-positive aerobes (*Streptococcus pneumoniae*, *Staphylococcus aureus*), Gram-negative aerobes (*Klebsiella* species, *Pseudomonas* species, *Hemophilus influenzae*), and anaerobes (*Bacteroides* species, *Peptostreptococcus*). Inadequate drainage of an empyema or the progressive development of loculations requires aggressive management with CT imaging and further intervention. Intrapleural installation of thrombolytics such as streptokinase has been associated with successful lysis of loculations and improved drainage. Additional chest tube placement or insertion of smaller "pigtail" catheters is reported to have a 60% to 90% success rate. Surgical options include decortication and open drainage.

Figure 123-1

Hemothorax

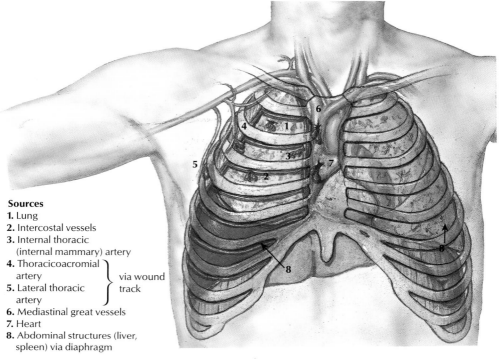

Sources
1. Lung
2. Intercostal vessels
3. Internal thoracic (internal mammary) artery
4. Thoracicoacromial artery ⎫
5. Lateral thoracic artery ⎭ via wound track
6. Mediastinal great vessels
7. Heart
8. Abdominal structures (liver, spleen) via diaphragm

Degrees and management

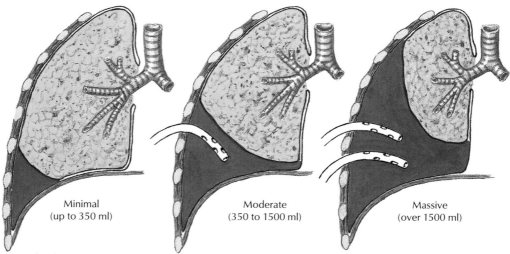

Minimal
(up to 350 ml)

Blood usually resorbs spontaneously with conservative management. Thoracentesis rarely necessary

Moderate
(350 to 1500 ml)

Thoracentesis and tube drainage with underwater-seal drainage usually suffices

Massive
(over 1500 ml)

Two drainage tubes inserted since one may clog, but immediate or early thoracotomy may be necessary to arrest bleeding

Figure 123-2

Cryptococcosis (Torulosis)

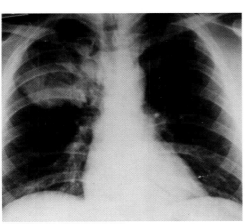

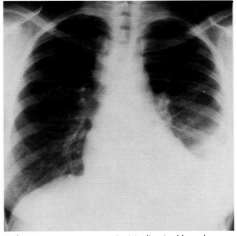

Pulmonary cryptococcosis presenting as a large masslike lesion, easily mistaken for carcinoma

Pulmonary cryptococcosis. Mediastinal lymph nodes enlarged and pleural effusion on left

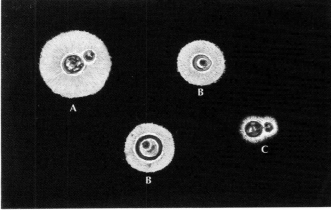

India ink preparation showing *C. neoformans*

A. Budding organism with thick capsule

B. Nonbudding organisms

C. Unencapsulated form (budding)

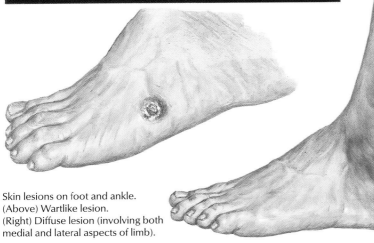

Skin lesions on foot and ankle.
(Above) Wartlike lesion.
(Right) Diffuse lesion (involving both medial and lateral aspects of limb).

Tuberculous pleural effusions are rare; typically, they present as an acute illness. PPD skin test results are reportedly negative in approximately one third of patients. Fluid examination reveals lymphocyte-predominant exudate. Mesothelial cells and eosinophils are uncommon. Typically, the fluid protein is >5 g/dL, LDH is mildly elevated, and the glucose is <60 mg/dL. The acid-fast bacteria smear or the culture results are rarely positive. Pleural biopsy is reported to have a high diagnostic yield. Most tuberculous effusions resolve spontaneously; however, treatment with standard tuberculous therapy is given to prevent recurrent disease. Serial thoracentesis has not been shown to improve outcome.

Malignant pleural effusions are due most commonly to lung (30%) and breast (25%) cancer. Lymphoma is responsible for 20% of malignant effusions. Mechanisms for these effusions include direct pleural involvement by tumor, reduced pleural pressure associated with bronchial obstruction, pulmonary embolism, or sequelae of chemotherapy or radiation therapy. Malignant effusions are usually moderate in size and associated with dyspnea, show a lymphocyte predominance, and have RBC counts >1,000,000/ mm. Large tumor burden is associated with a low pH (<7.30) and glucose (<60 mg/dL) as well as shortened survival time. Pleural fluid cytology is diagnostic in approximately 65% of cases. The yield can increase when 3 separate fluid specimens are submitted. Closed pleural biopsy is only diagnostic in approximately 50% of cases. Thoracoscopy is diagnostic in 93% of cases. Treatment options include treating the underlying cancer, drainage with "pigtail catheter" or chest tube, and chemical pleurodesis.

Chylothorax is characterized by a milky-white effusion with an elevated triglyceride level due to the accumulation of chyle in the pleural space from disruption of the thoracic duct. The most common cause of chylothorax is lymphoma (37% of cases). Other causes include metastatic cancer, surgical or nonsurgical trauma, lymphangiomyomatosis, and cirrhosis. Conservative therapy includes bowel rest, parenteral nutrition, and treatment of underlying disorder. Definitive therapy involves repair of the thoracic duct.

Hemothorax is defined as a pleural fluid hematocrit exceeding 50% of the serum value. Trauma and iatrogenic vascular injury are the most common causes, but it is seen with a variety of disorders including arteriovenous malformations, ascites, malignancy, coagulopathy, endometriosis, neurofibromatosis, pneumothorax, retroperitoneal hemorrhage, sequestration, and vascular anomalies. Treatment involves large bore chest tube thoracostomy and thoracotomy when the bleeding persists.

Pneumothorax

Pneumothorax reflects air escaping into the pleural space. Pneumothoraces can be divided into spontaneous (without antecedent trauma) and traumatic (result of direct or indirect trauma). *Spontaneous pneumothoraces* are further divided into primary (in otherwise healthy individuals) and secondary (as complication of underlying lung disease). *Primary spontaneous pneumothoraces* are caused by rupture of apical subpleural blebs. Most *secondary spontaneous pneumothoraces* are due to chronic obstructive lung disease although they have been associated with a variety of disorders (Table 123-2).

Dyspnea and pleuritic chest pain are the most common symptoms. If pneumothorax is suspected, obtain an end-expiratory chest radiograph. Simple observation will suffice as treatment for asymptomatic patients with small (<15% of

Table 123-2
Diseases Associated with Secondary Spontaneous Pneumothorax

Alveolar proteinosis
Asthma
Berylliosis
Chronic obstructive airways disease
Cystic fibrosis
Histiocytosis X
Idiopathic pulmonary hemosiderosis
Lung cancer
Metastatic sarcoma
Lymphangiomyomatosis
Marfan's syndrome
Ehlers-Danlos syndrome
Paragonimiasis
Pneumocystis carinii pneumonia
Primary biliary cirrhosis
Sarcoidosis
Scleroderma
Silicosis
Tuberculosis
Rheumatoid lung disease

Figure 123-3

Tension Pneumothorax

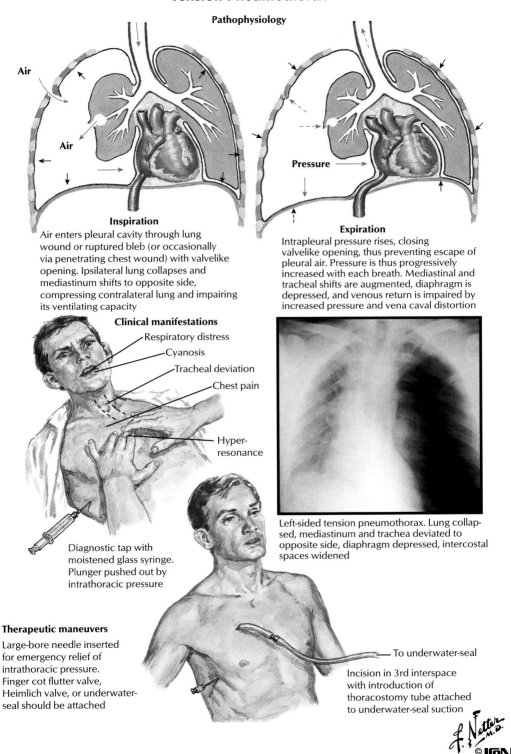

Pathophysiology

Air

Air

Pressure

Inspiration

Air enters pleural cavity through lung wound or ruptured bleb (or occasionally via penetrating chest wound) with valvelike opening. Ipsilateral lung collapses and mediastinum shifts to opposite side, compressing contralateral lung and impairing its ventilating capacity

Expiration

Intrapleural pressure rises, closing valvelike opening, thus preventing escape of pleural air. Pressure is thus progressively increased with each breath. Mediastinal and tracheal shifts are augmented, diaphragm is depressed, and venous return is impaired by increased pressure and vena caval distortion

Clinical manifestations

Respiratory distress

Cyanosis

Tracheal deviation

Chest pain

Hyper-
resonance

Diagnostic tap with moistened glass syringe. Plunger pushed out by intrathoracic pressure

Left-sided tension pneumothorax. Lung collapsed, mediastinum and trachea deviated to opposite side, diaphragm depressed, intercostal spaces widened

Therapeutic maneuvers

Large-bore needle inserted for emergency relief of intrathoracic pressure. Finger cot flutter valve, Heimlich valve, or underwater-seal should be attached

To underwater-seal

Incision in 3rd interspace with introduction of thoracostomy tube attached to underwater-seal suction

hemithorax) primary spontaneous pneumothoraces. Supplemental oxygen accelerates the rate of air absorption. Needle aspiration is the initial treatment for symptomatic primary spontaneous pneumothorax. If it is unsuccessful, chest tube thoracostomy should be performed. Chest tube thoracostomy is the treatment of choice for secondary spontaneous pneumothoraces.

Tension pneumothorax, a one-way valve mechanism that results in a progressive rise in pleural pressure, occurs in 3% to 5% of patients with spontaneous pneumothorax and in 5% to 15% of those with barotrauma (patients on mechanical ventilation) (Figure 123-3). Contralateral displacement of the trachea and mediastinum occurs and venous return is impaired resulting in cardiopulmonary distress. Placement of a large bore needle or an angiocatheter will decompress the tension. Mortality is about 30% if treatment is delayed.

FUTURE DIRECTIONS

The workup of pleural effusions is often a lengthy process fraught with pitfalls, particularly when dealing with malignant pleural effusions. Several studies suggest that thoracoscopy increases the diagnostic yield in patients with benign and malignant pleural disease when thoracentesis and closed pleural biopsy (CPB) results are nondiagnostic. Thoracoscopy is a minimally invasive and relatively safe procedure that will likely supplant CPB in the diagnostic workup of malignant pleural effusions.

REFERENCES

Light RW. *Pleural Diseases.* 4th ed. Philadelphia, Pa: Lippincott Williams & Wilkins; 2001.

Sahn SA. Management of complicated parapneumonic effusions. *Am Rev Respir Dis.* 1993;148:813-817.

Sahn SA. State of the art: the pleura. *Am Rev Respir Dis.* 1988;138:184-234.

Section XV

DISORDERS OF THE IMMUNE SYSTEM, CONNECTIVE TISSUE, AND JOINTS

Chapter 124

Calcium Pyrophosphate Dihydrate Deposition Disease

Robert G. Berger

Calcium pyrophosphate dihydrate deposition disease (CPPD; pseudogout) is caused by precipitation of the phlogistic crystals of CPPD within the synovial, tenosynovial, or cartilaginous spaces. *Phlogism* is the capability of a biological compound to produce inflammation when present in its crystalline form. In the musculoskeletal system, phlogistic crystals include sodium urate, calcium pyrophosphate, calcium hydroxyapatite, and calcium oxalate. Each crystal produces a distinct clinical syndrome. Unlike uric acid crystals, which almost always produce clinical inflammation, CPPD crystals may deposit in cartilaginous tissue, particularly in elderly patients, and produce no apparent clinical symptoms. These deposits appear within the joint spaces on routine radiographs of knees or wrists in approximately 30% of patients older than 80 and in 10% of patients between the ages of 60 and 75. Only a small percentage of these patients will exhibit any of the clinical manifestations that are described in this chapter.

ETIOLOGY AND PATHOGENESIS

The biochemical mechanism or defects producing the articular deposits of CPPD have yet to be established. The search for the metabolic basis of CPPD depostion disease has concentrated on studying those mechanisms that increase pyrophosphate synthesis or decrease its elimination in articular cartilage or synovium. Increased pyrophosphate concentration in the synovial fluid may be a by-product of increased synthesis of proteoglycans or collagenous and noncollagenous proteins. Decreased elimination of pyrophosphate may result from aberrant activity of enzymes associated with adenosine triphosphate pathways within the articular space.

Despite the lack of understanding of the pathophysiology of CPPD depostion disease, certain diseases have an absolute association with the entity, and should be pursued as coexisting whenever a patient first presents with clinical manifestations of CPPD depostion. These can be remembered as the 5 Hs: hyperparathyroidism, hemochromatosis, hypothyroidism, hypomagnesemia, and hypophosphatasia. Early appearance of the disease (before age 40) may be associated with any of these conditions, or in some cases, the result of a rare inherited familial form.

CLINICAL PRESENTATION
Acute Pseudogout

Classical acute CPPD depostion disease is known as *pseudogout* because of the abrupt clinical presentation of an acute monoarthritis or oligoarthritis. This form of the disease affects older women preferentially and usually occurs in the knees, shoulders, or wrists (Figure 124-1). Its presentation mimics that of gout (although it rarely affects the toes and fingers) and septic arthritis.

On physical examination, as in gout, the patient usually cannot move the affected joint without severe pain. Large tense joint effusions are common in knees or shoulders during the acute attack. Patients will have redness and heat over the joint and may have a low-grade fever.

Laboratory findings during the acute attack may include an elevated WBC count with a left shift, elevated sedimentation rate, and increased levels of other acute phase reactants such as ferritin and C-reactive protein. Synovial fluid will be mildly to moderately inflammatory, containing mostly polymorphonuclear neutrophils, but may appear grossly purulent. Radiographs may or may not show chondrocalcinosis within the involved joint (Figure 124-2).

Osteoarthritic Calcium Pyrophosphate Deposition Disease

Patients present with a chronic, sometimes deforming, arthritis primarily affecting the knees, wrists, shoulders, and MCP joints. They may describe episodic acute attacks of swelling, redness, and pain in the involved joints or a more indolent history of chronic non-inflammatory pain. Physical examination reveals changes consistent with osteoarthritis with joint crepitus, deformities, and decreased range of motion. The knee may have valgus deformities ("windswept knees") instead of the more common varus deformities seen in pure osteoarthritis. The wrist is almost never involved in pure osteoarthritis; therefore, when wrist deformities are present in a patient with other osteoarthritic joints, the diagnosis of CPPD depostion disease should be considered.

Laboratory evaluation is not helpful. Sedimentation rate is normal. Radiographs of involved joints usually show osteoarthritis, although the presence of chondrocalcinosis, particularly in the wrist ulnar triangular fibrocartilage, may be helpful to discriminate this form of the disease from routine osteoarthritis.

Pseudo-Rheumatoid Calcium Pyrophosphate Deposition Disease

This rare form can mimic rheumatoid arthritis. The presentation is a symmetrical acute or chronic polyarthritis, particularly of the hands and wrists. Serum rheumatoid factor may sometimes be positive. Occasionally, patients with this form of the disease may be quite ill, with fever, polyarticular inflammation, and sedimentation rates above 100 mm/hr (Westergren). Radiographs (particularly of the hands) may discriminate this entity from classical rheumatoid arthritis.

DIAGNOSTIC APPROACH

Diagnosis of any of the forms of pseudogout can only be made by demonstration of weakly positively birefrigent, rhomboidal-shaped, CPPD crystals in synovial fluid obtained by aspiration of the involved joints. Most commercial laboratories have the facility for examination of synovial fluid under cross-polarized compensated microscopy, but unlike uric acid crystals, CPPD crystals will remain observable in synovial fluid samples for only 48 to 72 hours before re-dissolving. These crystals are much smaller than uric acid crystals (approximately one fourth the diameter of a neutrophil) and may be shed into the synovial fluid as a result of another process that is primarily responsible for the joint inflammation. For this reason, the presence of calcium pyrophosphate crystals (even intracellular) in synovial fluid cannot entirely rule out the possibility of coexistent infectious arthritis. If a high clinical index of suspicion for infectious arthritis is present, the patient should be treated for bacterial arthritis until culture results return. Serum calcium, phosphate, and thyroid-stimulating hormone (TSH) levels should be obtained on all patients with the first presentation of CPPD depostion disease and genetic markers for hemochromatosis should be pursued in the appropriate clinical situation.

MANAGEMENT AND THERAPY
Acute Pseudogout

The most effective, least toxic therapy for acute pseudogout involving one or two joints is local intra-articular corticosteroid injection with a long-acting steroid preparation such as triamcinolone hexacetonide. These crystalline-branched chain esters of cortisol will be present and have anti-inflammatory effects within the synovial space for 2 to 3 months. Patients with acute polyarticular pseudogout should be treated with rapidly acting NSAIDs. Long-acting NSAIDs with delayed time to steady state concentrations (piroxicam and nabumetone) should be avoided. The newer COX2-selective NSAIDs have not been studied for use in acute pseudogout. Low-dose oral prednisone with subsequent rapid taper may be used when NSAIDs are contraindicated. Oral colchicine does have some beneficial effect in acute pseudogout but should be reserved for the rare patient who cannot receive any of the other therapies.

Osteoarthritic Calcium Pyrophosphate Deposition Disease

Patients with osteoarthritic CPPD depostion disease are treated similarly to those with osteoarthritis. Because of the inflammatory basis of the arthropathy, NSAIDs (not acetaminophen) should be used as first-line agents. Oral corticosteroids are usually not effective, and surgical joint replacement may be required if severe joint destruction is present.

Figure 124-1

Pseudogout

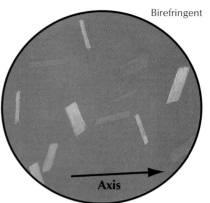

Birefringent

Axis

Acute Pseudogout

Abrupt clinical onset, usually in older women. Typically a mono or oligoarthritis affecting knees, shoulders, or wrists.

Osteoarthritic Form

Chronic, deforming arthritis primarily affecting knees, shoulders, and wrists. M-P joints may also be involved

Hand may be involved in osteoarthritic and pseudorheumatoid forms

Diagnosis made on basis of demonstration of weakly positive birefringent, rhomboid-shaped calcium pyrophosphate dihydrate crystals in synovial fluid aspirate of involved joints

Pseudo-Rheumatoid Form

Rare - mimics rheumatoid arthritis as symmetrical acute or chronic polyarthritis particularly of hands and wrists

Many patients exhibit radiographic evidence of CPPD deposition but are clinically asymptomatic

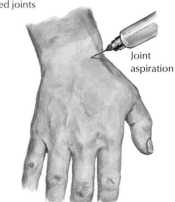

Joint aspiration

Commonly affected joints

Wrist involvement is common in pseudogout, but rare in osteoarthritis and helps to differentiate the two conditions

Associated Conditions
(The 5 "H"s)

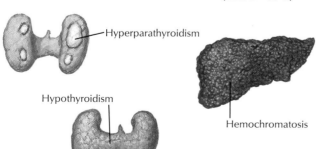

Hyperparathyroidism

Hypothyroidism

Hemochromatosis

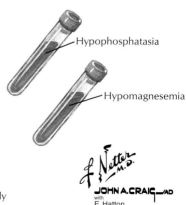

Hypophosphatasia

Hypomagnesemia

Certain conditions show an absolute association and should be pursued as coexisting when patients first presents with clinical manifestations – especially in patients younger than age 40.

JOHN A.CRAIG—MD
with
E. Hatton
© ICON

Figure 124-2

Articular Chondrocalcinosis (Pseudogout)

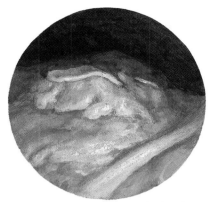

Crystalline synovitis. Biopsy disclosed calcium pyrophosphate crystals seen under polarized light microscopy.

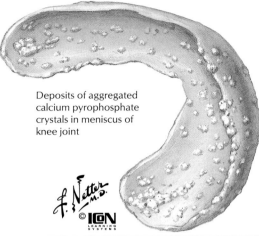

Deposits of aggregated calcium pyrophosphate crystals in meniscus of knee joint

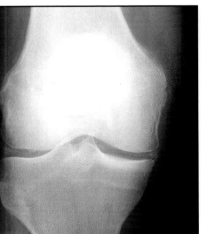

Anteroposterior radiograph of knee reveals densities due to calcific deposits in menisci

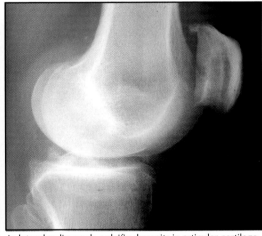

In lateral radiograph, calcific deposits in articular cartilage of femur and patella appear as fluffy white opacities

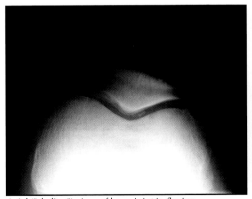

Axial ("skyline") view of knee joint in flexion demonstrates calcinosis of articular cartilages of patella and femur

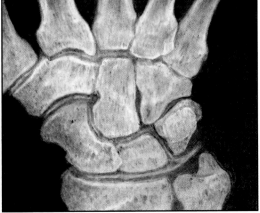

Drawing of radiograph shows calcific deposits in articular cartilages of carpus as fine lines between carpal bones and in radiocarpal joint

Pseudo-rheumatoid Calcium Pyrophosphate Deposition Disease

These patients may try an NSAID as initial therapy, but frequently require moderate doses of oral corticosteroids for control of the joint disease. Unlike true rheumatoid arthritis, this form of the disease tends to occur in the form of acute attacks that spontaneously resolve after weeks to months, allowing for episodic use of corticosteroids.

FUTURE DIRECTIONS

The therapies for control of CPPD depostion disease are less than optimal because the biochemical defects that result in the formation of CPPD crystals are unknown and no preventative pharmacologic agents are available for this condition. Ongoing research into the underlying biochemistry and physical chemistry should result in effective control of this disease, similar to what has already been achieved in the management of gout.

REFERENCES

Agudelo CA, Wise CM. Crystal-associated arthritis. *Clin Geriatr Med.* 1998;14:495-513.

Halverson PB. Calcium crystal-associated diseases. *Curr Opin Rheumatol.* 1996;8:259-261.

Reginato AJ, Tamesis E, Netter P. Familial and clinical aspects of calcium pyrophosphate deposition disease. *Curr Rheumatol Rep.* 1999;1:112-120.

Rosenthal AK. Calcium crystal-associated arthritides. *Curr Opin Rheumatol.* 1998;10:273-277.

Chapter 125

Gout

Robert G. Berger

Gout is a disease caused by precipitation of the phlogistic crystals of sodium urate within the synovial or tenosynovial spaces. *Phlogism* is the capability of a biologic compound to produce inflammation when present in its crystalline form. In the musculoskeletal system, phlogistic crystals include sodium urate, calcium pyrophosphate, calcium hydroxyapatite, and calcium oxalate. Each crystal produces a distinct clinical syndrome. The cumulative incidence of gout over a 20-year follow-up period is approximately 8% with a male predominance. The risk of an acute attack of gout relates to the level of the serum uric acid; the risk increases as the serum urate level rises. At a serum urate level of 9 mg/dL, the risk of developing gout is approximately 5 times that of a person with a "normal" serum uric acid level. Although most patients have an elevated serum uric acid level, this value may be falsely low particularly during an acute exacerbation of the disease, when uric acid is being consumed within the synovial spaces by the crystallization process.

ETIOLOGY AND PATHOGENESIS

Uric acid forms as a consequence of the purine breakdown biochemical pathway and is eliminated primarily by renal excretion and secretion. An elevation of the serum uric acid concentration and resultant gout occurs by one of the following etiologies.

Under-excretion by the kidney causes 85% to 90% of clinical gout. It occurs primarily from a presumed genetic defect in renal handling of uric acid but may also occur as a result of tubular renal disease (with normal creatinine clearance) or any disease that results in a decrease in overall renal function. Drugs and ingestions decreasing renal excretion of uric acid, such as thiazide and loop diuretics, cyclosporine, ethambutol, alcohol, lead, and low-dose aspirin, may also produce hyperuricemia.

Genetic defects in the purine elimination pathway resulting in overproduction of uric acid cause 5% of clinical gout (Figure 125-1). Increased activity of 5'-phosphoribosyl-1-pyrophosphate (PRPP) synthetase (alcohol use also results in increased activity of this enzyme), or partial or complete deficiency of the purine "scavenge pathway" enzyme hypoxanthine guanine phosphoribosyltransferase (HGPRT) are the most common enzyme abnormalities causing this mechanism of hyperuricemia. Complete deficiency of the HGPRT enzyme results in the Lesch-Nyhan syndrome with its neurologic sequelae and is seen almost exclusively in the pediatric population.

High cell turnover states can result in the overproduction of uric acid in patients with normal purine pathway biochemistry (secondary gout). Such states occur in the presence of hematologic malignancies, particularly in multiple myeloma in the elderly population, during chemotherapy of hematologic malignancies or metastatic carcinoma, during the onset of treatment of pernicious anemia, or in exfoliative skin disorders such as psoriasis.

CLINICAL PRESENTATION
Acute Gout

Classical acute gout usually involves the metatarsal-phalangeal (MTP) joint of the great toe. This acute monarthritis, known as *podagra*, occurs with an abrupt onset usually in the early morning hours. Erythema, warmth, and acute pain occur over the dorsal aspect of the joint and may involve the extensor tendons and surrounding tissue. The pain is usually out of proportion to findings from the clinical examination, and patients frequently describe podagra as the "worst pain they have ever experienced." They may not be able to tolerate a thin bed sheet or cool air moving over the top of the involved joint. Without treatment, the attack may last from 5 to 7 days, and resolve with scaling of the superficial dermis over the involved areas. Recurrent attacks

Figure 125-1   **Purine Elimination Biochemical Pathway**

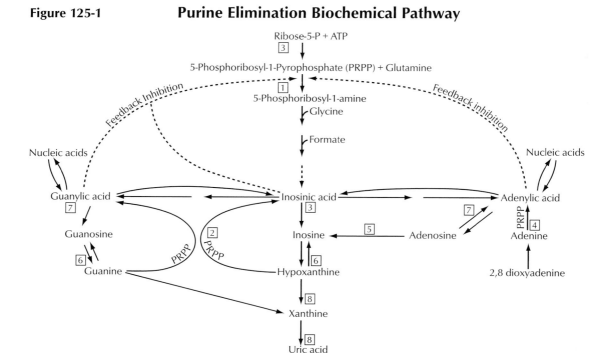

are common, and may occur as frequently as monthly or sporadically, with attacks every few years.

Acute gout may affect any joint in the body. The knees, wrists, shoulders, MTP, and proximal or distal interphalangeal finger or toe joints are the most commonly involved. The axial skeleton, including the hips, is less commonly affected, but acute gout has been reported in the sacroiliac joints and the sternoclavicular joints. Attacks may be limited to tenosynovial sheaths alone and may be confused with other causes of "tendonitis," particularly overuse musculoskeletal syndromes. Polyarticular attacks involving two or more joints or tendons are not uncommon and may mimic other systemic rheumatic diseases. Fever and malaise are common in polyarticular acute gout, but less so in monoarticular attacks.

On physical examination, the patient usually cannot move the affected joint or tendon without severe pain. Tendon involvement can be elicited by stretching the suspected muscle-tendon unit without moving the underlying joint. Large tense joint effusions are common in knees, shoulders, or ankles during the acute attack. Occasionally, a

posterior popliteal cyst (Baker's cyst) may form as a result of acute gout in the knee, rupture down the posterior calf, and mimic the physical findings of a DVT.

Laboratory findings during the acute attack may include an elevated WBC count with a left shift, elevated sedimentation rate (sometimes greater than 100 mm/hr, Westergren), and increased levels of other acute phase reactants such as ferritin and C-reactive protein. Synovial fluid contains large numbers of polymorphonuclear neutrophils (PMNs) and may appear grossly purulent. Serum uric acid may be normal and is of no value in the diagnosis of gout. Radiographs are almost always normal, other than illustrating soft tissue swelling and effusion in the larger joints, unless the involved joint has had damage from recurrent attacks or the patient has chronic gout.

Chronic Gout

Patients with *chronic gout* present with a chronic, sometimes deforming arthritis affecting hands, wrists, feet, knees, and shoulders (Figure 125-2). It can produce ulnar deviation, swan neck deformities, and other hand and foot deformities. As a result, chronic gout may occasionally be misdiagnosed as rheumatoid arthritis. Patients may describe episodic acute attacks of swelling, redness, and pain in the involved joints or a more indolent history of chronic swelling and pain. Physical examination shows a chronic synovitis most commonly involving the hands and feet and is usually asymmetric (unlike rheumatoid arthritis). In addition, joint deformities and decreased range of motion may be present.

Laboratory evaluation compounds the confusion with rheumatoid arthritis as 20% to 25% of patients with chronic gout have a positive serum rheumatoid factor test result. Serum uric acid is usually elevated but may be normal. Sedimentation rate is modestly elevated. Radiographs show erosive destructive disease similar to rheumatoid arthritis, but an experienced bone radiologist may discern more cystic periarticular erosions with new bone formation that help distinguish the findings of chronic gout from rheumatoid arthritis.

Tophaceous Gout

In some patients, almost always with the chronic form of gout, subcutaneous deposits of uric acid known as *tophi* develop. These deposits form nodules, usually over the extensor surfaces of the elbows, in the Achilles tendons, extensor surfaces of the hands and feet, and within the pinnae of the ears (Figure 125-3). Their appearance on physical examination is identical to that of rheumatoid nodules and can only be distinguished by the presence of uric acid crystals on cross-polarized compensated microscopy done on aspirate or biopsy specimens of the nodules. A severe form of tophaceous gout known as *saturnine gout* may develop in patients who abuse homemade alcohol "moonshine" made by using older model automobile batteries containing lead.

DIAGNOSTIC APPROACH

Diagnosis of any of the forms of gout can only be made by demonstration of negatively birefringent needle-shaped uric acid crystals in synovial, tenosynovial, or nodule fluid obtained by aspiration of the involved joints, tendons, or subcutaneous nodules. In acute gout, these crystals are both extracellular and intracellular within PMNs. In chronic and tophaceous gout, free uric acid crystals may be present without any inflammatory cell reaction. Most commercial laboratories are able to examine synovial fluid under cross-polarized compensated microscopy. Uric acid crystals will remain observable in synovial fluid samples for up to 7 days. Planar bone radiography may be helpful in establishing a diagnosis of gout.

MANAGEMENT AND THERAPY
Acute Gout

Nonsteroidal antiinflammatory drugs (NSAIDs) remain the mainstay of treatment of the acute attack. Indomethacin was the first of this group to be used for acute gout. The initial dose, between 100 and 200 mg/day orally in divided doses (depending on the severity of the attack and the weight of the patient), should produce some relief of symptoms within 2 hours. The dosage should be decreased gradually over 3 to 4 days as the acute gout resolves. Other NSAIDs such as naproxen (500 mg 2 to 3 times daily) or ibuprofen 800 mg 4 times daily are also effective. Aspirin is contraindicated because it produces an increased serum uric acid level at the onset of usage. Long-acting NSAIDs with delayed time to steady state concentration (piroxicam and nabumetone) should be avoided. NSAIDs should not be used in patients with preexisting renal disease in whom hyperkalemia and deterioration of renal function may be precipitated because of altered renal hemodynamics. The newer COX2-selective NSAIDs have not been studied for use in acute gout.

If NSAIDs are contraindicated, patients can receive oral colchicine. There is no current role for intravenous administration of colchicine for acute gout. Colchicine is effective in acute gout and a clear response to this drug may be valuable in supporting the diagnosis. However, doses close to toxic levels are needed and the following regimen is usual: 1.2 mg initially, followed by 0.6 mg every 2 hours until there is either diarrhea or vomiting or the patient obtains relief of pain. The total dose required usually ranges between 4 and 8 milligrams. Relief may not occur for some hours after the toxic features have developed and may not be complete.

Intra-articular injection of steroids can be used when colchicine and NSAIDs are contraindicated. Oral steroids may also be considered for those patients who have too many joints involved for intra-articular injections.

Figure 125-2

Gouty Arthritis
Natural History

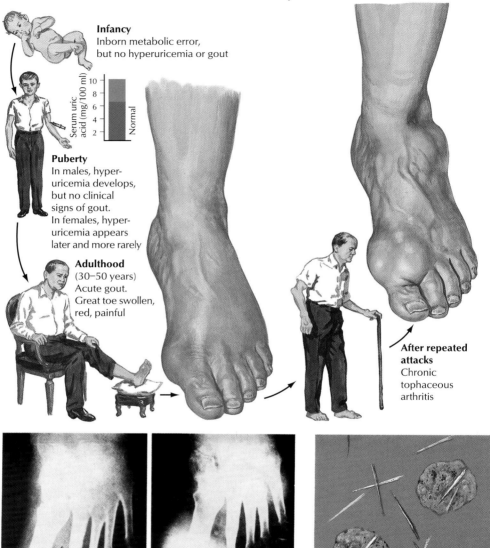

Infancy
Inborn metabolic error,
but no hyperuricemia or gout

Serum uric acid (mg/100 ml)

Normal

Puberty
In males, hyper-
uricemia develops,
but no clinical
signs of gout.
In females, hyper-
uricemia appears
later and more rarely

Adulthood
(30–50 years)
Acute gout.
Great toe swollen,
red, painful

After repeated attacks
Chronic tophaceous arthritis

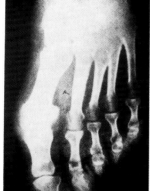

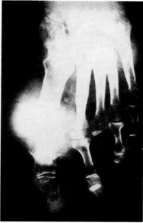

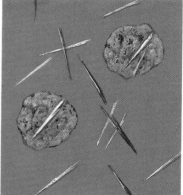

Early tophaceous gouty arthritis

Same patient 12 years later, untreated

Free and phagocytized monosodium urate crystals in aspirated joint fluid seen on compensated polarized light microscopy

Figure 125-3

Tophaceous Gout

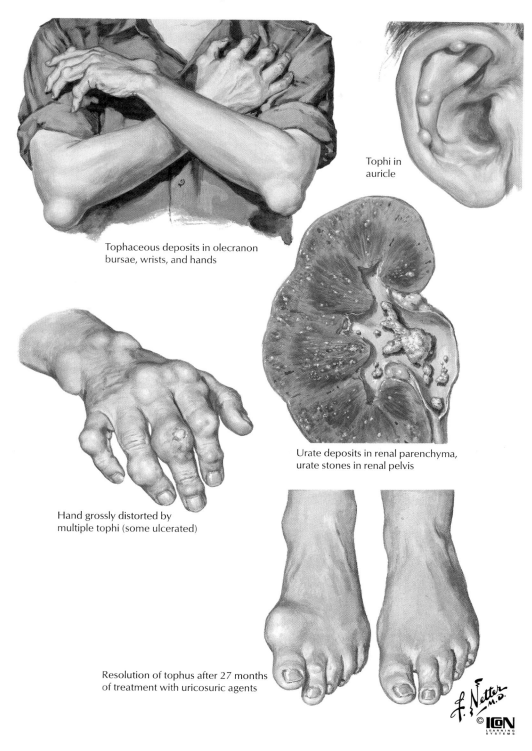

Tophi in auricle

Tophaceous deposits in olecranon bursae, wrists, and hands

Urate deposits in renal parenchyma, urate stones in renal pelvis

Hand grossly distorted by multiple tophi (some ulcerated)

Resolution of tophus after 27 months of treatment with uricosuric agents

Chronic Gout and Recurrent Acute Gout

Patients with chronic gout or episodic recurrent acute gout should receive prophylactic treatment with agents that lower serum uric acid. The decision to use these drugs in episodic acute gout should be based on an individual patient's desires, because some patients will tolerate 4 to 5 attacks yearly and use only NSAIDs during each attack, while others prefer long-term prophylaxis. Low purine diets are unpalatable and rarely tolerated as a method to lower serum uric acid. Uric acid-lowering agents should never be started during an acute attack because they will worsen and prolong the course of the attack. Patients with episodic acute gout should be asymptomatic for at least 4 to 6 weeks before uric acid–lowering agents are begun. Patients with chronic gout should be taking a NSAID or daily colchicine (0.6 mg twice daily) when prophylactic treatment is started.

The choice of prophylactic agent is based on whether the patient is an under-excretor or over-producer of uric acid. Ninety percent of patients with gout are under excreters of uric acid and should receive the less toxic uricosuric agents. Allopurinol is reserved for over-producers of uric acid. A 24-hour urine collection for uric acid will establish which group the patient is in, and therapy should be based on this value. A serum uric acid level should be drawn at the onset of prophylaxis and used as a guide to adjust dosing of the drug chosen, with a goal for lowering the serum uric acid to the range of 5 to 7 mg/dL. Historically, colchicine (0.6 mg twice daily) has been added to any prophylactic regimen to prevent any "breakthrough" attacks.

Probenecid, the original uricosuric agent, is used as initial therapy in patients who under-excrete uric acid. It acts by inhibiting reabsorption of urate from the renal tubule and thus increasing urinary urate excretion. It is contraindicated in patients with nephrolithiasis and is not effective in patients with decreased renal function. Its effect is decreased by the concurrent administration of aspirin. The initial dose is 500 mg twice daily and the drug is available in a combination form with 0.6 mg of colchicine. Sulfinpyrazone (200 mg twice daily) is also an effective uricosuric drug that may be used in lieu of probenecid.

Allopurinol, which is rapidly metabolized to oxypurinol, acts by inhibiting the enzyme xanthine oxidase, thereby reducing the production of uric acid. It should be used only in over-producers of uric acid or when uricosuric agents are contraindicated or ineffective. The initial dose should be 100 mg/day, and depending on the risk of precipitating acute gout, this can then be increased each week by 100 mg/day until a dose of 300 mg/day is reached. Occasionally, dosages approaching 600 mg/day are required in patients who have genetic causes for over-production of uric acid. The main complications of its use are allergic reactions, which may range from a minor skin rash to a severe, life-threatening toxic epidermolysis with interstitial nephritis. A rash may develop in approximately 30% of patients beginning allopurinol. If this occurs, the drug should be immediately discontinued. The dose should be reduced in the presence of renal insufficiency (by approximately 100 mg/day for a 30 mL/minute decrease in creatinine clearance).

Tophaceous Gout

The goal of therapy is to reduce serum uric acid and mobilize and dissolve the nodular deposits of uric acid. This is accomplished by using uricosuric agents with allopurinol in patients who can tolerate this regimen. These patients do not require 24-hour urine collection for uric acid because both classes of drugs are used in combination. Allopurinol is instituted first with a 6-week interval before beginning the uricosuric agent. Once the tophaceous deposits have disappeared (this may take years), the uricosuric agent may be stopped.

FUTURE DIRECTIONS

The development of new drugs that decrease uric acid production will remain a focus of pharmacutical research. The hope is to make available agents with fewer side effects than allopurinol.

REFERENCES

Agudelo CA, Wise CM. Crystal-associated arthritis. *Clin Geriatr Med.* 1998;14:495–513.

Davis JC Jr. A practical approach to gout. Current management of an 'old' disease. *Postgrad Med.* 1999;106:115–116, 119–123.

Pascual E. Gout update: from lab to the clinic and back. *Curr Opin Rheumatol.* 2000;12:213–218.

Simkin PA. Gout and hyperuricemia. *Curr Opin Rheumatol.* 1997;9:268–273.

Chapter 126

Low Back Pain in Adults

Timothy S. Carey

Low back pain is a common and remitting ailment for most adults; approximately 80% have an episode sufficiently severe that they cannot do their usual daily activities for at least 1 day at some time in their lives. Approximately 8% of adults have an episode in a given year and approximately 3% to 4% have the very disabling syndrome of chronic low back pain. The majority of patients with low back pain can be treated at the primary care level.

ETIOLOGY AND PATHOGENESIS

Adult vertebrae are complex anatomic and biomechanical structures (Figure 126-1). Usually, these structures function extraordinarily well under various loads, postures, torque, and after mild-to-moderate trauma. Most back pain occurs in the lumbar area, and 95% of intervertebral disc problems occur at the L-2 through L-5 areas.

The "pain generator" for most cases of back pain is unclear. The annulus fibrosus of the intervertebral disc is richly innervated, and many cases of back pain are undoubtedly discogenic. Facet joints, ligaments, and muscles can all cause chronic back pain. Leg pain is more likely to be related to pressure on the intervertebral disc, but can occur as a result of bone spurs or pressure on the nerve roots related to spinal stenosis. *Sciatica* is generally defined as radiation of pain to the level of the knee or below. Classic discogenic pain is more prominent in the leg than in the back. In *spinal stenosis*, a variation of sciatica, the patient's thigh pain becomes worse on walking or prolonged standing (pseudoclaudication). The pathogenesis of pseudoclaudication appears to relate to a congenitally narrow spinal canal combined with bony overgrowth around the facet joints.

Over 85% of cases of acute back pain are not related to sciatica, spinal stenosis, or serious causes such as malignancy, abdominal aortic aneurysm, etc. Cases of nonspecific chronic back pain are usually the most difficult to manage and require a great deal of skill in both communicating with patients and coordinating care.

CLINICAL PRESENTATION

Because most patients will have a relatively nonspecific diagnosis, it is important to identify the minority of patients who do have a specific cause of their back pain. Patients with acute back pain generally present after 2 weeks of symptoms. Often they are fearful that the cause of their back pain is serious and will result in chronic pain or permanent disability. Eliciting these fears by asking, "What do you think is causing your back pain?" can lead to productive reassurance.

DIFFERENTIAL DIAGNOSIS

The history should include a search for "red flag" factors relating to the patient's back pain.

Cauda Equina Syndrome

In the *cauda equina syndrome*, the acute onset of urinary retention or fecal incontinence, loss of anal sphincter tone and perianal anesthesia are typical and may occur with bilateral leg weakness. Immediate MRI and referral to an orthopedic surgeon or neurosurgeon is indicated. The etiology is most commonly related to a metastatic malignancy, and rarely to a large central disc herniation.

Infectious Discitis/Osteomyelitis

Back pain associated with fever, sweats, and weight loss may occur with infectious discitis/osteomyelitis. These patients will generally have an elevated erythrocyte sedimentation rate and may be immunocompromised or have a nidus of infection, such as a chronic urinary tract infection. Plain film radiographs may only have a 70% sensitivity in the early phases of discitis.

Figure 126-1

Lumbosacral Spine and Ligaments

Lateral view

Posterior view

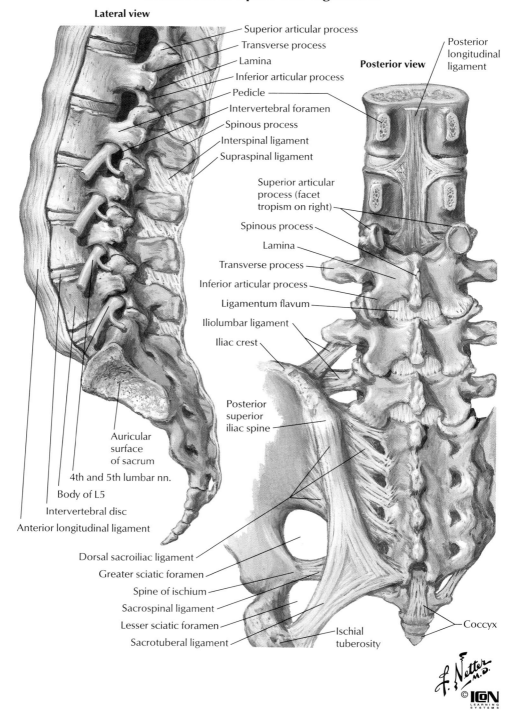

- Superior articular process
- Transverse process
- Lamina
- Inferior articular process
- Pedicle
- Intervertebral foramen
- Spinous process
- Interspinal ligament
- Supraspinal ligament
- Posterior longitudinal ligament
- Superior articular process (facet tropism on right)
- Spinous process
- Lamina
- Transverse process
- Inferior articular process
- Ligamentum flavum
- Iliolumbar ligament
- Iliac crest
- Posterior superior iliac spine
- Auricular surface of sacrum
- 4th and 5th lumbar nn.
- Body of L5
- Intervertebral disc
- Anterior longitudinal ligament
- Dorsal sacroiliac ligament
- Greater sciatic foramen
- Spine of ischium
- Sacrospinal ligament
- Lesser sciatic foramen
- Sacrotuberal ligament
- Ischial tuberosity
- Coccyx

Metastatic Cancer

Progressive and unrelenting back pain can be a sign of prostate, breast, or lung cancer. Multiple myeloma may initially present as back pain. A history of non-skin cancer in the previous 5 to 10 years requires plain film radiographs, measurement of ESR, and/or advanced imaging such as bone scan, MRI, or CT scan.

Trauma

Trauma, especially in a patient with or at risk for osteoporosis, should raise concern regarding fracture.

Ankylosing Spondylitis and Other Syndromes

Pain made worse with morning stiffness in younger men and relieved by exercise may be indicative of early disease.

Back pain may occasionally present as referred pain from an abdominal or retroperitoneal source. These may include the burning pain of early shingles (herpes zoster), back pain secondary to an abdominal aortic aneurysm, or pyelonephritis.

These "red flags" are important because some causes of back pain may lead to an irreversible neurologic deficit. The chance of a patient presenting with back pain having one of these serious "red flag" problems is low, but will vary substantially depending on the practice setting.

A brief evaluation for "yellow flags" is also indicated. These social factors include litigation through personal injury or workers' compensation, intense preoccupation with the pain, or anger toward the employer, all of which may indicate a worse prognosis from back pain. The presence of one of these factors should not at all indicate that the patient is malingering. The physician's perspective should be attuned to encouraging improved functioning and psychosocial support.

DIAGNOSTIC APPROACH

The physical examination can be brief in most cases. Examination of the abdomen may pick up bruits or pulsating masses in cases of abdominal aneurysm; this is especially important in males over the age of 50 with a heavy smoking history and other signs of atherosclerosis. Palpation of the back can sometimes find tender areas or trigger points. Usually, these are quite nonspecific; however, it is important to touch the part of the patient that hurts.

Examination of the knee jerk and ankle reflexes can pick up nerve root impingement (Figures 126-2, 126-3, and 126-4). Testing of dorsiflexion foot strength can assess the L-4 to L-5 nerve root. The ankle jerk reflex assesses L-5 to S-1. Over 90% of nerve root impingements occur at 1 of these 2 levels. The dorsum of the foot may have hypoesthesia in impingement of the L-4 to L-5 disc space.

The straight leg raising sign is relatively specific but not very sensitive for nerve root impingement. If positive, pain on the affected side radiates to the level of the knee or below. The leg is elevated passively.

Rectal examination is indicated when there is concern about carcinoma of the prostate gland (prolonged pain, older men) or potential cauda equina syndrome (bilateral leg weakness, incontinence, or retention of urine or stool).

Exaggerated pain behavior, reproduction of pain by pressing on the top of the head (axial loading, which transmits essentially zero force to the lumbar spine) is associated with a strong psychologic component to pain. These patients tend to do poorly with surgery and require greater attention to psychosocial issues.

The majority of patients do not require immediate imaging studies. Lumbar spine radiographs are indicated when there is concern regarding trauma, in the presence of "red flags," or if the patient has not attained functional recovery within 4 to 6 weeks. There is no consensus regarding indications for advanced techniques such as CT or MRI. Such tests should be urgently performed when there is concern regarding metastasis or infection. In general, such advanced imaging techniques are indicated only when a "red flag" is present or an operation is under active consideration. While highly sensitive, herniated discs may be found in 20% to 30% of asymptomatic individuals. MRI evidence of spinal stenosis has been demonstrated in over 20% of individuals over age 60 without symptoms.

MANAGEMENT AND THERAPY

When a serious cause of low back pain is found (metastatic malignancy, discitis), specific treatment is urgently indicated. However, most cases of back pain can be divided into three broad categories: nonspecific back pain, nerve root impingement related to herniated disc, and spinal stenosis.

Figure 126-2

Sensory and Motor Innervation of Lower Limb
Sensory (dermatomes)

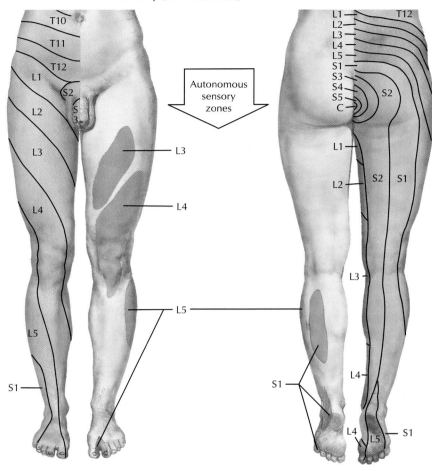

Autonomous sensory zones

Motor

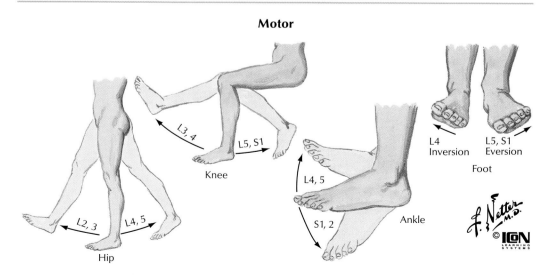

Figure 126-3

Clinical Features of Herniated Lumbar Nucleus Pulposus

Level of Herniation	Pain	Numbness	Weakness	Atrophy	Reflexes
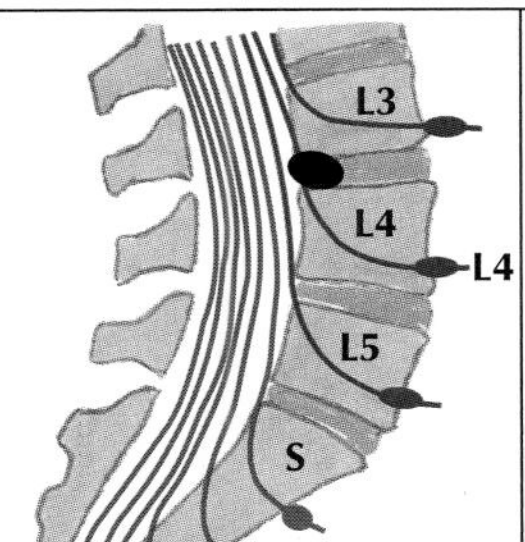 L3-4 disc; 4th lumbar nerve root	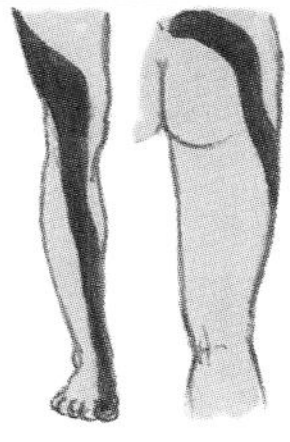 Lower back, hip, posterolateral thigh, anterior leg	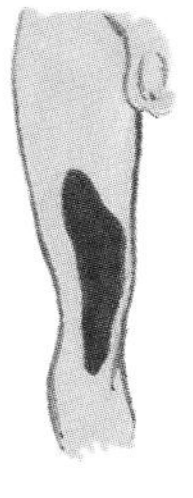 Antero-medial thigh and knee	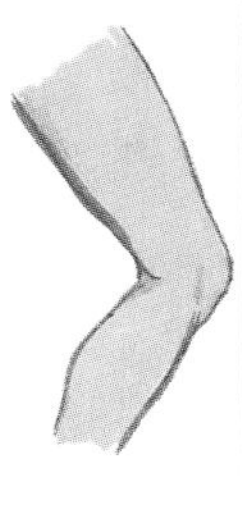 Quadriceps	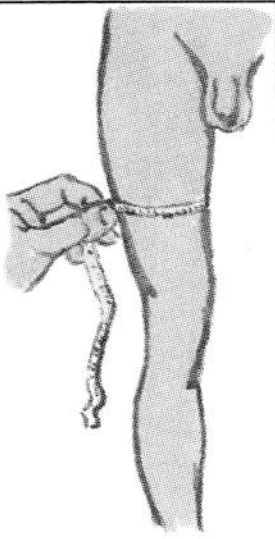 Quadriceps	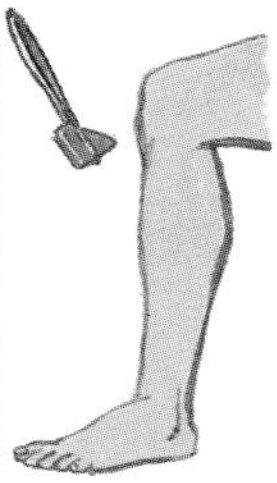 Knee jerk diminished
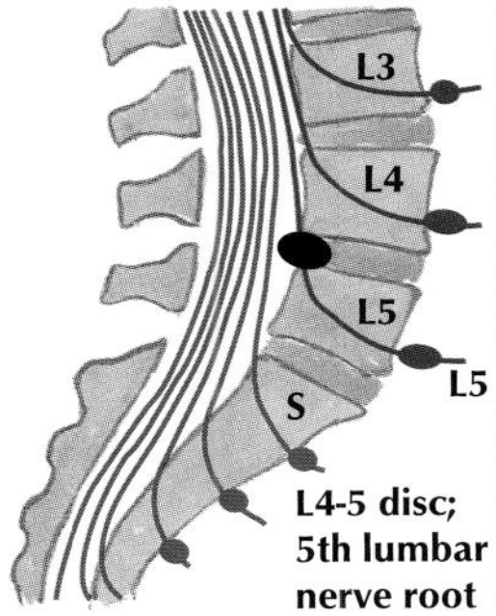 L4-5 disc; 5th lumbar nerve root	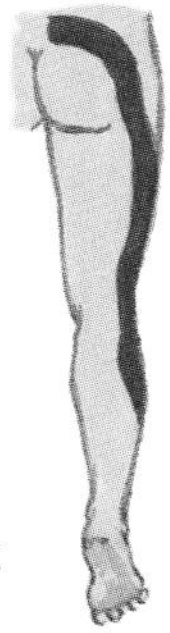 Over sacro-iliac joint, hip, lateral thigh and leg	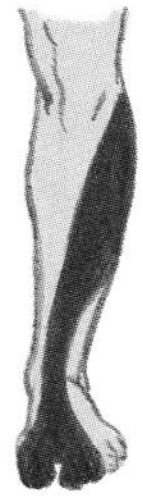 Lateral leg, web of great toe	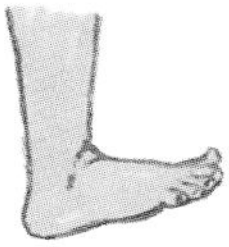 Dorsifexion of great toe and foot; difficulty walking on heels; foot drop may occur	Minor	Changes uncommon (absent or diminished posterior tibial reflex
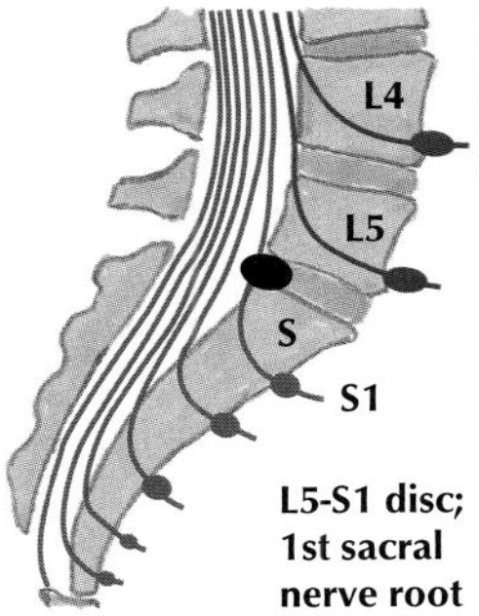 L5-S1 disc; 1st sacral nerve root	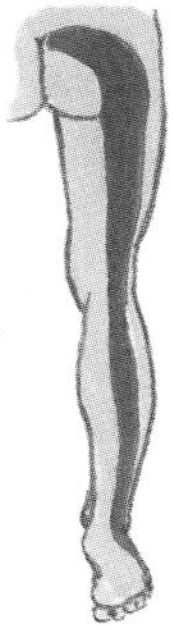 Over sacro-iliac joint, hip, postero-lateral thigh and leg to heel	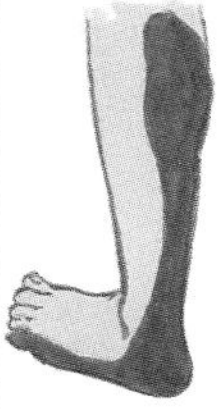 Back of calf; lateral heel, foot and toe	Plantar flexion of foot and great toe may be affected; difficulty walking on toes	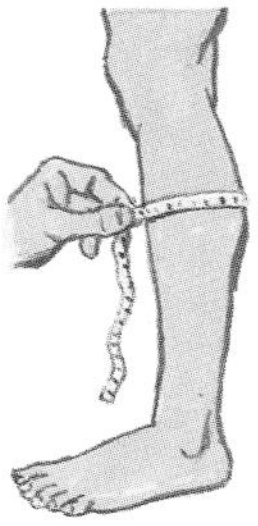 Gastrocne-mius and soleus	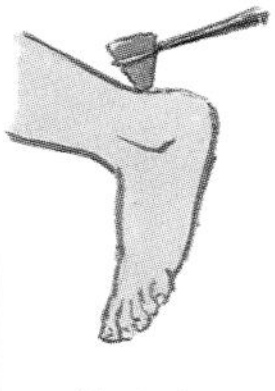 Ankle jerk diminished or absent
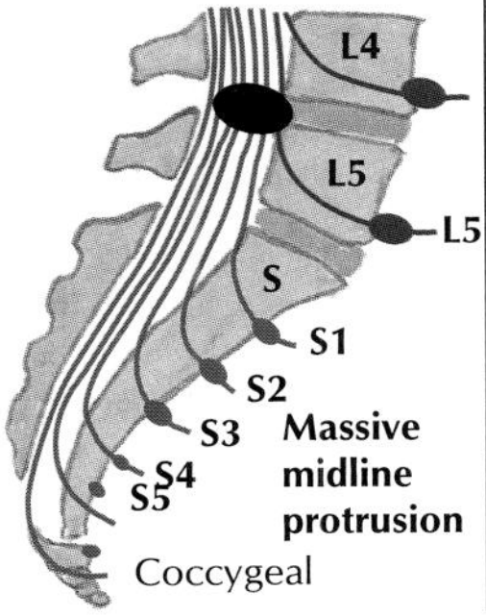 Massive midline protrusion	Lower back, thighs, legs, and/or perineum depending on level of lesion; may be bilateral	Thighs, legs, feet, and/or perineum; variable; may be bilateral	Variable paralysis or paresis of legs and/or bowel and bladder inconti-nence	May be extensive	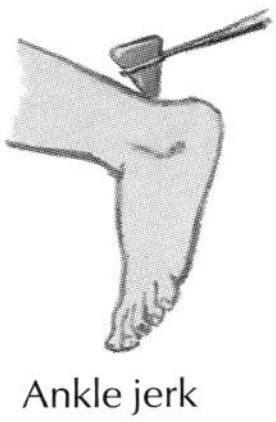 Ankle jerk diminished or absent

F. Netter M.D.

© ICON
LEARNING
SYSTEMS

Figure 126-4

Pain Patterns in Lumbar Disease

Radicular pain due to nerve root compression

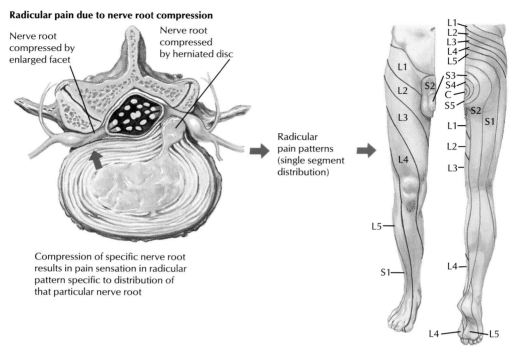

Nerve root compressed by enlarged facet

Nerve root compressed by herniated disc

Radicular pain patterns (single segment distribution)

Compression of specific nerve root results in pain sensation in radicular pattern specific to distribution of that particular nerve root

Nonradicular, referred pain due to facet or disc disease

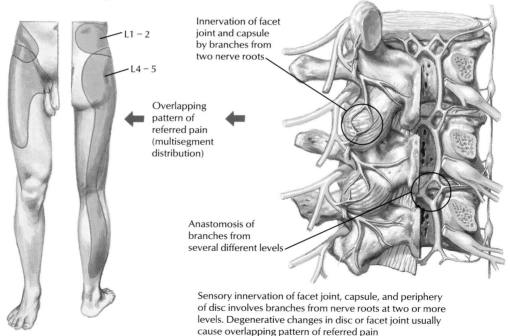

L1 – 2

L4 – 5

Innervation of facet joint and capsule by branches from two nerve roots

Overlapping pattern of referred pain (multisegment distribution)

Anastomosis of branches from several different levels

Sensory innervation of facet joint, capsule, and periphery of disc involves branches from nerve roots at two or more levels. Degenerative changes in disc or facet joint usually cause overlapping pattern of referred pain

JOHN A. CRAIG—MD

C. Machado—M.D.

© ICON

Nonspecific Low Back Pain

Over 80% of patients present with nonspecific or mechanical low back pain. This lack of specificity is often frustrating for both doctors and patients. Providing patients with an explanatory model of what is going on with their back so that they can live with their symptoms until the fortunate natural history of back pain allows them to improve is important. Patients often relate well to phrases such as "it's like a flu in your back," or "strained ligaments."

Ninety-five percent of patients with nonspecific acute back pain (less than 2 months of symptoms) return to their usual daily functioning within 3 months of conservative treatment. Reassurance, appropriate analgesia, and advice to resume usual daily activities as quickly as possible are the most effective treatments. Bed rest for more than 48 hours appears to be counterproductive. Acetaminophen, NSAIDs, and, possibly, a muscle relaxant provide adequate symptom relief for most patients. Those with very severe initial symptoms may benefit from a short course of a narcotic analgesic. Encourage patients to return to work as quickly as possible. A note or conversation with a patient's supervisor regarding avoiding heavy lifting or awkward postures for a designated period is often indicated. Prolonged time off work, such as prolonged bed rest, appears to worsen rather than improve back-related disability. Patients often benefit from a telephone call or return office visit within 2 weeks. If the patient is off work at 2 weeks, more specific treatment such as a physical therapy referral may be in order. Spinal manipulative therapy may be performed by doctors of chiropractic medicine, osteopathic physicians, and some physical therapists. Randomized trials of spinal manipulation have yielded somewhat conflicting results; more recent studies have demonstrated marginal, if any benefit when compared with conventional conservative medical therapy.

Herniated Lumbar Disc

Diagnostic clues include true sciatica and presence of suggestive neurologic findings (Figure 126-5). In the absence of "red flags," a supportive approach is indicated. Ninety percent of patients with sciatica improve with conservative therapy over a 3-month period. Some patients benefit from a brief (1 to 2 days) period of bed rest. Patients often are quite fearful of resuming usual activities, and a physical therapy referral may be helpful to coach the patient to maintain activities such as walking, even when uncomfortable. If a patient has persistent predominant leg pain as the primary back symptom, especially if combined with asymmetric reflexes or mild weakness in dorsiflexion of the foot, limited evidence suggests that the patient may benefit from an advanced imaging technique and consideration of operative microdiscectomy.

Spinal Stenosis

Cohort studies have demonstrated that, over several years, one third of patients stay the same and one third worsen. Some patients become severely impaired with near constant pain and limited ambulation. Analgesics and physical therapy may offer only modest benefit. Because walking is often limited by the nature of the disease, swimming or stationary bicycling may be helpful. Surgical decompression appears to offer substantial relief of leg symptoms and improved walking distance, although most patients will continue to have back pain and some limitation in walking distance. Older age leads to greater risk of cardiac complications at the time of surgery.

Chronic Back Pain

Many patients with chronic low back pain have no radiculopathy or anatomical abnormalities that clearly explain their symptoms. Patients with 2 months of continuous symptoms have over a 50% chance of having significant back symptoms 1 to 2 years later. No single therapy appears to be beneficial for their symptoms. Lumbar spinal fusion may provide some relief, but it is a significantly morbid procedure with high failure rates, which provides relief of symptoms in less than half of patients.

Intensive exercise regimens reduce pain and improve functioning. Reinforcement of exercise needs to take place on an ongoing basis. Tricyclic antidepressant medications and anti-seizure medications such as gabapentin are useful adjuncts. Long-term opioid therapy is favored by some authorities. One small, randomized trial showed that opioids reduced pain; however, activity levels were not improved. Patients with disabling chronic pain may benefit from referral to a multidisciplinary pain center.

Figure 126-5

Intervertebral Disc

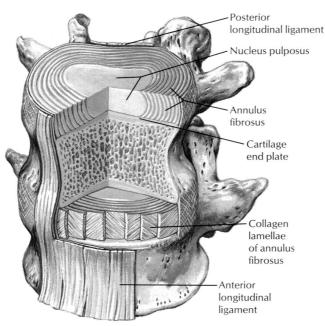

Posterior
longitudinal ligament

Nucleus pulposus

Annulus
fibrosus

Cartilage
end plate

Collagen
lamellae
of annulus
fibrosus

Anterior
longitudinal
ligament

Intervertebral disc composed of central nuclear zone
of collagen and hydrated proteoglycans surrounded
by concentric lamellae of collagen fibers

Pump mechanism of disc nutrition

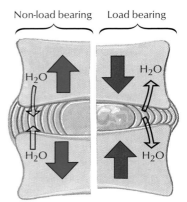

Non-load bearing   Load bearing

H_2O H_2O

H_2O H_2O

Movement-driven pump mechanism
alternately compresses and relaxes
pressure on disc, pumping water
and waste products out and water
and nutrients in. Baseline turgor
maintained by hydrophilic proteins.
Failure of pump mechanism may
result in biochemical changes,
causing back pain

JOHN A. CRAIG—MD
C. Machado—M.D.
© ICN

Disc rupture and nuclear herniation

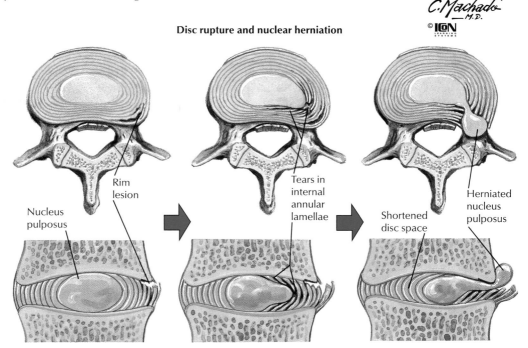

Nucleus
pulposus

Rim
lesion

Tears in
internal
annular
lamellae

Shortened
disc space

Herniated
nucleus
pulposus

Peripheral tear of annulus fibrosus and cartilage end plate (rim lesion) initiates sequence of events
that weaken and tear internal annular lamellae, allowing extrusion and herniation of nucleus pulposus

FUTURE DIRECTIONS

The use of an initial clinical diagnostic evaluation and a stepped care approach to back pain can reduce provider and patient frustration and result in improved outcomes, including improved functional status and earlier return to work. Basic research in identifying the pain generator in a larger portion of cases will improve diagnosis and better guide treatment. Randomized trials, currently under way, will give clinicians better information about which patients may benefit from discectomy, spinal fusion, and spinal decompressive surgery.

REFERENCES

Cherkin DC, Deyo RA, Battie M, Street J, Barlow W. A comparison of physical therapy, chiropractic manipulation, and provision of an educational booklet for the treatment of patients with low back pain. *N Engl J Med.* 1998;339:1021–1029.

Deyo RA, Weinstein JN. Low back pain. *N Engl J Med.* 2001;344:363–370.

Jamison RN, Raymond SA, Slawsby EA, Nedeljkovic SS, Katz NP. Opioid therapy for chronic noncancer back pain. A randomized prospective study. *Spine.* 1998;23:2591–2600.

Katz JN, Lipson SJ, Chang LC, Levine SA, Fossel AH, Liang MH. Seven- to 10-year outcome of decompressive surgery for degenerative lumbar spinal stenosis. *Spine.* 1996;21:92–98.

Chapter 127
Osteoarthritis

Joanne M. Jordan

Osteoarthritis (OA) is the most common form of arthritis, affecting approximately 21 million adults in the United States. Symptomatic knee and hip OA is the leading cause of joint replacement surgery, disability, and diminished quality of life among older individuals. Onset is unusual before the fifth decade, and prevalence increases with age. Below the age of 50 years, men with OA outnumber women, but after this age, women are more likely to have OA than men, particularly of the hand and knee.

OA may be the final common pathway of many different disease processes. Although commonly defined radiographically, radiographic change can exist without corresponding symptoms. The causes of pain and disability from OA are complex and include co-morbid conditions, muscle weakness, and psychosocial factors, as well as radiographic severity.

ETIOLOGY AND PATHOGENESIS

Formerly regarded as primarily a disorder of articular cartilage, OA affects the entire joint, including cartilage, subchondral bone, ligaments, synovium, and surrounding muscle. The earliest pathologic changes are increased hydration and loss of proteoglycan content of cartilage, with subchondral bony thickening or sclerosis (Figure 127-1). With progression, cartilage frays or fibrillates with the development of focal ulcerations sometimes leading to exposure of subchondral bone. Growth of bony osteophytes, a hallmark of the condition, occurs at joint margins, and mild synovitis may also ensue (Figure 127-2). Laxity of ligaments and weakness of surrounding muscle, formerly believed to be the result of disuse, may actually precede some of these disease processes.

The cause of these events is unknown, but certain risk factors for the occurrence and progression of OA have been identified, although their relative importance varies for different populations and for different joints. For example, increased body mass index is associated with knee and hand OA, but less strongly with hip OA. Furthermore, these associations may be stronger in women, in whom weight loss has been shown to decrease the risk of symptomatic knee OA. The

role of hormonal status and bone mineral density in OA is complex, with the incidence of OA in women increasing greatly with the onset of menopause. Genetics may account for as much as 65% of OA. Other risk factors include joint injury, occupational and sports physical demands, and possibly quadriceps weakness.

CLINICAL PRESENTATION

OA has a characteristic joint distribution; symptoms depend on the joint involved. The most commonly involved joints are the knees, hands, feet, hips, and spine. The usual presenting complaint in OA is pain, initially activity-related, with pain at rest occurring with advanced pathology. Stiffness after inactivity (gel phenomenon) is prominent, but morning stiffness is of shorter duration and intensity than in systemic inflammatory arthropathies.

On clinical examination, the affected joint demonstrates hard, bony enlargement with or without soft tissue swelling, crepitus, tenderness, and limited range of motion. Synovial fluid, when present, is typically noninflammatory or only mildly inflammatory, and may have associated calcium pyrophosphate crystals.

Knee OA is characterized by insidious onset of pain, "gelling," limited motion and difficulty in walking, transferring, and stair climbing (Figure 127-3). Physical examination reveals crepitus and bony enlargement with pain along the medial and/or lateral joint line with or without effusion. Varus deformity is not uncommon, with flexion deformity and joint instability signs of severity. Quadriceps weakness may occur early and may contribute to progression.

Figure 127-1

Early Joint and Articular Changes

Normal joint and articular surface

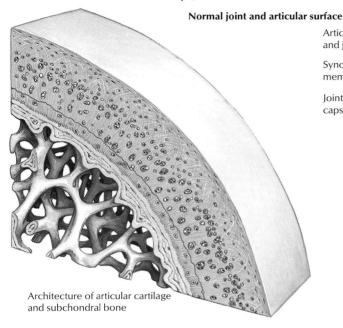

Architecture of articular cartilage
and subchondral bone

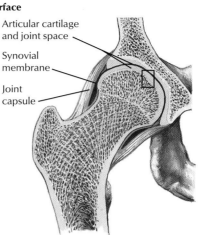

Articular cartilage
and joint space

Synovial
membrane

Joint
capsule

Joint with normal space and
cartilage-covered articular
surfaces

Early degenerative changes

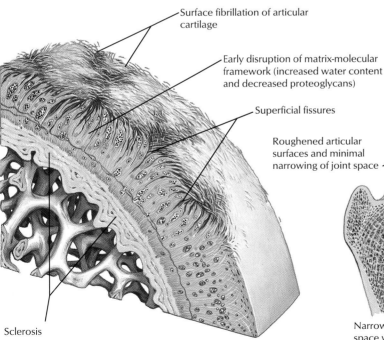

Surface fibrillation of articular
cartilage

Early disruption of matrix-molecular
framework (increased water content
and decreased proteoglycans)

Superficial fissures

Roughened articular
surfaces and minimal
narrowing of joint space

Sclerosis

Sclerosis (thickening) of subchondral
bone, an early sign of degeneration

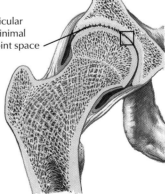

Narrowing of upper portion of joint
space with early degeneration of
articular cartilage

JOHN A.CRAIG—MD

C.Machado
—M.D.

©ICON
LEARNING
SYSTEMS

Figure 127-2

Advanced Joint and Articular Changes

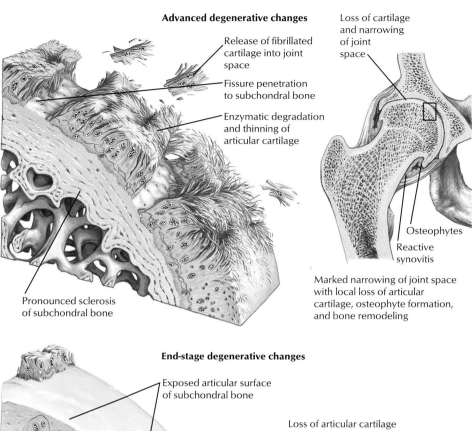

Advanced degenerative changes

Release of fibrillated cartilage into joint space

Fissure penetration to subchondral bone

Enzymatic degradation and thinning of articular cartilage

Pronounced sclerosis of subchondral bone

Loss of cartilage and narrowing of joint space

Osteophytes

Reactive synovitis

Marked narrowing of joint space with local loss of articular cartilage, osteophyte formation, and bone remodeling

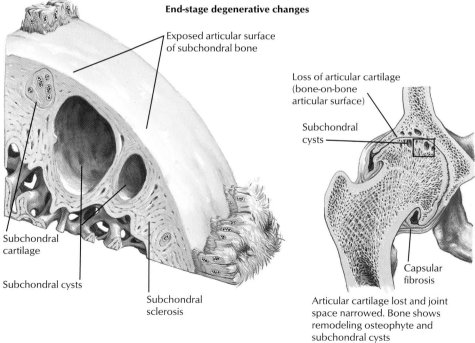

End-stage degenerative changes

Exposed articular surface of subchondral bone

Subchondral cartilage

Subchondral cysts

Subchondral sclerosis

Loss of articular cartilage (bone-on-bone articular surface)

Subchondral cysts

Capsular fibrosis

Articular cartilage lost and joint space narrowed. Bone shows remodeling osteophyte and subchondral cysts

JOHN A.CRAIG—AD
C.Machado
M.D.
©ICN

Figure 127-3

Clinical Findings

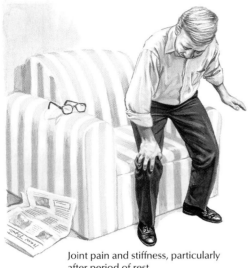

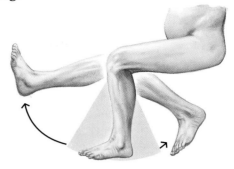

Limited range of motion in affected joint on both active and passive testing

Joint pain and stiffness, particularly after period of rest

In severe cases, disuse leads to muscle atrophy

Osteophytes visible or palpable

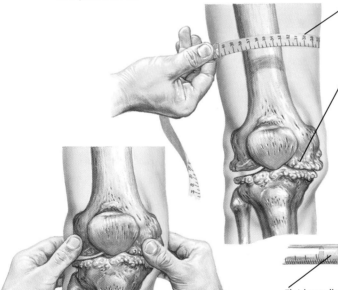

Joint palpation reveals osteophytes and crepitus (grinding sensation) on joint movement

Fluid usually clear to amber with low cell count. May contain cartilage fragments

Arthrocentesis most useful for ruling out other joint disorders

JOHN A. CRAIG—MD
C. Machado
—M.D.
© ICN
LEARNING
SYSTEMS

Hip OA usually presents with groin pain, but pain can be felt in the thigh, buttock, or knee. Pain and limitation of motion in walking, bending, and transfer can be severe. On examination, painful limitation of internal rotation can be an early sign. Deformity and limitation of hip flexion indicate advanced disease.

OA of the hand causes bony enlargement of the distal interphalangeal joints (Heberden's nodes) and proximal interphalangeal joints (Bouchard's nodes). It can begin with an acute inflammatory phase, but the joints may become less symptomatic after the initial inflammation has subsided. Involvement of the first carpometacarpal joint can be associated with significant pain and limited function (Figure 127-4). Bilateral involvement of multiple joints within and across joint groups is frequent. Metacarpophalangeal joints are affected less commonly; prominent involvement of these joints in the OA process should prompt consideration of secondary causes.

Radiographic evidence of OA in the cervical and lumbar spine, frequently with degenerative disk disease, is very common in those over the age of 45, but may not be associated with symptoms. Clinical symptoms in the cervical spine can include pain in the neck and occiput, with radiation down the arm, weakness, or paresthesia occurring from compression of cervical nerves from osteophytic encroachment on intervertebral foramina. An analogous process can occur in the lower thoracic and lumbosacral spine.

DIFFERENTIAL DIAGNOSIS

Diagnosis of OA is usually made clinically, but other disorders need to be considered, depending upon the joint(s) involved. OA in individuals younger than 45 frequently has an antecedent cause, such as hereditary conditions, previous trauma, or congenital or developmental conditions such as Legg-Perthes disease. OA typically has an insidious onset; an acute onset should prompt investigation for crystal arthropathies, infection, or trauma. OA does not have systemic inflammatory features or prolonged morning stiffness. If these are present, systemic inflammatory arthropathies such as rheumatoid arthritis, malignancy, or infection should be considered.

Patients may mistakenly refer to the lumbar spine, pelvis, or greater trochanter as the "hip." The differential diagnosis of hip OA thus includes fracture, avascular necrosis, inflammatory arthropathies, and pathologies involving the lumbar spine/pelvis or surrounding structures. Trochanteric bursitis is characterized by discomfort in the hip region, particularly with stair climbing and lying on the offending side. Palpation over the greater trochanter reproduces the patient's pain, and groin pain and painful limitation of hip rotation are absent. Low back pain with radiation, weakness, numbness, and paresthesia helps differentiate hip OA from lumbar spine disorders. Hip fracture usually presents acutely following trauma, but in the frail and osteoporotic patient, can occur without such history. Clinical suspicion should be high in such patients, particularly if severe pain on hip motion or a posture of hip flexion and external rotation is present. Avascular necrosis of the hip should be considered in the patient with sickle cell disease, diabetes mellitus, or a history of corticosteroid or alcohol use.

Because hand OA is common, especially in women, hand complaints should be evaluated with the purpose of eliminating an accompanying, superimposed inflammatory condition. Involvement of the metacarpophalangeal joints with significant soft tissue swelling should suggest an inflammatory arthropathy, such as rheumatoid arthritis or calcium pyrophosphate dihydrate deposition. Involvement of the metacarpophalangeal joints with bony enlargement can occur in hand OA, but such findings may also indicate other disorders, such as hypothyroidism, hemochromatosis, hyperparathyroidism, or calcium pyrophosphate dihydrate deposition.

Involvement of the first metatarsophalangeal joint in the foot may mimic gout if sufficient erythema and swelling exist. Involvement of multiple metatarsophalangeal joints may indicate an inflammatory arthropathy, such as rheumatoid arthritis, particularly if accompanied by prolonged morning stiffness and involvement of the small joints of the hands.

DIAGNOSTIC APPROACH

There are no definitive tests for OA, and the diagnosis is clinical. A thorough history and physical examination to elicit the presence of other conditions should be performed. Unless

Figure 127-4

Hand Involvement in Osteoarthritis

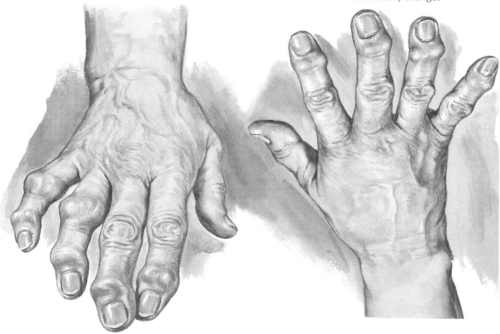

Early Heberden nodes
with inflammatory changes

Chronic Heberden nodes. 4th and 5th
proximal interphalangeal joints also
involved in degenerative process.

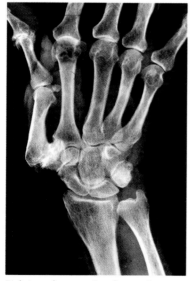

End-stage degenerative changes in
carpometacarpal articulation of thumb

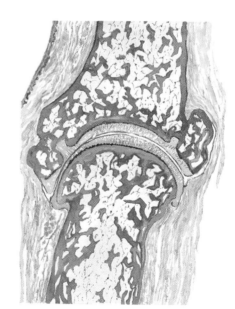

Section through distal interphalangeal joint
shows irregular, hyperplastic bony nodules
(Heberden nodes) at articular margins of
distal phalanx

clinical suspicion exists for a systemic inflammatory arthropathy or systemic autoimmune conditions, there is little purpose in measuring rheumatoid factor, antinuclear antibodies, or other serologic tests.

Assessment of complete blood cell count, electrolytes with glucose and creatinine, and liver function tests should be checked before beginning pharmacologic therapy, especially in the older individual with co-morbid medical conditions. In cases of atypical appearance of the hands, particularly with involvement of the metacarpophalangeal joints, evaluation for hypothyroidism and hemochromatosis may be warranted.

Radiographs typically show osteophytes, joint space narrowing, sclerosis of subchondral bone, cysts, and joint deformity. They can confirm a diagnosis and exclude others, particularly in those cases with an unclear clinical picture or where other diagnoses, such as inflammatory arthropathy, hip fracture, avascular necrosis, infection, or malignancy may exist. Radionuclide scans, magnetic resonance imaging, and other modalities may be useful in certain situations, but are not routinely needed.

MANAGEMENT AND THERAPY

There is no cure for OA, nor are there pharmacologic agents available to affect the underlying pathologic process.

Medical management consists of non-pharmacologic modalities and pharmacologic agents to relieve pain and improve function and health-related quality of life, with the goal of avoiding complications of therapy. In more severe cases, surgical intervention, particularly joint replacement, can be effective.

Non-pharmacologic Therapy

Assessment of gait disturbances, leg length discrepancy, functional and other difficulties is critical in developing an individualized treatment plan. Ambulatory aids, orthotics, and splints can alleviate pain and improve function. Instruction in joint protection and energy-saving techniques, aerobic exercise, muscle strengthening, and range-of-motion exercises can help the patient regain, maintain, or improve function. Weight loss should be prescribed for overweight OA patients.

Pharmacologic Therapy

If the above measures prove insufficient, pharmacologic therapy (oral, intra-articular, and topical) can be considered.

Oral and Topical Therapy

Acetaminophen and non-opioid analgesics can be helpful in the patient with mild-to-moderate or intermittent pain. NSAIDs can be used when acetaminophen is ineffective. However, the potential for serious side effects, including gastrointestinal ulceration and bleeding, exacerbation of hypertension, renal dysfunction, and fluid retention, particularly in older individuals with co-morbidities, may limit their use. Selective cyclooxygenase 2 inhibitors can provide analgesia similar to traditional NSAIDs with less likelihood of gastrointestinal ulceration and bleeding, but they do not spare the kidney, limiting their use in patients with renal pathology. Opioids should be reserved for those with severe pain that cannot be controlled otherwise. Glucosamine and chondroitin, nutraceuticals that have demonstrated possible symptom and disease modifying properties in OA, are popular supplements currently under study. Topical methylsalicylate, capsaicin, and NSAIDs can be useful as adjunctive or sole therapy in some patients.

Intra-articular Therapy

Intra-articular corticosteroid therapy can relieve pain and inflammation in patients with OA. Need for repeated corticosteroid injections should prompt re-evaluation of the medical regimen and consideration of surgical intervention. Intra-articular hyaluronan is administered in a series of injections for knee OA; although no definite disease modification has been shown for such agents, there may be a pain-relieving effect that can last several months.

FUTURE DIRECTIONS

Therapy in OA at this time modifies symptoms without altering the underlying disease process, which may have progressed considerably by the time symptoms occur. The goals of research are to develop better means to identify individuals at increased risk of OA for early intervention and to develop pharmaceuticals to influence the disease process. Avenues for exploration in this regard include genetics, advanced imaging, and bio-markers in serum, urine, synovial fluid, and others. For those in whom OA has already progressed, research also endeavors to improve techniques and materials for joint replacement and to develop new ways to grow, modify, and implant cartilage into diseased joints.

REFERENCES

Recommendations for the medical management of osteo-arthritis of the hip and knee: 2000 update. American College of Rheumatology Subcommittee on Osteoarthritis Guidelines. *Arthritis Rheum.* 2000;43:1905–1915.

American College of Rheumatology Web site. Available at: http://www.rheumatology.org. Accessed March 2, 2003.

Arthritis Foundation Web site. Available at: http://www.arthritis.org. Accessed March 2, 2003.

Felson DT, Lawrence RC, Dieppe PA, et al. Osteoarthritis: new insights. Part 1: the disease and its risk factors. *Ann Intern Med.* 2000;133:635–646.

Felson DT, Lawrence RC, Hochberg MC, et al. Osteoarthritis: new insights. Part 2: treatment approaches. *Ann Intern Med.* 2000;133:726–737.

Chapter 128

Polymyalgia Rheumatica and Giant Cell Arteritis

Mary Anne Dooley

Polymyalgia rheumatica (PMR) and giant cell arteritis (GCA) are linked conditions affecting individuals over age 50 and more often women than men. Prevalence increases with age. The incidence varies with ethnicity: high-risk populations include Scandinavians and people of Northern European descent. The incidences of PMR and GCA are 20 to 53/100,000 and 15 to 25/100,000, respectively, of the population older than 50 in these groups compared to 1 to 2/100,000 in African American and Hispanic populations. PMR can also develop in up to one half of patients with GCA, but GCA develops in only 15% with PMR. Both conditions can coexist in the same individual or develop sequentially with delayed onset of symptoms described up to 10 years after the initial illness. In both conditions, ESR is typically elevated. Elevations in interleukin-6 (IL-6) and association with human leukocyte antigen–DR4 have also been found.

ETIOLOGY AND PATHOGENESIS

The etiology of PMR and GCA is not known. Several potential mechanisms including infections, local degenerative processes, genetic susceptibility, and endocrinopathy have been proposed as instigators of a cellular autoimmune process. Specific autoantibodies, hypergammaglobulinemia, or the presence of B cells in vascular lesions have not been found. GCA is a vasculitis of medium and large vessels most commonly affecting the cranial branches of the arteries originating from the aortic arch. The vasculitis is transmural with mononuclear cell infiltrate, destruction of the internal and external elastic lamina, and intimal proliferation. Multinucleated giant cells and granuloma formation may be absent.

CLINICAL PRESENTATION
Polymyalgia Rheumatica

Symptoms are severe aching and stiffness in the neck, shoulders, and hip girdles. Myalgias are symmetric, often begin in the shoulders, and may have abrupt onset. Constitutional symptoms including weight loss, malaise, and depression can be present; spiking fevers are rare. Muscle strength is normal, but it can appear diminished due to pain. Active rather than passive motion is limited by pain. There is often a disparity between the severity of myalgias reported and the clinical findings.

Giant Cell Arteritis

Signs and symptoms of vascular insufficiency or signs of systemic inflammation may predominate in subsets of patients with GCA. Cranial arteritis presents with headaches of variable intensity localized to the temporal or occipital area in two thirds of patients. Temporal artery tenderness or decreased pulsation with scalp tenderness is often but not always present (Figure 128-1). Jaw claudication is very specific for GCA but found in only up to one half the patients. It can present with trismus rather than fatigue of the masseters. Tongue claudication also occurs and throat soreness may be noted during swallowing.

Constitutional symptoms are more frequent than in PMR and are present at onset in up to 50% of patients with GCA. A syndrome of fever of unknown origin with high-grade spiking fevers is seen in 15% of patients with GCA. Anorexia, weight loss, night sweats, chills, and depression may be presenting complaints.

Visual symptoms are varied and include blurry vision, diplopia, eye pain, visual hallucinations, partial visual loss, and amaurosis fugax. Bilateral or unilateral blindness, often without any previous visual symptoms, occurs in 15% to 20% of patients. If untreated in one eye, the contralateral eye may become affected. Ischemic optic neuropathy due to arteritis of the posterior ciliary ophthalmic arteries is seen on funduscopic examination.

Figure 128-1

Giant-Cell (Temporal) Arteritis, Polymyalgia Rheumatica

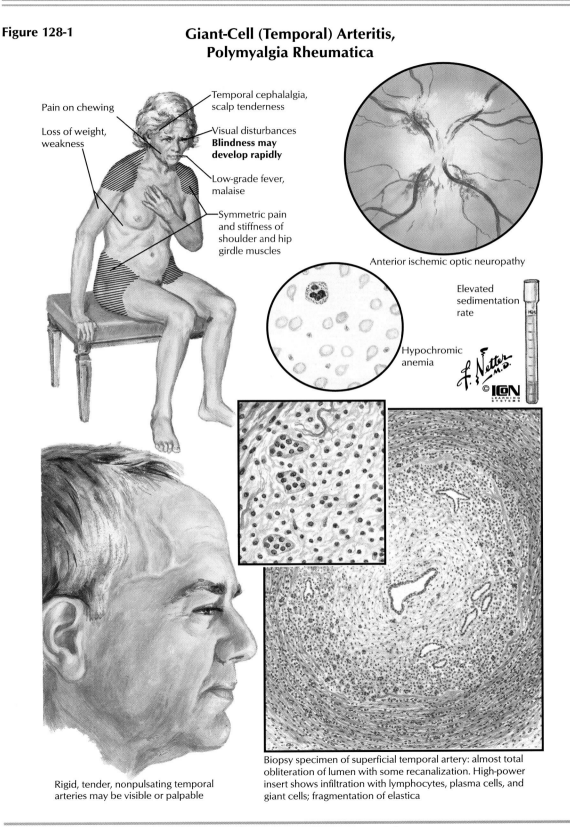

Pain on chewing

Temporal cephalalgia, scalp tenderness

Loss of weight, weakness

Visual disturbances **Blindness may develop rapidly**

Low-grade fever, malaise

Symmetric pain and stiffness of shoulder and hip girdle muscles

Anterior ischemic optic neuropathy

Elevated sedimentation rate

Hypochromic anemia

Biopsy specimen of superficial temporal artery: almost total obliteration of lumen with some recanalization. High-power insert shows infiltration with lymphocytes, plasma cells, and giant cells; fragmentation of elastica

Rigid, tender, nonpulsating temporal arteries may be visible or palpable

Neurologic manifestations including transient ischemic attacks, stroke, and neuropathies are present in 30% of patients. Large vessel vasculitis, presenting with arm claudication, pulselessness, or Raynaud's phenomenon may be present with evidence of occlusion or aneurysm. Thoracic aortic aneurysm has been reported as a late complication and may be up to 17 times more likely in patients with GCA. Fatalities from myocardial infarction (coronary arteritis) or ruptured aortic aneurysm, although rare, may occur.

Differential Diagnosis

Underlying infection and malignancy need to be excluded. Hepatitis C, subacute bacterial endocarditis, Lyme disease, and other chronic infections such as tuberculosis or brucellosis may cause diagnostic confusion. Multiple myeloma may present similarly to PMR; however, patients with myeloma usually have a paraprotein on serum and urine electrophoresis. Amyloidosis, including jaw or arm claudication, can mimic GCA and should be excluded.

Hypothyroidism, spondyloarthropathy, polymyositis, and, rarely, amyotrophic lateral sclerosis can present similarly to PMR. Polymyositis usually produces muscle weakness and, less commonly, muscle pain. An elevated creatine kinase level, findings on electromyography, and muscle biopsy findings confirm the diagnosis. Early rheumatoid arthritis (RA) may mimic PMR, but the synovitis is usually more pronounced and symmetric. Resolution of the synovitis of PMR is complete on low dose steroids, while this may not be the case in RA. Erosive disease is seen with RA but not PMR.

DIAGNOSTIC APPROACH

The diagnosis of GCA should be considered in patients older than 50 who present with symptoms of new or changing headaches, vision loss, PMR, or arterial occlusion in the extracranial vascular territory. There should be minimal delay in obtaining confirmation of arteritis. The superficial temporal artery site is easily accessible and most frequently biopsied. PMR is a clinical diagnosis supported by nonspecific laboratory findings.

The temporal artery biopsy specimen is abnormal in up to 80% to 90% of GCA but rare in PMR. It is used to diagnose GCA but not PMR. As the lesions of GCA are patchy, this biopsy should be between 3 and 5 cm optimally and if negative, contralateral biopsy should be strongly considered to yield the best results. The temporal artery biopsy specimen shows fragmentation of the elastica lamina, luminal narrowing and intimal edema, granulomas with multinucleated giant cells, and monocellular infiltrate.

Magnetic resonance angiography and angiography are used to assess vessel involvement, particularly large vessel involvement in GCA. Noninvasive vascular studies have been used, but identify only patients with pronounced luminal narrowing.

There is no single diagnostic test for PMR or GCA. ESR is usually, but not always, elevated over 40 mm/h. Some authors suggest that up to 25% of patients with positive results on temporal artery biopsy may have a normal ESR. Other acute phase reactants may also be elevated such as C-reactive protein. Other findings include normochromic normocytic anemia, thrombocytosis, and abnormal liver function tests, particularly alkaline phosphatase and elevated von Willebrand factor. Determinations of rheumatoid factor, antinuclear antibodies, and other autoantibodies such as antineutrophil cytoplasmic antibodies are negative. Complement levels are typically not decreased.

MANAGEMENT AND THERAPY

Systemic steroids are the drugs of choice in the treatment of GCA and PMR. Side effects are more likely to occur at higher daily or cumulative doses over time.

They include cushingoid facies and habitus, skin bruising and fragility, electrolyte disturbance, elevated serum glucose, osteoporosis and osteonecrosis, increased susceptibility to infections, increased appetite, and salt and water retention causing weight gain. Both PMR and GCA respond dramatically and rapidly to corticosteroids. In GCA, initial doses of prednisone at 1 mg/kg or 60 mg per day are used in the first month. Prednisone can usually be tapered by 10% every 1 to 2 weeks thereafter, but the patient should be maintained on low dose therapy for at least 1 to 2 years. Disease relapse or appearance of PMR are common when tapering steroids. ESR and C-reactive protein do not always reflect disease activity, and recurrence of symptoms should be taken seriously. In PMR, response to lower doses of prednisone is common; at onset only one third of patients receive doses above 20 mg daily. Typically, patients can taper the dosage by 5-mg increments every 2 to 4 weeks, with slower taper below 7.5 mg doses. While PMR is generally a self-limited process, prednisone is usually not discontinued for 1 year and may be continued in some patients for 2 years or longer. Some patients may require 1 to 2 mg doses long-term to avoid relapse; symptoms, not just laboratory results, guide steroid taper. Symmetric additive polyarthritis progressing to seronegative RA will develop in some patients and may require therapy to avoid erosive arthritis. NSAIDs can be used in conjunction with steroids in mild PMR. Side effects include gastrointestinal intolerance and bleeding, hepatic and renal toxicity, and allergic reactions.

The efficacy of methotrexate and azathioprine has not been clearly demonstrated in either PMR or GCA. They have been used in conjunction with steroids as steroid-sparing agents, but data are lacking to document significant response. Two recent trials of methotrexate as a steroid-sparing agent in GCA reached opposite conclusions. Cyclophosphamide, an immunosuppressive agent, has been used in large vessel vasculitis, and there are case reports of use in severe GCA.

Patients should be monitored closely for PMR and GCA because they can occur together or separately in the same individual. Advise patients with a history of either PMR or GCA to report any symptoms of GCA immediately whether or not they are receiving treatment. Prophylaxis for steroid osteoporosis such as calcium and vitamin D supplementation should be given. Monitor bone densitometry and consider antiresorptive therapy such as bisphosphonates. Monitor patients for steroid-associated complications of diabetes or hypertension.

Polymyalgia Rheumatica

Use the lowest dose of corticosteroids to control symptoms. The initial dose of prednisone should be between 7.5 and 20 mg/day. Once symptoms are controlled for 2 to 4 weeks and ESR is normalized, reduce dose by 10% every 2 to 4 weeks until 10 mg/day is reached. Then the dose should not be reduced faster than 1 mg per month. If there is not a marked clinical improvement within 1 week of initiation of steroid therapy the diagnosis should be reconsidered. Treatment is usually necessary for 2 years at least but rarely more than 5 years. Treatment adjustment is predominantly based on clinical judgment of symptoms, although ESR can be a useful parameter to observe for response to therapy. Relapses are common on tapering the prednisone.

Giant Cell Arteritis

GCA is a medical emergency because it can lead to blindness. Treatment helps prevent visual complications, although blindness while on treatment has been reported. Do not delay corticosteroid treatment until after the temporal artery biopsy, which should be performed within days to increase the likelihood of obtaining a positive biopsy result. When visual symptoms are present, corticosteroid therapy should be no lower than 60 mg daily of prednisone equivalent. Recovery of vision loss with high-dose methylprednisolone has been described in case reports, but vision loss is usually irreversible.

FUTURE DIRECTIONS

Genetic and immunologic studies are the focus of current investigation. Certain HLA-DR4 haplotypes are associated with increased risk of disease, but HLA polymorphisms do not associate with differential disease expression in GCA. The interaction between macrophages, multinucleated giant cells, and endothelial injury response and repair processes may play important roles in clinical expression of GCA. New biomarkers of disease activity may arise. Serum IL-6 levels may be more sensitive in detecting ongoing inflammation than CRP or ESR.

REFERENCES

American College of Rheumatology Web site. Available at: http://www.rheumatology.org. Accessed March 2, 2003.

Arthritis Foundation Web site. Available at: http://www.arthritis.org. Accessed March 2, 2003.

Hunder GG. Giant cell arteritis and polymyalgia rheumatica. *Med Clin North Am.* 1997;81:195-219.

Jover JA, Hernandez-Garcia C, Morado IC, Vargas E, Banares A, Fernandez-Gutierrez B. Combined treatment of giant-cell arteritis with methotrexate and prednisone: a randomized, double-blind, placebo-controlled trial. *Ann Intern Med.* 2001;134:106–114.

Koopman WJ, ed. *Arthritis and Allied Conditions: A Textbook of Rheumatology.* 14th ed. Philadelphia, Pa: Lippincott Williams & Wilkins; 2001.

National Institute of Arthritis and Musculoskeletal and Skin Diseases Web site. Available at: http://www.niams.nih.gov. Accessed March 2, 2003.

Ruddy S, Harris ED Jr, Sledge CB, Sergent JS, Budd RC, eds. *Kelley's Textbook of Rheumatology.* 6th ed. Philadelphia, Pa: WB Saunders Co; 2001.

Spiera RF, Paget S, Spiera H. Methotrexate in giant-cell arteritis. *Ann Intern Med.* 2001;135:1006–1007.

Weyand CM, Goronzy JJ. Arterial wall injury in giant cell arteritis. *Arthritis Rheum.* 1999;42:844–853.

Chapter 129
Rheumatoid Arthritis

Beth L. Jonas and Robert A.S. Roubey

Rheumatoid arthritis is a multisystem inflammatory disorder with a worldwide prevalence rate in the population of approximately 1%. The peak age of onset is between 40 and 50 years, with females being affected significantly more often than males; however, with increasing age, the male to female ratio equilibrates.

ETIOLOGY AND PATHOGENESIS

The etiology of rheumatoid arthritis (RA) has not been established, and it is likely to be multifactorial. It is clear that genetic makeup, the immune responses of the individual, and an inciting agent, possibly of bacterial or viral origin, all play a role. RA is associated with a conserved sequence in the hypervariable region of the human leukocyte antigen (HLA) DR gene; the so-called shared epitope. The presence of the shared epitope has been shown to be associated with both susceptibility to and severity of RA in some populations. A putative arthrogenic antigen has not been elucidated, although it is likely that numerous exogenous or endogenous antigens may trigger the disease.

CLINICAL PRESENTATION

The diagnosis of rheumatoid arthritis is an important one, particularly now that early treatment with disease-modifying anti-rheumatic drugs (DMARDs) and the newer biologic agents is recommended. The diagnostic criteria of the American College of Rheumatology are shown in Table 129-1. Eventually, a symmetric inflammatory polyarthritis with small joint involvement develops in all patients. The majority of patients present with an insidious onset over weeks to months, but some patients (approximately 10%) have an acute onset over a few days. The small joints of the hand and wrist are most commonly involved early but some patients may present with a monoarthritis. The diagnosis can be difficult in the early stages, and patients with chronic joint pain need to be reviewed on a regular basis.

Signs and symptoms include joint pain; joint swelling with synovitis (synovial thickening and fluid); joint stiffness, worse in the mornings; joints that are usually warm, and occasionally erythematous; limited range of motion; nodule formation on the extensor aspect of the forearm; low-grade fever in some cases; and malaise and fatigue (Figure 129-1). Extra-articular manifestations occur in patients with more severe disease and may include Sjögren's syndrome, episcleritis or scleritis, pleurisy, pulmonary nodules, pulmonary fibrosis, pericarditis, rheumatoid vasculitis, and Felty's syndrome (Figure 129-2).

Initial laboratory test results may be normal, but can show a thrombocytosis, leukocytosis, mild anemia (normochromic, normocytic or microcytic), raised erythrocyte sedimentation rate, and high C-reactive protein. IgM rheumatoid factor is present in approximately 50% of cases at presenta-

Table 129-1
Criteria for the Classification of Rheumatoid Arthritis* (revised 1987)

1. Morning stiffness lasting greater than 1 hour

2. Arthritis in 3 or more joint areas

3. Arthritis of the hand joints

4. Symmetric arthritis

5. Rheumatoid nodules

6. Serum rheumatoid factor

7. Radiographic changes: erosions or unequivocal periarticular osteopenia

*Patients are said to have RA if they satisfy 4 of the 7 criteria.
Adapted from Arnett FC, Edworthy SM, Bloch DA, McShane DJ, et al. The American Rheumatism Association 1987 revised criteria for the classification of rheumatoid arthritis. *Arthritis Rheum.* 1988; 31:315–24. Reprinted with permission of Wiley-Liss, Inc., a subsidiary of John Wiley & Sons, Inc.

tion, and in 70% to 75% of cases over time. Aspiration of inflammatory fluid from the joint often reveals a high white cell count with polymorphonuclear leukocytes predominating. Synovial fluid analysis is particularly important in early disease to rule out crystalline arthropathies, or in the case of a monoarthritis to rule out infection.

DIFFERENTIAL DIAGNOSIS

The differential diagnosis includes:

- Seronegative spondyloarthropathies: particularly psoriatic arthritis, but also ankylosing spondylitis, reactive arthritis, and the arthritis of inflammatory bowel disease
- Polyarticular gout or calcium pyrophosphate crystal deposition disease
- Early stages of diffuse connective tissue diseases, such as systemic lupus erythematosus, scleroderma, polymyositis
- Hemochromatosis
- Arthritis associated with the hemoglobinopathies or hemophilia
- Infectious arthritis (parvovirus B_{19}).
- Bacterial endocarditis
- Arthritis associated with thyroid disease (hypothyroidism or hyperthyroidism)
- Osteoarthritis
- Polymyalgia rheumatica
- Rheumatic fever
- Sarcoidosis

DIAGNOSTIC APPROACH

Patients with recent onset of inflammatory polyarthralgia or polyarthritis should have a complete history and physical examination. Although RA is very common, attention should be paid to elements of the history or physical examination that might suggest another cause. Swollen or tender joints should be surveyed to document true synovitis and to form a baseline examination to assess progress in future visits. Radiographs are often normal in early disease. The presence of periarticular osteopenia can sometimes be helpful in differentiating inflammatory from noninflammatory causes of joint pain. Radiographs of the hands (and feet if clinically indicated) can be useful in patients with disease duration of 6 months or more. The presence of erosions on the baseline radiograph is a poor prognostic factor and indicates the need for an aggressive approach.

Synovial fluid analysis is performed to document the inflammatory nature of the joint disease and rule out other causes of synovitis, including gout, calcium pyrophosphate deposition disease, and septic arthritis. Other laboratory tests include a rheumatoid factor, complete blood cells count, chemistry profile, and some acute phase reactants such as WESR or C-reactive protein.

MANAGEMENT AND THERAPY
Disease-Modifying Agents

The most commonly used disease-modifying antirheumatic drugs include hydroxychloroquine, sulfasalazine, methotrexate, and leflunomide. The mechanism of action of these drugs is complex, but they all inhibit inflammatory responses and suppress synovitis. Hydroxychloroquine is useful in very early and mild disease. As it is laid down in pigment tissue, ophthalmologic assessment is still recommended. There is little or no risk of long-term ocular sequelae if standard dose regimens are adhered to (200 to 400 mg daily). Sulfasalazine is given orally; the dosage should be increased slowly from 500 mg to 2 g daily. Some patients might require a trial of up to 4 g daily for 4 to 6 weeks if there is no response. Side effects include indigestion, abnormal liver function tests, leukopenia, anemia, and skin rashes. Complete blood cell count and liver function tests should be monitored on a regular basis, at least for the first 3 months of therapy. Methotrexate, the most commonly used member of this group, is given orally in a dose of 7.5 to 25 mg once a week. Side effects include indigestion, oral ulcers, hair loss, occasional blood dyscrasias, and abnormal liver function tests. The risk of hepatic fibrosis with long-term administration now seems sufficiently small to preclude routine liver biopsy. Great care should be taken in prescribing to patients who have a regular moderate alcohol intake, history of liver disease, diabetes or obesity; it is contraindicated in pregnancy. The addition of folic acid, 1 mg daily is recommended to reduce toxicity. Monitoring of blood cell counts and liver function tests is recommended every 8 weeks. Leflunomide, a newer agent, is given orally in a dose of 20 mg daily after a 3-day loading dose of 100 mg daily. It has been shown to slow the radiographic progression of disease. Common side effects include diarrhea, elevated transaminase levels,

Figure 129-1

Early and Moderate Hand Involvement
in Rheumatoid Arthritis

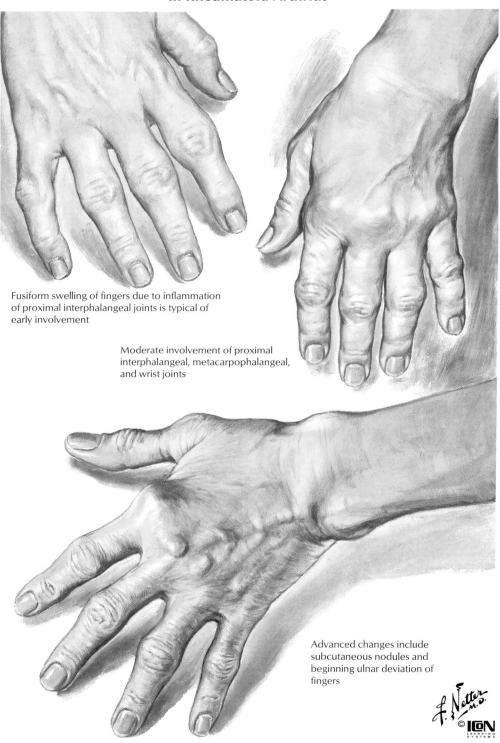

Fusiform swelling of fingers due to inflammation
of proximal interphalangeal joints is typical of
early involvement

Moderate involvement of proximal
interphalangeal, metacarpophalangeal,
and wrist joints

Advanced changes include
subcutaneous nodules and
beginning ulnar deviation of
fingers

Figure 129-2

Extra-articular Manifestations in Rheumatoid Arthritis

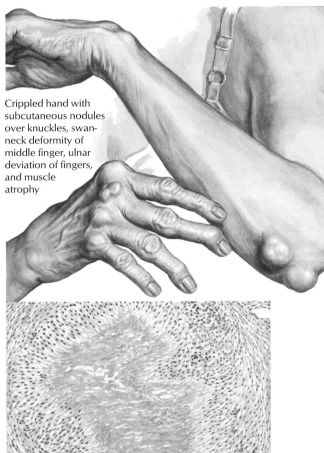

Crippled hand with subcutaneous nodules over knuckles, swan-neck deformity of middle finger, ulnar deviation of fingers, and muscle atrophy

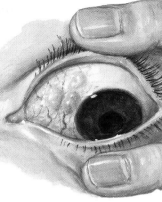

Nodular episcleritis with scleromalacia

Subcutaneous nodule just distal to olecranon process, and another in olecranon bursa

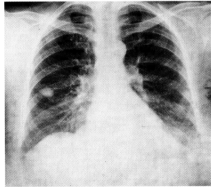

Section of rheumatoid nodule. Central area of fibrinoid necrosis surrounded by zone of palisading mesenchymal cells and peripheral fibrous tissue capsule containing chronic inflammatory cells.

Radiograph shows rheumatoid nodule in right lung. Lesion may be misdiagnosed as carcinoma until identified by biopsy or postsurgical pathologic analysis.

reversible alopecia, and rash. Leflunomide is teratogenic in animals. Women who wish to become pregnant or men who want to father a child must first discontinue the drug and take cholestyramine (8 grams 3 times daily for 11 days) to eliminate the drug. Leflunomide in reduced dose (10 mg daily) may be used in combination with methotrexate, but long-term safety has not been established. Monitoring of blood cell counts and liver function tests is recommended every 8 weeks. Gold compounds include sodium aurothiomalate, aurothioglucose, and auranofin. Sodium aurothiomalate and aurothioglucose are given by intramuscular injection in doses of 20 to

50 mg once a week (following a test dose). Side effects include bone marrow suppression, skin rash, glomerulonephritis, colitis, and pneumonitis. Mouth ulcers also occur frequently. A full blood cell count and urinalysis should be done before each injection. If side effects occur, the dosage should be reduced or ceased. Other agents still in use include azathioprine, D-penicillamine, cyclosporin A, and rarely cyclophosphamide.

Biologic Response Modifiers

Etanercept is a recombinant dimeric fusion protein of the soluble human tumor necrosis factor (TNF) receptor. Etanercept, 25 mg subcutaneously twice weekly, has been shown to be effective in RA that has been refractory to other DMARDs. Injection site reactions are common, but rarely limit therapy. Infections, some life-threatening, have been reported and warrant caution in debilitated patients. Infliximab is a monoclonal antibody that binds TNF and neutralizes its activity. Like Etanercept, it is indicated in RA unresponsive to traditional DMARDs. It is given by IV infusion at weeks 0, 2, and 6 and then every 8 weeks. Infusion reactions may occur, but are usually mild. Severe infections have been reported, particularly tuberculosis. Therefore, a pretreatment PPD is recommended for patients starting anti-TNF therapy. The newest anti-TNF agent, adalimumab, is a fully humanized monoclonal antibody given subcutaneously, 40 mg every other week.. The FDA has approved Anakinra, IL1-receptor antagonist, for RA. It is given subcutaneously 100 mg daily. Efficacy appears to be moderate, but it may be an option for patients who have not responded to TNF inhibition. Injection site reactions can be severe, but usually wane after 4 to 6 weeks of therapy.

Corticosteroids

Systemic corticosteroids are very effective in the treatment of rheumatoid arthritis, but significant short- and long-term toxicity limits their use. Doses of prednisone should be kept below 10 mg daily if possible, and the majority of the dose given in the morning. Corticosteroids should be aggressively tapered once effective DMARDs have been instituted if at all possible. Intra-articular injections can be extremely useful in modifying inflammation in individual joints. However,

they should not be given at intervals of less than 3 months and are contraindicated in the presence of local sepsis.

Nonsteroidal Anti-inflammatory Drugs (NSAIDs)

Nonsteroidal anti-inflammatory drugs (NSAIDs) interfere with the production of prostaglandins and therefore reduce pain and inflammation. NSAIDs produce a plethora of adverse reactions, the most common being peptic ulceration. The newer selective COX-2 inhibitors have a significant advantage over traditional NSAIDs because the relative risk of GI ulceration is lower. All NSAIDs have significant renal adverse effects, particularly in the elderly, including acute renal failure and fluid retention. As a rule, NSAIDs should be used as an adjunct to DMARD therapy and never as monotherapy in patients with established RA.

Drug Therapy

NSAIDs are suitable for first-line agents for management of active disease. Consider low-dose prednisone (10 mg daily) in patients who are not adequately controlled on NSAIDs, at least until effective DMARD therapy can be achieved. Most patients with rheumatoid arthritis will require DMARDs. These drugs should be commenced once the diagnosis of rheumatoid arthritis is established. Delay will lead to irreversible joint destruction in most patients with moderate or severe disease activity. Patients may not respond to disease-modifying antirheumatic drug therapy for up to 3 months once a therapeutic dose is achieved. Disease activity should be monitored frequently to evaluate efficacy. If there is no evidence of disease suppression, then the drug should be changed. Periodic radiographic assessment is recommended even in those patients with an adequate clinical response, as progression of erosive disease warrants intensification of therapy. When response to methotrexate is incomplete, combinations of methotrexate with other agents such as sulfasalazine, leflunomide, or a TNF-inhibitor may be beneficial. If general control is achieved but individual joints continue to show active inflammation, intra-articular corticosteroid injections can be considered. These might need to be repeated on occasions but probably no more than 4 times per year in weight-bearing joints. A joint requiring more frequent injections may need other treatment such as yttrium or dysprosium synovectomy, surgical treatment, or another disease-modifying drug.

Surgical Treatment

The major reason for surgery is pain relief or restoration of function. Surgical options include synovectomy (of joint or tendons), arthroplasty, and arthrodesis. Synovectomy can be performed on the knees, wrists, metacarpophalangeal joints, or other joints unresponsive to other therapies. The synovium might well grow back into the joint if disease activity continues, but patients can be given some pain relief for a number of years. Arthroplasty with joint replacement is commonly used in the hips, knees, and metacarpophalangeal and interphalangeal joints. Shoulder and elbow joint replacements are now gaining acceptance; wrists and ankles are still in their infancy. Use of new prosthetic materials and cementless prostheses is likely to improve long-term morbidity. Although joint replacement should be put off as long as possible, great relief can be afforded appropriate patients. Intractuble wrist or ankle disease can be treated with arthrodesis.

Avoiding Treatment Errors

The diagnosis of inflammatory joint disease should be confirmed. Whether the pain is due to active synovitis or to secondary degenerative changes should be determined. This is particularly important in those patients with chronic disease where the question of disease modifying antirheumatic drug therapy is raised. It is especially important to be aware of potential drug interactions and to continually reassess patients and change drugs or other treatments if there is no response to treatment. Referring patients to a rheumatologist on diagnosis is advisable, particularly for educational purposes. Also consider referral if there is deteriorating function; when the patient appears generally ill and systemic corticosteroids are contemplated; if there is persistent inflammation in a joint (this could lead to deformity); or if a surgical procedure is contemplated.

Optimum Treatment

Psychologic factors are very important in a patient who has chronic pain and inflammatory joint disease. These need to be addressed and demand a combined approach with allied health professionals such as the physiotherapist, occupational therapist, social worker, nurse, and, of course, the patient's family. Patient education and self-management skills are extremely important.

FUTURE DIRECTIONS

Research in RA has made significant strides in the past 10 years with the understanding of the role of genetic factors in disease onset and progression, the cytokine profile in active disease, and the introduction of targeted therapies based on these discoveries. The TNF inhibitors have made a huge contribution to our armamentarium of antirheumatic therapies. There are a number of new biologic compounds on the horizon. The next decade will bring further work on mechanisms of inflammation that may contribute to disease activity and the development of novel therapeutic targets.

REFERENCES

Albers JM, Paimela L, Kurki P, et al. Treatment strategy, disease activity, and outcome in four cohorts of patients with early rheumatoid arthritis. *Ann Rheum Dis.* 2001;60:453−458.

Boers M. Rheumatoid arthritis. Treatment of early disease. *Rheum Dis Clin North Am.* 2001;27:405−414.

Gabriel SE. The epidemiology of rheumatoid arthritis. *Rheum Dis Clin North Am.* 2001;27:269−281.

Kremer JM. Rational use of new and existing disease-modifying agents in rheumatoid arthritis. *Ann Intern Med.* 2001;134:695−706.

Chapter 130

Scleroderma

Fathima Kabir and Mary Anne Dooley

Scleroderma (hard skin) is a chronic disorder of the connective tissue characterized by inflammation, fibrosis and degenerative changes in the skin, blood vessels, joints, skeletal muscle, and certain internal organs such as the gastrointestinal tract, heart, kidney, and lungs (Figure 130-1). In the United States, the incidence is approximately 20 to 30 new cases per million people annually. The female-to-male incidence ratio is 3:1, and the peak age of onset is 40 to 60 years. No significant racial differences have been found. Systemic sclerosis is classified into 3 major clinical subtypes: *diffuse cutaneous scleroderma* (dcSSc), *limited cutaneous* (lcSSc), and *overlap*. These subtypes are distinguished from each other on the basis of extent and degree of skin involvement primarily.

ETIOLOGY AND PATHOGENESIS

The etiology of scleroderma remains unclear. Prior investigation suggests that it is a multigenic, complex disorder. An individual with a susceptible genetic background may encounter an inciting factor such as infection, organic solvents, drugs, or environmental agents. Implicated environmental agents include silica dust exposure, but several retrospective studies do not show increased risk in women with silicone breast implants. Clinical expression includes vascular, fibrotic, and immunologic features. Pathogenetic events include endothelial cell injury and vascular obliteration, increased matrix deposition by dermal and visceral fibroblasts, and activation of cellular and humoral immune responses. Genetic factors play a role in disease susceptibility, but no single major histocompatibility complex allele is associated with increased risk of scleroderma in all ethnic groups. Microchimerism (the persistence of fetal cells in the maternal circulation) may contribute to immune activation in this autoimmune disorder.

CLINICAL PRESENTATION
Diffuse Cutaneous Scleroderma

Widespread skin fibrosis affects distal and proximal extremities (proximal to elbow), trunk, and face. There is a tendency to rapid progression of skin thickening and early occurrence of visceral disease affecting the gastrointestinal tract, lung, heart, and kidneys. Palpable tendon friction rubs and flexion contractures are fre-

quently associated. Ten-year survival is usually less than 70%.

Limited Cutaneous Scleroderma

There is restricted skin fibrosis affecting the distal extremities and face and occasional late development of pulmonary arterial hypertension, pulmonary fibrosis, or small bowel malabsorption. The CREST syndrome that presents with findings of calcinosis, Raynaud's phenomenon, esophageal dysfunction, sclerodactyly, and telangiectasia is closely analogous to limited cutaneous scleroderma (lcSSc). Ten year survival is >70%.

Overlap

There is either diffuse or limited skin fibrosis and typical features of one or more of the connective tissue diseases such as rheumatoid arthritis, systemic lupus erythematosus, polymyositis, dermatomyositis, or Sjögren's syndrome.

Scleroderma sans Sclerodactyly

Some patients with scleroderma may have no detectable skin thickening and present with pulmonary fibrosis, or renal, cardiac, or gastrointestinal disease. Raynaud's phenomenon may be present.

Raynaud's Phenomenon

Raynaud's phenomenon, an episodic and reversible vasospasm precipitated by cold exposure or emotional stress, occurs in approximately 95% of scleroderma patients at some time during the disease. It is accompanied by color changes of pallor (white), acrocyanosis (blue), and reperfusion hyperemia (red). Typically, it affects the fingers, toes, nose, and ears but can also affect the heart, lungs, and kidneys. Ischemic necrosis may occur, leading to ulceration of the fingertips. Gangrene or superinfection may occur at these sites.

Skin

Early in the disease, patients may complain of puffy, edematous hands (edematous phase). This is replaced with thickening and tightening over subsequent weeks to months (indurative phase). Hypopigmentation and hyperpigmentation of the skin may occur. Over several years, the skin may revert to normal thickness or become thin (atrophic phase). Perioral involvement leads to thinning of the lips, puckering, and reduced oral aperture. In *early diffuse cutaneous scleroderma* (dcSSc), skin sclerosis progresses rapidly, peaking in the first 2 years. It is closely associated with progression of visceral disease and development of joint contractures. In lcSSc, skin thickening is minimal over several years and does not correlate with development of visceral disease. Calcinosis from intracutaneous or subcutaneous calcific deposition of hydroxyapatite is commonly present on the digital pads, and extensor surface of the forearms, elbows, and knees. Occasionally, it is more widespread. Telangiectasias, most typical of lcSSc, are usually present on the fingers, face, lips, and anterior chest. On nail-fold capillary microscopic examination, dilated loops of capillaries are seen in both diffuse and limited subsets of scleroderma. In dcSSc, a paucity of nail-fold vessels or "drop out" may be seen.

Musculoskeletal

Arthralgias and joint stiffness may affect the small and large joints of the body. Tendon friction rubs commonly palpated over the flexor or extensor tendons due to fibrinous tenosynovitis and tendinitis are specific for dcSSc. They are associated with increased skin thickness, renal involvement, and reduced survival. A small number of patients develop proximal muscle weakness that is associated with electromyographic and pathologic evidence of myositis.

Gastrointestinal Tract

Esophageal dysfunction eventually develops in approximately 80% of patients. The most fre-

quent symptoms are heartburn and substernal dysphagia. Conventional barium swallow shows hypomotility of the distal portions of the esophagus. Classic manometric findings consist of an incompetent lower esophageal sphincter and low amplitude contractions in the distal smooth muscle portion of the esophagus. Small bowel dysfunction has been reported in 20% to 60% of patients. Reduced peristalsis leads to stasis and intestinal dilatation, which favors bacterial overgrowth, causing fat malabsorption and eventually malnutrition. Pseudo-obstruction is a rare complication that presents with severe postprandial bloating and cramps. Hypomotility of the small intestine results in a functional ileus with symptoms simulating a mechanical obstruction. Impaired peristalsis of the colon may produce constipation, either alone or alternating with diarrhea. Patchy atrophy of the muscular wall leads to development of wide-mouthed diverticula on the antimesenteric border of the transverse and descending colon. The liver, biliary tract, and pancreas are rarely involved. Primary biliary cirrhosis (PBC), the liver disorder seen most frequently with limited cutaneous scleroderma, is strongly associated with the presence of the antimitochondrial antibody.

Lung

Pulmonary involvement occurs in over 70% of patients with systemic sclerosis (diffuse cutaneous scleroderma) and is the most common cause of disease-related mortality (Figure 130-2). Interstitial lung disease (ILD) and pulmonary vascular disease leading to pulmonary hypertension are the main clinical manifestations. The most common symptoms for interstitial lung disease are dyspnea on exertion and dry cough. Dry, bibasilar end inspiratory rales may be heard, and chest radiographs show reticular interstitial changes or fibrosis, most prominent in the lower lung fields. A restrictive ventilatory defect is commonly noted. High-resolution CT identifies a "ground-glass" appearance representing active alveolitis. Bronchoalveolar lavage (BAL) is used to determine active disease. Alveolitis is characterized by an overall increase in alveolar macrophages and granulocytes recovered by BAL, as well as an increased percentage of granulocytes (neutrophils >3% and/or eosinophils >2.2% of total cells). Interstitial alveolitis may

Figure 130-1

Progressive Systemic Sclerosis (Scleroderma)

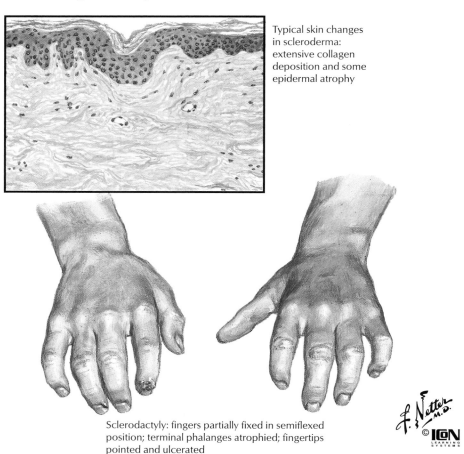

Typical skin changes in scleroderma: extensive collagen deposition and some epidermal atrophy

Sclerodactyly: fingers partially fixed in semiflexed position; terminal phalanges atrophied; fingertips pointed and ulcerated

progress to fibrosis with irreversible scarring, secondary pulmonary hypertension, and hypoxia. Individuals at highest risk for severe restrictive disease are black race, male gender, younger age patients with diffuse cutaneous disease and anti-topoisomerase I antibody. Pulmonary hypertension characterized by rapidly progressive dyspnea and accentuation of the pulmonic component of the second heart sound occurs in approximately 5% of patients with lcSSc, typically 10 to 30 years after onset of Raynaud's phenomenon. Occasionally, it is seen in patients who have anti-U3RNP antibody. The diffusing capacity is severely reduced, and ECG shows evidence of right heart dysfunction. Prognosis is poor; median survival of less than 2 years may be impacted by intravenous prostacyclin vasodilation.

Heart

Clinically symptomatic pericardial disease is infrequent (5% to 16%). The echocardiogram can detect small effusions in approximately 41% of asymptomatic patients with scleroderma. Large pericardial effusions (>200 mL) can lead to cardiac tamponade and is a marker for poor outcome with increased risk of subsequent renal crisis. Myocarditis is rare but has been documented in patients with systemic scleroderma and concomitant skeletal myositis with systolic and/or diastolic dysfunction occurring as a result of myocardial fibrosis. Approximately 37% of patients (both diffuse and limited cutaneous) have abnormalities on resting EKG. Supraventricular and ventricular arrhythmias are found more frequently in patients with diffuse cutaneous scle-

Figure 130-2

Progressive Systemic Sclerosis
(PSS; Scleroderma); Lung Involvement

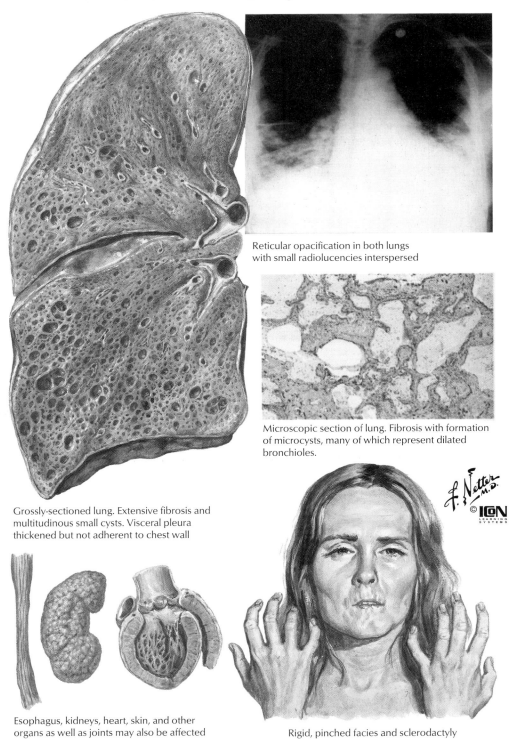

Reticular opacification in both lungs
with small radiolucencies interspersed

Microscopic section of lung. Fibrosis with formation
of microcysts, many of which represent dilated
bronchioles.

Grossly-sectioned lung. Extensive fibrosis and
multitudinous small cysts. Visceral pleura
thickened but not adherent to chest wall

Esophagus, kidneys, heart, skin, and other
organs as well as joints may also be affected

Rigid, pinched facies and sclerodactyly

roderma. Cardiac arrhythmias are strongly associated with mortality and are related to the severity of cardiopulmonary and renal involvement.

Kidney

Twenty-five percent of patients with dcSSc may develop renal crisis in contrast to only 1% of patients with lcSSc. Scleroderma renal crisis (SRC) is defined as the new onset of accelerated hypertension and rapidly progressive oliguric renal failure. These patients also have elevated plasma rennin activity and an active urinary sediment (microscopic hematuria, proteinuria). Microangiopathic hemolytic anemia and thrombocytopenia are prominent hematologic features. Some patients present with congestive heart failure, ventricular arrhythmias, or large pericardial effusions. Factors helpful in identifying patients with dcSSc at risk for developing SRC are rapid progression of skin thickening, disease duration less than 4 years, anti-RNA polymerase III antibody, antecedent high dose steroid use (>20 mg daily), and serum creatinine ≥3 mg/dL, or they are poor prognostic signs.

DIFFERENTIAL DIAGNOSIS

The differential diagnosis should exclude scleroderma-like disorders. These include localized scleroderma with fibrosis involving distinct areas, different levels of the skin, and sometimes the underlying soft tissue, muscle, or bone, more commonly occurring in women and in children. Subtypes include isolated or generalized morphea, linear scleroderma, nodular (keloid) scleroderma, and, rarely, localized bullous lesions. Diffuse scleroderma with eosinophilia (eosinophilic fasciitis) is associated with swelling, stiffness, and restricted range of motion, but usually spares the hands and face. A history of precipitating trauma may be obtained.

Other disorders may mimic systemic scleroderma (SSc). Sclerodactyly and fibrosis of the palmar fascia are seen in insulin-dependent diabetes mellitus, particularly juvenile-onset, a condition called *diabetic chiropathy*. Chronic graft-versus-host disease, particularly after bone marrow grafts, may produce many common clinical, biochemical, and histologic features of SSc. Environmental exposures (inhalation of epoxy resins, vinyl chloride, silica dusts, organic solvents and pesticides;

ingestion of toxic rape seed cooking oil; or injection of paraffin, or bleomycin) may produce features of SSc. Miscellaneous/rare conditions include Sézary syndrome, scleredema, carcinoid syndrome, Werner's syndrome, porphyria cutanea tarda, progeria, phenylketonuria, local lipodystrophies, and POEMS syndrome (Plasma cell dyscrasia, polyneuropathy, organomegaly, monoclonal spikes, and scleroderma-like skin changes).

DIAGNOSTIC APPROACH

The diagnosis of systemic scleroderma is approached systematically by evaluating the patient for evidence of autoantibody formation and the major target organs for evidence of early involvement. Features of other connective tissue disorders such as lupus or dermatomyositis should be elicited. Antinuclear antibodies are relatively specific for scleroderma. Autoantibodies associated with diffuse cutaneous scleroderma disease are anti-topoisomerase I (Scl 70) or anti–RNA polymerase I and III antibodies. Anti-centromere antibody is found in up to 90% of patients with limited cutaneous systemic scleroderma and 5% of those with diffuse cutaneous scleroderma. Additional assessment tests include radiographs of the hands (acral osteolysis and calcification), chest (bibasilar pulmonary fibrosis), and esophagus (barium swallow showing hypomotility). Pulmonary function testing demonstrating decreased diffusion capacity with a restrictive pattern and high resolution chest CT showing ground glass opacities are more sensitive indicators of early lung disease. A skin biopsy in an affected area that demonstrates a progressive increase in dermal collagen with loss of appendages can establish the diagnosis.

MANAGEMENT AND THERAPY

There is no proven therapy for scleroderma. The primary focus is preservation of end organ function to prolong survival, and to enhance quality of life.

Skin

In the early stages, pruritus may be treated with antihistamines, topical doxepin, 1% hydrocortisone cream, or PUVA therapy. Later, topical emollients help to lubricate sclerotic skin. A recent placebo-controlled study of therapeutic D-penicillamine versus low dose D-penicillamine failed to show a difference in skin score or mortality rate. Considering the toxic side effect profile, late onset of action, and lack of proven efficacy, enthusiasm for D-penicillamine treatment in scleroderma has diminished.

Raynaud's Phenomenon

The most effective method of preventing Raynaud's Phenomenon (RP) is avoidance of cold exposure. Patients should wear warm protective clothing and avoid tobacco use. Long-acting calcium channel blockers (nifedipine, amlodipine, felodipine) are safe and effective vasodilators. Other vasodilators such as nitrates and prazosin are used alone or in combination with calcium channel blockers. One coated aspirin (81 mg daily) is recommended to inhibit platelet activation and occlusion. Intravenous prostaglandins (epoprostenol, iloprost), which reduce the severity of RP and may prevent digital ulceration, are effective when given acutely for critical digital ischemia. Selective digital sympathectomy has been successful in cases that are not responsive to medical management. Oral antibiotics with good staphylococcal coverage are indicated if lesions become infected. Treat deeper soft tissue infections or osteomyelitis with intravenous antibiotics, debridement of devitalized tissue, and, if necessary, amputation.

Calcinosis

Colchicine (7- to 10-day course) can be used for suppression of local inflammation surrounding the calcinosis.

Gastrointestinal Disease

Esophageal dysfunction symptoms can be minimized with small, frequent meals, elevation of the head of the bed, and use of proton pump inhibitors. Patients with persistent symptoms should be evaluated with upper GI endoscopy for stricture or Barrett's metaplasia. Small bowel dysmotility symptoms can be managed with increasing dietary fiber, avoidance of drugs that affect motility (narcotics) and empiric antibiotic therapy for bacterial overgrowth. Octreotide has been used as a small bowel prokinetic agent with variable results. In refractory disease, parenteral hyperalimentation may be needed to improve nutrition.

Pulmonary Hypertension

Conventional therapies such as vasodilators, diuretics, and anticoagulation are recommended. Epoprostenol (prostacyclin) administered by continuous intravenous infusion has been demonstrated to improve the clinical and hemodynamic measurements in patients with scleroderma.

Interstitial Lung Disease

Patients with active alveolitis had improvement or stabilization in lung function when treated with oral or monthly intravenous cyclophosphamide for 12 to 18 months. The current practice is to repeat bronchoalveolar lavage 4 to 8 weeks later and, if alveolitis is still present, to repeat the cycle. Supplemental oxygen should be administered when there is resting or exertional hypoxia.

Renal Disease

Scleroderma renal crisis represents a medical emergency. A rapid-acting ACE inhibitor should be titrated to normalize blood pressure promptly. Some patients may not respond and progress to renal failure requiring dialysis. Patients requiring dialysis for 12 to 18 months for SRC may recover renal function with continued ACE inhibitor therapy.

Musculoskeletal Disease

NSAIDs may help associated arthralgias. A regular exercise program can improve joint range of motion. Active myositis is treated with methotrexate, azathioprine, or other immunosuppressive agents.

FUTURE DIRECTIONS

There are no proven effective therapies to treat systemic scleroderma. Recent trials of methotrexate and cyclosporin A have not shown convincing efficacy. A large multicenter trial of relaxin (an insulin-like protein secreted by the corpus luteum during pregnancy that decreases collagen synthesis by fibroblasts) did not demonstrate improvement in skin score. New therapies under investigation include an oral endothelin-1 inhibitor (bosentan), subcutaneous infusion of prostacyclin, and intravenous IFN-gamma infusion.

REFERENCES

American College of Rheumatology Web site. Available at: http://www.rheumatology.org. Accessed March 2, 2003.

Arthritis Foundation Web site. Available at: http://www.arthritis.org. Accessed March 2, 2003.

Koopman WJ, ed. *Arthritis and Allied Conditions: A Textbook of Rheumatology.* 14th ed. Philadelphia, Pa: Lippincott Williams & Wilkins; 2001.

National Institute of Arthritis and Musculoskeletal and Skin Diseases Web site. Available at: http://www.niams.nih.gov. Accessed March 2, 2003.

Poormoghim H, Lucas M, Fertig N, Medsger TA Jr. Systemic sclerosis sine scleroderma: demographic, clinical, and serologic features and survival in forty-eight patients. *Arthritis Rheum.* 2000;43:444–451.

Ruddy S, Harris ED Jr, Sledge CB, Sergent JS, Budd RC, eds. *Kelley's Textbook of Rheumatology.* 6th ed. Philadelphia, Pa: WB Saunders Co; 2001.

Sanchez-Guerrero J, Colditz GA, Karlson EW, Hunter DJ, Speizer FE, Liang MH. Silicone breast implants and the risk of connective-tissue diseases and symptoms. *N Engl J Med.* 1995;332:1666–1670.

Chapter 131

Spondylarthropathies

Beth L. Jonas and Robert A.S. Roubey

The spondyloarthropathies are a group of systemic inflammatory disorders with similar musculoskeletal findings, extra-articular manifestations, and immunogenetic associations. The major conditions and syndromes are *ankylosing spondylitis* (AS), *reactive arthritis* (formerly Reiter's syndrome), *enteropathic arthritis, psoriatic arthritis*, and *juvenile spondyloarthropathy*. While these diagnostic entities are useful and important, it may be more useful to regard the spondyloarthropathies not so much as a group of four or five distinct entities, but as arthropathies characterized by combinations including: *sacroiliitis*, with or without spondylitis; *peripheral inflammatory arthritis*, which is often asymmetrical and affects the lower limbs predominantly; *enthesopathy*, especially at the heels and around the pelvis; certain *extraarticular features*, including iritis, and some mucocutaneous lesions; *absence of rheumatoid factor*; and *familial aggregation* and *increased prevalence of human leukocyte antigen* (HLA)-B27.

ETIOLOGY AND PATHOGENESIS

Most of the spondyloarthropathies are associated with inheritance of the HLA-B27 histocompatibility antigen (Table 131-1). HLA-B27 is particularly associated with spondylitis, sacroiliitis, and eye involvement. Epidemiological data and transgenic animal models support the role of HLA-B27 in disease pathogenesis. There appears to be a close association of HLA-B27 diseases with intestinal bacteria and/or inflammation. Reactive arthritis is associated with Yersinia, Salmonella, Shigella, and Campylobacter gastrointestinal infections, as well as with Chlamydia genitourinary infection. Although intact organisms are not present in inflamed joints, bacterial antigens have been identified in affected synovium. In inflammatory bowel disease, increased intestinal permeability and exposure to normal intestinal flora may play a role in the development of enteropathic arthritis. Microscopic and usually asymptomatic gastrointestinal inflammation is present in patients with ankylosing spondylitis and venereally acquired reactive arthritis.

CLINICAL PRESENTATION

The musculoskeletal features that characterize the spondyloarthropathies as a group include inflammatory back pain, axial arthritis, and enthesopathies.

Inflammatory back pain and axial arthritis are characterized by an insidious onset, radiation of pain to the buttocks and thighs that sometimes

Table 131-1
HLA-B27 Frequency in Spondyloarthropathies

Disorder	HLA-B27 frequency
Ankylosing spondylitis	90%
With uveitis or aortitis	nearly 100%
Reactive arthritis	50%–80%
With sacroiliitis or uveitis	90%
Juvenile spondyloarthropathy	80%
Inflammatory bowel disease	Not increased
With peripheral arthritis	Not increased
With spondylitis	50%
Psoriasis	Not increased
With peripheral arthritis	Not increased
With spondylitis	50%
Unaffected whites	6%–8%

alternates from side to side, prominent stiffness, and relief with activity rather than rest. Initially, pain is worse in the low back, but later may involve the thoracic and cervical areas, sometimes with pain around the thoracic cage. In established disease, there may be loss of normal lumbar lordosis, restriction of lumbar movements in all directions, restriction of chest expansion, and sacroiliac joint and sternal tenderness.

Enthesopathy is inflammation at the site of ligamentous attachments to bone (the enthesis). In spondyloarthropathy, enthesopathy commonly causes plantar fasciitis, Achilles tendinitis, and pain at other sites including the attachment of the thigh adductors at the pelvis, intercostal muscle insertions, ischial tuberosities, and pelvic brim.

Clinical Features of Individual Syndromes
Ankylosing Spondylitis

Ankylosing spondylitis usually presents with inflammatory back pain and stiffness in a young adult, although 20% present with peripheral joint involvement, and more than 50% have joints other than the spine affected at some stage. The disease is 3 times more common in males than females (Figures 131-1 and 131-2).

Enthesopathy is a common association as previously described.

Iritis (uveitis) occurs in 25% to 30% and may present with severe throbbing pain, usually unilateral, associated with lacrimation, photophobia, and blurring of vision (Figure 131-2).

Cardiac involvement occurs in 1% to 4% and includes aortic insufficiency, conduction defects, and pericarditis (Figure 131-2).

HLA-B27 is present in 90% of patients (nearly 100% of patients with uveitis or aortitis).

Reactive Arthritis

Nonseptic arthritis and often sacroiliitis develop after an acute infection with certain venereal or dysenteric organisms (Figure 131-3). The number of affected males is even greater than that in ankylosing spondylitis. HLA-B27 is positive in 60% to 80%. Onset is usually abrupt, with urethritis, conjunctivitis, and diarrhea, followed 1 to 3 weeks later by arthritis. Knees and ankles are usually affected but radiologic sacroiliitis occurs in approximately 20% to 40%, and 10% develop a condition indistinguishable from ankylosing spondylitis.

Mucocutaneous lesions, including keratoderma blenorrhagica and circinate balanitis, may occur. Conjunctivitis is common. Cardiac disease develops in 5% to 10%.

Psoriatic Arthritis

Some form of psoriatic arthropathy develops in approximately 5% of patients with psoriasis (Figure 131-4). There are several patterns of arthritis:

Mono- or oligoarticular disease is the most common (70% to 80%). The distribution is asymmetric, affecting a large joint, such as the knees, and/or a few scattered distal interphalangeal joints, proximal interphalangeal joints, and metacarpophalangeal joints. There may be diffuse swelling of one or more involved fingers and toes ("sausage digits").

Symmetrical polyarthritis may resemble rheumatoid arthritis. Arthritis mutilans, a particularly aggressive form of the disease with osteolysis of affected joints, occurs in approximately 5% of patients with psoriatic arthritis.

Spondyloarthropathy occurs in approximately 10% of patients. Sacroiliitis may be less symmetrical than that of ankylosing spondylitis, and unilateral spinal changes may be seen.

HLA-B27 is present in approximately 60% of patients with spondylitis. It is not associated with psoriasis or with peripheral psoriatic arthritis (Figure 131-4).

Enteropathic Arthritis

Both peripheral and axial involvement can occur in patients with inflammatory bowel disease (ulcerative colitis and Crohn's disease). Peripheral arthritis occurs in 10% to 20% of patients. Joint disease may precede the onset of bowel symptoms and the diagnosis of inflammatory bowel disease, particularly in Crohn's disease. Arthritis may be acute and migratory. Knees, ankles, and feet are most frequently affected.

Spondylitis and sacroiliitis occur in approximately 10% of patients with inflammatory bowel disease. They may resemble ankylosing spondylitis and are occasionally asymptomatic.

HLA-B27 is present in 50% of patients with axial disease and is not associated with inflammatory bowel disease alone or with peripheral arthritis.

Juvenile Spondyloarthropathy

A subgroup of patients with juvenile-onset arthritis presents with pauciarticular onset, often later than other forms. The age of onset is about 10 years, affecting boys more than girls. Hips, knees, and ankles are affected. Acute iritis is common, and HLA-B27 is usually positive.

Figure 131-1

Ankylosing Spondylitis

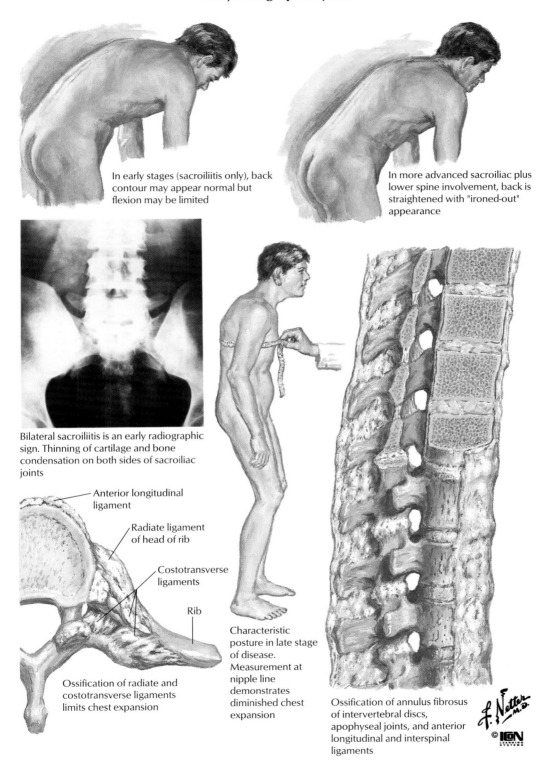

In early stages (sacroiliitis only), back contour may appear normal but flexion may be limited

In more advanced sacroiliac plus lower spine involvement, back is straightened with "ironed-out" appearance

Bilateral sacroiliitis is an early radiographic sign. Thinning of cartilage and bone condensation on both sides of sacroiliac joints

Anterior longitudinal ligament

Radiate ligament of head of rib

Costotransverse ligaments

Rib

Ossification of radiate and costotransverse ligaments limits chest expansion

Characteristic posture in late stage of disease. Measurement at nipple line demonstrates diminished chest expansion

Ossification of annulus fibrosus of intervertebral discs, apophyseal joints, and anterior longitudinal and interspinal ligaments

Figure 131-2   **Ankylosing Spondylitis**

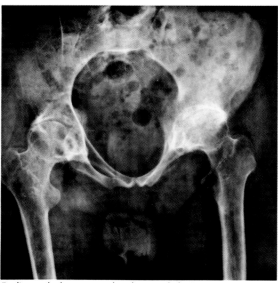

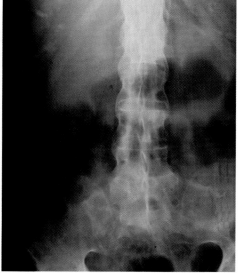

Radiograph shows complete bony ankylosis
of both sacroiliac joints in late stage of disease

"Bamboo spine." Bony ankylosis of joints
of lumbar spine. Ossification exaggerates
bulges of intervertebral discs

Complications

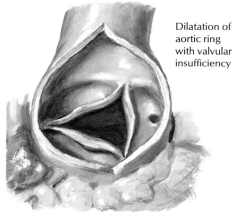

Dilatation of
aortic ring
with valvular
insufficiency

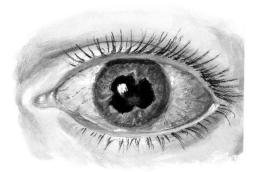

Iridocyclitis with irregular pupil due
to synechiae

Ankylosing spondylitis develops in approximately half of these patients in young adult life.

DIFFERENTIAL DIAGNOSIS
Spondylitis and Sacroiliitis

Mechanical low back pain may be difficult to differentiate. Features suggestive of inflammatory back pain and the spondyloarthropathies include an insidious onset, younger age, pain lasting longer than 3 months, and improvement with exercise.

Lumbosacral disk disease may have similar clinical characteristics, however, neurologic signs of nerve root compression are uncommon in the spondyloarthropathies.

Figure 131-3

Reactive Arthritis

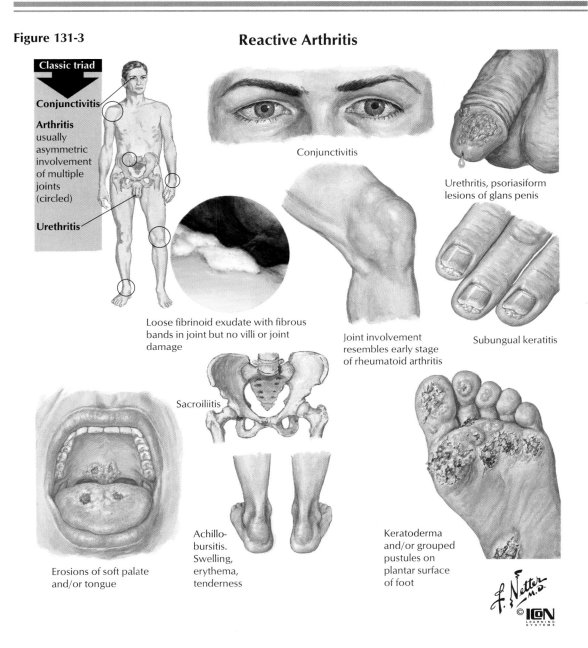

Classic triad

Conjunctivitis

Arthritis usually asymmetric involvement of multiple joints (circled)

Urethritis

Conjunctivitis

Urethritis, psoriasiform lesions of glans penis

Loose fibrinoid exudate with fibrous bands in joint but no villi or joint damage

Joint involvement resembles early stage of rheumatoid arthritis

Subungual keratitis

Sacroiliitis

Erosions of soft palate and/or tongue

Achillo-bursitis. Swelling, erythema, tenderness

Keratoderma and/or grouped pustules on plantar surface of foot

Osteoarthritis occurs in older patients and can usually be differentiated radiographically.

Diffuse idiopathic skeletal hyperostosis occurs in older patients and may involve all levels of the spine. This disease is characterized by large spurs and ossification along the anterolateral aspect of multiple contiguous vertebrae.

Peripheral Arthritis

Acute monoarthritis should be differentiated

from septic arthritis, gout, or pseudogout by synovial fluid examination. Psoriatic arthritis resembling rheumatoid arthritis may be differentiated by distal and asymmetric interphalangeal joint involvement, the absence of rheumatoid factor, and the presence of psoriatic skin and/or nail lesions.

Distinguishing between different types of spondyloarthropathy may be difficult, especially early in the course of the disease. For example, spondylitis preceding the development of inflam-

Figure 131-4

Psoriatic Arthritis

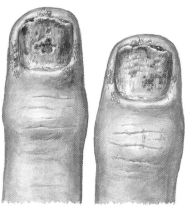

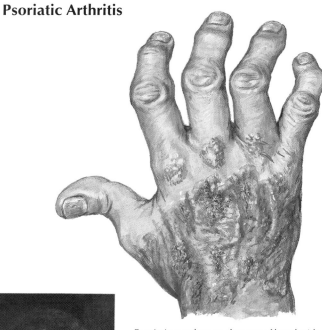

Pitting, discoloration, and erosion of fingernails with fusiform swelling of distal interphalangeal joints

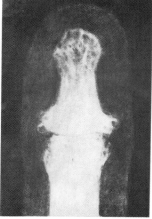

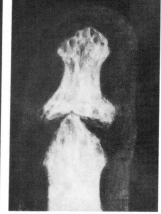

Psoriatic patches on dorsum of hand with swelling and distortion of many interphalangeal joints and shortening of fingers due to loss of bone mass

Radiographic changes in distal interphalangeal joint. Left: in early stages, bone erosions seen at joint margins. Right: in late stages, further loss of bone mass produces "pencil point in cup" appearance

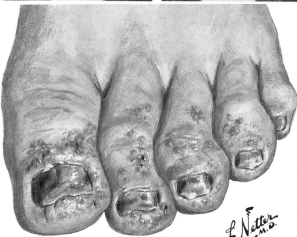

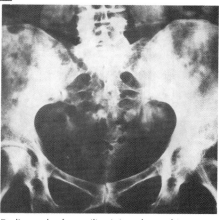

Toes with sausagelike swelling, skin lesions, and nail changes

Radiograph of sacroiliac joints shows thin cartilage with irregular surface and condensation of adjacent bone in sacrum and ilia

matory bowel disease may be indistinguishable from ankylosing spondylitis. Cutaneous lesions of reactive arthritis may be indistinguishable from pustular psoriasis. The presence of other extra-articular manifestations of reactive arthritis is helpful.

DIAGNOSTIC APPROACH

The diagnosis of the spondyloarthropathies is largely based on the history, physical examination, and radiography. Laboratory tests rarely make or refute the diagnosis.

The patient's history is helpful. Characteristic features include inflammatory back pain in younger patients, asymmetric peripheral arthritis, pain at one or more entheses, extraarticular features and/or precipitation of the arthritis by enteric or sexually acquired infection, and a positive family history.

In the physical examination, there may be no obvious physical signs of spondylitis in early or mild disease. Forward flexion can be measured by Schober's test in which the examiner marks 2 points on the patient's back, one at the lumbosacral junction (sacral dimples) and one 10 cm above. Forward flexion in normal individuals increases the distance between the 2 points by at least 5 cm. Any loss of lumbar lordosis should be noted. Costovertebral involvement is manifested by decreased chest expansion (< 5 cm chest expansion on inspiration, measured at the nipple line). Tenderness over the sacroiliac joints and other signs of sacroiliitis such as pelvic compression and Gaenslen's sign (pain on involved side hip hyperextension with the opposite hip in flexion) may be helpful, but are not uniformly reliable. Enthesitis at one or more sites (e.g., plantar fasciitis, Achilles tendinitis, epicondylitis) may be present. A thorough search for extra-articular manifestations should be done including examination of skin, nails, genital lesions, heart, and eyes.

Radiographic evidence of sacroiliitis or spondylitis with syndesmophytes may be present. Periostitis and new bone formation may be seen at sites of enthesitis and/or around affected joints. Radiographic features of psoriatic arthritis include asymmetrical erosions of interphalangeal joints, including the distal interphalangeal joints, and "pencil-in-cup" appearance of the distal interphalangeal joints (Figure 131-4). Synovial fluid analysis is nonspecific but useful in excluding infection

and crystal-induced arthritis. Tests for rheumatoid factor and antinuclear antibodies are characteristically negative. HLA-B27 testing is generally not necessary. In selected cases, it may be useful in decreasing the uncertainty of the diagnosis. The test does not help distinguish between ankylosing spondylitis and other spondyloarthropathies. In reactive arthritis, identification of persistent pathogens by urethral and stool culture or polymerase chain reaction (e.g., Chlamydia) is recommended.

MANAGEMENT AND THERAPY

It is important to identify the active elements in the disease (spondylitis, peripheral arthritis, enthesopathy) because their relative activity and severity affect both the treatment and prognosis. Management has two main arms: drugs to control pain, stiffness, and synovitis; and physical therapy to prevent range of motion limitation and maintain muscle power.

The diagnosis and prognosis should be discussed with the patient, stressing that the majority of these diseases are mild, that there is effective but noncurative treatment, and that the long-term prognosis is generally good.

NSAIDs are important in controlling symptoms of spondylitis and peripheral arthritis. Indomethacin (25 to 50 mg 3 to 4 times daily) is usually effective. The extended release capsule or a nighttime suppository may be given to counter early morning stiffness. Several agents may be tried to find the best tolerated drug.

Sulfasalazine is effective in treatment of the peripheral arthritis of spondyloarthropathy. Side effects include nausea, rash, reversible reduction in sperm count, and, rarely, agranulocytosis. Regular hematologic monitoring is required, at least in the early stages. Despite side effects, it is a useful drug (at a dose of 2 to 3 g daily in divided doses) if NSAIDs have failed. Some reports suggest benefit in spondylitis also.

Intra-articular corticosteroid injections are useful for selected peripheral joints. Systemic corticosteroids are not indicated.

Methotrexate is an effective treatment for the skin and joint manifestations of psoriasis. Typically, therapy is initiated with a single weekly oral dosage of 7.5 mg. The weekly dosage may be gradually increased in 2.5- or 5.0-mg increments to 30 mg per week. Methotrexate may also be useful in other forms of spondyloarthropathy (e.g., ankylosing spondylitis).

Antibiotics should be given to patients with proven Chlamydia urethritis. A number of studies also suggest that antibiotics may decrease the duration of disease in patients with Chlamydia-induced reactive arthritis. The use of antibiotics in post-dysenteric reactive arthritis is controversial.

Initial reports suggest that inhibition of tumor necrosis factor-α (TNF-α) may be useful in the spondyloarthropathies not responsive to other agents. Limited data indicate that infliximab was effective in several cases of in spondyloarthropathy associated with Crohn's disease, and in a small open-label trial involving patients with Crohn's disease, ankylosing spondylitis, psoriatic arthritis, and undifferentiated spondyloarthropathy. Etanercept was beneficial in a placebo-controlled study in patients with psoriatic arthritis.

In axial disease, the major aims of early therapy are to relieve pain and stiffness and to maintain normal posture and mobility. The inflamed painful spine may feel more comfortable in the flexed position, but fusion in this position can be functionally disastrous. Physical therapy aims to reduce rigidity and ensure that, if ankylosis does occur, the spine is in a nonflexed position. Regular supervision is usually required and participation in classes may be helpful. Various modalities, such as ultrasound, may be helpful in relieving pain due to enthesopathy.

Appropriate orthotic devices may be helpful (e.g., insoles for plantar fasciitis). Uveitis, cardiac, pulmonary, and severe cutaneous involvement should be assessed by appropriate specialists.

FUTURE DIRECTIONS

Ongoing investigations in the seronegative spondyloarthropathies include studies of the pathophysiology of the diseases, specifically with respect to the role of pathogenic bacteria, the immunogenetics of the diseases, and the role of the new biologic response modifiers in the treatment of severe spondyloarthropathies.

REFERENCES

Alvarez I, Lopez de Castro JA. HLA-B27 and immunogenetics of spondyloarthropathies. *Curr Opin Rheumatol.* 2000;12:248–253.

Calin A, Taurog JD, eds. *The Spondylarthritides.* Oxford, England: Oxford University Press; 1998.

McGonagle D, Khan MA, Marzo-Ortega H, O'Connor P, Gibbon W, Emery P. Enthesitis in spondyloarthropathy. *Current Opin Rheumatol.* 1999;11:244–250.

Patel S, Veale D, FitzGerald O, HcHugh NJ. Psoriatic arthritis—emerging concepts. *Rheumatology (Oxford).* 2001;40:243–246.

Rosenberg AM. Juvenile onset spondyloarthropathies. *Curr Opin Rheumatol.* 2000;12:425–429.

Chapter 132
Systemic Lupus Erythematosus

Mary Anne Dooley

Systemic lupus erythematosus (SLE) is a chronic inflammatory autoimmune disease involving multiple organ systems. It is characterized by the production of non-organ–specific autoantibodies, including antinuclear (ANA), anti-double–stranded DNA (anti-dsDNA), anti-phospholipid antibodies, and a marker autoantibody (anti-Sm). Significant health consequences include renal failure, vasculitis, arthritis, and neuropsychiatric complications including seizures and psychosis. The clinical course of SLE involves periods of flares and remissions, and therapy may include extensive use of corticosteroids and other immunosuppressants. The disease has a striking female predominance. Peak incidence occurs during reproductive years usually ages 15 to 40 with women affected up to 10 times more frequently than men. Among children and postmenopausal patients, the female-to-male ratio is 2:1 to 3:1. There is a genetic component; concordance in monozygotic twins is as high as 25%. African Americans have a 3-fold increased incidence of SLE, experience disease at younger ages, and have increased mortality when compared with whites. Mortality rates from SLE have been relatively stable among whites since the 1970s, but they have increased among African Americans. Hispanics and Asians have an increased prevalence of SLE and nephritis. Despite investigative attention, racial differences in lupus expression remain poorly understood.

SLE is one of several forms of lupus. Other forms include *chronic cutaneous lupus* (without systemic features), *drug-induced lupus* (a self-limited form of lupus that resolves when the offending drug is discontinued), *subacute cutaneous lupus*, and *neonatal lupus* (a transient rash or congenital heart block noted at delivery due to maternal anti-Rho antibody crossing the placenta).

ETIOLOGY AND PATHOGENESIS
The cause of SLE is unknown. The clinical syndrome of lupus is likely to result from the interaction of several differing susceptibility genes and potential environmental triggers including endogenous factors, such as sex hormone metabolism, stress, or diet; and exogenous triggers, such as silica or sunlight exposure, infections, or environmental toxins. Abnormalities in function include hyperactivity of B cells resulting in increased immunoglobulin production, recognition of self-antigens, and autoantibody formation with failure of normal tolerance. T cell defects include excessive T cell helper function and defects in cell-mediated immunity.

CLINICAL PRESENTATION
Musculoskeletal Disease
Musculoskeletal involvement is one of the earliest and most frequent manifestations of SLE. Arthralgia and tendinitis are more frequent than swelling from synovitis. Jaccoud's arthritis is a nonerosive but deforming arthropathy (due to ligamentous laxity) that may develop. Myositis is infrequent (<15%), and mild to moderate in severity. Myopathy may also develop due to therapy with corticosteroids or, rarely, antimalarials. Osteonecrosis (avascular necrosis), frequently affecting the femoral heads bilaterally, may develop in up to 5% to 10% of SLE patients. Raynaud's phenomenon, small vessel vasculitis, fat emboli, and anticardiolipin antibodies, while often related to the duration and peak of corticosteroid exposure, have also been implicated.

Cutaneous Disease
The mucocutaneous system is affected in 80% to 90% of patients. *Discoid lupus* is most common, affecting 15% to 30% of SLE patients. The specific LE skin findings are seen in the context of acute cutaneous LE (with malar erythema or a generalized bullous or photosensitive rash). The nonspecific features are protean and range from a florid cutaneous vasculitis (small vessel) to panniculitis or livedo reticularis.

Cardiopulmonary Disease

Pleuritis is most frequently encountered. A syndrome of progressive loss of lung volume (shrinking lung) due to diaphragmatic dysfunction is increasingly recognized. It is now apparent that the second part of the recognized bimodal curve of lupus mortality is due to accelerated arteriosclerotic disease. The ongoing inflammatory process appears to be an independent risk factor separate from comorbidities of hypertension, hypercholesterolemia, corticosteroid therapy, and diabetes. Lupus patients have also been shown to have elevated serum homocysteine levels as another risk factor (Figure 132-1).

Renal Disease

Renal involvement is highly variable in histologic presentation (Figure 132-2). Lupus nephritis can range from mild asymptomatic proteinuria to rapidly progressive glomerulonephritis associated with end-stage renal disease. Nephritis develops more often in affected African Americans. The progression of diffuse proliferative nephritis to end-stage renal disease occurs more quickly in African Americans compared to whites, even with comparable cytotoxic therapy, and is independent of age, duration of lupus, history of hypertension or control of hypertension, and activity or chronicity indices on renal biopsy. Early onset of renal disease from the time of presentation is a poor prognostic indicator. Other prognostic features of a poorer outcome are youth, male gender, persistent azotemia, and high activity and chronicity scores on renal biopsy. SLE is not a contraindication to renal transplantation because lupus patients do not differ from others in frequency of rejection or graft maintenance. The risk of recurrence of lupus nephritis in the transplant is less than 10%.

Neuropsychiatric Disease

Manifestations are protean and include acute and chronic neurologic disease. All levels of the central and peripheral nervous systems may be involved. Headaches, seizures (focal and diffuse), and various aberrations of the psyche (affective disorders, psychoses, and organic brain disease) are the most common problems. Secondary mechanisms, infection, uremia, and drugs (particularly corticosteroids), must be excluded.

Pregnancy

Fertility in uncomplicated SLE is normal. Lupus flares have not been found to be uniformly more frequent or severe during pregnancy; however, there is an increased frequency of midtrimester abortions (15%), increased prematurity (20%), and stillbirth (5%). Lupus activity at the time of conception is a predictor of pregnancy outcome. The neonatal lupus syndrome may be associated with rash, complete heart block, or transient thrombocytopenia. Heart block is irreversible. Mothers may have anti-Rho without a clearly definable connective tissue disorder. Contraception for lupus patients should take into account the increased risk of thrombosis seen with antiphospholipid antibodies. If present, estrogen-containing contraceptives should be avoided. The safety of oral contraceptives in young women with SLE is the focus of an ongoing trials sponsored by the National Institutes of Health.

DIFFERENTIAL DIAGNOSIS AND DIAGNOSTIC APPROACH

The criteria for classification of SLE, as revised in 1982 and in 1997 by the American College of Rheumatology, are shown in Table 132-1. These criteria allow comparison of patients across clinical studies and are not diagnostic clinical criteria. Patients may present with fewer than 4 features and clearly have SLE without other clinical or serologic features; patients with primary antiphospholipid antibody syndrome may meet 4 or more criteria and not have SLE.

Antinuclear antibodies are the most sensitive screening test because more than 95% of patients with lupus will have positive results when the test is performed using a substrate containing human nuclei such as HEP-2 cells. A positive test result for ANA is not specific for SLE; positive ANA results may occur in normal individuals with increased frequency with age so that 15% older than 65 have a positive ANA test result, usually at low titer. It is important to exclude other autoimmune diseases that may be confused with SLE, particularly those associated with a positive ANA test result such as rheumatoid arthritis; Sjögren's syndrome or scleroderma; isolated Raynaud's phenomenon; or organ-specific autoimmune diseases, including idiopathic thrombocytopenic purpura, autoimmune thyroid disease, and

Figure 132-1

Lupus Erythematosus of the Heart

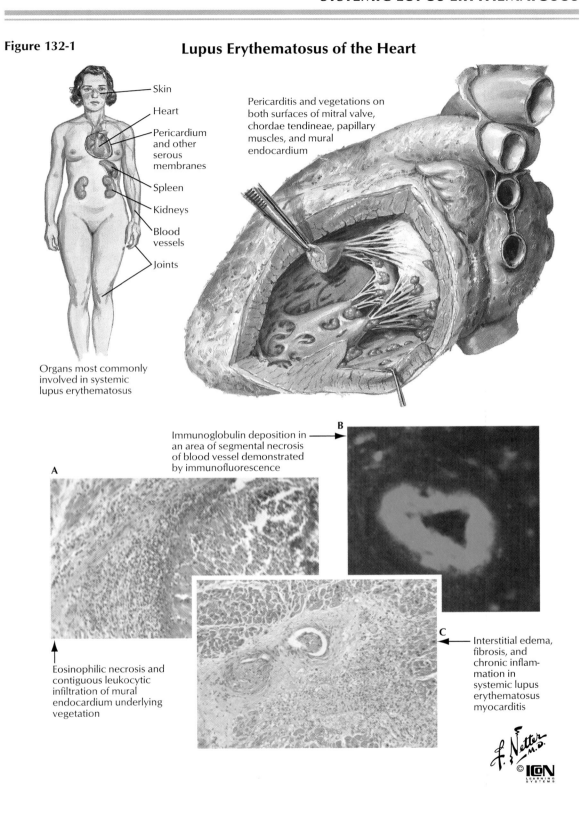

Skin

Heart

Pericardium and other serous membranes

Spleen

Kidneys

Blood vessels

Joints

Organs most commonly involved in systemic lupus erythematosus

Pericarditis and vegetations on both surfaces of mitral valve, chordae tendineae, papillary muscles, and mural endocardium

B

Immunoglobulin deposition in an area of segmental necrosis of blood vessel demonstrated by immunofluorescence

A

Eosinophilic necrosis and contiguous leukocytic infiltration of mural endocardium underlying vegetation

C

Interstitial edema, fibrosis, and chronic inflammation in systemic lupus erythematosus myocarditis

Table 132-1
The 1997 Revised American College of Rheumatology
Criteria for Systemic Lupus Erythemtosus

1. Malar rash	Fixed malar erythema, flat or raised
2. Discoid rash	Erythematous raised patches with keratotic scaling and follicular plugging; atrophic scarring may occur in older lesions
3. Photosensitivity	Skin rash as an unusual reaction to sunlight, by patient history or physician observation
4. Oral ulcers	Oral or nasopharyngeal ulcers, usually painless, observed by physician
5. Arthritis	Nonerosive arthritis involving two or more peripheral joints, characterized by tenderness, swelling, or effusion
6. Serositis	a. Pleuritis (convincing history of pleuritic pain or rub heard by physician or evidence of pleural effusion) OR b. Pericarditis (documented by ECG or rub or evidence of pericardial effusion)
7. Renal disorder	a. Persistent proteinuria >0.5 g/day or >3+ OR b. Cellular casts of any type
8. Neurologic disorder	a. Seizures (in the absence of other causes) b. Psychosis (in the absence of other causes)
9. Hematologic disorder	a. Hemolytic anemia b. Leukopenia (<4,000/mm^3 on 2 or more occasions) c. Lymphopenia (<1,500/mm^3 on 2 or more occasions) d. Thrombocytopenia (<100,000/mm^3 in the absence of offending drugs)
10. Immunologic disorder	a. Anti-dsDNA OR b. Anti-Sm OR c. Positive finding of anti-phospholipid antibodies based on 1) An abnormal serum level of IgG or IgM anti-cardiolipin antibodies, OR 2) A positive test result for lupus anticoagulant using a standard method, OR 3) A false-positive serologic test for syphilis known to be positive for 6 months and confirmed by Treponema pallidum immobilization or fluorescent treponemal antibody absorption test
11. Antinuclear antibody	An abnormal titer of ANA by immunofluorescence or an equivalent assay at any time and in the absence of drugs known to be associated with drug-induced lupus syndrome

With permission from Tan EM, Cohen AS, Fries JF, et al. The 1982 revised criteria for the classification of systemic lupus erythematosus (SLE). *Arthritis and Rheum.* 1982; 25:1271-7 and Updating the American College of Rheumatology revised criteria for the classification of systemic lupus erythematosus (letter). *Arthritis Rheum.* 1997; 40:1725. Reprinted with permission of Wiley-Liss, Inc., a subsidiary of John Wiley & Sons, Inc.

Figure 132-2

Renal Lesions
in Systemic Lupus Erythematosus (SLE)

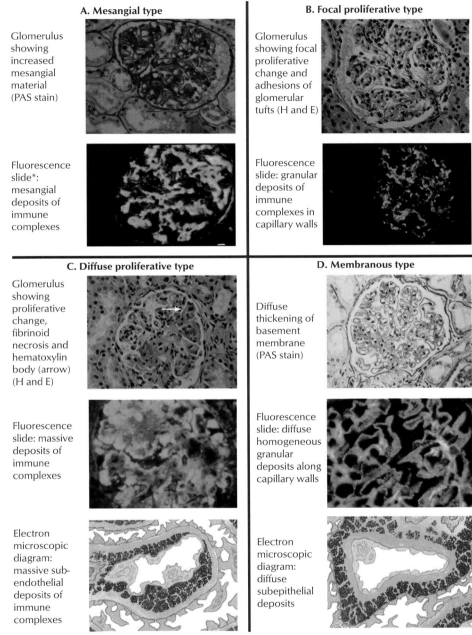

A. Mesangial type

Glomerulus showing increased mesangial material (PAS stain)

Fluorescence slide*: mesangial deposits of immune complexes

B. Focal proliferative type

Glomerulus showing focal proliferative change and adhesions of glomerular tufts (H and E)

Fluorescence slide: granular deposits of immune complexes in capillary walls

C. Diffuse proliferative type

Glomerulus showing proliferative change, fibrinoid necrosis and hematoxylin body (arrow) (H and E)

Fluorescence slide: massive deposits of immune complexes

Electron microscopic diagram: massive sub-endothelial deposits of immune complexes

D. Membranous type

Diffuse thickening of basement membrane (PAS stain)

Fluorescence slide: diffuse homogeneous granular deposits along capillary walls

Electron microscopic diagram: diffuse subepithelial deposits

* All fluorescence slides stained with fluorescein-labeled rabbit antihuman gamma globulin

hemolytic anemia. Family members of SLE patients will frequently have a positive ANA test result without clinical features of SLE. Many autoimmune diseases may have overlapping features, making strict classification difficult. The presence of antibodies to the Sm antigen, although found in only 30% of patients, is pathognomonic for a diagnosis of SLE.

Drug-induced lupus may be associated with a number of medications, most frequently procainamide or hydralazine. More recently, minocycline, alpha interferon, and tumor necrosis factor-α (TNF-α) blockers are also associated with ANA and anti-dsDNA antibody formation.

MANAGEMENT AND THERAPY

Lupus is a clinically heterogenous disorder with some patients experiencing troubling skin or joint complaints and others life-threatening renal or neurologic compromise. The focus of treatment is on individual clinical manifestations. It is essential to determine the activity and severity of the disease, (e.g., active or in remission) and potential involvement of vital organs to choose appropriate therapy. Evidence for an inflammatory process may prompt immunosuppressive therapy versus anticoagulation for thrombotic or embolic events. Patient education about the spectrum of disease and long-term outcomes is essential to recruit the patient as an active partner in recognizing clinical changes and important risks.

Patients should be instructed to avoid excessive ultraviolet light exposure, for example, with use of high level (30+) sunscreen or screening of fluorescent lighting sources. Lupus patients are at increased risk of infection even in the absence of corticosteroids; fevers should be fully assessed rather than attributed initially to SLE. Fatigue is common and can be severe. Excluding other causes such as thyroid disease, coexisting fibromyalgia, adrenal insufficiency following steroid tapering, or depression is important. Regular long-term follow-up should be provided, including urinalyses, because renal involvement can be asymptomatic until well established. Lupus patients have an increased risk of premature cardiovascular disease from their underlying inflammatory disease. Patients should be encouraged to pay rigorous attention to minimizing traditional risk factors. Lupus is associated with an increased risk of osteoporosis even without steroid therapy, and prevention or treatment of bone loss is important.

Pharmacologic Agents

Nonsteroidal antiinflammatory drugs (NSAIDs) are useful in controlling joint symptoms (arthralgia, arthritis), pleuritis, pericarditis, and headaches. The selective COX-2 inhibitors have not been studied specifically in SLE, but are likely to show the same decreased GI toxicity demonstrated in other patient populations. The side effects of COX-2 as well as nonselective cyclooxygenase inhibitors include adverse effects on kidney, liver, and CNS function that may mimic increased SLE activity.

Many of the clinical features of SLE respond to corticosteroids, which may be given orally, parenterally by intramuscular injection, intra-lesional injection for skin lesions, intra-articular injection for arthritis, or by pulse (intravenous) administration.

The long -term risks include increased susceptibility to infection, cataracts, hypertension, diabetes, and osteoporosis.

Antimalarial drugs may be helpful and include hydroxychloroquine or, more rarely, chloroquine or quinacrine. These agents are most useful when cutaneous, joint, pleural, or pericardial features are predominant. Regular ophthalmology examinations for monitoring possible toxicity are essential. The risk of ocular toxicity with hydroxychloroquine is low if the recommended doses are used. Benefits include lipid-lowering and possible anti-thrombotic effects.

Immunosuppressive drugs (e.g., azathioprine, cyclophosphamide, mycophenolate mofetil, and cyclosporin A) are used for severe disease and for their steroid-sparing effects. Their potential toxicities make close monitoring mandatory. Methotrexate has been increasingly used for severe arthritis or skin disease, again with appropriate monitoring. Close attention to contraception is required during therapy given the risk of teratogenicity.

Key points in the management of SLE include the following:

SLE is a disease of remissions and exacerbations. Patients who are in clinical remission should not receive therapy. Cyclophosphamide should not be used in non-life–threatening situations due to the severity of its side effects, which include gonadal ablation, alopecia, bladder hemorrhage, and malignancy. Plasma exchange (plasmapheresis) has not shown benefit in severe lupus nephritis, but has shown anecdotal responses in treating acute life-threatening situations (e.g., widespread vasculitis). In patients with concurrent thrombotic thrombocytopenic purpura, this therapy can be life-saving.

FUTURE DIRECTIONS

Previous investigators demonstrated an association between lower socioeconomic status measures and higher morbidity and mortality in SLE. This relationship is complex and a focus of long-term assessment in the Lumina cohort. Environmental risks for developing lupus have been addressed in the Carolina Lupus study, a case-controlled population-based study of lupus patients in the southeastern United States. Exposure to silica was a strong risk. Surprisingly, although lupus has a striking female predominance, women with SLE had less endogenous or exogenous estrogen exposures and breast-feeding was protective.

Several new agents are under investigation for SLE therapy. Mycophenolate mofetil is presently in a US trial sponsored by the FDA to compare response to this agent versus intermittent intravenous cyclophosphamide as initial therapy for proliferative glomerulonephritis. Monoclonal antibodies are directed to inhibit costimulatory pathways for T-cell-B-cell activation including anti-CD40 ligand and BLYS. Down-regulation of production of anti-dsDNA antibodies by an oral tolerogen (LPJ 394) has shown initial promise in delaying renal flare in patients with high-titer, high-affinity anti-dsDNA antibody levels. While a low number of patients have been treated with autologous hematopoietic stem cell transplantation, 7 SLE patients were disease-free at a median follow-up of 25 months. Durability of response remains unknown. Immunoablative high-dose cyclophosphamide without stem-cell transplant, thus decreasing the risk of graft-versus-host disease, is under study for therapy of severe refractory SLE.

REFERENCES

Alarcon GS, Roseman J, Bartolucci AA, et al. Systemic lupus erythematosus in three ethnic groups: II. Features predictive of disease activity early in its course. LUMINA Study Group. Lupus in minority populations, nature versus nurture. *Arthritis Rheum.* 1998;41:1173–1180.

American College of Rheumatology Web site. Available at: http://www.rheumatology.org. Accessed March 2, 2003.

Arthritis Foundation Web site. Available at: http://www.arthritis.org. Accessed March 2, 2003.

Buyon JP. Neonatal lupus syndromes. *Am J Reprod Immunol.* 1992;28:259–263.

Cooper GS, Dooley MA, Treadwell EL, St Clair EW, Gilkeson GS. Hormonal and reproductive risk factors for development of systemic lupus erythematosus: results of a population-based, case-control study. *Arthritis Rheum.* 2002;46: 1830–1839.

Hochberg MC. Updating the American College of Rheumatology revised criteria for the classification of lupus erythematosus. *Arthritis Rheum.* 1997;40:1725.

Koopman WJ, ed. *Arthritis and Allied Conditions: A Textbook of Rheumatology.* 14th ed. Philadelphia, Pa: Lippincott Williams & Wilkins; 2001.

Lockshin MD, Reinitz E, Druzin ML, Murrman M, Estes D. Lupus pregnancy. Case-control prospective study demonstrating absence of lupus exacerbation during or after pregnancy. *Am J Med.* 1984;77:893–898.

National Institute of Arthritis and Musculoskeletal and Skin Diseases Web site. Available at: http://www.niams.nih.gov. Accessed March 2, 2003.

Ruddy S, Harris ED Jr, Sledge CB, Sergent JS, Budd RC, eds. *Kelley's Textbook of Rheumatology.* 6th ed. Philadelphia, Pa: WB Saunders Co; 2001.

Tan EM, Cohen AS, Fries JF, et al. The 1982 revised criteria for the classification of systemic lupus erythematosus. *Arthritis Rheum.* 1982;25:1271–1277.

Chapter 133

Vasculitis

Raymond L. Kiser and Ronald J. Falk

The vasculitides are a heterogeneous group of disorders characterized by inflammation of blood vessel walls. The inciting events causing inflammation vary among disease groups and are largely unknown. In general, infectious and immunologic abnormalities are the predominant cause. Blood vessels of all sizes are involved, from the large vessels (aorta) to the tiniest of venules (post-capillary venules). Consequently, a myriad of clinical and pathologic presentations occurs. While specific diseases may have a predilection for certain organs (e.g., Kawasaki's disease), most vasculitides (especially the small vessel vasculitides) affect virtually any vascular bed. The clinical diagnosis involves careful clinical assessment, specific laboratory and radiographic tests, and tissue samples of targeted organs. In 1994, a consensus conference formulated a nomenclature that has gained international acceptance. (Table 133-1)

Causes of Vasculitis

Direct infection of vessels

Immunological injury
· Immune complex—mediated
· Direct antibody attack—mediated
· Anti-neutrophil cytoplasmic autoantibody associated and possibly anti-neutrophil cytoplasmic antibody—mediated
· Cell-mediated

Unknown

The most significant recent advance has been the discovery and clinical utilization of anti-neutrophil cytoplasmic antibodies (ANCA) and serological markers of small vessel vasculitis (SVV). These have been especially useful in the diagnosis of Wegener's granulomatosis, microscopic polyangiitis, and Churg-Strauss syndrome.

ETIOLOGY AND PATHOGENESIS

The unifying feature of all vasculitides is the activation of inflammatory mediators within vessel walls. Virtually all components of the effector arm of the immune system may be impugned. For instance, T cell–mediated inflammation has been implicated as a causative feature in giant cell arteritis and Takayasu's arteritis. Yet, the reason for T cell activation remains unknown. In *immune complex–mediated vasculitides*, circulating antibody-antigen complexes deposit within the vessel wall or form within the vessel wall itself (in situ immune complex formation). Direct antibody binding to antigens integral to vessel walls occurs in *Goodpasture's syndrome* due to anti-glomerular basement antibodies, and in *Kawasaki's disease* due to anti-endothelial antibodies. Regardless of how they are deposited within the vascular immune complex, complement, coagulation, and kinin systems act as phlogistic stimulants for neutrophils and monocytes. These cells then release toxic oxygen metabolites and enzymes that damage the vasculature.

Pauci-immune vasculitides are characterized by lack of immune complexes or direct antibody binding to the vessel wall. They are closely associated with ANCA; although the role of ANCA is not certain, evidence suggests that they are pathogenic agents (Figure 133-1).

This may occur by several mechanisms. In the presence of stimulatory cytokines, ANCA antigens are translocated to the surface of neutrophils and monocytes, allowing binding of ANCA to their target antigens. Alternatively, release of these antigens from leukocytes and endothelial cells may result in damage from immune-complex formation with ANCA or by the direct effect of leukocyte serine protein, causing endothelial cell death.

CLINICAL PRESENTATION

Most patients present with constitutional symptoms including fever, weight loss, and arthralgias.

Figure 133-1

Vasculitis

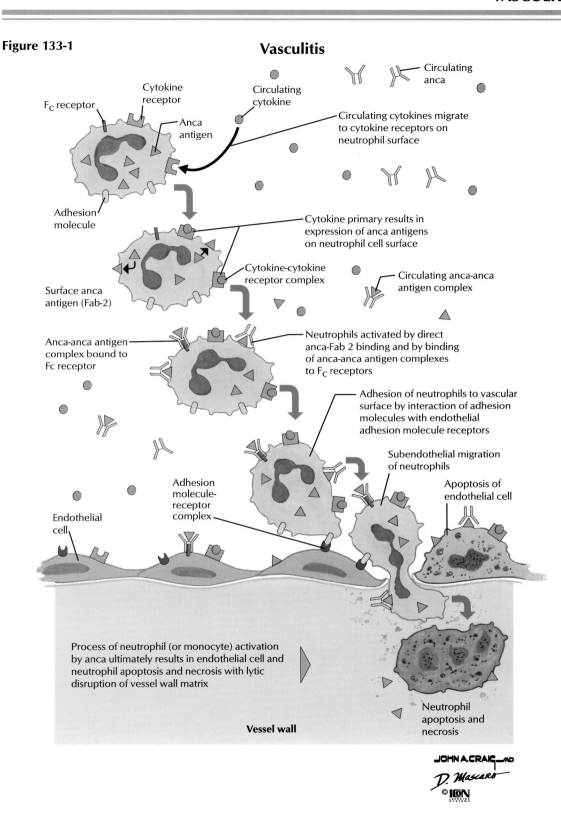

Circulating anca

F_C receptor

Cytokine receptor

Circulating cytokine

Anca antigen

Circulating cytokines migrate to cytokine receptors on neutrophil surface

Adhesion molecule

Cytokine primary results in expression of anca antigens on neutrophil cell surface

Surface anca antigen (Fab-2)

Cytokine-cytokine receptor complex

Circulating anca-anca antigen complex

Anca-anca antigen complex bound to Fc receptor

Neutrophils activated by direct anca-Fab 2 binding and by binding of anca-anca antigen complexes to F_C receptors

Adhesion of neutrophils to vascular surface by interaction of adhesion molecules with endothelial adhesion molecule receptors

Subendothelial migration of neutrophils

Apoptosis of endothelial cell

Adhesion molecule-receptor complex

Endothelial cell

Process of neutrophil (or monocyte) activation by anca ultimately results in endothelial cell and neutrophil apoptosis and necrosis with lytic disruption of vessel wall matrix

Neutrophil apoptosis and necrosis

Vessel wall

JOHN A. CRAIG—MD

D. Mascaro

© ICON

Table 133-1
Names and Definitions of Vasculitis Adopted by the Chapel Hill Consensus Conference on the Nomenclature of Systemic Vasculitis

Name	Large Vessel Vasculitis*
Giant cell (temporal arteritis)	Granulomatous arteritis of the aorta and its major branches, with a predilection for the extracranial branches of the carotid artery. Often involves the temporal artery. Usually occurs in patients older than 50 and often is associated with polymyalgia rheumatica.
Takayasu arteritis	Granulomatous inflammation of the aorta and its major branches. Usually occurs in patients younger than 50.
	*Medium-Sized Vessel Vasculitis**
Polyarteritis nodosa (classic polyarteritis nodosa)	Necrotizing inflammation of medium-sized or small arteries without glomerulonephritis or vasculitis in arterioles, capillaries or venules. Kawasaki disease arteritis involving large, medium-sized, and small arteries and associated with mucocutaneous lymph node syndrome. Coronary arteries are often involved. Aorta and veins may be involved. Usually occurs in children.
	*Small Vessel Vasculitis**
Wegener's granulomatosis[†,††]	Granulomatous inflammation involving the respiratory tract and necrotizing vasculitis affecting small to medium-sized vessels, e.g., capillaries, venules, arterioles, and arteries. Necrotizing glomerulonephritis is common.
Churg-Strauss syndrome[†,††]	Eosinophil-rich and granulomatous inflammation involving the respiratory tract and necrotizing vasculitis affecting small to medium-sized vessels and associated with asthma and blood eosinophilia.
Microscopic polyangiitis (microscopic polyarteritis)[†,††]	Necrotizing vasculitis with few or no immune deposits affecting small vessels, i.e., capillaries, venules, or arterioles. Necrotizing arteritis involving small and medium-sized arteries may be present. Necrotizing glomerulonephritis is very common. Pulmonary capillaritis often occurs.
Henoch-Schönlein purpura[††]	Vasculitis with IgA-dominant immune deposits affecting small vessels, i.e., capillaries, venules, or arterioles. Typically involves the skin, gut, and glomeruli and is associated with arthralgias or arthritis.
Essential cryoglobulinemic vasculitis[††]	Vasculitis with cryoglobulin immune deposits affecting small vessels, i.e., capillaries, venules, or arterioles, and associated with cryoglobulins in serum. Skin and glomeruli are often involved.
Cutaneous leukocytoclastic angiitis	Isolated cutaneous leukocytoclastic angiitis without systemic vasculitis or glomerulonephritis.

* Large artery refers to the aorta and the largest branches directed toward major body regions (e.g., to the extremities and the head and neck); medium-sized artery refers to the main visceral arteries (e.g., renal, hepatic, coronary, and mesenteric arteries); and small artery refers to the distal arterial radicals that connect with arterioles (e.g., renal arcuate and interlobular arteries). Note that some small and large vessel vasculitides may involve medium-sized arteries; but large and medium-sized vessel vasculitides do not involve vessels smaller than arteries.
† Strongly associated with anti-neutrophil cytoplasmic autoantibodies (ANCA).
†† May be accompanied by glomerulonephritis and can manifest as nephritis or pulmonary-renal vasculitic syndrome.
Adapted from Jennette JC, Falk RJ, Andrassy K, et al. Nomenclature of systemic vaculitides. Proposal of an international consensus conference. *Arthritis Rheum.* 1994;37:187-192 with permission of Wiley-Liss, Inc., a subsidiary of John Wiley & Sons, Inc.

Organ-specific manifestations can occur concurrently, but may lag for weeks. The clinical features are markedly variable and depend on the type of vasculitis, the size of involved vessels, and the organs affected.

The *large vessel vasculitides* are typically manifest by ischemia of the involved tissues. The most common symptom seen with Takayasu's arteritis is claudication, particularly in the upper extremities, with absent or asymmetric pulses and bruits. Renovascular hypertension develops in 40% of patients. Important epidemiologic features include the predominance of Takayasu's arteritis in women and in those younger than 50. Giant cell arteritis is usually seen in patients older than 50 who have headache, jaw claudication, swollen and tender temporal arteries, and vision loss. Approximately half of patients with giant cell arteritis have polymyalgia rheumatica.

Medium vessel vasculitides often manifest with infarctions of affected organs. Polyarteritis nodosa causes ischemia involving the vasa nervosum resulting in mononeuritis multiplex. Aneurysms and infarctions of the renal circulation result in renal insufficiency and hypertension, while disease in other vascular beds, such as the mesentery, results in symptoms of bowel ischemia (Figure 133-2).

Many cases of polyarteritis nodosa are associated with hepatitis B. *Kawasaki disease*, occurring almost exclusively in children, is characterized by involvement of the axillary, iliac, and coronary vessels. It is accompanied by the mucocutaneous lymph node syndrome with cardinal features including fever, conjunctivitis, adenopathy, mucosal lesions, and desquamatory rash.

Small vessel vasculitis is most common and can be classified as immune complex etiologies (e.g., systemic lupus erythematosus, Henoch-Schönlein purpura) and as pauci-immune disorders. The *pauci-immune disorders* are a consequence of the paucity or lack of immune complex deposition viewed by indirect immunofluorescence microscopy of affected tissues. These diseases are typically associated with ANCA and include Wegener's granulomatosis, Churg-Strauss syndrome, and microscopic polyangiitis. Patients present with inflammation of single or multiple organs. For example, many patients present with skin disease due to *leukocytoclastic vasculitis*. The cutaneous manifestations of dermal vasculitis are numerous and include purpura, livido reticularis, nodules, ulcers, and hives. Similarly, many patients present with kidney disease due to glomerulonephritis. Glomeruli are small capillaries that are inflamed by many types of SVV. Glomerular inflammation results in hematuria, proteinuria, hypertension, and rapidly progressive renal insufficiency.

The most common cause of the renal-dermal vasculitic syndrome is the ANCA-SVV, especially microscopic polyangiitis. A common systemic vasculitis that causes a renal-dermal vasculitic syndrome is *Henoch-Schönlein purpura*, most commonly seen in children after a respiratory tract infection. It is characterized by cramping abdominal pain, purpura, and arthralgias (Figure 133-3). Cryoglobulinemia, another cause of renal dermal vasculitic syndrome, has been attributed recently to hepatitis C found in the cryoprecipitate.

Glomerulonephritis and pulmonary disease is found in Goodpasture's syndrome (Figure 133-4), Wegener's granulomatosis, Churg-Strauss syndrome, and microscopic polyangiitis. Respiratory symptoms range from fleeting pulmonary infiltrates to gross hemoptysis. Pulmonary involvement in Wegener's granulomatosis results in nodules and cavities. Churg-Strauss syndrome is also characterized by pulmonary symptoms, but only rarely has renal involvement. Asthma is one of the disease-defining findings, and allergic rhinitis is common. Many patients with small vessel vasculitis, especially Wegener's granulomatosis, have upper respiratory symptoms, including sinus pain, epistaxis, and occasional stridor from tracheal involvement.

Signs and Symptoms of Necrotizing Small Vessel Vasculitis

- Cutaneous purpura, nodules, and ulcerations
- Peripheral neuropathy (mononeuritis multiplex)
- Abdominal pain and blood in stool
- Hematuria, proteinuria, and renal insufficiency
- Hemoptysis and pulmonary infiltrates or nodules
- Necrotizing (hemorrhagic) sinusitis
- Myalgias and arthralgias
- Muscle and pancreatic enzymes in blood
- Iritis and uveitis

DISORDERS OF THE IMMUNE SYSTEM, CONNECTIVE TISSUE, AND JOINTS

Figure 133-2 Renal Involvement in Classical Form of Polyarteritis Nodosa

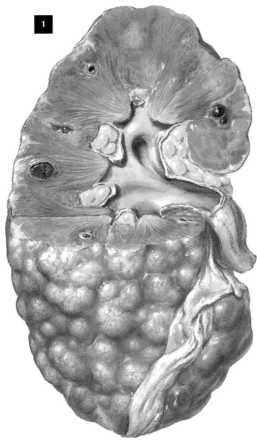

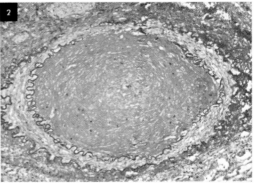

Almost complete obliteration of lumen of arcuate renal artery by intimal fibrosis; fragmentation of internal elastic membrane and medial fibrosis (elastic Van Gieson stain, X 100)

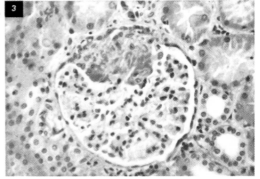

Focal glomerular lesion: Segment of glomerular tuft destroyed by necrotic process with much fibrin and some cellular reaction; patient died from intestinal perforation (H. & E. stain, X 200)

Coarsely nodular, irregularly scarred kidney: Cut section reveals organizing infarcts and thrombosed aneurysms in corticomedullary region

DIFFERENTIAL DIAGNOSIS

The systemic inflammatory nature of the vasculitic process may represent a diagnostic dilemma. Diseases in the differential diagnosis include systemic infections such as endocarditis, bacteremia with sepsis, and other connective tissue forms of vascular illness including lupus and malignancies.

Many of the features in the vasculitides are nonspecific. Purpura, considered a classic sign, may be seen in meningococcemia, viral illnesses, and thrombocytopenic disorders. Pulmonary abnormalities can be difficult to differentiate from respiratory infections. Glomerulonephritis can be seen with primary renal diseases such as membranoproliferative glomerulonephritis and IgA nephropathy. Mononeuritis multiplex is one of the more specific findings in vasculitis, and only rarely can be mimicked by asymmetric presentations of other neuropathies such as diabetic neuropathy.

DIAGNOSTIC APPROACH

A clinical history and examination remain the most helpful diagnostic tools. The physician must ascertain which organ system is affected. The major advance in diagnostic testing is a serological

Figure 133-3

Nephropathy in Anaphylactoid Purpura
(Henoch-Schönlein Disease)

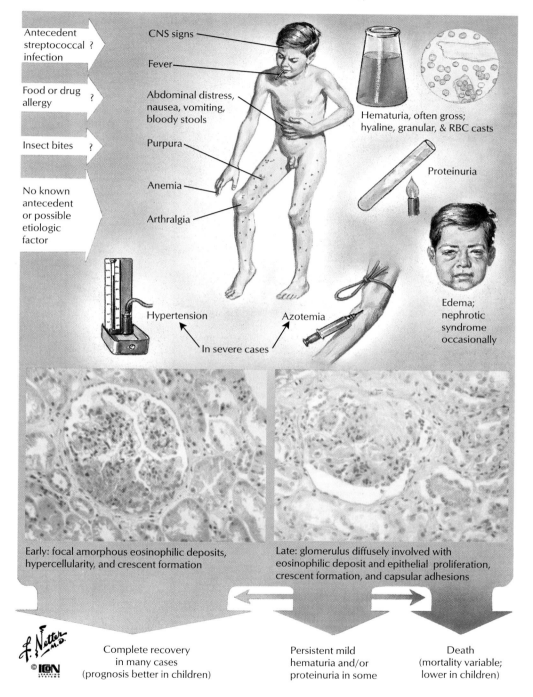

Antecedent streptococcal ? infection

Food or drug allergy ?

Insect bites ?

No known antecedent or possible etiologic factor

CNS signs

Fever

Abdominal distress, nausea, vomiting, bloody stools

Purpura

Anemia

Arthralgia

Hematuria, often gross; hyaline, granular, & RBC casts

Proteinuria

Hypertension

Azotemia

In severe cases

Edema; nephrotic syndrome occasionally

Early: focal amorphous eosinophilic deposits, hypercellularity, and crescent formation

Late: glomerulus diffusely involved with eosinophilic deposit and epithelial proliferation, crescent formation, and capsular adhesions

Complete recovery in many cases (prognosis better in children)

Persistent mild hematuria and/or proteinuria in some

Death (mortality variable; lower in children)

Figure 133-4

Lung Purpura with Nephritis
(Goodpasture's Syndrome)

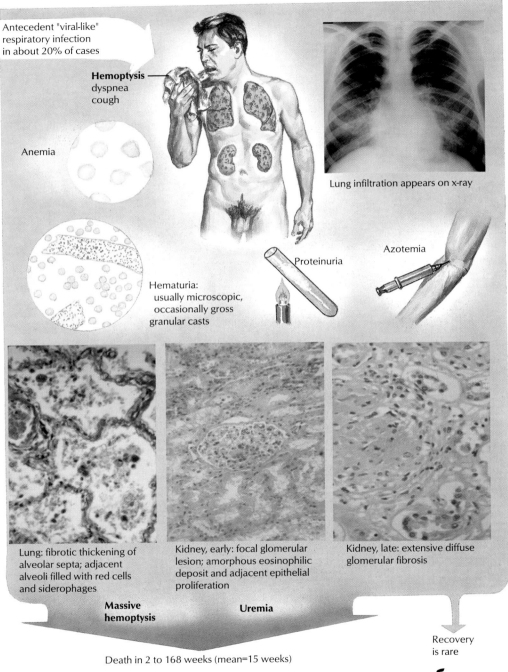

Antecedent "viral-like" respiratory infection in about 20% of cases

Hemoptysis dyspnea cough

Anemia

Lung infiltration appears on x-ray

Azotemia

Proteinuria

Hematuria: usually microscopic, occasionally gross granular casts

Lung: fibrotic thickening of alveolar septa; adjacent alveoli filled with red cells and siderophages

Kidney, early: focal glomerular lesion; amorphous eosinophilic deposit and adjacent epithelial proliferation

Kidney, late: extensive diffuse glomerular fibrosis

Massive hemoptysis

Uremia

Recovery is rare

Death in 2 to 168 weeks (mean=15 weeks)

marker, anti-neutrophil cytoplasmic autoantibodies that can react to normal constituents of neutrophils and monocytes. Cytoplasmic ANCA, or C-ANCA, react with the serine protease known as proteinase 3, while perinuclear ANCA, or P-ANCA, react with myeloperoxidase (MPO-ANCA). Other serologic tests that may be useful include those for hepatitis B and C, antinuclear antibody (ANA), anti-glomerular basement membrane (GBM) antibodies, cryoglobulins, and evaluation of complement components C3 and C4. A urinalysis looking for hematuria remains a crucial part of the assessment.

Radiographic studies also have a valuable role in the diagnosis of vasculitides. Chest radiographs may demonstrate infiltrates or hemorrhage. CT scans are often needed for better resolution of nodules and cavities. For large- and medium-vessel vasculitides, angiography may be useful, although magnetic resonance angiography may allow a noninvasive diagnosis. Demonstration of aneurysms is critical in confirming the diagnosis of polyarteritis nodosa when no specific evidence of small vessel vasculitis can be found.

Biopsy of the affected organs is one of the most important tests. Biopsy specimens of purpuric skin lesions typically demonstrate leukocytoclastic vasculitis. Although this confirms the presence of vasculitis, it does not differentiate between diseases. Biopsy of the lungs or kidneys can be very helpful, especially if immunohistology is performed. Immune-mediated vasculitides will demonstrate granular deposits of immunoglobulin, such as in IgA or Henoch-Schönlein purpura, or linear staining such as in Goodpasture's syndrome. ANCA-associated diseases generally demonstrate vascular necrosis without the presence of immune complexes.

MANAGEMENT AND THERAPY

Treatment must be designed for each patient based on the severity of disease and the specific diagnosis. The natural history of each vasculitis varies considerably. For instance, some vasculitides are mild in nature and never cause any major end organ damage. In contrast, patients with ANCA-SVV require glucocorticoid and cytotoxic therapy to prevent morbidity or mortality.

Takayasu's and giant cell arteritis generally respond to high-dose corticosteroids. Prednisone, at 1 mg/kg daily, is used for the acute phase and then tapered over several months. Some patients may require maintenance low-dose prednisone. Steroid-resistant disease may be treated with methotrexate.

Henoch-Schönlein purpura usually requires only supportive care. NSAIDs may be used for associated arthralgias, and steroids for severe abdominal pain and glomerulonephritis. Unlike most vasculitides, Kawasaki disease is not treated with steroids due to worsening of coronary artery disease. The standard treatment for Kawasaki's disease is high-dose aspirin and pooled intravenous gamma globulin.

ANCA-associated vasculitis is treated with high-dose steroids and a cytotoxic agent such as cyclophosphamide. Induction therapy involves pulse IV methylprednisolone 7 mg/kg (maximum 500 mg) IV every day for 3 days. In the case of pulmonary bleeding, plasmapheresis should be included as induction therapy. Prednisone is then given orally at 1 mg/kg daily for the first month, and then tapered to alternate-day therapy by the end of the second month. If remission is maintained, glucocorticoids are gradually removed over the next 2 to 3 months. Cyclophosphamide is given IV once a month, beginning at 0.5 g/m² body surface area (BSA). The dose is increased to 1 g/m² BSA based on nadir white blood cell counts. These are drawn 2 weeks after each dose, with a goal of 3,000 to 5,000. An alternative is oral cyclophosphamide used at 2 mg/kg per day, although this regimen exposes the patient to a higher cumulative dose and may have increased side effects.

Goodpasture's syndrome is treated similarly to the ANCA-associated vasculitides. However, plasmapheresis is used as induction therapy. If cryoglobulinemia is caused by hepatitis C, treatment for cryoglobulinemic vasculitis should consist of alpha-interferon and ribavirin. High-dose corticosteroids, cytotoxic agents, and plasmapheresis have been used for severe disease. Treatment of vasculitides associated with other systemic diseases should generally be directed at the underlying disease. A host of other treatments are being tried (for example, methotrexate, mycophenolate mofetil, soluble tumor necrosis factor (TNF) receptor blockers), although none of these treatments has become the standard of care.

Figure 133-5

Distribution of Specific Vasculitis Syndromes

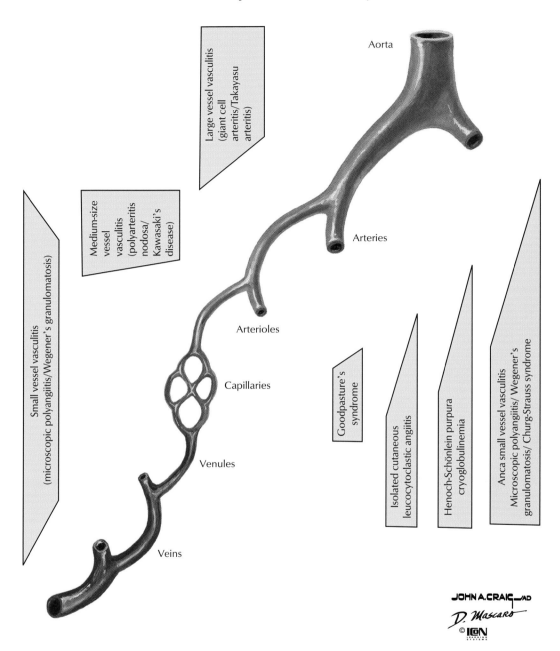

Aorta

Arteries

Arterioles

Capillaries

Venules

Veins

Large vessel vasculitis (giant cell arteritis/Takayasu arteritis)

Medium-size vessel vasculitis (polyarteritis nodosa/ Kawasaki's disease)

Small vessel vasculitis (microscopic polyangiitis/Wegener's granulomatosis)

Goodpasture's syndrome

Isolated cutaneous leucocytoclastic angiitis

Henoch-Schönlein purpura cryoglobulinemia

Anca small vessel vasculitis Microscopic polyangiitis/ Wegener's granulomatosis/ Churg-Strauss syndrome

JOHN A. CRAIG—AD

D. Mascaro

©ICN

FUTURE DIRECTIONS

Ideally, research should be aimed at prevention of vascular inflammation to avoid any end organ damage. Detecting populations at risk using genetic markers may allow for close scrutiny of specific individuals. Until appropriate detection tools are avail-able, early diagnosis of disease before end-organ damage occurs should be the overriding goal. This requires education of patients and physician to consider the spectrum of vasculitis and order the appropriate laboratory tests (Figure 133-5). Once the diagnosis is made, early treatment with drugs that specifically target pathogenetic forces without suppressing the entire immune system should be the goal.

REFERENCES

Guillevin L, Lhote F, Cohen P, et al. Polyarteritis nodosa related to hepatitis B virus. A prospective study with long-term observation of 41 patients. *Medicine (Baltimore)*. 1995;74:238–253.

Jennette JC, Falk RJ. Small-cell vasculitis. *N Engl J Med*. 1997;337:1512–1523.

Jennette JC, Falk RJ, Andrassy K, et al. Nomenclature of systemic vaculitides. Proposal of an international consensus conference. *Arthritis Rheum*. 1994;37:187–192.

Myklebust G, Gran JT. A prospective study of 287 patients with polymyalgia rheumatica and temporal arteritis: clinical and laboratory manifestations at onset of disease and at the time of diagnosis. *Br J Rheumatol*. 1996;35:1161–1168.

Saulsbury FT. Henoch-Schonlein purpura in children. Report of 100 patients and review of the literature. *Medicine (Baltimore)*. 1999;78:395–409.

Section XVI
OCULAR DISEASES

Chapter 134
Diabetic Retinopathy

Travis A. Meredith

Diabetic retinopathy, the most significant cause of visual loss in working-age adults in the United States, develops in nearly all persons with a duration of diabetes of 20 years or more. This is a startling statistic because as many as 16 million patients in the United States are affected with diabetes mellitus. Diabetic retinopathy becomes more common with increased duration of the disease. The Early Treatment Diabetic Retinopathy Study (ETDRS) developed a classification scheme which recognizes a number of discrete stages that culminate in visual loss. The earliest stages, *non-proliferative retinopathy*, are subdivided into mild, moderate, moderately severe, and severe. *Proliferative retinopathy*, a later stage, occurs when abnormal blood vessels grow on the surface of the retina or the optic nerve. It is differentiated into early and high-risk phases.

ETIOLOGY AND PATHOGENESIS

The precise sequence of events in diabetic retinopathy is complex and, despite multiple studies, is not entirely understood. Hyperglycemia is the major force in the development of the many abnormalities that ultimately result in visual loss in untreated patients. With increased blood glucose, hemoglobin A1C, growth hormone, and intracellular sorbitol levels increase. Capillary basement membranes develop thickening, and there is a selective loss of the mural cells (pericytes). Endothelial cells proliferate in some capillaries, while others become acellular. With disease progression, some areas deteriorate to a non-perfused capillary bed consisting of acellular strands of thickened basement membrane. Microaneurysms, small, round, red dots in the retina created by outpouchings of the capillary wall, develop in other areas of the retina. Eventually, microaneurysms become hypercellular, obliterated, and sometimes thrombosed.

Blood flow within the retina changes as the disease progresses. Retinal blood vessels are not directly regulated by the autonomic nervous system but are governed by an autoregulation process that is lost as the disease progresses. Systemic hypertension is associated with an increased risk of diabetic retinopathy incidence, progression, and visual loss and often further damages the retinal vascular system.

As focal hypoxia occurs, two significant concomitant processes begin to involve the retina.

Vascular endothelial growth factor (VEGF) contributes to a breakdown of the blood retinal barrier in early diabetic retinopathy; VEGF kinase inhibitors have been shown to decrease this VEGF-induced blood retinal barrier breakdown. Increased permeability of the vascular capillaries leads to *macular edema*. When this edema involves the central macular area, mild-to-moderate visual loss begins to occur.

The second major process is the development of abnormal new blood vessels called *proliferative diabetic retinopathy* or neovascularization. These new vessels are most often seen on the optic nerve and on the retinal surface, but in extreme cases, may grow on the iris, producing neovascular glaucoma in eyes with marked retinal ischemia. VEGF has been shown to be sufficient for the development of retinal neovascularization, and induced expression of VEGF in the retina results in neovascularization. When VEGF kinase inhibitors are administered in an experimental setting, retinal neovascularization is blocked.

CLINICAL PRESENTATION

Microaneurysms are the earliest manifestation of diabetic retinopathy (Figure 134-1). Injection of a fluorescent dye into the antecubital veins allows photographs of the inner eye to light up these areas of microaneurysms and demonstrate that more are present than can be seen through simple fundus ophthalmoscopic examination. Small intraretinal hemorrhages, dot and blot hemorrhages, are the

Figure 134-1

Diabetic Retinopathy

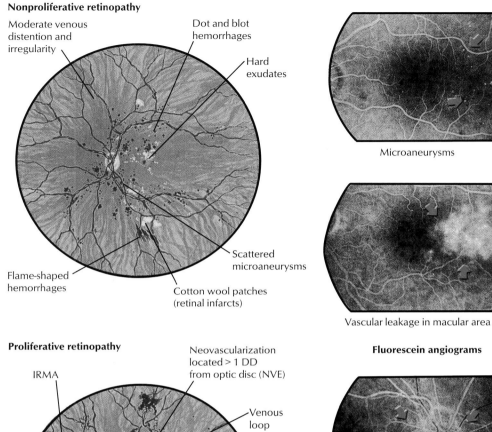

Nonproliferative retinopathy

Moderate venous distention and irregularity

Dot and blot hemorrhages

Hard exudates

Scattered microaneurysms

Flame-shaped hemorrhages

Cotton wool patches (retinal infarcts)

Microaneurysms

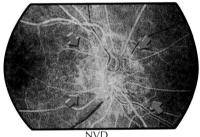

Vascular leakage in macular area

Proliferative retinopathy

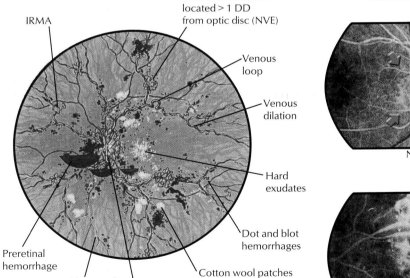

IRMA

Neovascularization located > 1 DD from optic disc (NVE)

Venous loop

Venous dilation

Hard exudates

Dot and blot hemorrhages

Preretinal hemorrhage

Narrowed arteriole

Neovascularization of optic disc (NVD)

Cotton wool patches

Fluorescein angiograms

NVD

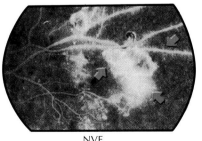

NVE

JOHN A. CRAIG—AD
© ICON

next manifestation. These circular hemorrhages tend to occur in the middle retinal layers. Closer to the optic nerve, where the nerve fiber layers are tightly packed, the hemorrhages may be more superficial, and by following the nerve fiber layer assume a flame-shaped appearance.

As capillary permeability further breaks down, fluid accumulates within the retina. It typically occurs in the middle retinal layers and is seen as a thickening of the retina. When the thickening involves the macula, the central area takes on a cystic appearance (*cystoid macular edema*) and is associated with mild-to-moderate visual loss. Greater degrees of altered permeability cause deposition of lipoprotein in the middle retinal layers called *hard exudates*, patchy yellow accumulations within the retina often associated with areas of thickening and edema.

At the later stages (often associated with severe systemic hypertension), focal infarcts called *cotton wool patches*, soft white superficial changes in the retina with fluffy indistinct borders, develop. When a fluorescein angiogram is performed, these areas correspond to areas of capillary obstruction and capillary dropout. As ischemia develops, the veins take on multiple focal areas of irregularity called *beading*. Arteries become narrowed and, on a gross level, loops may occur in the major veins. Smaller intraretinal changes at the small vessel and capillary level consist of dilation of microvasculature called *intraretinal microvascular abnormalities* (IRMA).

The development of hypoxia then leads to elaboration of vasogenic factors including VEGF, which stimulates the formation of neovascular tufts on the retinal surface and optic nerve surface (Figure 134-2). These small new abnormal vessels break through from the retinal surface and begin to grow on the posterior hyaloid face using the hyaloid as a scaffold. As vessels grow more exuberantly, they begin to be accompanied by fibrous tissue in their development. The hyaloid then contracts, elevating the fibrovascular tissue and sometimes exerting sufficient force on the retina to produce *traction retina detachment*. Vision may be lost either from the hemorrhaging, blocking access of visual images to the retina, or by the detachment of the macula by the fibrovascular proliferation. Typically, many of these findings are in the fundus at one time. The precise findings, their severity, and their extent throughout the fundus are combined into the grading scale used in clinical studies.

MANAGEMENT AND THERAPY

Management of diabetic retinopathy encompasses three strategies: 1) systemic control of diabetes and its complications to prevent the occurrence and progression of diabetic retinopathy; 2) regular ocular examinations to detect lesions that become vision threatening; and 3) direct ocular management including laser photocoagulation and pars plana vitrectomy surgery.

The Diabetes Control and Complications Trial (DCCT) and the *United Kingdom Prospective Diabetes Study* (UKPDS) demonstrated conclusively that intensive glycemic control in patients with type 1 and type 2 diabetes has beneficial effects for preventing vision loss due to diabetic retinopathy. Patients placed on intensive insulin therapy in the DCCT had a slight initial worsening of retinopathy, which reversed after 18 months. Subsequently, patients with intensive glycemic control fared considerably better on every measurement with a 76% risk reduction in onset of retinopathy, a 63% reduction of progression of retinopathy, and a 56% reduction in need for laser treatment. These benefits persisted 4 years after the period when intensive control was instituted. In a study of type 2 patients, the UKPDS demonstrated a reduction in aggregate microvascular endpoints with improved glycemic control.

An association between hypertension and diabetic retinopathy has been demonstrated in multiple studies. In the UKPDS, intensive blood pressure control significantly reduced the need for photocoagulation, the risk of diabetic retinopathy progression, and moderate visual loss. Elevated total cholesterol, high-density lipid, and triglyceride levels have been associated with the faster development of hard exudates in the retina; more extensive hard exudates are correlated with a higher risk of moderate visual loss. Definite improvement of retinopathy by administration of lipid-lowering agents has not been demonstrated, but it seems reasonable in view of the positive effects on cardiovascular morbidity for these individuals.

Regular ocular examinations are important

Figure 134-2   ## Complications of Proliferative Diabetic Retinopathy

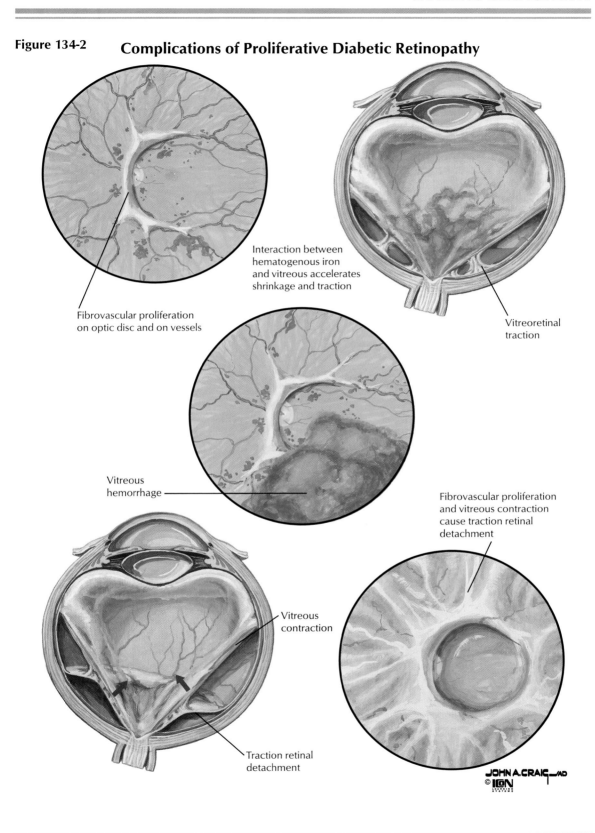

Fibrovascular proliferation
on optic disc and on vessels

Interaction between
hematogenous iron
and vitreous accelerates
shrinkage and traction

Vitreoretinal
traction

Vitreous
hemorrhage

Fibrovascular proliferation
and vitreous contraction
cause traction retinal
detachment

Vitreous
contraction

Traction retinal
detachment

JOHN A. CRAIG—MD
© ICON

to detect diabetic retinopathy in its early stages and allow early intervention when high-risk characteristics occur. Earliest intervention has a strong correlation with a better prognosis for avoiding moderate visual loss. Numerous studies indicate that only 60% of the American population is being appropriately screened at regular intervals.

Laser photocoagulation performed as an office procedure is the mainstay of treatment of proliferative diabetic retinopathy and diabetic macular edema (Figure 134-3). Small laser burns are placed in the retina using a fundus contact lens. Typical burn sizes are between 100 μ and 500 μ. The light energy is absorbed into the small vascular structures, as in the case of argon wavelengths, or into the pigment epithelium in the case of argon and krypton wavelengths. Heat is produced creating a burn. In the case of direct treatment of microaneurysms, this burn seals the micro-aneurysm and decreases the leakage.

When abnormal blood vessels proliferate on the optic nerve surface or the retinal surface, a panretinal or full scatter photocoagulation is carried out. In this treatment, approximately 1,200 to 1,600 laser burns are randomly placed throughout the peripheral parts of the ocular fundus avoiding the nerve, the macula, and large vessels. Visual loss correlates with the number of risk factors present. When 1 or 2 risk factors are present, the 2-year risk of severe visual loss is reduced from 7% to 3%. When 3 or 4 risk factors are present, the risk of severe visual loss is reduced from 26% to 11%.

Diabetic macular edema has been defined as 1) retinal thickening within 500 μ of the fovea, 2) hard exudates associated with thickening within 500 μ of the fovea, or 3) a disc area of edema within one disc diameter of the fovea (Figure 134-4). The decision for treatment is made on the basis of the thickening noted on ophthalmoscopic examination. Treatment is directed at leaking microaneurysms within 500 μ of the center of the fovea. Most physicians now will treat even 20/20 eyes if the position of the aneurysm seems favorable and the risk of treatment can be minimized. Appropriate and timely laser photocoagulation for macular edema can reduce the risk of severe visual loss by more than 95% and reduce the risk of moderate visual loss from 25% to 12%.

When early treatment of proliferative disease is not carried out or is ineffective, vitreous hemorrhage or traction retinal detachment may develop. Surgical intervention is then indicated with the goals of removing the blood, reattaching the retina, and arresting the proliferative process. When necessary, intraocular photocoagulation can be performed once the retina is visualized and reattached. Because of the success in controlling the proliferative process, surgical intervention is sometimes indicated before vision is lost when fibrovascular proliferation is growing in a particularly aggressive fashion.

FUTURE DIRECTIONS

The management of diabetic retinopathy will center on improved early detection, medical management of the systemic condition, development of medications that control vascular proliferation and vascular permeability, and improved laser and surgical strategies, particularly for macular edema. Efforts are underway to assure that a higher percentage of diabetic patients are screened so that early disease may be detected and managed properly. These include mandated screening programs by health maintenance organizations and special screening initiatives put forward through a collaboration of Medicare and eye care provider organizations. Telemedicine screening initiatives are being studied in which photographs may be taken through non-dilated pupils and referred to expert reading centers where detection of retinopathy can be achieved without actual dilated examination by a trained ophthalmic examiner.

Improved cooperation between internists and ophthalmologists will undoubtedly lead to better management of diabetic retinopathy. The end-organ effects of hypertension and elevated lipid levels may be viewed directly in the fundus examination by the ophthalmologist who can then emphasize to the patient and the treating physician the importance of better control of these parameters. Patients will often value the advice of a second physician who reinforces the diabetic care provider's recommendations regarding the importance of good blood glucose control.

Compounds that block the VEGF pathways may reduce the progression of retinopathy to the proliferative stage and reduce the vascular

Figure 134-3

Photocoagulation

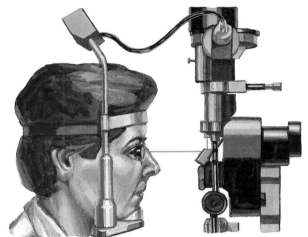

Laser beam directed into eye by slit lamp delivery system

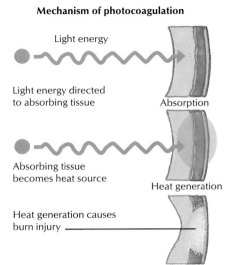

Mechanism of photocoagulation

Light energy

Light energy directed to absorbing tissue — Absorption

Absorbing tissue becomes heat source — Heat generation

Heat generation causes burn injury — Burn injury

Wavelength (nm)	Light energy emission by source (nm)				Light energy absorption		
	Xenon	Argon	Ruby	Krypton	Hemoglobin	Xanthophyll	Melanin
Ultraviolet <400							
Violet 400–450							
Blue 450–480				478			
B-green 480–510		488					
Green 510–550		514		530			
Y-green 550–565							
Yellow 565–590				568			
Orange 590–630							
Red 630–700			694	647			
Infrared >700							

Vascular photocoagulation

Laser — Thermal injury — Burn

Abnormal or leaking vessels sealed or destroyed by light wavelengths absorbed by hemoglobin (argon, 514 nm, or krypton, 568 nm)

Retinal photocoagulation

Laser — Thermal injury — Burn

Retinal areas destroyed by light wavelengths absorbed by melanin and retinal xanthophyll (argon, 488 nm and 514 nm)

JOHN A. CRAIG—AD
© ICON

Figure 134-4 ## Focal Photocoagulation for Macular Edema

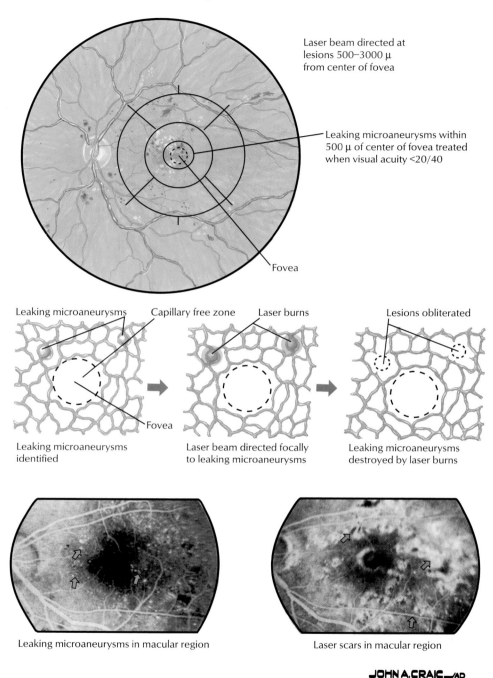

Laser beam directed at lesions 500–3000 μ from center of fovea

Leaking microaneurysms within 500 μ of center of fovea treated when visual acuity <20/40

Fovea

Leaking microaneurysms Capillary free zone Laser burns Lesions obliterated

Fovea

Leaking microaneurysms identified

Laser beam directed focally to leaking microaneurysms

Leaking microaneurysms destroyed by laser burns

Leaking microaneurysms in macular region

Laser scars in macular region

JOHN A. CRAIG—AD
© ICON

permeability and are currently under study in clinical trials. Macular edema continues to be the main cause of visual loss from diabetic retinopathy, and new strategies are being devised for its management. At this time, direct injection of intraocular steroids, implantation of intraocular steroid devices, sustained-release intraocular steroid devices, and surgery removing the internal hyaloid membrane are investigational approaches to achieve better control and reduction of macular edema.

REFERENCES

Diabetic retinopathy. American Diabetes Association. *Diabetes Care.* 1998;21:157-159.

The effect of intensive treatment of diabetes on the development and progression of long-term complications in insulin-dependent diabetes mellitus. The Diabetes Control and Complications Trial Research Group. *N Engl J Med.* 1993;329:977-986.

Photocoagulation for diabetic macular edema. Early Treatment Diabetic Retinopathy Study report number 1. Early Treatment Diabetic Retinopathy Study Research Group. *Arch Ophthalmol.* 1985;103:1796-1806.

Photocoagulation treatment for proliferative diabetic retinopathy. Clinical application of Diabetic Retinopathy Study (DSR) findings. DRS Report Number 8. The Diabetic Retinopathy Study Research Group. *Ophthalmology.* 1981;88:583-600.

Aeillo LP, Cahill MT, Wong JS. Systemic considerations in the management of diabetic retinopathy. *Am J Ophthalmol.* 2001;132:760-776.

Chapter 135

Glaucoma

Sandra M. Johnson

Glaucoma is defined as a characteristic optic neuropathy with associated visual field defects, often associated with elevated intraocular pressure (IOP).

Glaucoma is a leading cause of blindness in the United States and the world. It is estimated that 80,000 Americans are blind due to glaucoma, and it is the leading cause of blindness in African Americans. *Primary open angle glaucoma* (POAG) is the most common form. Referral of at-risk patients for early detection and treatment is essential because only advanced and irreversible vision loss is recognized by an afflicted patient. Risk factors include African American ancestry, family history of the disease, elevated intraocular pressure, and age. Ocular parameters such as baseline cup-to-disc ratio and corneal thickness are gaining importance. The disease is also associated with the vascular risk factors of diabetes mellitus and hypertension, as well as myopia, or nearsightedness. Glaucoma cases are increasing due to the aging population in the United States.

ETIOLOGY AND PATHOGENESIS

As we age, intraocular pressure characteristically elevates within the normal range of 10 to 21 mm Hg. IOP level is primarily determined by the rate of aqueous production and the resistance to outflow across the trabecular meshwork (Figure 135-1). Elevated IOP is usually caused by increased resistance to outflow, but glaucoma without elevated IOP does exist. Because patients can have both pressure dependent and pressure-independent glaucoma, other poorly understood factors are thought to predispose optic nerve axons to damage. Factors under consideration include structure of the lamina cribrosa and optic nerve blood flow.

In primary open angle glaucoma, the anterior segment angle structures all appear normal. The angle, which is the junction between the cornea and iris, contains the trabecular meshwork. It is viewed using special lenses, a technique referred

to as gonioscopy. In *secondary open angle glaucomas*, the angle is open, but a cause of malfunction or obstruction is detected on examination or in the history. For example, corticosteroid use may increase resistance to outflow in approximately one third of patients, with a minority demonstrating a clinically significant rise in IOP. A higher percentage of glaucoma patients will demonstrate elevation of IOP. Elevated episcleral pressure, which may be idiopathic or secondary, causes a secondary open angle glaucoma. Conditions leading to elevated episcleral venous pressure include carotid-dural fistulas, Sturge-Weber syndrome, thyroid ophthalmopathy, a retrobulbar tumor, or superior vena cava syndrome. Likewise, trauma may lead to malfunction of an open angle.

Closed angle, as defined by gonioscopy, is the other major category of glaucoma. This may result from anatomical changes with aging, which lead to pupillary block. *Angle closure* may also be secondary to a disease process that pulls the iris over the trabecular meshwork, as in neovascular glaucoma or a process such as an intraocular tumor that pushes the iris forward causing obstruction of the angle.

CLINICAL PRESENTATION

There is some variation in the presentation of glaucoma. In significant open angle glaucoma, the presentation is one of painless vision loss. A patient with acute angle closure glaucoma will present dramatically with a red painful eye, blurred vision, and nausea and vomiting (Figure 135-2). Neovascular glaucoma secondary to retinal vascular disease such as proliferative diabetic retinopathy may present much the same as acute angle closure. Both of these glaucomas involve angle closure and acute elevation of IOP, which results in their shared symptoms. An infant may

Figure 135-1

Intraocular Pressure

Normal

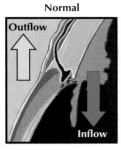

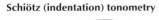

Dynamic equilibrium
between aqueous
production and
drainage

Increased

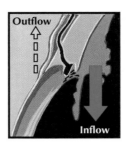

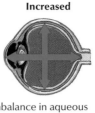

Imbalance in aqueous
production and drainage

Schiötz (indentation) tonometry

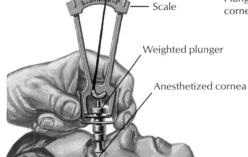

Scale

Weighted plunger

Anesthetized cornea

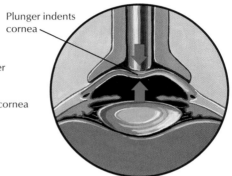

Plunger indents
cornea

Intraocular pressure measured by amount of corneal indentation produced by known weight

Goldmann (applanation) tonometry

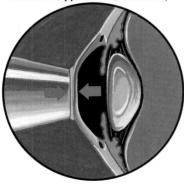

Intraocular pressure determined by
amount of force needed to flatten
constant surface area of cornea

Overlap

Correct endpoint

Inadequate force
(reads low)

Excess force
(reads high)

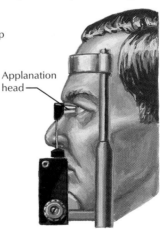

Applanation
head

JOHN A.CRAIG—AD
©ICN

Figure 135-2

Primary Closed Angle Glaucoma

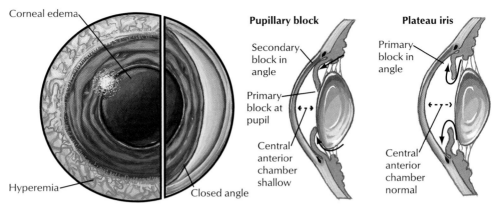

Pupillary block

Secondary block in angle

Primary block at pupil

Central anterior chamber shallow

Plateau iris

Primary block in angle

Central anterior chamber normal

Corneal edema

Hyperemia

Closed angle

Acute angle closure results in marked increase in intraocular pressure with conjunctival hyperemia, corneal edema, and fixed middilated pupil. Subacute and chronic forms may be relatively asymptomatic.

Angle closure may result from primary pupillary block with bulging iris or from less common plateu iris (primary occlusion at periphry of iris)

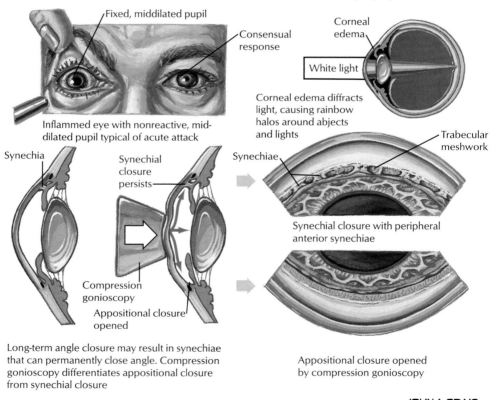

Fixed, middilated pupil

Consensual response

Inflammed eye with nonreactive, mid-dilated pupil typical of acute attack

Corneal edema

White light

Corneal edema diffracts light, causing rainbow halos around abjects and lights

Synechia

Synechial closure persists

Compression gonioscopy

Appositional closure opened

Long-term angle closure may result in synechiae that can permanently close angle. Compression gonioscopy differentiates appositional closure from synechial closure

Synechiae

Trabecular meshwork

Synechial closure with peripheral anterior synechiae

Appositional closure opened by compression gonioscopy

Figure 135-3

Optic Disc and Visual Field Changes in Glaucoma

Early

Right eye
nasal side

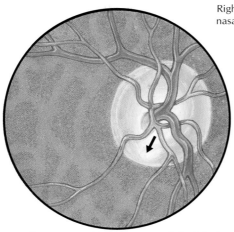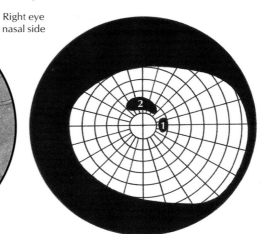

Funduscopy: notching of contour of physiologic cup in optic disc with slight focal pallpr in area of notching; occurs almost invariably in superotemporal or inferotemporal (as shown) quadrants

Perimetry: slight enlargment of physiologic blind spot (1) development of secondary, superonasal field defect (2) which corresponds to nerve fiber damage in area of inferotemporal notching

Minimally advanced

Right eye
nasal side

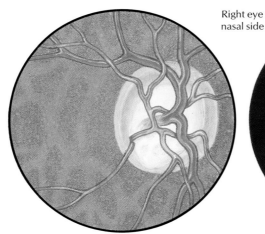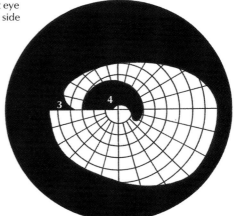

Funduscopy: increased notching of rim of cup; thinning of rim of cup (enlargement of cup); deepening of cup; lamina cribrosa visible in deepest areas.

Perimetry: localized constriction of superonasal visual field (3) because of progessive damage to inferotemporal fibers; superior arc-shaped scotoma (Bjerrum's scotoma) develops (4)

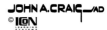
JOHN A. CRAIG—AD
© ICN

Table 135-1
Commonly Used Topical Medicines for Management of Glaucoma

Drug Class	Members	Major Systemic Interactions	Common Ocular Side Effects*
Beta blockers	timolol, metipranolol, carteolol, betaxolol, levobunolol	bradycardia, exacerbate lung ds., depression, malaise	nonspecific
Prostaglandin analogs	latanoprost, travoprost, bimatoprost, unoprostone	rare	lash thickening/darkening, caution in inflammation, Iris darkening
Topical carbonic anhydrase inhibitors	dorzolamide brinzolamide	avoid in true sulfa allergy	non-specific
Adrenergic agents	brimonidine iopidine	hypotension, sleepiness, dry mouth	allergy, including lids

*All eyedrops can cause ocular irritation manifested by foreign body sensation, hyperemia, or stinging/burning.

be born with a developmental defect in the outflow system leading to congenital glaucoma with characteristic photophobia, tearing, and a cloudy cornea.

DIFFERENTIAL DIAGNOSIS

The differential diagnosis of glaucoma based on a patient's symptoms can be quite broad. A patient with painless loss of vision could have retinal detachment, macular degeneration, cataract, or artery occlusion. The differential of acute angle closure is that of a red eye. Conditions such as infectious keratitis, conjunctivitis, orbital cellulitis, and uveitis can present in a similar manner.

The differential diagnosis of glaucoma based on ocular examination includes other optic neuropathies, including acute ischemic optic neuropathy, toxic optic neuropathies such as vitamin B[12] deficiency, and previous optic neuritis.

Pituitary adenomas can cause optic nerve and visual field defects that resemble glaucoma. In general, other optic neuropathies display more pallor than cupping compared to glaucoma, where loss of ganglion cells leads to cupping or thinning of the neuroretinal rim much more than pallor.

DIAGNOSTIC APPROACH

The diagnosis requires a complete eye examination, including gonioscopy and automated visual field testing. Gonioscopy determines whether a glaucoma is an open or a closed angle type or is likely to progress to a closed angle. Examination of the various intraocular structures establishes whether a patient has a secondary cause of glaucoma. Intraocular pressure is measured, and the optic nerve is closely inspected. Automated visual field testing is done to assess the function of the optic nerve and to measure relative scotomas not detected on confrontational visual field testing. The type of correlation seen between the disc features and visual field findings are depicted in Figure 135-3.

MANAGEMENT AND THERAPY

Most glaucoma cases in the United States are treated with medically tolerated topical drug therapy (Table 135-1), followed by laser, then incisional surgery. The principle that guides the aggressiveness of treatment is the concept of *target IOP*. Once the clinical assessment is complete, the ophthalmologist chooses a treatment goal that is the level of IOP that he or she believes will not cause further glaucomatous damage. The overall choice of treatment involves noting the patient's medical history and taking quality of life issues into account.

Once the IOP has been decreased as much as possible by medications, the management of angle closure glaucoma is *laser peripheral iridotomy* (LPI). This procedure uses a laser to create an opening in the superior peripheral iris to permit an alternate route of aqueous flow from the posterior to anterior chambers.

For open angle glaucoma, laser trabeculoplasty is used. Trabeculoplasty treatment, like LPI, is an office procedure, with minimal pain and high success rate, although its effect can last from months to years. In some patients, multiple treatments per eye can be given. Patients who have failed their maximum tolerated medical therapy and trabeculoplasty often progress to incisional surgery. In the most common filtering surgery, *trabeculectomy*, a small hole is created through which aqueous fluid can flow from the anterior chamber to the subconjunctival space. The fluid collection, most often under the upper lid, is termed a *bleb*. The bleb wall is thinned conjunctiva. In many circumstances, it is a thin barrier against penetration of bacterial organisms that can gain access to the intraocular space and result in significant infection. Thus, any patient who has had filtration surgery and in whom a red eye develops should have prompt evaluation. The other major filtering procedure used for patients with conjunctival scarring involves placing a plate in a superior quadrant with a small tube placed into the anterior chamber that shunts aqueous fluid to the plate and then into the subtenon's space. These devices are made of silicone and polymethylmethacrylate and are called glaucoma shunts or tube implants.

Developmental glaucoma in infants is a surgical disease like acute angle closure. Surgery is done after some stabilization of pressure by medications. Angle surgery, called *goniotomy* or *trabeculotomy*, is usually the first-line procedure and curative in most infants.

FUTURE DIRECTIONS

Research in glaucoma includes identifying the genetics of the disorder and more elegantly understanding the process by which the trabecular meshwork develops sclerosis, and whether there are optic nerve structural or vascular characteristics that are inherited and predispose individuals to glaucomatous optic neuropathy. One gene, present in approximately 16% of POAG, has been identified, and a screening test can now be used clinically in select cases. Another large area of study is optic nerve head blood flow, which, given its anatomic location and number of vascular supplies, has been difficult to image to date. Multiple technologies are evolving to image the retinal ganglion cell layer and the optic nerve, to reliably screen for the disease, and to follow its progression more precisely and objectively. Great strides are being made in understanding the cascade leading to ganglion cell death, which may lead to pharmacologic neuroprotection. This research area overlaps with other neurobiology studies of diseases such as stroke and Alzheimer's disease.

The emphasis on medical therapy is compliance through simpler medical regimens and newer pharmacologic agents, such as the prostaglandin analogs, which only require daily dosing; most other topical agents can now be used twice daily. Studies are focusing on combination drugs, such as an adrenergic agent and beta blocker or a prostaglandin analog and beta blocker.

REFERENCES

Colomb E, Nguyen TD, Bechetoille A, et al. Association of a single nucleotide polymorphism in the TIGR/MYOCILIN gene promoter with the severity of primary open-angle glaucoma. *Clin Genet.* 2001;60:220-225.

Cantor LB, ed. Section 10: glaucoma. In: *Basic and Clinical Science Course 2002.* San Francisco, Calif: American Academy of Ophthalmology; 2002.

Kass, et al. The Ocular Hypertension Treatment Study: A randomized trial determines that topical ocular hypotensive medication delays or prevents the onset of primary open-angle glaucoma. *Arch Ophthalmol.* 2002; 120:701-13

Sommer A, Tielsch JM, Katz J, et al. Relationship between intraocular pressure and primary open angle glaucoma among white and black Americans. The Baltimore Eye Survey. *Arch Ophthalmol.* 1991;109:1090-1095.

Wigginton SA, Higginbotham EJ II. Glaucoma diagnosis and management. *Ophthalmol Clin North Am.* 2000;13.

Chapter 136

Myopia and Common Refractive Disorders

Thomas S. Devetski

All ocular refractive disorders, or *ametropias,* are defined as aberrant focusing of entering light rays away from the optimal plane of the retinal macula. Ametropias include myopia, hyperopia, astigmatism, and presbyopia. These conditions represent a significant public health issue in the United States. A 1980 survey of vision correction in the United States estimates that over half of the population older than 3 years have refractive errors corrected with spectacles or contact lenses.

ETIOLOGY AND PATHOGENESIS

In basic optical terms, the human visual system is made up of the cornea, crystalline lens, and ocular axial length. Each of these anatomical components must develop in precise balance to produce sharp optical focus on the retina.

Emmetropia (Figure 136-1) is vision devoid of optical defects, and *emmetropization* is the developmental process of growth and integration of ocular components, which optimally leads to normal vision. Until age 3, cornea and lens curvatures (refractive powers) are adjusted through a poorly understood mechanism to correlate with changes in axial length. The result is that greater than 95% of eyes end up with a refraction close to emmetropia (between +4 and −4 diopters of refractive error).

Myopia (nearsightedness) *(Figure 136-1)* is the most common refractive error with a prevalence of 80% of ametropias. It is a disorder in which light from distant objects is focused anterior to the retina. The refractive power of the eye is too strong for its axial length. Myopia can be classified as *simple* juvenile-onset, *adult-onset,* and *degenerative.*

Simple myopia accounts for more than 85% of all myopia. It is estimated that 15% to 25% of the US population has or will have juvenile-onset myopia. Typically, it begins after age 5 with gradual increases in severity until around 16 when 75% stabilize in correction. The rest may continue to experience an increase in severity into their 20s and 30s. Increases of −.25 to −.75 per year are common, but higher rates are not unusual.

Generally, earlier onset of myopia leads to higher refractive error at the endpoint. There is evidence of gender difference, as girls tend to begin progression of myopia and stabilize 1 or 2 years before boys. Positive family history is the primary risk factor for developing simple myopia. Studies indicate that children of parents who both have myopia have a 33% to 60% prevalence of myopia, and when only one is afflicted, a 23% to 40% prevalence. If neither parent has myopia, there is only a 6% to 15% chance of developing myopia. Research involving prediction of myopia indicates that at third-grade age, 60% of individuals with a cycloplegic refraction of +.5 (hyperopia) or less will become myopic by eighth grade.

Adult-onset myopia begins at approximately 20 years. Typically, it affects individuals, such as graduate students, in a high near-point stress environment. The disorder has an unpredictable endpoint in terms of time and severity, but it usually ends in low-to-moderate myopia. It is possible for previously stable myopic individuals to experience an increase in severity years later at times of increased near-point activity. It has been hypothesized that a new process of emmetropization occurs, developing an optical focus for near, which induces myopic progression.

Degenerative myopia is rare (1% to 2% of all myopia) and a far more serious form in which the eye elongates at a rapid and pathological rate. As the eye elongates, the retina thins, increasing the incidence of retinal degeneration and detachment. Typically, tears in the retina occur at the level of Bruch's membrane with secondary hemorrhages and scarring at the macula leading to permanent visual distortion and blindness. Degenerative myopia is developmental in origin and progresses most rapidly at puberty.

Other causes of temporary myopic shifts are variations in blood sugar levels, nuclear sclerotic cataract progression, or introduction of various pharmaceutic agents (pilocarpine, tetracycline, adrenergic agents, phenothiazines, corticosteroids, oral contraceptives). These myopic tendencies are usually reversible.

Hyperopia (farsightedness) (figure 136-1) is characterized by a weaker than normal refractive power or a shorter axial length, both of which cause light to focus posterior to the retina in the unaccommodated eye. Its incidence is directly related to age. The majority of full-term infants begin life with low hyperopia. The percentage decreases rapidly with the emmetropization process of gradual flattening of lens and cornea in conjunction with growth-related elongation of the eye. The severity in individuals under 30 is often difficult to measure because of the accommodative system's ability to produce positive refractive power, in essence "correcting" hyperopia. This aberrant use of the accommodative system can bring with it other binocular integration and general eye disorders. The strong association between moderate-to-high hyperopia in childhood and development of amblyopia and strabismus (esotropia) is an example.

Astigmatism (figure 136-1) is a refractive disorder in which the cornea has a non-spherical shape, with different powers at individual meridians or axes. This causes entering light rays to focus at multiple locations instead of a single point. *Lenticular astigmatism* is an unusual variant caused by abnormal tilting of the crystalline lens. Astigmatism follows a course similar to myopia, manifesting around age 8 and stabilizing in the middle teen years. There is no gender difference, and both distance and near vision are affected. Astigmatism affects approximately 25% to 40% of the population and is commonly found in conjunction with myopia or hyperopia.

Presbyopia involves the progressive loss of accommodative ability in middle age leading to difficulty focusing on near objects. Accommodation, the ability to change shape and power of the crystalline lens by contraction of the ciliary body, develops maximum amplitude early in childhood. With advancing age, hardening of the crystalline lens reduces flexibility and increases accommodative effort. Although hyperopia is often confused with presbyopia, hyperopia is relatively uncommon, whereas presbyopia will cause noticeable effects in everyone by age 45. Other eye disorders such as accommodative insufficiency may cause identical symptoms at an earlier age.

CLINICAL PRESENTATION

The clinical presentation of all ametropias involves blurred vision at one or more viewing distances. In myopia, distance vision is affected while near vision remains intact. Frequently, an individual will seek eye care when having difficulty driving at night or watching television. Unfortunately, children often tolerate very poor vision without complaining, so attention should be given to apparent difficulty seeing the classroom blackboard or while playing sports. Frequently, individuals with myopia report that "squinting" (creating a pinhole effect) improves vision.

Hyperopia is less straightforward in presentation. Theoretically, it is the opposite of myopia, leading to the assumption of blurred near and intact distance vision, but that is rarely the case. The accommodative system is able to "correct" low amounts of hyperopia without much difficulty until ages 30 to 40. Individuals under this age are rarely aware of their refractive error and are resistant to the notion of refractive correction. Eventually, the accommodative system wanes, and the farsighted person has difficulty seeing at all distances and must resort to wearing spectacles or contact lenses.

Astigmatism is usually less visually disturbing unless it occurs along with another refractive error. Those afflicted can get along for years without correction, and as with myopia, squinting improves vision. Common complaints include visible halo effects while driving at night, or monocular diplopia.

Presbyopia is easily recognized in individuals 40 and over. It manifests as gradual and progressive loss of near focus ability, usually worse at the end of the day. As the accommodative demand for near work exceeds the accommodative

Figure 136-1

Myopia and Other Refractive Errors

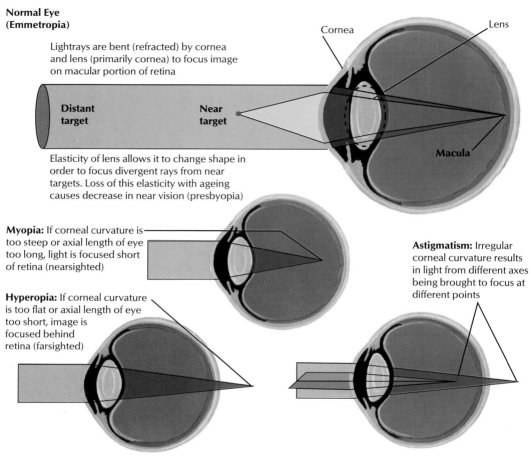

Normal Eye (Emmetropia)

Lightrays are bent (refracted) by cornea and lens (primarily cornea) to focus image on macular portion of retina

Cornea

Lens

Distant target

Near target

Macula

Elasticity of lens allows it to change shape in order to focus divergent rays from near targets. Loss of this elasticity with ageing causes decrease in near vision (presbyopia)

Myopia: If corneal curvature is too steep or axial length of eye too long, light is focused short of retina (nearsighted)

Hyperopia: If corneal curvature is too flat or axial length of eye too short, image is focused behind retina (farsighted)

Astigmatism: Irregular corneal curvature results in light from different axes being brought to focus at different points

Treatment Options

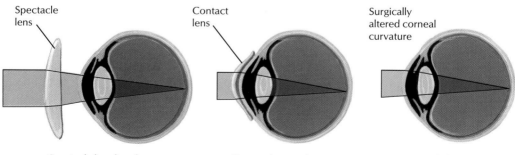

Spectacle lens

Contact lens

Surgically altered corneal curvature

Spectacle lens bends (refract) light rays to focus image on retina

Contact lens performs as a "corrected" corneal surface, focusing image on retina

Surgical alteration of abnormal corneal curvature allows clear focusing of image on retina

JOHN A.CRAIG—AD
with
E. Hatton
© ICON
LEARNING
SYSTEMS

reserve, blurred vision, headaches, fatigue, and eyestrain occur. Hyperopes typically have an earlier onset than myopes, and astigmatism can exacerbate symptoms.

DIAGNOSTIC APPROACH

Diagnosing refractive error is relatively straightforward and can be accomplished using Snellen or other visual acuity charts for near and far. The Snellen equivalent optotype system is based on a standard normal acuity measurement of 20/20, which equates to a letter height of 8.7 mm measured at 20 feet. All other sizes of letters for different acuity levels are extrapolated from this standard. The numerator in the acuity fraction corresponds to the distance a standard letter can be seen by a tested individual (usually 20 feet), and the denominator corresponds to the distance the same letter can be seen by a normal observer. An acuity level of less than 20/20 at distance, with normal acuity at near indicates some level of myopia. Normal acuity at distance with difficulty focusing at near indicates hyperopia. Astigmatism causes a generalized reduction of acuity at near and far, and presbyopia is similar to hyperopia in middle-aged or older individuals.

The most accurate method of measuring refractive error is to perform cycloplegic refraction to best-corrected acuity. This procedure requires instillation of pharmaceutic agents (e.g., cyclopentolate) for paralysis of the ciliary body and the accommodative system. Cycloplegia is especially important when assessing refractive error in children because of their high accommodative amplitude and its effortless use. In-office use of specialty ophthalmic equipment such as phoropter and automated refractor enable quick and efficient measurement of refractive error and simulates spectacle-corrected vision.

MANAGEMENT AND THERAPY

There are many treatments (Figure 136-1) available for correction of ametropias, running the gamut from very basic to extremely high-tech. Corrective methods are classified generally as either nonsurgical or surgical.

Non-surgical Methods

Non-surgical corrective options, including spectacles and contact lenses, are the most widely used and are reversible. Spectacles, the most common option, provide economical, safe, and exacting correction of all ametropias. Limitations include facial discomfort, lack of peripheral vision, and cosmesis. Nonetheless, with the advent of high-index materials, improved progressive bifocal designs, and newer frame designs, spectacle use has increased in popularity. Plastic polymers are the most widely used materials in the fabrication of ophthalmic lenses because they are lighter weight and safer than glass. Recent estimates of contact lens use in the United States are as high as 10% to 15%. Soft hydrogel contact lens wearers comprise 85% of the population wearing contact lenses with the remainder using rigid gas permeable or hard. With current technology, contact lenses can be used to correct virtually any refractive condition. Advantages include improved cosmesis, intact peripheral vision, and correction of irregular corneal disorders not correctable with spectacles (e.g., keratoconus). Disadvantages include expense, risk of infection or other pathology, and required diligence in care.

Surgical Methods

Current surgical corrective options include laser procedures and corneal implantation. Of these, the laser procedures are the most popular. Several techniques using various laser types have been developed to correct the majority of refractive disorders. Laser procedures offer an ever-expanding level of precision "sculpting" of the corneal tissues to provide refractive correction.

Photorefractive keratectomy (PRK) uses a computer-guided excimer laser (193 nm wavelength) to reshape the corneal stroma to a desired curvature for refractive correction. PRK requires removal of stromal tissue, so unusually thin corneas can limit the amount of correction. Because epithelial tissue must be disrupted for laser access to the stroma, a bandage contact lens is applied directly after surgery to decrease pain and protect healing epithelium. Mild-to-moderate discomfort may be reported for 2 to 3 days as re-epithelialization occurs. PRK usually takes only 1 to 2 minutes to perform and can currently be used to correct 1 to 12 diopters of myopia, 1 to 6 diopters of hyperopia, and up to 4 diopters of astigmatism. Approved by the FDA in 1995, PRK has proven most accurate in correction of low-to-moderate myopia (up to −6 diopters) with a post-operative acuity 20/40 or better in 90% to 95% of procedures. A major complication, besides under- or over-correction, is a transient visual disturbance described as foggy or hazy vision that is most noticeable at night.

Laser-assisted in-situ keratomileusis (LASIK) is a refractive procedure that combines PRK with the surgical creation of a corneal flap by an instrument called a microkeratome. This precise instrument cuts a thin, circular flap in the superficial layers of the cornea, leaving a hinge on one side. Once the flap is folded away, PRK is performed on the exposed stroma. The flap is then carefully placed back in its original position, completing the procedure. Like PRK, LASIK can be used to treat myopia, hyperopia, and astigmatism. The accuracy of postoperative correction is the same or slightly better than PRK. The advantages over PRK are faster vision rehabilitation and less discomfort. The major complications are loss of best-corrected acuity and reduced corneal sensitivity, which can lead to a chronic irritation similar to dry-eye syndrome. Both PRK and LASIK can be performed several times on the same eye ("enhancements") for refinement of surgical correction or naturally occurring refractive changes.

Corneal ring implantation is a non-laser refractive procedure for correcting low amounts of myopia (−1 to −3 diopters). This procedure involves implantation of two plastic, crescent-shaped segments into the cornea, causing flattening of the central cornea. The implanted segments are produced in different thicknesses, which determine the amount of correction. The procedure takes about 15 minutes and is reversible.

FUTURE DIRECTIONS

The future of refractive correction lies with several promising technologies. In the laser arena, "wave-front" technology is being used in an attempt to increase the accuracy of correction by identifying and compensating for high order optical aberrations. This customized correction has the potential to produce acuities far superior to current procedures.

Other non-laser surgical options on the horizon are phakic intraocular lenses and intracorneal contact lenses (inlays) for correction of myopia, hyperopia, and astigmatism, as well as scleral expansion and accommodative intraocular lenses for the correction of presbyopia. Of all the disorders, the permanent correction of presbyopia is the most difficult to achieve.

REFERENCES

Amos JF, ed. *Diagnosis and Management in Vision Care.* 2nd ed. Boston, Mass: Butterworth-Heinemann; 1998.

Aurell E, Norrsell K. A longitudinal study of children with a family history of strabismus: factors determining the incidence of strabismus. *Br J Ophthalmol.* 1990;74:589-594.

Goss DA, Jackson TW. Clinical findings before the onset of myopia in youth: 4. Parental history of myopia. *Optom Vis Sci.* 1996;73:279-282.

National Center for Health Statistics, Poe GS. *Eye Care Visits and Use of Eyeglasses or Contact Lenses, United States, 1979 and 1980.* Washington, DC: National Center for Health Statistics; 1984. DHHS publication (PHS) 84-1573.

Zadnik K, Mutti DO, Friedman NE, et al. Ocular predictors of the onset of juvenile myopia. *Invest Ophthalmol Vis Sci.* 1999;40:1936-1943.

Section XVII

PSYCHIATRIC DISORDERS

Chapter 137

Alcohol Dependence and Alcohol Abuse

J.C. Garbutt

Humans have used alcohol, ethanol or beverage alcohol, for thousands of years. Most cultures use alcohol or have prohibitions against its use. Physicians need to understand the consequences of the use of alcohol and be able to recognize when use becomes problematic and develops into an illness—alcoholism. In the United States, recent surveys indicate that approximately 65% of individuals report lifetime alcohol use and approximately 45% report drinking in the past year, whereas the lifetime prevalence rate of alcohol dependence is near 13% with a 12-month prevalence of around 4%. Men have higher rates of alcohol problems than women have. Problem drinkers are much more common in health care settings such as emergency rooms, burn units, psychiatry services, and general medical services. Surveys indicate that approximately 30% of men and 10% of women admitted to a general hospital have an alcohol-related disorder.

ETIOLOGY AND PATHOGENESIS

Alcoholism, as a disease syndrome, was described independently in 1785 by the American physician Dr. Benjamin Rush and the British physician, Dr. Thomas Trotter. The evolution of the disease concept of alcoholism has been important for destigmatizing alcohol problems and in advancing understanding of the nature of alcoholism and its treatment.

Adoption and twin studies suggest that genetic factors contribute on the order of 50% of the variance for liability for alcoholism in men and women. The gene(s) contributing to the development of alcoholism are not known.

Apart from genetic influences, significant advances have occurred in understanding the neurobiologic actions of alcohol and their possible relevance to the development of alcoholism (Chapter 146, Figure 146-1). Thus, the observation that alcohol, similar to other drugs of abuse, activates brain reinforcement centers, perhaps taking on behavioral significance for an individual, is an important finding. Evidence continues to build that chronic alcohol use alters brain reinforcement circuitry leading to a preoccupation with using the drug and the compulsion to use it even in the face of personal deterioration. Other factors that influence the development of alcoholism include comorbid psychiatric disorders (e.g., bipolar disor-

der), peer influences, familial and cultural drinking patterns, and the availability and cost of alcohol.

Alcoholism is a progressive, and not uncommonly, fatal illness. There may be attempts to control drinking by shifting the type of beverage and through periods of abstinence. The individual may have cycles of treatment and relapse, never receive treatment, or achieve significant improvement with, or even without, treatment.

CLINICAL PRESENTATION

The clinical presentation of alcoholism is extremely varied. In a general medical practice or hospital setting, the medical or traumatic consequences of alcoholism are the most common reasons an individual with an alcohol problem comes to a physician's attention. Alcohol has toxic effects on most organ systems, and individuals may present with any of a variety of medical problems (e.g., cirrhosis, pancreatitis) or behavioral problems, including depression and insomnia (Figure 137-1). A connection between alcohol use and the presenting physical symptoms is commonly not offered. However, many patients come to a physician requesting help with alcohol problems; so, the notion that alcoholism is always concealed is not correct.

Laboratory tests that should alert the clinician to consider heavy alcohol use in the differential diag-

Figure 137-1

Effects of Alcohol on End Organs

Cellular damage

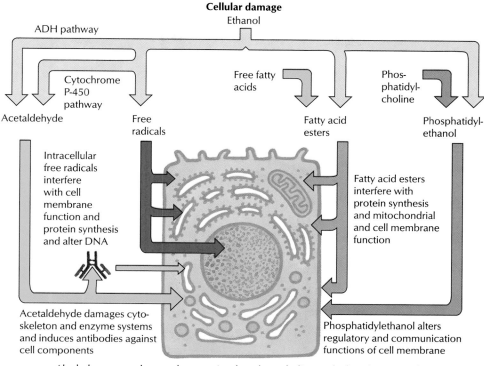

Ethanol

ADH pathway

Cytochrome P-450 pathway

Acetaldehyde

Free radicals

Free fatty acids

Fatty acid esters

Phos-phatidyl-choline

Phosphatidyl-ethanol

Intracellular free radicals interfere with cell membrane function and protein synthesis and alter DNA

Fatty acid esters interfere with protein synthesis and mitochondrial and cell membrane function

Acetaldehyde damages cyto-skeleton and enzyme systems and induces antibodies against cell components

Phosphatidylethanol alters regulatory and communication functions of cell membrane

Alcohol causes end organ damage via ethanol metabolites and ethanol-generated compounds, which alter structure and function of cell components

Organ damage

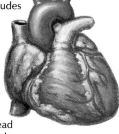

Cardiovascular damage includes arrhythmias and cardio-myopathy

Immune system suppression increases risk of infection and some cancers

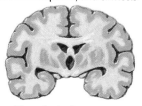

Hepatic damage includes fatty liver, alcoholic hepatitis, and cirrhosis

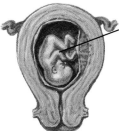

Teratogenic effects may lead to fetal alcohol syndrome

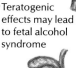

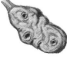

Neurologic damage ranges from Korsakoff dementia to subclinical cognitive defects

Increased risk of spontaneous abortion

Testicular atrophy and diminished libido

Anovulation and early menopause

JOHN A. CRAIG—AD
©ICN

Figure 137-2

Alcohol Dependence

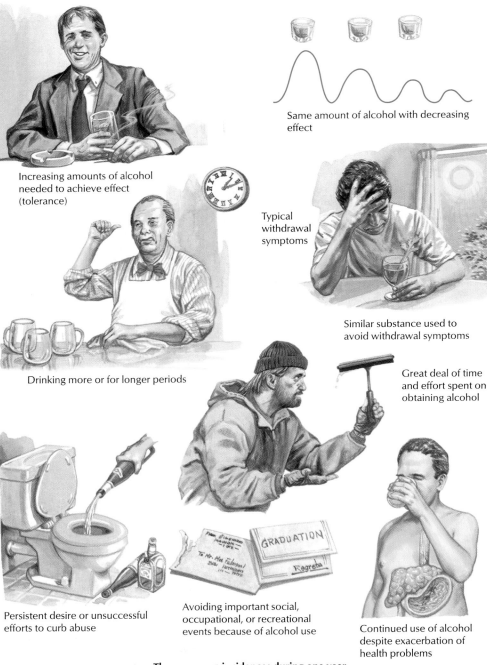

Same amount of alcohol with decreasing effect

Increasing amounts of alcohol needed to achieve effect (tolerance)

Typical withdrawal symptoms

Similar substance used to avoid withdrawal symptoms

Drinking more or for longer periods

Great deal of time and effort spent on obtaining alcohol

Persistent desire or unsuccessful efforts to curb abuse

Avoiding important social, occupational, or recreational events because of alcohol use

Continued use of alcohol despite exacerbation of health problems

Three or more incidences during one year indicate pattern of physical dependence

JOHN A. CRAIG—MD

C. Machado
—M.D.

© ICON

nosis include abnormal liver function tests showing increases in gamma-glutamyl transferase (GGT), aspartate aminotransferase (AST), alanine aminotransferase (ALT), and bilirubin; elevated mean corpuscular volume; elevated uric acid; and elevated triglycerides. Blood alcohol levels greater than 0.10 g/dL found during an emergency visit or a general medical visit are strongly suggestive of alcohol abuse or dependence.

DIFFERENTIAL DIAGNOSIS

The differential diagnosis of alcohol dependence can be conceptualized as separating the consequences of heavy alcohol use from the diagnosis of the core syndrome. Because many patients present with symptoms and signs of alcohol-related medical illnesses, the differential diagnosis includes medical illnesses such as viral hepatitis or peptic ulcer.

An important diagnostic issue is whether the patient's alcohol problems qualify as *primary alcoholism* versus alcohol abuse or even simply use. The diagnosis of *alcohol dependence* (alcoholism) as defined by the Diagnostic and Statistical Manual of Mental Disorders, Fourth Edition (DSM-IV) includes a maladaptive pattern of substance use, leading to clinically significant impairment or distress, as manifested by 3 or more of the following, occurring in the same 12-month period (Figure 137-2):

· Tolerance as evidenced by requiring more alcohol to achieve intoxication or less of an effect with continued use of the same quantity of alcohol.
· Withdrawal symptoms when alcohol is stopped.
· Alcohol is taken in greater quantities or for a longer time than intended.
· Persistent desire or unsuccessful efforts to reduce use.
· A great deal of time spent in using and recovering from alcohol.
· Important activities are given up or reduced because of alcohol use.
· Alcohol use is continued despite adverse consequences.

Alcohol abuse involves a recurrent pattern of harmful use of alcohol (e.g., driving while intoxicated, missing work), but does not involve the development of tolerance, withdrawal symptoms, or a compulsive use pattern. In fact, the compulsive quality of alcohol use is the hallmark sign of alcoholism. As one alcoholic stated, "When I wasn't occupied with drinking alcohol, I was preoccupied with it."

DIAGNOSTIC APPROACH

The diagnosis of alcoholism and alcohol abuse depends on the documentation of signs and symptoms (Figure 137-3). Because the diagnosis is based primarily on history, the approach involves gathering data on alcohol use patterns and related problems from the patient, as well as collateral sources of information such as a spouse.

The approach to the diagnosis can be conceptualized as a series of steps:

Consideration: Clinicians should be aware that many patients will have alcohol problems and that the first step in identification of alcoholism or alcohol abuse is to consider it as a possibility.

Screening Questions: These include how often the patient drinks alcohol, the average quantity of consumption, and the maximum quantity of consumption. Screening tests have been developed including the CAGE (4 questions), and the AUDIT (10 questions), which are easy to administer and provide good sensitivity for detection of alcohol problems.

Detailed History: Once evidence is obtained that an alcohol problem is likely, additional history should be gathered in an effort to establish whether the patient has alcoholism or alcohol abuse.

Update and Review: Clinicians should continue to review the alcohol history and current use patterns longitudinally to ascertain if there is improvement or deterioration.

Laboratory tests for alcoholism have suffered from a lack of specificity. For example, GGT is a reasonably sensitive test of recent heavy alcohol use but is not specific for alcohol use. Recently, carbohydrate deficient transferrin (CDT) has emerged as a test with improved specificity for heavy alcohol use, and it may develop into a useful clinical tool.

MANAGEMENT AND THERAPY

The treatment of alcoholism should involve a long-term management approach similar to the treatment of diabetes or hypertension. O'Brien and McLellan (1996) have articulated this perspective of a harm-reduction model viewing alcoholism as a chronic disease. In this model, the clinician is aware that there will be ups and downs in the

Figure 137-3

Signs Suggestive of Alcohol Abuse

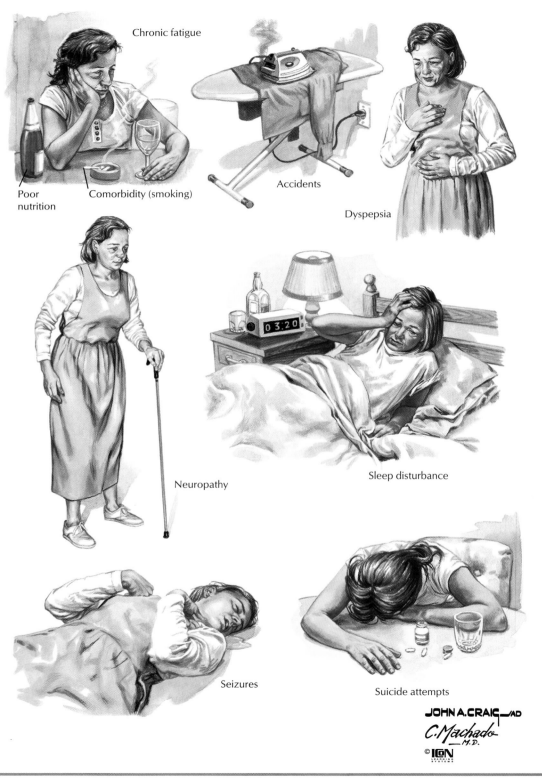

Chronic fatigue

Poor nutrition

Comorbidity (smoking)

Accidents

Dyspepsia

Neuropathy

Sleep disturbance

Seizures

Suicide attempts

JOHN A. CRAIG—AD

C. Machado—M.D.

© ICON
LEARNING SYSTEMS

course of treatment but that over time many patients will have significant reductions in their use of alcohol and fewer alcohol-related problems.

The initial step in alcoholism treatment is for the clinician to identify alcohol as a problem for the patient and attempt to work collaboratively with the patient on ways to modify drinking behavior. Most patients do not understand the nature of addiction, nor are they fully aware of the health-related consequences of heavy alcohol use; therefore, education is valuable.

The decision whether to medically detoxify a patient depends upon the risk of serious withdrawal (i.e., seizures, delirium tremens). Factors that increase the likelihood of serious withdrawal include history of seizures or delirium tremens (DTs), concomitant medical illness, old age, and to some extent, quantity/frequency of alcohol consumption. Patients who do not have risk factors can be monitored for signs of significant withdrawal—the *Clinical Institute Withdrawal Assessment of Alcohol Scale Revised* is a useful instrument to quantify withdrawal severity. Patients with risk factors or significant withdrawal symptoms require medical detoxification, and this should be completed in a residential medical setting unless an established outpatient detoxification program is available. The benzodiazepines have been recommended as the treatment of choice for alcohol withdrawal and are highly effective in reducing withdrawal symptoms and in reducing the risk of seizures or DTs. However, DTs develop in some patients despite benzodiazepine treatment. Thiamine should also be given to prevent the development of permanent memory impairment (Korsakoff's syndrome).

Detoxification has been referred to as the first step in alcoholism treatment. Many approaches have been tried to help the alcoholic or alcohol abuser to change his or her drinking behavior ranging from long-term residential care to brief outpatient visits. To date, no clear algorithms are available to guide the clinician on what specific form of treatment should be recommended for a given patient. However, patients with milder forms of alcohol problems may show improvement in a primary care setting with very brief interventions that provide education, feedback, and encouragement to alter drinking patterns. Patients with more severe alcohol problems usu-

ally require more specialized treatment that may include a period of residential care, intensive outpatient treatment, encouragement to attend Alcoholics' Anonymous (AA), and medication. The strategies employed in these settings include motivational therapy, cognitive-behavioral relapse prevention therapy, and engagement in the 12 steps of AA. An important element in working with the alcoholic patient is to provide care over time and to avoid therapeutic nihilism—"nothing is going to help anyway." In fact, outcome studies suggest that 50% or so of alcoholics will have at least a 50% reduction in alcohol use 6 months after treatment.

Medication management of alcoholism is in the midst of significant change that should enhance treatment. For years, the only medication to treat alcoholism was disulfiram, an inhibitor of aldehyde dehydrogenase, which produces an aversive reaction when alcohol is consumed and provides a psychologic deterrent to alcohol consumption. Its efficacy is related to compliance, and it may be particularly valuable in highly motivated patients or with supervised administration. In the United States, disulfiram is usually given as 250 mg/day once a patient is detoxified from alcohol.

Naltrexone represents a new class of medications for the treatment of alcoholism that do not act via aversive deterrence. Naltrexone is an opioid antagonist that has been shown to reduce the risk of relapse to heavy drinking and, possibly, enhance the likelihood of abstinence. Naltrexone is thought to work by counteracting the "high" experienced after drinking alcohol so that patients are less likely to lose control. Naltrexone is usually started after several days of sobriety and continued for weeks to months in combination with psychosocial treatment.

Acamprosate, another new agent, has been approved for alcoholism treatment in Europe. Acamprosate may modulate the N-methyl-D-aspartate receptor thought to be one site of alcohol's actions. It has been shown to reduce significantly the frequency of drinking and enhance the likelihood of abstinence. Because of the added value provided by medications and the overall positive risk/benefit ratio, clinicians should strongly consider the use of medications in the treatment of alcoholism.

FUTURE DIRECTIONS

The development of the disease concept of alcoholism was a great advance for the understanding and treatment of alcoholism. In the next 50 years, a more detailed understanding of the pathophysiologic basis of alcoholism may be described, and advances in treatment should occur with the development of new medications targeting specific forms of alcoholism. Hopefully, there will also be advances in prevention of alcohol problems and more effective government policy interventions to reduce the public health impact of alcohol.

REFERENCES

Ewing JA. Detecting alcoholism. The CAGE questionnaire. *JAMA.* 1984;252:1905–1907.

Fleming MF, Barry KL, Manwell LB, Johnson K, London R. Brief physician advice for problem alcohol drinkers. A randomized controlled trial in community-based primary care practices. *JAMA.* 1997;277:1039–1045.

Garbutt JC, West SL, Carey TS, Lohr KN, Crews FT. Pharmacological treatment of alcohol dependence: a review of the evidence. *JAMA.* 1999;281:1318–1325.

Grant BF. Prevalence and correlates of alcohol use and DSM-IV alcohol dependence in the United States: results of the National Longitudinal Alcohol Epidemiologic Survey. *J Stud Alcohol.* 1997;58:464–473.

Koob GF, Roberts AJ. Brain reward circuits in alcoholism. *CNS Spectrums.* 1999;4:23–37.

Mayo-Smith MF. Pharmacological management of alcohol withdrawal. A meta-analysis and evidence-based practice guideline. American Society of Addiction Medicine Working Group on Pharmacological Management of Alcohol Withdrawal. *JAMA.* 1997;278:144–151.

O'Brien CP, McLellan AT. Myths about the treatment of addiction. *Lancet.* 1996;347:237–240.

Prescott CA, Kendler KS. Genetic and environmental contributions to alcohol abuse and dependence in a population-based sample of male twins. *Am J Psychiatry.* 1999;156:34–40.

Saunders JB, Aasland OG, Babor TF, de la Fuente JR, Grant M. Development of the Alcohol Use Disorders Identification Test (AUDIT): WHO Collaborative Project on Early Detection of Persons with Harmful Alcohol Consumption—II. *Addiction.* 1993;88:791–804.

Sullivan JT, Sykora K, Schneiderman J, Naranjo CA, Sellers EM. Assessment of alcohol withdrawal: the revised Clinical Institute Withdrawal Assessment for Alcohol scale (CIWA-Ar). *Br J Addict.* 1989;84:1353–1357.

Chapter 138
Anxiety and Panic

Lea C. Watson and B. Anthony Lindsey

Most patients with psychiatric symptoms are seen in the general medical setting exclusively. This is particularly true for patients with anxiety disorders, in whom somatic symptoms predominate. Although detection of these disorders remains poor, the direct and indirect costs of untreated anxiety are enormous, and effective evidence-based treatments are available.

"Anxiety" is tension or apprehension that is disproportional to the actual stimulus (Figure 138-1). There are five principal anxiety disorders in adults: *panic disorder* (PD) with or without agoraphobia, *social phobia* (SP), *obsessive-compulsive disorder* (OCD), *generalized anxiety disorder* (GAD), and *posttraumatic stress disorder* (PTSD). Simple phobias (e.g., specific fear of storms or heights) are common also but rarely present in the primary care setting. In the general medical setting, panic disorder is the most prevalent of the principal disorders. The lifetime prevalence is approximately 1% to 2%, with a 2-fold increased risk for women, and onset in the 20s most frequently. Often, PD has a complicated medical presentation and a significant burden of comorbidities. The remaining principal disorders will not be covered in detail here. OCD (Chapter 144) usually requires early psychiatric referral. GAD, SP, and PTSD require multimodal therapies and are often too time-intensive to be exclusively managed in the general medical setting. Table 138-1 summarizes these disorders.

ETIOLOGY AND PATHOGENESIS

As with most psychiatric disorders, it is likely that psychologic and environmental triggers unmask a biologic predisposition to PD.

Neurobiological

There is an explosion of research in this area including the study of the "fear" and "anxiety" centers in the brain, such as the amygdala, locus ceruleus, and hippocampus. Preliminary neuroimaging studies highlight deficits in these neuroanatomical areas. Provocative agents including sodium lactate, carbon dioxide, caffeine, yohim-bine, m-chlorophenylpiperazine, fenfluramine, and cholecystokinin can induce panic states in patients with PD. Supporting neurochemical hypotheses is the fact that similar states cannot be induced in normal control subjects. No specific etiologic determinants have emerged in this likely heterogeneous disorder. Family studies also suggest that PD is familial, with increased risk for first-degree relatives of those with the disorder.

Cognitive-Behavioral

Progressive fear of recurrent attacks is a large part of PD, and even more important when *agoraphobia* (avoidance of activities secondary to fear of having an attack) occurs. Many believe that this conditioning leads to "catastrophic" misinterpretation of bodily sensations starting a cycle of escalating anxiety.

CLINICAL PRESENTATION

Most patients with PD (85%) make their initial contact in the medical setting, most in the emergency department, followed by visits to their primary care physician. PD usually manifests in the third or fourth decade. The criteria for a panic attack (Table 138-2) should be differentiated from panic disorder (Table 138-3). Panic attacks can occur in the context of multiple illnesses, and do not necessarily represent PD. The hallmark difficulty in recognizing PD is that patients usually do not complain of anxiety, but present with somatic symptoms, with estimates of 10 to 15 symptoms at presentation. The most common cluster of symptoms is cardiac, including chest pain and tachycardia. GI and pulmonary symptoms are also common, and nearly half of these patients will report neurologic symptoms (headache,

Figure 138-1

Panic Disorder

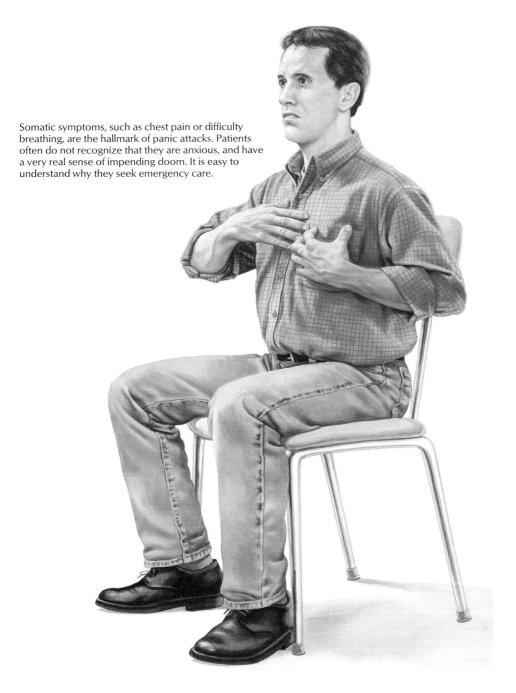

Somatic symptoms, such as chest pain or difficulty breathing, are the hallmark of panic attacks. Patients often do not recognize that they are anxious, and have a very real sense of impending doom. It is easy to understand why they seek emergency care.

Table 138-1
Other Common Anxiety Disorders

	Social Phobia	Generalized Anxiety Disorder	Posttraumatic Stress Disorder
Defining features	Excessive fear of public scrutiny in single or multiple situations; may have panic attacks	Unrealistic or excessive worry about common life circumstances; chronic autonomic hyperarousal	Status post threat to life or body -followed by intrusive memories, avoidance, and hyperarousal
Lifetime prevalence	5% to 13%	5% (2:1 female)	1% to 14% (Varies with specific trauma)
Common comorbidities	Depression, substance abuse	Depression, substance abuse, panic disorder	Substance abuse, depression, somatoform disorders
Treatment	*SSRI, †benzodiazepines, CBT	*SSRI, †benzos	*SSRI, anti-adrenergic agents (clonidine, propranolol)
Referral threshold	Low- therapy enhances medications	Depends on symptom severity and number of comorbidities	Low- patients are usually time intensive

Benzo, Benzodiazepines; CBT, Cognitive behavioral therapy; SSRI, selective serotonin reuptake inhibitor.
*See Table 138-4 for SSRI dosing.
†See Table 138-4 for benzodiazepine dosing.

Table 138-2
Panic Attack Diagnostic Criteria

A discrete period of intense fear or discomfort, in which 4 (or more) of the following symptoms developed abruptly and reached a peak within 10 minutes:

1. Palpitations, pounding heart, or accelerated heart rate
2. Sweating
3. Trembling or shaking
4. Sensations of shortness of breath or smothering
5. Feeling of choking
6. Chest pain or discomfort
7. Nausea or abdominal pain
8. Feeling dizzy, unsteady, lightheaded, or faint
9. Paresthesias (numbness or tingling sensations)
10. Chills or hot flushes
11. Derealization (feelings of unreality) or depersonalization (being detached from oneself)
12. Fear of losing control or going crazy
13. Fear of dying

Adapted from *The Diagnostic and Statistical and Manual of Mental Disorders*, fourth edition, text revision. Copyright © 2000 American Psychiatric Association.

Table 138-3
Panic Disorder Diagnostic Criteria

A. Both (1) and (2)

1. Recurrent unexpected panic attacks
2. At least one of the attacks has been followed by 1 month (or more) of one (or more) of the following:

   a. Persistent concern about having additional attacks
   b. Worry about the implications of the attack or its consequences (e.g., losing control, having a heart attack, going crazy)
   c. A significant change in behavior related to the attacks

B. The panic attacks are not due to the direct physiologic effects of a substance (e.g., a drug of abuse, a medication) or a general medical condition (e.g., hyperthyroidism).

C. The panic attacks are not better accounted for by another mental disorder, such as social phobia, specific phobia, obsessive-compulsive disorder, or posttraumatic stress disorder

Table 138-4
Agoraphobia Diagnostic Criteria

A. Anxiety about being in places or situations from which escape might be difficult (or embarrassing) or in which help may not be available in the event of having an unexpected or situationally predisposed panic attack or panic-like symptoms. Agoraphobic fears typically involve characteristic clusters of situations that include being outside the home alone, being in a crowd or standing in a line, being on a bridge, or traveling in a bus, train, or automobile.

B. The situations are avoided (e.g., travel is restricted) or else are endured with marked distress or with anxiety about having a panic attack or panic-like symptoms, or require the presence of a companion.

Adapted from *The Diagnostic and Statistical and Manual of Mental Disorders*, fourth edition, text revision. Copyright © 2000 American Psychiatric Association.

dizziness most frequent). PD may also be complicated by agoraphobia (Table 138-4).

DIFFERENTIAL DIAGNOSIS
Psychiatric

Major depression and bipolar disorder often present with predominant anxiety symptoms and should always be considered as a primary diagnosis in the differential diagnosis of the anxious patient. Depression also develops later in life in one third to one half of patients with PD. Many drugs of abuse, including cocaine, marijuana, amphetamines, and caffeine may also induce panic states independent of panic disorder.

Medical

PD and anxiety symptoms coexist with one third or more of several common conditions, including atypical chest pain, Parkinson's disease, irritable bowel syndrome, and chronic obstructive pulmonary disease. The diagnosis of PD should not be conceptualized as mutually exclusive from "medical" illness. Current medications, including sympathomimetic medications such as cold/allergy preparations, should also be investigated as causes of anxiety symptoms. Alcohol and other sedative withdrawal can also cause anxiety symptoms.

DIAGNOSTIC APPROACH

A high index of suspicion for PD and related disorders should be maintained for patients who are

Common Medical Conditions Associated with Anxiety/Panic Symptoms

Anemia, angina, arrhythmias, asthma, congestive heart failure, electrolyte disturbance, hyperthyroidism, hypoxia, hypoglycemia, myocardial infarction, parathyroid disorder, pulmonary embolism, seizures, transient ischemic attacks, vertigo.

young, have multiple somatic complaints, and visit the doctor frequently. A search for PD, depression, and substance abuse should be a priority. (PD sufferers are more than 4 times as likely to abuse alcohol.) If a primary anxiety disorder seems likely, defer extensive system-specific workups (endoscopy, cardiac catheterization, etc.). A thorough medical, psychiatric, family, and social history will usually lead to the correct diagnosis.

The medical workup includes physical examination, with thorough neurologic examination; medication history (include over-the-counter medications); ECG (if greater than 40, having current chest pain, or significant family history of heart disease.); and selected laboratory tests including: CBC, chemistry panel, thyroid stimulating hormone. If the patient is older than 40, non-psychiatric medical diagnoses should be suspected and excluded.

MANAGEMENT AND TREATMENT

Significant evidence has emerged to guide the treatment of anxiety disorders, specifically PD. The greatest challenge remains in detecting these disorders and in prescribing adequate treatment. (Table 138-5) Most importantly, clinicians must routinely consider the possibility of a PD diagnosis. Once detected, the goals of treatment include reduction of the frequency and intensity of symptoms, and management of the anticipatory anxiety associated with panic attacks. Both medications and behavioral therapy have proven equally efficacious in psychiatric populations. Pharmacotherapy in PD has been well studied, with similar monotherapeutic efficacy among the tricyclic antidepressants, the monoamine oxidase inhibitors, high potency benzodiazepines, and selec-

Table 138-5
First-line Medications for Panic Disorder

Class	Agent	Starting Dose	Maintenance
SSRI			
	citalopram	10 mg/day	20–40 mg/day
	fluoxetine*	5–10 mg/day	20–80 mg/day
	fluvoxamine	25 mg/day	50–300 mg/day
	paroxetine	10 mg/day	20–60 mg/day
	sertraline	25 mg/day	50–200 mg/day
Benzodiazepines			
	alprazolam	0.25–0.5 mg tid	2–6 mg/day total
	clonazepam	0.5 mg bid-tid	1–4 mg/day recommended max.
	lorazepam	0.5–1.0 mg bid-tid	2–10 mg/day total

*Fluoxetine has a long half life and may not be the best choice for a patient with known sensitivity to drug side effects.

tive serotonin reuptake inhibitors (SSRIs). However, side effects, potential drug interactions, dietary restrictions, and risk for dependence have limited the utility of the first three classes. SSRIs have supplanted these older agents for first-line therapy due to a more favorable side effect profile. The 3- to-4-week latency in response in SSRI treatment of depression may be shorter for panic disorder (2 to 3 weeks), but PD patients generally have greater sensitivity to side effects.

Benzodiazepines, which have a rapid onset of action, (several days) are best used adjunctively in the acutely ill patient to bridge delayed response to SSRIs. Alprazolam, clonazepam, and lorazepam have the most data supporting their use. Prescribe adequate *standing* doses of benzodiazepines as opposed to *as-needed* doses.

Cognitive behavioral therapy (CBT) (psychoeducation, symptom monitoring, breathing training, cognitive restructuring focusing on correction of catastrophic misinterpretations of bodily sensations, and exposure) designed to address panic symptoms has proven efficacy, but requires trained therapists and committed patients. This may be an important referral point for patients desiring a non-pharmacologic intervention. Patients should be informed that studies show that the best success is seen with the combination of medications and CBT.

Response rates vary, but controlled trials suggest that 60% to 80% patients become "panic free" during any proven treatment, with improved outcomes as treatment is extended. PD is a chronic illness usually requiring maintenance therapy and often characterized by residual symptoms. Optimal length of treatment has not been fully elucidated, and relapse is common, particularly without maintenance therapy. Agoraphobia and other psychiatric comorbidities are thought to be predictors of poorer outcomes. PD, particularly in association with depression and substance abuse, also places the patient at increased risk for suicide.

Optimal management of PD includes assessing for suicide risk, evaluating and acknowledging the degree of functional impairment, establishing and maintaining a therapeutic alliance, patient and family education, communicating with other physicians (which plays a large role in preventing unnecessary diagnostic tests), and helping the patient learn how to address early signs of relapse. Patient should be encouraged to limit consumption of caffeine and sympathomimetic drugs, and to abstain from use of illicit substances.

Use of SSRIs in the treatment of anxiety disorders should begin at the *lowest* possible dose, be titrated slowly, but assertively to the maximum dose necessary for symptom improvement, which is often higher than that required for depression (start low, go slow, but go. . . and go). Adequate duration of this dose is 6 weeks before determining medication failure.

Consider referral to a psychiatrist for diagnostic clarification (consultation); for suicidal patients;

after two trials of first-line treatment have failed; for treatment of agoraphobia; when psychotherapy is indicated (e.g., significant life stressors, limited support systems); when patients have psychiatric comorbidity that is unstable (e.g., unremitting depressive symptoms, active substance abuse); or when optimal management exceeds the time constraints of the primary care setting.

FUTURE DIRECTIONS

The complexity and challenge presented by anxious patients must be embraced and integrated into primary care. Researchers should continue their search for new therapeutic agents, especially given that 20% to 40% of patients may not respond to current therapies. Neuroimaging technologies are quickly evolving to help answer some of these questions, and psychotherapeutic principles are being equally explored. Efficient and feasible methods to detect these common disorders must also be further investigated. Interdisciplinary communication and multimodal interventions will continue to be crucial in the successful management of the anxious patient.

REFERENCES

Practice guideline for the treatment of patients with panic disorder. Work Group on Panic Disorder. American Psychiatric Association. *Am J Psychiatry.* 1998;155(suppl):1–34.

American Psychiatric Association. *Diagnostic and Statistical Manual of Mental Disorders.* 4th ed, text rev. Washington, DC: American Psychiatric Association; 2000.

Anxiety Disorders Association of America Web site. Available at: http://www.adaa.org. Accessed March 3, 2003.

Ballenger JC. Current treatments of the anxiety disorders in adults. *Biol Psychiatry.* 1999;46:1579–1594.

Ballenger JC. Panic disorder in the medical setting. *J Clin Psychiatry.* 1997;58(suppl 2): 3–19.

Goddard AW, Charney DS. Toward an integrated neurobiology of panic disorder. *J Clin Psychiatry.* 1997;58(suppl 2):4–12.

Katon W, Vitaliano PP, Russo J, Jones M, Anderson K. Panic disorder. Spectrum of severity and somatization. *J Nerv Ment Dis.* 1987;175:12–19.

National Alliance for the Mentally Ill Web site. Available at: http://www.nami.org. Accessed March 3, 2003.

National Institute of Mental Health (NIMH) Web site. Available at: http://www.nimh.nih.gov. Accessed March 3, 2003.

Chapter 139
Delirium

Michael A. Hill

A delirium (also known as acute organic brain syndrome, metabolic or toxic encephalopathy, toxic brain syndrome, or acute confusional state) is a global physiologic disturbance of cortical function associated with disturbances of consciousness, attention, cognition, and perception that develops acutely or subacutely and tends to fluctuate during the course of a day. It should be considered a life-threatening emergency, and the recognition of the condition and the search for and mitigation of causative factors should be the central treatment goals.

Historically, a lack of clear criteria for defining delirium has confounded prevalence estimates, but it is a common condition by any measure. Costs are estimated to be $8 billion annually. Delirium is very common in a hospital setting, occurring in 10% to 30% of all admissions, 30% to 40% of the elderly, 30% to 40% of AIDS patients, up to 50% of post-surgical patients, and in many burn unit patients. It is also common in patients with dementia (25% to 80% of hospitalized patients with delirium have dementia, and almost half of all dementia patients admitted will have a delirium.), in terminally ill patients (80%), and in nursing home patients (6% to 7%).

Risk factors include age, preexisting brain damage, CNS disease (especially dementia), and drug intoxication. Predictive risks for inpatients are use of physical restraints, malnutrition, more than 3 new medications, use of a bladder catheter, and/or any iatrogenic event.

ETIOLOGY AND PATHOGENESIS

Anything that can cause general cortical dysfunction can cause a delirium. Causes can be grossly classified as due to a general medical condition, substance abuse or withdrawal, or as having an unspecified etiology. The most common cause in a hospital setting is multifactorial.

Causes of delirium include the following:
- Drug-induced (neuroleptic malignant syndrome [NMS], anticholinergic delirium, idiosyncratic neurotoxicity, combination effects such as antihistamines + narcotics)
- Metabolic abnormalities (hypoxia, anemia, hypoglycemia, hepatic encephalopathy, uremia)
- Infectious processes (viral encephalopathy, meningitis)
- Seizures (partial status, delirium following electroconvulsive therapy (ECT), interictal states)
- Endocrine disorders (thyrotoxicosis)
- Sensory deprivation, REM sleep deprivation, temperature dysregulation (high fevers)
- Acute vitamin deficiencies (thiamine → Wernicke's encephalopathy)
- Toxins (organophosphates, CO, organic solvents)
- Intoxications (hallucinogens, stimulants, cocaine, anticholinergics)
- Withdrawal states (alcohol → delirium tremens, sedative-hypnotics, opioids)
- CNS disorders (tumors, strokes, degenerative conditions, head trauma, vasculitides)

CLINICAL PRESENTATION

The essential feature of delirium is a reduced level of consciousness with impaired ability to sustain, shift, or focus (concentrate) attention. The condition often develops quickly and usually fluctuates over time. Because of this impaired "condition" of the brain, a number of other signs and symptoms can be expected, including the following:
- Disorientation to time, place, and situation with nighttime worsening ("sundowning")
- Impaired recent memory, visuospatial impairments, dysarthria, aphasia, dysgraphia, dysnomia
- Perceptual disturbances (misinterpretations, illusions, hallucinations [especially visual])
- Disorganized thinking with rambling speech,

DELIRIUM

irrelevant answers, and/or delusions
- Emotional lability, fearfulness
- Psychomotor disturbances including hyperactivity (often with psychotic symptoms), hypoactivity (with somnolence), or mixed presentations
- EEG with generalized slowing (except in alcohol/sedative-hypnotic withdrawal syndromes)
- Sleep-wake cycle disturbances
- Findings on physical examination reflecting specific causative factors such as cranial nerve palsies with Wernicke's encephalopathy and asterixis with hepatic encephalopathy

The onset may be acute or subacute, with prodromal symptoms of restlessness, anxiety, irritability, distractibility, and/or sleep disturbance progressing to delirium over 24 to 72 hours. Symptoms may last from less than 1 week to many months, with most resolving within 10 to 12 days, though 15% last longer than 30 days. Symptoms often persist after discharge. Persistent cognitive deficits after maximal recovery are quite common in elderly patients and in patients with AIDS and may represent an unmasking of dementia. Delirium in the medically ill is associated with significant morbidity such as pneumonia, decubitus ulcers, longer hospital stays, and increased postoperative complications. Twenty-five percent of patients with delirium die within 6 months, and the mortality rate for hospitalized patients with delirium is 3 to 7 times higher than for those patients without delirium (matched for age and illness severity). Quiet (hypoactive) delirium is no less serious and, in at least one study, was associated with higher mortality rates.

DIFFERENTIAL DIAGNOSIS

The differential diagnoses for a sudden cognitive mental status change include the following:
- An evolving or progressing dementia
- A delirium alone
- A primary psychiatric disorder with thought process impairments (pseudodelirium*)
- A delirium superimposed on dementia; this latter circumstance is so common that all acute mental status changes in a person with dementia should be considered a delirium until proven otherwise.

*Psychosis with severe cognitive disorganization can look like a delirium with disorientation, memory impairments, and general confusion. However, a decrease in level of consciousness is not seen with psychosis alone.

DIAGNOSTIC APPROACH

All patients with delirium of uncertain cause require blood chemistries (electrolytes, glucose, calcium, magnesium, PO_4, albumin, BUN, aspartate aminotransferase, alanine aminotransferase, bilirubin, alkaline phosphatase), CBC with differential, ECG, chest radiograph, measurement of O_2 saturation or arterial blood gases, urinalysis with culture and sensitivity, and urine drug/toxicology screen.

When clinically indicated, other specific tests should be considered: VDRL or FTA, heavy metal screen, B_{12} and folate, ANA, urine porphyrins, blood ammonia, HIV, thyroid stimulating hormone, blood cultures, medication blood levels (e.g., digoxin, lithium, phenobarbital, diphenylhydantoin, theophylline, tricyclics), lumbar puncture, neuroimaging (CT or MRI), and EEG.

MANAGEMENT AND THERAPY

Early recognition of delirium may offer significant opportunities to prevent disability and irreversible deterioration. Psychiatric symptoms should not be allowed to cause reduced medical surveillance. Delirium should always be considered in all acute mental status changes. By one estimate, 32% to 67% of all deliria go undetected.

Medications

Medications useful in controlling symptoms or in increasing patient comfort include the following:

Antipsychotics

Antipsychotics are useful for psychosis, agitation, and emotional lability. They are shown to be superior to benzodiazepines in effectiveness (except in sedative-hypnotic/alcohol withdrawal syndromes) with fewer side effects in head-to-head studies. The most commonly used agents include:
- *Haloperidol* (1 to 2 mg every 4 hours [0.25 to 0.50 mg for elderly]) with titration to higher doses as indicated for continued symptoms. Can be given orally, IM or IV. Extrapyramidal symptoms are less severe with IV dosing. IV dosing should be no more than 5 mg/min to reduce cardiac complications)
- *Droperidol* has a more rapid onset of action, is more sedating, and has similar dosing guidelines
- *Risperidone* (0.25 to 1 mg every 4 hours orally)

General Treatment Strategies

- Identify causative factors and mitigate if possible.
- Ensure safety and comfort of the patient and others.
- Avoid restraints if possible, but use if necessary for safety.
- Improve function/decrease symptoms (consider medications for severe symptoms).
- Reduce factors that may exacerbate delirium (such as anticholinergic medicines).
- Provide an optimal level of environmental stimulation by ensuring that the room is adequately lighted, including the use of night-lights in the evening.
- Avoid over- or under-stimulation. Keep exposure to chaotic environments to a minimum because many delirious patients are hyperresponsive to stimuli.
- Reduce sensory impairments (let patients use glasses and hearing aids if the clinical state allows).
- Provide environmental cues to facilitate orientation (each room should have a large, easily seen calendar and clock).
- Remind the patient of the day, date, and situation frequently. Reminders of who people are may be necessary as well.
- Bring familiar items from home into the room if possible.
- Encourage frequent interactions with staff and family.
- Consider telling the patient that he or she is confused and disoriented.
- Eliminate nonessential medications and ensure adequate hydration and nutrition.

Antipsychotics should not be used in NMS. If QTc > 450 msec, cardiac status should be further assessed before beginning or continuing use of these agents. Antipsychotics should also be avoided in anticholinergic delirium.

Benzodiazepines

These agents can be useful for agitation and/or fearfulness. They are used as monotherapy for sedative-hypnotic and alcohol withdrawal deliria or adjunctively with antipsychotics if antipsychotics alone are not working for agitation. Lorazepam is the drug of choice because it is short-acting and has no active metabolites. Benzodiazepines should be avoided in patients with hepatic encephalopathy. Remember that benzodiazepines can promote amnesia and respiratory depression.

Other Treatments

Anticholinesterases (physostigmine, donepezil, rivastigmine) are useful in anticholinergic delirium, but may work for other types of deliria as well since underactivity in brainstem cholinergic neurons is common. In alcohol withdrawal the problem may be catecholaminergic overactivation). An example of dosing is the following: physostigmine: 1 to 2 mg IV or IM or continuous IV infusion at 3 mg/hr, or donepezil: 5 to 10 mg p.o. once daily. *Thiamine* is used in Wernicke's encephalopathy. *ECT* may be useful for refractory NMS or prolonged delirium.

FUTURE DIRECTIONS

For delirium, as for many of the reversible causes of dementia, the improvement in treatment will parallel advances in the recognition and management of the medical conditions that are causal. Investigations are underway to examine whether memory-enhancing agents that work through cholinergic mechanisms to reverse the symptoms of anticholinergic delirium can be beneficial in other types of deliria as well. Excitotoxic neuromodulators such as memantine are also being investigated for both dementia and delirium as a way of limiting damage that results from the brain's intrinsic attempts to compensate for degenerating systems.

REFERENCES

Practice guideline for the treatment of patients with delirium. American Psychiatric Association. *Am J Psychiatry.* 1999; 156(suppl):1–20.

American Academy of Neurology Web site. Available at: http://www.aan.com. Accessed March 4, 2003.

American Association of Geriatric Psychiatry Web site. Available at: http://www.aagpgpa.org. Accessed March 4, 2003.

The American Geriatrics Society Web site. Available at: http://www.americangeriatrics.org. Accessed March 4, 2003.

American Psychiatric Association Web site. Available at: http://www.psych.org. Accessed March 4, 2003.

Coffey CE, Cummings JL, eds. *The American Psychiatric Press Textbook of Geriatric Neuropsychiatry.* 2nd ed. Washington, DC: American Psychiatric Press; 2000.

Lipowski ZJ. Delirium in the elderly patient. *N Engl J Med.* 1989:320:578–582.

Chapter 140
Dementia

Michael A. Hill

Dementia is an acquired syndrome characterized by multiple cognitive deficits that include short-term memory impairment and at least one of the following:

Aphasia: language impairments (especially naming or word-finding problems).

Apraxia: motor memory impairments (e.g., dressing difficulties).

Agnosia: sensory memory impairments (especially impaired visuospatial skills and recognition)

Abstract thinking or executive function impairments: planning and organizing deficits.

These deficits must be sufficient to cause impairment in social or occupational functioning and must not be explainable by another medical or psychiatric disorder.

The prevalence of dementia increases dramatically with age. It is estimated that between 2 million and 4 million people in the United States suffer from dementia. As consensus has developed on the diagnostic criteria, the numbers have begun to stabilize into the ranges shown in Table 140-1.

Dementias can be classified as *primary versus secondary* on the basis of the pathophysiology leading to damaged brain tissue (e.g., primary degenerative dementias versus vascular dementias); *cortical versus subcortical,* depending on the cerebral location of the primary deficits (e.g., Alzheimer's dementia versus the dementia of Parkinson's disease) (Table 140-2); *reversible versus irreversible,* depending on optimal treatment expectations; and *early-onset versus late-onset* (before age 65 versus after age 65).

The concept of irreversibility is a nebulous one. Many formerly "irreversible" dementias such as the dementia of Alzheimer's disease may in fact be "arrestable" or at least slowed down. Some reversible dementias (such as that caused by vitamin B_{12} deficiency) may in fact lead to irreversible brain damage if allowed to progress untreated. Many of these dementias are better thought of as "modifiable" rather than as fully reversible. Still, the concept of reversibility is a useful one as it directs the workup of patients with dementia symptoms.

COMMON DEMENTIAS

The dementia caused by Alzheimer's disease is the most common form, accounting for 50% to 75% of all dementias. The pathophysiology consists of higher than expected concentrations of neuritic plaques (abnormal insoluble amyloid protein fragments) and neurofibrillary tangles (disturbed tau-microtubule complexes), especially in the hippocampal and the posterior temporoparietal areas. There is cholinergic system degeneration, with decreased acetylcholine levels and significant loss of neurons in certain areas (such as in the nucleus basalis of Meynert) (Figure 140-1). Degeneration may begin in the entorhinal cortex and progress to other limbic structures. Risk factors include age, family history, Down's syndrome, head trauma, female gender, genetics (apolipoprotein E-4 [APO E-4] allele on chromosome 19 for late-onset disease, autosomal dominant gene mutations on chromosomes 1, 14, and 21 for early-onset disease), ethnicity (African Americans > whites), late-onset depression, and depressive pseudodementia (Figure 140-2). Protective factors

Table 140-1
Prevalence Estimates for Dementia

Age (y)	Prevalence Estimates for Dementia*	Age (y)	Incidence Estimates for Dementia
>65	5%–10%	65-74	0.5%–1%
>75	10%–20%	75-84	2%–4%
>85	25%–50%	85+	6%–8%
>95	40%–70%†		

* Lower prevalence estimates often reflect the exclusion of mild dementias
† Limited data suggest prevalence may level off or decline after age 100

Table 140-2
Less Common Dementias

Primary Degenerative Dementias

Lewy body dementias (may account for 7% to 26% of dementias)
Frontotemporal dementias (Pick's disease, Amyotrophic lateral sclerosis dementias, Huntington's disease)

Neurologic Disorders Associated with Dementia

Progressive supranuclear palsy (profound apathy, downward eye gaze, paralysis)
Dementia due to Parkinson's disease (20% to 60% of patients) (Figure 140-4)
Normal-pressure hydrocephalus (dementia, incontinence, ataxia)
Neoplasms (frontal and temporal tumors especially)
Head trauma (e.g., dementia pugilistica)
Subdural hematoma (chronic), CNS vasculitis, lupus cerebritis
Demyelinating disorders such as MS

Infectious Causes of Dementia

Neurosyphilis, Lyme disease
Viral, parasitic, bacterial, and fungal meningitis or encephalitis
Postencephalitic dementia (especially following herpes encephalitis)
Opportunistic infections or brain abscess
Human prion disease (transmissible spongiform encephalopathies including Creutzfeldt-Jakob disease [CJD], variant CJD ["mad-cow disease"], and kuru)

General Medical Causes of Dementia

Thyroid and adrenal disease
Vitamin deficiency states (thiamine, niacin, or B_{12})
Metabolic derangements (dialysis dementia, hepatic encephalopathy, hypercalcemia, glucose dysregulation, electrolyte disturbances, posthypoxia)
Medications (sedatives, antihypertensives, cardiac drugs, narcotics, anticholinergics)
Whipple's disease, sarcoidosis, Wilson's disease
Toxins (heavy metals, organic poisons)

include education, anti-inflammatory agents, estrogen replacement therapy, smoking, and APO E-3.

Vascular dementias (15% to 20%) include Binswanger's dementia, multi-infarct dementia, and dementias caused by anoxic damage, coronary artery bypass graft surgery, and inflammatory diseases. Age, hypertension, diabetes, and hyperlipidemia are the documented risk factors.

General alcohol-related dementias are common. Korsakoff's dementia is comparatively uncommon.

HIV dementia is the most common dementia in those under the age of 55.

CLINICAL PRESENTATION

Dementia is always associated with cognitive disturbances (memory and language) and functional impairments. Visuospatial impairments and behavioral disturbances are usually seen as well. Specific symptoms vary by type of dementia and include the following:

Memory impairments: difficulty learning or retaining new information (repeated conversations), information retrieval deficits (being unable to recall names), personal episodic memory impairment (misplacing items), and problems

Figure 140-1   Microscopic Pathology in Alzheimer's Disease

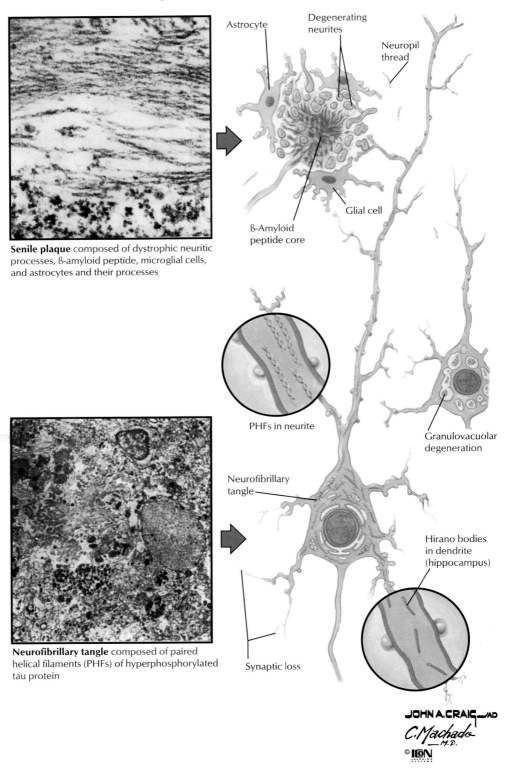

Senile plaque composed of dystrophic neuritic processes, ß-amyloid peptide, microglial cells, and astrocytes and their processes

Astrocyte

Degenerating neurites

Neuropil thread

Glial cell

ß-Amyloid peptide core

PHFs in neurite

Granulovacuolar degeneration

Neurofibrillary tangle

Hirano bodies in dendrite (hippocampus)

Synaptic loss

Neurofibrillary tangle composed of paired helical filaments (PHFs) of hyperphosphorylated tau protein

JOHN A.CRAIG___AD

C.Machado
___M.D.

© ICN
LEARNING
SYSTEMS

Figure 140-2

Possible Factors in Development and Progression of Alzheimer's Disease

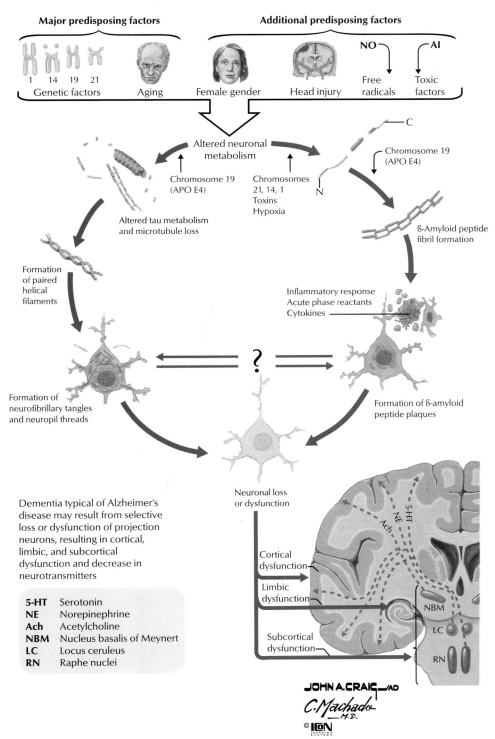

Major predisposing factors

1 14 19 21
Genetic factors — Aging

Additional predisposing factors

Female gender — Head injury — NO → Free radicals — AI → Toxic factors

Altered neuronal metabolism

Chromosome 19 (APO E4)

Chromosomes 21, 14, 1
Toxins
Hypoxia

C

Chromosome 19 (APO E4)

Altered tau metabolism and microtubule loss

ß-Amyloid peptide fibril formation

Formation of paired helical filaments

Inflammatory response
Acute phase reactants
Cytokines

?

Formation of neurofibrillary tangles and neuropil threads

Formation of ß-amyloid peptide plaques

Neuronal loss or dysfunction

Dementia typical of Alzheimer's disease may result from selective loss or dysfunction of projection neurons, resulting in cortical, limbic, and subcortical dysfunction and decrease in neurotransmitters

Cortical dysfunction

Limbic dysfunction

Subcortical dysfunction

5-HT	Serotonin
NE	Norepinephrine
Ach	Acetylcholine
NBM	Nucleus basalis of Meynert
LC	Locus ceruleus
RN	Raphe nuclei

NBM
LC
RN

JOHN A. CRAIG AD
C. Machado M.D.
© ICN

with declarative (or semantic) memory (what) more so than with procedural memory (how).

Language deficits: list-generation deficits (seen especially in Alzheimer's disease), word-finding problems, and use of less complex sentence structure. Auditory comprehension is usually preserved.

Visuospatial impairments: visual recognition impairments (not recognizing relatives), spatial deficits (getting lost in familiar surroundings), and 3-D drawing deficits.

Functional impairment and performance on cognitive testing may not correlate strongly early in the course of dementia; an individual may function reasonably well in many areas despite deficits on testing early in the illness. The rate and specific pattern of loss will vary by individual. Deficits appear first in instrumental activities of daily living (IADLs) such as managing finances, driving, using the telephone, shopping, working, taking medications, and keeping appointments. Eventually deficits appear in self-maintenance skills or activities of daily living (ADLs) such as feeding, grooming, dressing, eating, and toileting.

Behavioral symptoms: Behavioral symptoms are nearly universal and often are the main focus of families' concerns and complaints. Caregivers' inability to manage these types of symptoms is highly correlated with the need for institutional placement of the patient. *Personality change* commonly occurs early. Symptoms include passivity (e.g., apathy, social withdrawal), disinhibition (e.g., inappropriate sexual behavior or language), and self-centered behaviors (e.g., childishness and loss of generosity). *Agitation* is very common and frequently worsens as the illness progresses. It includes agitated speech (25%), physical aggression (30%), and nonaggressive behaviors such as wandering and pacing (25% to 50%). Aggression strongly correlates with caregiver burnout, especially when wandering is also present.

Associated features of dementia include depression (40% to 50% of patients with Alzheimer's disease; percentage may be higher in vascular dementia); psychotic delusions (30% to 40%), typically paranoia about theft and infidelity; perceptual disturbances, often visual (20% to 40% in Alzheimer's disease, possibly higher in *Lewy body dementia*); and sleep disturbances (>50%) such as insomnia and sleep-wake cycle disruptions.

Course and Staging of Dementia

Most dementias have an insidious onset, with progressive worsening over many years. Some dementias have a more fulminant course (e.g., the dementia accompanying Creutzfeldt-Jakob disease), and others may remit spontaneously or with treatment (e.g., dementias caused by B_{12} deficiency, and hypothyroidism).

Alzheimer's dementia has a predictable progression that can be staged. Cognitive and social skills are often lost in the reverse order in which they were developed. Individuals may appear to function well on a superficial social level long after they have become unable to handle complex decision-making tasks such as financial planning. Alzheimer's patients typically live 8 to 10 years after diagnosis, and diagnosis often occurs 3 to 4 years after symptoms appear. *Vascular dementias* may show a stepwise progression and are often associated with focal neurologic findings (Figure 140-3). They often have a shorter course than Alzheimer's type dementia. Alzheimer's disease can coexist with vascular dementia, a condition that is referred to as a *mixed dementia*. There is some evidence that the clinical symptoms of Alzheimer's disease may correlate with the extent of underlying cerebrovascular disease in both Alzheimer's and mixed-type dementias. Common causes of death in late-stage dementia include aspiration pneumonia, sepsis from stasis ulcers, and urinary tract infections.

DIFFERENTIAL DIAGNOSIS

The differential diagnoses for memory impairment include:

Amnestic syndrome: short-term memory impairment without significant or new impairments in other cognitive domains (e.g., alcohol amnestic syndrome)

Delirium: impairments of consciousness and attention that lead to a host of cognitive deficits including (but not limited to) those seen in dementia.

Mental retardation: impaired intellectual capacities, present before the age of 18, that may or may not affect memory

Pseudodementia (also known as the *dementia syndrome of depression*): Cognitive impairment that occurs in the context of another psychiatric disorder (such as depression), often caused by decreased concentration and/or poor effort during

Figure 140-3

Clinical Characteristics of Vascular (Multiinfarct) Dementia

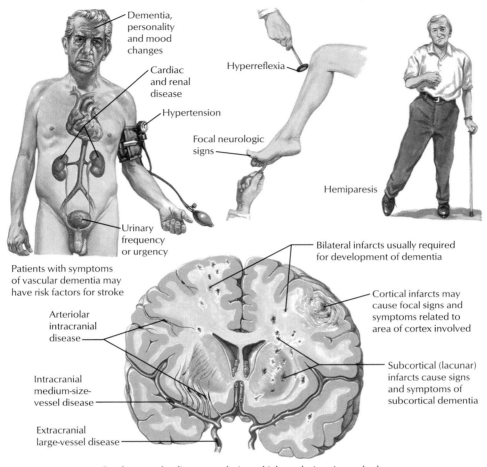

Dementia, personality and mood changes

Cardiac and renal disease

Hypertension

Urinary frequency or urgency

Hyperreflexia

Focal neurologic signs

Hemiparesis

Patients with symptoms of vascular dementia may have risk factors for stroke

Arteriolar intracranial disease

Intracranial medium-size-vessel disease

Extracranial large-vessel disease

Bilateral infarcts usually required for development of dementia

Cortical infarcts may cause focal signs and symptoms related to area of cortex involved

Subcortical (lacunar) infarcts cause signs and symptoms of subcortical dementia

Cerebrovascular disease results in multiple occlusions in cerebral vascular tree, causing scattered cortical and subcortical infarcts

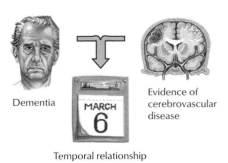

Dementia

MARCH 6

Temporal relationship

Evidence of cerebrovascular disease

Triad of characteristics that suggests vascular etiology

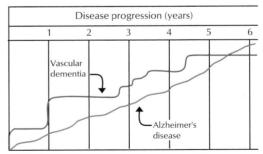

Disease progression (years)

Vascular dementia

Alzheimer's disease

Clinical progression. Vascular dementia exhibits abrupt onset and stepwise progression in contrast to gradual onset and progression of Alzheimer's disease

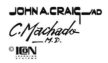

JOHN A. CRAIG—MD

C. Machado —M.D.

© ICN

Figure 140-4

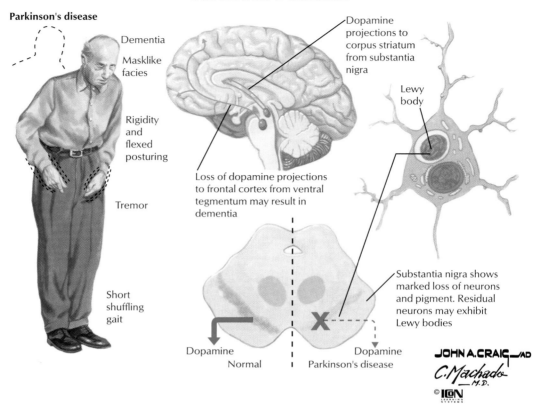

Subcortical Dementias

Parkinson's disease

Dementia

Masklike facies

Rigidity and flexed posturing

Tremor

Short shuffling gait

Dopamine projections to corpus striatum from substantia nigra

Lewy body

Loss of dopamine projections to frontal cortex from ventral tegmentum may result in dementia

Substantia nigra shows marked loss of neurons and pigment. Residual neurons may exhibit Lewy bodies

Dopamine Normal

Dopamine Parkinson's disease

JOHN A. CRAIG—MD
C. Machado—M.D.
© ICON

testing. Among elderly patients with depressive pseudodementia (regardless of response to antidepressants), 50% will develop an irreversible dementia within 3 to 5 years.

Age-related cognitive decline: Age-associated memory impairment (AAMI), mild cognitive impairment (MCI) and benign senescent forgetfulness are mild impairments in memory that are not associated with significant functional impairments. However, the incidence of progression to dementia in these conditions is about 10% per year.

Receptive aphasia: impaired cognitive functioning due to failure to understand speech.

DIAGNOSTIC APPROACH

A careful history from the patient and a reliable informant is critical for early detection of dementia. Screening includes a physical examination, with particular focus on the neurologic exam and cognitive testing. Cognitive testing tools are helpful for screening for dementia and for monitoring progression. Available cognitive tests include the

Mini Mental State Exam (MMSE—scores below 24 to 27 can be significant depending on patients' premorbid abilities), the 6-Item Blessed Orientation-Memory-Concentration Test (BOMC), and functional assessment tools such as the Functional Activities Questionnaire (FAQ). Full neuropsychologic assessment should be considered when cognitive testing and functional assessment results are at odds; early dementia is strongly suspected in a high-IQ individual with a normal MMSE (or equivalent tool); or mild impairment is seen in those with low IQ, limited education, difficulty with English, or minority racial or ethnic background. Also consider neuropsychologic testing when impairments are mild and of less than 6 months' duration, there are no functional impairments, or competency must be determined or legal puposes. (Table 140-3)

Diagnostic Workup

A diagnostic workup should be done to rule out disorders other than dementia, to identify

Table 140-3
Dementia Types and Diagnosis

Dementia Type	Suggested by	Dementia Type	Suggested by
Alzheimer's disease	· Insidious onset and progressive worsening · Prominent memory retention deficits early in course · Onset after age 60, no focal signs or gait disturbances · Exclusion of reversible dementias · Anosmia	Vascular dementia	· Relatively abrupt onset and stepwise or fluctuating course · Prior history of stroke, or hypertensive nephropathy · Focal neurologic signs and/or symptoms · Emotional lability, depression · Somatic complaints, with relative preservation of personality
Lewy body dementia	· Executive function impairments > memory impairments early on · Fluctuating deficits day-to-day · Visual hallucinations (well-formed images) · Mild parkinsonism	Dementia syndrome of depression (pseudodementia)	· Memory/concentration impairments without apraxia, agnosia, and aphasia · Apathy, low motivation, and other neurovegetative signs of depression · Exaggerated complaints of memory impairment, poor effort in testing
Frontotemporal dementia	· Prominent early personality changes, with apathy and antisocial behavior · Peculiar behavior and verbal stereotypes such as "Let's go, let's go" · Preserved visuospatial skills	HIV/AIDS dementia	· Forgetfulness, psychomotor slowing, poor concentration, impaired problem solving, apathy · Neurologic signs, e.g., tremor, ataxia, hyperreflexia, frontal release signs, impaired rapid repetitive movements
Subcortical dementia (Figure 140-4)	· Psychomotor slowing, frontal systems dysfunction, short-term memory impairment · Depression and apathy · Neurologic findings, e.g., parkinsonism, ataxia, urinary incontinence · Language difficulties less pronounced until late in course	Delirium (as opposed to dementia)	· Acute or subacute onset · Impaired consciousness and attention · Fluctuating course · Disorganized thinking · Medical illness · Mental status change in patient with preexisting dementia

reversible (13%) or treatable dementias (such as those due to normal-pressure hydrocephalus, thyroid disease, or psychiatric disorders), and to clarify the specific dementia syndrome. Routine assessment includes CBC with differential, serum electrolytes, calcium, glucose, BUN/CR, LFTs, TFTs, B_{12} and folate, U/A, and syphilis serology. Sedimentation rate, HIV testing, CXR, 24-hour urine for heavy metals, toxicology screen, neuroimaging, lumbar puncture, EEG, functional imaging, Lyme titers, endocrine studies (other than thyroid), and rheumatologic studies should be obtained when indicated. Consider neuroimaging in all new cases, although in individuals

Table 140-4
Cholinesterase Inhibitors

Drug	Starting Dose	Target Dose	Notes
Tacrine	10 mg qid	120–160 mg/day	Not currently used because of qid dosing and LFT elevations
Donepezil	5 mg qd	10 mg qd	Maintain starting dose for 4-6 weeks to minimize side effects. May be increased to 10 mg after 4–6 weeks
Rivastigmine	1.5 mg bid	6–12 mg/day	Similar side effects to tacrine, donepezil, and galantamine: nausea, vomiting, bradycardia
Galantamine	4 mg bid	8–12 mg bid	Reversible anticholinesterase inhibitor plus modulation of receptors to increase acetylcholine release

over age 60 with no focal symptoms or signs, seizures, or gait disturbances, it can be considered optional. *Lumbar puncture* is indicated for CNS infection, reactive serum syphilis serology, hydrocephalus, dementia in an individual under age 55, rapidly progressive dementia, immunosuppression, and suspicion of metastatic cancer or CNS vasculitis. *EEG* may be helpful in distinguishing delirium from dementia, diagnosing Creutzfeldt-Jakob disease, and identifying or evaluating seizure disorders. If available, *functional imaging* (SPECT, PET, MRS) can clarify the type of dementia. *The Ischemia Scale* can help differentiate Alzheimer's disease from vascular dementia but may overdiagnose vascular dementia when both are present. Staging identifies current care needs and predicts future requirements. Functional assessment scales help to track responses to interventions. Psychosocial assessment includes patient issues (competency, safety, and appropriateness of current living situation), caregiver issues (support network, depression, financial planning), and environmental issues (Should the patient be driving? Is the home environment optimized?)

MANAGEMENT AND THERAPY
Primary Symptoms

Treatment strategies attempt to mitigate or reverse the effects of the dementia on mental functioning. Cholinergic deficits are obvious in Alzheimer's dementia, but functional cholinergic deficits may be relevant to other dementias as well. Strategies to reverse symptoms may include specific therapies to reverse an underlying disease process (such as vitamin B_{12} or thyroid replacement). Cholinergic strategies for Alzheimer's disease include precursors (such as lecithin), cholinergic agonists (not currently available), and cholinesterase inhibitors (Table 140-4). Gene therapy and tissue transplantation are experimental at present.

Strategies to prevent progression include controlling risk factors (hypertension/diabetes management, stroke prevention strategies), treating underlying medical causes aggressively, and implanting cerebral shunts for normal pressure hydrocephalus. There is evidence that antioxidants (vitamin E [400 to 1000 IU twice daily], ginkgo biloba, selegiline), anti-inflammatory agents (NSAIDs), and other neuroprotective agents (acetyl carnitine) may be useful in progressive dementias. Vitamin E has the best evidence and is the least toxic. Current evidence is not strong enough to recommend ginkgo or acetyl carnitine.

Strategies to enhance CNS function (or to promote compensatory mechanisms) include estrogen replacement, which may delay onset of Alzheimer's disease in postmenopausal women and ergoloid mesylates which may be useful in high doses and are well tolerated. Anticholinergic medications and sedatives should be avoided.

Figure 140-5

Pharmacologic Management Options in Alzheimer's Disease

Cholinergic approaches

Cholinergic therapies attempt to boost cholinergic function diminished by loss of cholinergic projections from basal forebrain to frontal cortex, amygdala, and hippocampus

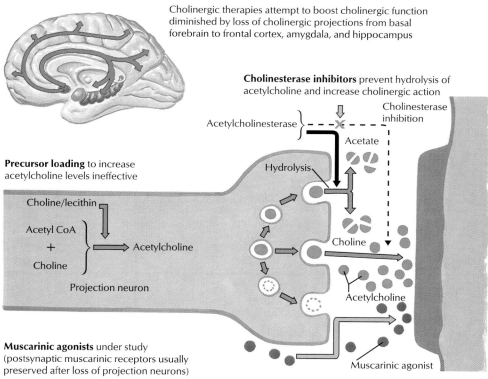

Cholinesterase inhibitors prevent hydrolysis of acetylcholine and increase cholinergic action

Cholinesterase inhibition

Acetylcholinesterase

Acetate

Precursor loading to increase acetylcholine levels ineffective

Hydrolysis

Choline/lecithin

Acetyl CoA + Choline → Acetylcholine

Choline

Projection neuron

Acetylcholine

Muscarinic agonists under study (postsynaptic muscarinic receptors usually preserved after loss of projection neurons)

Muscarinic agonist

JOHN A. CRAIG—MD
C. Machado—M.D.
©ICN

Secondary or Associated Symptoms

Treatment strategies are often necessary for managing secondary symptoms of dementia such as depression (see Chapter 114), psychosis, agitation, wandering, and insomnia. These symptoms result from the disease process because of its effects on memory and other cognitive abilities such as judgment, mood, social inhibition, and executive functioning. The primary goal is to ensure the safety of the patient and the family, to improve the quality of life of the patient and the primary caregivers, and ultimately to prevent caregiver burnout and forestall institutionalization of the patient. The first treatment principle is to do a careful medical evaluation, especially for sudden mental status changes, new-onset or worsen-ing psychosis, and/or agitation. A medical evaluation should also be considered for mood changes. When new or ongoing medical problems are being addressed appropriately, specific symptomatic treatments can be started.

Psychosis

If the patient is in little distress or danger, calm reassurance and distraction may be all that are required. Avoid traditional antipsychotics because of their association with extrapyramidal side effects, tardive dyskinesia, orthostasis, anticholin-ergic effects, and QTc effects. Low-dose chlorpro-mazine (12.5 to 50 mg) may be useful for insom-nia in some situations. Atypical antipsychotics are the current drugs of choice (Table 140-5).

Table 140-5
Atypical Antipsychotics

Atypical Agent	Useful for	Pros	Cons*	Dose Range
Risperidone	Agitation, psychosis	Well studied, generally well tolerated	EPS common in elderly, prolactin elevations	0.25–2 mg bid
Olanzapine	Mania, psychosis, agitation	Weight gain can be a plus for some patients	Weight gain, hyperglycemia, anticholinergic, increased lipids	2.5–10 mg qd
Quetiapine	Psychosis, agitation, insomnia	Low doses useful for insomnia. Not anticholinergic	Sedating, complicated dosing	25–200 mg bid
Ziprasidone	Psychosis	Low sedation and weight gain	Prolongs QTc interval	20–60 mg bid
Clozapine	Refractory psychosis (not for first-line use)	Parkinson's disease patients may benefit	Sedation, bone marrow suppression, highly anticholinergic	12.5–300 mg qd

*Potential orthostasis and high cost are problems with all these agents.

Agitation

Try to respond to the patient in a direct and calm manner; redirection may be helpful; arguing is usually not. Determine what is upsetting the patient (is the patient psychotic, disoriented, anxious, in pain). Medications can sometimes be helpful. Target specific conditions first (e.g., antidepressants for agitation in the context of depression). Antiagitation medications include antipsychotics, anticonvulsants, benzodiazepines, anticholinesterases, trazodone, and buspirone.

Wandering

When possible, accommodate the patient in a secure, well-lit environment. Consider dementia-proof locks and environmental barriers such as grid patterns on the floor. Determine whether the patient is anxious or restless.

Insomnia

Educate patients/caregivers about sleep hygiene measures (avoid stimulants, minimize daytime naps, etc.). Determine whether this symptom is a manifestation of another disorder such as depression. Avoid benzodiazepines because of associated ataxia and amnesia. Consider trazodone (50 to 100 mg) or quetiapine (25 to 50 mg) if medications are needed. Zolpidem (5 to 10 mg) may be useful for short periods.

Caregiver Issues

There is a high incidence of depression (50%) and other stress-related disorders among those who care for patients with dementia. Refer caregivers to support groups such as the Alzheimer's Association (www.alz.org). Provide legal referrals for handling competency issues.

FUTURE DIRECTIONS

Much excitement is being generated about potential new treatments for Alzheimer's disease, the most common and increasingly prevalent form of dementia. Antiamyloid vaccines, secretase inhibitors, anti-inflammatory strategies (such as COX-2 inhibitors), and more-specific memory-enhancing agents are all being tested, with encouraging early results. Gene replacement techniques and surgical implantation techniques are being investigated as well. As more successful treatment strategies are identified, the need for accurate early detection methods becomes paramount and the development of a safe, easy-to-use, and reliable screening test for Alzheimer's disease (and other degenerative dementias) will be a high priority. Currently, functional imaging, CSF markers, and genetic testing hold the most promise.

REFERENCES

Practice guideline for the treatment of patients with Alzheimer's disease and other dementias of late life. American Psychiatric Association. *Am J Psychiatry.* 1997; 154(suppl):1-39.

Practice parameter for diagnosis and evaluation of dementia (summary statement). Report of the Quality Standards Subcommittee of the American Academy of Neurology. *Neurology.* 1994;44:2203-2206.

Alzheimer's Association Web site. Available at: http://www.alz.org. Accessed March 4, 2003.

Alzheimer Research Forum Web site. Available at: http://www.alzforum.org. Accessed March 4, 2003.

American Academy of Neurology Web site. Available at: http://www.aan.com. Accessed March 4, 2003.

American Association of Geriatric Psychiatry Web site. Available at: http://www.aagpgpa.org. Accessed March 4, 2003.

The American Geriatrics Society Web site. Available at: http://www.americangeriatrics.org. Accessed March 4, 2003.

American Psychiatric Association Web site. Available at: http://www.psych.org. Accessed March 4, 2003.

Barclay L, ed. *Clinical Geriatric Neurology.* Philadelphia, Pa: Lea & Febiger; 1993.

Coffey CE, Cummings JL, eds. *The American Psychiatric Press Textbook of Geriatric Neuropsychiatry.* 2nd ed. Washington, DC: American Psychiatric Press; 2000.

Hachinski VC, Iliff LD, Zilhka E, et al. Cerebral blood flow in dementia. *Arch Neurol.* 1975;32:632-637.

Mayeux R, Sano M. Treatment of Alzheimer's disease. *N Engl J Med.* 1999;341:1670-1679.

Small GW, Rabins PV, Barry PP, et al. Diagnosis and treatment of Alzheimer disease and related disorders. Consensus statement of the American Association for Geriatric Psychiatry, the Alzheimer's Association, and the American Geriatrics Society. *JAMA.* 1997;278:1363-1371.

Chapter 141

Depression

John J. Haggerty

The word depression signifies a common and non-pathologic emotional experience. It also signifies a specific biopsychologic disorder. The two are not the same. Depression, the illness, is a coherent syndrome with a constellation of specific signs, symptoms, and features. A lifelong recurrent disorder, it occurs in 10% to 20% of the population worldwide. It interferes with work, family life, and has a mortality rate of 15%.

ETIOLOGY AND PATHOGENESIS

Depression results from disturbances in monoamine neurotransmission, serotonin, norepinephrine, and dopamine in particular. It may be maintained by secondary neurohormonal changes involving the thyroid and adrenal cortical axes. These combined changes ultimately result in altered nucleic acid transcription. The strongest etiologic factor is inheritance. Risk for depression can also be acquired through early life trauma, which may "wire-in" exaggerated neurohormonal stress responses. Other medical illnesses or interventions may cause a secondary depressive syndrome, most notably hypothyroidism, and medications such as antihypertensive agents that affect central monoamine neurotransmission. A variety of substances may also induce secondary depression during intoxication or withdrawal, most notably alcohol, cocaine, and stimulants.

CLINICAL PRESENTATION

Although clinically evident depression presents in the third or fourth decade typically, the initial onset of depression can occur at any point in the life cycle, including early childhood. The presentation varies from individual to individual and across the life cycle, but the core features are always present during an episode (Figures 141-1 and 141-2). As codified in the *Diagnostic and Statistical Manual-IV* (DSM-IV), these include depressed mood, or anhedonia (required); increased or decreased appetite; increased or decreased sleeping; slowed activity; fatigue; exaggerated self-criticalness, worthlessness, or guilt; decreased libido; mental slowing, decreased memory, or inattention; recurrent thoughts of death or suicide. DSM-IV requires 5 signs or symptoms concurrently for at least 2 weeks for an unequivocal diagnosis, but most clinicians recognize that patients can qualify for the diagnosis with as few as 3 to 4 symptoms. Depressed mood is not always the most prominent symptom, and may even be absent. Often the presenting symptom will be insomnia, nervousness, or memory change. Depression is often accompanied by anxiety, and may be complicated by striking symptoms of psychosis such as auditory hallucinations and delusions of impoverishment or guilt. Depressive episodes may occur with or without evident stressors, and reported stressors often are actually the result of incipient depression rather than the cause.

DIFFERENTIAL DIAGNOSIS
Adjustment Disorder

In adjustment disorder, depressed mood follows clearcut stressors, but the full depressive syndrome is not present or is transient (less than 2 weeks). Adjustment disorder does not respond to antidepressant medication.

Bipolar Disorder, Depressed Phase

Approximately 20% of individuals who present with depression actually have unrecognized bipolar mood disorder. The recognized forms of bipolar disorder, bipolar I and bipolar II, differ primarily in the severity of the manic phase. Bipolar I requires the occurrence of full-blown mania at some point in the life cycle. Bipolar II requires only the occurrence of hypomania. Because hypomania is often transient and non-dysfunctional, it can be easily overlooked. Because the depressed phase of bipolar disorder is usually indistinguishable from simple depressive disorder (unipolar), bipolar II disorder can easily masquerade as unipolar depression. This distinction is important because bipolar disorder

Figure 141-1

The Face of Depression

"Doctor, what's wrong with me?"

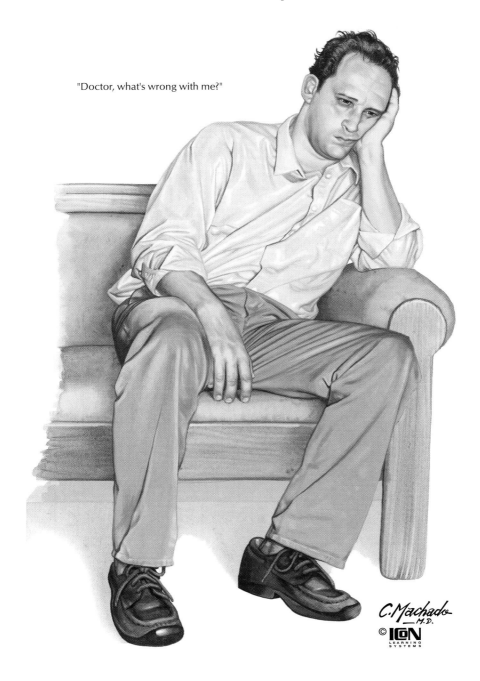

Figure 141-2

Depression (Unipolar)

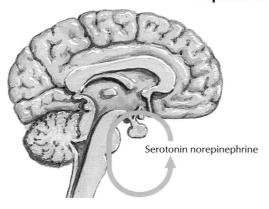

Serotonin norepinephrine

Depression is a biochemically mediated
state most likely based on abnormalities in
metabolism of serotonin and norepinephrine

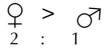

Female gender predominates

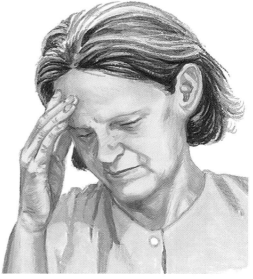

Clinical syndrome characterized by withdrawal,
anger, frustration, and loss of pleasure

Associated Symptoms and Comorbidities

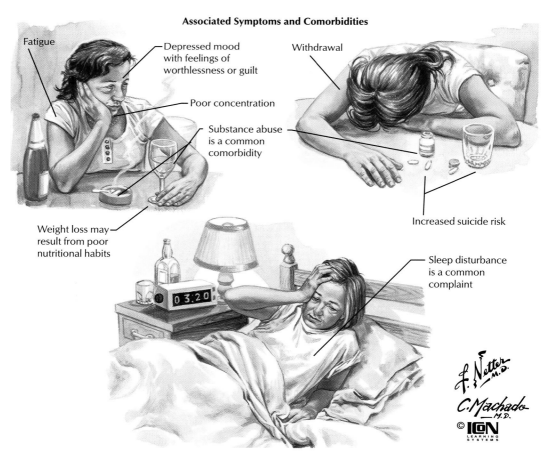

Fatigue

Depressed mood
with feelings of
worthlessness or guilt

Poor concentration

Substance abuse
is a common
comorbidity

Weight loss may
result from poor
nutritional habits

Withdrawal

Increased suicide risk

Sleep disturbance
is a common
complaint

requires a different treatment approach, emphasizing mood stabilizers over antidepressants.

Substance-Induced Depression

Substance-induced depression can be a direct result of substance use, but it can also exist as an independent co-morbid condition complicating substance abuse. Depression that is purely secondary to a substance clears within several days to a week of substance discontinuation. If depression does not resolve within this time frame, it requires treatment in its own right.

Depression Secondary to Medical Illness

Depression secondary to a medical condition should be considered whenever depressive mood changes accompany a medical condition known to be associated with depression. A partial list includes hypothyroidism, Addison's or Cushing's disease, pancreatic cancer, AIDS, tuberculosis, multiple sclerosis, stroke, Alzheimer's disease, Parkinson's disease, and diabetes mellitus. Sometimes depression may be the first manifestation of undetected systemic illness, and for this reason medical history and reasonable medical assessment should be part of the standard evaluation of all new cases of depression.

DIAGNOSTIC APPROACH

Consider depression not just in patients who present with depressed mood, but also in those who complain of insomnia, anxiety, decreased energy, or cognitive changes primarily. The diagnosis is established purely on the basis of history and observation of symptoms and signs consistent with the diagnostic criteria. Excellent self-administered screening tools such as the Zung or Beck depression inventories are available. Information from family members or close associates is invaluable in substantiating the diagnosis when the onset of symptoms has been insidious. Diagnostic evaluation must include enumeration of the frequency and timing of prior episodes, and an exploration for past episodes of elevated mood. This information is necessary for later treatment planning, including decisions about the duration of treatment. Every evaluation must include queries about suicide risk. The simplest way to begin this inquiry is to ask, "Have you had thoughts of death or of harming yourself in any way?" Thoughts of dying or committing suicide are extremely common in depression. Most frequently they remain at the thought level and can be managed on an outpatient basis. However, in a significant minority of patients, thoughts are accompanied by intent or specific suicidal plans. Rapid psychiatric consultation or hospitalization is required. History of suicide attempt and presence of psychosis, substance use, or significant isolation raise the risk for suicide.

MANAGEMENT AND THERAPY

The most important principle for the management of depression is to view it as a lifelong disorder that recurs at a rate of at least 50% following a single episode. The recurrence rate climbs with each subsequent episode, as does the rate of chronic residual symptoms between major episodes. Treatment planning must take this into account in terms of patient education and duration of treatment. Medication treatment of an episode of depression should extend at least 6 to 12 months, and indefinite maintenance treatment should be considered following severe or recurrent episodes. The second most important principle is that, while all antidepressant agents have similar efficacy rates overall, there is significant variability in terms of response and tolerance among patients. Many patients will have to try more than one antidepressant before finding one that works for them.

Initial medication treatment usually starts with a member of the serotonin-specific reuptake inhibitor (SSRI) class of antidepressants, which includes fluoxetine, sertraline, paroxetine, and citalopram. If there is a personal or family history of preferential response to a particular antidepressant of any class, then this should be the first choice. A generic member of the older tricyclic class of antidepressants is an equally good choice if cost is an issue. Sixty percent to 70% of patients will respond to the initial choice. Evidence-based algorithms exist to guide treatment when it is necessary to move beyond this step. The usual sequence is to 1) increase dose every 1 to 2 weeks as tolerated; 2) add either lithium or tri-iodothyronine (25 to 50 µg) as an augmenting agent; 3) switch to a different member of the same class or switch to a member of a different class (bupropion, venlafaxine, mirtazapine, nefazodone, tricyclic, monoamine oxidase inhibitor [MAOI]); 4) combine antidepressants

(SSRI + bupropion or tricyclic; venlafaxine + mirtazapine); and 5) consider electroconvulsive therapy (ECT), which has the highest response rate of all somatic treatments for depression.

Psychotherapy is equally as effective as medication in mild-to-moderate depression, but not in severe depression. Psychotherapies specifically designed for depression, cognitive behavioral therapy and interpersonal psychotherapy in particular, have been shown to have the highest effectiveness. A combination of psychotherapy plus medication provides the best coverage.

FUTURE DIRECTIONS
Further Delineation of Pathogenesis and Inheritance

Research utilizing functional brain imaging and molecular biology will significantly improve our understanding of the neural circuitry of depression and of what happens between the synapse and the cell nucleus during initiation, maintenance, and recovery from depression.

Development of Antidepressant Treatments with Novel Mechanisms of Action

There are many individuals who do not respond to available treatments, all which tend to focus on synaptic activity. Examples of treatments under investigation include agents that block the exaggerated hypothalamic-pituitary-adrenal axis in depression, transcranial magnetic stimulation, and vagal nerve stimulation.

Public Education and Stigma Reduction

Failure to seek treatment is the single most important impediment to reducing morbidity and mortality in depression. Public education about depression lags far behind health information efforts for other common illnesses. Investment of public resources in the development of organized, ongoing screening and health education programs for depression will have an impact on the burden of depression that is equal to if not greater than biological advances.

REFERENCES

American Psychiatric Association. *Diagnostic and Statistical Manual of Mental Disorders.* 4th ed, text rev. Washington, DC: American Psychiatric Association; 2000.

Greenberg AM, Goldstein RD. Depressive disorders. In: Tasman A, Lieberman JA, eds. *Psychiatry.* Philadelphia, Pa: WB Saunders Co; 1997.

Haggerty JJ Jr. Depression. In: Dornbrand L, Hoole AJ, Fletcher RH, eds. *Manual of Clinical Problems in Adult Ambulatory Care: With Annotated Key References.* 3rd ed. Philadelphia, Pa: Lippincott-Raven; 1997.

Chapter 142

Emotional and Behavioral Problems Among Adolescents and Young Adults

Carol A. Ford and Linmarie Sikich

Emotional and behavioral problems among youth are associated with substantial morbidity, mortality, and health-care costs. Adolescents and young adults experiencing these problems are more likely to participate in behaviors leading to negative outcomes such as injuries, sexually transmitted infections, and unwanted pregnancy. Frequently, such problems herald the onset of psychiatric disorders including major depression, bipolar affective disorder, and schizophrenia, which will require lifelong treatment. Emotional and behavior problems may complicate management of chronic illness in youth by influencing choices about adherence to treatment plans. In all of these situations, individuals' life trajectories may be affected by the establishment of maladaptive patterns of behavior and negative influences on major life decisions about education, work, and family. Adolescents and young adults with emotional and behavioral problems are at increased risk for suicide and homicide, the second and third leading causes of death in this age group.

ETIOLOGY AND PATHOGENESIS

There is a broad spectrum of emotional and behavioral problems seen among adolescents and young adults (Figure 142-1). The etiology of most problems appears multifactorial with genetic, biologic, social, and developmental factors contributing to varying degrees.

CLINICAL PRESENTATION

Many adolescents and young adults with emotional and behavioral problems first present in medical rather than mental health-care settings. Routine examination should include a psychosocial history, asking about family and peer relationships, school/vocation, alcohol and other drug use, sexual behaviors, emotional health, and body image. Common presentations include 1) physical symptoms directly related to underlying mental health problems; 2) mental status changes that raise questions about underlying medical versus mental illness; 3) negative health outcomes of behaviors precipitated by underlying mental health problems; and 4) concerning symptoms elicited during routine health care.

Youth experiencing emotional or behavioral problems that are seriously impacting their life and functioning are usually not "just going through a phase" of normal development, and evaluation must include assessment for psychiatric disorders.

Depressive Disorders

The prevalence of major depressive disorder (MDD) in adolescence is estimated at 4% to 8% with a male-female ratio of 1:2. Symptoms include at least 2 weeks of marked change in mood and/or loss of interest and pleasure, as well as significant changes in patterns of appetite, weight, sleep, activity, concentration, energy level, or motivation. To be significant, symptoms must impair relationships or performance of activities. Comorbid psychiatric conditions including anxiety disorders, learning problems, attention deficit–hyperactivity disorder (ADHD), and substance abuse are common. Adolescents tend to display more irritability and behavioral problems and fewer neurovegetative symptoms than adults with MDD. Hallucinations are also more frequent. Clinical variants include atypical depression with increased sleep and weight gain, seasonal affective disorder, and dysthymia with very chronic changes in mood and motivation but few neurovegetative symptoms. Approximately 25% of youth with major depression will attempt suicide within 5 years.

Anxiety Disorders

There are several different anxiety disorders seen in youth with estimated prevalence ranging from 0.3% to 4.6%. These include *panic disorder* (0.6%

Figure 142-1

Emotional and Behavioral Problems Among Adolescents and Young Adults

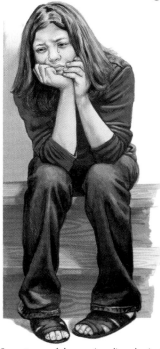

Panic disorder is characterized by the presence of panic attacks with at least four of the following symptoms: palpitation, dyspnea, nausea, dizziness, sweating, paresthesia, and gastrointestinal discomfort

Symptoms of depressive disorder include: at least 2 weeks of marked change in mood and/or loss of interest and pleasure; and significant changes in patterns of appetite, weight, sleep, activity, concentration, energy level, or motivation

Refusal to maintain weight at or above a minimally normal weight or failure to gain weight during a period of expected growth; intense fear of gaining weight; disturbance in body image; and the absence of at least 3 spontaneous menstrual cycles in post-menarcheal females are symptoms/signs of anorexia nervosa

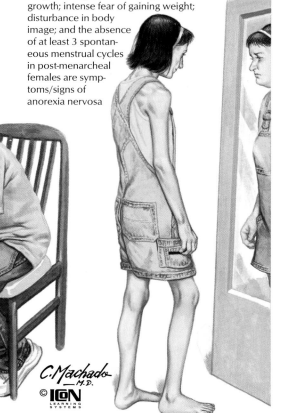

The most common features of substance use disorder among adolescents are impairment in psychosocial and academic functioning. This disorder increases the risk for suicide if associated with other psychiatric disorders

prevalence), *posttraumatic stress disorder* (PTSD) (~1%), *generalized anxiety disorder* (4.6%), *obsessive-compulsive disorder* (1.9%), and various phobias. Distribution by gender varies by disorder and age of onset. In each disorder, unwanted, disturbing thoughts or worries negatively impact functioning. Panic disorder is characterized by the presence of panic attacks with at least 4 somatic symptoms including palpitations, dyspnea, nausea, dizziness, sweating, paresthesias, and gastrointestinal discomfort. Early onset of panic disorder is associated with greater morbidity. Youth with PTSD often have experienced recurrent traumas and may have difficulty identifying a clear precipitant.

Bipolar Affective Disorder

The overall prevalence of *bipolar affective disorder* (BPAD) is 2%, with one third of adults reporting onset during adolescence. There are no significant gender differences. The diagnosis requires the presence of at least one episode with manic symptoms that include significantly elevated, expansive, or irritable mood associated with functional impairment and pressured speech, racing thoughts, grandiosity, and decreased need for sleep. Mixed manic and depressed episodes are common. Youth tend to have more frequent, but shorter, episodes with more severe psychotic symptoms than adults. Youth with bipolar disorder are at even greater risk for suicide than those with major depression. They are also likely to be involved in dangerous sexual and physical activities with numerous health risks.

Substance Use Disorders

Substance use is very common among adolescents and young adults, especially the use of alcohol. To be considered a problem, substance use must produce dysfunction in one or more domains of a patient's life and cause clinically significant levels of distress or impairment. The most common features among adolescents are impairment in psychosocial and academic functioning. Substance use disorders are often associated with other psychiatric disorders and significantly increase the risk for suicide in those disorders.

Eating Disorders

Estimates of the lifetime prevalence of *anorexia nervosa* range from 0.5% to 3.7% and of *bulimia*

nervosa range from 1.1% to 4.2%. Eating disorders are more common in females (male-female ratio of 1:6 to 1:10), and onset usually occurs during adolescence and young adulthood. Symptoms of anorexia nervosa include 1) refusal to maintain weight at or above a minimally normal weight or failure to gain weight during a period of expected growth; 2) intense fear of gaining weight; 3) disturbance in body image; and the absence of at least 3 spontaneous menstrual cycles in postmenarchal females. Symptoms of bulimia nervosa include 1) recurrent episodes of binge eating characterized by eating large amounts of food in a short period and inability to control eating; 2) recurrent inappropriate compensatory behavior to prevent weight gain (e.g., self-induced vomiting, misuse of medications, fasting, or excessive exercise); 3) both binge eating and inappropriate compensatory behaviors that have occurred at least twice a week for 3 months; and 4) self-evaluation unduly influenced by body shape and weight.

Patients with anorexia nervosa often present to medical settings with weight loss or amenorrhea. Patients with either disorder may present with complications of severe electrolyte disturbances. Occasionally, patients present with constipation or esophageal tears. Rates of comorbid psychiatric diagnosis among patients with eating disorders are high (50% to 75%). Mortality rates vary according to age of onset, length of disease, and presence of purging behaviors. Death is typically from cardiac arrhythmia or suicide. In general, younger adolescents have the best outcomes and adults have the worst.

Schizophrenia Spectrum Disorders

Schizophrenia affects 1% of the adult population; 60% have symptoms during adolescence. Equal numbers of males and females are affected, although males typically have earlier onset with more severe symptoms. At least 2 of the following symptoms are required for diagnosis: 1) delusions; 2) hallucinations; 3) disorganized or illogical speech; 4) catatonia or grossly disorganized behavior; or 5) negative symptoms (social withdrawal, apathy, and poverty of speech). Frank symptoms are often preceded by transient hallucinations or delusions, social isolation, or deterioration in social and academic functioning. Substance use may trigger symptoms in biologically vulnerable individuals or may reflect efforts to self-medicate. Youth tend to have less systematized delusions and more complex hallucinations than adults. The main variant is schizoaffective disorder with intermittent affective symptoms but persistent psychotic symptoms. One in 10 individuals with schizophrenia commits suicide.

Attention Deficit–Hyperactivity Disorder

The estimated prevalence of *attention deficit–hyperactivity disorder* (ADHD) is 5% in the school-age population with male-female ratios ranging from 4:1 to 9:1. As many as 80% will have symptoms persisting into adolescence and 65% into adulthood. Infrequently, ADHD will be diagnosed in adolescents and young adults, although there should be a history of attentional difficulties in childhood. Symptoms may be predominately inattention, predominately hyperactivity with impulsiveness, or a combination of both. Typically, symptoms are present in situations that are unstructured, boring, or require sustained mental effort. Adolescents often complain of restlessness rather than hyperactivity. Other psychiatric illnesses such as major depression and schizophrenia may also reduce attention.

DIFFERENTIAL DIAGNOSIS

When evaluating emotional and behavioral disorders in youth, it is important to recognize that the same symptoms may occur in different disorders. For instance, striking changes in appetite and weight may be seen in anorexia nervosa, major depression, schizophrenia, and substance abuse. Generally, the diagnosis is dependent upon the constellation of symptoms observed and their developmental course. It is also essential to consider nonpsychiatric etiologies such as medical illness or reactions to medications.

DIAGNOSTIC APPROACH

The evaluation and management of adolescents and young adults should be conducted in a developmentally appropriate manner. Issues to consider include age, cognitive development, psychosocial development, and parental relationships. Youth often provide more accurate reports about their affective state, anxieties, and cognitive processes than their parents, but may have diffi-

culty recognizing behavioral, functional, and social problems. Legal, ethical, and professional guidelines have been developed for managing confidentiality when providing health care to minor adolescents.

The general approach to diagnosis includes 1) taking a complete history with additional information from family and other sources (e.g., school personnel); 2) physical examination, including a detailed neurologic examination; 3) the judicious use of laboratory tests to exclude primary medical conditions; and 4) consultation with or referral to a mental health professional as needed. All patients should be assessed for risk of suicide. Factors that place youth at highest risk for suicide include male gender, previous suicide attempt, substance abuse, MDD, agitation, and psychosis.

MANAGEMENT AND THERAPY

The American Academy of Child and Adolescent Psychiatry has recently published a series of practice parameters guiding the treatment of adolescents with depressive disorders, anxiety disorders, substance use, schizophrenia, attention-deficit–hyperactivity disorder, and suicidal behavior. In addition, the American Psychiatric Association recently published a revised practice guideline for treatment of patients with eating disorders.

General management strategies encourage the adolescent or young adult to take an active role in treatment. Health-care providers and families should provide support and guidance. Treatment often includes individual cognitive, behavioral and/or supportive therapy, family therapy, education and psychopharmacology.

Cognitive therapy has been demonstrated to be particularly effective in the treatment of anxiety disorders and milder cases of depression. Behavior therapy is often essential for the treatment of eating disorders, substance abuse disorders, ADHD and BPAD. Education about the illnesses and their treatments is essential in all disorders.

Medication treatments are largely based on data from adults. Serotonin reuptake inhibitors are the first line of treatment for major depression (SRIs) and anxiety disorders, and they may also be useful in the treatment of some eating disorders. Some of the newer antidepressants may be alternatives. Tricyclic medications have been established to be ineffective antidepressants in youth. Mood stabilizers including lithium, valproic acid, carbamazepine and many newer anti-epileptic agents are the cornerstone of treatment for BPAD. Each of these agents can have significant systemic side effects including renal, liver, and hematological changes.

Antipsychotic medication is essential for youth with psychotic symptoms, whether associated with depression, BPAD, or schizophrenia. The newer antipsychotics have significantly fewer extrapyramidal side effects, but some may cause considerable weight gain and increased risk of diabetes mellitus and lipid abnormalities. Many of the antipsychotics also lead to prolactin elevations that may cause gynecomastia, galactorrhea, amenorrhea, and increased risks of osteopenia. Stimulants such as methylphenidate, which increase central nervous system norepinephrine and dopamine, may offer substantial benefits to patients with ADHD, including better concentration and an increased attention span.

Management of patients who are at high risk for suicide includes measures to assure their acute safety and treatment for associated emotional disorders. Those at highest risk may need to be hospitalized. Those who do not require hospitalization need to have adequate supervision and support from a responsible adult and a safe home environment. It is essential that they and their families remove access to firearms and medications.

All adolescents and young adults with emotional and behavioral problems should continue receiving routine health care to monitor for possible health consequences of psychotropic medications and to assess emerging health needs.

FUTURE DIRECTIONS

A recent national survey in the United States found that adolescents and young adults with psy-chiatric disorders are much less likely to be identified and treated than older adults. Better identification depends upon improving community education about major mental illnesses in youth, recognition in schools, and diagnosis by primary care physicians. Research needs to focus on prevention, early intervention, and treatment of emotional and behavioral disorders specifically in adolescent and young adult populations. Focus on mental health issues in this age group has potential to substantially reduce morbidity, mortality, health-care costs, and the individual/societal burden of psychiatric illness among youth and across the life cycle.

REFERENCES

American Academy of Child & Adolescent Psychiatry web site. Summary of practice parameters. Available at: http://www.aacap.org/clinical/parameters.html. Accessed March 20, 2003.

Confidential health services for adolescents. Council on Scientific Affairs, American Medical Association. *JAMA.* 1993; 269:1420-1424.

Practice guideline for the treatment of patients with eating disorders (revision). American Psychiatric Association Work Group on Eating Disorders. *Am J Psychiatry.* 2000; 157(suppl):1-39.

Kessler RC, Olfson M, Berglund PA. Patterns and predictors of treatment contact after first onset of psychiatric disorders. *Am J Psychiatry.* 1998;155:62-69.

National Institute on Drug Abuse Web site. NIDA InfoFacts: high school and youth trends. Available at: http://www.nida.nih.gov/infofax/hsyouthtrends.html. Accessed March 4, 2003.

Ozer E, Brindis CD, Millstein S, Knopf DK, Irwin CE Jr. *America's Adolescents: Are They Healthy?* San Francisco, Calif: University of California, National Adolescent Health Information Center; 1998.

US Preventive Services Task Force. *Guide to Clinical Preventive Services.* 2nd ed. Baltimore, Md: Lippincott Williams & Wilkins; 1996.

Wolraich ML, ed. *The Classification of Child and Adolescent Mental Diagnoses in Primary Care: Diagnostic and Statistical Manual for Primary Care (DSM-PC) Child and Adolescent Version.* Elk Grove Village, Ill: American Academy of Pediatrics; 1996.

Chapter 143
Grief

Burton R. Hutto

The loss of a love object triggers a complex set of biologic, psychologic, and social reactions. Definitions vary, but, generally, *grief* refers to the psychological response, *bereavement* to the loss itself, and *mourning* to the social expression of grief. Social expressions differ widely among cultures and families, and grief can vary depending on the bereaved person's psychologic makeup and the nature of the lost relationship. Grief can also be a psychologic reaction to any loss. A person may grieve misspent youth and missed opportunities or the loss of any cherished object such as a pet or even an inanimate object. Grieving the loss of a loved person typically evokes more pronounced and clinically relevant responses, but other losses should not be dismissed.

CLINICAL PRESENTATION
Normal Grief

Initial responses to a death often include a sense of shocked disbelief and numbness. The bereaved person engages in "searching" behaviors that include seeing the lost loved one, hearing his or her voice, or feeling his or her touch (Figure 143-1). Such hallucinatory experiences may last weeks or sometimes months, and are not considered pathologic. Following the initial shock, a period of intense anguish and emotionality ensues. All conceivable emotions can be experienced with rapid fluctuation. Many of the neurovegetative symptoms of depression such as low energy, loss of appetite with weight loss, and insomnia can last for months. The final stage of grief includes a reorganization of the psychologic life that may take years. Although most bereaved people await "closure" and a return to normal, some losses lead to psychologic changes that last a lifetime.

Generally, experts agree on such a stage model of grief, yet the individual variance is so wide that boundaries of normal grief can be hard to define. The time frame cannot be specified or predicted for any individual, and attenuated experiences of any of the stages, or nonlinear progression through them, do not always signify pathology. Stage models provide a broad outline that does not account for the variables of psychologic differences, personal history, or cultural expectations. Most people avoid pain and will attempt to suppress expressions of grief. What emerges is a

compromise between this suppression and the underlying pain. Such partial expressions of the depth of the pain can be perceived not only as unwanted but also as "out of the blue."

Anniversary reactions can reawaken earlier stages of grief, and they can occur not only at the anniversary of the loss but also around significant holidays or other reminders of the loss. When a bereaved person reaches the age at which a parent died, often there is some pause of grief. Such anniversary reactions can be unconscious to the person who experiences only the symptoms without understanding their context.

Biologic changes can accompany grief. There is evidence to suggest numerous physiologic changes such as impairment of immunity, increased adrenocortical activity, increased prolactin, and increased growth hormone. The clinical significance of such changes is not clear.

Pathologic Grief

Grief has pathologic forms marked by abnormalities of time course or intensity. *Absent grief* or rigid denial occurs when expression of grief is much less than expected. *Delayed grief* is another abnormality of time course in which the expression of grief is somehow postponed or suspended. The grief may follow a typical course after the delay. *Chronic grief* can continue for years, remain extremely intense, and block personal growth and the establishment of new attachments. Pathologic grief characterized by such abnormalities of time course or intensity can border

Figure 143-1

Grief

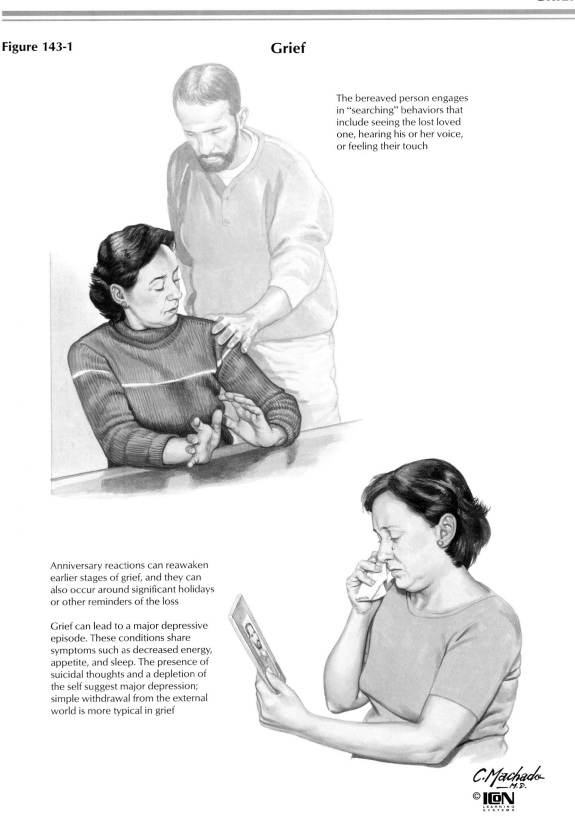

The bereaved person engages in "searching" behaviors that include seeing the lost loved one, hearing his or her voice, or feeling their touch

Anniversary reactions can reawaken earlier stages of grief, and they can also occur around significant holidays or other reminders of the loss

Grief can lead to a major depressive episode. These conditions share symptoms such as decreased energy, appetite, and sleep. The presence of suicidal thoughts and a depletion of the self suggest major depression; simple withdrawal from the external world is more typical in grief

on normal grief and is distinguished by the degree of functional impairment.

Grief can also lead to a *major depressive episode*, and because grief and depression share some symptoms including decreased energy, appetite, and sleep, differentiating the two can be difficult. Symptoms characterized by a depletion of the self, such as the presence of undue guilt, suicidal thoughts, or feelings of worthlessness suggest a major depression. Simple withdrawal from the external world is more typical of normal grief. Severe psychomotor retardation and hallucinations, other than brief "contacts" with the lost one, suggest a possible depressive episode complicating the grief. The number of depressive symptoms present at 1 month after the loss is a strong predictor of an unremitting depression. In addition, sleep studies may distinguish depression from grief. Medications, alcohol, and illicit substances can be abused in the effort to avoid painful effects of grief. Substance abuse requires aggressive treatment to prevent its progression and the development of further consequences.

Somatic expressions of grief can be psychologically mediated or related to the biologic response to loss. Grieving patients commonly seek medical advice for vague symptoms of somatic distress such as dull aching pains. Studies of relative risk for diagnosable morbidity following grief have been inconclusive. Several studies have demonstrated an increased relative risk for mortality in bereaved spouses, but the absolute risk remains low.

Risk Factors for Pathologic Outcomes

The risk of pathologic outcome in grief is increased by factors related to the loss and by factors related to the psychology of the grieving person. Sudden, unanticipated, and untimely deaths are more likely to be associated with adverse outcomes. If such losses are horrific (e.g., violent deaths, deaths in disaster or accidents), the bereaved person may suffer post-traumatic stress symptoms that interfere with grief. Other types of losses are more difficult to bear. The loss of a spouse or child, or the loss of a parent during childhood or adolescence, are major life events that are often traumatic. Multiple losses, suicide, or murder-related deaths add to the complications of grief. *Concurrent life crises and stresses*

such as accidents, illness, separation from family, relationship difficulties, unemployment, or the consequences of trauma may be so severe that the bereaved person is completely occupied with psychologic survival and may not have the energy to withstand the process of grief.

Some individuals may be more vulnerable to pathologic grief. A perceived lack of social support worsens outcomes. A history of psychiatric disorder and a history of suicidal behavior specifically should alert the clinician to monitor closely for difficulty in the process of grief. The nature of the relationship that is lost can also contribute to pathology in grief. The loss of ambivalent or dependent relationships can be problematic. With ambivalence, acknowledgment of satisfaction with the death of the person who is also beloved can provoke extreme guilt. The loss of either partner of a dependent relationship requires an unusual degree of sudden development towards independence and autonomy. Such persons may instead quickly establish new similar relationships before completing a process of grief.

MANAGEMENT AND THERAPY

Most commonly, grief will run its own course with little need for intervention by a clinician. Inquiry about perceived supports and education to help the patient anticipate the process of grief are almost always justified. Sensitivity to the circumstances and psychologic meaning of the particular loss will guide further management.

Medication is not part of the management of normal or pathologic grief unless specific indications exist. If sedation is initiated, it should be prescribed for a few nights while support and counseling are also provided. Sedation can impair the memory of important events such as viewing the body, family gatherings, or funeral services that may provide the patient comfort in the future. If major depression develops, antidepressant medication is indicated.

The role of any caregiver is to facilitate normal grief and not to intervene in any way that might interfere with grief such as giving ill-conceived advice, religious or other prescriptive formulas for grieving, or inappropriate medication for normal reactive processes. Nor should a clinician prevent the bereaved from undertaking adaptive tasks such as viewing the deceased or attending the funeral or memorial service. Availability and sensitivity will facilitate uncomplicated grief. When a complication occurs or is anticipated, more specific measures can be taken. One intervention that may be indicated is a more involved level of counseling.

Bereavement Counseling

The goal of bereavement counseling is to facilitate the grieving process or to convert pathologic grief to normal grief. Bereavement counseling has been established as being effective in a number of studies. Key elements include having the patient review: 1) the period leading up to the death and the immediate afterward, including perceptions, rituals, and reactions; 2) the history of the lost relationship, including its good and bad aspects; 3) what has happened since the loss, including social responses and support, and other stressors; 4) the impact on and needs of other family members and their relationship to the bereaved person; and 5) relevant experience and coping, including earlier losses and personal styles. Such explorations are designed to assist the bereaved person in expressing grief and reassessing the lost relationship, two important aspects of the resolution process. If a grieving person is unwilling or unable to move forward from the loss, an exploration of the block he or she is experiencing such as trauma, depression, or dependent needs may be necessary. Some bereaved people need permission from a perceived authority to stop mourning after sufficient expression of grief.

Other Interventions

Information, education, books, and videos about grief may help the bereaved anticipate their reactions. The opportunity to explore concrete memories, places, and objects associated with the deceased (e.g., by looking at and discussing photographs or visiting the gravesite) may help overcome resistance to grieving. Self-help associations for general bereavement or the specific form of loss (Sudden Infant Death Association, Compassionate Friends [for loss of a child], Stillbirth and Neonatal Death Support Groups, and spousal support groups) can provide support, education, role models, and practical assistance. Writing about the loss (e.g., keeping a diary or journal) or giving testimony builds mastery and may be of value for some bereaved people. Referral to a psychiatrist with skills in this area is sometimes appropriate. Indications include severe, unremitting grief; a traumatic loss (especially if the bereaved develops symptoms of post-traumatic stress disorder); major depression or suicidal ideation; and children who have lost a parent or sibling, especially if a surviving parent is depressed.

REFERENCES

Biondi M, Picardi A. Clinical and biological aspects of bereavement and loss-induced depression: a reappraisal. *Psychother Psychosom.* 1996;65:229–245.

Parkes CM. Bereavement in adult life. *BMJ.* 1998;316:856-859.

Raphael B. *The Anatomy of Bereavement.* New York, NY: Basic Books; 1983.

Rozenzweig A, Prigerson H, Miller MD, Reynolds CF III. Bereavement and late-life depression: grief and its complications in the elderly. *Annu Rev Med.* 1997;48:421–428.

Woof WR, Carter YH. The grieving adult and the general practitioner: a literature review in two parts (part 1). *Br J Gen Pract.* 1997;47:443–448.

Chapter 144

Obsessive-Compulsive Disorder

Linda M. Nicholas

Obsessive-compulsive disorder (OCD) is a well defined, often debilitating illness characterized by obsessions, compulsions, or both. First described 150 years ago, the conceptualization of OCD has undergone profound changes over the past 2 decades. Once considered a rare psychogenic syndrome with treatment based on the exploration of early childhood conflict, OCD is now understood as a prominent, neuropsychiatric disease with abnormal brain circuitry and neurotransmitter dysfunction. Unfortunately, OCD continues to be a hidden, often unrecognized illness with an average 5- to 10-year lag from onset of symptoms to appropriate diagnosis and treatment. Because effective treatment is highly specific and nonspecific treatments are ineffective, many are left to suffer needlessly.

OCD affects 2% to 3% of the US population, and cross-national studies have found a remarkably similar prevalence across diverse geographical and cultural sites. Men and women are equally likely to be affected. Age of onset is typically during late adolescence or early adulthood, although childhood onset is not uncommon, with as many as one third of patients recalling the emergence of symptoms before age 15 years. Males tend to have an earlier age of onset than females.

ETIOLOGY AND PATHOGENESIS

Remarkable advances have been made in our understanding of the genetic and neurologic underpinnings of OCD. The observation that the tricyclic antidepressant, *clomipramine*, a serotonin reuptake inhibitor (SRI), is effective in treating patients with OCD, while antidepressants with primarily noradrenergic reuptake activity (e.g., desipramine) are not, led to the hypothesis that serotonin plays a major role in the mediation of OCD. Results of neuroendocrine, metabolite, and platelet binding studies also suggest dysregulation of serotonin function in OCD.

Studies using modern neuroimaging techniques strongly implicate basal ganglia circuitry in the mediation of OCD symptoms. Corticostriatal pathways involve both serotonergic and dopaminergic neurons. Several structural studies have found decreased basal ganglia volumes in OCD patients compared with those in healthy controls. Functional studies utilizing positron emission tomography (PET) have shown increased resting activity in the frontal lobes, basal ganglia, and cingulum of patients with OCD with normalization of these findings following successful pharmacologic or behavioral intervention. Neuropsychologic and neurosurgical studies are also consistent with the importance of the basal ganglia in OCD.

Family and twin studies indicate a genetic contribution to the etiology of OCD. There is increased risk of OCD in first-degree relatives of affected patients, as well as increased concordance in monozygotic compared with dizygotic twins.

CLINICAL PRESENTATION

The clinical description of OCD has changed little over the past 150 years. The core clinical symptoms are obsessions or compulsions that are either time-consuming or cause functional impairment or distress, and are not due to another psychiatric or medical illness.

Obsessions are persistent thoughts, images, or impulses that are experienced as intrusive, distressing, and inappropriate. Most studies have found that the most common obsessional theme in both adults and children is that of contamination, typified by fear of dirt, germs, toxins, environmental hazards, or bodily secretions (Figure 144-1). Patients may fear spreading disease or contracting an illness, and such worries are often associated with elaborate and time-consuming washing or bathing compulsions. Other obsessions include pathologic doubt, whereby one worries that his or her actions may cause harm or

Figure 144-1

Obsessive Compulsive Disorder

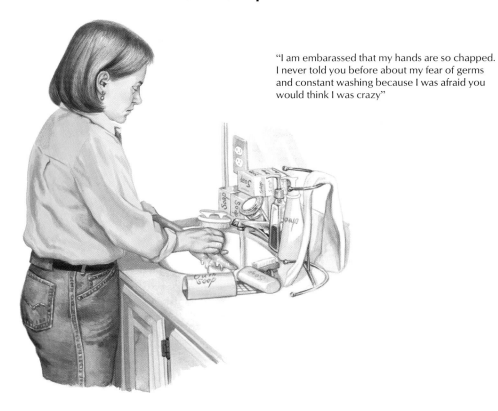

"I am embarassed that my hands are so chapped. I never told you before about my fear of germs and constant washing because I was afraid you would think I was crazy"

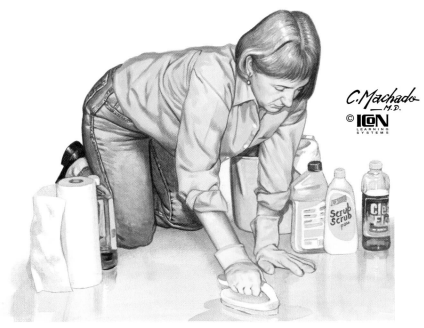

disastrous consequences; somatic obsessions; sexual or aggressive thoughts and images; and need for symmetry, order, or exactness.

Compulsions are repetitive behaviors or mental acts that an individual feels driven to perform to reduce anxiety or to prevent some dreaded event or outcome, even though the event may be totally unrelated to the behavior. Common compulsions are checking, washing (often associated with contamination obsessions), counting, needing to ask or confess, repeating, hoarding, and ordering or arranging. In clinical samples, the presence of pure obsessions or compulsions is rare. Often patients who appear to have only obsessions also have covert reassurance rituals or mental compulsions, such as repeating or praying rituals.

Traditionally, the obsessions and compulsions in OCD have been characterized as "ego-dystonic" (i.e., patients typically view their thoughts and behaviors as senseless and excessive). However, more recent studies and field trials have reported a subset of patients who at times lack insight and display conviction about the reasonableness of their obsessions and necessity of their rituals. It is more likely that insight in OCD may span a spectrum from good to delusional thinking.

Several studies have found that approximately two thirds of OCD patients have a lifetime diagnosis of a comorbid psychiatric disorder. Major depression is very common (50% to 67%) as are other anxiety disorders, including social anxiety disorder, specific phobia, panic disorder, and generalized anxiety disorder. OCD rarely occurs with mania. Some patients with schizophrenia have co-existing obsessions and compulsions, and concurrent OCD may be associated with poorer outcome of schizophrenia.

There is a high degree of bidirectional overlap between tic disorders and OCD. Close to 25% of patients with tic disorders met full criteria for OCD and, conversely, 20% of OCD patients have a lifetime history of multiple tics, with 5% to 10% having a lifetime history of Tourette's syndrome (TS). Patients with tics and obsessive-compulsive symptoms have an earlier average age of onset and strong family histories of OCD and TS. Psychostimulants (e.g., methylphenidate or dextroamphetamine) may exacerbate both tics and obsessive-compulsive symptoms in susceptible individuals.

Recent research has focused on the concept of an "obsessive-compulsive spectrum," based on the observation that a series of possibly related disorders are similar in phenomenology, associated features (age of onset, clinical course, neurobiology), familial transmission, and clinical response to specific pharmacologic and behavioral interventions. These include eating disorders, certain somatoform disorders (hypochondriasis, body dysmorphic disorder), and disorders of impulse control (trichotillomania, pathologic gambling).

DIFFERENTIAL DIAGNOSIS

There are a number of medical disorders that can produce syndromes resembling OCD, including diseases of the basal ganglia, such as Huntington's disease, certain tumors, post-encephalitic conditions, and traumatic brain injury. Because OCD characteristically presents in the teens and 20s, new onset of symptoms in an older individual should raise questions considering the possibility of neurologic contributions.

Swedo and colleagues observed a high prevalence of obsessions and compulsions in children in whom Sydenham's chorea developed. Sydenham's chorea is a neurologic variant of rheumatic fever following a Group A beta-hemolytic streptococci infection. Because there is evidence that Sydenham's chorea may be an autoimmune response involving antibodies to the basal ganglia, this association has led to intriguing work on this phenomenon that has come to be called pediatric autoimmune neuropsychiatric disorder associated with Streptococcus (PANDAS) and treatment with immunologic interventions, such as plasmapheresis or intravenous immunoglobulin therapy. This syndrome tends to present more acutely, in contrast to the more insidious onset in other cases of childhood OCD.

The clinician must also rule out other psychiatric conditions in which obsessive-compulsive behavior might be found. Major depressive disorder is frequently comorbid with OCD and may be characterized by obsessive ruminations. The two conditions may be differentiated by the course of illness. Obsessive symptoms associated with a depression are only present during the depressive episode, while true OCD symptoms will persist independently of a depressive episode. Additionally, depressed patients do not see their thoughts as absurd or senseless. It can also be difficult to distinguish OCD from the worry and anxious apprehension seen in generalized anxiety disorder (GAD). In patients with GAD, the content of the anxious thoughts is realistic, although the worry is excessive. OCD is often confused with obsessive- compulsive personality disorder (OCPD). Although patients with OCD may display perfectionism and indecisiveness, they are no more likely than healthy controls to exhibit the features characteristic of OCPD, such as rigidity, restricted ability to express warmth, or excessive devotion to work.

Psychotic symptoms may sometimes result in obsessions and compulsions that are difficult to distinguish from OCD with poor insight. In most instances, however, patients with OCD will be able to acknowledge the unreasonable nature of their symptoms. Additionally, psychotic disorders, such as schizophrenia, are characterized by other symptoms that are not present in OCD, such as hallucinations, disorganized speech, or flattened affect.

DIAGNOSTIC APPROACH

The failure to properly diagnose OCD is most likely due, in part, to the shame and humiliation that many patients feel about the symptoms and the fear that they will be seen as "crazy." Adults and children can be very secretive about their symptoms, and often OCD is not apparent until secondary symptoms (e.g., dermatological problems from excessive washing and cleaning) reveal themselves or until families complain. However, lack of suspicion on the part of clinicians, as well as failure to ask appropriate screening questions, also play a role in the failure to recognize this disorder. The primary method of establishing a diagnosis is a clinical interview with specific questions designed to elicit a history of intrusive thoughts or behavioral rituals.

Because OCD typically presents in adolescence or early adulthood, screening questions should be asked of any patient in this age group who presents with anxiety, depression, secondary symptoms, or whose family complains of odd rituals and preoccupations. Sample questions might include, "Do you experience thoughts or images that you find disturbing but cannot seem to keep out of your head?" and "Are there actions you feel you must do over and over even though you don't want to?" A patient-administered diagnostic

instrument, as well as relevant information about OCD is available on the *Obsessive Compulsive Foundation* website.

MANAGEMENT AND THERAPY

Pharmacotherapeutic advances have revolutionized the treatment of OCD. SRIs, including clomipramine and the selective serotonin reuptake inhibitors (SSRIs), are the first-line treatment for OCD. Treatment of OCD is specific; other antidepressants are ineffective. Additionally, the therapeutic lag time is longer (8 to 16 weeks) and higher doses are often needed for patients with OCD compared to those with other conditions.

A case report in 1967 provided the first hint that clomipramine might be effective for OCD. Its effectiveness was later confirmed by multicenter placebo-controlled trials. Clomipramine also has norepinephrine and dopamine reuptake properties and is associated with the adverse effects typical of tricyclic antidepressant agents, including anticholinergic, antihistaminergic, alpha-adrenergic side effects, quinidine-like cardiac properties, sexual dysfunction, increased risk of seizures, and lethality in overdose. SSRIs are better tolerated than clomipramine and are also effective in treating obsessive-compulsive spectrum disorders. Fluvoxamine, sertraline, fluoxetine, and paroxetine have been shown to be effective in large, multicenter, placebo-controlled trials. There is also evidence that citalopram, the most selective of the SSRIs, is effective. Additionally, SRIs may effectively treat comorbid mood and anxiety disorders.

A review of studies suggests that 65% to 70% of OCD patients have a clinically significant response to initial SRI treatment and that as many as 90% of patients respond with sequential trials. Thus, patients who do not respond to one SRI may respond to a different one. Generally, treatment provides a 30% to 60% relief of symptoms but does not induce a full remission. Symptoms tend to re-emerge upon discontinuation of therapy, thus requiring long-term treatment for most patients. Long-term data suggest that efficacy is maintained and may even increase over time.

Because as many as 40% to 60% of patients do not have an adequate response to SRI treatment, augmentation strategies are important in managing OCD. A number of pharmacologic agents, including a second SRI, lithium, buspirone, clonazepam, and trazodone, have been used to augment SSRIs, but data confirming their usefulness are limited. Dopamine antagonists, such as haloperidol, have been found to be helpful, particularly in patients with comorbid tic disorders or poor insight. More recently, the combination of an SRI and risperidone seems to hold some promise. Electroconvulsive therapy has not been shown to be effective. Neurosurgery, particularly cingulotomy, has been effective in treating severe, refractory OCD.

Behavioral therapy has consistently been shown to be helpful in reducing the symptoms of OCD. Techniques are based on exposure and response prevention. Patients are increasingly exposed to the feared situation or avoided stimuli and prevented from performing the associated rituals. Compulsions are more amenable to behavioral treatment than obsessions. Because traditional psychodynamic psychotherapy is not effective for OCD, patients should be referred to a mental health professional trained in these techniques. A combination of pharmacotherapy and behavioral therapy has been found to be very effective and is associated with earlier response and reduced risk of relapse.

FUTURE DIRECTIONS

As our understanding of the brain continues to advance, the exact nature of the pathogenesis and etiology of OCD should become more apparent, enabling more precise detection and treatment. More work should be done identifying subtypes of OCD, as well as exploring alternative and adjunctive treatment for patients with treatment resistance. Exciting developments clarifying this important disorder will certainly continue over the coming years.

REFERENCES

Attiullah N, Eisen JL, Rasmussen SA. Clinical features of obsessive-compulsive disorder. *Psychiatr Clin North Am.* 2000; 23:469–491.

Hollander E, Kaplan A, Allen A, Cartwright C. Pharmacotherapy for obsessive-compulsive disorder. *Psychiatr Clin North Am.* 2000;23:643–656.

Obsessive-Compulsive Foundation Web site. Available at: http://www.ocfoundation.org. Accessed March 4, 2003.

Stein DJ. Advances in the neurology of obsessive-compulsive disorder. Implications for conceptualizing putative obsessive-compulsive and spectrum disorders. *Psychiatr Clin North Am.* 2000;23:454–562.

Swedo SE, Leonard HL, Garvey M, et al. Pediatric autoimmune neuropsychiatric disorders associated with streptococcal infections: clinical description of the first 50 cases. *Am J Psychiatry.* 1998;155:264–271.

Chapter 145
Schizophrenia

John H. Gilmore

Schizophrenia describes a heterogeneous group of chronic relapsing psychotic disorders with a lifetime incidence of approximately 1% worldwide. Schizophrenia has a significant impact on the functioning of an individual. The overt clinical symptoms typically present in late adolescence or early adulthood, at a time when one is establishing independence from family, beginning higher education or employment, and establishing adult relationships. Males have an earlier onset, more severe symptoms, poorer treatment response, and a more chronic course. Childhood-onset schizophrenia is a rare, more severe form of the adult-onset illness. Approximately 10% of new-onset psychosis occurs after the age of 40 to 45 years, designated as late-life schizophrenia.

Schizophrenia is, at its core, a disorder of altered reality perception, characterized by hallucinations and delusions (Figure 145-1). However, its onset, presentation, clinical course, and presumably its causes are remarkably heterogeneous. The course is characterized by acute episodes of psychotic symptoms with intervening periods of relative stability that have a varying degree of residual symptoms and functional impairment. The chronic course is variable. In some individuals, symptoms are minimal between acute psychotic episodes, and there is little functional impairment. At the opposite extreme, hallucinations and delusions persist, and there is profound functional impairment.

ETIOLOGY AND PATHOGENESIS

There is clearly a genetic component to schizophrenia. The incidence in the first-degree relatives of an affected individual is approximately 10%. The concordance rate in monozygotic twins is approximately 45%. The search for genes that confer risk for schizophrenia has been disappointing because it is becoming evident that the contribution of any single gene to risk for schizophrenia is small. Regions on several chromosomes have been identified and it is most likely that schizophrenia is a polygenic disorder with multiple susceptibility genes.

Environmental factors contribute to risk for schizophrenia. Prenatal exposure to maternal infection, perinatal hypoxia, and other obstetrical complications increase risk. Birth in an urban area and late winter–early spring birth are more frequent in people in whom schizophrenia develops, perhaps a result of toxic, nutritional, or infectious exposures.

Structural neuroimaging studies find subtle abnormalities of the brain, including mild enlargement of the lateral and third ventricles, and gray matter reductions in the frontal and temporal lobes, as well as in the hippocampus. There is emerging evidence that white matter is also abnormal. Functional imaging studies such as positron emission tomography (PET), MRI, and magnetic resonance spectroscopy also reveal abnormalities in frontal cortex and temporal structures, including the hippocampus. Abnormalities in the cerebellum, thalamus, and striatum have been described.

Postmortem studies reveal subtle abnormalities as well including: changes in neuron number, alteration of various synaptic protein densities, and reduced density of dendritic spines. Abnormalities in several neurotransmitter systems have been implicated by postmortem, PET, and preclinical studies, as well as by the mechanism of action of anti-psychotic medications. The dopamine, glutamate, and serotonin systems are all of importance in schizophrenia.

Currently, schizophrenia is conceptualized with a "two-hit" model in which genetic risk factors interact with perinatal environmental risk factors to cause subtle abnormalities in brain structure and connectivity between neurons. Age-dependent neurodevelopmental events during adolescence such as synaptic pruning and myelination "unmask" abnormal functional circuits in the brain and give rise to clinical symptoms.

Figure 145-1

Schizophrenia

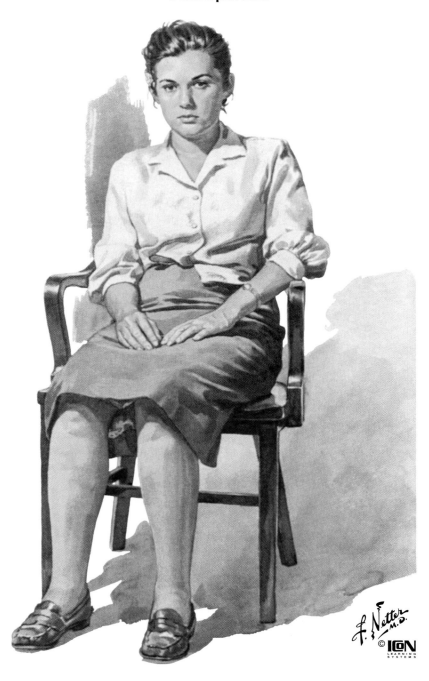

Schizophrenia is a heterogeneous disorder with a wide range of symptomatology. This patient demonstrates the flat affect that is common in schizophrenia. She appears to be responding to internal stimulation—perhaps attending to auditory hallucinations. Alternatively, she may have significant negative symptoms including anhedonia, amotivation, and poverty of speech. Finally, she may have parkinsonism secondary to anti-psychotic medication.

CLINICAL PRESENTATION

There are 3 main domains of symptoms associated with schizophrenia: 1) positive symptoms, 2) negative symptoms, and 3) cognitive dysfunction. *Positive symptoms* are the classic symptoms of psychosis and include delusions and hallucinations. Delusions, false beliefs that are held with conviction despite evidence to the contrary, are present in more than 90% of patients. Delusions can take many forms; paranoid, persecutory, and religious are common. Hallucinations, perceptual disturbances that can occur in any sensory modality, are present in approximately 50% of patients. Of these, auditory and visual hallucinations are the most common.

Negative symptoms are abnormalities of volition and include restricted or flat affect, anhedonia, poverty of speech, apathy, amotivation, and asociality. Approximately 25% of patients with schizophrenia have the "deficit syndrome" or primary negative symptoms, which may be a true subtype of schizophrenia. In other patients, negative symptoms, although common, are secondary to the positive symptoms (i.e., a paranoid person would be asocial and amotivated), depression, anxiety, demoralization, an understimulating environment, or side effects of the medication used to treat psychosis.

Patients typically have *cognitive dysfunction*, which is increasingly recognized as a major reason for functional impairment. A variety of neurocognitive functions including attention, memory, and executive function are impaired. Patients often present with disorganized thinking and speech, due to cognitive dysfunction, as well as positive and negative symptoms.

DIFFERENTIAL DIAGNOSIS

The differential diagnosis of psychosis is long and begins with substance abuse (amphetamines, cocaine, phencyclidine, hallucinogens) or withdrawal (alcohol, sedative-hypnotic). Psychosis is often seen in a hospital setting in the form of delirium resulting from a variety of causes. Medical conditions include acute intermittent porphyria, Cushing's syndrome, hypocalcemia and hypercalcemia, hypoglycemia, hypothyroidism and hyperthyroidism, hepatic encephalopathy, and paraneoplastic syndromes. Neurologic conditions include partial complex seizures, brain tumors, multiple sclerosis, degenerative disorders (Alzheimer's,

Pick's, Huntington's), infections (HIV, neurosyphilis, herpes simplex), lupus cerebritis, strokes, and Wilson's disease. Nutritional deficiencies of folate, niacin, thiamine, and vitamin B_{12} can present with psychosis. Many prescribed medications, heavy metals and other toxic agents can cause psychotic symptoms. Psychotic symptoms are present in other psychiatric disorders including mania, severe depression, brief psychotic disorder, delusional disorder, and schizoaffective disorder.

DIAGNOSTIC APPROACH

The diagnosis is a clinical one based on symptoms present during an interview and by history. Diagnostic criteria for schizophrenia include the presence of 2 of the following for 1 month: delusions, hallucinations, disorganized speech, grossly disorganized or catatonic behavior, and negative symptoms. In addition, significant social/occupational impairment and duration of symptoms of at least 6 months are needed to make a diagnosis of schizophrenia. Symptoms that meet criteria for schizophrenia but have not lasted as long as 6 months are designated as schizophreniform disorder. Patients often believe that their psychotic experiences are real and do not recognize that they are ill. Acutely psychotic patients are frequently disorganized, responding to internal stimuli, and unable to attend to questions. Therefore, it is necessary to get collaborative history from a friend or family member.

New-onset psychosis requires a careful workup, including a physical and neurologic examination to rule out medical and neurologic causes, and substance abuse. Basic laboratory tests include a drug screen, CBC, blood chemistries including calcium, thyroid function tests, HIV, VDRL, and measurement of vitamin B_{12} and folate levels. Additional laboratory work including ceruloplasm, heavy metals, and auto-antibody titers, is pursued based on history, physical examination, and clinical suspicion. Neuroimaging (CT, MRI) is typically done in the workup to rule out a brain tumor and other CNS abnormalities.

MANAGEMENT AND THERAPY

Hospitalization is indicated when the patient is disorganized and is unable to care for himself or herself, or unable to participate in treatment as an outpatient. Suicidal ideation is common. As many as 50% attempt suicide and 10% are successful. Less frequently, patients with schizophrenia harbor homicidal thoughts based on their delusions. The presence of suicidal and homicidal ideation should be carefully assessed. Hospitalization is indicated when the patient is a danger to himself or herself or to others.

The mainstay of treatment is antipsychotic medications. There are a number of antipsychotic medications, now designated as the older "typical" antipsychotics or the newer "atypical" antipsychotics. While antipsychotics have different receptor binding profiles, all have dopamine D2 receptor antagonist properties that are thought to underlie their antipsychotic action. All antipsychotics are equally efficacious in the treatment of psychosis; choice is based on side effect profile, prior treatment response, and physician or patient preference. Clozapine has shown to be more effective than other antipsychotics in patients with treatment-resistant schizophrenia (those who have failed 2 other antipsychotic trials of adequate dose and duration). Cognitive dysfunction and disorganization may make it difficult for a patient to consistently take medication. In these situations, long-acting injectable antipsychotics can be given every 2 to 4 weeks.

Antipsychotic side effects represent a significant challenge in the management of schizophrenia. Acute extrapyramidal syndromes such as parkinsonism, dystonias, akathisia, and acute dyskinesia are most common. Tardive dyskinesia is a long-term effect consisting of involuntary choreoathetoid movements of the mouth, hands, or trunk. Neuroleptic malignant syndrome, a rare but potentially fatal syndrome, is characterized by fever, muscular rigidity, and mental status changes, and can also include autonomic instability, leukocytosis, and elevated creatinine kinase. Other side effects include sedation, orthostatic hypotension, ECG changes (especially prolongation of the Q-T interval), agranulocytosis, hyperprolactinemia, and sexual dysfunction. As more experience with the newer "atypical" antipsychotics is gained, significant weight gain; elevation of glucose, cholesterol, and triglycerides; and the development of type II diabetes mellitus are increasingly recognized as serious long-term side effects.

Patients frequently have co-morbid psychiatric disorders that need to be recognized and treated to improve the course of schizophrenia and a patient's overall functioning. The most common are substance abuse, depression, and obsessive-compulsive disorder.

While medication is the foundation of treatment, other psychosocial treatment modalities play an important role in helping a patient deal with the impact of schizophrenia on his or her life. Supportive, psychoeducational, and cognitive-behavioral therapies, as well as family psychoeducation and intensive community-based outreach programs, all improve outcome and level of functioning in patients. Rehabilitative strategies are used to help patients compensate for deficits in cognitive and social functioning.

Management of Medical Illness in Patients with Schizophrenia

Medical illness is common in patients with schizophrenia, and the recognition and treatment of medical illness presents a challenge to clinicians. Individuals with schizophrenia have high rates of morbidity and mortality related to a variety of medical conditions including cardiovascular disease, infections, endocrine disorders, and cancer. This high rate of morbidity and mortality is probably related to the side effects of antipsychotic medications, high rates of smoking, low physical activity, poor nutrition, and high levels of chronic stress.

Psychiatrists and other physicians fail to diagnose medical conditions in one third to one half of patients with schizophrenia and a comorbid medical disorder. Psychotic symptoms and cognitive dysfunction, as well as elevated pain thresholds associated with schizophrenia, interfere with symptom recognition, symptom reporting, and seeking help on the part of the patient. From the physician's perspective, a frightening, unhygienic patient with imaginary voices and delusions may be assumed to have imaginary medical problems. Physicians must be alert to high rates of unreported and unrecognized medical illness in patients with schizophrenia. Once a medical illness is diagnosed, it is important to anticipate how the positive and negative symptoms and cognitive dysfunction of schizophrenia might impact a patient's ability to participate in treatment.

FUTURE DIRECTIONS

There is a clear need for improved pharmacologic treatment of schizophrenia. Only 35% to 45% of patients with schizophrenia have their positive symptoms well controlled by antipsychotic medication, and an estimated 33% are considered to be treatment-resistant. In addition, available antipsychotics have potentially serious side effects. Medications that treat negative symptoms and cognitive dysfunction have the potential to improve functional outcome. There is new interest in recognizing and treating schizophrenia before the onset of gross psychotic symptoms with the hope of preventing the progression of the illness and improving long-term outcome. Continuing advances in understanding brain development and functioning from basic neuroscience studies will ultimately improve our ability to define the causes and pathogenesis of schizophrenia and should lead to improved preventive and therapeutic efforts.

REFERENCES

Hirsch SR, Weinberger DR, eds. *Schizophrenia*. 2nd ed. Malden, Mass: Blackwell Publishing; 2003.

Hwang MY, Bermanzohn PC, eds. *Schizophrenia and Comorbid Conditions*. Washington, DC: American Psychiatric Press; 2001.

Lewis DA, Lieberman JA. Catching up on schizophrenia: natural history and neurobiology. *Neuron.* 2000;28:325-334.

Lieberman JA, Murray RM, eds. *Comprehensive Care of Schizophrenia: A Textbook of Clinical Management*. London, England: Martin Dunitz; 2001.

Shriqui CL, Nasrallah HA, eds. *Contemporary Issues in the Treatment of Schizophrenia*. Washington, DC: American Psychiatric Press; 1995.

Chapter 146
Substance Abuse

Robert E. Gwyther and John M. Thorp Jr

The abuse of licit, illicit, and prescription drugs is common. At least 15% of outpatient visits, 25% to 40% of inpatient admissions, and more than 50% of some specialty unit patients (e.g., psychiatry, burn units) have a substance abuse problem. Alcohol and tobacco abuse cause a majority of these encounters; however, the abuse of other drugs, including stimulants (e.g., cocaine, amphetamines), opioids (e.g., heroin, oxycodone), depressants (e.g., benzodiazepines, barbiturates), and hallucinogens (e.g., lysergic acid, phencyclidine) is substantial. Drug abuse is associated with many diseases and should be considered as a causative factor in every patient encounter.

ETIOLOGY AND PATHOGENESIS

The unifying feature of all drugs of abuse is that they directly stimulate or enhance the effect of endogenous neurotransmitters in a sequence of CNS nuclei that constitute the reinforcement (or pleasure) pathway (Figure 146-1). These subcortical nuclei normally reinforce specific behaviors, such as eating and reproduction. Drug abusers seek positive reinforcement from using drugs. Drug use is often accompanied by negative consequences (physical, psychologic, social, etc.). Patients who continue to use drugs in spite of negative consequences are said to be dependent (*Diagnostic and Statistical Manual of Mental Disorders-VI* [DSM-IV]) or addicted (World Health Organization, American Society of Addiction Medicine).

Specific drugs have toxic effects on the body, commonly harming the brain, liver, heart, and/or blood vessels. Some problems are due to direct effects, for example, respiratory depression from opiates. Some are due to the method of use, such as acquiring HIV by sharing contaminated needles. Other problems occur when pharmacologically dependent patients are deprived of their drugs and withdrawal syndromes develop. The severity of withdrawal depends on the quantity and duration of use of a drug. Other toxicities are due to interactions between abused drugs and other substances ingested (e.g., necrotizing vasculitis caused by cocaethylene, a byproduct of using cocaine and alcohol together).

Drug toxicity is related to the blood level achieved and duration of action. Given a drug's mechanism of metabolism, these factors depend on 1) size of the dose; 2) time taken for the dose to become active on the brain; 3) dilution in the bloodstream before reaching the brain; and 4) whether first pass metabolism in the liver occurs. In general, oral administration yields a low blood level and has a relatively long effect. Transmucosal and subcutaneous routes also yield low blood levels and have a long effect. Intravenous administration yields higher blood levels, but shorter duration of action, and drugs inhaled into the lungs yield the highest blood levels, but have the shortest duration of action. Another factor in drug effect is purity. Street drugs are uncontrolled; they have varying concentrations or may be "cut" with additives, which can lead to complications (e.g., talc granulomas; overdose from heroin).

CLINICAL PRESENTATION

Drug-related diseases have numerous presentations and can mimic many other problems. The following are some drugs and their common, toxic presentations:

Stimulants: tachycardia, increased blood pressure, ischemia of brain or heart, delusions, grandiose behavior

Opioids: bradycardia, decreased respiratory rate, miotic pupils, decreased consciousness.

Sedative-hypnotic drugs: bradycardia, hypotension, decreased respiratory rate, decreased consciousness, ataxia

Hallucinogens: hallucinations, disorientation, anxiety, psychosis

Signs and symptoms of drug withdrawal are

Figure 146-1

Brain Reward Circuit

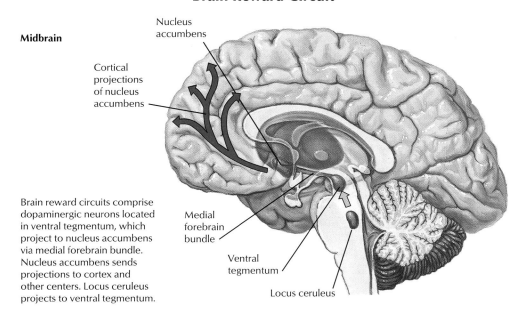

Midbrain

Nucleus accumbens

Cortical projections of nucleus accumbens

Brain reward circuits comprise dopaminergic neurons located in ventral tegmentum, which project to nucleus accumbens via medial forebrain bundle. Nucleus accumbens sends projections to cortex and other centers. Locus ceruleus projects to ventral tegmentum.

Medial forebrain bundle

Ventral tegmentum

Locus ceruleus

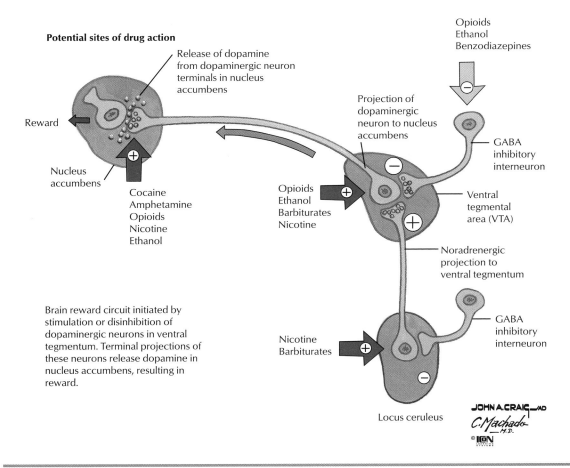

Potential sites of drug action

Release of dopamine from dopaminergic neuron terminals in nucleus accumbens

Reward

Nucleus accumbens

Cocaine
Amphetamine
Opioids
Nicotine
Ethanol

Opioids
Ethanol
Benzodiazepines

Projection of dopaminergic neuron to nucleus accumbens

GABA inhibitory interneuron

Opioids
Ethanol
Barbiturates
Nicotine

Ventral tegmental area (VTA)

Noradrenergic projection to ventral tegmentum

Nicotine
Barbiturates

GABA inhibitory interneuron

Brain reward circuit initiated by stimulation or disinhibition of dopaminergic neurons in ventral tegmentum. Terminal projections of these neurons release dopamine in nucleus accumbens, resulting in reward.

Locus ceruleus

JOHN A. CRAIG—AD
C. Machado
M.D.
© ICN

commonly the opposite of their toxicities. For instance, people withdrawing from phenobarbital, a sedative-hypnotic, may appear agitated and have hypertension or tachycardia. Drug abusers may dislike some effects of their primary drug and use other drug(s) to counteract them. For example, sedative-hypnotic and/or opioid drugs may be used to counteract undesirable effects of cocaine. Acutely, patients may demonstrate the net effect of several drugs and, because the half-lives of different drugs vary widely, they may demonstrate simultaneous, toxic manifestations of some drugs and withdrawal effects from others.

Signs and symptoms of drug intoxication and withdrawal may mimic other diseases (Figures 146-2, 146-3 and 146-4). For instance, seizures are a feature of sedative-hypnotic drug withdrawal (including alcohol), but can also occur because of head trauma or intracranial bleeding. Patients who use drugs are prone to automobile crashes and falls, so physicians should not assume that a known alcohol abuser who presents with seizures is in alcohol withdrawal. A comprehensive list of presenting signs and symptoms of drug abuse is not useful because of the large number of agents and their association with numerous diseases. "Red flags" for substance abuse include the following:

Historical factors: Violence, trauma, hematemesis, acute mental status changes, acute psychosis, previous drug abuse, homelessness, criminal behavior, financial deterioration, job loss, seeking a specific controlled substance.

Physical findings: Increased or decreased pulse, respirations or blood pressure; poor hygiene; odor of alcohol; jaundice, splinter hemorrhages, needle tracks or spider hemangiomata; miosis or mydriasis; perforated nasal septum; new heart murmur; ataxia, hyperreflexia; combativeness, decreased consciousness; findings inconsistent with the stated level of pain.

Diagnostic test results: Positive drug screen; elevated liver enzymes; positive cardiac enzymes in a young person; ECGs showing rapid rhythms; evidence of MI in a young person; CT or MRI evidence of stroke in a young person.

DIFFERENTIAL DIAGNOSIS

Drugs may be the underlying cause of disease in patients not previously known to be abusers. Because known drug abusers are often malnour-

ished, have underlying organ damage, and experience events such as falls or tracheal aspiration while intoxicated, it is common for them to develop other mental and physical illnesses. Drug abuse should be listed in most differential diagnoses. Some general considerations for drug-related problems are: 1) when the working diagnoses are ruled out, think about drugs; 2) when young patients suffer ischemia (e.g., transient ischemic attacks or MI), consider cocaine and/or the combination of cocaine and alcohol; 3) when treating a substance abuser (e.g., delirium in a withdrawal syndrome) without getting the expected response, look for a complication (e.g., subdural hematoma); 4) toxic manifestations of one drug (e.g., agitation, tachycardia in cocaine intoxication) mimic the withdrawal symptoms of another (e.g., agitation, tachycardia in barbiturate withdrawal); 5) drug use is associated with perinatal problems (e.g., premature labor, placental abruption with cocaine abuse) and newborn complications (e.g., HIV, opiate withdrawal in infants of heroin-addicted mothers).

DIAGNOSTIC APPROACH

Drug abuse diagnoses follow the criteria established in the DSM-IV, which includes categories for intoxication, withdrawal, dependence, and related disorders for numerous drugs and drug categories. Basically, a patient must have used a specific drug for a time, suffered untoward effects, and in the case of dependence, continued to abuse the drug. The diagnosis of "addiction" defined by the American Society of Addiction Medicine is similar to dependence under DSM-IV criteria.

Drug abuse may be diagnosed during any physician encounter. In a non-judgmental fashion, ask the patient about the type, amount, and frequency of substances used. After determining use, its consequences should be explored, including physical symptoms, relationship and employment problems, and emotional/psychologic issues. Input from partners, close family members, and friends may help define the magnitude of the patient's problem, especially for patients who deny problems.

The CAGE screening test, developed for alcohol use, is composed of 4 questions and may be used as a quick drug abuse screen for routine encounters.

A "yes" response to 2 items is a positive screen,

CAGE Screening Test

Cut down—Have you felt the need to cut down on your drinking or drug use?

Annoyed—Have people annoyed you by criticizing your drinking or drug use?

Guilty—Have you ever felt guilty about your drinking or drug use?

Eye-opener—Do you need to have an eye-opener to get started in the morning?

Adapted from Mayfield DL, McLeod G, Hall P. The CAGE Questionaire. *JAMA.* 1984; 252:1905–07.

necessitating further information to make a DSM-IV diagnosis. CAGE accurately identifies 80% to 90% of male alcoholics and its accuracy varies in other circumstances. Its applicability to pregnant women is unclear. The MAST (Michigan Alcohol Screening Test) and DAST (Drug Abuse Screening Test), longer questionnaires that contain weighted items, are prone to false-positive results and should be administered concomitantly to detect poly-substance abuse. ASI (Addiction Severity Index), a multifactorial diagnostic instrument, provides a way to assess the impact of substance use on a patient's life.

Drug abuse diagnoses are most often obtained from a good history. Sometimes, laboratory testing is helpful, although laboratory tests may be normal in someone with drug problems. Blood testing for drugs is quantitatively accurate and necessary for managing critical problems but has the diagnostic disadvantage of a relatively narrow window of positivity. Urine drug screens are qualitatively accurate and offer a longer window of positivity (e.g., 48 to 72 hours for cocaine users, 2 to 4 weeks for regular marijuana users). Hair testing is helpful in documenting remote use and use over time. However, it is not quantitatively accurate or readily available, and hair testing is expensive.

Laboratory testing may be necessary to make diagnoses; properly manage patients' medical conditions; monitor patients in addiction treatment; screen job applicants; and monitor federal personnel involved in the Departments of Transportation (e.g., pilots, truck drivers) and Defense (e.g., the Army). The federal screening panel includes amphetamines, cannabinoids, cocaine, opioids, and phencyclidine. Laboratories are regulated by strict criteria;

certified medical review officers interpret positive results, taking patient histories into account.

Legal and ethical dilemmas of laboratory drug testing include the following:

Informed consent: Ideally, patients should understand the ramifications of getting tested for drug use. Yet, some patients are unconscious on presentation and cannot give consent. Others are minors living in states where parents can demand tests even though the child refuses. Some refusals may be ignored, especially when a patient is intoxicated and not competent to refuse. Inevitably, drug tests sometimes are performed without patient consent.

Criminal/civil justice: Negative consequences may avail from positive tests. For a drug test to be admissible in a criminal court the following must happen: 1) a chain of custody must be established from the time the sample is collected until the results are introduced into evidence; and, 2) the methodology required by the state's courts must be used.

Medicolegal liability: There is legal risk for physicians treating drug abusers without definitive diagnoses. If a patient suffers a bad outcome from a medical condition caused by use of illicit drugs (defined in most states as the fault of the user), but the drug use was never documented, the treating physician might be held responsible.

MANAGEMENT AND THERAPY

Once the diagnosis of drug abuse is made, one should follow an appropriate course of action, guided by the clinical scenario. A common sense sequence is the following: 1) treat urgent medical problems first; 2) if the patient is an alcohol abuser, give thiamine to prevent encephalopathy; and 3) psychiatric problems should be considered, diagnosed, and treated. If dangerous to self or others, the patient may warrant commitment. Person(s) being threatened by the drug abuser must be informed and appropriate authorities notified; 4) if the patient is pharmacologically dependent on a drug (e.g. heroin addict admitted with a fractured femur), administer an appropriate substitution or detoxification regimen (e.g., methadone) to prevent withdrawal; 5) if a pharmacologically dependent patient wishes to stop using drugs, detoxify the patient; 6) determine the patient's motivation and resources to support addiction treatment and involve social workers and/or drug

Figure 146-2

Opioid Withdrawal

Signs and Symptoms

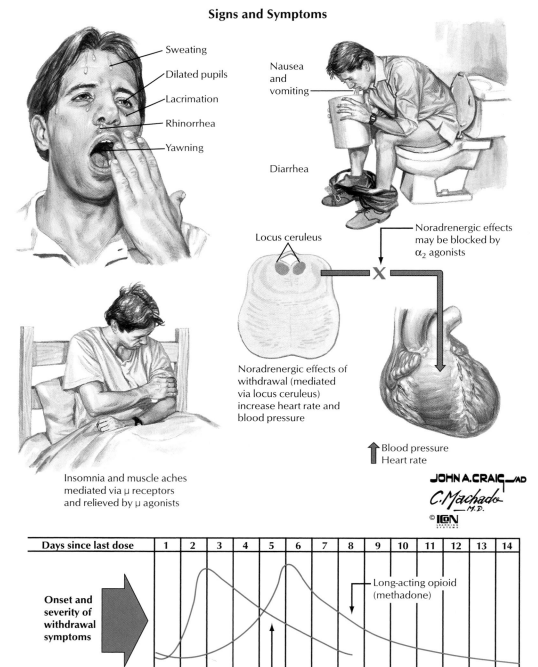

Sweating

Dilated pupils

Lacrimation

Rhinorrhea

Yawning

Nausea and vomiting

Diarrhea

Locus ceruleus

Noradrenergic effects may be blocked by α_2 agonists

Noradrenergic effects of withdrawal (mediated via locus ceruleus) increase heart rate and blood pressure

Blood pressure
Heart rate

Insomnia and muscle aches mediated via μ receptors and relieved by μ agonists

JOHN A. CRAIG—AD
C. Machado
—M.D.
©ICN

Days since last dose	1	2	3	4	5	6	7	8	9	10	11	12	13	14

Onset and severity of withdrawal symptoms

Long-acting opioid (methadone)

Short-acting opioids (morphine, hydromorphone)

Severity of opioid withdrawal varies with dose and duration of opioid use. Onset and duration of symptoms after last drug dose depend on half-life of particular drug

Figure 146-3

Alcohol Withdrawal

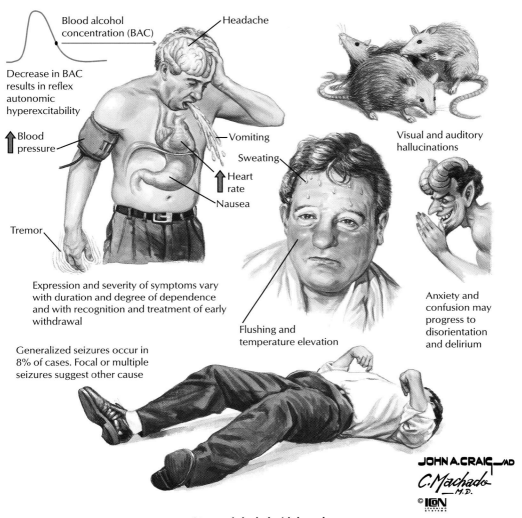

Blood alcohol concentration (BAC)

Headache

Decrease in BAC results in reflex autonomic hyperexcitability

↑ Blood pressure

Vomiting

Sweating

↑ Heart rate

Nausea

Visual and auditory hallucinations

Tremor

Expression and severity of symptoms vary with duration and degree of dependence and with recognition and treatment of early withdrawal

Flushing and temperature elevation

Anxiety and confusion may progress to disorientation and delirium

Generalized seizures occur in 8% of cases. Focal or multiple seizures suggest other cause

JOHN A. CRAIG—MD
C. Machado—M.D.
© ICN LEARNING SYSTEMS

Stages of alcohol withdrawal

	Stage 1	Stage 2	Stage 3
Hours after alcohol consumption	24 36 (peak) 48	(48–72)	(72–105)
Symptoms	Mild-to-moderate anxiety, tremor, nausea, vomiting, sweating, elevation of heart rate and blood pressure, sleep disturbance, hallucinations, illusions, seizures	Aggravated forms of Stage 1 symptoms with severe tremors, agitation, and hallucinations	Acute organic psychosis (delirium), confusion, and disorientation with severe autonomic symptoms

Stage 1 withdrawal usually self-limited. Only small percentage of cases progress to stages 2 and 3. Progression prevented by prompt and adequate treatment

Figure 146-4

Benzodiazepine Withdrawal

High-dose withdrawal

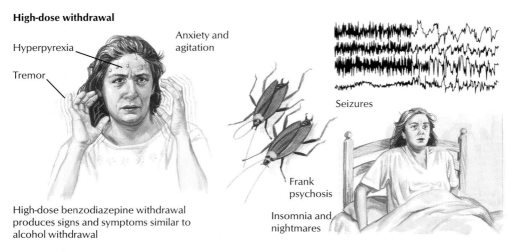

Hyperpyrexia

Tremor

Anxiety and agitation

Seizures

Frank psychosis

Insomnia and nightmares

High-dose benzodiazepine withdrawal produces signs and symptoms similar to alcohol withdrawal

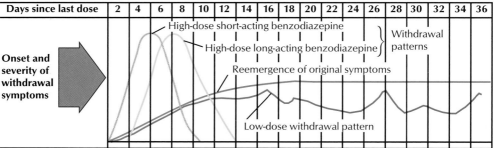

Days since last dose	2	4	6	8	10	12	14	16	18	20	22	24	26	28	30	32	34	36

Onset and severity of withdrawal symptoms

High-dose short-acting benzodiazepine

High-dose long-acting benzodiazepine

Withdrawal patterns

Reemergence of original symptoms

Low-dose withdrawal pattern

Low-dose (therapeutic) withdrawal

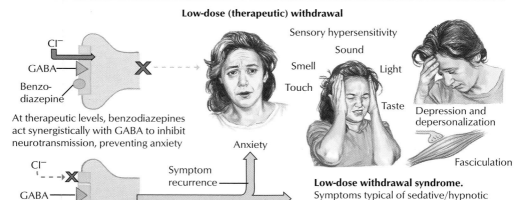

Cl⁻

GABA

Benzo-diazepine

At therapeutic levels, benzodiazepines act synergistically with GABA to inhibit neurotransmission, preventing anxiety

Cl⁻

GABA

Benzodiazepine

Symptom recurrence

Anxiety

Low-dose withdrawal syndrome

Sensory hypersensitivity

Sound

Smell

Light

Touch

Taste

Depression and depersonalization

Fasciculation

Low-dose withdrawal syndrome. Symptoms typical of sedative/hypnotic withdrawal, fluctuating hypersensitivity to sensory input, muscle twitching, depression, and depersonalization.

Withdrawing long-term benzodiazepine causes loss of synergism with GABA inhibition, resulting in recurrence of original symptoms and low-dose withdrawal syndrome

JOHN A. CRAIG—MD

C. Machado—M.D.

© ICON
LEARNING
SYSTEMS

counselors in these assessments as appropriate; 7) addiction treatment should be initiated at the earliest feasible stage. Options include:

Brief Intervention: Brief interventions are used for patients diagnosed as "risky users." This involves educating the patient about the pros and cons of drug use, discussing options for changing behavior, obtaining patient commitment to reduce consumption, and follow-up.

Pharmacotherapies: Substitution involves prescribing the same drug (e.g., nicotine patches for cigarette smokers) or a cross-tolerant drug (e.g., methadone for heroin addicts) to ease or prevent a withdrawal syndrome. Blocking uses antagonistic drugs to block the desirable effects of abused drugs (e.g., naltrexone for opiate abusers). If patients take the abused drug, they are unable to perceive its positive effects. Aversion involves taking disulfiram, to precipitate a noxious physical reaction if a patient subsequently drinks alcohol.

"12-Step" Programs: Inpatient or outpatient addiction treatment, which endeavors to educate patients about addiction and using "self-help" groups (e.g., Narcotics Anonymous) to maintain sobriety.

Aversion Therapy: Using classical conditioning principles, therapists either administer electric shock to patients' arms while the (drug addicted) patients use simulated drugs in the usual fashion; or, administer emetics, then have alcoholic patients drink and subsequently regurgitate alcoholic beverages.

Cognitive-Behavioral Treatment: Patients and therapists work to identify the pros and cons of drug use and make rational decisions about behavior change.

"Self-Help" Groups: Beginning with Alcoholics Anonymous (AA) during the 1930s, a variety of therapeutic organizations have been developed to change addictive behaviors, including Narcotics Anonymous (NA) and Cocaine Anonymous focus on drug addiction. Overeaters Anonymous and Gamblers Anonymous are other similar programs. These programs have long-term success rates as high or higher than other therapies, especially for members who stay involved at least a year.

Finally, most clinicians have "recovering patients" in their practices. Physicians should follow these principles in their treatment: use appropriate, non-pharmacologic therapies when possible. Be wary of treating anxiety, insomnia, pain, and allergies with sedative-hypnotic drugs, opioids, and antihistamines, which may provoke relapse. Treat depression and anxiety with drugs that are usually not addictive (e.g., selective serotonin reuptake inhibitors [SSRIs], buspirone). If a recovering drug abuser needs an analgesic, contract specifically for pain relief. If opioids are required, offer to detoxify the patient with methadone as an inpatient. Offer ongoing support for the patient's recovery.

FUTURE DIRECTIONS

It is widely acknowledged that the "War on Drugs" is not working. The price and purity of available illicit drugs have not been adversely affected by federal spending. The government and the courts are looking increasingly to drug treatment rather than incarceration for drug users, so physicians will increasingly be asked to treat or refer patients.

The number of patients with substance abuse, specifically opiate abuse, overburdens the federally controlled network of methadone programs. Additionally, programs are located such that many patients must drive hours each day to participate. While methadone maintenance has been shown to be cost-effective, it is not meeting the needs of the nation. Two possibilities are being considered for the future: LAAM (levo-alpha-acetylmethadol), a long-acting substitute for opiate dependence, is already available in a few methadone programs. It can be administered 3 times per week, rather than the daily. Buprenorphine, a long-acting opioid agonist, has been approved by the FDA for use in outpatient treatment of opioid addicts by certified physicians. Similar authorization for LAAM and methadone is being studied.

REFERENCES

Brown RL. Identification and office management of alcohol and drug disorders. In: Fleming MF, Barry KL, eds. *Addictive Disorders.* St Louis, Mo: Mosby-Year Book Inc; 1992.

Fleming MF, Barry KL. Clinical overview of alcohol and drug disorders. In: Fleming MF, Barry KL, eds. *Addictive Disorders.* St Louis, Mo: Mosby-Year Book Inc; 1992.

Moore RD, Bone LR, Geller G, Mamon JA, Stokes EJ, Levine DM. Prevalence, detection, and treatment of alcoholism in hospitalized patients. *JAMA.* 1989;261:403–407.

Steindler EM. Appendix B: ASAM addiction terminology. In: Graham AW, Schultz TK, eds. *Principles of Addiction Medicine.* Chevy Chase, Md: American Society of Addiction Medicine; 1998.

Section XVIII

DISORDERS OF THE SKIN

Chapter 147
Alopecia

Heidi T. Jacobe and David S. Rubenstein

Hair loss results from a number of pathological and physiological processes (Figure 147-1). Identification of the causative agents of hair loss enables the clinician to design a rational approach to treatment. This chapter will briefly familiarize the reader with the basic diagnostic tools and treatment options for common causes of hair loss (Table 147-1).

NON-SCARRING ALOPECIA

Non-scarring alopecia is hair loss in the setting of a normal-appearing scalp. The hair pull test will differentiate breaking from shedding.

The hair pull test is performed by taking 50 to 100 hairs and gently pulling from the scalp out. Repeat this several times all over the scalp. If more than a few hairs come out from the roots, the test result is positive. The hair bulbs should be examined under the microscope to determine if the hairs are anagen or telogen hairs. This will help differentiate between different causes of non-scarring alopecia.

In the patient with brittle hair the hair pull test will reveal broken off hair with no visible bulb. Patients with brittle hair should be questioned regarding hair care. Improper hair care is the most common cause of brittle hair in adults. Treatment is gentle hair care. Brittle hair in children, in the absence of tinea capitis, can be the result of a heritable structural defect of the hair shaft. These patients should be referred to a dermatologist.

ALOPECIA AREATA
Etiology and Pathogenesis

The precise etiology of alopecia areata is unknown. However, a genetic predisposition and autoimmunity appear important. Alopecia areata is associated with a number of autoimmune disorders including atopy, autoimmune thyroid disease, vitiligo, diabetes mellitus, Addison's disease, pernicious anemia, lupus erythematosus, and rheumatoid arthritis.

Clinical Presentation

Alopecia areata is most common in children and young adults. Patients note a sudden loss of hair in oval patches (Figure 147-2). Non-scalp hair-bearing areas are rarely affected. Re-growth occurs after 1 to 3 months. Hair loss may occur in new areas while re-growth occurs.

Examination reveals 1 to 4 cm oval patches of alopecia with a smooth scalp or short stubs of hair (exclamation point hairs). Nail pitting occurs in 3% to 30% of patients.

Diagnostic Approach

The diagnosis is usually clinical. The hair pull test shows dystrophic anagen and telogen hairs. Serological testing should be performed to rule out syphilis. Biopsy is rarely necessary. The differential diagnosis includes secondary syphilis.

Management and Therapy

Limited alopecia areata frequently resolves spontaneously and treatment is not always necessary. The therapy of choice is intradermal injection of triamcinolone acetonide repeated every 4 weeks until re-growth is achieved. Atrophy is the major side effect. Potent topical steroids (clobetasol propionate) in cycles of 2 weeks on and 1 week off are an alternative, particularly in widespread disease or for children.

ANDROGENETIC ALOPECIA
Etiology and Pathogenesis

This polygenic disorder predisposes affected individuals to lose hair from androgen-sensitive follicles on the scalp.

Clinical Presentation

Affecting men and women equally, hair loss begins in the 20s and is fully expressed by middle age. Two thirds of affected women have andro-

Figure 147-1

Hair Loss

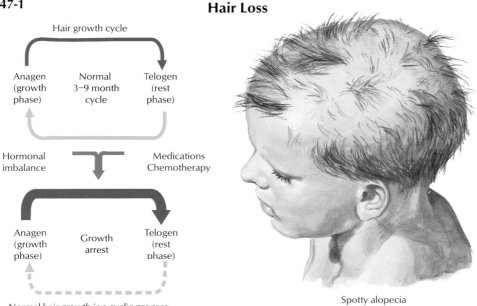

Hair growth cycle

Anagen (growth phase) — Normal 3–9 month cycle — Telogen (rest phase)

Hormonal imbalance — Medications Chemotherapy

Anagen (growth phase) — Growth arrest — Telogen (rest phase)

Normal hair growth is a cyclic process. Conditions that upset the grow-rest cycling may delay replacement of normal hair loss, resulting in alopecia. Such conditions are usually reversible.

Spotty alopecia

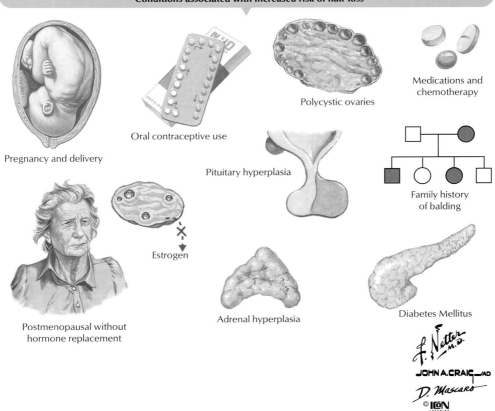

Conditions associated with increased risk of hair loss

Pregnancy and delivery

Oral contraceptive use

Polycystic ovaries

Medications and chemotherapy

Pituitary hyperplasia

Family history of balding

Postmenopausal without hormone replacement

Estrogen

Adrenal hyperplasia

Diabetes Mellitus

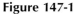

TABLE 147-1
Evaluation of the Patient with Hair Loss

History

Determine if the hair loss is abnormal. Hair counts distinguish pathologic from physiologic hair loss. Have patients collect shed hairs for 7 days for the evaluation. Loss of more than 50 to 100 hairs per day indicates pathologic processes.

Determine the timing of hair loss. Is it acute or gradual? Has it been present since birth?

Identify associated symptoms such as pain, tenderness, and pruritus.

Determine if there are other skin complaints.

Elicit a history of recent illness, stress, or medication use.

Identify associated medical problems.

Identify affected family members.

Clinical Exam

Determine if the hair loss is scarring or non-scarring. Scarring alopecias are characterized by the permanent loss of hair follicles within the foci of alopecia.

Determine if the process is inflammatory or non-inflammatory. Inflammatory processes present with erythema, pruritus, or pain.

Assess the presence or absence of scale, pustules, and adenopathy .
Determine the pattern of hair loss. Is it restricted to focal areas of the scalp, or does it involve other hair-bearing regions?

Laboratory Examination

The hair pull test identifies pathologic hair loss. Approximately 50 hairs are gently pulled from the base of the hairs. Release of 2 or more hairs is abnormal.

Examine the bulbs of the released hairs microscopically to determine the phase of the hair cycle. Telogen hairs have rounded, non-pigmented bulbs. Anagen hairs have a cylindrical or tapered pigmented bulb (Figure 147-3).

Hair shaft examination identifies traumatic or genetic causes for hair loss.

Punch biopsy aids in identifying underlying pathology, particularly in cases of scarring or permanent hair loss.

Potassium hydroxide preparation and fungal cultures are performed for suspected cases of tinea capitis.

Figure 147-2 Alopecia Areata

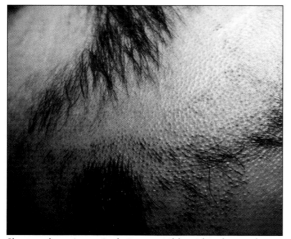

Short exclamation point hairs are visible within the patches of non-scarring hair loss.

genetic alopecia. Men have frontal recession, proceeding to loss of hair in the crown and sometimes to total hair loss in the central scalp. The terminal scalp hairs become vellus hairs. In advanced cases, the scalp is shiny and smooth. Women have miniaturized hairs, increased space between individual hairs, and preservation of the frontal hairline.

Diagnostic Approach

A thorough history and examination are usually adequate. The differential diagnosis includes other causes of non-scarring alopecia. A careful medication history will exclude drug-induced alopecia. Medications associated with hair loss include anticoagulants, ACE inhibitors, beta-blockers, lithium, oral contraceptives, retinoids, valproic acid, and vitamin A excess. In women,

Table 147-2
Causes of Telogen Effluvium

Psychological stress

Physical stress-systemic illness, surgery

Anemia

Endocrine: postpartum, peri- or postmenopausal states, hypo- or hyperthyroidism, oral contraceptives

Nutritional: protein/calorie deprivation, essential fatty acid deficiency, zinc deficiency, biotin deficiency, iron deficiency, vitamin A excess

Medications

signs of a hyperandrogenetic state should prompt endocrinological evaluation.

Management and Therapy

Minoxidil, applied twice a day to a dry scalp, is the mainstay of therapy. It prevents further hair loss and provides moderate regrowth at the vertex of the scalp in 30% of patients. Results take at least 3 months to become evident. It must be used continually to preserve the beneficial effect. In men, finasteride (1 mg/day) used continuously to preserve regrowth is effective for hair loss at the crown. Decreased libido and erectile dysfunction occur in less than 2% of men. Finasteride is contraindicated in women. Minoxidil and finasteride may be used in combination. Advanced hair loss requires surgical intervention (hair transplant or scalp reduction).

TELOGEN EFFLUVIUM
Etiology and Pathogenesis

A traumatic event (Table 147-2) can induce a large number of hairs to prematurely enter catagen, then telogen. Telogen hairs are shed 2 to 3 months after the event with 50% of the hair affected.

Clinical Presentation

Telogen effluvium occurs in both sexes and all age groups with an abrupt onset of diffuse shedding. A precipitating event 3 months before the onset of the hair loss usually can be identified. Physical examination may appear unremarkable.

Differential Diagnosis

The main differential diagnosis is anagen efflu-

Figure 147-3

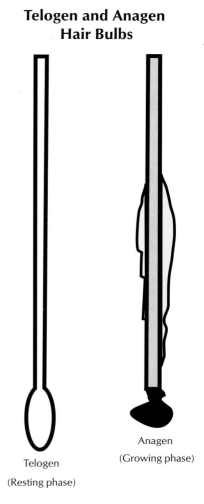

Telogen and Anagen Hair Bulbs

Anagen
(Growing phase)

Telogen
(Resting phase)

vium, which occurs after chemotherapy. Anagen effluvium begins within 2 to 4 weeks after drug exposure, produces much more marked hair loss, and is characterized by the presence of anagen hairs on the hair pull test.

Diagnostic Approach

The characteristic history in a patient with a normal scalp is usually adequate. The hair pull test is positive, revealing non-dystrophic telogen hairs. Biopsy is not indicated.

Management and Therapy

This condition spontaneously resolves in 6 months.

Figure 147-4   Discoid Lupus Erythematosus

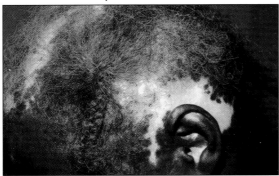

Note areas of scar formation and complete absence of hair follicles.

TINEA CAPITIS
Etiology and Pathogenesis

Tinea capitis is a contagious infection of the scalp and hair caused by superficial fungi (*Trichophyton tonsurans*, *Microsporum canis*) common in children and in patients chronically using topical corticosteroids in the scalp. Replication of fungi within and around the hair shaft leads to breakage as it exits the hair follicle resulting in non-scarring hair loss. A vigorous inflammatory reaction called a kerion may develop. Chronic inflammation from the kerion or from secondary bacterial infection can lead to scalp fibrosis and permanent hair loss.

Clinical Presentation

Tinea capitis presents as single or multiple dry scaling patches, with numerous hairs broken off as they exit the follicle (black dot ringworm), with or without an inflammatory border. Kerions are characterized by boggy indurated plaque(s) with pustules; pre-auricular, post-auricular, and cervical adenopathy are often present.

Diagnostic Approach

Potassium hydroxide (KOH) preparation of plucked hairs and skin scrapings from the border of the lesion identifies spores within (endothrix) or outside (ectothrix) the hair shaft and hyphal elements, respectively. Fungal cultures are helpful in identifying suspicious KOH-negative cases. A punch biopsy with periodic acid-Shiff stain can demonstrate fungi. The differential diagnosis includes seborrheic dermatitis.

Management and Therapy

Griseofulvin, itraconazole, or terbinafine with adjunctive daily use of ketoconazole shampoo decreases the risk of infecting contacts. Concomitant use of systemic corticosteroids may reduce the inflammation and risk of fibrosis associated with kerion.

SCARRING (CICATRICIAL) AND PERMANENT ALOPECIAS

Processes that lead to scarring and permanent alopecia result in irreversible hair loss. True scarring results in loss of elastic tissue; non-scarring permanent alopecias retain elastic tissue. Non-scarring permanent hair loss is due to atrophy or infiltrative replacement of follicular structures. End-stage disease is characterized by loss of hair follicles. It may be difficult to clinically distinguish advanced stages of scarring and permanent alopecias. Histological analysis is helpful in identifying the specific disease process.

Discoid Lupus Erythematosus
Etiology and Pathogenesis

Discoid lupus erythematosis (DLE) is an autoimmune disorder of unclear etiology. Five percent to 10% of patients with DLE have or will have signs and symptoms of systemic lupus.

Clinical Presentation

Early lesions are erythematous to violaceous patches and plaques with adherent scales. A hair pull test may reveal anagen hairs. With progression, patients develop hypopigmentation, atrophy, telangiectasias, and fibrosis/scar (Figure 147-4). Similar appearing cutaneous lesions can be found in areas other than the scalp. Often there are superficial ulcerations of the palate as well as proximal nail-fold erythema and telangiectasias.

Differential Diagnosis

The differential diagnosis includes lichen planopilaris and Pseudopelade of Brocq. Experts debate whether pseudopelade represents a single entity or common end-stage scarring for diseases such as lupus erythematosus and lichen planopilaris.

Diagnostic Approach

A punch biopsy specimen from the lesion border will demonstrate superficial and deep perivascular lymphocytic infiltrate, interface dermatitis, follicular plugging, and increased mucin deposition.

Management and Therapy

Focal lesions can be treated with ultrapotent or superpotent topical corticosteroids or with intralesional corticosteroids to the active inflammatory borders. Widespread disease often requires the use of systemic agents (hydroxychloroquine, quinacrine, chloroquine, or acitretin). End-stage fibrotic lesions are not amenable to medical treatment. Cosmetics may be useful in masking the atrophic hypopigmented patches of end-stage lesions.

Lichen Planopilaris
Etiology and Pathogenesis

Lichen planopilaris is a progressive, scarring inflammatory hair loss that may represent an autoimmune process.

Clinical Presentation

This condition typically affects middle-age adults and is more common in women. Patients present with focal patches of hair loss with inflammatory violaceous to brown keratotic papules at the lesion periphery. Tufts of 3 or more hairs may remain within scarred foci. A hair pull test is positive for anagen hairs. Clinical lesions of lichen planus may be seen at sites other than the scalp, including the mucous membrane (lacy white reticulated Wickham striae of oral cavity), skin (violaceous polygonal flat-topped papules and plaques), and nail changes (pterygium).

Differential Diagnosis

Histological studies can aid in distinguishing lichen planopilaris from lupus.

Diagnostic Approach

Punch biopsy specimens reveal a lichenoid perifollicular lymphocytic infiltrate. Giemsa stain demonstrates decreased or absent perifollicular elastic fibers. Direct immunofluorescence studies show globular deposits of IgM and IgA at the follicular basement membrane referred to as cytoid bodies.

Management and Therapy

High-potency topical corticosteroids or systemic corticosteroids for 3 months, followed by gradual taper, may be effective in slowing or halting hair loss. Patients often experience relapse after discontinuation of therapy.

Figure 147-5   Sarcoid

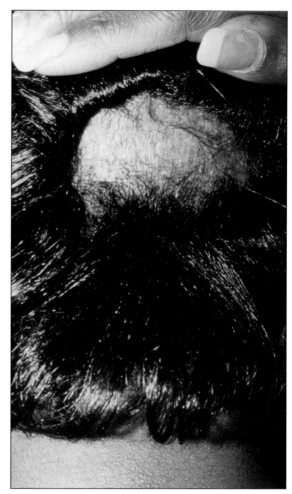

No hair follicles are discernable in this plaque of alopecia.

Morphea
Etiology and Pathogenesis

Morphea is a poorly understood slowly progressive process of increased hyalinization of dermal collagen fibers. Early stages may clinically and histologically demonstrate a mild inflammatory reaction. Clinical similarity with *Borrelia*-associated acrodermatitis chronic atrophicans suggests an inciting infectious event.

Clinical Presentation

Examination reveals a non-inflammatory or violaceous thickened or atrophic-bound down plaque with hair loss and decreased or absent hair follicles. A typical finding, the "En coup de sabre" refers to linear scalp lesions that are thought to resemble the scar resulting from a saber wound.

Differential Diagnosis

This permanent alopecia should be distinguished from true scarring alopecias.

Diagnostic Approach

A punch biopsy specimen will demonstrate loss of hair follicles, but normal elastic fibers.

Management and Therapy

Potent topical corticosteroids have been reported to have some benefit as have intralesional corticosteroids.

Dissecting Cellulitis
Etiology and Pathogenesis

This may represent an aberrant immune response to *Staphylococcus aureus* or *Propionibacterium acnes*; however, the etiology remains unknown.

Clinical Presentation

Active lesions present as a vigorous inflammatory reaction characterized by pustules, fluctuant abscesses, and sinus tracts. This painful, chronic, progressive, suppurative process commonly affects young African American men and eventually results in true scarring and permanent hair loss. When cultured, pustules are typically sterile or grow skin commensals.

Differential Diagnosis

Dissecting cellulitis may appear clinically similar to kerion and furunculosis.

Diagnostic Approach

Perform a culture to rule out fungal and bacterial pathogens. Punch biopsy specimens demonstrate follicular abscesses containing neutrophils. Lymphocytes, plasma cells, and foreign body giant cells may also be present. Late stage lesions show destruction of follicles with true scarring. Special stains for microbial pathogens should be performed. Secondary bacterial infection is not uncommon.

Management and Therapy

Tetracyclines, doxycycline, minocycline, or isotretinoin are the mainstays of treatment.

Sarcoid
Etiology and Pathogenesis

Granuloma formation may represent an immune response to a persistent antigen.

Clinical Presentation

This slowly progressive hair loss is more common in African American women. Sarcoid has variable morphologies and may present as papules, plaques, atrophic patch, ulcerations, with or without crust/scale often in association with pulmonary sarcoid and other cutaneous sarcoidal lesions (erythema nodosum). Sarcoid causes true scarring (Figure 147-5), although non-scarring sarcoidal alopecia has also been reported.

Differential Diagnosis

Sarcoid should be distinguished from discoid lupus erythematosus, morphea, and necrobiosis lipoidica diabeticorum.

Diagnostic Approach

A punch biopsy specimen reveals non-caseating granulomas and true scarring with decreased elastic fibers. Workup includes a full body examination for other cutaneous manifestations of sarcoid and chest radiographs to look for pulmonary disease.

Management and Therapy

Ultrapotent topical corticosteroids, intralesional corticosteroids, systemic prednisone, hydroxychloroquine, or low-dose methotrexate are effective treatments.

Primary or Metastatic Neoplasm
Etiology and Pathogenesis

Infiltrating tumor cells result in the destruction of normal skin architecture including hair follicles.

Clinical Presentation

Examination reveals a firm nodule, plaque, or space-occupying mass that visibly replaces cutaneous appendageal structures.

Differential Diagnosis

Common malignancies that infiltrate the scalp to cause hair loss include cutaneous T or B cell lymphomas and metastatic breast, lung, and prostate carcinoma.

Diagnostic Approach

Punch or incisional biopsy is essential to demonstrate the malignant histology.

Management and Therapy

Treatment includes local excision and treatment of the underlying malignancy.

FUTURE DIRECTIONS

Recent work by Fuchs and colleagues has implicated the *Wnt* signaling pathway in hair follicle development. This observation raises the intriguing possibility that drugs could be designed to stimulate new hair growth by activation of *Wnt* signaling. Such therapies would be useful in treating non-scarring hair loss, particularly androgenetic alopecia.

REFERENCES

American Academy of Dermatology Web site. Available at: http://www.aad.org. Accessed March 4, 2003.

Cotsarelis G, Sun TT, Lavker RM. Label-retaining cells reside in the bulge area of pilosebaceous unit: implications for follicular stem cells, hair cycle, and skin carcinogenesis. *Cell.* 1990;61:1329–1337.

Gat U, DasGupta R, Degenstein L, Fuchs E. De Novo hair follicle morphogenesis and hair tumors in mice expressing beta-catenin in skin. *Cell.* 1998;95:605-614.

Headington JT. Cicatricial alopecia. *Dermatol Clin.* 1996;14:773–782.

National Alopecia Areata Foundation Web site. Available at: http://www.alopeciaareata.com. Accessed March 4, 2003.

Olsen EA, ed. *Disorders of Hair Growth: Diagnosis and Treatment.* New York, NY: McGraw-Hill; 1994.

Van Neste D, Fuh V, Sanchez-Pedreno P, et al. Finasteride increases anagen hair in men with androgenetic alopecia. *Br J Dermatol.* 2000;143:804–810.

Society for Investigative Dermatology Web site. Available at: http://www.sidnet.org. Accessed March 4, 2003.

Chapter 148
Bullous Skin Disease

David S. Rubenstein and Luis A. Diaz

Blisters are classified by etiology or location; intraepidermal, dermal-epidermal junction, or subepidermal. Primary causes of blistering include inherited defects in cell adhesion proteins or diseases in which cell adhesion proteins are the target antigens for autoimmune responses. Autoimmune bullous skin disease typically presents in adults and tends to persist in the absence of clinical intervention. Secondary causes include infectious, traumatic, and inflammatory processes. Blistering as a secondary event is often acute in onset, transient, and resolves with treatment of the underlying disease.

The clinical manifestations of bullous genodermatoses are apparent at birth or shortly thereafter and similarly affected family members may be identified. Laboratory examination is critical to making a correct diagnosis and should include biopsy for 1) routine histology to determine the plane of cleavage within the skin and the presence/absence and nature of the inflammatory infiltrate, and 2) direct immunofluorescence to identify the nature and location of immunoreactants in the skin. Additional diagnostic studies include indirect immunofluorescent studies, Western blot analysis, immunoprecipitation, enzyme-linked immunosorbent assay, and immunoelectronmicroscopy (Table 148-1).

BULLOUS PEMPHIGOID
Etiology and Pathogenesis

Bullous pemphigoid (BP) is an autoimmune disease in which IgG autoantibodies target the basal keratinocyte hemidesmosome proteins BP180 (BP antigen 2) and BP230 (BP antigen 1). Passive transfer of BP180 IgG to neonatal mice causes subepidermal blister formation, demonstrating that the antibodies are pathogenic (Figure 148-1).

Clinical Presentation

BP typically affects adults in the fifth to sixth decades of life with tense bullae on either a non-inflammatory or an erythematous base (Figure 148-2). BP may be localized or widespread. An urticarial phase may precede the development of frank blisters by 2 to 4 weeks. BP may resolve spontaneously within 2 to 6 years.

Table 148-1
Differential Diagnosis of Bullous Skin Disease

Infection
- Herpes simplex
- Herpes zoster
- Bullous impetigo
- Staphylococcal scalded skin syndrome
- Bullous tinea pedis

Injury/Trauma
- Burn (thermal, solar)
- Cryoinjury
- Friction
- Ischemia
- Pressure

Inflammatory
- Acute allergic contact dermatitis
- Dyshidrotic eczema
- Lichen planus
- Toxic epidermal necrolysis

Bullous Genodermatoses
- Epidermolysis Bullosa Simplex
- Junctional Epidermolysis Bullosa
- Dystrophic Epidermolysis Bullosa
- Hailey-Hailey (Benign Familial Pemphigus)

Autoimmune
- Erythema multiforme
- Bullous Pemphigoid
- Cicatricial Pemphigoid
- Herpes Gestationis
- Linear IgA Bullous Dermatoses
- Epidermolysis Bullosa Acquisita
- Pemphigus Vulgaris
- Pemphigus Foliaceus
- Paraneoplastic Pemphigus
- Dermatitis Herpetiformis

Figure 148-1

Autoantibody Mediated Blisters
Location of Cleavage Plane

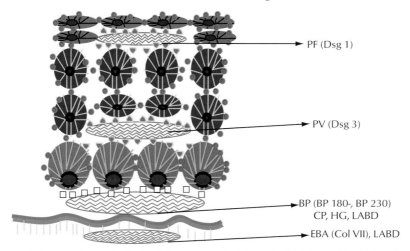

→ PF (Dsg 1)

→ PV (Dsg 3)

→ BP (BP 180-, BP 230)
CP, HG, LABD

→ EBA (Col VII), LABD

PF, pemphigus foliaceous; PV, pemphigus vulgaris; BP, bullous pemphigoid; CP, cicatricial pemphigoid; HG, herpes gestationalis; LABD, linear IgA bullous dermatosis; EBA (epidermolysis bullosa acquisita; Dsg 1, desmoglein; Dsg 3 desmoglein 3, Col VII, type VII collagen.

Figure 148-2 **Bullous Pemphigoid**

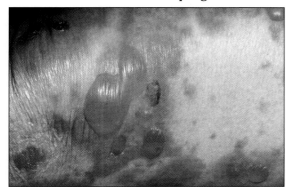

Tense bulla and urticarial plaques in bullous pemphigoid (courtesy of Dr. Walter Barkey).

Differential Diagnosis

BP can be distinguished from other bullous dermatoses, particularly epidermolysis bullosa acquisita (EBA), by immunofluorescent studies on salt split skin (Figure 148-1).

Diagnostic Approach

Punch biopsy should be performed for routine histologic studies and direct immunofluorescence. Histologic analysis of BP demonstrates a subepidermal blister with an eosinophilic infiltrate. Direct immunofluorescence demonstrates linear staining of the basement membrane with IgG and C3. In BP, immunoreactants localize to the blister roof on salt split skin. Approximately 80% of patients with active disease will demonstrate immunoreactants by indirect immunofluorescence.

Management and Therapy

Localized BP may respond to ultrapotent topical or intralesional corticosteroids. Initial management should utilize systemic corticosteroids with the subsequent addition of a steroid-sparing agent such as azathioprine. Higher doses of prednisone or additional immunosuppressive agents such as cyclosporine may be necessary to control severe disease. Some patients respond to tetracycline and niacinamide. This is particularly useful in the elderly patient with focal stable disease and medical problems exacerbated by prednisone.

BULLOUS PEMPHIGOID-LIKE DISEASES

Related autoimmune diseases in which autoantibodies target the hemidesmosome complex include cicatricial pemphigoid (CP), herpes gestationis (HG), and linear IgA bullous dermatoses (LABD). CP is a group of chronic, progressive diseases in which autoantibodies target the β4 integrin subunit, BP 180, or laminin 5. HG is an autoimmune blistering disease of pregnant women. In LABD, a disease of adults and children, IgA antibodies to BP 180 and to type VII collagen have been described. These processes present as subepidermal blistering diseases. The workup should include biopsies for routine histological analysis and for direct immunoflourescence. Immunosuppressive agents including prednisone, azathioprine, and cyclophosphamide are used for treatment. For CP, aggressive therapy with high-dose systemic corticosteroids and adjunctive agents (azathioprine or cyclophosphamide) should be considered due to the risk of blindness with ocular disease and stenosis with esophageal and laryngeal disease. Less aggressive disease should be treated with minimal mucosal involvement with dapsone or ultra-potent topical corticosteroids. HG resolves postpartum; therefore, the goal of therapy is symptom relief and decreased blister formation. Mild disease can often be controlled with antihistamines and topical corticosteroids. Aggressive disease may require systemic corticosteroids. LABD is often self-limited in children, spontaneously resolving within several years. In adults, the disease may persist for many years. Dapsone or systemic corticosteroids can be used to control disease. Mucosal disease, particularly involving the eyes, should be treated aggressively.

EPIDERMOLYSIS BULLOSA ACQUISITA
Etiology and Pathogenesis

In this autoimmune process, patients make antibodies against type VII collagen, which is the major protein component of anchoring fibrils.

Clinical Presentation

EBA is a disease of middle-aged adults characterized by non-inflammatory vesicles, bullae, and erosions on trauma prone areas (knees, elbows, extensor hands/fingers, sacrum). It heals with scar and milia formation. Permanent nail dystrophy or loss and scarring alopecia may result. A bullous pemphigoid-like variant of EBA presents with blisters and vesicles on an inflammatory base.

Differential Diagnosis

Porphyria cutanea tarda can be distinguished by the presence of photoexacerbation, hirsutism,

and positive urine porphyrins. Bullous lupus can present with vesicles and bullae identical to those seen in EBA. However, in addition to collagen VII autoantibodies, patients have a positive antinuclear antigen (ANA) and other more typical lupus erythematosus (LE) lesions. The BP-like variant of EBA is distinguished from BP by immunofluorescence on salt split skin.

Diagnostic Approach

Biopsy specimens reveal a subepidermal blister in which the presence of an inflammatory infiltrate is variable. Direct immunofluorescence demonstrates linear staining of IgG with or without C3, IgA, and IgM along the basement membrane zone. Incubating perilesional skin biopsies in 1M NaCl (salt split skin) results in separation of the epidermis from the dermis by cleavage formation within the lamina lucida. In EBA, immunoreactants localize to the dermal side of salt split skin. In BP, the immunoreactants localize to the epidermal side. Indirect immunofluorescence is positive in greater than 50% of patients with EBA. Immuno-electron microscopy demonstrates the localization of immunoreactants below the lamina densa.

Management and Therapy

Immunosuppressive therapy does not alter the course. Avoidance of trauma, hot environments, and wound care are beneficial.

PEMPHIGUS VULGARIS
Etiology and Pathogenesis

Pemphigus vulgaris (PV) is an autoimmune disease in which autoantibodies target the desmoso-

Figure 148-3 Pemphigus Vulgaris

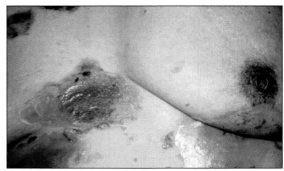

Flaccid vesicles and erosions of pemphigus.

mal cadherin desmoglein-3 (dsg-3). Passive transfer of anti dsg-3 PV IgG to neonatal mice reproduces the clinical and histologic findings of PV, demonstrating that the IgG is pathogenic.

Clinical Presentation

Patients in their 50s and 60s present with flaccid vesicles, bullae, and erosions of the skin with prominent mucosal lesions (Figure 148-3). Examination for ocular lesions is imperative; scarring can result in loss of vision. Most patients have oral lesions, often as the initial presentation. Lesions are painful, but not usually pruritic. Severe oral pain can lead to decreased oral intake and dehydration. Loss of skin barrier function places these patients at risk for secondary infection and fluid and electrolyte disturbances. Skin fragility is demonstrated by Nikolsky's sign in which minimal mechanical traction causes lateral movement of the epidermis relative to the underlying structures.

Differential Diagnosis

Histologic studies and immunofluorescence distinguish PV from erythema multiforme major and toxic epidermal necrolysis.

Diagnostic Approach

Biopsy specimens reveal suprabasal acantholysis, which is a loss of cell-cell adhesion just above the basal layer (Figure 148-1). Direct immunofluorescence demonstrates IgG outlining keratinocyte cell membranes.

Management and Therapy

PV is life-threatening. Untreated, the mortality approaches 60%. Rapid therapeutic response necessitates high-dose systemic corticosteroids. Consider adjunctive steroid-sparing agents (azathioprine or cyclophosphamide). Mycophenolate mofetil, as a single agent or as a steroid-sparing agent, is successful in treating PV, pemphigus foliaceus (PF), and paraneoplastic pemphigus (PNP). Ocular involvement should be managed with an ophthalmologist.

PEMPHIGUS FOLIACEUS
Etiology and Pathogenesis

In this autoimmune disease, autoantibodies target desmoglein-1 (dsg-1), a major component of suprabasal keratinocyte desmosomes. Anti-dsg-1

Figure 148-4   Pemphigus Foliaceus

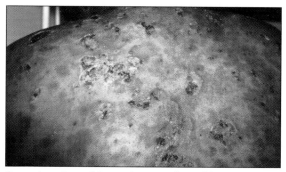

Crusted erosions of the trunk in pemphigus foliaceus.

PF IgG is pathogenic; passive transfer to neonatal mice reproduces the clinical and histologic findings of PF. Endemic PF, *Fogo selvagem*, occurs in native populations of Brazil. Both hereditary susceptibility and environmental factors likely combine to incite the production of autoantibodies in susceptible individuals.

Clinical Presentation

Acantholysis in the upper epidermis results in fragile vesicles that are often not identified clinically. Examination reveals painful or burning, scaling, and crusted erosions of the scalp, face, and trunk (Figure 148-4).

Differential Diagnosis

PF is distinguished from exfoliative dermatitis by histologic studies and direct immunofluorescence.

Diagnostic Approach

Biopsy specimens reveal acantholysis in the subcorneal and granular layers of the epidermis (Figure 148-1). Direct immunofluorescence shows IgG outlining keratinocyte cell membranes. Indirect immunofluorescence on skin substrates demonstrates anti-keratinocyte IgG in 80% to 90% of patients. A highly sensitive and specific ELISA is available to detect anti-dsg-1 IgG in PF sera.

Management and Therapy

Local disease is managed with potent topical corticosteroids. Widespread disease is managed with systemic prednisone. Steroid-sparing agents (azathioprine or cyclophosphamide) are added to lower the prednisone dose or if patients fail to respond adequately to prednisone alone.

PARANEOPLASTIC PEMPHIGUS
Etiology and Pathogenesis

PNP is a blistering disease associated with an underlying lymphoproliferative disorder. The autoantibody response may represent an immune response to tumor antigens and includes antibodies to desmoplakin I (250 kDa), desmoplakin II, bullous pemphigoid antigen 1 (230 kDa), envoplakin (210 kDa), periplakin (190 kDa), dsg-3, and dsg-1. Passive transfer experiments show that the anti-dsg-3 IgGs cause acantholysis.

Clinical Presentation

PNP aggressively involves the oral and ocular mucosa. Pulmonary and esophageal epithelia may be similarly affected. Patients present with painful oral erosions and ulcerations and a variety of cutaneous lesions that may mimic the flaccid bullae and erosions of PV, the crusted plaques of PF, the dusky targetoid lesions of erythema multiforme, or even the widespread erythema and skin necrosis of toxic epidermal necrolysis.

Differential Diagnosis

PNP is distinguished from PV, PF, ulcerative oral lichen planus, erythema multiforme major, and toxic epidermal necrolysis by indirect immunofluorescence on bladder epithelia and by immunoprecipitation studies.

Diagnostic Approach

Biopsy specimens demonstrate variable features including suprabasilar acantholysis; keratinocyte necrosis, a dense lichenoid infiltrate at the dermoepidermal junction; and subepidermal blistering. Direct immunofluorescence shows IgG and C3 staining of keratinocyte cell membranes. Features consistent with BP include IgG or C3 staining of the basement membrane zone. Differentiation of PNP from other variants of pemphigus is made by 1) indirect immunofluorescence of patient sera on rat bladder epithelium substrates (positive in 75% to 85% of PNP patients, but unusual in PV and PF); and 2) the presence of periplakin and envoplakin autoantibodies in PNP, but not PV nor PF. PNP can affect the palms and soles, which is unusual in PV.

Management and Therapy

Patients with PNP should be evaluated for the presence of an underlying neoplasm. Surgical exci-sion for benign tumors often results in clearing of the disease within 6 to 18 months. When associated with malignancy, PNP is difficult to treat. Numerous therapies have been tried, including treatment of the underlying malignancy, prednisone, azathioprine, cyclophosphamide, cyclosporine, dapsone, and plasmapheresis. However, none is uniformly successful. Most patients with PNP and malignant neoplasms die within 2 years of the onset of PNP. Involvement of the pulmonary epithelium can result in respiratory failure.

DERMATITIS HERPETIFORMIS
Etiology and Pathogenesis

Dermatitis herpetiformis (DH) is an autoimmune blistering disease associated with gluten sensitive enteropathy; IgA autoantibodies can be identified in the papillary dermis.

Clinical Presentation

DH is a chronic disease that typically affects people in the second to fourth decades and presents as extremely pruritic, grouped vesicles symmetrically distributed on extensor surfaces, typically the scalp, back, elbows, knees, and buttocks. Scratching often makes it difficult to find intact vesicles on physical examination. Examination may reveal only secondary grouped, crusted lesions.

Differential Diagnosis

DH is differentiated from linear IgA disease, bullous pemphigoid, herpes gestationis, scabies, and erythema multiforme by histologic and immunofluorescent studies.

Diagnostic Approach

Biopsy specimens reveal a subepidermal vesicle with papillary dermal neutrophils and variable numbers of eosinophils. Direct immunofluorescence shows granular deposits of IgA at the tips of the dermal papilla.

Management and Therapy

Dapsone is the treatment of choice. Patients respond within 1 to 2 days with decreased pruritus and no new lesion formation. Once control is achieved, the dose should be titrated down to the lowest level that controls disease. The risk of agranulocytosis necessitates monitoring the complete blood cell count when initiating therapy. Dapsone can cause hemolysis and methemoglobinemia, which can be severe in glucose-6-phosphatase–deficient (G6PD) deficient patients. For this reason, G6PD status should be determined before beginning dapsone. Patients on dapsone should be monitored for the development of peripheral neuropathy. Sulfapyridine is an alternative to dapsone. Clearing of DH lesions can occur with gluten-free diets; however, most patients do not tolerate restrictive diets and may take up to 1 year for the skin to clear.

FUTURE DIRECTIONS

Current research on autoimmune blistering disease is aimed at 1) determining the mechanism by which autoantibodies cause loss of keratinocyte adhesion, 2) developing treatments that prevent the loss of cell adhesion without the need for global immunosuppression, and 3) identifying the triggers that incite the autoantibody response. Ongoing studies of *fogo selvagem*, the endemic forms of pemphigus foliaceus, have revealed close associations between certain environmental triggers that lead to host cross-reactive immune responses. Studies of *fogo selvagem* are likely to yield insights into the biology of autoimmunity that extend far beyond cutaneous pathology.

REFERENCES

American Academy of Dermatology Web site. Available at: http://www.aad.org. Accessed March 4, 2003.

Anhalt GJ, Diaz LA. Prospects for autoimmune disease: Research advances in pemphigus. *JAMA*. 2001;285:652-654.

Anhalt GJ, Kim SC, Stanley JR, et al. Paraneoplastic pemphigus. An autoimmune mucocutaneous disease associated with neoplasia. *N Engl J Med*. 1990;323:1729-1735.

Diaz LA, Guidice GJ. End of the century overview of skin blisters. *Arch Dermatol*. 2000;136:106-112.

Dystrophic Epidermolysis Bullosa Research Association of America (DebRA) Web site. Available at: http://www.debra.org. Accessed March 4, 2003.

International Pemphigus Foundation Web site. Available at: http://www.pemphigus.org. Accessed March 4, 2003.

Society for Investigative Dermatology Web site. Available at: http://www.sidnet.org. Accessed March 4, 2003.

Stanley JR. Pemphigus and pemphigoid as paradigms of organ-specific, autoantibody-mediated diseases. *J Clin Invest*. 1989;83:1443-1448.

Woodley DT, Briggaman RA, Gammon WR. Acquired epidermolysis bullosa. A bullous disease associated with autoimmunity to type VII (anchoring fibril) collagen. *Dermatol Clin*. 1990;8:717-726.

Chapter 149

Eczema and Other Common Dermatoses

Dean S. Morrell and David S. Rubenstein

Eczema is a term broadly applied to many inflammatory skin conditions with dermatoses characterized by the presence of pruritus, erythema, scaling, macules, papules, plaques, and/or vesicles. Evaluation includes a thorough history focusing on onset (acute versus chronic), inciting and exacerbating factors, associated medical conditions, and family history of similar or related diseases. On physical examination, attention should be paid to individual lesion morphology, pattern, and distribution. A potassium hydroxide preparation of skin scrapings is often helpful in differentiating superficial fungal infection from other causes of scaling dermatitides. A punch biopsy is helpful in identifying specific dermatoses.

ATOPIC DERMATITIS
Etiology and Pathogenesis

Atopic dermatitis is an immune-mediated disease. Most patients have a personal or family history of atopic disease (allergic rhinitis, asthma, and atopic dermatitis). In affected areas, a predominance of T-helper type 2 cells produce interleukins that cause elevated IgE and eosinophil levels. Controversy exists on the role of potential food and other environmental allergens upon the pathogenesis of atopic dermatitis.

Clinical Presentation

The major feature is pruritus. In adults, chronic flexural involvement with lichenified erythematous plaques is common (Figure 149-1). The plaques are distributed symmetrically on the face, neck, and antecubital and popliteal fossae. Significant involvement of the dorsal hands and feet can occur. Exacerbations typically occur during dry weather and episodes of stress. Even during periods of relative remissions, individuals usually have dry and sensitive skin. Secondary bacterial or viral infections involving affected areas should always be considered during acute exacerbations.

Differential Diagnosis

The intense pruritus and symmetrical distribution usually distinguish atopic dermatitis from other scaling eruptions. Seborrheic dermatitis, irritant dermatitis, and contact dermatitis should be considered.

Figure 149-1   Atopic Dermatitis

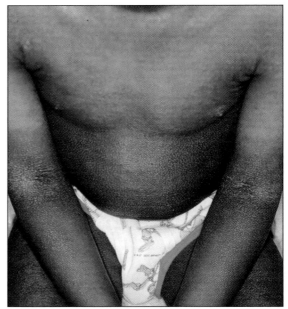

Lichenified plaques of the antecubital fossa are typical.

Diagnostic Approach

Bacterial and viral cultures dictate therapy in secondarily infected plaques.

Management and Therapy

Affected skin has an impaired barrier to transcutaneous water loss. Therefore, efforts to improve and maintain skin hydration are helpful. Daily bathing can be useful if the use of soap is minimized and post-bathing emollient use is maximized. Thicker moisturizers such as petrolatum are effective during winter months, while lighter products are better tolerated in warmer weather.

Oral antihistamines are quite effective in controlling episodes of pruritus. Awareness of possible sedation with the use of these products is important.

Topical corticosteroids are the mainstay of treatment. The location and thickness of the plaque guide the choice of an agent. They are best used in pulsed applications such that a particular agent significantly improves the area in 1 to 2 weeks. This pulsing avoids the chronic use of topical steroids and reduces the risk of steroid atrophy. Low-to-medium potency steroids can be used intermittently on the face and neck. Potent and ultrapotent steroids are occasionally necessary for thickened, lichenified plaques on extremities.

Crusted and weeping lesions frequently have secondary bacterial infection. Topical soaks or compresses with aluminum acetate are indicated for these lesions followed by steroid application. Oral antibiotics (anti-staphylococcal, anti-streptococcal) may be necessary for multiple areas of infection.

Tacrolimus, a recent advance in topical immunomodulatory therapy, is indicated in extensive, severe, and recalcitrant cases. Topical pimecrolimus, an agent that inhibits T-lymphocyte activation, should be considered in patients with disease resistant to corticosteroid therapy. Phototherapy, photochemotherapy (PUVA), and cyclosporine should be considered if topical therapies fail to improve the quality of life.

CONTACT DERMATITIS
Etiology and Pathogenesis

Allergic contact dermatitis represents a cell-mediated immune response to haptens, small molecules that modify endogenous macromolecules in the skin. These modified antigens are taken up and presented by Langerhans cells, the resident antigen-presenting cells in the skin. T-helper type 1 cells, which secrete the cytokines IL-2 and interferon alfa, are the predominant subclass of T cells that mediate the immune response in allergic contact dermatitis. Re-exposure to antigen results in repeated bouts of cutaneous inflammation due to the generation of antigen-specific memory T-cells. In contrast, irritant contact dermatitis represents a response to a non-immune

mediated injury to the skin from prolonged or repeated exposures to noxious substances. Soaps, detergents, and organic solvents are typical agents that cause irritant contact dermatitis.

Clinical Presentation

Acute contact dermatitis is a very pruritic eruption characterized by erythema, papules, vesicles, and bullae corresponding to the pattern and exposure of the contactant (Figure 149-2). An acute vesicular eruption in a geometric pattern is essentially pathognomonic for acute contact dermatitis. Chronic contact dermatitis presents as lichenified, scaling, erythematous, hyperpigmented and/or hypopigmented, papules and/or plaques. The clinical spectrum of irritant contact dermatitis is broad ranging from acute erythema and vesiculation to lichenified, scaling, fissured hyperpigmented and/or hypopigmented, papules and/or plaques.

Differential Diagnosis

Contact dermatitis should be distinguished from other eczematous dermatitides including atopic dermatitis, nummular eczema, seborrheic dermatitis, and lichen simplex chronicus.

Diagnostic Approach

The onset, distribution, and pattern of the reaction are helpful in identifying responsible contactants. Biopsy is rarely indicated.

Figure 149-2   Contact Dermatitis

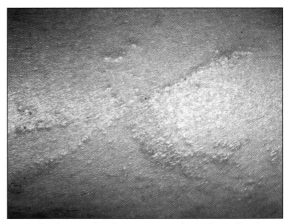

Linear distribution of erythematous papules and vesicles characterizes contact dermatitis to poison ivy.

Management and Therapy

Identification and removal of the offending agent is necessary. This requires eliciting an extensive history to determine the relationship of the patient's exposures to the onset, exacerbations, and ameliorations of the dermatitis. An astute clinician may discern the responsible agent from the pattern and distribution of the rash. For example, eyelid dermatitis is often an allergic contact dermatitis to nail polish (patients rub the eyelids), and ear lobe involvement is often due to nickel in earrings. Patch testing may identify potential allergic contactants. Topical corticosteroids, emollients, and antihistamines resolve the condition once the exposure has been identified and eliminated. For vigorous, generalized, acute contact dermatitis, such as that seen in response to poison ivy, systemic corticosteroids may be indicated. Prednisone tapered over 2 to 3 weeks prevents flares seen after discontinuation experienced with the use of corticosteroid dose packs.

SEBORRHEIC DERMATITIS
Etiology and Pathogenesis

Individuals appear to have increased numbers of *Pityrosporum ovale* in lesional skin; however, the exact role of this organism in the pathogenesis is unclear.

Clinical Presentation

Seborrheic dermatitis is a chronic inflammatory disease with periods of remissions and exacerbations. It is characterized by waxy scale overlying erythematous patches involving the eyebrows, nasal bridge, and nasolabial folds. Extension to forehead and post-auricular areas is often seen (Figure 149-3). On the scalp, diffuse dry scale (dandruff) is common. Intertriginous areas can have sharply demarcated erythematous patches with yellowish, "greasy," or waxy scale. Rarely, progression to generalized erythematous exfoliation is seen.

Differential Diagnosis

Psoriasis, intertrigo, candidal infection, and atopic dermatitis should be considered.

Diagnostic Approach

Cultures of intertriginous lesions will differentiate seborrhea dermatitis from candidal intertrigo.

Figure 149-3   Seborrheic Dermatitis

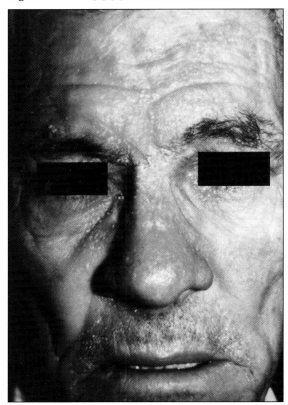

Erythema and greasy yellow scale of the forehead, eyebrows, nasal bridge, and nasolabial folds.

Management and Therapy

Seborrheic dermatitis is more responsive to treatment than psoriasis is. Treatment for 3 to 5 days is usually adequate to control flares. Shampooing with zinc pyrithione selenium sulfide 1% to 2.5%, salicylic acid, or ketoconazole decreases scalp scale. Facial and intertriginous areas respond to periodic application of hydrocortisone 1 to 2.5%, ketoconazole, or sulfur-based products. Resistant cases may need brief application (bid, 5-7 days) of medium potency corticosteroids and should be evaluated for possible secondary bacterial or fungal infections.

STASIS DERMATITIS
Etiology and Pathogenesis

Poor venous return leads to edema, which increases the diffusion barrier of oxygen and nutrients to the epidermis. These chronic changes result in inflammation and often in secondary ulceration.

Clinical Presentation

Stasis dermatitis occurs on the lower extremities of elderly patients as a bilateral, pruritic, erythematous, scaling macular, and sometimes papular eruption. Pitting edema is present. Chronic stasis dermatitis results in pigment deposition from hemosiderin. Ulceration can occur.

Differential Diagnosis

Potassium hydroxide preparation of skin scrapings differentiates stasis dermatitis from dermatophytosis. Cellulitis is unilateral and acute in onset. Constitutional symptoms and elevated white counts may be present.

Diagnostic Approach

The clinical presentation is quite characteristic. When ulceration is present, other causes of ulcer formation should be considered including arteriolar disease, vasculitis, infection, malignancy, and pyoderma gangrenosum. If clinically warranted, biopsy may be helpful in excluding non-stasis entities.

Management and Therapy

Decreasing lower extremity edema by leg elevation, compression stockings, and medical management of underlying cardiovascular disease is essential. Low-to-middle potency topical corticosteroids reduce cutaneous inflammation and pruritus. Frequent emollients aid in preventing exacerbations after the inflammation has resolved. Stasis ulcers respond well to a medicated compression dressing.

DERMATOPHYTOSIS
Etiology and Pathogenesis

Superficial mycoses are caused by fungi that can be classified in three genera: *Epidermophyton, Microsporum,* and *Trichophyton.* Fungi are transmitted from soil, animals, and humans. Genetic susceptibility and immunosuppression promote dermatophytosis. Once infected, the incubation period can be as little as 2 to 4 days before skin lesions are evident. Tinea capitis is most commonly caused by *Trichophyton tonsurans. T. rubrum, T. mentagrophytes,* and *Microsporum canis* cause tinea faciei. Tinea corporis can be secondary to any of the dermatophytes. Tinea pedis is most frequently caused by *T. rubrum.* Infection of the nails (onychomycosis) can be seen from a variety of fungi.

Figure 149-4   Tinea Faciei

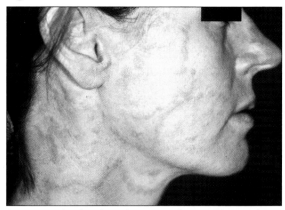

Serpiginous bordered, eyrthematous plaque with central clearing.

Clinical Presentation

Tinea faciei (facial) and corporis (body) present similarly with annular, erythematous, scaling patches, and plaques (Figure 149-4). The borders are active with more erythema and elevation while the centers tend to be clear and flat. Tinea pedis can be quite inflammatory with weeping and vesiculation or non-inflammatory with dry, scaling, and erythematous patches. Onychomycosis presents as a thickened nail plate with subungual debris. The plate often separates from the underlying nail bed.

Tinea capitis is unusual after adolescence. Inflammatory lesions develop into boggy, indurated, erythematous plaques called kerions. Non-inflammatory lesions present with scaling papules and patches with broken-off hairs.

Differential Diagnosis

Tinea faciei can be confused with lupus erythematosus, seborrheic dermatitis, contact dermatitis, and atopic dermatitis. Onychomycosis must be distinguished from psoriasis, atopic or contact dermatitis, lichen planus, chronic paronychia, and trachyonychia. Tinea capitis should be differentiated from pediculosis, atopic dermatitis, seborrheic dermatitis, psoriasis, and bacterial infection.

Diagnostic Approach

A potassium hydroxide preparation of the scale, hair, or nail from affected lesions is essential. Nail plates can be clipped and fixed in formalin for dermatopathic evaluation with periodic acid-Schiff staining. Skin biopsies are rarely needed.

Management and Therapy

Multiple antifungal drugs are available. Localized tinea faciei, corporis, pedis, and cruris can be treated effectively with topical agents (clotrimazole, miconazole, econazole, oxiconazole, ketoconazole, terbinafine, naftifine, ciclopirox, and butenafine) twice per day for 1 week after the eruption resolves. Extensive skin disease is more effectively treated with oral therapy (terbinafine, itraconazole, fluconazole). Regular use of antifungal powders can prevent recurrences of tinea cruris and pedis. Erosive tinea pedis can be secondarily infected with gram-negative organisms; therefore, topical or oral antibacterial therapy should be considered as an adjunct to antifungal therapy.

Hair or nail involvement requires systemic therapy. Griseofulvin remains the drug of choice for childhood tinea capitis. The newer allylamines (terbinafine) and triazoles (itraconazole, fluconazole) may replace griseofulvin with easier dosing and shorter treatment duration. Onychomycosis requires 3 to 4 months of therapy (terbinafine, itraconazole). Rare cases of hepatic failure and exacerbation of congestive heart failure have been reported with several of the oral antifungal agents. For this reason, patients should be screened for underlying hepatic and cardiac disease before the use of these systemic medications. Recurrences are not unusual and preventive measures (antifungal cream or powder) are probably helpful after a course of oral therapy. Recently, topical therapy has been approved for onychomycosis (Penlac). Daily application in conjunction with regular nail hygiene for 1 year clears infection in approximately 12% of individuals.

FUTURE DIRECTIONS

Corticosteroids have been the therapeutic mainstay for the treatment of eczema and dermatitis. However, chronic steroid use results in dermal atrophy and tachyphylaxis. Non-steroid drugs are being developed that target specific components of the immune response. One such agent is tacrolimus, which inhibits signaling downstream of the T-cell receptor and has been released as a topical agent for the treatment of atopic dermatitis. Ascomycin, another compound that interferes with downstream components of the T-cell receptor signaling cascade, is being developed for the treatment of dermatitides. Numerous bioengineered macromolecules are being developed to modify immune cell responses by disrupting antigen presentation and cytokine secretion profile and will likely broaden the therapeutic options available to treat eczema and dermatitis.

REFERENCES

Alaiti S, Kang S, Fiedler VC, et al. Tacrolimus (FK506) ointment for atopic dermatitis: a phase I study in adults and children. *J Am Acad Dermatol*. 1998;38:69–76.

American Academy of Dermatology Web site. Available at: http://www.aad.org. Accessed March 5, 2003.

Griffiths CE. Ascomycin: an advance in the management of atopic dermatitis. *Br J Dermatol*. 2001;144:679–681.

Reitamo S, Wollenberg A, Schopf E, et al. Safety and efficacy of 1 year of tacrolimus ointment monotherapy in adults with atopic dermatitis. The European Tacrolimus Ointment Study Group. *Arch Dermatol*. 2000;136:999–1006.

Rietschel RL, Fowler JF Jr, eds. *Fisher's Contact Dermatitis*. 5th ed. Philadelphia, Pa: Lippincott Williams & Wilkins; 2001.

Society for Investigative Dermatology Web site. Available at: http://www.sidnet.org. Accessed March 5, 2003.

Van Leent EJ, Graber M, Thurston M, Wagenaar A, Spuls PI, Bos JD. Effectiveness of the ascomycin macrolactam SDZ ASM 981 in the topical treatment of atopic dermatitis. *Arch Dermatol*. 1998;134:805–809.

Chapter 150
Psoriasis

Heidi T. Jacobe

Psoriasis is a chronic, relapsing disorder of the skin characterized by sharply demarcated, red plaques with silvery scale in a characteristic distribution. It occurs in 1% to 3% of the population. The lesions are usually very distinctive, allowing diagnosis based on physical findings alone. Arthropathy is the only non-cutaneous manifestation.

ETIOLOGY AND PATHOGENESIS

The pathogenesis of psoriasis is not understood. Evidence of a genetic predisposition includes 1) increased incidence in relatives and children of affected patients, 2) high rate of concordance in monozygotic twins, and 3) the association of major histocompatibility antigens with disease expression. The presence of this genetic predisposition along with the appropriate environmental triggers (bacteria/drugs) produce the excessive, but controlled cellular proliferation and inflammation that is the hallmark of psoriasis.

CLINICAL PRESENTATION

Psoriasis affects men and women equally. It usually begins in the third decade, but can develop at any age. It is clinically distinctive. Psoriasis begins as red, scaly papules that coalesce to form sharply demarcated plaques with adherent silvery white scale (Figure 150-1). The extent of scaling varies with the body part involved and treatment. Scaling can be quite thick in the scalp and minimal in intertriginous areas and treated sites (Figure 150-2). The plaques are deep red underneath the scale.

Psoriasis has a predilection for certain cutaneous sites including elbows, knees, gluteal cleft, scalp, fingernails, and toenails (Figure 150-3). Nail involvement most commonly appears as pits in the surface of the nail plate; less commonly, oil stains (brown discoloration), onychodystrophy, and onycholysis occur (Figure 150-4). It has a tendency to spread to sites of skin trauma (Koebner's phenomenon). Lesions may be asymptomatic or extremely pruritic. Most disease is limited to the sites listed above, but there are many other clinical presentations of psoriasis (Table 150-1).

Psoriatic arthritis follows the onset of the cutaneous manifestations most commonly but may occur at any time. It usually presents as asymmetric arthritis involving one or more joints of the fingers and toes. The affected digit is acutely hot and swollen and eventually develops soft tissue swelling producing the so-called "sausage digit." There is a 5% incidence of psoriatic arthritis in the psoriatic population; men and women are affected equally. The usual age of presentation is between 20 and 40. Approximately 80% of patients have nail involvement. Psoriatic arthritis can be progressive and deforming. Rheumatoid factor and ANA test results are usually negative.

DIFFERENTIAL DIAGNOSIS

The differential diagnosis often depends on the morphology of the psoriatic lesions. Classic plaque psoriasis is quite distinctive, but may occasionally be difficult to distinguish from nummular eczema, mycosis fungoides, atopic dermatitis, or tinea corporis. Guttate psoriasis should be differentiated from secondary syphilis, pityriasis lichenoides et varioliformis, or pityriasis rosea (Figure 150-3). Scalp psoriasis can be confused with seborrheic dermatitis or eczema. One distinguishing characteristic of scalp psoriasis is its tendency to move onto the forehead. Inverse psoriasis resembles seborrheic dermatitis, tinea, or candidal infection.

DIAGNOSTIC APPROACH

Classic plaque psoriasis is usually diagnosed clinically. Guttate psoriasis is differentiated from secondary syphilis through serologic testing. Pityriasis rosea is excluded by history and histologic examination. When tinea or candida is suspected, potassium hydroxide preparation of scale is helpful. In

Figure 150-1

Plaque Psoriasis

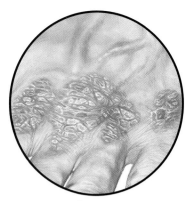

Typical appearance
of cutaneous lesions
(plaque lesion)

Section of Skin Lesion

Histopathologic features

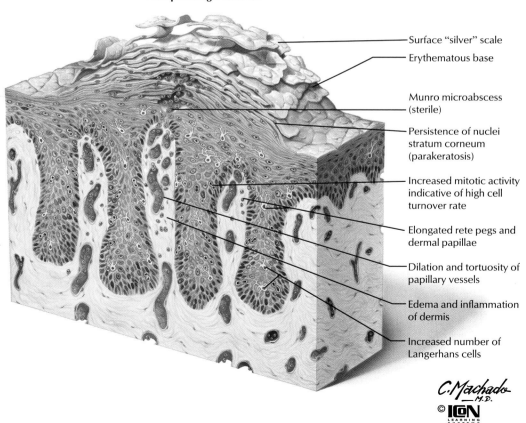

Surface "silver" scale

Erythematous base

Munro microabscess
(sterile)

Persistence of nuclei
stratum corneum
(parakeratosis)

Increased mitotic activity
indicative of high cell
turnover rate

Elongated rete pegs and
dermal papillae

Dilation and tortuosity of
papillary vessels

Edema and inflammation
of dermis

Increased number of
Langerhans cells

Figure 150-2

Psoriasis in the Genital Area

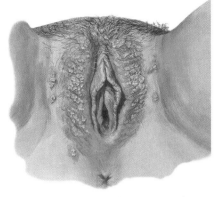

Typical appearance of intertriginous lesion. Note minimal scale.

Figure 150-4

Psoriatic Nail Involvement

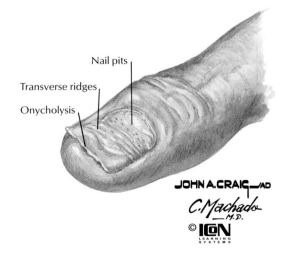

Nail pits

Transverse ridges

Onycholysis

JOHN A. CRAIG—AD

difficult cases, a punch biopsy can be done for histologic examination. HIV type 1 should be considered in patients with a particularly explosive onset of widespread psoriasis infection, including assess-

Figure 150-3   **Psoriasis**

Typical distribution

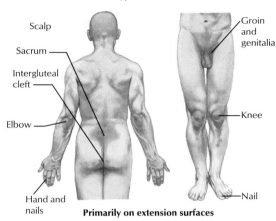

Scalp

Sacrum

Intergluteal cleft

Elbow

Hand and nails

Groin and genitalia

Knee

Nail

Primarily on extension surfaces

Table 150-1
Clinical Presentations of Psoriasis

· Chronic plaque psoriasis
· Guttate psoriasis-acute eruptive psoriasis following streptococcal pharyngitis
· Pustular psoriasis
· Erythrodermic psoriasis
· Psoriasis of the palms and soles
· Inverse psoriasis (flexural areas)

ment of risk factors for HIV infection. HIV testing should be offered to all these patients.

MANAGEMENT AND THERAPY

Management of psoriasis is determined by several factors.

Amount of body surface area involved: Generally, patients with less than 20% body surface area involvement can be treated topically; greater than 20% body surface area involvement requires treatment with UV light or systemic therapy.

Area of involvement: Select topical medications based on where they will be applied. Potency is guided by the characteristics of the skin being treated. Some topical preparations (calcipotriene and tazarotene) can irritate the face or intertrigi-

Table 150-2
Steroid Potency in Psoriasis

Group I Super High	Clobetasol proprionate 0.05% (cream, ointment, scalp solution)
Group II High	Fluocinonide 0.05% (cream, ointment, scalp solution)
Group III Intermediate	Betamethasone diproprionate 0.05% (cream) Betamethasone-17-valerate 0.1% (ointment)
Group IV Intermediate	Fluocinolone acetonide 0.025% (ointment, scalp solution)
Group V	Hydrocortisone butyrate 0.1% (cream)
Group VI Low	Desonide 0.05% (cream, lotion)
Group VII Very low	Hydrocortisone 1, 2.5% (cream, ointment)

nous areas. Systemic therapy is also guided by the distribution of lesions. For example, ultraviolet light therapy is not a good choice for intertriginous or scalp psoriasis.

Degree of plaque inflammation: Extremely angry, red plaques are irritated and worsened by certain topical therapies including tar, anthralin, and calcipotriene.

Patient health/mental status: Some patients are unable or unwilling to follow a complicated regimen that includes multiple topical medications. Other patients may not be candidates for systemic therapy. It is important to tailor treatment to the individual needs of the patient.

Topical Therapy Options

Topical steroids offer the advantage of quick response with rapid improvement in inflammation and itching. Tolerance develops fairly quickly, and patients who did very well initially will note decreasing efficacy over time. This often leads to overuse of the preparation in an attempt to recapture the initial dramatic improvement. Patients should be educated regarding this aspect of steroid use. The specific steroid preparation needs to be tailored to the area where it will be applied and the thickness of the psoriatic plaque. Treat the face and intertriginous areas with a class V to VII steroid cream or ointment (Table 150-2).

The extremities and trunk can be treated with class IV to I steroid creams or ointments depending on the thickness of the plaques. Hands and feet have thick skin and usually require a class I or II steroid ointment. Ointments have better absorption, making them more effective, but are less well tolerated. Scalp psoriasis can be treated with a class IV to I steroid solution. Most topical steroids are designed for twice a day use. Class I steroids can induce atrophy and striae very quickly and cause adrenal axis suppression if applied to a large body surface area. Most practitioners use a class I steroid for 2 weeks alternating with a 1-week rest period. As patients improve, they can taper the frequency of steroid use. Long-term steroid use should be discouraged. Application twice a week for maintenance is acceptable. Systemic steroids should not be used for psoriasis. Although they rapidly control the disease, withdrawal produces a rebound effect and potential conversion to pustular psoriasis, which requires hospitalization.

Vitamin D analogues (calcipotriene ointment, cream, and solution): Calcipotriene inhibit the proliferation of keratinocytes and normalize their maturation. Vitamin D analogues are effective as single agents but better results are achieved when they are used along with a potent topical steroid. A typical regimen begins with once a day applica-

Figure 150-5

Psoriatic Arthritis

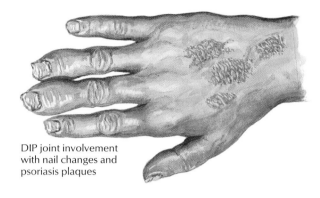

Distal
interphalangeal
(DIP)

DIP joint involvement
with nail changes and
psoriasis plaques

Wrist

Psoriatic arthritis may
present as monoarticular or
oligoarticular involvement

JOHN A. CRAIG — MD
C. Machado
— M.D.
© ICON
LEARNING
SYSTEMS

tion of calcipotriene and of a class I steroid, which is continued until the plaques begin to thin, usually 2 to 3 weeks. Subsequently, calcipotriene is applied twice a day Monday through Friday, and the class I steroid is applied twice a day on the weekend. This phase can be continued for several weeks or even months. The goal is to use calcipotriene once or twice a day for maintenance as a single agent. Calcipotriene benefits include reduced time to clearance, decreased steroid use, less tolerance to steroids, and prolonged improvement. The most common side effect is irritation at the site of application, and it should not be used on the face and intertriginous areas. There have been no reported effects on bone or calcium metabolism if less than 100 g a week is used. Acidic substances such as salicylic acid should be avoided because they inactivate calcipotriene.

Tazarotene (0.05% or 0.1% gel) is a retinoid developed specifically for use in psoriasis. It can be irritating and should only be used in non-inflamed stable plaque psoriasis. Topical steroids can be used to help decrease inflammation. Tazarotene is rated pregnancy category X and should not be used in pregnant women. Use in intertriginous sites should be avoided. The advantages of Tazarotene are that it is a once daily dosage that can be used on the scalp, it decreases steroid use, and it often provides a prolonged response.

Keratolytics: Psoriatic plaques frequently develop thick, adherent scale that limits the absorption and efficacy of topical medications, particularly on the scalp. Keratolytics including salicylic acid, urea, and lactic acid are available to debride the scale. A lotion or cream containing one of these agents can be applied to psoriatic plaques either concomitantly with other topical medications or separately. The scalp responds well to a lotion or solution containing a keratolytic applied under a shower cap overnight followed by a shampoo in the morning and the application of corticosteroid solution. Improvement within 1 to 2 weeks is typical, allowing for the discontinuation of the keratolytic. Patients should then be instructed to restart keratolytics whenever scale starts to build up.

Special Considerations

Patients with scalp psoriasis should use medicated shampoos in addition to the agents discussed above. Formulations with additives such as salicylic acid, zinc pyrithione, selenium sulfide, or coal tar can be helpful. Psoriasis in intertriginous sites is frequently superinfected with candida. The addition of a topical antifungal with yeast coverage is helpful in these patients.

Patients with psoriasis are prone to bacterial superinfection, manifested by honey-colored crusting. Oral antibiotics with good staphylococcal coverage provide improvement.

There is a correlation between the severity of psoriasis and the degree of stress the patient is experiencing. Minimizing stress can also improve psoriasis.

Certain drugs including lithium, beta-blocking drugs, antimalarials, and systemic steroids can exacerbate psoriasis and should be avoided.

If the patient has greater than 20% body surface area involvement or remains unresponsive to topical therapy, consider referral to a dermatologist. Dermatologists use ultraviolet light, methotrexate, acitretin, cyclosporin, and a variety of other systemic medications to control severe, widespread psoriasis.

FUTURE DIRECTIONS

Innovative treatments for psoriasis are constantly under development. Recombinant-immunomodulatory drugs such as etanercept and infliximab are currently in trials, as are anti-CD4 monoclonal antibodies, monoclonal anti-IL-8 antibodies, and a fusion protein DAB389 IL-2. Flash lamp pulsed dye laser and photodynamic therapy have also been reported to offer some benefit.

REFERENCES

American Academy of Dermatology Web site. Available at: http://www.aad.org. Accessed March 5, 2003.

Camisa C. *Handbook of Psoriasis*. Malden, Mass: Blackwell Science; 1998.

Fitzpatrick TB. Psoriasis. IN: Freedberg IM, Eisen AZ, Wolff K, et al, eds. *Fitzpatrick's Dermatology in General Medicine*. 5th ed. New York, NY: McGraw-Hill; 1999.

National Psoriasis Foundation Web site. Available at: http://www.psoriasis.org. Accessed March 5, 2003.

Chapter 151
Scabies and Pediculosis

Heidi Jacobe, MD

SCABIES

Scabies is a contagious disease characterized by extreme pruritus and widespread inflammatory papules. It can be endemic among school-aged children and institutionalized patients, particularly those in nursing homes. Scabies occurs in all age groups and both sexes.

Etiology and Pathogenesis

Scabies results from the infestation of the skin with the mite *Sarcoptes scabiei* var. *hominis*. The mite goes through its entire life cycle on human skin. The female mite burrows through the stratum corneum, laying 3 to 4 eggs a day for up to a month. The eggs hatch and the larvae mature, perpetuating the cycle.

The mite is transmitted through close skin-to-skin contact. It is difficult to transmit scabies through bedding and clothing.

Skin lesions result from a delayed hypersensitivity reaction to the mite, feces, and larvae in the skin. There is usually a 2-week delay between infestation and the onset of pruritus and skin lesions. This delayed hypersensitivity reaction is the reason most patients itch for 2 to 4 weeks after the mite is eradicated.

Clinical Presentation

Patients complain of pruritus that is usually worse at night. A history of other itchy people at home is particularly suggestive.

Physical examination reveals widespread inflammatory papules, often excoriated. These have predilection for the lateral aspects of the fingers, webspaces, wrists, elbows, anterior axillary folds, umbilicus, girdle area, and feet. The penis is usually involved (Figure 151-1). Pruritic papules and nodules on the penis should be considered scabies until proven otherwise. The pathognomonic burrow is a 2- to 5-mm dirty white, slightly scaling thread-like line found on the hands. Occasionally a black dot representing the mite is seen at the end of the burrow. Secondary impetiginization and eczematous change are common.

Scabies in infants and young children presents as a widespread, pruritic eruption often involving the face, palms, and soles. Unlike adults, vesicles, pustules, and nodules in addition to papules develop in infants. The elderly are less likely to develop a brisk inflammatory response and frequently present with pruritus and few skin lesions. It is easy to miss scabies in patients with good personal hygiene because the lesions are sparse and burrows are practically non-existent. Norwegian (crusted) scabies occurs in the immunologically compromised host. This is a psoriasiform eruption of the hands and feet accompanied by nail dystrophy and generalized hyperkeratosis and scaling. Pruritus is frequently absent.

Differential Diagnosis

In patients with few skin lesions, scabies can be misdiagnosed as neurotic excoriations. Crusted scabies is often misdiagnosed as a papulosquamous disorder. Scabies can be confused with other pruritic conditions, including atopic dermatitis, papular urticaria, insect bites, and dermatitis herpetiformis.

Diagnostic Approach

The diagnosis of scabies is made by identifying the mite, egg, or feces from a skin scraping (Figure 151-1). Skin biopsy is unnecessary in most cases.

Management and Therapy

Use of topical scabicides is the mainstay of therapy (Figure 151-2). The quantity prescribed must be limited as patients frequently overuse the medication in an effort to get relief, which results in scabicide-induced dermatitis, which can be confused with continued infestation.

Figure 151-1

Dermatoses Secondary to Ectoparasites

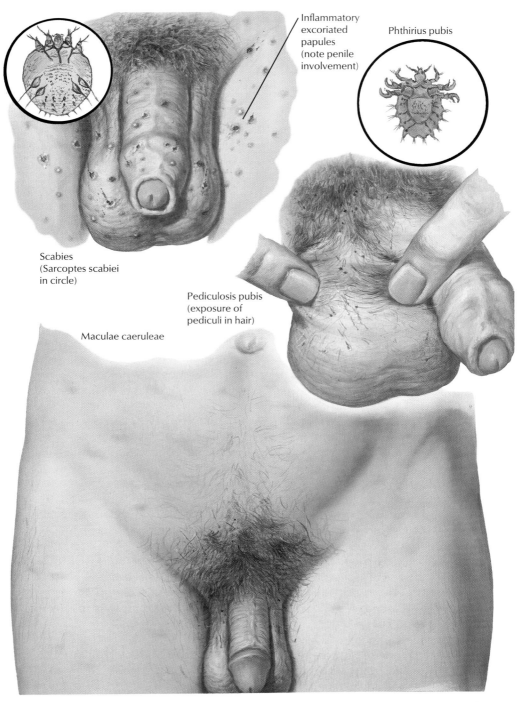

Inflammatory
excoriated
papules
(note penile
involvement)

Phthirius pubis

Scabies
(Sarcoptes scabiei
in circle)

Pediculosis pubis
(exposure of
pediculi in hair)

Maculae caeruleae

Figure 151-2

Sexually Transmitted Ectoparasites

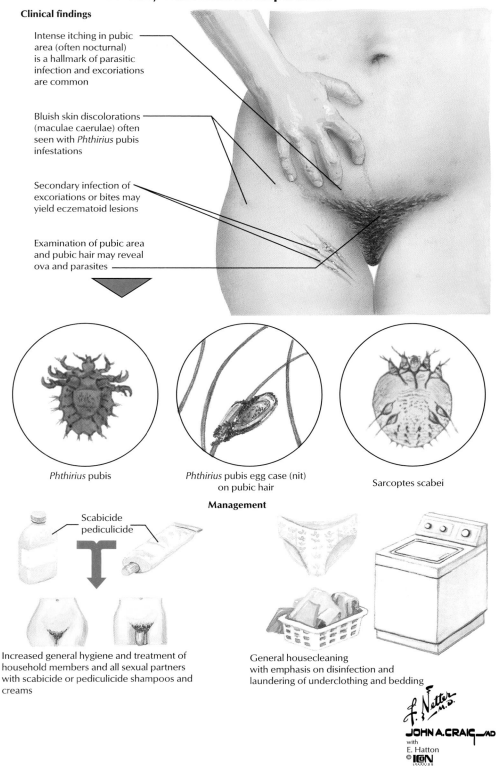

Clinical findings

Intense itching in pubic area (often nocturnal) is a hallmark of parasitic infection and excoriations are common

Bluish skin discolorations (maculae caerulae) often seen with *Phthirius* pubis infestations

Secondary infection of excoriations or bites may yield eczematoid lesions

Examination of pubic area and pubic hair may reveal ova and parasites

Phthirius pubis

Phthirius pubis egg case (nit) on pubic hair

Sarcoptes scabei

Management

Scabicide pediculicide

Increased general hygiene and treatment of household members and all sexual partners with scabicide or pediculicide shampoos and creams

General housecleaning with emphasis on disinfection and laundering of underclothing and bedding

F. Netter M.D.

JOHN A. CRAIG—MD
with
E. Hatton
© ICON

Scabicides should be applied in a thin layer from the neck down after bathing with special attention to the area between the fingers and toes, under the nails, the umbilicus, genitalia, and between the buttocks. The medication should be washed off after 8 to 10 hours. After therapy, all linens, towels, bedclothes, and underwear should be washed in a washing machine with hot water. Children's plush toys, if not washable, should be put out of human contact for 72 hours, allowing the mite to die. Some clinicians advocate a second treatment 1 week later, although there is no conclusive evidence that this improves response.

Permethrin 5% cream is the first choice in topical scabicides because of its high efficacy and low potential for toxicity. Resistance has not been reported. Permethrin cannot be used in infants less than 2 months old or in pregnant and lactating women.

Lindane 1% cream is as effective as permethrin, but has much higher potential for central nervous system toxicity. Lindane should not be used in infants, young children, pregnant or lactating women, patients with underlying neurological disorders, or those with the potential for misuse of the medication.

Precipitated 6% sulfur is the alternative for infants less than 2 months old and pregnant or lactating women. Ivermectin, an oral antiparasitic agent used extensively in veterinary practice, is safe and efficacious in the treatment of scabies.

Oral antihistamines and medium potency topical steroids provide symptomatic relief of the pruritus that often persists for up to 1 month after therapy.

PEDICULOSIS

Pediculosis is an infestation by *Pediculosis capitis* (head louse), *Pediculosus humanus* (body louse), or *Pthirius pubis* (pubic louse). Although infestation still commonly occurs, improved hygiene and treatment have resulted in control of the major louseborne diseases such as trench fever. Consequently, pediculosis is predominantly associated with itching and skin changes today.

Head Lice

Head lice affect all levels of society and all races, with the exception of African Americans in whom incidence is fairly low. Children are predominantly affected. The louse is transmitted by hair-to-hair contact or through shared towels or hair-grooming instruments. Head lice infestations are a growing problem.

Clinical Presentation

The hallmark of head lice is intense scalp pruritus. Physical examination reveals scaling and erythema of the scalp with erythematous papules on the posterior neck. Excoriations are frequently present. Intense scratching leads to secondary infection of the scalp, producing honey-colored crusting over matted hair and lymphadenopathy. Close examination of the hair shaft reveals innumerable gray, oval egg capsules (nits) adhering firmly to the hair shaft (Figure 151-2).

Diagnosis

Diagnosis is confirmed by plucking a few hairs and examining them microscopically. Nits are identified by their adherence to the hair shaft and the presence of a breathing aperture at the superior aspect of the egg casing. The presence of nits alone does not confirm active infection. Live lice or viable eggs confirm the presence of active head lice infestation.

Differential Diagnosis

Other causes of scalp pruritus such as tinea capitis should be considered, especially in children.

Management and Therapy

Permethrin cream rinse 1% and synergized pyrethrins are available. They are highly efficacious with a low toxicity profile. After treatment, nits are removed with a fine-toothed comb. A second treatment is necessary if adult lice are observed 1 week after the initial treatment.

Following therapy, all clothing, towels, bed linens, hair ribbons, and clothes must be machine washed and dried or dry-cleaned. Plush toys should be put in plastic bags in a warm place for 2 weeks. Hair-grooming implements should be washed in hot, soapy water for 20 minutes. Thorough vacuuming of floors and furniture is important to remove any shed hairs with viable eggs. Some practitioners advocate treatment of the entire household; others treat only those family members with signs of active infection.

The use of lindane has decreased due to reports of CNS toxicity in patients who overused or misused the product. There are also reports of resistance to permethrin and synergized pyrethrin. This has led to the emergence of alternative therapies including petrolatum occlusion and trimethoprim/sulfamethoxazole.

Body Lice

Body lice are found where poor hygiene and crowded living conditions predominate. In the United States, body lice are usually seen in homeless people. The louse is spread through infested clothing and bedding.

Clinical Manifestations

The primary symptom is severe pruritus. These patients frequently have numerous linear excoriations over the trunk and neck due to intense scratching. Secondary bacterial superinfection is common. Close examination may reveal a few macules or papules at the sites where the louse has fed. Lice are rarely present on the patient, but can be found in the clothing.

Diagnosis

The diagnosis should be suspected in indigent patients with severe pruritus and few primary skin lesions. Although the louse is rarely present on the infested individual, nits are present on the clothing, particularly the seams near the body folds. The identification of nits or live lice in the clothing confirms the diagnosis.

Differential Diagnosis

Pediculosis corporis can easily be misdiagnosed as neurotic excoriations, unless the clothing is examined.

Management and Therapy

The mainstay of therapy is good hygiene, clean clothes and bedding, and adequate nutrition. The patient's clothing, towels, and bed linens should be laundered with hot, soapy water, dry-cleaned, or boiled. A single application of 5% permethrin cream should be used to treat the patient as described in the management of scabies.

Pubic (Crab) Lice

Pediculosis pubis is a sexually transmitted disease. It is common among homosexual men, where it has a tendency to recur. Presence of pubic lice should elicit increased vigilance for other sexually transmitted diseases.

Clinical Manifestations

Pubic lice most commonly affect the pubis, but the short hair in the inguinal area, perianal area, thighs, and trunk can also be affected. In children, the eyelashes and periphery of the scalp hair can be involved. Patients complain of pruritus in the affected area.

Physical examination reveals excoriations, which may lead to secondary infection with lymphadenopathy. Close examination reveals nits cemented to the pubic and perianal hair (Figure 151-2). The characteristic maculae caeruleae are infrequently present on the trunk and thighs.

Diagnosis

Diagnosis is confirmed by plucking an affected hair and examining it microscopically. Presence of nits is diagnostic. It is important to examine all hair-bearing sites in infected patients, as sites outside the pubic area are frequently involved.

Management and Therapy

Treatment consists of topical application of various preparations. The entire pubic area should be treated as well as the thighs, trunk, and axillary region. Sexual partners should be treated simultaneously. Unaffected household members do not require therapy. Following therapy, all underwear, clothing, linens, and towels that came into contact with the infested person should be washed in hot, soapy water.

The most commonly used agents are synergized pyrethins. A fine-toothed comb is used to remove nits and lice. A second treatment after 7 to 10 days is often necessary.

Eyelashes should be treated with petrolatum applied twice daily for a week followed by removal of any remaining nits.

REFERENCES

Headlice.org Web site. Available at: http://www.headlice.org. Accessed March 5, 2003.

Meinking TL, Taplin D, Hermida JL, Pardo R, Kerdel FA. The treatment of scabies with ivermectin. *N Engl J Med.* 1995; 333:26–30.

Orkin M, Maibach HI, Dahl MV, eds. *Dermatology.* Norwalk, Conn: Appleton & Lange; 1991.

Schachner LA. Treatment resistant head lice: alternative therapeutic approaches. *Pediatr Dermatol.* 1997;14:409–410.

Chapter 152
Urticaria

Nancy E. Thomas

Urticaria can be a source of great frustration to the patient and physician because, although the source of reported associations are extensive, many patients have idiopathic urticaria. It can be recalcitrant to treatment, leading to therapeutic trials of many agents.

ETIOLOGY AND PATHOGENESIS

Urticaria results from fluid transudation from tiny cutaneous blood vessels, often with mast cells and histamine acting as mediators. It can be subclassified as immunologic and non-immunologic. Physical urticaria is non-immunologic, whereas urticaria due to food, drugs, or insect stings often is immunologic. The most common allergic mechanism is the type I hypersensitivity state mediated by IgE. Urticaria can also be induced by type III (immune complex) reactions with activation of classic or alternative complement cascades, as in serum sickness. In non-immunologic urticaria, physical factors or substances cause nonspecific histamine release from mast cells. Genetic factors may predispose individuals to urticaria as evidenced by the hereditary syndromes in Table 152-1. Angioedema is similar to urticaria but involves deeper dermal and subcutaneous tissues. The plasma kinin generating system may be important in types of angioedema. Recently, autoimmune chronic urticaria has been identified, occurring in up to 48% of patients with chronic idiopathic urticaria. In this condition, an anti-IgE antibody of the IgG class or antiFcεRIα cross links adjacent mast cell receptors or IgE molecules. Disorders and substances reported, but not necessarily proven, to be associated with urticaria or angioedema are listed in Tables 152-1 and 152-2. In chronic urticaria, an etiologic diagnosis is established in less than 10% of patients.

CLINICAL PRESENTATION

Intensely itching wheals with smooth, elevated, usually white centers and surrounding erythema characterizes urticaria (Figure 152-1). The lesions can range in size from pinpoint to several centimeters and can be circular, annular, or serpigi-nous (Figure 152-2). Typically, lesions appear in widely distributed crops over the body surface. Variations in presentation of the physical urticarias are given in Table 152-3. Chronic urticaria and physical urticaria can co-exist. Contact urticaria is most prominent where the inciting substance has contacted the skin. Adrenergic urticaria presents with a halo of white skin around a small papule and can be associated with stress. A single wheal tends to last less than 24 hours. Usually no constitutional symptoms are present but urticaria can have accompanying nausea, vomiting, abdominal cramping, headache, salivation, wheezing, and syncope.

Angioedema is an area of painful swelling, often initially around the eyelids, lips, or on a limb, which can persist for several days. In hereditary angioedema, an autosomal dominant condition, episodes of nonpruritic swelling occur either spontaneously or after minor trauma. Erythema may be present before the swelling occurs, but typically urticaria is absent. Laryngeal edema, which is often life threatening, and gastrointestinal involvement can occur.

DIFFERENTIAL DIAGNOSIS

If individual lesions last more than 24 hours, have a violaceous hue, show hyperpigmentation, are painful, non-blanching, or are associated with signs and symptoms of a rheumatologic disease, a biopsy is indicated to rule out *urticarial vasculitis*. In urticaria pigmentosum/mastocytosis, patients can get pruritic urticarial-type wheals at the site of the mast cell infiltrates in the skin. The skin lesions, however, are often persistent red-brown papules or macules that can urticate with stroking (Darier's sign). Pruritic urticarial papules and plaques of pregnancy (PUPPP) typically seen in the third

Table 152-1
Disorders Associated with Urticaria or Angioedema

Acquired angioedema
Adrenergic urticaria
Atopy
Autoimmune anti-IgE or anti FceRI
Bacterial infections
Dental abscess
Genitourinary infection
Helicobacter pylori
Mycoplasma infection
Sinus infection
Streptococcal infections
Endocrine disorders
Hyperthyroidism
Progesterone
Fungal infections
Candida
Dermatophytosis
Hematologic disorders
Iron-deficiency /anemia
Paraproteinemia

Infestation and Parasites
Amebiasis
Ascaris
Filariasis
Giardiasis
Hookworm
Malaria
Scabies
Schistosomiasis
Strongyloides
Trichomonas
Hereditary/syndromes
Arthritis-hives-angioedema
C3b inactivator deficiency
Hereditary angioedema
Muckle-Wells syndrome
(urticaria, deafness,
amyloidosis)
Erythropoietic protoporphyria
Schnitzler's syndrome

Malignancy
Carcinoma
Leukemia
Lymphoma
Myeloma
Polycythemia vera
Rheumatologic disorders
Necrotizing vasculitis
Polymyositis
Rheumatoid arthritis
Rheumatic fever
Sjögren's syndrome
Still's disease
Systemic lupus erythematosus
Viral infections
Coxsackie
Cytomegalovirus
Epstein-Barr virus
ECHO virus
Hepatitis B and C
HIV
Mononucleosis

Figure 152-1   Urticaria

Figure 152-2   Annular and Aerpiginous Urticaria

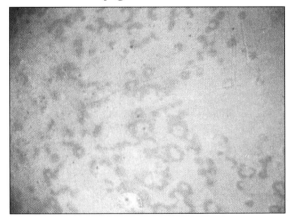

Figure 152-3   Cholinergic Urticaria

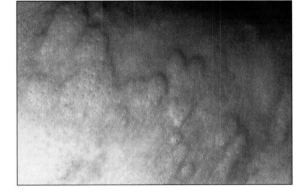

Figure 152-4   Solar Urticaria

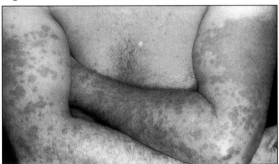

DISORDERS OF THE SKIN

Table 152-2
Substances Associated with Urticaria or Angioedema

Blood products	Dextran	Shellfish
Contactants	Diuretics	Tomatoes
Animal dander and saliva	Isoniazid	**Food additives**
Arthropods	Nonsteroidal anti-inflammatory	Sulfites
Foods	drugs	Tartrazine
Latex	Opioids	**Implants**
Marine forms	Penicillins	Amalgam fillings
Medications (topical)	Polymyxin B	Intrauterine devices
Plants	Quinidine	Orthodontic bands
Textiles	Sulfa drugs	Platinum
Toiletry items	Radiographic contrast media	Tantalum staples
Drugs*	Vancomycin	**Insect/ arthropod stings and bites**
Anesthetics	**Foods**	**Inhalants**
Angiotensin-converting enzyme	Berries	Animal dander
inhibitors	Cheese	Cigarette smoke
Anti-epileptic agents	Chocolate	Dusts
Aspirin	Eggs	Flour
Bromides	Fish	Mold
Cephalosporins	Milk	Pollen
Chloroquine	Nuts	

*Almost any prescription or over-the-counter medication can cause urticaria.

trimester, are characterized by pruritic erythematous papules and urticarial plaques with onset typically in the striae distensae of the abdomen. In *papular urticaria*, a hypersensitivity syndrome, lesions are more persistent, typically on the lower extremities, and thought to be due to insect bites. *Erythema multiforme* and the urticarial phase of *bullous pemphigoid* are often also considered in the differential diagnosis. *Serum sickness* occurs 8 to 10 days after administration of a foreign protein. In addition to urticaria, fever, lymphadenopathy, arthralgias or arthritis, splenomegaly, and nephritis can be present. Laboratory tests can show leukopenia, hypocomplementemia, and albuminuria.

DIAGNOSTIC APPROACH

A thorough history and review of systems is key with emphasis on timing of attacks, provoking factors, and associated signs and symptoms. The timing of urticaria along with a list of exposures is helpful in determining an underlying cause. Often a diary of food intake and exposures will help determine any associations. Urticaria can be caused by almost any medication, so trials off medication may be necessary. A wheal can be circled and observed to see if it lasts more than 24 hours, as would be expected in urticarial vasculitis. A skin biopsy, done at the edge of a wheal, will clarify the diagnosis. If a particular allergen is suspected, scratch, intradermal, or radioallergosorbent testing may be valuable. Aeroallergens, dermatophytes, foods, and candida can be tested. Allergy to aeroallergens should be considered if there is a history of rhinitis or asthma.

Urticaria is considered chronic if it is present for 6 weeks or longer. The laboratory workup for chronic urticaria includes a CBC with differential, sedimentation rate, urinalysis and urine culture, thyroid-stimulating hormone, liver function tests, hepatitis B and C, and a chest radiograph. Additional tests, based on history and physical examination, may include thyroid autosomal antibodies, antinuclear antibody, complement levels, serum IgE, streptococcal throat culture, monospot, stool for parasites, and vaginal smears for *Candida* and *Trichomonas*. If serum sickness is present, urinalysis, CBC and sedimentation rate should be done.

In hereditary angioedema, C4 levels, which remain depressed between attacks, are a reliable screening test. An IgE-mediated allergic or drug reaction, or parasitic infection should be considered if eosinophilia or elevated IgE is present. An elevated

Table 152-3
Physical Urticarias

Type of Urticaria	Clinical Appearance	Method to Test for Presence
Aquagenic	Small punctate pruritic wheals in a follicular pattern on an erythematous background	Wet compresses at 35° to 36°C for 30 minutes
Cholinergic	Small (2-3 mm) very pruritic papules on a large erythematous background (Figure 152-3)	Use methacholine skin test or immerse in hot bath of 42°C, raising body temperature 0.7°
Cold	Wheal assumes the shape of the stimulus with surrounding erythema	Wheal and flare within 10 to 15 minutes at the site of application of an ice cube, maintained for 5 minutes
Dermatographism	Linear cutaneous wheal greater than 3 mm long, surrounded by a flare	Stroke skin on back firmly with tongue blade or dermatographometer
Delayed pressure	Raised painful erythematous deep-seated swellings develop in areas 4 to 8 hours after pressure exposure	15 pounds of weight slung over the shoulder for 15 minutes with the patient walking during the test.
Local heat	Eythema, pruritus, urticaria	Apply warm compress to forearm
Solar	Urticaria in exposed areas (Figure 152-4)	Expose skin to defined wavelengths of light
Vibration-induced angioedema	Pruritus, erythema, and local swelling in the area confined to application of a vibratory stimulus	Gently apply lab vortex to forearm for 4 minutes

erythrocyte sedimentation rate (ESR) suggests a systemic disease or urticarial vasculitis. Testing for physical urticaria can be done as noted in Table 152-3. In cold urticaria, laboratory testing may include cryoglobulins, cryofibrinogens, VDRL, cold hemolysis, and α-1 antitrypsin. Adrenergic urticaria is diagnosed by intracutaneous injection of noradrenaline (0.5×10^{-6} M).

MANAGEMENT AND THERAPY

Ideally, the cause of the urticaria is determined and eliminated. In physical urticaria, the associated physical factor should be avoided. Because aspirin and nonsteroidal anti-inflammatory medications can function as histamine releasers and cause exacerbation, they should be discontinued. Patients should be warned that in physical urticaria, such as cold urticaria, intense exposure to the inciting agent (such as diving into a cold pool) can result in massive angioedema and anaphylaxis.

Acute urticaria is usually treated with antihistamines and, if severe, with corticosteroids. An acute episode of urticaria accompanied by asthma, laryngeal edema, or circulatory collapse is treated as a medical emergency with epinephrine, systemic corticosteroids, oxygen, intravenous fluids, or even possible airway intubation. Adrenaline emergency packs should be prescribed for patients with a history of severe urticaria or angioedema.

H1 blockers are often the first-line treatment (Table 152-4). Tricyclic antidepressants, especially doxepin, are used to take advantage of its combination of H1 and H2 blockade. Alternatively, there may

Table 152-4
Antihistamines Used for Pruritus

· Cetirizine 10 mg once daily
· Cyproheptidine 4 mg every 8 hours
· Diphenhydramine 25 to 50 mg every 6 hours
· Doxepin 25 mg every 12 to 24 hours
· Fexofenadine 60 mg every 12 hours
· Hydroxyzine 10 to 25 mg every 6 hours
· Loratadine 10 mg once daily

be some value in adding an H2 blocker such as ranitidine (150 mg orally every 12 hours) or cimetidine (300 mg orally every 8 hours) to an H1 blocker.

For chronic urticaria, it is best to avoid giving the patient corticosteroids whenever possible. Other treatments that may have value are attenuated anabolic steroids, nifedipine, dapsone, sulfasalazine, colchicines, NSAIDs, methotrexate, hydroxychloroquine, ultraviolet B, and psoralen plus ultraviolet light of A wavelength. Some clinicians use estrogen therapy for autoimmune progesterone urticaria. In patients with autoimmune thyroiditis, urticaria has been reported to respond to thyroxine, even when the patient is euthyroid.

Cyproheptadine can be effective for cold urticaria. In physical urticaria, induction of tolerance is sometimes possible. Adrenergic urticaria responds to β-blocker therapy.

Hereditary angioedema is treated with attenuated androgens for chronic control. Use purified C1 inhibitor for acute episodes and as prophylaxis for surgery. Systemic corticosteroids and antihistamines are not helpful in controlling this condition.

FUTURE DIRECTIONS

The recent discovery of autoimmune chronic urticaria represents a significant advance and may provide a classification for a significant proportion of chronic urticaria that was previously deemed to be idiopathic. Also, whether proposed disease associations such as chronic urticaria and *Helicobacter pylori* are real or merely coincidental remains to be determined. In a recent study, the prevalence of *H. pylori* infection was not elevated among urticaria patients compared to controls. Latex allergy is important as a cause of urticaria and anaphylaxis. The future should bring better control of its presence in our environment and preventive measures to avoid sensitization of individuals.

New antihistamines are undergoing testing and may result in improved treatments. In addition, modulators of non-antihistaminic mediators, such as leukotriene receptor antagonists, may prove to be of value for treating urticaria. Recently, two distinct mast cell populations have been identified, and their homeostasis between inhibition and activation is under study. These studies may lead to drugs directed against these subtypes.

REFERENCES

Crawford MB. Urticaria [emedicine Web Site]. July 17, 2002. Available at: http://www.emedicine.com/emerg/topic628.htm. Accessed March 5, 2003.

Greaves MW. Chronic urticaria. *N Eng J Med.* 1995;332:1767–1772.

Hook-Nikanne J, Varjonen E, Harvima RJ, Kosunen TU. Is *Helicobacter pylori* infection associated with chronic urticaria? *Acta Derm Venereol.* 2000;80:425-426.

Leung DY, Diaz LA, DeLeo V, Soter NA. Allergic and immunologic skin disorders. *JAMA.* 1997;278:1914-1923.

Litt JZ. *Drug Eruption Reference Manual.* 9th ed. Boca Raton, Fla: CRC Press; 2000.

Metzger WJ. Urticaria, angioedema, and hereditary angioedema. IN: Grammer LC, Greenberger PA, eds. *Patterson's Allergic Diseases.* 6th ed. Philadelphia, Pa: Lippincott Williams & Wilkins; 2002.

Nettis E, Dambra P, Loria MP, et al. Mast-cell phenotype in urticaria. *Allergy.* 2001;56:915.

toxic. *See* Delirium
En coup de sabre lesion, 994
Endarterectomy, 175
Endocarditis, **474–480**
   antimicrobial therapy for, 477*t,* 478
   clinical presentation of, 474, 478*f,* 520
   culture-negative, 478
   diagnosis of, 474–480
   differential diagnosis of, 867
   embolic effects of, 474, 479*f*
   enterococcal, antimicrobial therapy for, 477*t*
   fungal, 476, 478
   gram-negative, 476
   HACEK, 474, 476, 478
     antimicrobial therapy for, 477*t*
   infective, 374
     antibiotic prophylaxis for, 103
     and aortic regurgitation, 105
   meningitis caused by, 520*t*
   noninfectious, 478
   pathogenesis of, 474
   portals of bacterial entry in, 474, 475*f*
   prophylaxis, 478
   prosthetic valve, 478
   staphylococcal, 476, **553**
     advanced lesions of, 555*f*
     antimicrobial therapy for, 477*t*
     early lesions of, 555*f*
   streptococcal, 476
     antimicrobial therapy for, 477*t*
   subacute bacterial, and fever of unknown origin, 481, 482*f*
   surgical management of, 478
     advances in (future directions for), 478
   valves involved in, 474, 475*f*
Endolimax nana, 310*f*
Endoluminal radiation, for peripheral vascular disease, 175
Endolymphatic hydrops, 725
   clinical presentation of, 727
   treatment of, 732
Endometriosis, **614–618**
   clinical presentation of, 615
   diagnosis of, 617
   differential diagnosis of, 617
   dissemination of, 614
   epidemiology of, 614
   etiology of, 614
   genetics of, 614–615
   and immune response, 614
   implantation sites of, 614, 616*f*
   and infertility, 632
   laparoscopic findings in, 615*f,* 617, 618, 631*f*
   pathogenesis of, 614–615
   recurrence of, after therapy, 617
   treatment of, 646
     advances in (future directions for), 618
     medical, 617
     surgical, 618
Endometritis, postpartum, and disseminated intravascular coagulation, 374
End-organ damage, in elderly, hypertension and, 135
Endoscopic balloon dilatation, in peptic ulcer disease, 345–346

Endoscopic retrograde cholangiopancreatography, 277–278, 335, 339
Endoscopy
   in anorectal disorders, 287, 289, 292
   in colorectal cancer, 434, 434*t,* 436*f,* 437
   in diarrhea, 301
   in esophageal cancer, 466*f,* 467*f,* 469–471
   in gastric cancer, 469
   in gastroesophageal reflux disease, 306, 307*f*
   in giardiasis, 311
   in *Helicobacter pylori* infection, 316*f,* 317–318
   immediate, in uninvestigated dyspepsia, 317
   in inflammatory bowel disease, 320, 324*f*
   in lung cancer, 443
   in oral and oropharyngeal cancer, 429
   in pancreatitis, 335, 339
   in peptic ulcer disease, 341, 345*f,* 345–346
   screening, 472
   therapeutic, 282, 308
   in uninvestigated dyspepsia, 317
Endothelial dysfunction
   in metabolic syndrome, 185
   in peripheral vascular disease, 167
Endovascular stenting, for peripheral vascular disease, 175
End-stage renal disease. *See also* Renal failure, chronic
   costs of, 748
   epidemiology of, 748
   etiology of, 748
   pathogenesis of, 748, 749*f*
   renal artery stenosis and, 144
Enema
   barium, 331
     in colorectal cancer, 434*t*
   for inflammatory bowel disease, 325
Enhanced external counterpulsation, 91
Enoxaparin, for myocardial infarction, 163
Entacapone, 692
Entamoeba coli, 310*f*
Entamoeba dispar, 534
Entamoeba histolytica, 310*f,* 311, 320, 328, 530, 534. *See also* Amebiasis
   traveler's diarrhea caused by, 500
Enteric fever. *See* Typhoid fever
Enteric sensory neurons, in irritable bowel syndrome, 329*f*
Enterobiasis, 525, 526*f*
Enterocele, 744*f*
Enterocutaneous fistula, in Crohn's disease, 320, 322*f*
Enteromonas hominis, 310*f*
Enterotoxins, 299
Enthesopathy, in spondyloarthropathy, 880
Entrapment neuropathy, 699*f*
   treatment of, 699
Entrapment syndromes, diabetes mellitus and, 185
Enzyme-linked immunoabsorbent assay
   in antiphospholipid syndrome, 379
   in *Helicobacter pylori* infection, 316*f,* 317, 317*t*
Eosinophilic granuloma, and hypogonadism, 232
Epicosapentaenoic acid, 118
Epidemic louse-borne typhus, physical findings in, 499*t*
Epidermal growth factor-receptor inhibitors
   for colorectal cancer, 441
   for head and neck cancer, 431
Epidermal inclusion cysts, 69

Other Netter Products Available From

Netter's Obstetrics, Gynecology and Women's Health
2002, 578 pages, casebound, ISBN 1-929007-25-6

Netter's Concise Atlas of Orthopaedic Anatomy
2002, 320 pages, paperback, ISBN 0-914168-94-0

Atlas of Human Anatomy, 3rd Edition
2003, 640 pages, paperback, ISBN 1-929007-11-6
casebound with CD, ISBN 1-929007-21-3

Netter's Anatomy Charts
2003, 12-chart set, 20" x 26," flexible lamination,
ISBN 1-929007-36-1

Netter's Anatomy Flashcards
2002, 331 cards, 4" x 6," ISBN 1-929007-08-6

Netter's Atlas of Human Embryology
2002, 267 pages, paperback, ISBN 0-914168-99-1

Netter's Atlas of Human Physiology
2002, 223 pages, paperback, ISBN 1-929007-01-9

The Netter Presenter: Human Anatomy Collection
CD, Institutional Version, ISBN 0-914168-98-3

The Netter Presenter: Human Embryology Collection
CD, Institutional Version, ISBN 1-929007-10-8

The Netter Presenter: Human Physiology Collection
CD, Institutional Version, ISBN 1-929007-09-4